OBSTETRICS AND GYNECOLOGY

Fourth Edition

CHARLES R.B. BECKMANN, M.D., M.H.P.E.
Director of Medical Education
Department of Obstetrics and Gynecology
Albert Einstein Medical Center
Philadelphia, Pennsylvania

Department of Obstetrics and Gynecology
Jefferson Medical College
Thomas Jefferson University
Philadelphia, Pennsylvania

FRANK W. LING, M.D.
UT Medical Group Professor and Chair
Department of Obstetrics and Gynecology
University of Tennessee College of Medicine
Memphis, Tennessee

DOUGLAS W. LAUBE, M.D., M.ED.
Professor and Chairman
Department of Obstetrics and Gynecology
University of Wisconsin Medical School
Madison, Wisconsin

ROGER P. SMITH, M.D.
Professor and Vice Chair
Department of Obstetrics and Gynecology
University of Missouri at Kansas City
Kansas City, Missouri

BARBARA M. BARZANSKY, PH.D., M.H.P.E.
Secretary, Council on Medical Education
The American Medical Association

WILLIAM N.P. HERBERT, M.D.
Professor and Chairman
Department of Obstetrics and Gynecology
University of Virginia
Charlottesville, Virginia

OBSTETRICS AND GYNECOLOGY

Fourth Edition

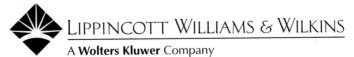

LIPPINCOTT WILLIAMS & WILKINS

A **Wolters Kluwer** Company

Philadelphia • Baltimore • New York • London
Buenos Aires • Hong Kong • Sydney • Tokyo

Editor: Neil Marquardt
Managing Editor: Bridget Hilferty
Marketing Manager: Aimee Sirmon
Production Editor: Christina Remsberg
Compositor: Shepherd, Inc.
Printer: Data Reproduction Corp.

351 West Camden Street
Baltimore, Maryland 21201-2436 USA

530 Walnut Street
Philadelphia, PA 19106

Printed in the United States of America

First Edition, 1992
Second Edition, 1995
Third Edition, 1998

Library of Congress Cataloging-in-Publication Data

LOC data has been applied for and is available.

The publishers have made every effort to trace the copyright holders for borrowed material. If they have inadvertently overlooked any, they will be pleased to make the necessary arrangements at the first opportunity.

To purchase additional copies of this book, call our customer service department at (800) 638-3030 or fax orders to (301) 824-7390. International customers should call (301) 714-2324.

Visit Lippincott Williams & Wilkins on the Internet: http://www.LWW.com. Lippincott Williams & Wilkins customer service representatives are available from 8:30 am to 6:00 pm, EST.

02 03 04 05
1 2 3 4 5 6 7 8 9 10

CONTENTS

Foreword *xi*
Preface *xiii*
Acknowledgments *xv*
Contributors *xvii*
How to Use This Book *xix*
APGO Educational Objectives *xxi*

UNIT I

Approach to the Patient

Chapter 1
Health Care for Women 2

Chapter 2
Ethics in Obstetrics and Gynecology 32

Chapter 3
Embryology, Anatomy, and Reproductive Genetics 39

UNIT II

Obstetrics

SECTION A

NORMAL OBSTETRICS

Chapter 4
Maternal–Fetal Physiology   63

Chapter 5
Antepartum Care   78

Chapter 6
Intrapartum Care   98

Chapter 7
Abnormal Labor   115

Chapter 8
Intrapartum Fetal Surveillance   131

Chapter 9
Immediate Care of the Newborn   145

Chapter 10
Postpartum Care   151

SECTION B

ABNORMAL OBSTETRICS

Chapter 11
Isoimmunization   165

Chapter 12
Postpartum Hemorrhage   173

Chapter 13
Postpartum Infection   182

Chapter 14
Abortion   191

Chapter 15
Ectopic Pregnancy   202

Chapter 16

Medical and Surgical Conditions of Pregnancy   216

Chapter 17

Hypertension in Pregnancy   260

Chapter 18

Multifetal Gestation   270

Chapter 19

Fetal Growth Abnormalities   276

Chapter 20

Third-Trimester Bleeding   285

Chapter 21

Postterm Pregnancy   296

Chapter 22

Preterm Labor   304

Chapter 23

Premature Rupture of Membranes   313

SECTION C

PROCEDURES

Chapter 24

Obstetric Procedures   319

UNIT III

Gynecology

SECTION A

GENERAL GYNECOLOGY

Chapter 25

Contraception   327

Chapter 26

Sterilization   347

Chapter 27
Vulvitis and Vaginitis   356

Chapter 28
Sexually Transmitted Diseases   366

Chapter 29
Pelvic Relaxation, Urinary Incontinence, and Urinary Tract Infection   384

Chapter 30
Endometriosis   396

Chapter 31
Dysmenorrhea and Chronic Pelvic Pain   407

SECTION B

BREASTS

Chapter 32
Disorders of the Breast   417

SECTION C

PROCEDURES

Chapter 33
Gynecologic Procedures   433

UNIT IV

Reproductive Endocrinology and Infertility

Chapter 34
Reproductive Cycle   444

Chapter 35
Puberty   455

Chapter 36
Amenorrhea and Dysfunctional Uterine Bleeding   464

Chapter 37
Hirsutism and Virilization 472

Chapter 38
Menopause 482

Chapter 39
Infertility 494

Chapter 40
Premenstrual Syndrome 508

UNIT V

Neoplasia

Chapter 41
Cell Biology and Principles of Cancer Therapy 518

Chapter 42
Gestational Trophoblastic Disease 524

Chapter 43
Vulvar and Vaginal Disease and Neoplasia 533

Chapter 44
Cervical Neoplasia and Carcinoma 547

Chapter 45
Uterine Leiomyoma and Neoplasia 568

Chapter 46
Endometrial Hyperplasia and Cancer 577

Chapter 47
Ovarian and Adnexal Disease 590

UNIT VI

Human Sexuality

Chapter 48
Human Sexuality 608

UNIT VII

Violence Against Women

Chapter 49
Sexual Assault and Domestic Violence   *618*

Study Questions   *625*
Index   *863*

FOREWORD

The publishing of a fourth edition of a medical text is a clear indication of the value and acceptance of previous editions. This fourth edition is more, much more, than just a revision and an updating, with current information and a new format that makes it user friendly.

The material is organized to relate to APGO Objectives. The use of case studies and discussion questions will prove most valuable to the student for self-evaluation and review. These qualities are further enhanced by a new section containing questions in standard format along with correct answers. The material is presented in a concise, well-organized, and readable fashion which makes it a valuable resource not only for students but for women's health care providers at all levels.

All authors have a special interest and skills in medical education and are to be congratulated in producing a medical text based on sound educational principles. I enthusiastically recommend this new edition and am confident that it will solidify its place as the number one text for clerkships in obstetrics and gynecology.

Martin L. Stone, M.D.
Professor and Chairman (Emeritus)
Department of Obstetrics and Gynecology
SUNY at Stony Brook, New York

PREFACE

Obstetrics and Gynecology in its *4th Edition* is again written specifically for medical students taking their clerkship in obstetrics and gynecology. The goals of the book with respect to medical school education are to provide the basic information about obstetrics and gynecology that medical students need to complete an obstetrics and gynecology clerkship successfully and to pass the national standardized examinations in this content area.

Obstetrics and Gynecology, 4th Edition, also provides the basic, practical information in obstetrics, gynecology, and general women's health needed by physicians and advanced practice nurses in the areas of family medicine, emergency medicine, adolescent medicine and pediatrics, and internal medicine. Family physicians will find this book especially useful in their board and recertification examinations. Nurse midwives will likewise find this book useful for many practice issues.

Great effort has been made to make each chapter short and concise, written in clear and unambiguous prose, including only the basic information needed and no more. Whenever possible, clear, concise summary tables and figures which teach and illustrate are used. The index has been revised and expanded to facilitate learning.

Obstetrics and Gynecology, 4th Edition, is unique in several important ways:

1. This textbook was written to facilitate *efficient, focused learning* and is based on the "Instructional Objectives for a Clinical Curriculum in Obstetrics and Gynecology, *7th Edition*" of the Association of Professors of Gynecology and Obstetrics. These national standards are used to organize most Ob-Gyn clerkships in the United States and Canada, and they are used as a guideline in the development of national standardized examinations. Effort has been made to address all the content of these objectives, as the objectives cover basic information that any health care provider engaged in the primary care of women should know.
2. Each chapter begins with reference to the objectives primarily covered in the chapter as well as concise descriptions of the objectives.
3. Each chapter ends with a series of case studies and discussion questions covering the content of the chapter.

These studies challenge the learner to use the information in the chapter.

4. At the end of the book there is a separate section containing clinically oriented questions in standardized examination formats, organized by chapter. These questions provide a rapid yet comprehensive review of all the information covered in the chapter. The answers are provided in small boxes at the bottom of each page to avoid annoying page shuffling during review.

Obstetrics and Gynecology, 4th Edition, was written by professional medical educators. Five authors are experienced obstetrician-gynecologists who have expertise and interest in medical education, including additional degrees in education, experience as clerkship and residency program directors, national leadership positions in the areas of primary care, and involvement in the preparation of national standardized examinations. The other author is a professional educator and anatomist with extensive experience in curriculum development and evaluation. With the exception of special sections and one chapter that was written by special contributors, the entire book was written, reviewed, and revised by these six individuals.

Basic medical school textbooks often contain large amounts of information more useful to advanced practitioners than to medical students and those providing primary women's health care. In contrast, *Obstetrics and Gynecology, 4th Edition,* focuses specifically on the basic information medical students need for the primary and obstetric-gynecologic care of women, the same information medical students need during the 6- to 8-week Ob-Gyn clerkship. *Obstetrics and Gynecology, 4th Edition,* written by professional educators according to sound educational principles, accomplishes these goals. The concise and easy-to-read chapters, correlated with national learning objectives and self-evaluation sections for measuring progress, fulfill our intention to provide the fundamental information about obstetrics and gynecology required for the basic care of women.

ACKNOWLEDGMENTS

We extend our appreciation to Elizabeth Nieginski, Julie Scardiglia, Amy Dinkel, Darrin Kiessling, Becky Himmelheber, Katie Levitt, Chrissy Remsberg, and Tim Satterfield at Lippincott Williams & Wilkins for their seemingly tireless help and encouragement during the arduous preparation of *Obstetrics and Gynecology, 4th Edition.* Likewise, we continue to be grateful for the innovative art provided by Joyce Lavery which adds so much to the usefulness of the book. We again extend a special thanks to Carol-Lynn Brown, our first editor, for her foresight and support in the early development of this book.

We also extend our special thanks to our ever patient families and secretaries who have kept their good spirits in the face of revision after revision. We wish to make a special acknowledgment of the work of Martha Mitchum, whose coordination of the efforts of the authors and attention to detail was instrumental in the completion of our work. We also extend special thanks to Charles Dunton, MD, Director of Gynecologic Oncology, and David Jaspan, DO, Assistant Clerkship Director, Department of Obstetrics and Gynecology, Albert Einstein Medical Center, Philadelphia, for their review of Bethesda 2001 in chapter 44.

CONTRIBUTORS

JOANNA M. CAIN, M.D.
Coauthor, Chapter 2
Professor and Chair
Department of Gynecology and Obstetrics
Oregon Health & Sciences University
Portland, Oregon

OWEN P. PHILLIPS, M.D.
Contributor, Chapter 3
Associate Professor of Obstetrics
    and Gynecology
Clerkship Director
Director of the Center for Women's Health
    Improvement
Department of Obstetrics and Gynecology
University of Tennessee at Memphis

HOW TO USE THIS BOOK

Obstetrics and Gynecology, 4th Edition, is specifically written for the medical student in a basic clerkship in obstetrics-gynecology. The book will help you study and review for national standardized examinations. The following suggestions will maximize your use of the book.

TO STUDY A TOPIC FOR THE FIRST TIME

First read the APGO Objectives that begin a chapter to orient you and focus your study. Then read the chapter, paying extra attention to the tables and figures. Next, attempt to answer the questions for the chapter at the end of the book. These questions are designed to ensure that you have learned the main points. If you missed certain questions, go back and reread the relevant points of the chapter. You also should answer the questions included in the case studies at the end of the chapter. Try to apply the material in the chapter to a specific patient you have encountered. See how the content relates to that specific case.

In this book, important terms are defined only once. When you are studying a topic, make sure you understand all the terms that are used. If you are not familiar with a specific term, use the subject index to find the place where the term is defined. Also, many chapters contain references to content that is included in other parts of the book. To get a thorough understanding of the topic, read these relevant pages as well (you can find them by using the subject index).

After you have studied the chapter and can answer the questions, go back and reread the relevant APGO Objectives. Make sure that you understand all the information that is included in the objectives.

TO REVIEW FOR EXAMINATIONS AFTER THE CLERKSHIP

For the review you may want to reread entire sections of the book. The study questions in the back of the book are similar in format to those used in the national standardized examinations. Try to answer the questions in a short time frame, as you would for the actual test. Do not check your answers until you have finished the questions for a whole chapter or section of the book. If you find you have answered questions incorrectly, go back and reread the specific pages in the chapter, and the related content elsewhere in the book.

APGO EDUCATIONAL OBJECTIVES

Below are the titles of each of the APGO Objectives, the "Instructional Objectives for a Clinical Curriculum in Obstetrics and Gynecology, 7th Edition" of the Association of Professors of Gynecology and Obstetrics. Each chapter begins with a short description of the objectives emphasized in the chapter.

Unit One: Approach to the Patient

1 HISTORY
2 EXAMINATION
3 PAP SMEAR AND CULTURES
4 DIAGNOSIS AND MANAGEMENT PLAN
5 PERSONAL INTERACTION AND COMMUNICATION SKILLS
6 LEGAL ISSUES IN OBSTETRICS AND GYNECOLOGY
7 ETHICS IN OBSTETRICS AND GYNECOLOGY
8 PREVENTIVE CARE AND HEALTH MAINTENANCE

Unit Two: Obstetrics

Section A: Normal Obstetrics

9 MATERNAL–FETAL PHYSIOLOGY
10 PRECONCEPTION
11 ANTEPARTUM CARE
12 INTRAPARTUM CARE
13 IMMEDIATE CARE OF THE NEWBORN
14 POSTPARTUM CARE
15 LACTATION

Section B: Abnormal Obstetrics

16 ECTOPIC PREGNANCY
17 SPONTANEOUS ABORTION
18 MEDICAL AND SURGICAL CONDITIONS IN PREGNANCY
19 PREECLAMPSIA–ECLAMPSIA SYNDROME
20 ISOIMMUNIZATION
21 MULTIFETAL GESTATION
22 FETAL DEATH
23 ABNORMAL LABOR
24 THIRD TRIMESTER BLEEDING
25 PRETERM LABOR
26 PREMATURE RUPTURE OF MEMBRANES
27 INTRAPARTUM FETAL SURVEILLANCE
28 POSTPARTUM HEMORRHAGE
29 POSTPARTUM INFECTION
30 ANXIETY AND DEPRESSION
31 MORTALITY
32 POSTTERM PREGNANCY
33 FETAL GROWTH ABNORMALITIES

Section C: Procedures

34 OBSTETRICS PROCEDURES

Unit Three: Gynecology

Section A: General Gynecology

35 CONTRACEPTION
36 STERILIZATION

37 ABORTION
38 VULVAR AND VAGINAL DISEASE
39 SEXUALLY TRANSMITTED DISEASES
40 SALPINGITIS
41 PELVIC RELAXATION AND URINARY INCONTINENCE
42 ENDOMETRIOSIS AND ADENOMYOSIS
43 CHRONIC PELVIC PAIN

Section B: Breasts
44 DISORDERS OF THE BREASTS

Section C: Procedures
45 GYNECOLOGIC PROCEDURES

Unit Four: Reproductive Endocrinology, Infertility, and Related Topics
46 PUBERTY
47 AMENORRHEA
48 HIRSUTISM AND VIRILIZATION
49 NORMAL AND ABNORMAL UTERINE BLEEDING

50 DYSMENORRHEA
51 CLIMACTERIC
52 INFERTILITY
53 PREMENSTRUAL SYNDROME

Unit Five: Neoplasia
54 GESTATIONAL TROPHOBLASTIC NEOPLASIA
55 VULVAR NEOPLASMS
56 CERVICAL DISEASE AND NEOPLASIA
57 UTERINE LEIOMYOMAS
58 ENDOMETRIAL CARCINOMA
59 OVARIAN NEOPLASMS

Unit Six: Human Sexuality
60 SEXUALITY
61 MODES OF SEXUAL EXPRESSION
62 PHYSICIAN SEXUALITY

Unit Seven: Violence Against Women
63 SEXUAL ASSAULT
64 DOMESTIC VIOLENCE

UNIT I

Approach to the Patient

1

HEALTH CARE FOR WOMEN

*Obstetrics and Gynecology as Specialty
and Primary-Preventive Health Care*

CHAPTER OBJECTIVES

This chapter deals primarily with APGO Objective(s):

PART 1   Health Care for Women

OBJECTIVE 8   Preventive Care and Health
Maintenance

A. Describe the indications and appropriate intervals for the following screening procedures that are part of routine health surveillance: Pap smear, mammogram, blood pressure monitoring, blood lipid profiles, occult fecal blood, sigmoidoscopy.

B. Describe the appropriate patient education associated with the following: contraception, sexually transmitted diseases, diet, exercise, stress management, smoking, immunization, substance abuse, seat belt use, sun exposure, local specific risks, and depression.

C. Discuss the costs and benefits of routine health surveillance.

D. Explain prevention guidelines for disease of the breast, cervix, colon, cardiovascular system, skin, bones, eyes.

PART 2   Evaluation and Management

OBJECTIVE 1   History

Take a thorough obstetric–gynecologic history, which includes chief complaint, present illness, menstrual history, obstetric history, gynecologic history, contraceptive history, sexual history, family history, and social history. Utilizing culturally and age appropriate communications skills, gain the patient's confidence and transmit the results of the history in written and oral form.

OBJECTIVE 2   Examination

A. Perform a thorough obstetric–gynecologic examination (breasts, abdomen, external genitalia, pelvic examination) utilizing culturally and age appropriate communication skills and attention to patient comfort and modesty, gaining her confidence and cooperation, and transmit the results in written and oral form.

B. Teach and explain breast and external genital self-examination to the patient.

OBJECTIVE 3   Pap Smear and Cultures

Obtain and properly handle specimens for a Pap smear and cultures to detect sexually transmitted diseases and explain the purpose of these tests to the patient.

OBJECTIVE 4   Diagnosis and Management Plan

Based on the results of the patient history and physical examination, generate a problem list, identify likely diagnosis, form a diagnostic impression, and develop a management plan considering patient values and economic issues

(Continued)

(laboratory and diagnostic studies, patient education plan, and plans for continuing care and treatment).

OBJECTIVE 5   Personal Interaction and Communication Skills

A. Establish rapport and work dependably with patients.

B. Work cooperatively and dependably with other members of the health care team.

C. Recognize personal limitations.

OBJECTIVE 62   Physician Sexuality

A. Demonstrate awareness of the influence of the physician's own sexuality on his/her interactions with patients.

B. Describe the behavior patterns of seductive patients.

C. Describe the appropriate boundaries of physician behavior.

PART 3   The Physician—Patient "Contract"

OBJECTIVE 6   Legal Issues in Obstetrics and Gynecology

A. Demonstrate a knowledge of the elements of informed consent: right to refuse care, outcomes, options/alternatives, capacity to choose, surrogate decision making.

B. Describe the following legal obligations to protect patient interests: advance directives, confidentiality, abandonment, contractual medical benefits, fraud, local laws concerning the reporting of suspected child abuse and domestic violence.

Although obstetrician–gynecologists provide specialty care for women, they also serve as the primary care physician for over one half of women in the United States. As "specialists," they provide obstetric and gynecologic care. As primary care physicians for women, obstetrician–gynecologists assume responsibility for primary-preventive health care (health promotion and disease prevention), including treatment of some nongynecologic problems and for other problems by appropriate diagnosis and referral. The annual gynecologic examinations are enhanced to become periodic health evaluations timed and tailored to address the important causes of morbidity and mortality in each age group of women.

To be successful with these diverse but important responsibilities, the obstetrician–gynecologist must understand the wide range of issues encompassed by the primary-preventive health care responsibility as

TABLE 1.1.	Leading Causes of Morbidity in Women in the United States			

| Cause of Morbidity | Age | | | |
	12–18	**19–39**	**40–64**	**>65**
HEENT conditions	+	+	+	+
URI	+	+	+	+
Infection (viral, parasites, bacterial)	+	+		
Sexual abuse	+			
Accidental injury	+	+		+
Digestive tract conditions	+			
Acute urinary conditions	+	+		
Osteoporosis/arthritis			+	+
Hypertension			+	+
Orthopedic conditions			+	
Heart disease			+	+
Hearing and vision impairments			+	+
Urinary incontinence				+

HEENT = head, ears, eyes, nose, and throat; URI = upper respiratory infection.

well as the specialty of obstetrics and gynecology, must be able to establish a good professional relationship with patients, and must be able to perform an excellent general and woman's health history, review of systems, and physical examination. In addition, the obstetrician–gynecologist must understand the differences between consultation and referral and when and how to perform and receive each.

PART I: OBSTETRICS AND GYNECOLOGY
Primary and Specialty Care for Women

Obstetrics was originally a separate branch of medicine and gynecology, a division of surgery. Obstetrics and gynecology merged into a single specialty as knowledge of the pathophysiology of the female reproductive tract led to a natural integration of the two. In the United States, obstetrics is now somewhat indistinctly divided into general obstetrics (dealing with uncomplicated pregnancy) and maternal–fetal medicine (dealing with complicated, or high-risk, pregnancy as well as reproductive genetics). Likewise, gynecology now includes general gynecology (dealing with nonmalignant disorders of the reproductive tract and associated organ systems), urogynecology and pelvic reconstructive surgery, gynecologic oncology, and reproductive endocrinology-infertility.

To facilitate the primary-preventive health care responsibility, the Task Force on Primary and Preventive Health Care of the American College of Obstetricians and Gynecologists (1993) published *The Obstetrician-Gynecologist and Primary-Preventive Health Care,* which contains guidelines for this care. By means of screening testing, counseling and patient education, behavioral intervention, and/or consultation, the obstetrician–gynecologist is able to address the major causes of morbidity (Table 1.1) and mortality (Table 1.2; Figure 1.1). Recommendations for screening testing (Table 1.3) are associated with high-risk situations and conditions; recommendations for immunization (Table 1.4) complete the tasks.

TABLE 1.2. Ten Leading Causes of Female Death in the United States, 1992

| Cause 0–14 | Age | | | |
	15–34	35–54	55–74	≥75
1. Diseases of infancy	Accidents	Cancer	Cancer	Heart disease
2. Congenital anomalies	Cancer	Heart disease	Heart disease	Cancer
3. Accidents	Homicide	Accidents	COPD	Cerebro-vascular disease
4. Cancer	Suicide	Cerebro-vascular disease	Cerebro-vascular disease	Pneumonia, influenza
5. Heart disease	HIV	Suicide	Diabetes	COPD
6. Homicide	Heart disease	Cirrhosis of liver	Pneumonia, influenza	Diabetes
7. Pneumonia, influenza	Cerebro-vascular disease	HIV	Accidents	Accidents
8. Septicemia	Congenital anomalies	Diabetes	Cirrhosis	Arterio-sclerosis
9. HIV	Pneumonia, influenza	COPD	Disease of arteries	Alzheimer's disease
10. Cerebral palsy	Diabetes	Homicide	Nephritis	Nephritis

COPD = chronic obstructive pulmonary disease; HIV = human immunodeficiency disease.

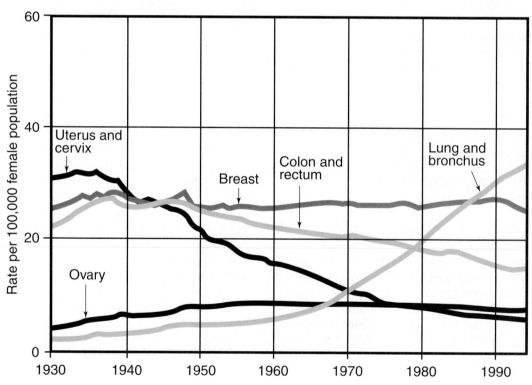

FIGURE 1.1. Age-adjusted cancer mortality for women in the United States, 1930–1995.

TABLE 1.3. Recommended Screening Testing and Health Care Interventions for Women

Risk Factor/Condition	Screening Test Recommendation or Intervention
Cervical dysplasia/cancer (high risk: immunosuppression, AIDS, multiple STDs or sexual partners, smokers)	Pap annually from onset of sexual activity or age 18; physician and patient discretion after three consecutive normal Paps after age 19
Skin cancer (high risk: extensive sun exposure, family/personal history of skin cancer, suspicious lesions)	Physical examination; counseling about sun exposure; consultation for suspicious lesions
Anemia (high risk: Caribbean, Latin American, Asian, Mediterranean, or African descent or history of menorrhagia)	Hemogram/sickle-cell preparation; hemoglobin electrophoresis
Hypercholesterolemia, coronary artery disease (high risk: elevated cholesterol; patient or sibling with cholesterol 240 mg/dl or higher; sibling, parent, or grandparent with coronary artery disease, especially at age 55 or under; smoking; diabetes mellitus)	Cholesterol/lipid profile every 5 years from age 19, every 3 to 4 years from age 65
Breast cancer (high risk: first-degree relative with breast cancer, especially if diagnosed premenopausally)	Screening mammography every other year from age 40, every year from age 50; yearly physician breast examination; self-breast examination instruction
Lung cancer, coronary artery disease	Counseling about smoking; regular blood pressure screening
Colorectal cancer	Sigmoidoscopy every 3 to 5 years after age 40; fecal occult blood test at physician discretion
Thyroid disease/risk for autoimmune disease (high risk: family history of thyroid disease, autoimmune disease)	TSH every 3 to 5 years after age 65
TB (high risk: patients with AIDS, who are immunosuppressed, or have close contact with those with TB; alcoholics and drug users; inmates of residential care facilities and prisons)	TB skin testing
Sexually transmitted diseases	As indicated by history/physical examination: "wet mount" from vaginal fluids, cultures for gonorrhea and chlamydia; RPR/VDRL; hepatitis; HIV; counseling about risk behaviors, safe sex practices
Diabetes mellitus (high risk: family history of diabetes; obesity; personal history of gestational diabetes mellitus)	Fasting blood glucose as indicated
Osteoporosis	Diet and exercise counseling combined with menopausal hormone-replacement therapy and calcium supplementation

AIDS = acquired immune deficiency syndrome; HIV = human immunodeficiency virus; RPR/VDRL = rapid plasma reagin/Venereal Disease Research Laboratory; STDs = sexually transmitted diseases; TB = tuberculosis; TSH = thyroid-stimulating hormone.

TABLE 1.4.   Immunization Recommendations

Immunization	Recommendations
Tetanus–diphtheria booster	Once between ages 14 and 16
Influenza vaccine	Every 10 years from age 19 to 64 for residents of chronic care facilities; persons with chronic cardiopulmonary disorders; and persons with metabolic diseases such as diabetes mellitus, hemoglobinopathies, immunosuppression, or renal dysfunction; annually for women 65 years old
Pneumococcal vaccine	Every 10 years from age 19 to 64 for women with medical conditions that increase the risk of pneumococcal infection (e.g., chronic cardiac or pulmonary disease, sickle-cell disease, nephrotic syndrome, Hodgkin's disease, asplenia, diabetes mellitus, alcoholism, cirrhosis, multiple myeloma, renal disease, or other immunosuppression)
Measles, mumps, rubella (MMR)	Rubella titer vaccine for women of childbearing age lacking evidence of immunity; a second measles immunization, preferably as MMR, for all women unable to show proof of immunity
Hepatitis B vaccine	Intravenous drug users; current recipients of blood products; persons in health-related jobs with exposure to blood or blood products; household and sexual contacts of hepatitis B virus carriers; prostitutes; persons with a history of sexual activity with multiple partners in the previous 6 months

Health promotion and disease and injury prevention by means of patient education is another significant component of the preventive care and health maintenance roles of the obstetrician–gynecologist. By means of history taking and discussion with the patient, and by use of prepared educational materials such as pamphlets, videos, and computer programs, issues such as contraception, prevention of sexually transmitted diseases, diet and exercise, stress management, tobacco, alcohol, and substance abuse, immunization, seat belt and car seat use, and sun exposure should be addressed.

By the first half of the 21st century, the number of older women in the United States will nearly double (Figure 1.2). The

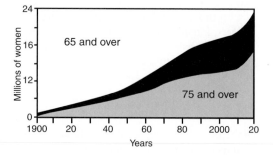

FIGURE 1.2.   Older women in the American population.

older women with their special health needs will comprise a significant part of the patients cared for by most general obstetrician–gynecologists, who will often be their primary physician as well. Their age specific needs will require a still wider range of knowledge and skills than heretofore expected of obstetrician–gynecologists. Obstetrician–gynecologists will continue to address issues such as hormone replacement therapy and screening for breast, cervical, uterine, and colorectal cancer, which have long been a part of obstetric–gynecologic care. In addition, they will have to provide care for some health issues (e.g., simple hypertension, thyroid disease) and will also need to address issues of safety and quality of living (e.g., vision and hearing, fall prevention, immunization, diet and exercise, emotional health and associated issues of cognitive change and social interaction). These older women and their families will expect their clinicians to help them maintain an active, healthy, and satisfying lifestyle for most of their lifetime, in addition to the identification and treatment of illness.

PART II: EVALUATION AND MANAGEMENT

Starting with the first interaction and continuing in each subsequent visit, the physician strives to establish and develop a professional relationship of mutual trust and respect with the patient. The physician gathers the historical and physical information needed for the patient's care, makes differential and presumptive diagnoses, identifies issues involving health promotion and maintenance and disease prevention, and formulates a management plan in cooperation with the patient. At the same time, the patient usually decides if the physician is knowledgeable and trustworthy and whether she will accept and follow the regimens and recommendations that are made.

The process begins with an appropriate greeting, which deserves special attention because of the importance of initial impressions. A handshake is commonly used. Surnames should generally be used. First names are more appropriate for friendship relationships; whereas the patient–physician relationship, although friendly, is profes-

sional. "What brought you to the office today?" or "How may I help you today?" are neutral opening questions that allow the patient to frame a response that includes her problems, concerns, and/or reasons for the visit.

Attentive, thoughtful listening is essential for accurate patient evaluation. What the patient says may be meaningfully understood only when considered in the context of her personal, emotional, or cultural situation. Sometimes issues are uncomfortably personal. A highly emotional response may be the first indication of an unstated problem that requires attention. Letting the patient know that your interest is not personal, but instead reflects your desire to learn what you need to know to help, often facilitates these difficult communications. When faced with a negative, perhaps hostile, response, the physician may use such a comment to resolve the conflict and reestablish a positive interaction. Ignoring a negative response usually dooms the professional relationship.

HEALTH EVALUATION: HISTORY, PHYSICAL EXAMINATION, AND COMPREHENSIVE HEALTH PLANNING
History
CHIEF COMPLAINT (AND OTHER PROBLEMS AND ISSUES)

The chief complaint is the reason for the patient's visit. Other health problems as well as issues of health maintenance and disease prevention may come directly from the stated chief complaint or may be derived from other history or specific questions about high-risk situations. This may be expressed and recorded as a quote or as a paraphrased statement, although care must be taken in the latter case to avoid obscuring the patient's true meaning with medical jargon. Establishing the chronology of a problem is important because chronological organization of symptoms may suggest a specific disorder. Care must be taken at the end of an encounter to address the chief complaint. Sometimes other problems or issues are discovered that are "more significant" (e.g., an asymptomatic pelvic mass) than the chief complaint. Nevertheless, the patient will correctly expect that her chief complaint, the reason she came in the first place, will be addressed; the clinician will be judged in part by whether this issue is addressed.

MENSTRUAL HISTORY

Menstrual history begins with *menarche,* the age at which menses began. The basic menstrual history should then include the duration of bleeding, the interval between the first day of menstrual flow and the first day of the next menstrual flow, the frequency of menses, and the *last menstrual period (LMP),* dated from the first day of the last normal period. Episodes of bleeding that are "light but on time" should be noted as such, because they may have diagnostic significance. Estimation of the amount of menstrual flow can be made by asking whether the patient uses pads or tampons, how many are used during the heavy days of her flow, and whether they are soaked or just soiled when they are changed. It is normal for women to pass clots during menstruation, but they should not normally be larger than the size of a dime. Asking the size of clots relative to coins is useful, because it provides patient and clinician with a standard reference. Specific inquiry should be made about irregular or intermenstrual bleeding or spotting and contact bleeding (postcoital or postdouching bleeding or spotting). Such abnormal bleeding must be correlated with information about contraceptive method, infections, concurrent gynecologic problems, and sexual practices.

The menstrual history may include perimenstrual symptoms (molimina) such as anxiety, fluid retention, nervousness, mood fluctuations, food cravings, variations in sexual feelings, and difficulty sleeping. Any medications used during this time should be noted. Crampy pain during the menses is common. It is abnormal when it interferes with daily activities or when it requires more analgesia than provided by plain aspirin, acetaminophen, or ibuprofen. Inquiry about duration, quality, radiation of the pain to areas outside the pelvis, and association with body position or daily activities completes the pain history.

The term *menopause* refers to the cessation of menses. The *climacteric* is the time of transition when ovarian function begins to wane. The climacteric history often begins with increasing menstrual irregularity and varying or decreased flow, associated with hot flashes, nervousness, mood changes, and decreased vaginal lubrication. The physician should ask the patient whether she has had or is undergoing *hormonal therapy* (estrogen replacement with or without progestin and/or other hormonal treatment) as well as other medical treatment such as psychoactive medications. A history of medical (radiation or chemotherapy) or surgical oophorectomy should be taken. *Postmenopausal bleeding* is abnormal; it is usually defined as bleeding six months after cessation of menses. It is an important historical fact that should be documented or stated as a pertinent negative because of its association with genital malignancy, especially endometrial carcinoma.

OBSTETRIC HISTORY

Obstetric history includes the number of pregnancies (*gravidity*) and outcome of each (*parity*). The following abbreviation may be used: gravida (G) a Para (P) b c d e, where

  a = number of pregnancies

  b = number of term pregnancies
    (≥ 37 weeks)

  c = number of preterm pregnancies
    (viability through 36 weeks)

  d = number of abortions (spontaneous
    or induced) and ectopic
    pregnancies

  e = number of living children

TABLE 1.5.	Obstetric Definitions
Gravida	A woman who is or has been pregnant
Primigravida	A woman who is in or who has experienced her first pregnancy
Multigravida	A woman who has been pregnant more than once
Nulligravida	A woman who has never been and is not now pregnant
Primipara	A woman who has delivered one pregnancy (regardless of the number of fetuses) that progressed beyond the gestational age of an abortion
Multipara	A woman who has delivered two or more pregnancies that progressed beyond the gestational age of an abortion
Nullipara	A woman who has never had a pregnancy progress beyond the gestational age of an abortion
Parturient	A woman currently in labor
Puerpera	A woman who has just recently given birth

Specific information about each item should be included. For term and preterm deliveries, determine the outcome, any complications, and mode of delivery. For abortions and ectopic pregnancies, determine any known causes, medical therapy and/or surgical procedure(s) done, complications, and feelings about these events. Some key obstetric terms are defined in Table 1.5.

GYNECOLOGIC HISTORY

The gynecologic history includes information about any *gynecologic disease and/or treatment* that the patient has had, including the diagnosis or as much as the patient can remember about her illness, the medical and/or surgical treatment, and the results. Questions about previous gynecologic surgery should include what surgery; reason for the surgery; when, where, and by whom the surgery was performed; the results as the patient understands them and whether they agreed with her expectations for the surgery; and the emotional and physical effects of the surgery.

Information about infectious and *sexually transmitted disease (STD)* should be obtained. Information about vaginitis should include frequency, duration, treatment, and effect of treatment. Vaginal discharge should be characterized by color, odor, consistency, quantity, association with rectal or urethral discharge, associated symptoms such as pain or pruritus, relationship to medication such as antibiotics and exogenous steroids, and relationship to exacerbations of diseases such as diabetes. Localized lesions or ulcerations should be characterized by date of recognition, location, growth, associated symptoms (pain, pruritus, bleeding, discharge), similar nonperineal lesions, treatment, and results of treatment. Pelvic inflammatory disease (PID) is a frequently encountered history. PID is classically characterized by fever, chills, abdominopelvic pain, and an appropriate response to oral or parenteral antibiotic therapy. PID is often confused with vaginitis, which may be differentiated by the different history of vaginal discharge and characterized by local symptoms such as pruritus or irritation. The patient should be asked specifically about a history of sexually transmitted and infectious diseases such as gonorrhea, herpes, chlamydia, warts (condylomata), hepatitis, acquired immune deficiency syndrome (AIDS), and syphilis as well as the use of intrauterine devices (IUDs) because these have been associated with PID. Finally, patients should be asked about behaviors that are high risk for the acquisition of human immunodeficiency virus (HIV) or hepatitis, including parenteral drug use, sexual relationships with drug users or bisexuals, transfusion before approximately 1980, and prostitution or promiscuity.

A history about *breast disease and breast cancer* should include previous known breast disease or cancer; previous breast biopsy; previous mammography or other imaging study; family history of breast cancer; and appreciation by the patient of a mass, discharge, or painful area. Correlation with the patient's age, menstrual status, and hormonal therapy should be made.

If a patient has a history of *infertility* (generally defined as failure to conceive for one year), questions concerning both partners should cover previous diseases or surgery that may affect fertility, previous fertility (previous children with the same or other partners), duration of time that pregnancy has been attempted, and a history of sexual practices.

Finally, *diethylstilbestrol (DES)* use by the patient's mother during her pregnancy should be noted, because it may be associated with infertility problems and/or vaginal adenosis or carcinoma in the daughter. A personal hygiene history should address the use of douching and vaginal "feminine sprays," deodorants, or self-medications. A history of gastrointestinal and urinary disorders completes the gynecologic history. If a history of urinary frequency or involuntary urine loss is elicited, consideration should be given to evaluation for urinary tract infection and/or evaluation for urogynecologic issues such as stress urinary incontinence. If a history of chronic constipation or water, blood, or mucus in the stool is elicited, consideration should be given to gastrointestinal evaluation.

SEXUAL AND CONTRACEPTIVE HISTORY

Taking a *sexual history* is facilitated by behaviors, attitudes, and direct statements by the physician that project a nonjudgmental manner of acceptance and respect for the patient's lifestyle. The initial questions are often the most difficult. A good opening question is, "Please tell me about your sexual partner or partners." This question is gender neutral, leaves the issue of number of partners open, and also gives the patient considerable latitude for response. In the final analysis, however, these questions must be individualized to each patient. If faced with an untoward emotional response, the physician should address the situation directly, assuring the patient that no disrespect or judgment was meant or implied and that the goal is solely to provide good health care. Data to be elicited should include age at first intercourse, the patient's present sexual partner(s) [including gender], types of sexual practices, and the patient's level of satisfaction with her sex life. Finally, questions regarding *child and/or adult sexual abuse and assault* should be asked. The patient may be asked, "Have you ever been touched against your will, either as a child or an adult?"

A patient's *contraceptive history* should include the contraceptive method currently used, when it was begun, any problems or complications, and the patient's and her partner's satisfaction with the method. Previous contraceptive methods should also be noted as well as the reasons they were discontinued. The history concludes with inquiry about the patient's future conceptive or contraceptive plans (Table 1.6).

Physical Examination

BREAST EXAMINATION

The breast examination by a physician remains the most cost-effective and reliable means of early detection of breast cancer when combined with appropriately scheduled mammography and regular breast self-examination. The results of the breast examination may be expressed by description or diagram or both, usually with reference to the quadrants and tail region of the breast or by allusion to the breast as a clock face with the nipple at the center (Figure 1.3). Development of the female breast

TABLE 1.6. The OB–GYN History and Physical Examination: Generalized Report Format

I. History
  A. Chief complaint
  B. Menstrual history
    1. Last menstrual period; previous menstrual period
    2. Menarche
    3. Usual menstrual duration; interval between first days of menstrual periods
    4. Menstrual flow
    5. Abnormal menses
    6. Pain
  C. Menopause
    1. Climacteric symptoms, if any
    2. Perimenopausal and postmenopausal history
    3. Postmenopausal bleeding
  D. Obstetric history
    1. Gravidity and parity
    2. Obstetric complications
  E. Gynecologic history
    1. Gynecologic diseases and treatment, including surgery and medical treatment
    2. Sexually transmitted diseases
      a. Vaginitis, vulvitis
      b. Local lesions
      c. Pelvic inflammatory disease
    3. Breast disease (history, biopsy information, any family history of breast carcinoma)
    4. Infertility
    5. Urinary tract/bowel complaints
    6. DES exposure
    7. Personal hygiene
  F. Sexual history (activity, problems, satisfaction)
  G. Sexual assault/abuse, adult and child
  H. Contraceptive history
    1. Present contraception
    2. Past contraception
    3. Conception plans
II. Physical examination
  A. Height, weight, and blood pressure
  B. Breast examination
  C. Examination of the abdomen, back, and lymphatics
  D. Pelvic examination
    1. Vulva
    2. Clitoris
    3. BUS (Bartholin's glands, urethra, Skene's glands)
    4. Vagina
    5. Cervix
    6. Uterus
    7. Adnexa
    8. Rectovaginal examination (guaiac determination, if needed)

DES = diethylstilbestrol.

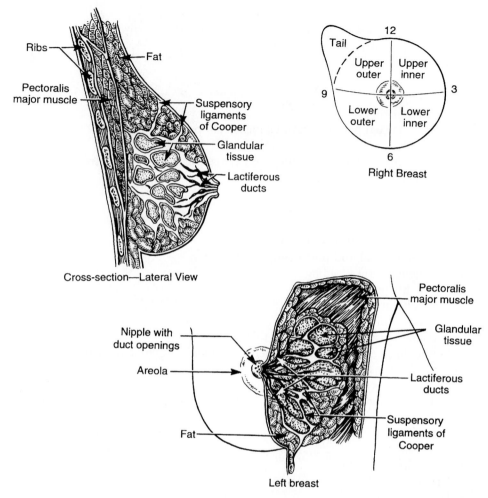

FIGURE 1.3. Clinical anatomy and associated examination schema of the breast.

as described in Tanner's sex maturity ratings is used in the description of the breast examination (Figure 1.4).

How to Do the Breast Examination (Figures 1.5 and 1.6)

The breasts are first examined by *inspection.* Inspection begins with the patient's arms at her sides and then with her hands pressed against her hips and/or with her arms raised over her head. If the patient's breasts are especially large and pendulous, leaning forward so that the breasts hang free of the chest may facilitate inspection. The patient's breasts are observed before and after these maneuvers, which alter the relations of the supportive fascia of the breast tissue as the arms move. Tumors often distort the relations of these tissues, causing disruption of the shape, contour, or symmetry of the breast or position of the nipple. Some asymmetry of the breasts is common, but marked differences or recent changes deserve further evaluation.

Discolorations and/or ulcerations of the skin of the breast or areola/nipple, or edema of the lymphatics, causing a leathery puckered appearance of the skin (like an orange skin, hence called peau d'orange), are abnormal. A clear or milky breast discharge (galactorrhea) requires evaluation. Bloody discharge from the breast is abnormal; it usually does not represent carcinoma but

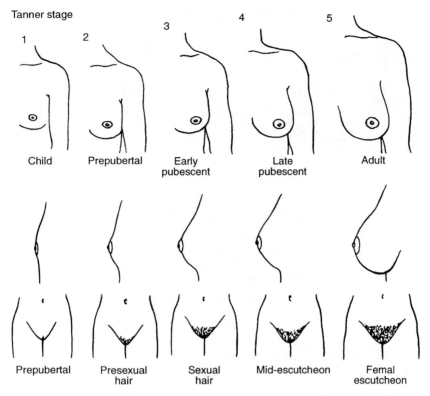

FIGURE 1.4.   Tanner's classification of sexual maturity: breasts and pubic hair.

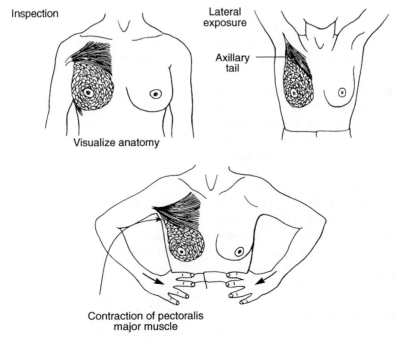

FIGURE 1.5.   Inspection of the breast.

Breast palpation techniques

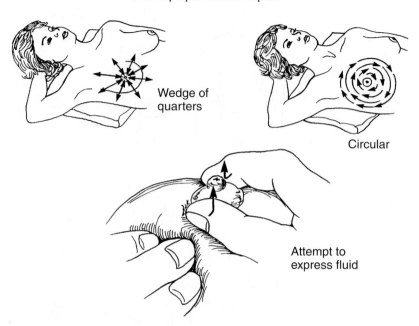

Wedge of quarters

Circular

Attempt to express fluid

FIGURE 1.6. Palpation of the breast.

rather inflammation of a breast structure. Pus usually indicates infection, although an underlying tumor may be encountered.

Palpation follows inspection, first with the patient's arms at her sides and then with the arms raised over her head. This is usually done in the supine position, although sometimes use of the sitting position with the patient's arm resting on the examiner's shoulder or over her head for examination of the most lateral aspects of the axilla is helpful. Palpation should be done with slow, careful maneuvers using the flat of the fingers and not the tips. The fingers are moved up and down in a wavelike motion, moving the tissues under them back and forth. By so doing breast masses are moved so that they may be more easily felt. A spiral or radial pattern is described over each breast to uniformly cover all of the breast tissue, including that of the axillary tail. If masses are found, their size, shape, consistency (soft, hard, firm, cystic), and mobility as well as their position should be determined. While there are many causes of "lumps," a comparison of the two that are especially common as well as carcinoma are presented in

Table 1.7. Women with large breasts may demonstrate a firm ridge of tissue found transversely along the lower edge of the breast. This is the inframammary ridge and is a normal finding. The examination is concluded with gentle pressure inward and then upward at the sides of the areola—a gentle "squeezing" action to express fluid. If fluid is noted on inspection or expressed, it should be sent for culture and sensitivity and cytopathology (fixed in the same manner as for a Pap smear) if indicated by its character and the clinical situation.

How to Teach the Breast Self-Examination (BSE)

Breast self-examination is an important part of women's health education. It is often not practiced regularly because of fear of what might be found, lack of confidence in how to do the examination, or belief that the examination will not help discover cancer. Good education about the examination and its benefits and how to do it on a regular basis should eliminate these barriers to good health care. An extra benefit may be derived: helping a woman assume a more

TABLE 1.7.   Characteristics of Common Breast Lumps

Characteristic	Fibrocystic Disorder	Fibroadenoma	Carcinoma
Incidence with age	25 to menopause, uncommon afterward	Puberty to menopause (peak 20–30)	Increases with age
Number	Usually multiple cysts	Usually one or two	Usually single
Shape and consistency	Well circumscribed cysts; "sheets" of dense tissue	Smooth, well circumscribed motile, "rubbery"	Irregular, poorly delineated from other tissue
Mobility	Mobile	Mobile	Mobility limited; often fixed to surrounding skin, tissue
Axillary involvement	No	No	May be present with metastatis
Nipple discharge	No	No	Often

active and beneficial role in her own health care, which may be translated in part to better "compliance" with health care plans.

It should be explained that BSE is like the breast examination provided by her clinician, having two parts—LOOKING and FEELING (Figure 1.7). The value of performing BSE on a monthly basis and reporting findings to the clinician should be emphasized, specifically including that the treatment of disease detected early in its course is much more likely to be successful compared to treatment started later after disease had had time to progress. It should be explained that a woman will become very expert in knowing her own breast and when something has changed. If something changes, it is then the task of the clinician to determine the significance, if any, of the change. LOOKING involves observation (inspection) of the breasts in a mirror with arms at the side and raised over the head. Changes in the way the breast or nipples look warrant discussion with the clinician. FEELING involves the systematic examination (palpation) of the entire breast (including up into the area under the armpit) using the flat part of the first three fingers. Lumps, bumps, changes in texture, or unusual discomfort warrant an examination by the clinician. Gentle squeezing of the nipples completes the BSR; if blood, fluid, or pus is expressed, an examination by the clinician is indicated.

PELVIC EXAMINATION

Despite advances in ultrasonography and other imaging technologies, *the pelvic examination remains a mainstay of clinical obstetrics and gynecology.* The results of the pelvic examination may be expressed by description or diagram or both.

How to Do the Pelvic Examination

Preparation for the pelvic examination begins with the patient emptying her bladder and donning an examination gown. An assistant should usually be present for the pelvic examination to assist in the preparation of specimens and act as a chaperon. It is important to thoroughly explain everything that is going to happen to a patient before it happens. The cardinal rule is "TALK BEFORE YOU TOUCH," because an unexpected touch is disconcerting.

Abdominal and especially pelvic examinations require relaxation of the muscles. An abrupt or stern command, such as "Relax now; I'm not going to hurt you," may raise the patient's fears, whereas a

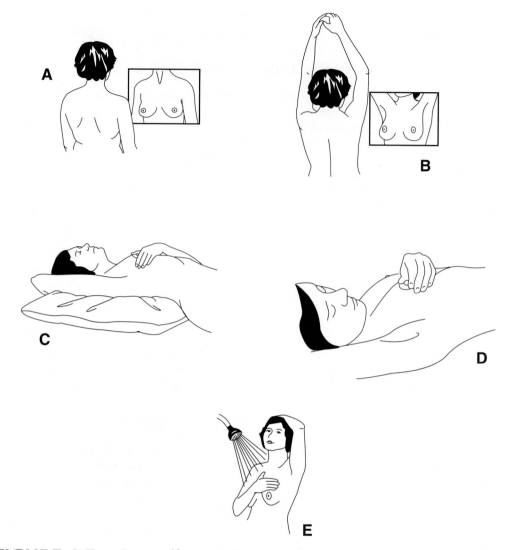

FIGURE 1.7.   Breast self-examination.

phrase such as "Try to relax as much as you can, although I know that it's a lot easier for me to say than for you to do" sends two messages: (1) that the patient needs to relax and (2) that you recognize that it is difficult, both of which demonstrate patience and understanding. A phrase such as "Let me know if anything is uncomfortable, and I will stop and then we will try to do it differently" tells the patient that there might be discomfort but that she has control and can stop the examination if discomfort occurs. If any maneuvers require deep palpation or may cause discomfort, the patient should be told what to expect before such

maneuvers are done. Few positions leave a woman with such a feeling of helplessness as the lithotomy position; returning a degree of control to her is most helpful. Using the word *we* also demonstrates that the examination is a cooperative effort, further empowering the patient and facilitating care. Techniques that help the patient to relax include encouraging the patient to breathe in and out gently and regularly rather than holding her breath and helping the patient to identify specific muscle groups (such as the abdominal muscle groups or the perineal muscle groups) that need to be relaxed.

The patient is asked to sit at the edge of the examination table and an opened, draping sheet is placed over the patient's knees. If a patient requests that a drape not be used, the request should be honored.

Positioning the patient for examination begins with the elevation of the head of the examining table to approximately 30° from horizontal. This serves three purposes: (1) it allows eye contact and facilitates communication between physician and patient; (2) it relaxes the abdominal wall muscle groups, making the examination much easier; and (3) it allows the clinician to observe the patient for responses to the examination, which may provide valuable information (e.g., wincing as evidence of pain on examination). The physician and/or an assistant should help the patient assume the lithotomy position. The patient should be asked to lie back, place her heels in the stirrups, and then slide down to the end of the table until her buttocks are flush with the edge of the table. After the patient is in the lithotomy position, the drape is adjusted so that it does not obscure the clinician's view of the perineum or obscure eye contact between patient and physician.

The physician should sit at the foot of the examining table with the examination lamp adjusted to shine on the perineum. The lamp is optimally positioned in front of the physician's chest a few inches or so below the level of the chin, just at the level of the perineum but at approximately an arm's length distance from it, allowing the examination maneuvers. The physician should glove both hands. This protects the patient's modesty and sense of privacy and also protects the clinician from sexually transmitted disease. After contact with the patient, there should be minimal contact with equipment such as the lamp.

The pelvic examination begins with the inspection and examination of the external genitalia. The physician begins by firmly placing the back of his hand on the patient's inner thigh, progressing to both hands touching the external genitalia, and thereafter to a sequential inspection and palpation of the external genitalia. Initial touching of the inner thigh begins the examination in a "personal and sensitive" area, although not as sensitive as the perineum. Throughout the pelvic examination, the examiner should make use of the bilateral symmetry of the body. Dissymmetry shows that one side is different from the other, perhaps because of disease, which then requires an explanation. All maneuvers should be performed gently yet with a firmness that is comfortable. Deliberate speed is important but do not be abrupt; neither linger beyond the time needed to do the task nor move too quickly, failing to gain the needed information.

Inspection should include the mons pubis, labia majora and labia minora, perineum, and perianal area. Inspection continues as palpation is performed in an orderly sequence, starting with the clitoral hood, which may be pulled back to inspect the glans proper. The labia are spread laterally to allow inspection of the introitus and outer vagina. The urethral meatus and the areas of the urethra and Skene's glands should be inspected. After forewarning the patient about the possible sensation of having to urinate, the forefinger is placed an inch or so into the vagina to gently milk the urethra. A culture should be taken of any discharge from the urethral opening. The forefinger is then rotated posteriorly to palpate the area of the Bartholin's glands between that finger and the thumb (Figure 1.8). The patient is then asked to bear down slightly as if she were going to have a bowel movement while the vaginal walls are inspected for cystocele or rectocele. Just as with the breast examination, women at different ages demonstrate different stages of development of the genitals and associated hair, as seen in Tanner's classification (see Figure 1.4).

The next step is the speculum examination. The parts of the speculum are seen in Figure 1.9. There are two types of specula in common use for the examination of adults. The Pederson speculum has flat and narrow blades that barely curve on the sides. The Pederson works well for most nulliparous women and postmenopausal women with atrophic, narrowed vaginas. The Graves speculum has blades that are wider, higher, and curved on the sides and is more appropriate for most

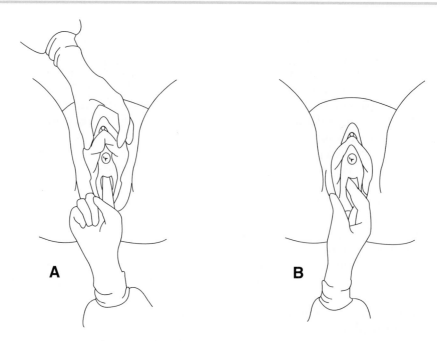

A

B

FIGURE 1.8. Palpation of the Bartholin's, urethral, and Skene's glands. (A) Palpation of urethral and Skene's glands and "milking" of urethra. (B) Palpation of Bartholin's glands.

parous women. Its wider, curved blades keep the looser vaginal walls on the multiparous women separated for visualization. A Pederson with extra narrow blades may be used for visualizing the cervix in pubertal girls.

First, the speculum is examined to be sure it is clean and in proper working order. If not already warm, the speculum should be warmed, because insertion of a cold speculum is unacceptable.

Speculum insertion and visualization of the vagina and cervix are performed in a stepwise manner (Figure 1.10). Moistening the speculum with warm water may help with insertion. Lubricants should not be used routinely because they interfere with cytologic and microbiologic specimens. Situations that require their use are encountered infrequently; examples include some prepubertal girls, some postmenopausal women, and patients with irritation or lesions of the vagina making manipulative examination uncomfortable.

Most physicians find the control of pressure and movement of the speculum facilitated by holding the speculum with the dominant hand. The speculum is held by the handle with the blades completely closed. The first two fingers of the opposite hand are placed on the perineum laterally and just below the introitus and pressure is applied downward and slightly inward until the introitus is opened slightly. If the patient is sufficiently relaxed, this downward pressure on the perineum results in an open introitus into which the speculum may be easily inserted. The speculum is initially inserted in a horizontal plane with the width of the blades perpendicular to the vertical axis of the introitus. The speculum is then inclined at approximately a 45° angle from horizontal; the angle is adjusted as the speculum is inserted so that the speculum slides into the vagina with minimal resistance. Inserting the speculum in a more vertical plane and then rotating the speculum is another method of introduction that is widely used. If the patient is not relaxed, posterior pressure from a finger inserted in the vagina sometimes relaxes the perineal musculature.

As the speculum is inserted, a slight continuous downward pressure is exerted so that distention of the perineum is used

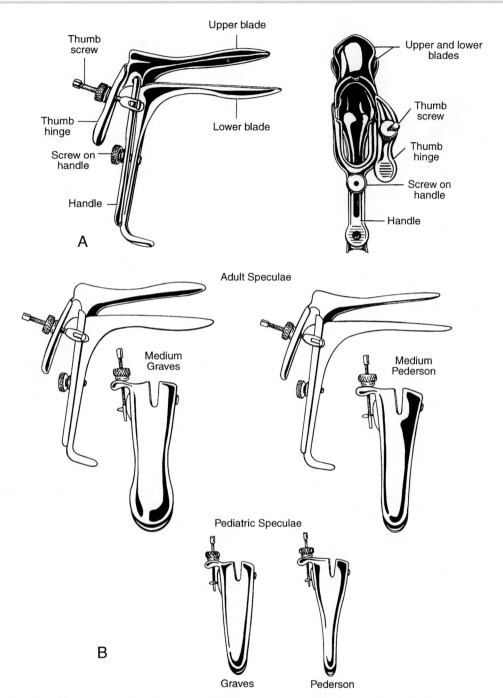

FIGURE 1.9.   The vaginal speculum. (*A*) Parts of the vaginal speculum. (*B*) Types of vaginal specula.

to create space into which the speculum may advance. Taking advantage of the distensibility of the perineum and vagina posterior to the introitus is a crucial concept for the efficient and comfortable manipulation of the speculum (and later for the bimanual and rectovaginal) examination. Pressure superiorly causes pain in the sensitive area of the urethra and clitoris. The speculum is inserted as far as it will go, which in most women means insertion of the entire speculum length.

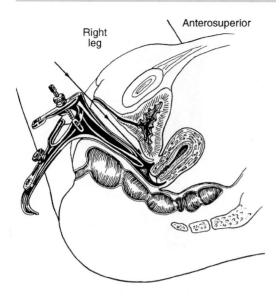

FIGURE 1.10.   Speculum insertion (note the angle of insertion).

The speculum is then opened in a smooth deliberate fashion. With slight tilting of the speculum, the cervix slides into view between the blades of the speculum. The speculum is then locked into the open position using the thumb screw. Failure to find the cervix most commonly results from not having the speculum inserted far enough. Keeping the speculum fully inserted while opening the speculum does not result in discomfort.

When the speculum is locked into position, it usually stays in place without being held. For most patients, the speculum is opened sufficiently by use of the upper thumb screw. In some cases, however, more space is required. This may be obtained by gently expanding the vertical distance between the speculum blades by use of the screw on the handle of the speculum.

With the speculum in place, the cervix and the deep lateral vaginal vault may be inspected. The Pap smear, "wet prep," and/or cultures may be taken at this time.

Before obtaining the Pap smear, the patient should be told that she may feel a slight "scraping" sensation but no pain. Specimens are collected to fully evaluate the transformation zone where cervical intraepithelial neoplasia is more likely to be

encountered. Most commonly, both an endocervical sample and an exocervical sample are obtained using appropriate sampling devices. The material is thinly smeared on a slide, avoiding large accumulations of mucus and other material. Thick accumulations of material cannot be accurately evaluated. *Immediate fixation* is important to avoid air drying artifacts, which compromise cytopathologic evaluation. Slides left in air longer than 10 seconds demonstrate a very high incidence of such artifacts (Figure 1.11). Other techniques for the acquisition of specimens for cytologic evaluation are also used, including placing the specimen in a liquid medium, which is spun down, and the cells obtained spread on a slide for evaluation (Thin Prep). This technique is suggested to have the advantage of a more uniform, easier to read slide while simultaneously bypassing the issues of even smearing of the slide and fixation artifacts. Finally, computer programs have been developed to assist in the reading of Pap smears, purporting the advantage of increased speed and accuracy and decreased cost. For the time, these systems will probably be used as an adjunct to standard Pap smear "reading" by cytologist/pathologist for purposes of quality assurance, although in the future their role may expand with greater experience in their use and refinement of the technology.

When specimen collection is completed, it is time for speculum withdrawal and inspection of the vaginal walls. After telling the patient that the speculum is to be removed and that she should not tighten her vaginal muscles on movement of the speculum, the blades of the speculum are opened very slightly by putting pressure on the thumb hinge and the thumb screw is completely loosened. Opening the speculum blades slightly farther before starting to withdraw the speculum avoids pinching the cervix between the blades. The speculum is withdrawn approximately 1 inch before pressure on the thumb hinge is slowly released. The speculum is withdrawn slowly enough to allow inspection of the vaginal walls. As the end of the speculum blades approaches the introitus, there should be no

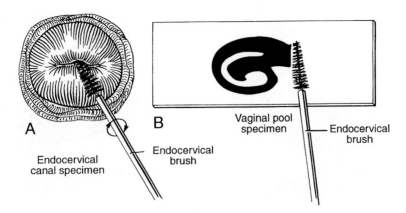

FIGURE 1.11. Pap smear. (*A*) Obtaining endocervical portion of Pap smear. (*B*) Strong specimen before fixation within 10 seconds.

pressure on the thumb hinge, otherwise the anterior blade can flip up, hitting the sensitive vaginal, urethral, and clitoral tissues.

The *bimanual examination* uses both hands (the "vaginal" hand and the "abdominal" hand) to entrap and palpate the pelvic organs. The bimanual examination begins by exerting gentle pressure on the abdomen approximately halfway between the umbilicus and the pubic hair line with the abdominal hand, while at the same time inserting one finger of the vaginal hand into the vagina to approximately 2 inches and gently pushing downward, distending the vaginal canal. The patient is asked to feel the muscles being pushed on and to relax them as much as possible. Then two fingers are inserted into the vagina until they rest at the limit of the vaginal vault in the posterior fornix behind and below the cervix. A great deal of space may be created by posterior distention of the perineum.

During the bimanual examination, the pelvic structures are "caught" and palpated between the abdominal and vaginal hands. Whether to use the dominant hand as the abdominal or vaginal hand is a question of personal preference. The most common error in this part of the pelvic examination is failure to make effective use of the abdominal hand. Pressure should be applied with the flat of the fingers, not the tips, starting midway between the umbilicus and the hairline, moving downward in conjunction with upward movements of the vaginal

hand. The bimanual examination continues with the circumferential examination of the cervix for its size, shape, position, mobility, and the presence or absence of tenderness or mass lesions. Cervical position is often related to uterine position. A posterior cervix is often associated with an anteverted or midposition uterus, whereas an anterior cervix is often associated with a retroverted uterus. Sharp flexion of the uterus, however, may alter these relations.

Bimanual examination of the uterus is accomplished by lifting the uterus up toward the abdominal fingers so that it may be palpated between the vaginal and abdominal hands. The uterus is evaluated for its size, shape, consistency, configuration, and mobility as well as masses or tenderness and for position (anteversion, midposition, retroversion, anteflexion, or retroflexion). The technique varies somewhat with the position of the uterus. Examination of the anterior and midposition uterus is facilitated with the vaginal fingers lateral and deep to the cervix in the posterior fornix. The uterus is gently lifted upward to the abdominal fingers and a gentle side-to-side "searching" motion of the vaginal fingers is combined with steady pressure and palpation by the abdominal hand to determine the characteristics of the uterus (Figure 1.12). Examination of the retroverted uterus is more difficult. In some cases the vaginal fingers may be slowly pushed below or at the level of the uterine

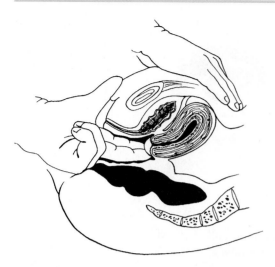

FIGURE 1.12. Bimanual examination of the uterus and adnexa.

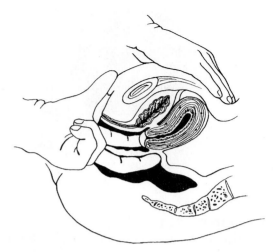

FIGURE 1.13. Rectovaginal examination.

fundus, after which gentle pressure exerted inward and upward causes the uterus to antevert or at least move "upward," somewhat facilitating palpation. Then palpation is accomplished as in the normally anteverted uterus. If this cannot be done, a waving motion with the vaginal fingers in the posterior fornix must be combined with an extensive rectovaginal examination to assess the retroverted uterus.

Bimanual examination of the adnexa to assess the ovaries, fallopian tubes, and support structures begins by placing the vaginal fingers to the side of the cervix deep in the lateral fornix. The abdominal hand is moved to the same side just inside the flare of the sacral arch and above the pubic hairline. Pressure is then applied downward and toward the symphysis with the abdominal hand while at the same time lifting upward with the vaginal fingers. The same movements of the fingers of both hands used to assess the uterus are used to assess the adnexal structures, which are brought between the fingers by these maneuvers to evaluate their size, shape, consistency, configuration, mobility, and tenderness as well as to palpate for masses. Special care must be taken when examining the ovaries, which are sensitive such that excessive pressure or sudden movements cause a deep visceral pain. It is important to note that

the ovaries are palpable in normal menstrual women approximately one half of the time, whereas palpation of ovaries in postmenopausal women implies the possibility of ovarian pathology usually requiring further evaluation.

The rectovaginal examination is an integral part of the complete pelvic examination on initial and annual examination as well as at interval examinations whenever clinically indicated. Full evaluation of the posterior aspect of the pelvic structures and of the support structures is possible only by this method in many patients. Because patients may have had bad experiences with this part of the pelvic examination, a careful explanation of the value of the examination and reassurance that the examination will be gently done is helpful.

The rectovaginal examination is begun by changing the glove on the vaginal hand and using a liberal supply of lubricant. The examination may be comfortably performed if the natural inclination of the rectal canal is followed: upward at a 45° angle for approximately 1 to 2 cm, then downward (Figure 1.13). This is accomplished by positioning the fingers of the vaginal hand as for the bimanual examination except that the index finger is also flexed. The second finger is then gently inserted through the rectal opening and inserted to the "bend" where the angle turns downward. The index (vaginal) finger is inserted into the vagina, and both fingers are inserted until the vaginal finger rests in the posterior fornix below the cervix and the rectal finger rests as far as it can go into the rectal canal. Asking the patient to bear down as the rectal finger is inserted is not necessary and may add to the tension for the patient. Palpation of the pelvic structures is then accomplished as in their vaginal palpation. The uterosacral ligaments are also palpated to determine if they are symmetrical, smooth, and nontender (as normally) or if they are nodular, slack, or thickened. The rectal canal is evaluated as are the integrity and function of the rectal sphincter. After palpation is complete, the fingers are rapidly but steadily removed in a reversal of the sequence of movements used on insertion. Care should be taken to avoid contamination of the vagina with fecal matter. A guaiac determination is made from fecal material collected on the rectal finger.

At the conclusion of the pelvic examination, the patient is asked to move back up on the table and thereafter to sit up. It is both good manners and helpful to offer a hand to the patient when she sits up. Discussion of the findings and recommendations for further care should be done after the patient has had a chance to clean herself, go to the washroom if needed, and dress.

Comprehensive Health Planning and Patient Management

Obstetrician–gynecologists promote good health, prevent disease, and manage specific disease states or medical conditions. The issues may fall within the scope of the obstetrician–gynecologist's practice or may require consultation or referral. Thus the obstetrician–gynecologist facilitates the health screening discussed earlier in this chapter, caring for identified problems (e.g., counseling about smoking cessation) or referral/consultation (e.g., for guaiac-positive stools). At times, the obstetrician–gynecologist provides care and at other times serves as the coordinator/facilitator of

care, the primary care responsibility. When a specific problem is identified, the classic schema of diagnosis and treatment facilitates care. Table 1.8 outlines the five tasks.

PART III: THE PHYSICIAN-PATIENT "CONTRACT"

The relationship between patient and physician should be one founded in mutual trust and respect with the joint goal of excellent, open, honest communication and joint decision making about all issues of care. The ages-old view of the relationship and responsibility of the physician as a sacred trust remains valid and should be a guiding principle in the physician's professional life.

The process of this relationship is found whenever there is contact between physician and patient, all or in part depending on the circumstances:

> Careful, empathetic listening to complaint or concern; identification of health promotion and disease prevention issues. Evaluation and identification or diagnosis of issues that need attention.
>
> Thorough explanation of the issues or diagnosis, and the proposed management—be it education, alteration of lifestyle, medication, surgery, or other. Included in this discussion is the presentation of not only the recommended course of action, but also alternative courses of action, the anticipated outcomes of the proposed action or inaction, and the risks and benefits of action or inaction.
>
> After all the questions of the patient are fully answered, she will select the course of action she finds appropriate and this decision should be honored in most circumstances. Continued contact (follow-up or periodic health maintenance care) allows evaluation of the efficacy of the chosen course of action, with alteration if needed using the same process to decide the nature of the alteration.

This process is often nowadays presented in the business/legal language of a "contract." Informed consent, for example, is the specific process used in preparation for some medical and most surgical managements.

TABLE 1.8. Generalized Patient Management Format

1. Formulation of differential diagnosis
   a. Formulate a differential diagnostic list of conditions that reasonably fit history and physical examination findings.
   b. Use to facilitate consideration of reasonably possible conditions and to provide a list for reconsideration if the presumptive diagnosis proves to be wrong.
2. Selection of laboratory testing
   a. Select tests that are necessary to confirm/rule out elements of the differential diagnosis and to select presumptive diagnosis.
   b. Tests should be valid and reliable, and present no unreasonable risks or cost relative to the value of the information to be obtained.
3. Selection of presumptive diagnosis
   a. Select a diagnosis that best fits information at hand.
   b. Remember that a patient may have more than one problem.
4. Development of management plan
   a. Develop a plan that provides proved, effective treatment for presumptive diagnosis.
   b. Benefits of proposed therapy should outweigh the risk of no treatment.
5. Follow-up management
   a. Follow-up on response to therapy to ascertain if the desired outcome is being or has been achieved. If not, the presumptive diagnosis and/or components of the therapy may be in error and reconsideration of both is required.
   b. This is an iterative process until the desired outcome is achieved.

An example is found in the section "The Decision for Sterilization" found in Chapter 26. Special situations such as sexual assault, domestic violence, and child abuse are governed by laws requiring reports to social service or legal authorities, and it is the responsibility of the physician to be aware of these responsibilities and to carry them out as required. As our medical technology becomes more and more powerful, many patients will wish to avail themselves of advance directives so that they are not subject to means of care that go beyond their desires. Using this process to help patients with these decisions is another important responsibility.

Health care is also an increasingly sophisticated and complicated business. Clinicians practice in different ways (e.g., solo practice, partnerships, as employees of health maintenance organizations or hospitals) and receive patients whose care is paid for by various kinds of health insurance organizations or who will require assistance to enter programs such as Medicare and Medicaid. The systems, in turn, often have

special "administrative requirements" for care, sometimes involving "permission" from a "gate-keeper"/primary care physician to whom the patient is assigned. The physician must understand how these systems affect patient care and how to work with them to assure that quality and appropriate care is rendered.

Several issues are of special importance. The first is clear and accurate documentation of history and physical examination findings and clinical management impressions (diagnoses) and plans. This facilitates good clinical communication with the obvious benefits that pertain. Second, the obstetrician–gynecologist may be the patient's primary care and obstetric–gynecologic clinician and will evaluate and treat accordingly. In the obstetric-gynecologic specialist role, patients will also be seen in consultation and referral, and the clinician must understand the rules for each kind of care. *Consultation* requires evaluation of the patient and the rendering of an opinion/recommendation, not care. Diagnostic procedures may be performed only with specific request as part of the consultation. *Referral* transfers care for a specific issue for a specific time, and includes treatment. Third, information about whatever kind of care is rendered must be used to create bills, which will allow reimbursement. Clinicians are usually reimbursed from third-party payers rather than directly by the patient. Many issues affect how much (what part) of the bill is paid and how, including which services are "covered" and "not covered" in the patient's contract with her third party payer, the specific policies and regulations of the third party payer's internal claims processing system, special "contractual" agreements between the physician and/or the physician's employer

and the third party payer, and government regulations. Additional issues often arise for patients covered by Medicaid and Medicare. What was done and why is translated into complex and often confusing numeric codes from the Health Care Financing Administration (HCFA), the American Medical Association's *Physician's Current Procedural Terminology (CPT)*, and the World Health Organization's *International Classification of Diseases (ICD-10)*. Unfortunately there is opportunity for illegal or unethical gain in this complex system, but also in theory the opportunity for appropriate compensation for needed care. Fraud, and such, should be anathema to the physician.

CASE STUDIES

Case 1A

A 68-year-old G4 P4004 comes to your office for her annual examination. She has been in good health except for some constipation, which she treats with Milk of Magnesia. She has been on hormone replacement therapy (Premarin 1.25 mg qd and Provera 2.5 mg qd) since menopause, approximately 15 years ago. She is widowed and lives in a retirement community in an efficiency apartment.

On physical examination her blood pressure, pulse, and weight are normal as is her general physical examination, including her breasts, chest, and abdomen. You note that her vulva and vagina are normal, although the latter is somewhat atrophic. Her uterus and cervix are surgically absent, and on questioning you learn that "they took my uterus out a long time ago because of tumors." Her rectovaginal examination is negative and her guaiac, positive.

Question Case 1A

Appropriate diagnostic studies include

A. Hemogram
B. Pap smear of vaginal vault
C. Coagulation profile
D. Sigmoidoscopy
E. Ultrasound of the pelvis

Answer: A, B, D

A hemogram in an elderly patient is always a useful measure of health but especially when there is the possibility of blood loss. A yearly Pap smear is also a routine screening test. Sigmoidoscopy is indicated because of the positive guaiac test. There is no history of a bleeding disorder warranting coagulation evaluation, and without physical findings or symptoms, ultrasound of the pelvis is likewise unnecessary.

(Continued)

Case 1B

An 18-year-old white G4 P1031 presents with a complaint of vaginal discharge for 3 weeks, which has not responded to an over-the-counter vaginal douche.

Question Case 1B

Although all the components of a new patient evaluation are important, the history so far makes which of the following lines of questioning especially pertinent?

A. Sexual history
B. Obstetric history
C. Contraceptive history
D. STD history
E. Social history

Answer: All

Questions about contraception and sexual practice are obvious, including the outcome of her four pregnancies. The complaint of vaginal discharge combined with multiparity at 18 years renders questions about frequency and number of partners and STDs pertinent. Her social situation, given her age and having a living child, is also important for the evaluation of her well-being as well as that of her child.

Case 1C

A 53-year-old Hispanic G4 P5014 comes to your office for a new patient visit. Her chief complaint is hot flashes and irritability that started about the same time her menses ceased, 13 months ago.

Personal Medical History			
	Medications	Glipizide	
	Medical	Diabetes, managed by her personal physician, an internist	
		Last "female examination" about 4 years ago; no history of STDs; all Pap smears have been normal; one mammogram at time last "female examination" also normal	
	Surgery	One ceasarean section; laparoscopic cholecystectomy about 3 years ago	
	Allergy	None	
FMHx			
	Father	Hypertension, s/p MI	
	Mother	Diabetes	
	Siblings	3 sisters, 4 brothers, all alive and well	
	Children	4, all alive and well	
PSFHx			
	Habits	Smoking	1 pack per week for 30–40 years
		Alcohol	Social only
		Drugs	None
	Social	Married for 39 years, husband Hector V. Hernandez, 58 and in good health; four children, three married and working, the last a senior in college	
	Employment/ Education	College graduate, works as senior teller in a local bank	

ROS	Constitutional	Pleasant articulate lady, oriented ×3
	Vision/Hearing	OK
	CV	No chest pain, SOB, DOE
	Resp.	No am cough, hemoptysis
	GI	No constipation or diarrhea, no bleeding
	GU	In last 4 months, some sense of urgency in urination; no urinary incontinence, no bleeding in urine
		Menses ceased abruply 13 months ago, although she has had some spotting in the last six weeks
		In last 6 months increasing difficulty with intercourse and disquiet for patient and husband; difficulty with intromission due to dry scratching feeling in her vagina as well as some decrease in his ability to maintain an adequate erection
	M/S	Some "stiffness" in joints, especially hands, in last two years; self-medicates with Motrin as needed
	Neuro	Negative
PE	Constitutional	Pleasant, well groomed, articulate bilingual Hispanic lady; oriented ×3; BP 140/80; P 60 and regular; R 16; Temp 98.4° F; 5 ft 8 in; 190 lbs
	HEENT	Normal; good dentition with repaired carries
	Neck	Supple, no thyroid enlargement
	Chest	Clear to auscultation and percussion
	CV	Normal heart sounds without murmurs; normal and symmetric pulses
	Back	Symmetric, no masses or tenderness
	Abdomen	No masses or organomegaly; scars appropriate to surgical history

	Pelvic	EG/Vulva	Normal; no lesions
		BUS	No abnormality
		Urethra	Normal
		Vagina	No lesions; somewhat dry; some decrease in rugae; 1 + cystocele, no rectocele, no enterocele, no uterine descent
			Wet Prep: pH 7.45; negative for clue cells, hyphae, trichomonads
		Cervix	Parous, no lesions; Pap smear and GC and *Chlamydia* cultures taken
		Uterus	Anteverted, anteflexed, normal size, shape, configuration, mobility
		Adnexa	Ovaries not palpated, no masses or tenderness
		Rectovaginal	Confirms above findings; guaiac negative

	M/S	No joint swelling or deformity, normal gait and posture as well as ROM
	Skin	No lesions
	Neurological	Normal
Laboratory		Dipstick urine in office negative for protein, one# glucose

(Continued)

Questions Case 1C

What is your initial problem list?

Answer:

Menopause, not on HRT
Postmenopausal bleeding
Sexual dysfunction—couple
Urinary urgency
1+ cystocele
Obesity
Smoking
Inadequate health screening
Diabetes, managed by internist,
1+ glucosuria on random sample

How will you address each item at the initial visit?

Answer:

Menopause, not on HRT: Initiate hormone replacement therapy (HRT, estrogen and progestin) after appropriate evaluation of PMPB; initiate calcium supplementation and exercise counseling and recommendations now.

Postmenopausal bleeding: Endometrial biopsy.

Sexual dysfunction—couple: Couple counseling, including discussion of sufficient stimulation (quality and quantity of foreplay, positions), use of lubricants; HRT will help with issues of vaginal tone, lubrication, and to some extent libido; husband may require referral to a urologist for evaluation, possible adjunct therapy associated with physiologic erectile dysfunction.

Urinary urgency: Most likely related to diabetes plus effects of estrogen deficiency; these may by addressed by, respectively, discussion with her internist and the initiation of HRT; there may also be a relationship to the cystocele.

Obesity: Counseling about diet and exercise; dietary and/or exercise program consultation as appropriate; discourage weight loss preparations and fad diets.

Smoking: Counseling and education about health risks; consultation to smoking cessation program if appropriate and requested.

Inadequate health screening—health promotion—preventive care: Mammogram on yearly basis; CVMS UA/C&S on yearly basis; Pap on yearly basis; STD screening now and on appropriate basis; flexible sigmoidoscopy now and every 3–5 years thereafter; cholesterol/lipid profile now and every 5 years until age 65, then every 3–4 years; pneumococcal and influenza vaccine now and in 10 years.

Diabetes, managed by internist, 1+ glucosuria on random sample: FBS or HgbA1c; coordinate care with internist.

Mrs Hernandez returns in two weeks, and the following laboratory data are available:

Pap: Satisfactory, negative
GC and *Chlamydia:* Negative
Mammogram: Normal (BiRad-2)
Pipelle endometrial biopsy: Scant tissue insufficient for diagnosis; suggest clinical correlation
CVMS UA/C&S: Normal except 1+ glucosuria; no growth
Flexible sigmoidoscopy consultation: Satisfactory study; normal
FBS: Normal
Cholesterol/Lipids: Normal
CBC: Normal Hgb and Hct, WBC count, platelets

What is the appropriate follow-up for the endometrial biopsy? Is HRT appropriate, and if so when?

Answer:

The PMPB is most likely from a denuded mucosal intrauterine surface bereft of endometrium as a result of estrogen deficiency. Thus, the endometrial biopsy is consistent with the clinically diagnosed estrogen deficiency. Hormone replacement therapy may be initiated and no further work-up is required at this time.

There are several options for estrogen replacement therapy, which starts by a thorough discussion of the benefits (vaginal dryness and tone, mood and libido, prevention of osteoporosis, and favorable effect on the cardiovascular lipid profile) and potential problems (association with breast carcinoma). There are several regimens involving oral conjugated estrogens or transdermal estradiols combined with a progestin, most commonly medroxyprogesterone. A commonly used regimen with high compliance and low risks is conjugated estrogen 0.625 and medroxyprogesterone acetate 2.5 mg daily. Other regimens are equally effective and may be more attractive to the patient.

Patients should be cautioned that the full effect of new estrogen replacement therapy regimens will not be fully realized for 60 to 120 days so that they will not be discouraged if they do not immediately realize all the "sought-after" benefits. Breast tenderness is a common but usually transient issue and not an undue source of concern if explained at the initial treatment. It is useful to see the patient about three months after initiating HRT to ascertain her satisfaction and response (altering the regimen if needed) and to ask any other questions that may have arisen in the interval. Thereafter, it is common to see patients either every six months or yearly for their annual health evaluation and education.

If PMPB continues for a clinically significant time, or changes quality or quantity in a significant manner, consideration may be given to further evaluation. Several options are available, the most commonly considered being repeat endometrial biopsy. Two methods are commonly used: repeat Pipelle endometrial biopsy and hysteroscopically directed endometrial biopsy. The former is a "random blind sample," but its reasonable sensitivity combined with low cost and high patient comfort make it a common choice. The latter is more specific, but also more costly and uncomfortable. D&C is no longer considered a useful option given its lack of advantage over the less expensive and uncomfortable office Pipelle endometrial biopsy.

C H A P T E R

ETHICS IN OBSTETRICS AND GYNECOLOGY

First Case: A Jehovah's Witness patient, hemorrhaging from a placenta previa, needs a cesarean section. Do we give blood against the patient's expressed wishes (a form of battery), even to save her life? Do we allow her to die while we deliver her child safely but motherless?

Second Case: A 33-year-old woman dying of cervical cancer has been given a high dose of morphine to try to abate her increasing and prolonged pain but her respirations have dropped to 3/minute. Should we give her a narcotic antagonist or let her die sooner with a side effect of the medication for her intractable pain?

Third Case: A markedly neurotic, child-abusing mother with several children refuses contraception. Should we require Norplant implants or Depo-Provera injections for this woman?

Fourth Case: A pregnant woman uses cocaine. Should the mother-to-be who uses cocaine be held accountable for the condition (including death) of her unborn child?

The ethical quandaries demonstrated in these four cases present a challenge to clarify the way we think about ethical problems in medicine in general and the specialty of obstetrics and gynecology in particular. There is a substantial literature that presents useful methods of thinking about ethical issues. By using this literature, you will not solely depend on your personal reaction to a problem or on your intuition. Instead, the use of ethical principles allows you to make better medical choices in a systematic manner rather than by either not dealing with them or reacting randomly based on emotions, personal bias, or social pressures.

How can you identify the basic ethical dilemmas of a confusing case? What sort of systematic approach is helpful? The answers to these questions are illustrated by detailed analysis of the first case.

A 24-year-old G2 P1001 Jehovah's Witness with a complete placenta previa is transferred from the antepartum care unit to labor and delivery with the onset of bleeding (2 cups of bright red blood in 10 minutes). Her husband, also a Jehovah's Witness, and her mother, who is not a member of that group, accompany her. She rapidly loses 1 liter of blood, and evidence of nonreassuring fetal status is found on the electronic fetal monitor. She reaffirms her absolute refusal of blood or blood products, even though an emergency cesarean section is proposed for her own and her fetus's survival. Her blood pressure is dropping despite rapid hydration. She becomes unconscious. The anesthesiologist says the patient will probably die with the insults of anesthesia and surgery without blood transfusion. The patient's mother demands that you give her daughter blood. The husband refuses. The fetal heart tracing demonstrates increasingly severe nonreassuring fetal status, consistent with impending in utero fetal demise, and you begin the cesarean section and deliver a healthy 7-lb girl with Apgar scores of 2 and then 8 with resuscitation. The patient survives the surgery, but in recovery her blood pressure drops to 50/0 postoperatively, and she remains unconscious and on a ventilator with a central venous pressure of 0. The patient's mother screams, "You are killing her! She is my only child!" Her husband firmly reminds you of the religious beliefs he and his wife share and warns you that his attorney is available if needed. What is the right thing to do?

The first step is to try to separate this emotional case into ethically separate concerns. An analytical scheme from the book *Clinical Ethics* is useful for this purpose (Table 2.1). Separating a case into four areas of concern allows us to fit each particular problem into a family of ethical issues that are associated with particular principles central to medical ethics. This process of systematic analysis and reflection is basic to medical ethics.

Considering this first case, we would ask, "What was the *medical indication* for the cesarean section?" Clearly, both child and mother would die without surgery. Continuing acute hemorrhage from placenta previa has no potential therapy other than surgical delivery and removal of the placenta. Support of the cardiovascular system with blood products is medically indicated. Yet this patient has clearly stated her *preference:* She will not accept blood products, both while no acute problem is present

TABLE 2.1. Areas of Concern and Associated Ethical Principles in Clinical Medical Ethics: A Functional Scheme for Clinical Ethical Decision Making

Ethical concern:	MEDICAL INDICATION What is the best treatment? What are the alternatives?	Ethical concern:	PATIENT PREFERENCES What does the patient want?
Ethical principle:	BENEFICENCE The duty to promote the good of the patient	Ethical principle:	AUTONOMY Respect for the patient's right to self-determination
Ethical concern:	QUALITY OF LIFE What impact will the proposed treatment or lack of it have on the patient's life?	Ethical principle:	CONTEXTUAL ISSUES What does the patient want? What are the needs of society?
Ethical principle:	NONMALEFICENCE The duty not to inflict harm or injury	Ethical principle:	JUSTICE The patient should be given what is his or her due.

or after. She believes that blood is directly opposed to God's will and that receiving blood, even against her wishes, will permanently and negatively affect her spiritual self. She does not feel life under such circumstances (i.e., after receiving blood) to be acceptable.

From her caregiver's viewpoint, blood transfusion is more likely to produce a better quality of life, that is, survival without neurologic or major organ sequelae. Without blood products, her survival is questionable, and even with survival, her risks for prolonged intensive care unit (ICU) stay, cardiac failure, renal failure, and hematologic sequelae are much greater.

Considering *contextual issues,* we wonder how this newborn child will do *without her mother.* In addition, what is the validity of the cost of care in an ICU for the sequelae resulting from the patient's choice when other patients need the ICU bed? What about the grandmother's concerns? Is the husband coercing the patient to not accept blood? Is he coercing the physician with comments about his attorney, or is that his

right to protect his wife? What would the law say if we gave the patient blood without permission?

The first case is complex, but it is clear that the patient's choice to refuse blood products is an underlying issue. Does this patient's autonomous refusal constitute a real choice, and if so, should we accept it? Although the law has much to say about the rights of individuals to choose or refuse care, the choice here not to give blood is based on the great respect caregivers must have for the right of patients to determine their care, which medical ethics has supported. There is much literature regarding autonomy and refusal of blood products that can be consulted to illuminate these choices.

In more general terms, the medical indications for a proposed management always need to be as clear and as "scientific" as possible. Is the benefit of what is proposed clearly greater than the harm that might be caused, or is the benefit at a level that makes the harm acceptable? Consider the second case: the 33-year-old dying slowly of cervical cancer. She is at risk from the pain medication needed to alleviate her suffering. Is the relief of pain so great a benefit that the decreased respiratory rate and potential respiratory arrest are acceptable? Consider the third case: the mother who refuses contraception yet abuses her children. Is Norplant medically indicated for the child-abusing patient? Does she have a medical contraindication to its use? Remember that before proceeding with a proposed treatment, the benefit to the patient must be clear. If the benefit is unclear but the treatment ongoing, the issues are still more complex.

Consider a variation in the case of the patient with cervical cancer. She is also unable to eat because of the pain, and the family requests total parenteral nutrition (TPN). It will make them "feel better about things." Many would consider TPN in this case to be medically futile and question the ethics of its continued use. The group of cases related to *medical indications* involves such concerns as benefit (or *beneficence*) and the related concept of *futility*.

The cases that can be categorized under *patient preferences* revolve around the principle of *autonomy,* the respect we hold for the patient's right to choose care. It is important to note that the physician–patient relationship emphasizes a relationship between the physician and the patient. Even in obstetrics, where the consequences of patient choices on another potential life can be significant, the primacy of the physician–patient (versus physician–fetus) relationship is paramount. What the patient wants and her capacity to make those choices are in question here. Consider the fourth case: Does the drug-using mother have the capacity to make decisions about her unborn child? By reason of the effect of the drugs, has she lost the capacity for acceptable decision making? Is society bound by her decision making? What about the rights of the unborn child? Consider the second case: Is the dying patient whose mentation is potentially clouded by impending death and the medications used for pain relief capable of decisions about her care?

Quality of life issues are always important. The absence of pain in a terminal cancer patient may significantly improve the quality of her living, even if the length of time is shortened. Some patients may consider the diminution of quality of life with potential permanent neurologic damage or loss of time with children arising as a result of blood loss (as in the first case) so significant that they will accept blood despite their religious beliefs. So, the harms of treatment or no treatment viewed in the context of a particular patient's life are what must be considered. In a sense, this deals with *nonmaleficence:* the duty not to harm patients while treating them. Harm clearly also must be viewed in the patient's framework. In the second case, prolonged life may not be valued if significant pain or a lengthy hospital stay constitute the quality of life that must be accepted. That becomes unacceptable "harm" to that patient. Yet, in the first case, the quality of life after blood transfusion may be acceptable to the patient because of the added time to be spent with her children and the diminished risk of major organ damage. The benefits of proposed therapy must be framed in the outcome of that therapy for good or ill.

Finally, all the *contextual and socioeconomic issues* that surround a particular case should be considered. It is here that the concerns of the children and mother and father and other relatives and concerns about legal issues and issues of cost are addressed. Threats to sue, angry families, and "dumping" of patients without health insurance or money to pay for health care, for example, can so overwhelm the health care team that the real ethical issues of a case (e.g., the capacity to choose, or futility) are not considered. Socioeconomic issues, although important in making final choices about care, in general should not override clear medical indications or clear patient preferences. When socioeconomic considerations are deeply divided from what is medically indicated or what a patient prefers, they cause problems. For example, imagine this in the second case: the 33-year-old mother cannot die at home near her children because of medical cost regulations; in the first case, the sequelae of refused blood products and prolonged ICU stay deny a bed to a patient with complications of leukemia therapy, so that this care has to be delivered in another institution away from trusted physicians. These outcomes appear unfair or unjust and illustrate cases dealing with the ethical principle of justice and how to determine allocation of resources.

What are the unique ethical problems of obstetrics and gynecology? Clearly, maternal and fetal conflicts and how we define procreation and family are uniquely poignant in obstetrics and gynecology. The primary concern of physicians is the best care of their patients. This has been true since Hippocrates admonished us "to do away with the suffering of the sick." Special-interest groups have variously defined the "rights" of the fetus so that, at times, the primacy of duty to the patient (mother) seems in question. Yet there never has been a time in the development of medical ethics or in the opinions expressed by the American College of Obstetricians and Gynecologists that the fetus has been considered to take precedence over the mother in considerations of medical care or the therapeutic alliance of physician and patient. This is valuable to keep in mind when considering these problems.

Abortion would be the first example of these considerations, one in which the controversy can be so emotional and damaging that an ethical discussion cannot occur. Consistent with our primary duty to the patient, those circumstances where survival of the mother would be seriously compromised by the maintenance of pregnancy are the least controversial. Clearly, preservation of the patient/mother's life and loss of the fetus would be supported by many viewers. As the "case" gets further away from this clearer situation, the discussion becomes more complex. To understand these controversies, it is valuable to explore what elements we use to define life as "human" before we define loss of a fetus as loss of a human life. What are the elements of humanness, and when are they achieved in pregnancy? Is ability to survive independent of the mother significant? Is the potential to achieve those elements defining human pertinent? These are important issues to explore

before considering, for example, a case such as elective abortion at 12 weeks or selective pregnancy reduction.

Defining these issues also helps in consideration of the "rights" of pregnant women to engage in behavior or activities that put the fetus at some risk, such as use of cocaine, alcohol, smoking, or refusal of cesarean section for fetal indications. At what level of human development or potential, if at all, does concern for fetal outcomes override the patient/mother's autonomous choices? In what sort of case might we reasonably override expressed patient wishes to preserve fetal life? For example, how does drug use interact with capacity to choose? Consider the fourth case: Is the drug-using mother's decision to continue to use drugs during pregnancy acceptable? What are the consequences of incarcerating such mothers as a solution? Is an acutely intoxicated mother's decision to refuse cesarean section for fetal indications acceptable?

In looking at the many changes in reproductive endocrinology, the idea of a clearest case, sometimes called a paradigm case, may help sort out the ethical discussions. What, for example, is the clearest set of relationships between parents and children? Biologically, the relationship between mother donating the egg and a father donating the sperm in vivo without augmentation is the paradigm case. The relationship of this family unit, with the parental responsibilities for financial support, history, culture, and education has been the traditional paradigm for family in our culture. How these elements change with a group of cases will vary. Adoption by a mother/father pair, adoption by a single parent, adoption by two mothers or two fathers, in vitro combination of egg from mother and father, in vitro combination of unrelated sperm with the maternal egg, and the varieties of gestational patterns with surrogacy and egg and sperm donation are all variations on the original theme. How far from our paradigm family is acceptable? Why? What do we do with the "extra" fertilized or harvested eggs from in vitro fertilization? How is this different or the same as the issue of humanness or potential for humanness that we raised when discussing abortion? What about the rejuvenation of the menopausal woman so that she can conceive and deliver? She and/or her partner may well not live through the maturation of their child. Who will then assume the parental responsibility, as well as the associated financial and logistic responsibilities? To whom does the child turn to seek redress if these responsibilities are not met, or are met unsatisfactorily?

SUMMARY

In obstetrics and gynecology, as in all medicine, there is potential to use the skills and concepts of medical ethics to help in the management of difficult situations. To do so requires using methods of systematic reflection to delineate the ethical problems and to analyze these problems further. The analytical framework shown in this chapter helps identify ethical issues, placing them in specific ethical areas, associating them with some principles and families of cases. Further analysis comparing a case to a paradigm case may be helpful. Finally, obtaining recent papers on the issues from MEDETHX in Medline or the medical library will bring together various authors' views on the ethical issues surrounding a given clinical situation.

CASE STUDIES

There are no clear answers in medical ethics, only questions to which we should apply a logical scheme for analysis to make the best decisions possible. Consider the following situations. Apply the decision matrix presented in this chapter to decide how you would analyze each.

Case 2A

Your patient is a 28-year-old G3 P3003 whose ethnic background and religious views place high value on a male offspring. She has had three girls. She is now 12 weeks' pregnant and requests you test for gender and abort a female pregnancy. She notes she must have a son for her husband and can barely afford a fourth child in any event.

Questions Case 2A

Do you do the test? Do you abort the pregnancy if it is female? If you do and she returns with another pregnancy, do you

continue the process to its logical conclusion: a male fetus or a complication so that further pregnancy is not possible? What if the husband insists? What if the mother is unsure? What if her attorney reminds you that it is her body, not yours, and her decision? What if your attorney reminds you that the public-relations outcome of this case stinks either way you choose?

Case 2B

A 26-year-old G7 P6006 arrives at an estimated 37 to 41 weeks' gestation in labor. She has had no prenatal care. She is an abuser of drugs and alcohol and is high on cocaine she ingested just before entering the hospital. When placed on an electronic fetal monitor with external probes, decelerations are noted, but the patient will not permit adjustment of the tocodynamometer to allow characterization of the decelerations, nor will she permit rupture of membranes for placement of a scalp electrode.

(Continued)

Questions Case 2B

What do you do? A cesarean section because you cannot evaluate the fetus effectively and it may be in distress? Wait and see if the patient will calm down and allow appropriate fetal assessment? Is the patient competent to make decisions, having just taken cocaine? Does the fetus have a right to a "good birth?" If you let the patient labor and deliver vaginally and the baby is brain damaged, are you liable? If you do a cesarean section and the baby is okay but the mother has a serious complication, are you liable?

Case 2C

A 15-year-old girl suffers a spontaneous abortion of her first pregnancy at 12 weeks' gestational age. She requires a suction curettage, which is performed without incident. At the time of discharge you offer a range of contraceptive options, emphasizing the value of contraception to avoid a further pregnancy while she continues her education. She refuses saying "birth control makes you fat," and "anyway, my boyfriend wants me to have a baby for him and I'm going to." The patient's mother is present, and she orders her daughter to use contraception, specifically Depo-Provera because she does not trust her to use oral contraceptives let alone a barrier method of contraception. She tells you that the boyfriend is 26 and that she will sue you if you do not "give" her minor daughter the "shot."

Questions Case 2C

Although emancipated while pregnant, the patient is now a minor, subject to her mother's decisions for most issues. Does that authority extend to contraception?

What about the patient's autonomy? Her opportunity to make good health decisions, hopefully building a pattern of same? What about the boyfriend? His age? What about the mother's comments? The mother's orders to the child? Her comments to you? Are they threats? Does she have an obligation to her minor daughter that should be discharged in this manner? Would referral of this situation to the court be likely to rectify the issues? Would such referral be appropriate or "ethical?"

Case 2D

A 39-year-old single mother of three is seen in your office for annual care. A breast lump and axillary nodes are found, and after evaluation she is found to have breast cancer with probable metastases. The patient declines referral for treatment, saying that, "it just isn't worth it as cancer cannot be cured." You carefully review the information about cancer therapy and the ability to cure often and extend quality life almost always, but she still declines further treatment. You point out that she is the single parent of three children ages 11, 13, and 15, and that they need her as long as possible. She still declines further care.

Questions Case 2D

You feel horrible, because you "know" she is shortening her life, leaving her children parentless earlier than needed. What should you do? Do you have any obligation to the children? Is this a kind of child abuse requiring referral to the social authorities? Are you liable later on, to the children or their estate? Do you have further obligations to the patient? How long and in what manner is it "ethical" to persist in trying to get her to have further care?

3

EMBRYOLOGY, ANATOMY, AND REPRODUCTIVE GENETICS

CHAPTER OBJECTIVES

Although there is no specific APGO objective that corresponds to the material in this chapter, this basic science material is critical as the basis for understanding of most of the chapters.

EMBRYOLOGY

A knowledge of the embryology of the female reproductive system is helpful in understanding both normal anatomy and the structural anomalies that can sometimes occur. Although this chapter concentrates on development in the female, comparisons with the development of the male reproductive system are made for illustration.

The genital system develops from embryonic intermediate mesoderm. With the folding of the embryo, the intermediate mesoderm comes to lie as two longitudinal rods on either side of the primitive aorta. In the trunk region, the rods are called nephrogenic cords (Figure 3.1A). There is a dorsal outgrowth of each nephrogenic cord, which bulges into the celomic cavity. These bulges, called the *urogenital ridges,* are covered with celomic epithelium. The urogenital ridges give rise to elements of both the urinary and the reproductive systems (Figure 3.1B).

In general, the elements of the reproductive system pass through an undifferenti-

ated stage in the early embryo; that is, development is identical in the male and female. Later, sex-specific differentiation occurs.

Development of the Ovary

Genetic sex, determined at fertilization, depends on whether the X-bearing oocyte is fertilized by an X- or Y-bearing sperm. However, early in development, the gonads are undifferentiated (i.e., the sex of the embryo cannot be determined from the appearance of the gonad).

The gonads begin to develop during the fifth week, when a portion of the urogenital ridge on the medial side of the mesonephric kidney thickens to form the *gonadal ridge.* The celomic epithelium divides to form finger-like bands of cells (the *primary sex cords*), which project into the underlying mesodermal mesenchyme of the gonadal ridge. In the female, it is the cortical area that predominates in the mature gonad, and it is this cortical tissue that contains the follicles. This growth results in the creation of a cortex and a medulla in the indifferent (undifferentiated) gonad.

During the fourth week, the *primordial germ cells* (which eventually give rise to the gametes) can be identified in the yolk sac. As the embryo folds, some of the yolk sac is incorporated into the embryo. During the sixth week, the primordial germ cells migrate into the mesenchyme of the gonadal ridge, where they become associated with the primary sex cords. In the female, the primordial germ cells become oogonia, which divide by mitosis during fetal life. No oogonia form after birth.

If a Y chromosome is present, the tunica albuginea of the testis begins to form in the mesenchymal tissue of the medulla during the eighth week. This is the first indication of the sex of the embryo. In the absence of a Y chromosome, the undifferentiated gonad develops into an ovary, which is identifiable by approximately the tenth week of development. In the ovary, the primary sex cords degenerate, and secondary sex cords (cortical cords) appear and extend from the surface epithelium into the underlying mesenchyme. The *oogonia* are incorporated into

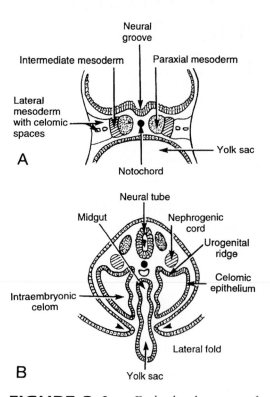

FIGURE 3.1. Early development of urogenital system.

them, and at approximately 16 weeks of development, the cortical cords organize into *primordial follicles*. Each follicle eventually consists of an oogonium, derived from a primary germ cell, surrounded by a single layer of squamous follicular cells, derived from the cortical cords. *Follicular maturation* begins when the oogonia enter the first stage of meiotic division (at which point they are called oocytes). Oocyte development is then arrested until puberty, when one or more follicles are stimulated to continue development each month (see Chapters 34 and 35).

Development of the Genital Ducts

In both the male and female, two pairs of ducts initially develop, the mesonephric (wolffian) and the paramesonephric (müllerian). As with the gonad, there is an indifferent (undifferentiated) stage in ductal development. During this stage, both sets of ducts are present in both the male and the female.

In the male, the *mesonephric ducts,* which drain the embryonic mesonephric kidneys, eventually form the *epididymis, ductus deferens,* and *ejaculatory ducts.* In the female, the mesonephric ducts almost completely disappear.

In the female, it is the *paramesonephric ducts* (or müllerian) that persist to form major parts of the reproductive tract (the *fallopian tubes, uterus,* and *parts of the vagina*). The paramesonephric ducts start to develop early in the sixth week, beginning as invaginations of the celomic epithelium in the vicinity of the mesonephric kidneys (Figure 3.2A). For each duct, the invagination fuses to form a tube. The cranial end of each duct opens into the celomic (future peritoneal) cavity. The ducts grow caudally, and the caudal segments fuse at approximately the eighth week of development into the Y-shaped *uterovaginal primordium* or *canal* (Figure 3.2B). The cranial (unfused) portion of each duct becomes a fallopian tube, and the fused portions become the uterus and parts of the vagina. This differentiation does not depend on the presence of ovaries.

When the two paramesonephric ducts fuse, two peritoneal folds are brought together. This creates the broad ligaments of the uterus (Figure 3.2C).

Development of the Vagina

Between weeks 5 and 7, the *primitive cloaca,* a pouch-like enlargement of the caudal end of the hindgut, is divided into the *urogenital sinus* (ventral) and the *anorectal canal* (dorsal). The contact of the caudally growing uterovaginal primordium with the urogenital sinus results in the formation of a solid mass of cells called the vaginal plate. The vaginal plate extends from the urogenital sinus into the caudal end of the uterovaginal

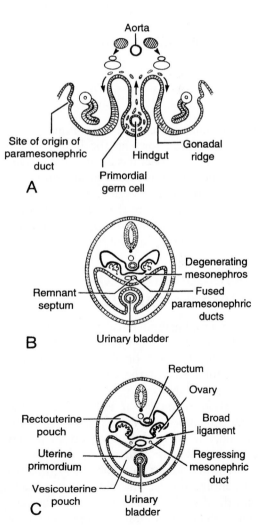

FIGURE 3.2. Formation of uterus.

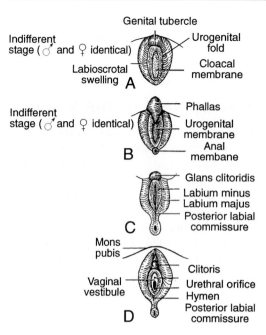

FIGURE 3.3.   Development of the external genitalia.

primordium. The central cells of the vaginal plate disappear, forming the lumen of the vagina. The peripheral cells of the plate persist as the vaginal epithelium. In addition to contributing to the vagina, the urogenital sinus also gives rise to the *epithelium of the urinary bladder*, the *urethra*, the *greater vestibular glands*, and the *hymen*.

Development of the External Genitalia

The external genitalia also pass through an indifferent stage. Early in the fourth week, the *genital tubercle*, or phallus, develops at the cranial end of the cloacal membrane. Soon after, labioscrotal swellings and urogenital folds appear at either side of the cloacal membrane (Figure 3.3A). The genital tubercle enlarges in both the male and the female (Figure 3.3B).

The division of the cloaca by the urorectal septum divides the cloacal membrane into the dorsal anal membrane and the ventral urogenital membrane. At approximately week 7, these membranes rupture.

At approximately 9 weeks, distinguishing sexual characteristics begin to appear, but the external genital organs are not fully formed until week 12. In the absence of androgens, the external genitalia are feminized (Figure 3.3C). The phallus develops into the relatively small *clitoris*. The unfused urogenital folds form the *labia minora* and the labioscrotal swellings become the *labia majora* (Figure 3.3D).

ANATOMY

This section first describes the normal anatomy of the female reproductive system. Anomalies, arising from defects in development, are then discussed.

Bony Pelvis

The bony pelvis is comprised of the paired *innominate bones* and the *sacrum*. The innominate bones are joined anteriorly to form the symphysis pubis, and each is articulated posteriorly with the sacrum through the sacroiliac joint (Figure 3.4).

The innominate bones are comprised of three portions—the *ilium*, the *ischium*, and the *pubis*—which become fused during adolescence. The three parts come together to contribute to the acetabulum. The sacrum is comprised of five or six sacral vertebrae, which are fused in adulthood. The sacrum articulates with the coccyx inferiorly and with the fifth lumbar vertebra superiorly.

The pelvis is divided into the pelvis major (*false pelvis*) and the pelvis minor (*true pelvis*), which are separated by the linea terminalis. The false pelvis, whose main function is to support the pregnant uterus, is bounded by the lumbar vertebrae posteriorly, an iliac fossa bilaterally, and the abdominal wall anteriorly. The true pelvis is formed by the sacrum and coccyx posteriorly and by the ischium and pubis laterally and anteriorly. Concern arises when its dimensions are inadequate to permit passage of the fetus.

There are *four pelvic planes:* the *pelvic inlet*, the *plane of the greatest diameter*, the *plane of the least diameter* (midplane), and the *pelvic outlet*. The pelvic inlet is bounded

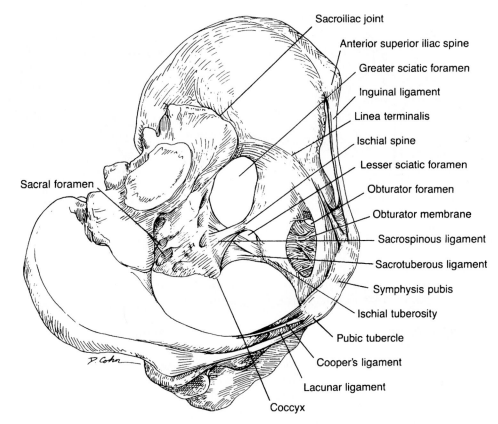

Sacroiliac joint
Anterior superior iliac spine
Greater sciatic foramen
Inguinal ligament
Linea terminalis
Ischial spine
Lesser sciatic foramen
Obturator foramen
Obturator membrane
Sacrospinous ligament
Sacrotuberous ligament
Symphysis pubis
Ischial tuberosity
Pubic tubercle
Cooper's ligament
Lacunar ligament
Coccyx
Sacral foramen

FIGURE 3.4.   View of the pelvis from above, showing bones, joints, ligaments, and foramina.

posteriorly by the promontory and alae of the sacrum, laterally by the linea terminalis, and anteriorly by the superior surface of the pubic bones. Thus the plane of the inlet separates the false pelvis and the true pelvis. The plane of the greatest diameter is bounded by the junction of the second and third sacral vertebrae posteriorly, the upper part of the obturator foramina laterally, and the midpoint of the pubis anteriorly. The plane of least diameter extends from the lower border of the pubis anteriorly to the lower sacrum at the level of the ischial spines. This plane is most important clinically, because arrest of fetal descent occurs most frequently at this point. The plane of the outlet is irregular, consisting of two intersecting triangles. It is bounded posteriorly by the tip of the sacrum, laterally by the ischial tuberosities and the sacrotuberous ligaments, and anteriorly by the lower border of the symphysis. There are certain key diameters of the pelvis that are important

in assessing the space available during fetal descent (Figure 3.5 and Table 3.1).

The female pelvis is classified into four basic types, according to the scheme of Caldwell and Moloy (Figure 3.6). The most common type is the *gynecoid,* occurring in approximately 40% to 50% of women. In this type, the inlet is rounded, the side walls are straight, the sacrum is well curved, and the sacrosciatic notch is adequate. In general, this gives the pelvis a cylindrical shape, which has adequate space along its length. The *platypelloid* pelvis occurs in only 2% to 5% of women. There is an oval inlet, the sacrum is normal, the side walls are straight, the sacrosciatic notch is narrower, and the interspinous and intertuberous diameters are increased compared with the other pelvic types. The *android* pelvis occurs in approximately 30% of all women but in only 10% to 15% of African-American women. There is a wedge-shaped inlet, the side walls

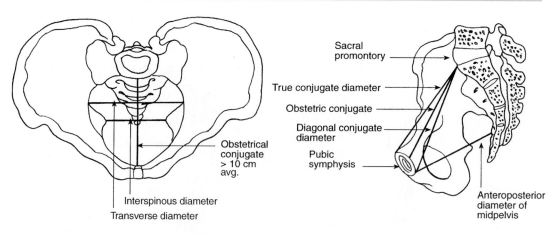

FIGURE 3.5. Pelvic diameters.

TABLE 3.1. Length of Pelvic Plane Diameters

Pelvic Plane	Diameter	Average Length (cm)
Inlet	True conjugate	10.5–11.5
	Obstetric conjugate	10.0–11.0
	Diagonal conjugate	12.5
	Transverse diameter	13.5
	Oblique diameter	12.5
Greatest diameter	Anterior–posterior	12.75
	Transverse	12.5
Midplane	Anterior–posterior	11.5–12.0
	Bispinous (interspinous)	10.0
Outlet	Anterior–posterior	11.5
	Bituberous	8.0–11.0

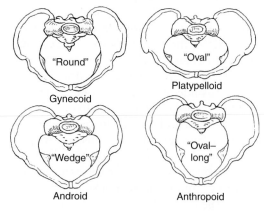

FIGURE 3.6. Caldwell-Moloy pelvic types.

converge, the sacrum is inclined forward, and the sacrosciatic notch is narrow. This pelvic type has limited space at the inlet, and the funnel shape results in even less space below. Fetal descent may be arrested at the midpelvis. The *anthropoid* type occurs in approximately 20% of all women and in approximately 40% of black women. The inlet is oval, long, and narrow; the side walls are straight (do not converge); the sacrum is long and narrow; and the sacrosciatic notch is wide. Both the interspinous and intertuberous diameters are somewhat smaller than in the gynecoid pelvis. Any individual may be of a pure or mixed pelvic type.

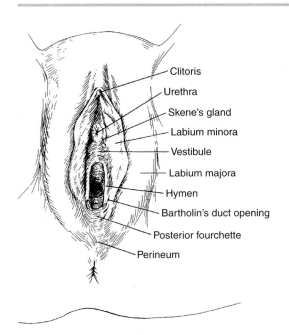

FIGURE 3.7.   Vulva and perineum.

Vulva and Perineum

The vulva contains the labia majora, labia minora, mons pubis, clitoris, vestibule, and ducts of glands that open into the vestibule (Figure 3.7). The labia majora are folds of skin with underlying adipose tissue; they are fused anteriorly with the mons pubis and posteriorly with the perineum. The skin of the labia majora contains hair follicles and sebaceous and sweat glands. The labia minora are narrow skin folds, which lie inside the labia majora. The labia minora merge anteriorly with the prepuce and frenulum of the clitoris and posteriorly with the labia majora and the perineum. The labia minora contain sebaceous and sweat glands but no hair follicles, and there is no underlying adipose tissue. The clitoris, which is located anterior to the labia minora, is the embryologic homolog of the penis. It consists of two crura (corresponding to the corpora cavernosa in the male) and the glans, which is found superior to the point of fusion of the crura. On the ventral surface of the glans is the *frenulum*, the fused junction of the labia minora. The *vestibule* lies between the labia minora and

is bounded anteriorly by the clitoris and posteriorly by the perineum. The urethra and the vagina open into the vestibule in the midline. The ducts of *Skene's (paraurethral) glands* and *Bartholin's glands* also empty into the vestibule.

The *muscles of the vulva* (superior transverse perineal, bulbocavernosus, and ischiocavernosus) lie superficial to the fascia of the urogenital diaphragm (Figure 3.8). The vulva rests on the triangular-shaped urogenital diaphragm, which lies in the anterior part of the pelvis between the ischiopubic rami. The urogenital diaphragm surrounds and supports the urethra and the vagina.

Vagina

The vagina is a muscular tube that extends from the vestibule to the uterus (Figure 3.9). The long axis of the vagina is approximately parallel to the lower portion of the sacrum. The uterine cervix projects into the upper portion of the vagina. Therefore, the anterior vaginal wall is approximately 2 cm shorter than the posterior wall. The area around the cervix, the fornix, is divided into four regions: the *anterior fornix*, two *lateral fornices*, and the *posterior fornix*. The posterior fornix is in close proximity to the peritoneum that forms the floor of the posterior pelvic cul-de-sac (pouch of Douglas). This allows access to the peritoneal cavity from the vagina (e.g., during culdocentesis).

At its lower end, the vagina traverses the urogenital diaphragm and is then surrounded by the two bulbocavernosus muscles. These act as a sphincter. The *hymen*, a fold of mucosal-covered connective tissue, somewhat obscures the external vaginal orifice in the child. The hymen is fragmented into irregular remnants with sexual activity and childbearing.

The major *blood supply* to the vagina is from the vaginal artery, a branch of the hypogastric artery. The veins follow the path of the arteries.

The *vaginal wall* consists of a mucous membrane and an external muscular layer. The lumen is lined by a stratified squamous

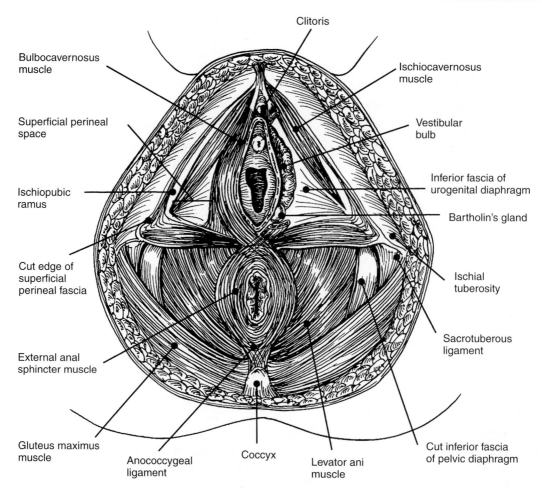

FIGURE 3.8.   Perineum and urogenital diaphragm.

epithelium. Beneath this is a submucosal layer of connective tissue, which contains a rich supply of veins and lymphatics. Submucosal rugae throw the lumen of the vagina into the characteristic H shape in the young; these folds become less prominent with age. The muscular wall has three layers of smooth muscle. The vaginal wall is extremely distensible, especially under hormonal influences during childbirth.

Uterus

The uterus is covered on each side by the two layers of the broad ligament, and it lies between the rectum and the bladder (see Figure 3.9). The close relation with structures in the broad ligament, especially the uterine arteries and veins and the ureters, has

important implications during surgery. The two major portions of the uterus are the *cervix* and the body (*corpus*), which are separated by a narrower isthmus. Before puberty, the length of the cervix and the body are approximately equal; after puberty, the ratio of the body to the cervix is between 2:1 and 3:1. The part of the body where the two uterine (fallopian) tubes enter is called the *cornu*. The part of the corpus above the cornu is termed the *fundus*. In the nonparous adult, the uterus is approximately 7 to 8 cm long and 4 to 5 cm wide at the widest part. The cervix is relatively cylindrical in shape and is 2 to 3 cm long. The corpus is generally pear shaped, with the anterior surface being flat and the posterior surface, convex. In cross section, the lumen of the corpus is triangular.

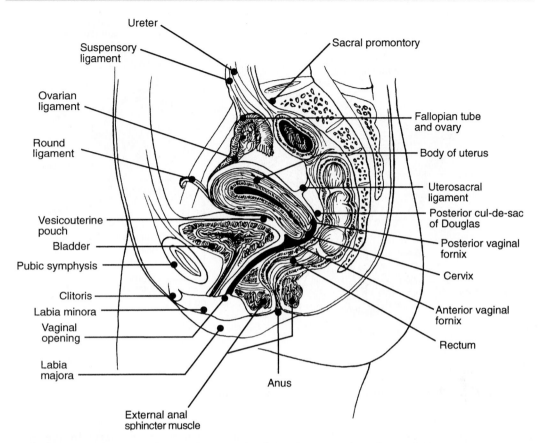

FIGURE 3.9. Midsagittal view of pelvic viscera and perineum.

The normal position of the uterus is variable. The angle between the long axis of the corpus and the cervix varies from *anteflexion* to *retroflexion,* and the angle between the cervix and the vagina varies from *anteversion* to *retroversion.* Unless caused by underlying pathology, these variations are normal. The uterus is supported by the following ligaments: *uterosacral, cardinal, round,* and *broad.* The *blood supply* to the uterus comes primarily from the uterine arteries and also from the ovarian arteries, whereas the venous plexus drains through the uterine vein.

The cervix joins the vagina at an angle between 45° and 90°. The opening to the vagina, the external os, is round to oval in nonparous women but is a transverse slit after childbirth. The portion of the cervix that projects into the vagina is covered with stratified squamous epithelium, which resembles the vaginal epithelium. The squamous epithelium changes to a simple columnar epithelium in the *transition* (transformation) *zone.* This zone is found at about the level of the external cervical os, although it is found higher in the endocervical canal in postmenopausal women. The importance of this zone in the process of neoplastic transformation is discussed in Chapter 44.

There are *three basic layers in the wall of the uterine body* (Figure 3.10). The inner mucosa (the endometrium) consists of the simple columnar epithelium with underlying connective tissue. The changes in the structure of this layer that occur during the normal menstrual cycle are described in Chapter 46. Beneath the mucosa is a thick muscular layer (the myometrium), covered by a peritoneal serosa. The muscle layer is continuous with the muscular walls of the vagina and the fallopian tubes.

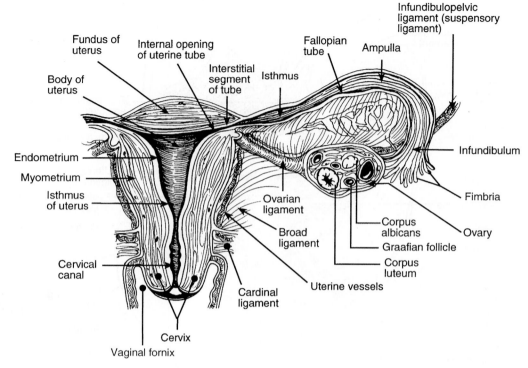

FIGURE 3.10. Frontal section of uterus and adnexa.

Fallopian Tubes

The fallopian tubes (the oviducts) average approximately 7 to 14 cm in length. Each tube can be divided into three portions: a narrow and straight isthmus, which adjoins the opening into the uterus; the ampulla, or central portion; and the infundibulum, which is fringed by the finger-shaped fimbriae. These surround the ovary and help to collect the oocyte at the time of ovulation. The fallopian tubes are supplied by the ovarian and uterine arteries. The epithelial lining of the fallopian tube is ciliated columnar. The cilia beat toward the uterus, assisting in oocyte transport.

Ovaries

Each ovary is approximately 3 to 5 cm long, 2 to 3 cm wide, and 1 to 3 cm thick in the menstrual years. The size decreases by approximately two thirds after menopause, when follicular development ceases. The ovary is attached to the broad ligament by the mesovarium, to the uterus by the ovarian ligament, and to the side of the pelvis by the suspensory ligament of the ovary (infundibulopelvic ligament), which is the lateral margin of the broad ligament (see Figure 3.10). The outer ovarian cortex consists of follicles embedded in a connective tissue stroma. The connective tissue medulla contains smooth muscle fibers, blood vessels, nerves, and lymphatics.

The ovaries are mainly supplied by the ovarian arteries, which are direct branches of the abdominal aorta, but there also is a blood supply from the uterine artery, a branch of the hypogastric artery (internal iliac artery; Figure 3.11). Venous return via the right ovarian vein is directly into the inferior vena cava, and from the left ovary into the left renal vein.

Anomalies of the Female Reproductive System

Anatomic anomalies arise from defects during embryologic development, and all occur very infrequently. Absence of the ovary is

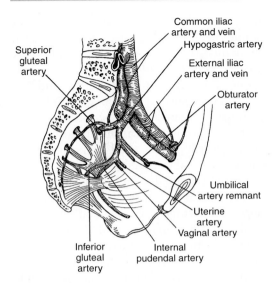

FIGURE 3.11. Arterial system of the female pelvis.

rare and usually associated with other genital tract anomalies. Ectopic ovarian tissue may occur, as supernumerary ovaries or as accessory ovarian tissue. In general, various kinds of uterine and vaginal malformations can arise from incomplete fusion of the paramesonephric ducts, incomplete development of one or both paramesonephric ducts, or incomplete canalization of the vaginal plate.

Absence of the uterus occurs when the paramesonephric ducts degenerate. This condition is associated with vaginal anomalies (such as absence of the vagina), because vaginal development is stimulated by the developing uterovaginal primordium. A double uterus (uterus didelphys) occurs when the inferior parts of the paramesonephric ducts do not fuse; this condition may be associated with a double or a single vagina. A bicornuate uterus results when lack of fusion is limited to the superior portion of the uterine body. If one of the paramesonephric ducts is poorly developed and fusion with the other duct does not occur, the result is a bicornuate uterus with a rudimentary horn. This horn may or may not communicate with the uterine cavity.

Absence of the vagina occurs when the vaginal plate does not develop. It is usually coupled with the absence of the uterus. If the vaginal plate does not canalize, the result is vaginal atresia. Imperforate hymen is a minor example of this.

REPRODUCTIVE GENETICS

Genetics is an integral part of obstetric and gynecologic care. Physicians must be able to identify women at increased risk for fetal abnormalities and to offer appropriate genetic screening and testing to patients based on their personal, family, and medical histories. In addition, physicians are responsible for assessing risk for their patients developing gynecologic or systemic disease. As molecular techniques permit better delineation of risk for malignancies and systemic diseases (e.g., hypercholesterolemia), gynecologists will remain at the forefront of providing appropriate screening and preventative health care. This section reviews current indications and techniques of genetic screening and testing applicable to the pregnant and gynecologic patient.

Genetic Counseling

Genetic counseling serves two important functions: (*1*) to obtain information from the patient in order to properly assess her risk for developing disease and for being delivered of an infant with congenital abnormalities; (*2*) to provide information to the patient regarding appropriate screening or diagnostic tests. Counseling should be in language understandable to the patient; complicated medical terms may not properly convey information to most patients and may create an atmosphere not conducive to an optimal exchange of information. Because this process may evoke anxiety, fear, or denial even in optimal situations, counselors should be prepared to repeat all or part of the communicated information.

Information gathering can be accomplished by several methods. Data forms, questionnaires, pedigree construction, and patient interviews are all effective methods for obtaining information concerning personal and family medical history, parental exposure to potentially harmful substances, or other issues that may impact on risk assessment. No single method or combination thereof is universally effective in obtaining all appropriate patient information. The specific methods used to gather information depend on the type of information required and the physician–patient relationship.

Genetic counseling should never be used to coerce a patient to undergo or forgo certain tests or pregnancy management decisions; information should be obtained and provided in a "nondirective" fashion. *Nondirective counseling* implies that the counselor acts in a completely objective manner, never interjecting personal opinions into the counseling session. It is essential to provide information in this manner so that patients arrive at reproductive decisions based on their own values, ethics, and desires and that the information provided by the counselor be both written and verbal. In addition to decisions concerning genetic screening or testing, counselors must be able to review alternative reproductive options (e.g., pregnancy termination, permanent sterilization, selective pregnancy reduction, donor insemination) with their patients in an empathetic yet nondirective manner.

The process of gathering information and reviewing diagnostic options is a critical one for obstetricians, gynecologists, and others, because they are responsible for determining which women are at increased risk for fetal abnormalities and for describing and offering appropriate prenatal screening or diagnostic tests. Gynecologists and other primary care physicians are responsible for not only providing screening and testing for gynecologic disorders but also nongynecologic conditions and systemic diseases.

Prenatal Diagnosis—Chromosome Abnormalities

In the United States, the most common indication for invasive prenatal diagnostic testing is increased risk for fetal chromosome abnormalities. Chromosome abnormalities (Table 3.2) also play an important role in spontaneous abortion and infertility; at least 50% to 60% of first-trimester spontaneous abortions, 5% of stillbirths, and 2% to 3% of couples experiencing multiple miscarriage or infertility will be found to have a structural or numerical chromosome alteration. Overall, 0.6% of all liveborns have a chromosome abnormality.

Couples who desire chromosome analysis because of a history of multiple miscarriage or infertility are evaluated by cytogenetic analysis of cultured lymphocytes obtained from peripheral blood (Figure 3.12). However, determination of fetal chromosome complement is not as simple or safe; obtaining fetal cells involves invasive procedures that increase fetal morbidity and mortality. Fetal chromosome analysis, either of continuing pregnancies or of spontaneous or induced abortions, is currently performed on cells obtained from amniotic fluid, placenta (chorionic villi), or fetal tissue. The procedures used to obtain these specimens are described later in this section.

Indications for Prenatal Cytogenetic Analysis
ADVANCED MATERNAL AGE

The most common indication for invasive prenatal diagnosis is advanced maternal age. The incidence of *Down syndrome* among newborns is approximately 1:800; however, the incidence of Down syndrome among newborns delivered to 35-year-old women is 1:385, and the incidence among 45-year-old women is 1:33. Down syndrome is not the only chromosome abnormality that increases in frequency with advanced maternal age; other autosomal trisomies and some sex chromosome polysomies (see Table 3.2) increase in incidence as parturients get older. In the United States, it is now standard obstetric practice to offer all women who are 35 years old or older at their estimated day of delivery invasive pre-

TABLE 3.2. Common Cytogenetic Abnormalities

Chromosome Abnormality	Livebirth Incidence	Characteristics
Trisomy 21 (Down syndrome)	1:800	Moderate to severe mental retardation; characteristic facies; cardiac abnormalities; increased incidence of respiratory infections and leukemia; only 2% live beyond 50 years
Trisomy 18 (Edwards syndrome)	1:8000	Severe mental retardation; multiple organic abnormalities; less than 10% survive 1 year
Trisomy 13 (Patau syndrome)	1:20,000	Severe mental retardation; neurologic, ophthalmologic, and organic abnormalities; less than 5% survive 3 years
Trisomy 16	0	Lethal anomaly occurs frequently in first-trimester spontaneous abortions; no infants are known to have trisomy 16
45,X	1:10,000	Occurs frequently in first-trimester (Turner syndrome) spontaneous abortions; associated primarily with unique somatic features; patients are not mentally retarded, although IQ of affected individuals is lower than siblings
47,XXX; 47,XYY; 47,XXY (Klinefelter syndrome)	Each approx. 1:900	Minimal somatic abnormalities; individuals with Klinefelter syndrome are characterized by a tall, eunuchoid habitus and small testes; 47,XXX and 47,XYY individuals do not usually exhibit somatic abnormalities, but 47,XYY individuals may be tall
del(5p)	1:20,000	Severe mental retardation, microcephaly, distinctive facial features, characteristic "cat's cry" sound (cri du chat syndrome)

natal diagnostic testing to detect fetal chromosome abnormalities.

The incidence of fetal chromosome abnormalities is higher at mid-trimester (e.g., sixteenth week of gestation) than at term because many chromosomally abnormal fetuses are aborted spontaneously after the sixteenth gestational week, resulting in a lower incidence of chromosome abnormalities in newborns than in fetuses evaluated at mid-trimester. It is, therefore, important to use consistently either mid-trimester or liveborn data when counseling patients concerning risks for fetal chromosome abnormalities.

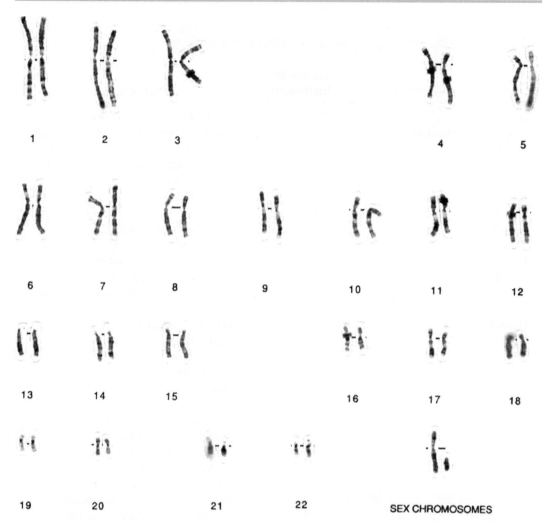

FIGURE 3.12. Normal (46,XY) metaphase spread of a cultured lymphocyte obtained from peripheral blood. Metaphases from other cell types have the same appearance.

PREVIOUS CHILD WITH CHROMOSOME ABNORMALITY

Women who have been delivered of a child with a numerical chromosome abnormality may be at increased risk for subsequent trisomy. If a woman is younger than 30 years old at the time of delivery, the recurrence risk for a subsequent trisomic newborn is estimated to be 1%–2%. However, if a woman is 30 years old or older and is delivered of a trisomic infant, the risk for subsequent trisomy is maintained at the estimated maternal age risk. The delivery of a trisomic abortus or stillbirth also confers a similar increased risk of chromosome abnormality; consideration of invasive prenatal testing in future pregnancies is warranted.

PARENTAL CHROMOSOME ABNORMALITY

Although an unbalanced parental chromosome complement is a rare occurrence, a balanced parental chromosome rearrangement is not uncommon. Approximately 4% of Down syndrome children are the result of an unbalanced robertsonian translocation between chromosome 21 and either chromosome 13, 14, 15, 21, or 22. Although 60% of these unbalanced translocations are

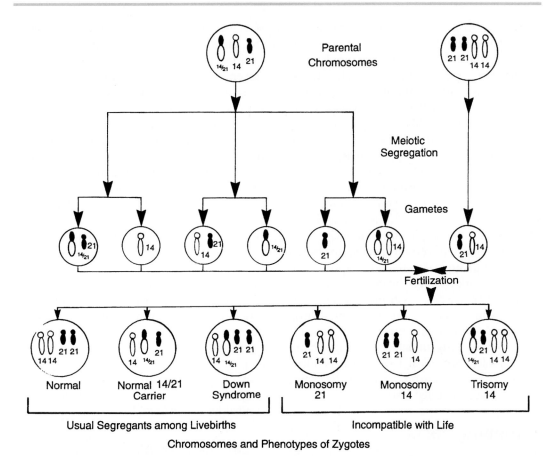

Meiotic Segregation

Gametes

Fertilization

Normal | Normal 14/21 Carrier | Down Syndrome | Monosomy 21 | Monosomy 14 | Trisomy 14

Usual Segregants among Livebirths

Incompatible with Life

Chromosomes and Phenotypes of Zygotes

FIGURE 3.13. Possible gametic products of a parental balanced translocation. Although theoretical risk for abnormal liveborns is 33%, the empiric risk is frequently lower.

the result of a *de novo* (i.e., new) rearrangement, the other 40% are the result of an *unbalanced* gamete inherited from a parent with a *balanced* chromosome rearrangement (Figure 3.13).

Three types of *parental chromosome rearrangements* that can result in chromosomally abnormal offspring are robertsonian translocations, reciprocal translocations, and inversions. *Robertsonian translocations* involve the two groups of acrocentric chromosomes, namely the D group (chromosomes 13, 14, and 15) and the G group (chromosomes 21 and 22); it is this type of balanced parental translocation that most frequently results in Down syndrome in offspring. The theoretical risk for a parent who has a balanced robertsonian translocation involving chromosome 21 to have a child with Down syndrome is 33%

(see Figure 3.13). However, the actual risk for Down syndrome in offspring is dependent on which parent has the translocation, the chromosomes involved, and the fact that many chromosomally abnormal pregnancies spontaneously abort. For example, if the mother carries a balanced robertsonian translocation involving chromosomes 14 and 21 [45,XX,–14,–21,+t(14q;21q)], the risk is approximately 10%, whereas if the father carries the same translocation, the risk is 1% or less. In addition, if the balanced translocation involves two number 21 chromosomes, the risk for Down syndrome in liveborns is 100%, irrespective of which parent carries the translocation.

Balanced reciprocal translocations may involve any chromosome and are the result of a reciprocal "trade" of chromosome material between two or more chromosomes.

This results in a rearranged complement characterized by the same amount of genetic material found in a "normal" complement. Similar to robertsonian translocations, empiric risk for newborn chromosome abnormality is less than the theoretical risk (33%). However, unlike robertsonian translocations, empiric risk of newborn chromosome abnormalities is approximately 11%, irrespective of which parent carries the translocation or the chromosomes involved.

Detection of a *parental inversion* resulting in fetal or newborn chromosome abnormalities is rare, despite the relatively common occurrence of certain specific inversions [e.g., inv9(p13;q21)] in the population. Such commonly occurring inversions do not apparently place couples at increased risk for chromosome abnormalities in offspring. Empiric data for unique inversions that result in chromosomally unbalanced progeny are unavailable; theoretical risks are dependent on whether the centromere is involved and the size of the inverted portion.

Screening Tests

A screening test is offered to individuals in a low risk population to determine who is at high risk and, therefore, candidates for invasive prenatal testing. Maternal age is a screen; however, it fails to detect 80% of pregnancies with Down syndrome (because younger women are having most of the babies). In order to detect chromosome abnormalities in younger women, maternal serum analyte screening is offered.

Currently, pregnancies are screened in the second trimester between 15 and 21 weeks. Several protocols are used. The most common involves measurement of maternal serum levels of α-fetoprotein (AFP), human chorionic gonadotropin (hCG), and unconjugated estriol (uE3). A risk profile is generated by a computer program taking into consideration the patient's age. If the patient-specific risk exceeds a given cut-off, the patient is considered a candidate for invasive testing (e.g., amniocentesis). Triple screening detects about 60% of fetal Down syndrome, and about 4% of all women screened will be categorized

screen-positive. Patients should be advised of the chance of a false-negative and false-positive result during counseling about the screen. Some laboratories include other analytes in second-trimester screening to increase the detection rate.

Because many children born with chromosome abnormalities have structural defects, ultrasonography can be used as an adjunctive screen. For example, the finding of a cardiac malformation on ultrasound carries a risk of 40% that the fetus may have a chromosome abnormality. Other findings, such as short femurs or kidney abnormalities, may increase the risk as well. Congenital anomalies on ultrasound are an indication for amniocentesis.

Studies are underway to evaluate the efficacy of screening for chromosome abnormalities in the first trimester. The advantages are obvious. The screening may employ maternal serum screening for certain analytes and ultrasonography. Preliminary studies show a detection rate for Down syndrome of 70%–80%.

MENDELIAN DISORDERS

Mendelian disorders result from mutations of specific genes. Expression of a disease or trait may result from expression of a single gene at a specific genetic locus on an autosomal chromosome (autosomal dominant; Figure 3.14) or may require expression of two genes at an autosomal locus (autosomal recessive; see Figure 3.14). In addition, those genes located on the X chromosome that result in specific disorders or traits are known as "X-linked;" X-linked conditions may also be dominant or recessive (see Figure 3.14). Because males have only one X chromosome, those males possessing a single X-linked gene that is associated with a recessive condition express that condition despite having only a single copy of the gene (hemizygosity; see Figure 3.14). Expression of the same condition in females requires two copies of the same gene.

A plethora of mendelian disorders and traits have been described, and a description

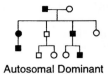

Autosomal Dominant

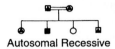

Autosomal Recessive

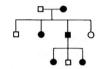

X-linked Dominant

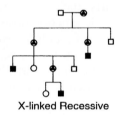

X-linked Recessive

□ Males
○ Females
■● Affected
□○ Unaffected but heterozygous
═ Consanguineous

FIGURE 3.14. Patterns of familial transmission expected for autosomal dominant, autosomal recessive, X-linked recessive, and X-linked dominant inheritance.

of them is beyond the scope of this section. Many mendelian disorders occur more frequently in certain groups (e.g., sickle-cell disease in blacks; cystic fibrosis in whites; Tay-Sachs, Gaucher's, and Neimann-Pick disease in Ashkenazic Jews; β-thalassemia in southern Europeans; and α-thalassemia in Asians) and usually have frequencies of less than 1:1000 in the at-risk group. Although screening for certain mendelian disorders is now available (e.g., sickle-cell disease, Tay-Sachs disease, thalassemia), couples found to be at risk for having children affected with most mendelian disorders are usually

discovered as a result of previously affected offspring or relatives. In addition, advanced paternal age (usually 50 years old or older) has been demonstrated to increase risk for certain mendelian disorders characterized by single gene mutations ("new mutations") associated with autosomal dominant conditions such as Marfan syndrome and achondroplasia. Counseling thus plays a critical role in determining risk for a couple having a child with a specific mendelian disorder. Information that better defines a couple's risk for affected offspring includes family history, specifically in regard to mendelian disorders or similar conditions, and the race, religion, and national origin of relatives. This information helps reassess risk and permits couples undergoing screening tests to further delineate their risk or, in appropriate situations, to undergo invasive prenatal testing.

Advances in technology, such as the polymerase chain reaction and gene sequencing have furthered our knowledge about human genetic disease. Genes responsible for many diseases have been located, and the mutations in those genes can be tested for. Examples include Tay-Sachs disease, hemophilia A, cystic fibrosis, sickle-cell disease, Duchenne's muscular dystrophy, and α-thalassemia. Directly testing for the mutation means that prenatal diagnosis is highly accurate and testing a proband is not always necessary.

The rarer the disease, the less likely that direct DNA testing is available. Indirect testing refers to the process of determining DNA sequences of specific length that are linked to the gene. These restriction fragment length polymorphisms (RFLPs) can be tested for by the Southern blot technique. The chromosome carrying the genetic mutation is tracked through the generations and can be tested for prenatally. Indirect testing is not as accurate as direct testing. However, for disorders where mutations causing disease have not been delineated (such as hemophilia B and cases of β-thalassemia), indirect testing is required.

Despite advances in molecular biology that have identified an increasing number of

RFLPs and gene mutations, certain disorders elude characterization by classical mendelian paradigms. Several nontraditional modes of inheritance have been recently described and explain why certain diseases did not "fit comfortably" in conventional mendelian inheritance patterns. Included in this group of nontraditional modes of inheritance are genomic imprinting, mitochondrial inheritance, and molecular expansion, which have helped delineate the genetics of disorders such as Prader-Willi and Angelman syndromes (genomic imprinting), Kearns-Sayre syndrome (mitochondrial inheritance), fragile X syndrome [CGG (cytosine-guanine-guanine) expansion], and Huntington disease [CAG (cytosine-adenine-guanine) expansion]. Of interest is that CGG expansion causes *deactivation* of the FMR-1 gene on the X chromosome and results in fragile X syndrome, whereas CAG expansion causes *activation* of the Huntington disease gene on chromosome 4 and expression of the disease. Increasing experience with human genome sequence will no doubt delineate new mechanisms of gene function and novel modes of heritability.

Fragile X is an X-linked disorder and the most common genetic cause of mental retardation. For affected boys, the IQ is similar to that of Down syndrome. For girls, the IQ may be normal or there may be mild developmental delay. All women who give a family history of boys with developmental delay, extreme hyperactivity, and speech and language problems should be offered fragile X carrier testing.

All DNA tests require recovery of DNA; this is accomplished by obtaining nucleated cells. For DNA analysis of newborns, children, or adults, nucleated cells are easily recoverable from peripheral blood samples. However, prenatal DNA analyses require fetal nucleated cells, and obtaining fetal cells is currently performed by chorionic villus sampling (CVS), amniocentesis, or percutaneous umbilical blood sampling (PUBS). As sequences of more genes are delineated, diagnosis of mendelian disorders heretofore undetectable will be possible.

POLYGENIC/MULTIFACTORIAL DISORDERS

Certain relatively common disorders result in a 2%–5% recurrence risk if first-degree relatives (parents, siblings, children) are affected. Such recurrence risks suggest a polygenic/multifactorial etiology in which undetermined genes and environmental stimuli are involved in disease expression. Many of these disorders are manifest by anatomic abnormalities. Some examples include cardiac anomalies such as ventricular and atrial septal defects and hypoplastic left heart syndrome; gastrointestinal anomalies including omphalocele, small bowel atresia, and diaphragmatic hernia; and urologic anomalies including renal agenesis and ureteropelvic junction obstruction.

An example of a polygenic/multifactorial disorder is neural tube defects, a group of disorders that occurs relatively frequently in both the United Kingdom and United States. The spectrum of neural tube defects ranges from anencephaly (absence of a portion or all of the forebrain) to spina bifida (spinal column closure defects). Neural tube defects occur in approximately 1 in 1500 births in the United States; however, in certain regions of the United States, neural tube defects occur more frequently (1 in 750 livebirths), whereas in some parts of the United Kingdom, the rate is 1 in 200 livebirths. Fetal neural tube defects are prenatally diagnosed by ultrasonography and AFP and acetylcholinesterase assays of amniotic fluid obtained by amniocentesis. However, approximately 85% of newborns with neural tube defects are born to women with no family or medication history that would have indicated them to be at increased risk and resulted in them being offered amniocentesis.

Folic acid has been shown to prevent recurrence and occurrence of neural tube defects. All women should be advised to take a prenatal vitamin that contains at least 0.4 mg of folic acid prior to conception. For women who have had a previous child with a neural tube defect, the recommended dose is 4 mg/daily.

Fortunately, we are now able to offer all low risk women, between 15 and 20 weeks' gestation, a screening blood test that measures maternal serum levels of α-fetoprotein (MSAFP), the fetal protein that is elevated in the amniotic fluid in cases of open fetal neural tube defect and that has been found to be elevated in the serum of most women carrying fetuses with open neural tube defects. However, like most screening tests, many women found to have elevated MSAFP levels are not carrying an affected fetus. Accordingly, physicians and health care professionals who provide MSAFP screening must inform their patients of possible false-positive and false-negative results, as well as availability of further diagnostic testing if screening results are abnormal.

INVASIVE PRENATAL DIAGNOSTIC PROCEDURES

Amniocentesis has been used for prenatal diagnosis for almost 20 years. The procedure involves removing, usually under concurrent ultrasound guidance, 20 to 40 cc of amniotic fluid. Traditionally, amniocentesis is performed between 15 and 20 weeks' gestation. Cytogenetic and DNA analyses of amniotic fluid specimens require culture of amniotic fluid cells, because most cells obtained from amniocentesis are not in metaphase and the number of viable cells is relatively small. Direct analysis of the amniotic fluid supernatant (amniotic fluid liquor) is possible for AFP and acetylcholinesterase assays; such analyses permit detection of fetal neural tube defects and other fetal structural defects (e.g., omphalocele, gastroschisis). In addition, some centers have begun to perform amniocentesis before 15 weeks' gestation; however, the safety and accuracy of "early amniocentesis" are still undetermined.

CVS was developed to provide early prenatal diagnosis. CVS is performed by transcervical or transabdominal aspiration of chorionic villi (immature placenta) under concurrent ultrasound guidance, usually between 10 and 12 weeks' gestation. Recent multicenter trials have demonstrated CVS to have similar safety and accuracy to that of "traditional" (i.e., performed at or after 15 weeks' gestation) amniocentesis. Another benefit of CVS is direct and, therefore, rapid cytogenetic and DNA analyses; this is possible because cytotrophoblasts obtained from first-trimester placentas are more likely to be viable and in metaphase than amniotic fluid cells. However, disorders that require analysis of amniotic fluid liquor, such as neural tube defects, are not amenable to prenatal diagnosis by CVS.

PUBS is usually performed after 20 weeks' gestation and is used to obtain fetal blood for blood component analyses (e.g., hematocrit, Rh status, platelets), as well as cytogenetic and DNA analyses. One major benefit of PUBS is the ability to obtain rapid (18 to 24 hours) fetal karyotypes. However, the safety of PUBS remains undetermined; accordingly, PUBS should not be used when amniocentesis or CVS can obtain similar diagnostic results in a timely fashion.

Other prenatal diagnostic procedures include *fetal skin sampling, fetal tissue (muscle, liver) biopsy, and fetoscopy*. These procedures are used only for the diagnosis of rare disorders not amenable to diagnosis by less invasive methods.

TERATOGENESIS

Teratogenesis is the development of fetal defects as a result of maternal exposure to specific compounds (agents) in the environment. Potential teratogenetic agents range from viruses and bacteria to heavy metals and organic compounds.

Teratology is the study of abnormal development of embryos and the causes of congenital malformations. Organs are most susceptible to teratogenic agents during periods of rapid cell division and differentiation. This organogenic period is from day 15 to day 60 (embryological age). Earlier actions may cause the death of the embryo and therefore end in spontaneous abortion.

The organ system's susceptibility depends on the timing of the exposure. The critical period for brain malformations is 3–16 weeks; however, the potential for damage extends throughout fetal development into the first

TABLE 3.3. Teratogenic Effects of Commonly Used Drugs	
Agent	**Effects**
Alcohol	Fetal alcohol syndrome, cardiac defects, mental retardation (50–80 IQ), microcephaly, facial anomalies
Phenytoin (anti-epileptic)	Broad nasal bridge, cleft lip and palate, microcephaly, average IQ of 71 in the full syndrome
Valproate (anti-epileptic)	Neural tube defects, craniofacial abnormalities
Warfarin	Depressed nasal bridge, stippled epiphyses, seizures, developmental delay, spontaneous abortion, stillborn neonatal hemorrhage

two years of life. For the neural tube it is 2–4 weeks (the tube is closed by day 28). The heart is vulnerable at 3–6 weeks. Insults beyond 9–10 weeks lead to functional defects and minor morphological abnormalities.

Pregnant women take an average of 4 drugs during pregnancy (excluding nutritional supplements). Forty percent of these women take a drug during the critical period of development. Fortunately, only a few drugs have been positively identified as teratogens. Listed in Table 3.3 are commonly used drugs with teratogenic effects.

Pregnant women should be advised to consult their physician before ingesting any medication during pregnancy. It is best to avoid using all medication during the first 8 weeks after conception, unless there is a strong medical indication. They should also be advised to discontinue all alcohol use and smoking.

Gynecology/Primary Care

As with the obstetrical patient, a careful family history provides the gynecologist with critical information that allows for appropriate screening and diagnosis for an ever expanding list of gynecologic and nongynecologic conditions. As with prenatal risk, racial and ethnic backgrounds provide important clues as to risk for certain diseases and appropriate screening paradigms.

Although gynecologists have historically been the central health care profes-sional in the screening of women for gynecologic malignancies (e.g., Pap smear and cervical cancer), advances in molecular technologies are permitting the inclusion of more disease states to this list. Although screening for breast and ovarian cancers by analysis of the BRCA gene family is not yet standard of care, such molecular screening may provide important information to selected women. Again, family and ethnic histories remain vital parts of the screening process, because BRCA genes may account for only 5% of malignancies in the general population but may account for 50% of breast-ovarian cancer cases, familial breast cancers, and a higher proportion in women with Eastern European (Ashkenazi) Jewish ancestry. In addition to the less than optimal specificity and sensitivity of BRCA analysis, such screening is further complicated by a lack of consensus regarding appropriate care following a positive or negative test result. Further work is thus needed and close consultation with geneticists is highly recommended.

Other nongynecologic conditions that are or may be soon amenable to molecular screening include cancer family syndrome, certain cholesterol/lipid abnormalities, clotting factor abnormalities (e.g., factor V-Leiden) that may increase risk for coronary vascular disease, and selected leukemias, lymphomas, and solid tumors. Again, close consultation with genetic professionals in your community is highly recommended.

CASE STUDIES

Case 3A

A 24-year-old G1 P0, *accompanied by her 27-year-old husband, presents with a history of 8 weeks of amenorrhea and the onset, earlier in the day, of cramping and bleeding. Clinical examination reveals an incomplete abortion and a suction and curettage is performed without incident. At the parents' request, the tissue is sent for genetic evaluation. She is Rh+ and in good health. Each has a negative family history of congenital anomalies and inherited disease and negative personal medical histories. Her physical examination is entirely normal.*

On her first office visit one week after the miscarriage, her course has been unremarkable, her physical examination is normal, and she feels well, although depressed. The couple questions what the significance of the miscarriage will be for future pregnancies.

Questions Case 3A

Your answer will include which of the following?

A. The likelihood of the next or subsequent pregnancies carrying to term is less than 35%
B. The likelihood of this pregnancy demonstrating a genetic disorder is less than 5%
C. The likelihood of their being able to conceive is reduced by 67% compared with couples who have had no miscarriage
D. All of the above
E. None of the above

Answer: E

Absent identified risk factors, the chances of conceiving and carrying the next pregnancy to term are not reduced. Provided the tissue obtained at suction and curettage is viable enough to permit culturing, the chances of a genetic anomaly are approximately 50%.

Three weeks later a genetic report is received indicating trisomy 16. You inform the patient and her husband of this information and suggest

A. They consider adoption
B. They consider sterilization of one or both partners and adoption
C. They continue with their plans to have another pregnancy in approximately 6 months
D. All of the above
E. None of the above

Answer: C

Trisomy 16 is associated with lethal outcomes in the first trimester. Your previous advice about future pregnancy remains valid.

Case 3B

A 31-year-old multigravida presents to your office upon referral from her primary care clinician. As part of an insurance evaluation, a BRCA analysis was performed, and subsequently her insurance application was denied because the test was positive. Her primary care clinician questions if prophylaxis is indicated, and if so what. Hysterectomy/ oophorectomy? Mastectomy? Chemotherapy? Questioning reveals no family history of carcinoma, specifically including breast and ovary. Physical examination is unremarkable in this thin healthy woman, specifically normal breast examination without masses or discharge and no palpable ovarian enlargement. Her clinician had a mammogram performed in preparation for consultation, and it is reported as negative.

(Continued)

Question Case 3B

Your recommendation is

A. Surgery
B. Chemotherapy
C. Routine annual care
D. Annual mammography and pelvic sonography
E. A modified annual evaluation regimen based on discussion with the patient

Answer: C, D, E

Present scientific evidence does not allow a clear answer to this perplexing question, certainly not one that will satisfy most clinicians or patients. Although this patient is at some increased risk of malignancy, the degree of risk and the effectiveness of increased screening is still uncertain. For now, a reasonable course is some increased level of screening (breast examination, mammography, pelvic examination, pelvic sonography), which seems "reasonable" to patient and clinician. Drastic steps such as surgery are not indicated in this case where there is no family history of malignancy or difficulty in physical examination.

UNIT II

Obstetrics

NORMAL OBSTETRICS

C H A P T E R

4

MATERNAL–FETAL PHYSIOLOGY

CHAPTER OBJECTIVES

This chapter deals primarily with APGO Objective(s):

OBJECTIVE 9 Maternal–Fetal Physiology

A. Explain the maternal physiologic changes associated with pregnancy and the physiology of the placenta and fetus.

B. Describe the effect of pregnancy on common diagnostic studies.

TABLE 4.1.	Key Gastrointestinal Changes in Pregnancy
Appetite	Usually increases, sometimes with unusual cravings (pica)
Gastric reflux	Results from cardiac sphincter relaxation and anatomic displacement
Gastric motility	Decreases
Intestinal transit time	Decreases
Liver	Does not change functionally; alkaline phosphatase increases
Gallbladder	Dilates
Bile composition	Does not change

There are many physiologic changes in pregnancy. Some mimic the signs, symptoms, or laboratory findings of disease in the nonpregnant patient yet are normal in pregnancy. Therefore, knowledge of normal maternal physiology helps avoid unnecessary diagnostic or therapeutic interventions.

MATERNAL PHYSIOLOGY
Dental Changes

The incidence of dental caries does not change with pregnancy, but that of gingival disease does. The gums become more edematous and soft during pregnancy and bleed easily with vigorous brushing. On occasion violaceous pedunculated lesions, which bleed easily, appear at the gum line. These are called *epulis gravidarum* during pregnancy (although they are actually just pyogenic granulomas), and they usually regress within two months of delivery. If they bleed excessively, they may need to be excised. Dental care is not contraindicated in pregnancy and indeed may be requisite to good maternal nutrition. Local anesthetics (preferably without epinephrine) and judicious use of x-rays (with pelvic shielding) are likewise acceptable.

Gastrointestinal Changes (Table 4.1)

One of the earliest symptoms of pregnancy is *nausea* and *vomiting,* or "morning sickness." Morning sickness typically begins between 4 and 8 weeks of gestational age and abates by the middle of the second trimester, usually by 14 to 16 weeks. Although the exact etiology of this nausea is unknown, it appears related to elevated levels of progesterone, human chorionic gonadotropin (hCG), and relaxation of the smooth muscle of the stomach. There are usually no significant nutritional deficits or weight loss associated with this distressing but transient symptom complex. Treatment consists primarily of reassurance, frequent small meals, and inclusion of bland foods (such as toast or crackers) as well as avoidance of those foods found to exacerbate the nausea and vomiting.

If the symptoms persist beyond the middle of the second trimester or if there is an associated weight loss, ketonemia, or electrolyte imbalance at any time, the diagnosis of *hyperemesis gravidarum* should be considered. Patients with this severe variety of nausea and vomiting in pregnancy must be hospitalized to receive parenteral fluid and electrolyte replacement. Environmental stressors and/or other psychological underpinning are common in these patients, and evaluation should attempt to assess these factors and reduce them, if possible.

Despite the gastrointestinal upset seen in early pregnancy, many patients report *dietary cravings* during pregnancy. Some may be the result of the patient's perception that a particular food may help with nausea and heartburn. *Pica* is an especially intense craving for such things as ice, laundry starch, or clay. Other patients develop dietary or olfactory aversions during pregnancy. *Ptyalism* is perceived by the patient to be the excessive production of saliva but

TABLE 4.2. Key Pulmonary Changes in Pregnancy

Increases	Does Not Change	Decreases
Oxygen requirement	Arterial pH	Carbon dioxide pressure
Oxygen pressure		Expiratory reserve volume
Tidal volume		Residual volume
Inspiratory capacity		Total lung capacity
Vital capacity		P_{CO_2}
Minute volume		Serum bicarbonate
P_{O_2}		

P_{CO_2} = partial pressure of carbon dioxide; P_{O_2} = partial pressure of oxygen.

probably represents the inability of a nauseated patient to swallow the normal amounts of saliva that are produced.

Most women increase their caloric intake by about 200 kcal/day, although the recommended dietary allowance in pregnancy is an additional 300 kcal/day. Energy requirements vary from individual to individual, however, so that clinical dietary management should be individualized for each pregnant patient.

In general, there is decreased *gastrointestinal motility* during pregnancy because of increasing levels of progesterone. Transit time in the stomach and small bowel increases significantly, 15%–30% in the second and third trimesters and more during labor. The *heartburn* experienced so commonly in pregnancy is *gastric reflux* associated with the increased emptying time, as well as reduced tone of the sphincter at the gastroesophageal junction and increased intra-abdominal pressure as gestational age increases.

Constipation is common in pregnancy and is associated with mechanical obstruction of the colon by the enlarging bowel, reduced motility as elsewhere in the gastrointestinal (GI) tract, and increased water absorption during pregnancy. Increased liquid intake and, when needed, bowel softeners and bulk expanders may be helpful.

Gallbladder emptying is also delayed in pregnancy, with the subsequent cholestasis resulting in an increased tendency to form gallstones. Liver function also changes in pregnancy, with alkaline phosphatase elevated as much as twofold during pregnancy. Serum cholesterol levels are increased during pregnancy whereas serum albumin decreases. Liver produced proteins such as fibrinogen rise as much as 50% compared to the nonpregnant state as do the levels of ceruloplasmin and the binding proteins for corticosteroids, sex steroids, thyroid hormones, and vitamin D.

Hemorrhoids are common in pregnancy and are caused by both constipation and elevated venous pressures due to increased pelvic blood flow and the effects of the enlarging uterus. The treatment of hemorrhoids during pregnancy is generally reassurance and topical medication for symptomatic relief; surgery is reserved for intractable cases.

Pulmonary Changes

Pregnancy-related changes of the respiratory system are the result of both anatomic and functional changes (Table 4.2). Mucosal hyperemia results in marked nasal stuffiness and an increased amount of nasal secretions. Patients often complain of allergy-like symptoms or chronic colds as a result of the symptoms associated with these changes. Anatomically, there are also pregnancy-induced accommodations for the enlarging uterus. The subcostal angle increases the chest circumference and the diameter increases slightly. There is increased diaphragmatic excursion and the diaphragm is elevated approximately 4 cm in late pregnancy.

Pulmonary functions are altered in pregnancy. There is a 30% to 40% increase in tidal volume. Inspiratory capacity increases approximately 5%, with respiratory rate, vital capacity, and inspiratory reserve remaining the same as in the non-pregnant state. The functional residual capacity, expiratory volume, and residual volume are all decreased by approximately 20%. The total lung capacity is also decreased by 5% with a resulting increase in minute ventilation of 30% to 40%. Arterial blood gases reflect this change in pulmonary function in the following ways: oxygen (PO_2) is increased, carbon dioxide (PCO_2) is decreased, and serum bicarbonate is reduced. An especially important change is decreased $PaCO_2$. Because of the increased minute ventilation in pregnancy, $PaCO_2$ levels fall to 27–32 mm Hg in the second half of pregnancy compared to the nonpregnant level of 40 mm Hg. This in turn causes an increase in the CO_2 gradient between fetus and mother, facilitating transfer of CO_2 from fetus to mother. Maternal arterial pH is maintained at normal levels (7.40–7.45) because the decreased PCO_2 is compensated by increased renal excretion of bicarbonate, yielding normal pregnancy bicarbonate levels of 18–31 mEq/L, which are significantly below nonpregnant normal values. In summary, there is a mild respiratory alkalosis, with the patient being aware of dyspnea, hyperventilation, and a relative decrease in exercise tolerance. This sensation of dyspnea (*dyspnea of pregnancy*) is experienced by nearly two thirds of women starting in the late first or early second trimester. The cause is unclear, perhaps related to some extent to reduced $PaCO_2$ and to an awareness of the increased tidal volume associated with pregnancy.

Cardiovascular Changes

The dramatic changes in the maternal cardiovascular system during pregnancy improve oxygenation and flow of nutrition to the fetus (Table 4.3). Cardiac output increases up to 50% in the first half of pregnancy as a result of increased stroke volume and in the latter half of pregnancy as a

TABLE 4.3. Key Cardiovascular Changes in Pregnancy

Increases	Decreases
Cardiac output	Systemic vascular resistance
Stroke volume	
Heart rate	Pulmonary vascular resistance
Left ventricular stroke work index	
	Colloid osmotic pressure
Mean arterial pressure (slight)	
Blood flow	
Uterus	
Kidney	
Breasts	
Skin	
Brain	

result of increased maternal heart rate as stroke volume returns to near normal prepregnancy levels. Late in pregnancy there may be a decrease in cardiac output when venous return to the heart is obstructed by the large gravid uterus. This at times near complete occlusion of the inferior vena cava is common in term pregnancy, especially in the supine position, with venous return from the lower extremities shunted primarily through the dilated paravertebral collateral circulation. Although most women do not become overtly hypotensive when lying supine, perhaps one in ten have symptoms that include dizziness, light-headedness, and syncope. This is often termed the *inferior vena cava syndrome* and may be related to some extent to the inability of these women to shunt via the paravertebral circulation. The distribution of the cardiac output also varies during pregnancy. The uterus receives about 2% of the cardiac output in the first trimester but up to 20% at term, mainly by means of a relative reduction of the fraction of cardiac output going to the splanchnic bed and skeletal muscle. The absolute blood flow to these areas is not changed, however, because of the increase in cardiac output in late pregnancy.

Because of the smooth muscle relaxing effect of increased levels of progesterone during pregnancy, *peripheral vascular resistance* is decreased. There is a decrease in arterial blood pressure during the first 24 weeks of pregnancy with a gradual increase returning to nonpregnant levels by term. Blood pressures higher than the nonpregnant values for a particular patient should be considered abnormal. Accurate serial blood pressure measurement during pregnancy is important. To do so, it is useful to remember that measured blood pressure is highest when a pregnant woman is seated, somewhat lower when supine, and lowest while lying on the side. In the lateral recumbent position the measured pressure in the superior arm is about 10 mm Hg lower than that simultaneously measured in the inferior arm.

Because the cardiovascular system is in a hyperdynamic state, normal physical findings on *cardiovascular examination* during pregnancy include an increased second heart sound split with inspiration, distended neck veins, and low-grade systolic ejection murmurs. These are often best heard over the left upper sternal border. Many normal pregnant women have an S_3 gallop, or third heart sound, after midpregnancy. Systolic ejection murmurs are believed to be caused by a normal increased blood flow across the aortic and pulmonic valves. Diastolic murmurs should not be considered normal findings in pregnancy.

Anatomically, the heart is displaced upward and to the left. Because the diaphragm is elevated and because the heart is in a more horizontal position, chest x-rays might appear to demonstrate cardiomegaly when no such abnormality exists.

During the course of labor, cardiac output increases approximately 40% above that in late pregnancy. Much of this is a result of pain and apprehension, because these findings are significantly reduced when a patient has an epidural anesthetic administered. Mean arterial blood pressure increases approximately 10 mm Hg during each contraction, unless adequate analgesia is provided. Cardiac output increases significantly immediately after delivery because obstruction of venous return to the heart caused by the gravid uterus is released and because extracellular fluid is quickly mobilized.

Hematologic Changes

Maternal *plasma volume* begins to increase as early as the sixth week of pregnancy and reaches a maximum at approximately 30 to 34 weeks, after which it is stable. The mean increase in plasma volume is approximately 50%; there is a greater increase in patients with multiple gestation. Similarly, larger babies are associated with a greater increase of maternal plasma volume, whereas a pregnancy complicated by intrauterine growth restriction is often associated with a less-than-normal increase in blood volume.

Red cell mass begins to increase later in pregnancy and increases to a lesser degree than does plasma volume. As a result, there is a "physiologic" anemia caused by dilution of approximately 15% compared with nonpregnancy levels. Whereas erythrocyte volume increases by approximately 18% without iron supplementation, it can increase up to 30% when iron supplements are used. After 30 to 34 weeks, the hematocrit (Hct) may increase somewhat, as erythrocyte volume continues to increase while plasma volume is stable (Table 4.4).

White blood cell (WBC) counts also increase slightly in pregnancy. During labor, the WBC count may further increase to 30,000/ml, with a return to nonpregnant levels during the puerperium. The increase in the WBC count is caused primarily by an increased number of granulocytes. Platelet counts during pregnancy may decline slightly but remain within the normal range of those of nonpregnant patients.

Pregnancy is considered a hypercoagulable state with an increased risk of *venous thromboembolism* both during pregnancy and the puerperium. The risk of thromboembolism is approximately 2 times normal during pregnancy and increases to 5.5 times normal during the puerperium. Fibrinogen (factor I) increases to a level of 400 to 500 mg/dl. There is an increase in

TABLE 4.4.   Key Hematologic and Biochemical Changes in Pregnancy

Increases	Does Not Change	Decreases
Plasma volume	Amylase	Hemoglobin concentration
Total erythrocyte volume	Lactic acid dehydrogenase	Hematocrit
Mean cell volume	(LDH)	Serum iron
Total iron-binding capacity	Glutamic oxaloacetic	Total protein
Erythrocyte sedimentation	transaminase (GOT)	Albumin
rate	Glutamic pyruvic	Osmolality
Alkaline phosphatase	transaminase (GPT)	

fibrin split products and in factors VII, VIII, IX, and X. Prothrombin (factor II) and factors V and XII remain unchanged during pregnancy. *Bleeding time* and *clotting time* do not change during a normal pregnancy.

The normal pregnant patient requires a total of 1000 mg of additional iron: 500 mg are used to increase maternal red cell mass, 300 mg are transported to the fetus, and the additional 200 mg are used to compensate for normal iron loss. Supplemental iron use in pregnancy is intended to prevent iron deficiency in the mother. It is not intended either to prevent iron deficiency in the fetus or to maintain maternal hemoglobin (Hb) concentration. Because iron is actively transported to the fetus, fetal hemoglobin levels are maintained despite maternal anemia. To supply her needs, 60 mg of elemental iron are recommended daily for the nonanemic patient. This is provided in 300 mg of ferrous sulfate. Patients who are anemic should receive twice this dose.

Renal Changes

Kidneys enlarge approximately 1 cm during pregnancy as measured on intravenous pyelography or ultrasonography. This is the result of an increase in interstitial volume as well as distended renal vasculature. Both the renal pelves as well as the ureters are dilated during pregnancy, because of the relaxing effect of progesterone. Typically, the right ureter is more dilated than the left. Mechanical compression of the ureters—by both the ovarian venous plexus and the enlarging uterus—contributes to dilation.

TABLE 4.5.   Key Renal Changes in Pregnancy

Increases	Does Not Change
Renal plasma flow	Urinary output
Glomerular	24-hour protein
filtration rate	excretion
Renin	
Angiotensin I and II	
Renin substrate	

Because progesterone also decreases *bladder* tone, there is increased residual volume and, with the dilated collecting system, urinary stasis results, predisposing to an increased incidence of pyelonephritis in patients with asymptomatic bacteriuria. There is also loss of urinary control as pregnancy advances. Because of the enlarging uterus, bladder capacity decreases, resulting in urinary frequency (Table 4.5).

Renal plasma flow (RPF) begins to increase early in the first trimester and increases to as much as 75% over nonpregnant levels at term. Similarly, *glomerular filtration rate* (GFR) increases to 50% over the nonpregnant state. Because of these changes, *creatinine clearance* is markedly increased in pregnancy, with 150 to 200 ml/min considered normal. Serum levels of creatinine, uric acid, and blood urea nitrogen (BUN) decrease in normal pregnancy. BUN falls about 25% to levels of 8–10 mg/dl at the end of the first trimester of pregnancy and is maintained at these levels for the remainder of the pregnancy. Likewise, serum creatinine values fall from a nonpregnant level of 0.8 mg/dl to pregnancy levels of 0.5–0.6 mg/dl by term. *Plasma osmolality* is decreased, primarily because of reduction in the serum *sodium concentration*. The tendency to lose sodium, as a result of the increased GFR, and the elevated levels of progesterone are compensated for by an increase in renal tubule reabsorption of sodium as well as by the increased levels of aldosterone, estrogen, and desoxycorticosterone. The plasma renin activity is up to 10 times that of the nonpregnant state. Similarly, renin substrate (angiotensinogen) and angiotensin are increased approximately fivefold. During pregnancy, the body retains approximately 1000 mEq of sodium in the fetus, placenta, and maternal intravascular and extracellular fluid spaces. Normal pregnant patients are relatively resistant to the hypertensive effects of the increased levels of renin-angiotensin-aldosterone, whereas patients with hypertensive disease of pregnancy are not.

Because of the increase in GFR, there is a greatly increased load of glucose presented to the renal tubules. As a result, *glucose excretion* increases in virtually all pregnant patients. Therefore, quantitative urine glucose measurements are not clinically useful in managing patients with diabetes, because they do not reflect blood glucose levels.

There is no significant increase in *protein loss* in the urine during pregnancy, the nonpregnant range of 100–300 mg/24 hours being equally valid in pregnancy. There are increases in urinary excretion of vitamin B_{12} and folate.

Skin Changes

During pregnancy, *vascular spiders* (spider angiomata) are most common on the upper torso, face, and arms. *Palmar erythema* occurs in more than 50% of patients. Both are caused by increased levels of circulating estrogen and regress after delivery. *Striae gravidarum* occur in over one half of pregnant women and can be either purple or pink initially and appear on the lower abdomen, breasts, and thighs. They are not related to weight gain but solely the result of the stretching of normal skin. There is no effective therapy to prevent these "stretch marks," nor can they be eliminated once they appear. They do eventually become white or silvery in color.

Hyperpigmentation is believed to be the result of elevated levels of estrogen and α-melanocyte-stimulating hormone (α-MSH) and a cross reaction with the structurally similar β-hCG. It commonly affects the umbilicus and perineum, although it may affect any skin surface. The lower abdomen linea alba darkens to become the linea nigra. The "mask of pregnancy," or *chloasma* (melasma), is also common. *Skin nevi* can increase in size and pigmentation but resolve after pregnancy. Removal of rapidly changing nevi is recommended during pregnancy. *Eccrine sweating* and *sebum production* are increased during normal pregnancy, with many patients complaining of acne. Melasma may never disappear completely.

Hair growth during pregnancy is maintained. The anagen (growth) phase normally lasts up to 6 years. Fewer follicles are in the telogen (resting) phase. Late in pregnancy, the number of hairs in telogen is approximately one half of the normal 20%, so that postpartum, the number of hairs entering telogen increases; thus there is significant hair loss 2 to 4 months after pregnancy. Hair growth typically returns to normal 6 to 12 months after delivery. Patients are often quite concerned about this "hair loss" until they are reassured that it is transient and that hair growth will renew in 6–12 months.

Breast Changes

The breasts increase in size during pregnancy, rapidly in the first 8 weeks and steadily thereafter. A total enlargement of 25%–50% is common and, in addition, the nipples become larger and more mobile and the areola larger and more deeply pigmented with enlargement of the Montgomery's glands. Blood flow increases to the breasts as they change to support lactation. Some patients may complain of breast or nipple tenderness and a tingling sensation. Estrogen stimulation also results in ductal growth, with alveolar hypertrophy being a result of progesterone stimulation. During the latter portion of pregnancy, a thick yellow fluid can be expressed from the nipples. This *colostrum* is more common in parous women. Ultimately, lactation depends on synergistic actions of estrogen, progesterone, prolactin, human placental lactogen, cortisol, and insulin.

Musculoskeletal Changes

As pregnancy progresses, a compensatory lumbar lordosis (anterior convexity of the lumbar spine) is apparent. This change is functionally useful as it helps keep the woman's center of gravity over the legs as the enlarging uterus would otherwise shift it quite anteriorly. But, as a result of the change, virtually all women complain of low back pain during pregnancy. Beginning early in pregnancy, the effects of relaxin and progesterone result in a relative laxity of the ligaments. The pubic symphysis separates at approximately 28 to 30 weeks. Patients often complain of an unsteady gait and may fall more commonly during pregnancy than during the nonpregnant state, as a result of both these changes and an altered center of gravity.

To provide for adequate calcium supplies to the fetal skeleton, mobilization of calcium stores occurs. Maternal serum ionized calcium is unchanged from the nonpregnant state, but maternal total serum calcium decreases. There is a significant increase in maternal parathyroid hormone, which acts to maintain serum calcium levels by increasing absorption from the intestine and decreasing the loss of calcium through the kidney. The skeleton is well maintained, despite these elevated levels of parathyroid hormones. This may be because of the effect of calcitonin. Although the rate of bone turnover increases, there is no loss of bone density during a normal pregnancy if adequate nutrition is supplied.

Ophthalmic Changes

The most common visual complaint of pregnant women is blurred vision. This is primarily caused by increased thickness of the cornea associated with fluid retention and decreased intraocular pressure. These changes are manifest in the first trimester and regress within the first 6–8 weeks postpartum. Changes in corrective lens prescriptions should, therefore, not be encouraged during pregnancy.

Reproductive Tract and Abdominal Wall Changes

The effects of pregnancy on the *vulva* are similar to the effects on other skin. Because of an increase in vascularity, *vulvar varicosities* are very common. These usually regress after delivery. An increase in vaginal transudation as well as stimulation of the vaginal epithelium result in a thick profuse *vaginal discharge*. The epithelium of the endocervix everts onto the ectocervix, with an associated mucous plug being produced. The *uterus* undergoes an enormous increase in weight from the 70-g nonpregnant size to approximately 1100 g at term, primarily through hypertrophy of existing myometrial cells. Similarly, the uterine cavity, which in the nongravid state has a volume of less than 10 ml, increases up to as much as 5 liters. Cardiac output to the uterus is less than 2% in the nongravid state but increases to 15% to 20% at term (i.e., 500 to 700 ml/min). There is also increasing pressure caused by intra-abdominal growth of the uterus, resulting in an exacerbation of *hernia defects,* most commonly seen at the umbilicus and in the abdominal wall (*diastasis recti,* a physiologic separation of the rectus abdominus muscles).

Endocrinologic Changes
CARBOHYDRATE METABOLISM

Several hormones secreted by the placenta are responsible for the *diabetogenic effect of pregnancy*. Human placental lactogen (HPL) increases the resistance of peripheral tissues and liver to the effects of insulin. Because HPL is secreted in proportion to placental mass, resistance to insulin increases as pregnancy progresses. Progesterone and estrogen also contribute to insulin resistance during pregnancy, and insulin is broken down by the placental production of insulinase. *Pregnancy is characterized by hyperglycemia, hyperinsulinemia, hypertriglyceridemia, and reduced tissue response to insulin.* The typical fasting glucose level is lower than that in the nonpregnant state, because the fetoplacental unit serves as a constant drain on maternal glucose levels. As a result, in response to maternal starvation, the patient demonstrates exaggerated hypoglycemia and hypoinsulinemia. Delivery of glucose from the mother to the fetus occurs by facilitated diffusion, and as a result, fetal glucose levels depend on maternal levels. The fetus does not, however, depend on the mother for insulin, because fetal insulin is apparent at 9 to 11 weeks of gestation (Table 4.6).

The major change in blood glucose levels in the pregnant woman is a lower fasting level with a prolonged elevation of glucose values after a glucose load is administered. The lower fasting levels result from the constant diffusion to the fetus, where glucose is used as the primary energy source. In addition, there is hypertrophy of the cells of the maternal pancreas, which secrete two to three times the nonpregnant level of insulin late in pregnancy.

THYROID FUNCTION

Several changes in the pregnant patient relate to thyroid function, with the net effect being that the normal pregnant woman is euthyroid. Estrogen induces an increased level of thyroxine-binding globulin (TBG), resulting in an increase in total thyroxine (T_4) and total 3,5,3'-triiodothyronine (T_3) beginning early in pregnancy. Free T_4 and free T_3, the active hormones, are unchanged from the normal range for nonpregnant patients (see Table 4.6).

TABLE 4.6.	Key Endocrine Changes in Pregnancy		
Gland/Organ	**Increases**	**Does Not Change**	**Decreases**
Thyroid	Total T_4		
	Total T_3	Free T_3	
	TBG	Free T_4	
Adrenal	CBG		
	Cortisol		
	Androstenedione		
	DOC		DHEAS
	Aldosterone		
Pituitary	Prolactin	TSH	FSH
	ACTH	Oxytocin	
Ovaries and placenta	Progesterone		
	17-Hydroxyprogesterone		
	Estradiol		
	Estriol		
	HPL		
	hCG (peak increase at 8–10 weeks' gestation)		

ACTH = adrenocorticotropic hormone; CBG = corticosteroid-binding globulin; DHEAS = dehydroepiandrosterone sulfate; DOC = deoxycorticosterone; FSH = follicle-stimulating hormone; hCG = human chorionic gonadotropin; HPL = human placental lactogen; T_3 = 3,5,3'-triiodothyronine; T_4 = thyroxine; TBG = thyroxine-binding globulin; TSH = thyroid-stimulating hormone.

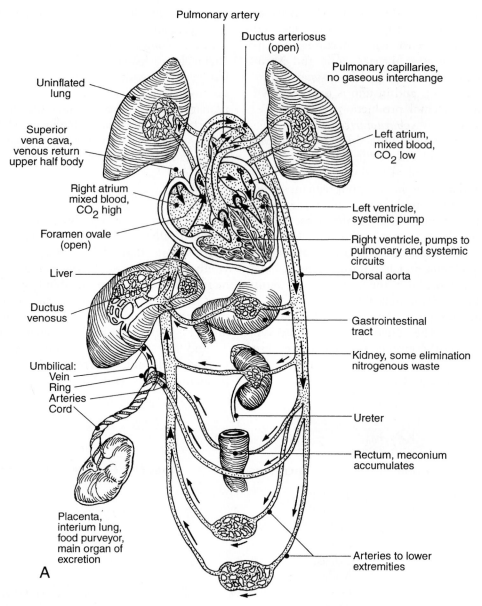

Pulmonary artery

Ductus arteriosus
(open)

Pulmonary capillaries,
no gaseous interchange

Uninflated
lung

Superior
vena cava,
venous return
upper half body

Left atrium,
mixed blood,
CO_2 low

Right atrium
mixed blood,
CO_2 high

Left ventricle,
systemic pump

Foramen ovale
(open)

Right ventricle, pumps to
pulmonary and systemic
circuits

Liver

Dorsal aorta

Ductus
venosus

Gastrointestinal
tract

Kidney, some elimination
nitrogenous waste

Umbilical:
Vein
Ring
Arteries
Cord

Ureter

Rectum, meconium
accumulates

Placenta,
interium lung,
food purveyor,
main organ of
excretion

Arteries to lower
extremities

A

FIGURE 4.1. Fetal circulation at term (A) and after delivery (B). Note the changes in function of the ductus venosus, foramen ovale, and ductus arteriosus in the transition from intrauterine to extrauterine existence. Stippling = deoxygenated blood; no stippling = oxygenated blood.

ADRENAL FUNCTION

During pregnancy, there is an estrogen-induced increase in the plasma concentration of corticosteroid-binding globulin (CBG), resulting in elevated levels of plasma cortisol. Like thyroid hormone, only the portion of cortisol that is unbound is metabolically active. Unlike thyroid hormone, however, the concentration of free plasma cortisol is elevated, progressively increasing from the first trimester until term. There is also increased plasma concentration of deoxycorticosterone (DOC), whereas dehydroepiandrosterone sulfate (DHEAS) is decreased (see Table 4.6).

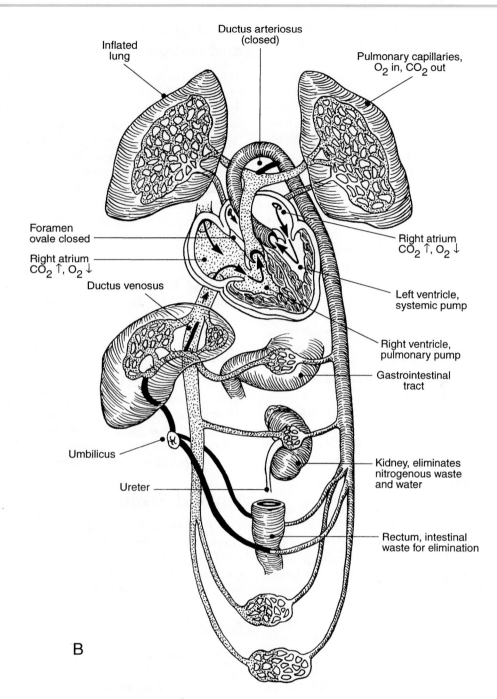

Ductus arteriosus (closed)

Inflated lung

Pulmonary capillaries, O_2 in, CO_2 out

Foramen ovale closed

Right atrium $CO_2 \uparrow, O_2 \downarrow$

Ductus venosus

Right atrium $CO_2 \uparrow, O_2 \downarrow$

Left ventricle, systemic pump

Right ventricle, pulmonary pump

Gastrointestinal tract

Umbilicus

Ureter

Kidney, eliminates nitrogenous waste and water

Rectum, intestinal waste for elimination

B

FIGURE 4.1. *(Continued)*

FETAL PHYSIOLOGY
Circulation (Figure 4.1)

The umbilical vein, which carries oxygenated blood (80% saturated) from the placenta, enters the portal system of the fetus and gives off branches to the left lobe of the liver. It then becomes the origin of the ductus venosus. Another branch joins blood flow from the portal vein that is flowing to the right lobe of the liver. Fifty percent of the umbilical blood supply goes through the ductus venosus. The blood flow from the left hepatic vein is mixed with the blood in the inferior vena cava and is directed toward the foramen ovale. Consequently, the well-oxygenated umbilical vein blood enters the left ventricle and supplies the carotid arteries. The relatively less oxygenated blood in the right hepatic vein, having entered the inferior vena cava, flows through the tricuspid valve into the right ventricle. Blood from the superior vena cava also preferentially flows through the tricuspid valve to the right ventricle. Blood from the pulmonary artery primarily flows through the ductus arteriosus into the aorta. Less than 10% of cardiac output goes to the lung, with blood flow through the foramen ovale accounting for approximately one third of the cardiac output.

The proximal aorta supplies highly saturated blood (65% saturated) to the brain and upper body. It is joined in its descending portion by the ductus arteriosus. The descending aorta then supplies blood to the lower portion of the fetal body, with a major portion of this blood being delivered to the umbilical arteries, which carry deoxygenated blood to the placenta.

Placenta

Glucose is the primary substrate for placental metabolism. It is estimated that as much as 70% of the glucose transferred from the mother is used by the placenta. The glucose that crosses the placenta does so by facilitated diffusion. Other solutes that are transferred from the mother to the fetus depend on the concentration gradient as well as on their degree of ionization, size, and lipid solubility. Fetal uptake of O_2 and excretion of CO_2 depend on the maternal and fetal blood-carrying capacities for these gases and on uterine and umbilical blood flows. There is active transport of amino acids, resulting in levels that are higher in the fetus than in the mother. Free fatty acids have very limited placental transfer, with resultant fetal levels that are lower than in the mother.

Hemoglobin and Oxygenation

Although the partial pressure of oxygen in fetal arterial blood is only 20 to 25 mm Hg, the fetus is adequately oxygenated because of its higher cardiac output and organ blood flow. In addition, the higher hemoglobin concentration in the fetus than in the adult and the higher oxygen saturation are responsible for the oxygenation of the fetus. At any given oxygen tension, the fetal blood has a higher oxygen saturation than does adult blood.

Kidney

The fetal kidney forms urine and, as a result, amniotic fluid. Fetal urine is hypotonic compared with that of a newborn.

Liver

The fetal liver is not fully functional even at term. Bilirubin is primarily eliminated through the placenta. It is this immaturity of function that accounts for the common practice of giving supplemental vitamin K to newborns to prevent bleeding problems.

Thyroid Gland

The fetal thyroid gland develops without direct influence from the mother. The placenta does not transport thyroid-stimulating hormone (TSH), and only minimal amounts of T_3 and T_4 cross the placenta.

Gonads

The primordial germ cells migrate during the eighth week of gestation from the endoderm of the yolk sac to the genital ridge. At this point, the gonads are undifferentiated. Differentiation into the testes occurs 6 weeks after conception, if the embryo is 46,XY. This testicular differentiation appears to depend on the presence of the H-Y antigen and the Y chromosome. If the Y chromosome is absent, however, an ovary develops from the undifferentiated gonad. Development of the fetal ovary begins at approximately 7 weeks. The development of other genital organs depends on the presence or absence of specific hormones and is independent of gonadal differentiation. If the fetal testes are present, testosterone and müllerian inhibitory factor (MIF) inhibit the development of female external genitalia. If these two hormones are not present, the female genitalia develop with regression of the wolffian ducts.

IMMUNOLOGY OF PREGNANCY

Although the maternal immune system is not altered in pregnancy, the antigenically dissimilar fetus is able to survive in the uterus without being rejected. This fetal allograft appears to be somehow protected in this privileged immunologic site.

The placenta serves as an effective interference between the maternal and fetal vascular compartments by keeping the fetus from direct contact with the maternal immune system. The placenta also produces estrogen, progesterone, hCG, and HPL, all of which may contribute to suppression of maternal immune responses on a local level. The placenta is, in addition, the site of origin for blocking antibodies and masking antibodies, which alter the immune response.

The mother's systemic immune system remains intact as evidenced by leukocyte count, B and T cell count and function, and immunoglobulin (Ig) levels. Because IgG is the only immunoglobulin that can cross the placenta, maternal IgG comprises a major proportion of fetal immunoglobulin both in utero and in the early neonatal period. It is in this fashion that passive immunity can be transferred to the fetus.

Fetal lymphocyte production begins as early as 6 weeks of gestation. By 12 weeks of gestation, IgG, IgM, IgD, and IgE are present and are produced in progressively increasing amounts throughout pregnancy.

CASE STUDIES

Case 4A

A 28-year-old G3 P2002 who has lived until recently in the deep South presents for prenatal care at 24 weeks of pregnancy. Her fundal height and gestational age correspond, and her general physical examination is normal. Her first two pregnancies were normal except for an anemia. She and her husband have negative past medical and family histories, and they are attorneys and have recently joined a firm in your town.

On receipt of her prenatal laboratory information, you notice a hemogram showing an Hb of 7.2, an Hct of 27, and hypochromic microcytic erythrocytes on smear.

Questions Case 4A

What additional laboratory tests would you order?
A. Repeat complete blood count (CBC)
B. Reticulocyte count
C. Serum Fe/total iron-binding capacity (TIBC)
D. Erythrocyte sedimentation rate (ESR)
E. Rapid plasma reagin (RPR)

Answer: B, C

An iron-deficiency anemia is documented with a low Fe and high TIBC.

Further questioning of the patient on her next visit should include specific questions about

(Continued)

A. Family history of iron-deficiency anemia
B. Family history of bleeding disorders
C. Personal history of bleeding disorders
D. Dietary history
E. History of prescription medicines in the last 2 years

Answer: C, D

Although a bleeding disorder is a possible cause of this anemia, there is no history of such. Diet may account for such an anemia, and indeed, deficient iron intake so as not to compensate for the increased iron use in pregnancy is the most common cause of iron deficiency anemia in pregnancy. However, on further questioning, the patient also tells of starch pica during each pregnancy and this one as well. Such a dietary craving is difficult at times to overcome, as its cause is presumed to be multifactorial, including components of taste cravings, social pressure, social and societal history, and "normal" behaviors, and a sense that such is "right." Intensive counseling combined with dietary assistance is often required.

Case 4B

A 32-year-old G1 P1001, *whom you followed through a normal pregnancy and delivery of a healthy boy approximately 2 weeks earlier, presents with concern about her hair falling out. On questioning, you learn that relatively large amounts of hair are coming loose during her normal morning hair-brushing routine. She has made no changes in shampoo, cosmetics, or diet. She is concerned and afraid that she has cancer.*

Question Case 4B

What are your next most appropriate actions?

A. Referral to a dermatologist for evaluation and treatment

B. Cortisone ointment to be applied to the scalp daily after meals
C. Reassurance, explaining that some permanent hair loss is part of being a mother and that she will probably keep enough hair to avoid using a wig
D. Reassure her that this is a normal occurrence, which will resolve

Answer: D

Some transitory hair loss in the second to fourth postpartum week is normal, but it resolves without permanent loss. Management consists of an explanation that this is a normal part of pregnancy and reassurance that the loss is only temporary and that the patient's previous hair distribution will return in time.

Case 4C

A 24-year-old G1 *comes to the office at 16 weeks' gestational age, terrified that she is developing "a bad heart" like her grandmother. Upon questioning, the symptom so frightening is an increasing sense of shortness of breath, even when she is resting, although it is most marked upon exercise. There is no history of pulmonary disease or recent upper respiratory infection, and her antepartum PPD was negative. She does not smoke nor does her husband. Her workplace has a good air-conditioning system and does not allow smoking. On physical examination, her vital signs are normal, her chest excursions are normal and easy, and her lung fields are clear to auscultation and percussion. Her nasopharynx is clear and her airway unobstructed.*

Question Case 4C

What is the appropriate management of this patient?

A. Chest x-ray, arterial blood gases, pulmonary function tests
B. Referral to a pulmonary specialist

C. Daily visiting nurse evaluation for one week to establish the pattern of dyspnea
D. Counseling

Answer: D

Dyspnea in pregnancy is a well recognized phenomena and benign in course, and in this case the history and physical examination are consistent with this diagnosis. Further laboratory evaluation or referral is not needed, and indeed may further frighten the patient. Instead, careful explanation and reassurance will suffice in most cases.

CHAPTER

ANTEPARTUM CARE

CHAPTER OBJECTIVES

This chapter deals primarily with APGO Objective(s):

OBJECTIVE 10   Preconception

Describe how pregnancy affects or is affected by medical conditions such as diabetes mellitus, chronic hypertension, vascular disease, heart disease, recurrent pregnancy loss, previous genetic abnormalities, maternal age over 35, substance abuse, medications, nutrition and exercise, immunizations, and the workplace including environmental hazards.

OBJECTIVE 11   Antepartum Care

A. Explain the initial and ongoing elements of antepartum care, including methods to diagnose pregnancy and establish gestational age; determination of obstetric risk status; techniques to access fetal growth, maturity, and well-being; appropriate diagnostic studies; antepartum patient education; antepartum nutritional needs; adverse effects of drugs and the environment.

B. Perform an obstetric physical examination.

C. Be able to answer commonly asked questions concerning pregnancy including issues of nutrition, drugs, and environmental concerns, and labor and delivery.

OBJECTIVE 31   Mortality

Define and describe the causes and the epidemiology rate for maternal death, fetal death, neonatal death, and perinatal death.

The purpose of antepartum care is to help achieve as good a maternal and infant outcome as possible. Complete obstetric care includes the correct diagnosis of pregnancy followed by an initial thorough assessment early in pregnancy; periodic examinations and screening tests as appropriate through the course of gestation; patient education addressing pregnancy care, labor and delivery, nutrition, exercise, and early infant care; and management of the patient during labor, delivery, and the postpartum period. Antepartum care ends with a final visit, generally six weeks following delivery.

Most pregnant women would deliver healthy infants without any prenatal care. Therefore, *obstetric care is designed to promote good health throughout the course of normal pregnancy, while screening for and managing any complications that may develop.* Specific conditions to which poor maternal and neonatal outcomes are often attributed include:

• Preterm or postterm delivery
• Perinatal infections
• Intrauterine growth restriction
• Hypertension
• Diabetes mellitus
• Birth defects

• Multiple gestation
• Abnormal placentation

Ideally, obstetric care should commence before pregnancy with a *preconception visit,* during which a thorough family and medical history for both parents and a physical examination of the prospective mother is done. Preexisting conditions that may affect conception and/or pregnancy are identified and appropriate management plans formulated with the goal of a "healthy" subsequent pregnancy.

Unfortunately, preconceptual counseling is not commonly used; instead, most women seek care only after one or more periods have been missed and pregnancy has already begun. All too many pregnant women have only episodic care, which contributes to increased perinatal and maternal morbidity and mortality. Educating patients on the benefits of regular, early care and motivating them to seek it is one of the most important public health goals of our time. For these reasons, obstetric care should be designed (*1*) to provide easy access to care, (*2*) to promote patient involvement, (*3*) to provide a team approach to ongoing surveillance and education for the patient and her fetus, and (*4*) to establish protocols for screening for high-risk conditions, along with an organized plan to address any complications that may arise.

DIAGNOSIS OF PREGNANCY

In a woman with regular menstrual cycles, a history of one or more missed periods (especially if associated with fatigue, nausea/vomiting, and breast tenderness) strongly suggests pregnancy. Urinary frequency caused by the enlarging uterus pressing on the bladder is another common finding.

The *diagnosis of pregnancy* should not be made based solely on the nonspecific symptoms and equivocal physical findings that are common in early pregnancy. A pregnancy test is used to make an accurate diagnosis. Once a positive pregnancy test is identified, the physician and patient must be aware of signs and symptoms of *spontaneous abortion, ectopic pregnancy,* and *trophoblastic disease,* which may complicate the early course of what is otherwise expected to be a normal intrauterine pregnancy.

On *physical examination,* softening and enlargement of the pregnant uterus become apparent six or more weeks after the last normal menstrual period. A *pelvic examination* in early pregnancy is one of the better ways to establish a due date [estimated date of confinement (EDC) or estimated date of delivery (EDD)]. Beginning at approximately 12 weeks of gestation (12 weeks from the onset of the last menstrual period), the uterus is enlarged sufficiently to be palpable in the lower abdomen. Other genital tract findings early in pregnancy include congestion and a bluish discoloration of the vagina (Chadwick's sign) and softening of the cervix (Hegar's sign). Increased pigmentation of the skin and the appearance of striae on the abdominal wall occur later in pregnancy. *Palpation of fetal parts and the appreciation of fetal movement and fetal heart tones* are diagnostic of pregnancy, but at a far more advanced gestational age. The patient's initial perception of fetal movement (called "quickening") is not usually reported before 16 to 18 weeks of gestation,

and often as late as 20 weeks in first time mothers.

Detection of *fetal heart tones* is also evidence of a viable pregnancy. With a traditional, nonelectronic fetoscope, auscultation of fetal heart tones is possible at or beyond 18 to 20 weeks' gestational age. The commonly used electronic Doppler devices can detect fetal heart tones at approximately 12 weeks of gestation. With this device, the patient and her family can also hear the fetal heart beat, a strong bonding experience that also can provide reassurance.

Several types of *urine pregnancy tests* are available, all of which measure *human chorionic gonadotropin* (hCG) produced in the syncytiotrophoblast of the growing placenta. Because hCG shares an α subunit with luteinizing hormone (LH), interpretation of any test that does not differentiate LH from hCG must take into account this overlap in structure. The concentration of hCG necessary to evoke a positive test result must, therefore, be high enough to avoid a false-positive diagnosis of pregnancy (i.e., a positive test result even though the patient is not pregnant). *Standard laboratory urine pregnancy tests become positive approximately four weeks following the first day of the last menstrual period* (i.e., around the time of the missed period). Home urine pregnancy tests have a low false-positive rate but a high false-negative rate (the test result is negative even though the patient is pregnant). All urine pregnancy tests are best performed on early morning urine specimens, which contain the highest concentration of hCG.

Serum pregnancy tests are more specific and sensitive because they test for the unique β subunit of hCG. This allows detection of pregnancy very early in gestation, even before the patient has missed a period. Further information about a pregnancy may be obtained by the quantification of hCG. Figure 5.1 is a graphic presentation of the normal quantitative values of β-hCG and the expected rate of production. This can help differentiate normal from abnormal pregnancies. These more reliable and sensitive serum tests are also more expensive and difficult to perform.

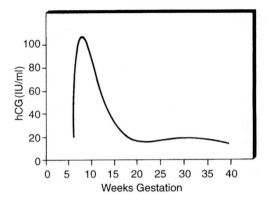

FIGURE 5.1. Human chorionic gonadotropin (hCG) concentrations in pregnancy.

Progesterone concentrations are also useful in determining pregnancy viability. Generally, serum progesterone levels less than 5 ng/ml are not consistent with a viable pregnancy, intrauterine or extrauterine, whereas levels greater than 25 ng/ml are usually consistent with a viable intrauterine pregnancy.

Ultrasound examination can detect pregnancy early in gestation. With abdominal ultrasound, a gestational sac is initially seen 5 to 6 weeks after the beginning of the last normal menstrual period (corresponding to β-hCG concentrations of 5000 to 6000 mIU/ml, second international standard). Transvaginal ultrasound can detect a pregnancy at 3 to 4 weeks' gestation (corresponding to β-hCG concentrations of 1000 to 2000 mIU/ml, second international standard). If the β-hCG concentration is greater than 4000 mIU/ml (second international standard), the embryo should be visualized by all techniques and cardiac activity usually detected.

INITIAL ANTENATAL EVALUATION

After the diagnosis of pregnancy has been established, a prenatal appointment is made, at which time a comprehensive history is taken, focusing on previous pregnancy outcome and any medical or surgical conditions that may affect pregnancy. The details of a recommended history include a history of past pregnancies, past medical history with specific attention to issues that may affect pregnancy, information pertinent to genetic screening, and information about the course of the current pregnancy. Special attention is also given to diet; the use of tobacco, alcohol, and medications; and substance abuse. Routine laboratory studies are ordered (Table 5.1), and the patient is given instructions concerning routine prenatal care, warning signs of complications, whom to contact with questions or problems, and nutritional and social service information. A complete physical examination is performed, including a Pap test and a cervical culture for *Neisseria gonorrhoeae* and *Chlamydia trachomatis.*

Risk assessment is an important part of the initial antenatal evaluation. Questions about past medical-surgical and obstetric history are asked as well as questions designed to learn about the patient's financial status, support mechanism (who will be able to help during and after pregnancy, specifically including the degree of involvement of the father), employment, transportation for antenatal care, ability to provide for the newborn, and social situation including the use of tobacco, alcohol, and drugs of abuse. Approximately 20% of pregnant women are victims of "battering" and will benefit from counseling and at times help in finding shelters and other social supports. Various evaluation systems are used by social service and third party payors to designate patients "at risk," and inclusion in this category may allow for provision of additional services and support during and after antepartum care. Inclusion in a "WIC" (women, infants, and children) program if qualified may also provide needed support for foodstuffs and other benefits postpartum and for some time into early childhood. In the United States, suicide, homicide, and trauma associated with auto accidents where seat belts were not used account for three fourths of maternal mortality. Questions about these risks and education about seat belt perinatal/health promotion activities are of great potential value. Finally, an increasing percent of

TABLE 5.1. Routine Obstetric Laboratory Tests

Test	Discussion
Initial Laboratory Tests—Routine	
1. Complete blood count	To determine hematologic status; to rule out anemia
2. Urinalysis and urine culture and sensitivity	To evaluate for UTI and renal function
3. Blood group, Rh	To determine blood type, Rh status, and risk of isoimmunization
4. Antibody screen	To detect maternal antibodies, which may damage fetus or make procurement of compatible blood for transfusion more difficult; the antibody screen is usually negative; anti-I and anti-Lewis are seen in approximately 1% of patients and are of no consequence to the fetus
5. Serologic test for syphilis (RPR, VDRL)	To detect previous/current infection; if positive, specific treponemal test required (e.g., FTA-ABS or MHA-TP)
6. Hepatitis B surface antigen	To detect carrier status or active disease; if positive, further testing indicated
7. Rubella titer	Approximately 85% of mothers have evidence of prior infection; if patient is seronegative, special precautions are needed to avoid infection, which can severely affect the fetus; vaccination is then required postpartum
8. Cervical cytology (Pap smear)	To screen for cervical dysplasia/cancer

(Continued)

women seeking antepartum care in the United States speak a language other than English, and provision for accurate translation by qualified professional translators is of great benefit.

INITIAL ASSESSMENT OF GESTATIONAL AGE: THE EDC

Every effort is made to assess accurately gestational age from which the EDC (due date or EDD) is calculated. This information is crucial to obstetric management, because it is needed to manage possible preterm labor or postdates pregnancy as well as the timing of evaluations (e.g.,

alpha-fetoprotein measurement, 1-hour glucose challenge testing). Initial assessment of gestational age is made by obtaining a thorough *menstrual history.* "Normal" pregnancy lasts 40 ± 2 weeks, calculated from the first day of the last normal menses (*menstrual or gestational age*). Calculation of the EDC is accomplished by adding 7 days to the first day of the last normal menstrual flow and counting back 3 months. In a patient with an idealized 28-day menstrual cycle, ovulation occurs on day 14, so that the *fertilization age* or *conception age* of the normal pregnancy is actually 38 weeks. The use of the first day of the last menses as a starting point for gestational age assignment is standard, and gestational, not conceptional, age is most commonly used.

TABLE 5.1. *(Continued)*

Test	Discussion
9. Cervical culture for *Neisseria gonorrhoeae*	To screen for infection; both cause neonatal and *Chlamydia trachomatis* conjunctivitis; association with premature labor and postpartum endometritis
10. Hemoglobin electrophoresis	To detect sickle-cell trait (HbSA), associated with higher risk for UTI, and sickle-cell disease (HbSS), at risk for multiple fetal and maternal complications
11. HIV titer by ELISA; Western blot if HIV+ by ELISA	Should be offered to all patients at risk (multiple sexual partners, drug use, or sexual contact with drug users); may be offered to all patients at physician's discretion
12. Glucose screening (usually 1-hour Glucola)	To screen for glucose intolerance in high-risk patients; usually at 28 weeks in low-risk patients
Subsequent Assessments	
13. MSAFP at 15 to 18 weeks (usually with hCG, estriol)	Elevated levels seen with neural tube defects, gastroschisis, and omphalocele; low levels associated with Down syndrome
14. Hematocrit at 25 to 28 weeks	To rule out anemia
15. Glucose screening (usually 1-hour Glucola) at 24 to 28 weeks	To screen for glucose intolerance

ELISA = enzyme-linked immunosorbent assay; FTA-ABS = fluorescent treponemal antibody absorption test; hCG = human chorionic gonadotropin; HIV = human immunodeficiency virus; MHA-TP = microhemagglutination assay-*Treponema pallidum;* MSAFP = maternal serum α-fetoprotein; RPR = rapid plasma reagin; UTI = urinary tract infection; VDRL = Venereal Disease Research Laboratory.

To establish an *accurate* gestational age, the date of onset of the last normal menses is crucial. A light bleeding episode should not be mistaken for a normal menstrual period. A history of irregular periods or taking medications that alter cycle length (e.g., oral contraceptives, other hormonal preparations, psychoactive medications) can confuse the menstrual history. If sexual intercourse is infrequent, or timed for conception based on basal body temperature readings, a patient may know when conception is most likely to have occurred, thus facilitating an accurate calculation of gestational age. Figure 5.2 contains portions of the American College of Obstetricians and Gynecologists Antepartum Records, which pertain to this information about dating, concisely organized as to be easily interpretable and useful.

Pelvic examination by an experienced examiner is accurate in determining gestational age within 1 to 2 weeks until the second trimester, at which time the lower uterine segment begins to form, thereby making clinical estimation of gestational age less accurate. From 16 to 18 weeks of gestation until 36 weeks of gestation, the fundal height in centimeters (measured from the symphysis to the top of the uterine fundus) is roughly equal to the number of weeks of gestational age in normal singleton pregnancies in the cephalic presentation within an anatomically normal uterus (Figure 5.3).

Part A

MENSTRUAL HISTORY

LMP ☐ DEFINITE ☐ APPROXIMATE (MONTH KNOWN) MENSES MONTHLY ☐ YES ☐ NO   FREQUENCY: Q _____ DAYS   MENARCHE _____ (AGE ONSET)

☐ UNKNOWN ☐ NORMAL AMOUNT/DURATION   PRIOR MENSES _____ DATE   ON BCP AT CONCEPT ☐ YES ☐ NO   hCG + ___/___/___

☐ FINAL _____

Part B

EDD CONFIRMATION	18–20-WEEK EDD UPDATE:
INITIAL EDD:	QUICKENING ____/____/____ +22 WKS = ____/____/____
LMP: ____/____/____ = EDD ____/____/____	FUNDAL HT. AT UMBIL. ____/____/____ +20 WKS = ____/____/____
INITIAL EXAM: ____/____/____ = _____WKS = EDD ____/____/____	FHT W/FETOSCOPE ____/____/____ +22 WKS = ____/____/____
ULTRASOUND ____/____/____ = _____WKS = EDD ____/____/____	ULTRASOUND ____/____/____ = ___WKS = ____/____/____
INITIAL EXAM: ____/____/____ INITIALED BY _____	FINAL EDD ____/____/____ INITIALED BY _____

FIGURE 5.2. Determining LMP and EDD ("dating"). This figure contains two portions of the American College of Obstetricians and Gynecologists Antepartum Records that pertain to dating of pregnancy. Part "A" is the section used to organize the information about the last menstrual period (LMP; menstrual history) collected at the time of the new obstetric evaluation. Part "B" is the section used to determine "final" estimated date of delivery (EDD; also called EDC, estimated date of confinement), collected over a period of time during antepartum care. These data head toward the setting of a final EDD based on the initial EDD derived from historical LMP, initial physical examination, and early obstetric ultrasound if performed, then modified by other data as noted in the 18–20 week EDD update. Clearly, the form is based on the ideal situation of initial prenatal care early in the first trimester but, unfortunately, care often starts later in gestation and the use of the form is adjusted as needed to compensate.

Obstetric ultrasound examination is the most accurate measurement available in the determination of gestational age. In the first trimester, transvaginal and transabdominal techniques allow gestational age determination with ± 1 to 2 weeks' accuracy by using measurements of the gestational sac and embryo/fetus. In the second trimester, accuracy is still high, in the ± 2-week range. In the latter portions of the third trimester, however, accuracy decreases to ± 2 to 3 weeks.

SUBSEQUENT ANTENATAL EVALUATION

For a patient with a normal pregnancy, *periodic antepartum visits* at 4-week intervals are usually scheduled until 32 weeks, at 2-week intervals between 32 and 36 weeks, and weekly thereafter (Figure 5.4). Patients with high-risk pregnancies or those with ongoing complications are usually seen more frequently, depending on the clinical

circumstances. At each visit, patients are asked about how they are feeling and if they are having any problems, such as vaginal bleeding, nausea/vomiting, dysuria, or vaginal discharge. After quickening, patients are asked if they continue to feel fetal movement and if it is the same or less since the last antepartum visit. Decreased fetal movement is a warning sign requiring further evaluation of fetal well-being.

The only routine laboratory test performed at every prenatal visit is *determination of glucosuria and proteinuria*. A trace of glucosuria is a normal finding in pregnancy and requires no further evaluation. Anything other than the presence of trace proteinuria should be considered abnormal and warrants further evaluation.

Maternal physical findings measured at each prenatal visit include blood pressure, weight, and assessment for edema. *Blood pressure* generally declines at the end of the first trimester, rising again in the third trimester. Compared with baseline levels,

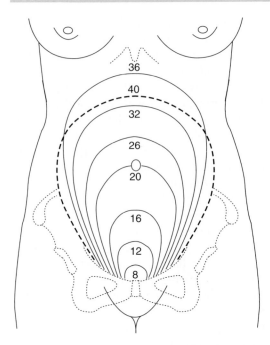

FIGURE 5.3. Fundal height. In a normal singleton pregnancy in the vertex presentation, fundal height roughly corresponds to gestational age between 16 and 36 weeks' gestational age. A convenient "rule of thumb" is 20 weeks equals 20 centimeters equals fundus at umbilicus in a woman with a normal body habitus. After 36 weeks, the fundal height either grows more slowly, or actually decreases as the uterus changes shape and/or the fetal head engages in the pelvis.

however, any increase in the systolic pressure of more than 30 mm Hg or any increase in the diastolic pressure of more than 15 mm Hg suggests pregnancy-associated hypertension. The *maternal weight* is compared with the pregravid weight and to the generally prescribed recommendation of a 25- to 35-pound weight gain through the course of pregnancy. There is usually a 3- to 4-pound increase between monthly visits. Significant deviation from this trend may require nutritional assessment and further evaluation. The presence of significant *edema* in the lower extremities and/or hands (*dependent edema*) is very common in pregnancy and, by itself, is not abnormal. Fluid retention can be associated with hypertension, however, so that blood pressure as well as weight gain and edema must be evaluated in the clinical context before the findings are presumed to be innocuous.

Obstetric physical findings made at each visit include assessment of the uterine size by pelvic examination or fundal height measurement, documentation of the presence and rate of fetal heart tones, and determination of the presentation of the fetus. Until 18 to 20 weeks, the *uterine size* is generally stated as *weeks* size, such as "12 weeks size," "16 weeks size," and so on. After 20 weeks of gestation (when the fundus is palpable at or near the umbilicus), the

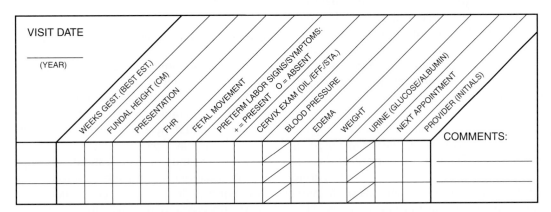

FIGURE 5.4. Antepartum visit record. This figure contains the flow sheet for antepartum visits from the Antepartum Record of the American College of Obstetricians and Gynecologists, summarizing succinctly the information requisite for each visit. This is often all that is needed for normal obstetric care, although additional notes are used when special information or management plans are part of care.

uterine size can be assessed with the use of a tape measure, which is the *fundal height measurement.* In this procedure, the top of the uterine fundus is identified and the zero end of the tape measure is placed at this uppermost part of the uterus. The tape is then carried anteriorly across the pregnant uterus to the level of the symphysis pubis.

Until 36 weeks in the normal singleton pregnancy, the number of weeks of gestation approximates the fundal height in centimeters. Thereafter, the fetus moves downward into the pelvis beneath the symphysis pubis ("lightening"), and fundal height measurement is less reliable. If the fundal height measurement is significantly greater than expected (i.e., "large for dates"), possible considerations include incorrect assessment of gestational age, multiple pregnancy, macrosomia (large fetus), hydatidiform mole, or excess accumulation of amniotic fluid (hydramnios). A fundal height measurement less than expected (i.e., "small for dates") suggests the possibility of incorrect assessment of gestational age, hydatidiform mole, fetal growth restriction, inadequate amniotic fluid accumulation (oligohydramnios), or even intrauterine fetal demise.

Fetal heart activity should be verified at every visit, by direct auscultation or by the use of a fetal Doppler ultrasound device. The normal fetal heart rate is 120 to 160 beats per minute (bpm), with higher rates found in early pregnancy; the maternal pulse may also be detected with the Doppler device, so that simultaneous palpation of maternal pulse and auscultation of fetal pulse may be necessary to differentiate the two. Deviation from the normal rate or occasional arrhythmias must be evaluated carefully.

Several determinations concerning the fetus can be made by *palpation of the pregnant uterus.* The most important of these is identifying the presentation, or "presenting part" of the fetus (i.e., what part of the fetus is entering the pelvis first). This is especially important after 34 weeks. Before that time, breech, oblique, or transverse presentations are not uncommon, nor are they significant, because they may vary from day to day. At term, more than 95% of fetuses are in the cephalic presentation (head down), with other presentations rather uncommon: breech (bottom first) approximately 3.5% and shoulder less than 1%. Unless the fetus is in a transverse lie (the long axis of the fetus is not parallel with the mother's long axis), the presentation will be either the head (vertex, cephalic) or the breech (buttocks).

The head is hard and well defined by ballottement, especially when the head is freely mobile in the fluid-filled uterus; the breech is softer, less round and, therefore, more difficult to outline. If a breech presentation is noted between 34 and 37 weeks, the option of external cephalic version (ECV) must be entertained and discussed with the patient. This procedure involves turning the fetus from the breech presentation to a vertex presentation, thereby avoiding the potential adverse consequences of a vaginal breech delivery.

SPECIFIC TECHNIQUES OF FETAL ASSESSMENT

Evaluation of the fetus can be conveniently categorized as assessment of fetal (1) growth, (2) well-being, and (3) maturity. The appropriate interpretation of these tests in light of the natural course of any antenatal problem provides a firm base on which decisions are made.

Assessment of Fetal Growth

Fetal growth can be assessed by fundal height measurement and ultrasonography. The increase in fundal height through pregnancy is predictable. Deviation of more than 2 cm in fundal height measurement from that expected at a particular gestational age between 18 and 36 weeks should prompt repeat measurement and may lead to further evaluation. A deviation of 4 cm or more is of great concern and requires further evaluation, including ultrasound assessment.

Ultrasonography is the most valuable tool in assessing fetal growth. In early pregnancy, determination of the gestational sac diameter and the crown-rump length correlates very closely with gestational age. Later in pregnancy, measurement of the biparietal diameter of the skull, the abdominal circumference, the femur length, and the cerebellar diameter can be used to assess gestational age and, using various formulas, to estimate fetal weight. The range of normal values for these measurements increases significantly as pregnancy advances so that a specific assessment of gestational age in the third trimester may be ± 3 weeks of the actual age. Earlier in pregnancy there is less deviation in normal values and the information derived is of greater accuracy. Measurements in the late first and early second trimesters are most reliable, generally ± 1 to 2 weeks.

Assessment of Fetal Well-being

Assessment of *fetal well-being* includes maternal perception of fetal activity and several tests using electronic fetal monitors and ultrasonography. Tests of fetal well-being have a wide range of uses, including *the assessment of fetal status at a particular time and prediction of fetal status for varying time intervals,* depending on the test and the clinical situation.

An active fetus is generally a healthy fetus, so that *quantification of fetal activity* is a common test of fetal well-being. A variety of methods can be used to quantify fetal activity, including the time necessary to achieve a certain number of movements each day, an average of the number of fetal movements in a given period of time repeated several times a day, or counting the number of movements in a given hour. If, for example, the mother detects more than four fetal movements while lying comfortably and focusing on fetal activity for 1 hour, the fetus is considered to be healthy. This type of testing has several advantages—it is reliable, it is inexpensive, and it involves the patient in her own care. For these reasons, fetal movement testing is frequently a part of routine obstetric care late in pregnancy, or earlier if high-risk conditions warrant. A useful qualitative measure

is to ask the question, "Is your baby moving more, less, or the same this week compared to last week?" An answer of "more" or "the same" is relatively reassuring, whereas "less" warrants further evaluation.

Techniques using *electronic fetal monitoring* and *ultrasonography* are more costly but also provide more specific information. The most common tests used are the nonstress test, the contraction stress test (called the oxytocin challenge test if oxytocin is used), and the biophysical profile.

The *nonstress test* (NST) measures the response of the fetal heart rate to fetal movement. With the patient in the left lateral position and the electronic fetal monitor transducer placed on her abdomen to record the fetal heart rate, the patient is asked to note fetal movement, usually accomplished by pressing a button on the fetal monitor, which causes a notation on the monitor strip. Interpretation of the nonstress test depends on whether the fetal heart rate accelerates in response to fetal movement. A *normal, or reactive, NST* occurs when the fetal heart rate increases by at least 15 bpm over a period of 15 seconds following a fetal movement (Figure 5.5A). Two such accelerations in a 20-minute span is considered reactive, or normal. The absence of these accelerations in response to fetal movement is a *nonreactive NST* (Figure 5.5B). A reactive NST is generally reassuring in the absence of other indicators of fetal stress. Depending on the clinical situation, the test is repeated every 3 to 4 days or weekly. A nonreactive NST is nonreassuring and must be immediately followed with further assessment of fetal well-being.

Whereas the nonstress test evaluates the fetal heart rate response to fetal activity, the contraction stress test (CST) measures the response of the fetal heart rate to the stress of a uterine contraction. With uterine contractions, uteroplacental blood flow is temporarily reduced. *A healthy fetus is able to compensate for this intermittent decreased blood flow, whereas a fetus that is compromised is unable to do so, demonstrating abnormalities such as fetal heart rate decelerations or bradycardia.* To perform a CST, a tocodynamometer is placed on the maternal

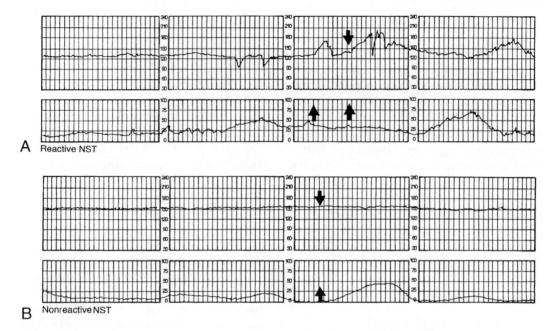

FIGURE 5.5. Nonstress testing. (*A*) Reactive nonstress test (NST); note fetal heart rate acceleration in response to fetal movement. (*B*) Nonreactive NST; note lack of fetal heart rate acceleration in response to fetal movement.

abdomen along with a fetal heart rate transducer. If contractions are occurring spontaneously, the test is known as a contraction stress test; if oxytocin infusion is required to elicit contractions, the test is called an *oxytocin challenge test* (OCT). The normal fetal heart rate response to contractions is for the baseline fetal heart rate to remain unchanged and for there to be no fetal heart rate decelerations. Decelerations, especially of the late variety (see Chapter 8), are nonreassuring. Repetitive decelerations following each contraction when three contractions occur in a 10-minute window constitute a positive, or abnormal, CST or OCT. This is usually an indication for expedited delivery.

Tests of fetal well-being have a significant incidence of false-positive results (i.e., the test suggests that the fetus is in jeopardy but the fetus is actually healthy). For this reason, these tests must be interpreted together with other assessments and are often repeated within 24 hours to verify the results. In addition, interpretations of the NST and OCT/CST are often combined. Because positive OCTs are common, fetal heart rate reactivity can have a significant impact on the final interpretation of the tests. If an OCT is positive, evidence for "reactivity" is sought (see Chapter 8). If the NST is reactive, the OCT result may be interpreted as a false-positive result. If, however, the positive OCT is accompanied by a nonreactive NST, the combination is considered especially worrisome, and a nonreassuring fetal status is likely to occur when labor begins.

The *biophysical profile* is a series of five assessments of fetal well-being, each of which is given a score of 0 or 2 (Table 5.2). The parameters include a reactive nonstress test, the presence of fetal breathing movements, the presence of fetal movement of the body or limbs, the finding of fetal tone (flexed extremities as opposed to a flaccid posture), and an adequate amount of amniotic fluid volume. Perinatal outcome can be correlated with the score derived from these five parameters. A score of 8 to 10 is considered normal, a score of 6 is equivocal requiring further evaluation, and a score of 4 or less is abnormal, usually requiring immediate intervention.

TABLE 5.2. Biophysical Profile

Biophysical Variable	Score	Explanation
Fetal breathing movements (FBM)	Normal = 2	At least 1 FBM of at least 30-seconds duration in 30 minutes
	Abnormal = 0	No FBM of at least 30-seconds duration in 30 minutes
Gross body movement	Normal = 2	At least 3 discrete body/limb movements in 30 minutes
	Absent = 0	2 or less discrete body/limb movements in 30 minutes
Fetal tone	Normal = 2	At least 1 episode of active extension with return to flexion of fetal limbs/trunk or opening/closing of hand
	Absent = 0	Either slow extension with return to partial flexion or movement of limb in full extension or no fetal movement
Reactive fetal heart rate	Normal = 2	Reactive NST
	Absent = 0	Nonreactive NST
Qualitative amniotic fluid volume	Normal = 2	At least 1 pocket of amniotic fluid at least 1 cm in two perpendicular planes
	Absent = 0	No amniotic fluid or no pockets of fluid greater than 1 cm in two perpendicular planes

NST = nonstress test.

The importance of adequate amniotic fluid volume is well established. Diminished amniotic fluid is thought to represent decreased fetal urinary output caused by chronic stress and shunting of blood flow away from the kidneys. The decreased amniotic fluid provides less support for the umbilical cord, which may be more frequently compressed, reducing blood flow and resulting in chronic fetal stress. Changes in fetal tone, breathing movements, and fetal movements are more likely to be signs of acute stress to the central nervous system.

Assessment of Fetal Maturity

In some high-risk obstetric situations, the maternal or fetal status is so grave that immediate delivery is required, regardless of gestational age; in others, a decision must be made as to whether the mother and fetus are at greater risk by continued antepartum management or whether delivery is best. If the pregnancy is viable but less than 36 weeks, the questions are, "How premature is the pregnancy?" and, more specifically, "Will the risk of prematurity-associated problems such as respiratory distress syndrome (RDS) be greater than those of continued intrauterine life?"

Because the respiratory system is the last fetal system to mature functionally, many of the *tests available to assess fetal maturity* focus on this organ system. Such tests, termed *direct tests* if they specifically measure substances associated with lung maturity, are routinely used, although not all tests are used in all hospitals. Other tests measure parameters from which the likelihood of maturity can be estimated; these are termed *indirect tests,* the most common being ultrasonography.

Neonatal RDS is the inability of the newborn to ventilate successfully because of the immaturity of the lungs. RDS results from lack of a group of phospholipids, collectively known as *surfactant*, which decreases the surface tension within alveolar sacs and thereby promotes easy ventilation by maintaining patency of these sacs. In utero, production of these phospholipids remains low until 32 to 33 weeks, after which production increases. There is a great variation in this process. Gestational age alone does not reliably predict surfactant production or lung maturity. RDS is manifest by signs of respiratory failure—grunting, chest retractions, nasal flaring, and hypoxia—possibly leading to acidosis and death. Management consists of skillful support of ventilation and correction of associated metabolic disturbances until the neonate can ventilate successfully without assistance. Recently, administration of synthetic or semisynthetic surfactant to the neonate offers additional hope for an improved outcome for these infants.

The fetus breathes in utero, and phospholipids enter the amniotic fluid where they can be obtained by amniocentesis and measured. Direct tests that measure components of surfactant are listed in Table 5.3. Use of fluid obtained vaginally after spontaneous rupture of membranes is not as common, although such fluid can be used for certain tests in some instances.

Ultrasonographic determination of gestational age and estimated fetal weight are common indirect tests performed to help assess maturity. Unfortunately, ultrasonographic assessment of gestational age and fetal size do not sufficiently correlate with maturity to allow for reliable prediction, especially in the marginal maturational period between 28 and 35 weeks of gestation. Performed correctly, any test that indicates fetal maturity is associated with the subsequent development of RDS in 5% or less of cases. The predictive value of these tests is much less helpful. Overall, only 50%

TABLE 5.3. Tests of Fetal Lung Maturity

Test	Endpoint for Maturity	Comment
Lecithin:sphingomyelin (L:S) ratio	≥ 2.0	Lecithin is the major component of surfactant; this test measures its production compared with sphingomyelin, a substance with constant production throughout pregnancy; the L:S ratio was the first reliable test of fetal lung maturity; the method is methodologically involved and labor intensive; it has been replaced by less costly tests in many laboratories
Phosphatidylglycerol (PG)	Present	A minor phospholipid that "appears" late in pregnancy; it can be measured by several methods, thus results are reported in different ways
Foam stability index (FSI)	≥ 47	Measures the ability of amniotic fluid surfactant to maintain foam at the meniscus of a solution of amniotic fluid and alcohol
Fetal lung maturity (FLM)	≥ 55	Involves fluorescence polarization; measures ratio of surfactant to albumin

of infants who are delivered shortly after test results indicate immaturity develop RDS.

ANTEPARTUM MANAGEMENT PLANS AND PATIENT EDUCATION

Plans for the antepartum, intrapartum, and postpartum periods are iteratively developed during the course of antepartum care and are associated with significant opportunity for patient education. The latter is crucial because it may provide new information for the patient or a good review of information already held, in either case necessary to allow informed decision making. Figure 5.6 contains the excellent summary "checklist" portion of the Antepartum Records of the American College of Obstetricians and Gynecologists. It is useful as a reminder of the issues to be discussed during antepartum care and the plans to be made, and as a record of what has been done and what remains to be done. Often, as in for example "labor signs," iterative education is important; in others such as "newborn car seat" a decision is needed, as many hospitals will not release a newborn unless the parent(s) have a car seat. Many clinicians will write the date tasks are done to help keep track of patient care.

OTHER CONSIDERATIONS AND COMMON QUESTIONS IN PREGNANCY

Employment

In normal pregnancy there are few restrictions concerning work, although it is beneficial to allow moderate activity and to allow for additional periods of rest. Strenuous work is best avoided. A physician's note asking employers to transfer pregnant patients to less physically demanding activities may be needed.

The traditional time designated for maternity leave is approximately 1 month before the expected date of delivery and extending until 6 weeks after birth. This may be modified, depending on complications of pregnancy, the work involved, the employer attitude, the rules of the health care system under which the patient receives care, and the wishes of the patient. Recent trends have shortened this time in many cases.

Exercise

Moderate exercise programs can be continued during pregnancy. During pregnancy regular, non-weight-bearing activity should be maintained on a three times a week schedule, if possible. Overly strenuous exercise, especially for prolonged periods, should be avoided. Patients unaccustomed to regular

---

PLANS/EDUCATION (COUNSELED ☐)

☐ ANESTHESIA PLANS _____	☐ TUBAL STERILIZATION _____
☐ TOXOPLASMOSIS PRECAUTIONS (CATS/RAW MEAT) _____	☐ VBAC COUNSELING _____
☐ CHILDBIRTH CLASSES _____	☐ CIRCUMCISION _____
☐ PHYSICAL/SEXUAL ACTIVITY _____	☐ TRAVEL _____
☐ LABOR SIGNS _____	☐ LIFESTYLE, TOBACCO, ALCOHOL _____
☐ NUTRITION COUNSELING _____	**REQUESTS** _____
☐ BREAST OR BOTTLE FEEDING _____	_____
☐ NEWBORN CAR SEAT _____	_____
☐ POSTPARTUM BIRTH CONTROL _____	**TUBAL STERILIZATION DATE INITIALS**
☐ ENVIRONMENTAL/WORK HAZARDS _____	CONSENT SIGNED ___/___/___ _____

FIGURE 5.6. Obstetric management plans and patient education. This figure contains the very useful management plan/patient education section from the Antepartum Records of the American College of Obstetricians and Gynecologists.

TABLE 5.4.   Recommended Weight in Pregnancy*

Maternal Classification	Weight Gain (kg)		Weight Gain (lb)	
	Total	Rate (4 weeks)	Total	Rate (4 weeks)
Prepregnant BMI†				
Underweight (< 19.8)	12.7–18.2	2.3	28–40	5.0
Normal weight (19.8–26.9)	11.4–15.9	1.8	25–35	4.0
Overweight (26.1–29.0)	6.8–11.4	1.2	15–25	2.5
Obese (> 29.0)	6.8	0.9	15	2.0
Twin gestation	15.9–20.4	2.7	35–40	6.0

Adapted from *Nutrition during Pregnancy,* Washington, DC, National Academy Press, 1990.
BMI = body mass index.
*Rate has been adjusted to second trimester.
†Pregnant weight (kg) ÷ height (cm) × 100.

exercise should not undertake vigorous new programs during pregnancy. Supine exercises should be discontinued after the first trimester to minimize circulatory changes brought on by pressure of the uterus on the vena cava. Any activity should be discontinued if discomfort, significant shortness of breath, or pain in the chest or abdomen appears. Changes in body contour and balance will alter the types of activities practical, and abdominal trauma should be avoided.

Nutrition and Weight Gain

Concerns about adequate nutrition and weight gain during pregnancy are common and appropriate. Poor nutrition, obesity, food faddism, and problems such as *pica* are associated with poor perinatal outcome. Concerns about the retention of weight gained during pregnancy are also common.

A complete nutritional assessment is an important part of the initial antepartum assessment, including history of dietary habits, special dietary issues or concerns, and weight trends. Regular weighing is an important part of antepartum care. Calculation of body mass index (BMI) is useful, because it relates weight to height, allowing a better indirect measurement of body fat distribution than is obtained with weight measurement alone.

Recommendations for total weight gain during pregnancy and the rate of weight gain per month appropriate to achieve it may be made based on a BMI calculated for the prepregnancy weight (Table 5.4). The "components" of an average weight gain in a normal singleton pregnancy are listed in Table 5.5. The maternal component of this weight gain starts in the first trimester and is most prominent in the first half of pregnancy. Fetal growth is most rapid in the second half of pregnancy, with the normal fetus tripling its weight in the last 12 weeks of pregnancy.

Published recommended daily allowances (RDAs) for protein, minerals, and vitamins are useful approximations. It should be kept in mind, however, that the RDAs are a combination of estimates and clinical research data and are not averages or means but, rather, values adjusted near the top of the normal ranges to encompass the estimated needs of most women. Thus many women have an adequate diet for their individual needs, even though it does not supply all the RDAs. RDAs are useful guidelines, but they must be considered in the light of individual nutritional assessment.

A balanced, adequate diet usually supplies all the vitamins needed in pregnancy. Vitamin supplementation is appropriate for specific therapeutic indication such as a patient's inability or unwillingness to eat a balanced, adequate diet or clinical demonstration of specific nutritional risk. Except for iron, mineral supplementation is likewise not required in otherwise healthy women.

TABLE 5.5. Components of Average Weight Gain in a Normal Singleton Pregnancy

Organ, Tissue, Fluid	Weight (kg)	Weight (lb)
Maternal		
Uterus	1.0	2.2
Breasts	.4	.9
Blood	1.2	2.6
Water	1.7	3.7
Fat	3.3	7.3
Subtotal	7.6	16.7
Fetal		
Fetus	3.4	7.5
Placenta	.6	1.3
Amniotic fluid	.8	1.8
Subtotal	4.8	10.6
Total	*12.4*	*27.3*

Financial problems and the inability to get to a grocery store may prevent some women from obtaining adequate foodstuffs. The WIC federal supplemental food program, food stamp programs, and Aid for Families with Dependent Children are resources that may help in these situations.

Breast-Feeding

Prenatal care is an excellent time to educate the patient about the benefits of breast-feeding, which include for the newborn excellent nutrition and provision of immunologic protection and for the mother more rapid uterine involution, economy, maternal-child bonding, and to some extent "natural child spacing." Indeed, these benefits are so great that women should be encouraged to consider breast-feeding, if not for an extended period of time, for at least the first few months of life. However, in balance it should be remembered that breast-feeding is not for everyone, and some women simply cannot breast-feed due to intolerant employment situations and similar constraints. Even in these unfortunate circumstances, however,

the use of breast pumps and milk storage may allow some degree of breast-feeding that is beneficial. In the event that breast-feeding is not possible or chosen, however, care must be taken not to suggest that "bottle-feeding" is somehow equivalent to "inadequate mothering," as adequate nutrition is also attainable by "bottle-feeding."

Tobacco

Smoking should be prohibited during pregnancy because of the established risks to both mother and fetus. In addition to the adverse maternal effects, metabolites from burning tobacco and paper covering are quickly transferred from the patient to her fetus. Infants born to women who smoke weigh less than those born to nonsmokers. Even exposure to passive smoking is associated with high levels of tobacco metabolites. At times, the gastrointestinal discomforts of early pregnancy are associated with a decreased interest in cigarette smoking. The patient should take advantage of this opportunity to cease smoking.

Sexual Intercourse

Sexual activity is not restricted during a normal pregnancy, although advice about more comfortable positions in later pregnancy may be appreciated (i.e., side-to-side, female superior). Sexual activity may be restricted or prohibited under certain "high-risk" circumstances such as known placenta previa, premature rupture of membranes, or actual or history of preterm labor (or delivery). Education of patient (and partner) about safe sex practices is as important in antepartum as in regular gynecologic care.

Travel

Travel is not prohibited during pregnancy, although it is customary and probably advisable for patients to avoid distant travel in the last month of pregnancy. This is not because of substantial risk to either mother or fetus but rather because of the likelihood that labor may ensue away from home and customary health care providers. If a long trip near term is planned, it is useful for the patient to carry a copy of her obstetric record in case she requires obstetric care. When traveling, patients are advised to avoid long periods of immobilization such as sitting. Walking every 1 to 2 hours, even for short periods, promotes circulation, especially in the lower legs, and decreases the risk of venus stasis and possible thromboembolism. Education about the regular use of a seat belt is especially important, with the seat belt worn under the abdomen as pregnancy advances.

Headaches

Headaches are common in early pregnancy and may be severe. The etiology of such headaches is not known. Treatment with acetaminophen in usual doses is recommended and generally adequate.

Nausea and Vomiting

The majority of pregnant women experience some degree of upper gastrointestinal symptoms in the first trimester of pregnancy. Classically, these symptoms are worse in the morning (the so-called morning sickness). However, patients may experience symptoms at other times or even throughout the day. Treatment consists of frequent small meals, avoidance of an "empty stomach" by ingesting crackers or other bland carbohydrates, and patience. Avoiding spicy or fatty foods may also be beneficial in reducing nausea. Medication specifically for nausea and vomiting during pregnancy (Bendectin) was removed from the market by the manufacturer several years ago because of growing litigation concerning congenital anomalies. This occurred even though the safety of the drug had actually been well established. Components of that drug—pyridoxine (vitamin B_6) and an antihistamine—have subsequently been used successfully to treat nausea and vomiting. A variety of other antinausea agents are sometimes used in patients unresponsive to conservative treatment. Hospitalization with fluid and electrolyte therapy may be required in extreme cases.

Heartburn

Heartburn (gastric reflux) is common, especially postprandially, and is often associated with eating too large meals or spicy or fatty foods. Patient education about smaller and more frequent meals and blander foods, combined with not eating immediately before retiring, is helpful. Antacids may be helpful and used judiciously in pregnancy.

Constipation

Constipation is physiologic in pregnancy, associated with increased transit time, increased water absorption, and often decreased bulk. Dietary modification including increased fluid intake and increased bulk with such foods as fruits and vegetables is usually helpful. Other useful interventions may include surface active bowel softeners such as *docusate* (Colace, 100 mg po bid) and the use of supplemental dietary fibers such as *psyllium hydrophilic mucilloid* (Metamucil).

Fatigue

In early pregnancy, patients often complain of extreme fatigue that is unrelieved by rest. There is no specific treatment, other than adjustment of the patient's schedule to the extent possible to accommodate this temporary lack of energy. Patients can be reassured that the symptoms disappear in the second trimester.

Leg Cramps

Leg cramps, usually affecting the calves, are common during pregnancy. A variety of treatments including oral calcium supplement have been proposed over the years, none of which is universally successful. Massage and rest are often advised.

Back Pain

Lower back pain is common, especially in late pregnancy. The altered center of gravity caused by the growing fetus places unusual stress on the lower spine and associated muscles and ligaments. Treatment focuses on heat, massage, and limited use of analgesia. A specially fitted maternal girdle may also help, as will avoiding shoes with high heels or platforms in favor of more sensible footwear.

Round Ligament Pain

Sharp groin pain, especially as pregnancy advances, is very common, often quite uncomfortable, and disturbing to patients who fear it represents preterm labor, labor, or "something is wrong." This pain is often more pronounced on the right side due to the usual dextrorotation of the gravid uterus. Reassurance that this represents stretching and spasm of the round ligaments (with an explanation of what round ligaments are) often suffices. Modification of activity, especially more gradual movement, is often helpful; analgesics are rarely indicated.

Varicose Veins and Hemorrhoids

Varicose veins are *not caused* by pregnancy but often first appear during the course of gestation. Besides the disturbing appearance to many patients, varicose veins can cause an aching sensation, especially when patients stand for long periods of time. Support hose can help diminish the discomfort, although they have no effect on the appearance of the varicose veins. Popular brands of support hose do not provide the relief that prescription elastic hose can. *Hemorrhoids* are varicosities of the hemorrhoidal veins. Treatment consists of sitz baths and local preparations. Varicose veins and hemorrhoids regress postpartum, although neither condition may abate completely. Surgical correction of varicose veins or hemorrhoids should not be undertaken for approximately the first 6 months postpartum, to allow for the natural involution to occur.

Vaginal Discharge

The hormonal milieu of pregnancy often causes an increase in normal vaginal secretions. These normal secretions must be distinguished from vaginitis, which has symptoms of itching and malodor, and spontaneous rupture of membranes, for which thin, clear fluid appears.

MEDICATIONS IN PREGNANCY

The number of medications available for a clinician's use increases every day, and with that increase comes an increase in complexity of accurate prescription. Dosages and schedules vary with indication, age, weight, and physiological parameters such as renal function; drug interactions are common, often with adverse results; drugs may be toxic, have serious or uncomfortable side effects, and may be contraindicated in pregnancy and/or breastfeeding. The Food and Drug Administration assigns medications a Pregnancy Risk Factor (PRF) based on extant information about the medication and its risk: benefit ratio. These PRFs help guide the appropriate use of medications in pregnancy, and are presented in Table 5.6. Pregnancy Category X is especially notable in that it indicates a teratogenic assocation and that the drug is contraindicated in pregnancy.

OBSTETRIC STATISTICS

The rates of maternal and fetal mortality are of importance in evaluating the natural history of disease and in the quality of obstetric care. Four statistics are commonly used for this purpose. *Maternal death* occurs during pregnancy; it is classified as *direct* if the cause of death is an obstetric disease and *indirect* if the cause of death is a disease made worse by pregnancy. If death is caused by accident, it is classified as *nonmaternal*. The *maternal death rate* is the number of deaths of obstetric cause per 100,000 live births. *Fetal death* is synonymous with *stillbirth* and is the number of infants born without any signs of life. It is expressed as the *fetal death rate,* or *stillbirth rate,* which is the number of stillbirths per 1000 infants born. *Neonatal death* refers to an infant's death within the first 28 days of life and is expressed as the

TABLE 5.6 Medications in Pregnancy and Breast Feeding: Pregnancy Risk Factors (PRF)

PRF Category	Description
A	Controlled human studies demonstrate no evidence of risk in pregnancy in any trimester and the possibility of fetal harm appears remote.
B	Animal-reproduction studies have not demonstrated fetal risk and there are no controlled human studies, or Animal—reproduction studies have demonstrated an adverse effect that was not confirmed in controlled human studies in the first trimester and there is no evidence of a risk in later trimesters
C	Animal-reproduction studies have demonstrated an adverse fetal effect and there are no controlled human studies or Animal-reproduction and human studies are not available so that drugs should be given only if the potential benefits justify the potential risk to the fetus
D	Positive evidence of human fetal risk exists but use may be acceptable despite the fetal risk if the drug is needed in a life-threatening situation, or for a serious disease for which safer drugs cannot be used or are ineffective.
X	Animal-reproductive and/or human studies demonstrate fetal abnormalities such that the risk of the use of the drug in pregnant women clearly outweighs any possible benefit. *Use of Class X drugs is contraindicated in women who are or may become pregnant.*

neonatal mortality rate (the number of neonatal deaths per 1000 live births). *Perinatal death* is the number of fetal deaths plus the number of neonatal deaths and is expressed as the *perinatal mortality rate* (deaths per 1000 total births).

More pleasant statistics are the *birth rate,* which is expressed as the number of births per 1000 people in the total population, and the *fertility rate,* which is expressed as the number of live births per 1000 females aged 15 to 45 in the population.

CASE STUDIES

Case 5A

A 14-year-old girl with an unknown interval of amenorrhea, a positive urinary pregnancy test, and morning sickness presents for prenatal care. Her uterus is not palpable on abdominal examination.

Questions Case 5A

All of the following questions are useful in determining her gestational age EXCEPT

A. If, and when, quickening was noted
B. Last menstrual period (LMP)
C. Contraceptive use, if any
D. Menstrual cycle regularity

Answer: A

Items B–D are important in establishing her EDC by dates. Quickening would suggest a pregnancy in the late first or early second trimester, at which time the uterus would be palpable abdominally.

What laboratory tests would be most useful to further ascertain her gestational age and EDC?

A. Qualitative β-hCG
B. Quantitative β-hCG
C. Obstetric ultrasound
D. Computed tomography (CT) scan

Answer: C

With a positive urinary pregnancy test, serum pregnancy tests are redundant. CT scans are not used in gestational age estimation. Ultrasound offers an excellent means to assess gestational age, especially when used early in pregnancy.

Case 5B

A 27-year-old G1 P0 at 37 weeks calls saying her baby is moving much less than it did a few days ago. On review of her antepartum record, you note no medical problems, normal fetal growth, and normal laboratory values as well as a normal obstetric ultrasound at 18 weeks.

Questions Case 5B

Your most appropriate action(s) is/are

A. Because she has an unremarkable antepartum record, reassure the patient that she is just inexperienced and that everything is okay
B. Suggest the patient come to the hospital for induction of labor
C. Suggest the patient come to the hospital for an NST
D. Suggest the patient come to the hospital for an OCT

Answer: C

Answer A will only raise the patient's concerns and does not address the problem of proper evaluation of decreased fetal movement. An NST is the least invasive and most cost-effective test. An OCT is also a good measure of fetal well-being but is more invasive and costly than is warranted in a patient with no risk factors. Induction of labor is done for maternal or fetal issues that make continued pregnancy of greater risk than the risk of induction, or it may be done electively at term if specific criteria are met and the patient fully understands the elective nature of the intervention and the risks that are involved. In this case none of these criteria are present based on the information available, and induction is not indicated, but rather further evaluation.

The patient comes to the hospital and receives an NST. It is nonreactive. Your most appropriate action is to suggest which of the following?

A. A biophysical profile
B. A repeat NST in 1 week
C. An induction of labor
D. A nutrition consult to avoid hypoglycemia-associated decreased fetal movement
E. Cordocentesis for fetal blood gas analysis

Answer: A

A biophysical profile is the least invasive and most cost-effective test of fetal well-being as follow-up to a nonreactive NST. An OCT would also serve as a test of fetal well-being, but it does not measure amniotic fluid volume and is more costly and invasive. Cordocentesis is likewise invasive, with significant maternal and fetal risks, and is not indicated. As before the NST, criteria for indicated induction of labor are absent and the patient is not at term so elective induction of labor is not appropriate.

INTRAPARTUM CARE

This chapter deals primarily with APGO Objective(s):

OBJECTIVE 12   Intrapartum Care

A. Describe the characteristics of true and false labor.
B. Describe the stages and mechanisms of normal labor.
C. Describe the initial labor assessment and the techniques to evaluate the progress of labor and the methods of monitoring of mother and fetus.
D. Describe intrapartum pain management.
E. Describe the management of normal labor and delivery (including episiotomy and vaginal repair of episiotomy and obstetric lacerations) and the immediate postpartum care of the mother.
F. Describe the indications for operative delivery.

Labor is the process by which products of conception (fetus, placenta, cord, and membranes) are expelled from the uterus. It is defined as the progressive effacement and dilation of the uterine cervix, resulting from rhythmic contractions of the uterine musculature. Cervical dilation that occurs without uterine contractions is not considered true labor. Uterine contractions without effacement and dilation of the cervix occur normally in the third trimester of pregnancy and are termed Braxton Hicks contractions, or false labor. Approximately 85% of patients undergo spontaneous labor and delivery between 37 and 42 weeks' gestation.

CHANGES BEFORE THE ONSET OF LABOR

As the patient approaches term, there is an increasing number of uterine contractions of greater intensity. Spontaneous uterine contractions, which are not felt by the patient, occur throughout pregnancy. Late in pregnancy they become stronger and more frequent, resulting in the patient's perception of discomfort. These Braxton Hicks contractions (false labor) are not associated with progressive dilation of the cervix, however, and therefore do not fit the definition of labor. It is frequently difficult for the patient to distinguish these often uncomfortable contractions from those of true labor, and as a result, it is difficult for the physician to determine the true onset of labor by history alone. Braxton Hicks contractions are typically shorter in duration and less intense than true labor contractions, with the discomfort being characterized as over the lower abdomen and groin areas. It is not uncommon for these contractions to resolve with ambulation.

True labor, on the other hand, is associated with contractions that the patient feels over the uterine fundus, with radiation of discomfort to the low back and low abdomen. These contractions become increasingly intense and frequent. The ultimate test of whether the contractions are those of true labor is if they are associated with cervical effacement and dilation.

Another event of late pregnancy is termed *lightening*. In this, the patient reports a change in the shape of her abdomen and the sensation that the baby has gotten less heavy, the result of the fetal head descending into the pelvis. The patient may also report that the baby is "dropping." The patient often notices that the lower abdomen is more prominent and the upper abdomen is flatter, and there may be more frequent urination as the bladder is compressed by the fetal head. The patient may also notice an easier time breathing, because there is less pressure on the diaphragm.

Patients often report the passage of blood-tinged mucus late in pregnancy. This *bloody show* results as the cervix begins thinning out (*effacement*) with the concomitant extrusion of mucus from the endocervical glands. Cervical effacement is common before the onset of true labor, as the internal os is slowly drawn into the lower uterine segment. The cervix is often significantly effaced before the onset of labor, particularly in the nulliparous patient. The mechanism of effacement and dilation is shown in Figure 6.1.

EVALUATION FOR LABOR

Instruction as to when to report to the hospital when labor is suspected is a routine part of antepartum care. *Patients are told to come to the hospital for any of the following reasons:* if their contractions occur approximately every 5 minutes for at least 1 hour, if there is a sudden gush of fluid or a constant leakage of fluid (suggesting rupture of membranes), if there is any significant bleeding, or if there is significant decrease in fetal movement. At the time of initial evaluation at the hospital, the *prenatal records* are reviewed to (*1*) identify complications of pregnancy up to that point, (*2*) confirm gestational age to differentiate preterm labor from labor in a term pregnancy, and (*3*) review pertinent laboratory information. A *focused history* helps in determining the nature and frequency of the patient's contractions, the possibility of

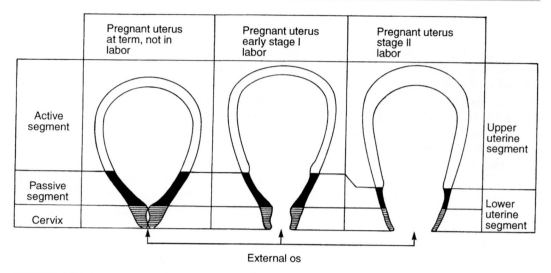

	Pregnant uterus at term, not in labor	Pregnant uterus early stage I labor	Pregnant uterus stage II labor	
Active segment				Upper uterine segment
Passive segment				Lower uterine segment
Cervix				

External os

FIGURE 6.1. Mechanism of effacement, dilation, and labor. With continuing uterine contractions, the upper uterus (active segment) thickens, the lower uterine segment (passive segment) thins, and the cervix dilates. In this way, the fetus is moved downward, into and through the vaginal canal.

spontaneous rupture of membranes or significant bleeding, or changes in maternal or fetal status. A *limited general physical examination* is performed (with special attention to vital signs) along with the abdominal and pelvic examinations. If contractions occur during this physical examination, they may be palpated for intensity and duration by the examining physician. Auscultation of the fetal heart tones is also of critical importance, particularly immediately following a contraction, to determine the possibility of any fetal heart rate deceleration.

The initial examination of the gravid abdomen may be accomplished using *Leopold maneuvers* (Figure 6.2), a series of four palpations of the fetus through the abdominal wall that helps accurately determine fetal lie, presentation, and position. *Lie* is the relation of the long axis of the fetus with the maternal long axis. It is longitudinal in 99% of cases, occasionally transverse, and rarely oblique (when the axes cross at a 45° angle, usually converting to a transverse or longitudinal lie during labor). *Presentation* is determined by the "presenting part" (i.e., that portion of the fetus lowest in the birth canal), palpated during the abdominal examination and when a vaginal examination is performed.

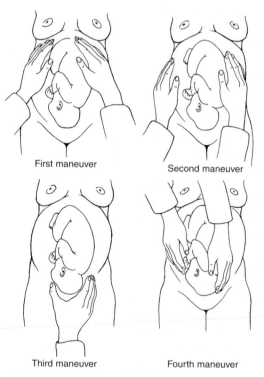

First maneuver   Second maneuver

Third maneuver   Fourth maneuver

FIGURE 6.2. Leopold maneuvers.

For example, in a longitudinal lie, the presenting part is either breech or cephalic. The most common cephalic presentation is the one in which the head is sharply flexed onto the fetal chest such that the occiput or vertex presents. *Position* is the relation of the

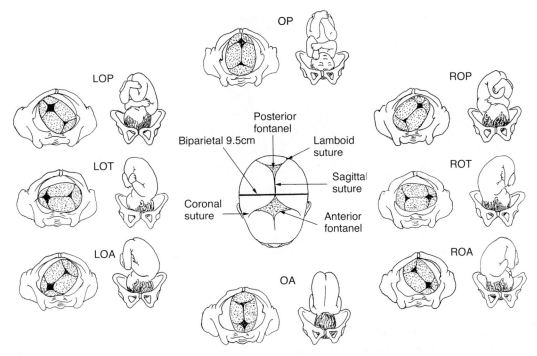

FIGURE 6.3. Various positions in vertex presentation. LOP = left occiput posterior; LOT = left occiput transverse; LOA = left occiput anterior; ROP = right occiput posterior; ROT = right occiput transverse; ROA = right occiput anterior.

fetal presenting part to the right or left side of the maternal pelvis (Figure 6.3). The fetal head may also be turned more or less toward the sacrum or symphysis, termed anterior and posterior *asynclitism,* respectively (Figure 6.4).

The *four Leopold maneuvers* (see Figure 6.2) include the following:

1. *Determining what occupies the fundus.* In a longitudinal lie, the fetal head is differentiated from the fetal breech, the latter being larger and less clearly defined.
2. *Determining location of small parts.* Using one hand to steady the fetus, the fingers on the other hand are used to palpate either the firm, long fetal spine or the various shapes and movements indicating fetal hands and feet.
3. *Identifying descent of the presenting part.* Suprapubic palpation identifies the presenting part as the fetal head, which is relatively mobile, or a breech, which moves the entire body. The extent to which the presenting part is felt to extend below the

symphysis suggests the station of the presenting part.
4. *Identifying the cephalic prominence.* As long as the cephalic prominence is easily palpable, the vertex is not likely to have descended to 0 station.

As part of the abdominal examination, palpation of the uterus during a contraction is helpful in determining the intensity of that particular contraction. The uterine wall is not easily indented with firm palpation during a true contraction, but may be indented during a Braxton Hicks contraction.

The *vaginal examination* should be performed using an aseptic technique. In the presence of significant bleeding, the vaginal examination should be done with extreme care, if at all, because of the risk of disrupting a placenta previa (see Chapter 20). If it is unclear whether or not membranes have been ruptured, a sterile speculum examination should be performed before any digital examination of the cervix to ascertain if spontaneous rupture of the membranes has occurred (see Chapter 23). Visualization of the cervix through the speculum also allows for better

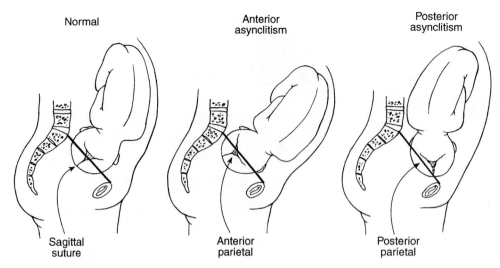

FIGURE 6.4. Asynclitism.

identification of the source of any bleeding. If membranes are ruptured and the patient is not in labor, digital cervical examination is often delayed until labor ensues. Or, intervention is vaginal. Both these strategies reduce the risk of uterine infection.

The digital portion of the vaginal examination allows the examiner to determine the consistency and degree of *effacement of the cervix*. *Effacement* is the degree to which the cervix has thinned and is expressed as a number of centimeters of cervical length where 4 centimeters is considered uneffaced, or as a percent of thinning from a perceived uneffaced state (Figure 6.5). A cervix that is not effaced, but is softened, is more likely to change with contractions than one that is firm, as it is earlier in pregnancy. If the cervix is not significantly effaced, it may also be evaluated for its *relative position* (i.e., anterior, midposition, or posterior in the vagina). A cervix that is palpable anterior in the vagina is more likely to undergo change in labor sooner than one found in the posterior portion of the vagina.

The cervix is also palpated for *cervical dilation*, described as centimeters of dilation. The individual examiner uses one or two fingers to identify the diameter of the opening of the cervix. Fetal *station* is also determined by identifying the relative level of the foremost part of the fetal presenting part relative to the level of the ischial spines. If the presenting part has reached the level

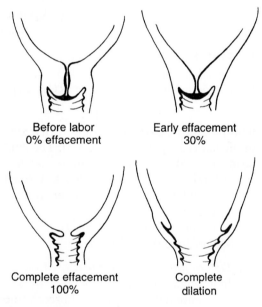

FIGURE 6.5. Effacement and dilation.

of the ischial spines, it is termed *0 station*. The distance between the ischial spines to the pelvic inlet above and the distance from the spines to the pelvic outlet below are divided into thirds, and these measurements are used to further define station. If the presenting part is palpable at the pelvic inlet, it is called −3 station, if it has descended one third of the way to the ischial spines, it is called −2 station, and so on. Descent of the fetal presenting part below the spines is sim-

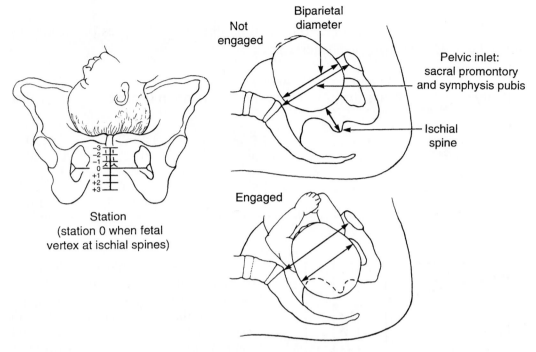

FIGURE 6.6.   Station and engagement of the fetal head.

ilarly defined as +1 station, +2 station, and so on (Figure 6.6). *The clinical significance of the fetal head presenting at 0 station is that the biparietal diameter of the fetal head, the greatest transverse diameter of the fetal skull, has negotiated the pelvic inlet.*

If the patient is found not to be in active labor (i.e., < 4 cm dilated) and there are no confounding medical or obstetric problems, she may be sent home to await the onset of true labor. If there is a question as to whether or not true labor has commenced, the patient may be reevaluated after approximately 1 hour. In some cases, patients are encouraged to ambulate to differentiate Braxton Hicks contractions (which may resolve) from true labor (which will continue). If the patient is in labor, she is admitted to the labor area of the hospital and active management of labor is undertaken.

STAGES OF LABOR

Although labor is a continuous process, it is divided into four functional stages. The *first stage* is the interval between the onset of labor and full cervical dilation (10 cm). The first stage is further divided into two phases.

The *latent phase* encompasses cervical effacement and early dilation. The second is the *active phase,* during which more rapid cervical dilation occurs, usually beginning at approximately 4 cm. The *second stage* encompasses complete cervical dilation through the delivery of the infant. The *third stage* begins immediately after delivery of the infant and ends with the delivery of the placenta. The *fourth stage* of labor is defined as the immediate postpartum period of approximately 2 hours after delivery of the placenta during which time the patient undergoes significant physiologic adjustment. Table 6.1 outlines the duration of various stages of labor, as suggested by Friedman, and Figure 6.7 represents this graphically.

MECHANISM OF LABOR

The mechanism of labor (also known as the cardinal movements of labor) refers to the changes of the position of the fetus as it passes through the birth canal. The fetus usually descends in a fashion whereby the occipital portion of the fetal head is the lower-most part in the pelvis and rotates toward the largest pelvic segment. This

TABLE 6.1. Mean Duration of the Various Phases and Stages of Labor with Their Distribution Characteristics

Parity	Latent Phase (hr)	Active Phase (hr)	Maximum Dilation (cm/hr)	Second Stage (hr)
Nulliparas				
Mean	6.5	4.5	3.0	1.0
Upper limit*	20.0	12.0	1.0	3.0
Multiparas				
Mean	5.0	2.5	6.0	0.5
Upper limit*	13.5	5.0	1.5	1.0

*5th or 95th percentile.

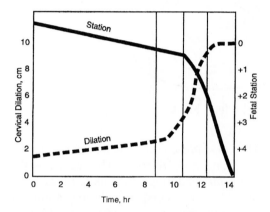

FIGURE 6.7. Graphic presentation of cervical dilation and station during the first and second stages of labor.

vertex presentation occurs in 95% of term labors. As a result, the cardinal movements of labor are defined relative to this presentation. How a fetus in the breech presentation moves through the birth canal is significantly different. To accommodate to the maternal bony pelvis, the fetal head must undergo several movements as it passes through the birth canal. These movements are accomplished by means of the forceful contractions of the uterus. *These cardinal movements of labor* do not occur as a distinct series of movements but rather as a group of movements that overlap as the fetus moves progressively through the birth canal. These are (*1*) engagement, (*2*) flexion, (*3*) descent, (*4*) internal rotation, (*5*) extension, and (*6*) external rotation (Figure 6.8).

Engagement is defined as descent of the biparietal diameter of the head below the pelvic inlet, suggested clinically by palpation of the presenting part below the level of ischial spines (0 station). Engagement is common days to weeks prior to labor in primigravidas, whereas in multigravidas it more commonly happens at the onset of labor. In any event, the importance of this event is that it suggests that the bony pelvis is adequate to allow significant descent of the fetal head. It is not uncommon for the fetal head to become engaged before the onset of true labor, particularly in nulliparous patients. *Flexion of the fetal head* allows for the smaller diameters of the fetal head to present to the maternal pelvis. *Descent of the presenting part* is a necessity for the successful completion of passage through the birth canal. The greatest rate of descent occurs during the latter portions of the first stage of labor and during the second stage of labor. Figure 6.7 is a graphic demonstration of fetal descent and dilation of the cervix. *Internal rotation*, like flexion, facilitates presentation of the optimal diameters of the fetal head to the bony pelvis, most commonly from transverse to either anterior or posterior. *Extension of the fetal head* occurs as it reaches the introitus. To accommodate to the upward curve of the birth canal, the flexed head now extends. *External rotation* occurs after delivery of the head as the head rotates to "face forward" relative to its shoulders.

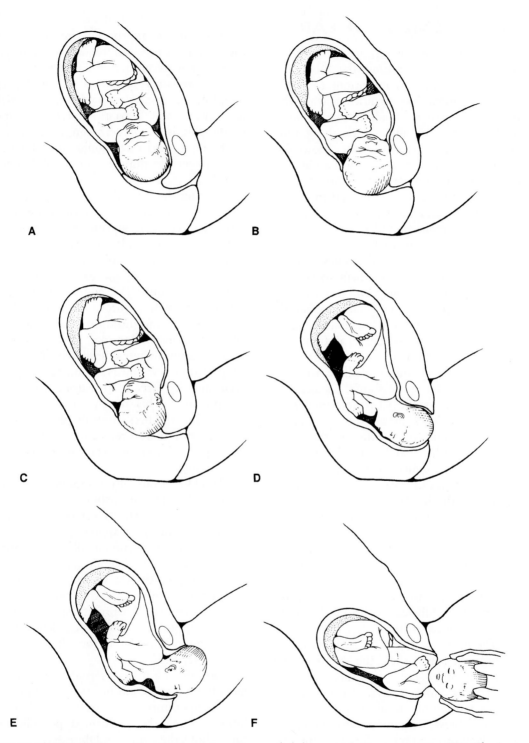

FIGURE 6.8. Cardinal movements of labor. (*A*) Engagement. (*B*) Flexion. (*C*) Descent and internal rotation. (*D*), (*E*) Extension. (*F*) External rotation.

MANAGEMENT OF LABOR

Although the patient may have undergone some education regarding the labor and delivery process, it is important to realize that the patient has significant fears that remain. The patient should not be left unattended for any significant length of time, and a support person may be allowed to remain with the patient throughout the labor and delivery process in most cases. Maternal vital signs should be taken at least every 30 minutes during the first stage of labor. The patient should be given nothing by mouth except for small sips of water, ice chips, clear liquids, or hard candies. Laboratory information, including hematocrit, type and screen, platelet count, and urinalysis for glucose and protein, are obtained when the patient is admitted to the hospital. An intravenous line (16- to 18-gauge) is frequently inserted during the active phase of labor to provide hydration and immediate access to the intravascular space should medications be necessary. As the gastrointestinal tract significantly slows in its function during labor, hydration by means of the intravenous line rather than by mouth is optimal.

During the course of labor, descent of the fetus causes the bladder to be elevated relative to the lower uterine segment and cervix. This often results in the patient having difficulty voiding. The patient should, therefore, be encouraged to void frequently. Catheterization may become necessary if the bladder becomes distended. The use of a cleansing enema to empty the lower colon may be used subject to the needs of the patient and local custom.

The *position* in which a woman labors depends on her wishes, the status of her pregnancy, and the plan for labor and delivery that she and her physician have developed. Laboring in sitting or reclining position at bed rest is common, with the lateral recumbent position often chosen to enhance uterine blood flow by taking the gravid uterus off the inferior vena cava. Other laboring positions (such as sitting in a rocking chair) or walking (ambulation) are also often beneficially employed. Indeed, the appropriate choice of labor positions at different stages of labor may increase maternal comfort and facilitate labor. At all times, there should be appropriate monitoring of the fetal heart rate and frequency and severity of uterine contractions. *Electronic fetal monitoring* is very common and often routine, but it is not necessary for the low-risk term pregnancy. If routine electronic fetal monitoring is not undertaken, auscultation of the fetal heart rate should be performed at least every 15 minutes, immediately after a uterine contraction.

During the second stage of labor, fetal heart rate auscultation should be performed after each uterine contraction. If electronic fetal monitoring is undertaken, either as routine or for patients who are considered at risk, an external tocodynamometer is initially used to assess uterine activity, providing information regarding the frequency and duration of contractions but not intensity. Internal pressure monitoring, using an intrauterine catheter, can be performed to measure intensity more accurately by directly measuring intrauterine pressure. This internal form of fetal monitoring requires rupture of the membranes and, therefore, cannot usually be accomplished until the cervix is at least 1 to 2 cm dilated.

Fetal heart rate can be monitored externally by Doppler ultrasound or internally using a direct fetal electrocardiogram, which is obtained by applying a scalp electrode. The latter technique allows for more detailed evaluation of subtle changes in fetal heart rate pattern (see Chapter 8). Whenever artificial rupture of the membranes is to be performed, the presenting part must be well applied to the cervix. This minimizes the risk of an iatrogenic umbilical cord prolapse.

Monitoring of maternal conditions, including pulse, blood pressure, respiratory rate, temperature, urine output, and fluid intake, should be performed periodically throughout the course of labor.

Because the latent phase of labor may be affected by *analgesic and anesthetic agents*, these should generally not be used until the active phase of labor. There is no evidence that either analgesics or anesthetics significantly affect the active phase of labor. Many patients have prepared for labor using childbirth education classes, during which time they are taught techniques of relaxation to deal with the pain of labor contractions. Some patients find the use of narcotic analgesics to be helpful adjuncts to these measures. In the doses typically given during labor, neonatal depression is not a major concern. Commonly used medications include the narcotic meperidine (Demerol; 5 to 20 mg slow IV p q 2–3 h or 25 to 75 mg IM q 3–4 h) and the synthetic opioid agonist-antagonist butorphanol tartrate (Stadol; 1 to 2 mg slow IV p q 3–4 h).

Any analgesic or anesthetic technique used during the labor and delivery process should take into account those sensory pathways involved and the points at which they may be affected. During the first stage of labor, pain results from contraction of the uterus and dilation of the cervix. This pain travels along the visceral afferents, which accompany sympathetic nerves entering the spinal cord at T10, T11, T12, and L1. As the head descends, there is also distention of the lower birth canal and perineum. This pain is transmitted along somatic afferents that comprise portions of the pudendal nerves that enter the spinal cord at S2, S3, and S4.

The anesthetic technique that provides pain relief during labor is the *epidural block*. The advantage of this technique is its ability to provide analgesia during labor as well as excellent anesthesia for delivery yet maintain the patient's sense of touch facilitating participation in the birth process. It can also be used in either vaginal or abdominal deliveries and in postpartum procedures such as tubal ligation. *Spinal anesthetic* is usually used for abdominal delivery, although on occasion it is performed for a difficult forceps delivery. A *pudendal block* with local anesthesia can be administered easily at the time of delivery to provide perineal anesthesia for a vaginal delivery (Figure 6.9). A *local block* (i.e., local injection of anesthetic) may be used at the area of an episiotomy or tear.

Epidural anesthesia is superior to spinal anesthesia in that it can be left as a continuous source of analgesia and anesthesia during both the labor and delivery process. It avoids the risk of spinal headache in the mother and reduces the risk of sympathetic blockade, which could lead to hypotension. There is also less motor blockade than with spinal anesthesia. Although the pudendal block is easy to perform and also has the least potential risk to the mother and fetus, its use is also the most limited. *General anesthesia* is reserved only for different operative deliveries and cesarean sections in selected cases. The potential risk of complications such as maternal aspiration reduces its more widespread use.

Evaluation of the patient's progress of labor is accomplished by means of a series of pelvic examinations. The number of examinations should be minimized to avoid the risk of chorioamnionitis. At the time of each vaginal examination, a sterile lubricant is used. Each examination should identify cervical dilation, effacement, station, position of the presenting part, and the status of the membranes. These findings should be noted graphically on the hospital record so that abnormalities of labor may be identified. During the latter portions of the first stage of labor, patients may report the urge to push. This may signify significant descent of the fetal head with pressure on the perineum. More frequent vaginal examinations during this time may be necessary. Similarly, in case of significant fetal heart rate decelerations, more frequent examinations may be necessary to determine whether or not the umbilical cord is prolapsed or if delivery is imminent.

In addition to rupturing the membranes to insert an intrauterine pressure catheter or a fetal scalp monitor, *artificial rupture of membranes* may be beneficial in other ways. The presence or absence of meconium (fetal stool) can be identified. Blood in the amniotic fluid may also have significance (see Chapter 20). Rupture of the membranes does, however, carry some risk, because the incidence of infection may be increased if labor is prolonged or umbilical cord prolapse may occur if rupture of the membranes is undertaken before engagement of the presenting fetal part. *Spontaneous rupture of membranes* has similar risks. The fluid should be observed for meconium and blood. Fetal heart tones should be assessed after membranes spontaneously rupture.

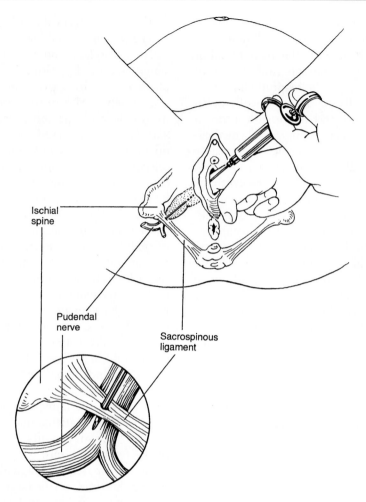

Ischial
spine

Pudendal
nerve

Sacrospinous
ligament

FIGURE 6.9. Pudendal block.

Once the *second stage of labor* has been reached (i.e., complete, or 10 cm of, cervical dilation), voluntary maternal effort (pushing) can be added to the involuntary contractile forces of the uterus to facilitate delivery of the fetus. With the onset of each contraction, the mother is encouraged to inhale, hold her breath, and perform an extended Valsalva maneuver. This increase in intra-abdominal pressure aids in fetal descent through the birth canal.

It is during the second stage of labor that the fetal head may undergo further alterations. *Molding* is an alteration in the relation of the fetal cranial bones, even resulting in partial bone overlap. Some minor degree is common as the fetal head adjusts to the bony pelvis. The greater the

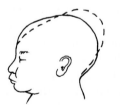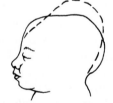

FIGURE 6.10. Molding of head.

disparity between the fetal head and the bony pelvis, the greater the amount of molding (Figure 6.10). *Caput succedaneum* is the edema of the fetal scalp caused by pressure on the fetal head by the cervix. An extended second stage may last as long as 2 to 3 hours, and the prolonged resistance encountered by the fetal vertex may prevent

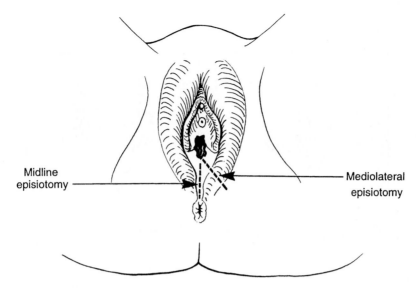

Midline
episiotomy

Mediolateral
episiotomy

FIGURE 6.11.   Episiotomy.

appropriate identification of fontanels and sutures. Both caput and molding resolve in the first few days of life. If identified before the second stage of labor, these changes should be noted on the pelvic examination and may indicate a significant problem in negotiation of the birth canal.

DELIVERY

The patient should be prepared for a well-controlled delivery of the fetal head. In general, nulliparous patients take a greater amount of time to deliver than multiparous patients, once the second stage of labor has started. The *dorsal lithotomy position* (*supine on back, legs bent at knees and elevated*) is a common position for vaginal delivery in the United States, both because of custom and preference of physicians who are commonly trained in delivery technique in this position. The position offers clear advantage for operative (forceps, breech) delivery and for the repair of more than minor obstetric lacerations. Other delivery positions (e.g., lateral, knee-chest, sitting) may also be used to advantage, especially for the normal spontaneous vaginal delivery, if desired by the patient and with a clinician skilled and comfortable in delivery in other positions. Vari-

ous delivery devices, such as a birthing chair or stool, may also be used to advantage under similar circumstances. With each successive contraction, the maternal force as well as uterine contractions cause more of the fetal scalp to be visible at the introitus with progressive thinning of the perineum and distention of the vaginal canal. With slow progressive labor and good control of the fetal head and body at delivery, the risk of obstetric laceration with a normal sized infant is low so that the need for episiotomy is low or even absent. However, if an episiotomy is needed, it should be performed only after the perineum has been thinned considerably by the descending fetal head (Figure 6.11). By enlarging the vaginal outlet, an episiotomy facilitates delivery and may be indicated in cases of instrumental delivery and/or protracted or arrested descent. Routine episiotomy is not a part of modern obstetric practice. If needed, episiotomies are usually cut midline or occasionally in a mediolateral direction. Advantages of the former include less pain, ease of repair, and less blood loss. The primary disadvantage is greater risk of extension into a third- or fourth-degree laceration, involving the rectal sphincter and rectal mucosa, respectively. Nonetheless, performing a mediolateral episiotomy is uncommon nowadays.

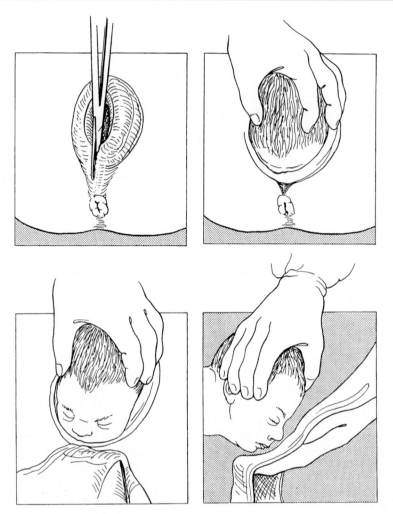

FIGURE 6.12.   Vaginal delivery with midline episiotomy assisted by modified Ritgen maneuver.

As the fetal head crowns (i.e., distends the vaginal opening), it is delivered by extension to allow the smallest diameter of the fetal head to pass over the perineum. This decreases the likelihood of laceration or extension of episiotomy. To facilitate this, the physician provides support to the perineal tissues and performs a modified *Ritgen maneuver* (Figure 6.12). In this, one hand is placed over the vertex while the other exerts pressure through the perineum onto the fetal chin. A sterile towel is used to avoid contamination of this hand by contact with the anus. The chin can then be delivered slowly, with control applied by both hands.

After the head is delivered, nasal and oral suction is performed with a bulb syringe. If meconium has been present, suctioning of the pharynx must also be accomplished. The neck should then be evaluated for the possible presence of a nuchal cord, which should be reduced over the fetal head if possible. If the cord is tight, it may be doubly clamped and cut. After delivery of the head, the shoulders descend and rotate to a position in the anteroposterior diameter of the pelvis. The attendant's hands are placed on the chin and vertex, applying gentle downward pressure, thus delivering the anterior shoulder. To avoid injury to the brachial plexus, care is taken not to put

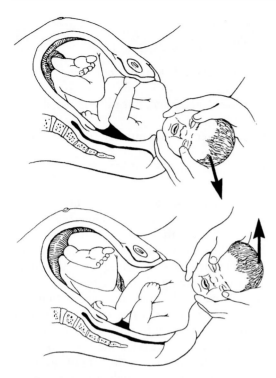

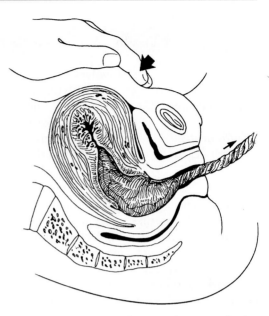

FIGURE 6.14. Delivery of the placenta.

FIGURE 6.13. Delivery of anterior and posterior shoulders.

excessive force on the neck. The posterior shoulder is then delivered by upward traction on the fetal head (Figure 6.13). Delivery of the body now occurs easily.

The fetus is then cradled in the attendant's arms, with the head down to maximize drainage of secretions to the oropharynx. Further suctioning is accomplished before clamping the umbilical cord. Heat loss should be minimized by rapid, thorough drying, then wrapping with warmed crib blankets is desirable. If the newborn is stable, he or she may remain with the mother to start bonding and/or first breast nippling. If the newborn is in some manner unstable, transfer to a radiant warmer and further pediatric care is indicated.

THIRD STAGE OF LABOR

Immediately after delivery of the infant, the uterus significantly decreases in size. Blood from the umbilical cord should be obtained and sent for type and Rh testing. Cord blood may also be obtained for arterial blood gases determination. Cord blood gas information is useful if problems develop in the immediate postpartum interval. *Delivery of the placenta* is imminent when the uterus rises in the abdomen, becoming globular in configuration, indicating that the placenta has separated and has entered the lower uterine segment; a gush of blood and/or "lengthening" of the umbilical cord also occur. These are the three classic *signs of placental separation.* Pulling the placenta from the uterus by excess traction on the cord should be avoided. This inappropriate application of force may result in *inversion of the uterus,* an obstetric emergency associated with profound blood loss and shock. Instead, it is appropriate to wait for spontaneous extrusion of the placenta, sometimes up to 30 minutes. As the placenta passes into the lower uterine segment, gentle downward pressure is applied to the fundus of the uterus, and the placenta is guided by very gentle traction on the umbilical cord (Figure 6.14).

If spontaneous placental separation does not occur, or as a routine for some physicians, the placenta may be removed

TABLE 6.2. Classification of Obstetric Lacerations

First degree	Involves the vaginal mucosa or perineal skin, but not the underlying tissue
Second degree	Involves the underlying subcutaneous tissue, but not the rectal sphincter or rectal mucosa
Third degree	Extends through the rectal sphincter but not into the rectal mucosa
Fourth degree	Extends into the rectal mucosa

manually. This is accomplished by passing a hand into the uterine cavity and using the side of the hand to develop a cleavage plane between the placenta and the uterine wall. The placenta can then be manually removed. Sufficient analgesia should be employed for this maneuver, and on occasion, anesthesia may be required. The umbilical cord should be evaluated for the presence of the expected two umbilical arteries and one umbilical vein.

After the placenta has been removed, the uterus should be palpated to ensure that it has reduced in size and become firmly contracted. Excessive blood loss at this or any subsequent time should suggest the possibility of uterine atony. The use of uterine massage as well as oxytocic agents such as oxytocin, Methergine (methylergonovine maleate), or prostaglandins may be routinely used.

Inspection of the birth canal should be accomplished in a systematic fashion. The introitus and vulvar areas, including the periurethral area, should be evaluated for lacerations. Ring forceps are commonly used to hold and evaluate the cervix. Lacerations, if present, are most commonly found at the 3 o'clock and 9 o'clock positions on the cervix. Lacerations of the vagina and/or perineum and extensions of the episiotomy are also evaluated. Repair is accomplished with an absorbable suture. Obstetric lacerations are classified in Table 6.2.

Vacuum extraction is sometimes used in lieu of obstetric forceps. Because traction is applied only to the instrument, some believe that the delivery is more physiologic and has less potential for trauma than forceps although bruising or trauma to the fetal scalp may occur.

Cesarean section now accounts for up to 15%–30% of births in some obstetrical units. The rate of cesarean section was stable at less than 5% until 1965. Cesarean section rates have increased since that time for various reasons. One of the major reasons often cited is the ready availability of neonatal intensive care units, in which infants have a significantly greater survival rate than what was once the case. Another factor in the increase in the rate of cesarean sections is its use in the delivery of fetuses in breech presentations. Cesarean sections are also performed if there are signs of nonreassuring fetal status or dystocias and as a repeat procedure.

An increasing number of cesarean sections are being done for dystocia and uterine inertia. In addition, increased sophistication for fetal surveillance provides more information about the possibility of nonreassuring fetal status. As a result, more cesarean sections can be attributed to cases of fetal distress. For many years, it was felt that a previous cesarean section mandated that all future deliveries would also have to be abdominal. With the increasing tendency to attempt vaginal birth after cesarean section (VBAC) with success rates of 70%–75%, fewer cesarean sections are now being performed for this indication.

Deciding on cesarean delivery has important ramifications, because the maternal mortality rate associated with cesarean delivery is two to four times that of a vaginal birth (i.e., 1 per 2500 to 1 per 5000 operations). Cesarean section can be performed through various incisions in the uterus. An incision through the thin lower uterine segment allows for subsequent trials at VBAC. An incision through the thick, muscular upper portion of the uterus, a classical cesarean section, carries a greater risk for subsequent uterine rupture if labor occurs so that repeat cesarean sections for these patients is still recommended.

FOURTH STAGE OF LABOR

For the first hour or so after delivery, the likelihood of serious postpartum complications is the greatest. Postpartum uterine hemorrhage occurs in approximately 1% of patients. It is more likely to occur in cases of rapid labor, protracted labor, or uterine enlargement (large fetus, polyhydramnios). Immediately after the delivery of the placenta, the uterus is palpated to determine that it is firm. Uterine palpation through the abdominal wall is repeated at frequent intervals during the immediate postpartum period to ascertain uterine tone. Perineal pads are applied and the amount of blood on these pads as well as pulse and blood pressure are monitored closely for the first several hours after delivery to identify excessive blood loss.

CASE STUDIES

Case 6A

A 22-year-old G1 at term comes to the labor unit complaining of increasingly severe and frequent uterine contractions for 10 hours and a gush of fluid 1 hour ago. Her prenatal records show an unremarkable antepartum course, with dating by last menstrual period (LMP) and second trimester ultrasound, normal fetal growth, and normal prenatal laboratory findings. Maternal examination including blood pressure are normal.

Questions Case 6A

The initial fetal management should consist of

A. Auscultation or Doppler evaluation of fetal heart rate (FHR)
B. Placement of fetal scalp electrode for evaluation of FHR
C. Palpation or tocodynamometer evaluation of uterine contractions
D. Placement of intrauterine pressure catheter (IUPC) for evaluation of uterine contractions
E. Leopold maneuvers to ascertain presentation and lie

F. Complete obstetric ultrasound to ascertain lie, presentation, and position (fetal status)
G. Speculum examination and evaluation of fluid, if present, by Nitrazine and slide evaluation
H. Pelvic examination

Answer: A, C, E, G, H

Auscultation, palpation, and Leopold maneuvers suffice as initial methods of evaluation of lie, fetal heart rate, and uterine contractions. Internal monitoring and ultrasound require more indication. Fluid should be examined to check for pH and ferning—signs of rupture of membranes—because the gush of fluid may well have been urine. Pelvic examination at term is acceptable to determine if the patient is in labor.

Leopold maneuvers show a normal-size fetus in cephalic presentation, palpation shows strong uterine contractions every 3 minutes, fluid examination is consistent with urine, and pelvic examination shows 3 cm and 100%, intact membranes, and a

(Continued)

cephalic part at –1 station. FHR is 145. What stage of labor is she in?

A. First stage
B. Second stage
C. Third stage
D. Fourth stage

Answer: A

Continued management includes

A. External electronic fetal monitor (EFM)
B. Internal EFM
C. Obstetric ultrasound
D. Induction of labor
E. Augmentation of labor

Answer: A

The patient is evidently in normal early labor with a normal pregnancy. External electronic monitoring is sufficient, and indeed, intermittent auscultation would be as satisfactory.

Labor continues for 5 hours, and cervical examination shows dilation to 4 cm. FHR remains normal. Then spontaneous rupture of membranes occurs with meconium fluid noted. Continued management includes

A. Fetal scalp electrode (FSE)
B. Amnioinfusion
C. IUPC
D. Obstetric ultrasound
E. Augmentation of labor

Answer: A, B, maybe C

With the unexpected presence of meconium-stained amniotic fluid, an FSE to evaluate fetal heart rate variability and an amnioin-fusion to decrease the risk of meconium aspiration are appropriate. An IUPC can be placed but is not required if external monitoring is sufficient and cervical change is progressing near the expected 1.5 cm/hr.

Case 6B

A 35-year-old G2 P0010 at term has been pushing in second stage for 3 hours; fetal heart tones are reassuring, but the patient is exhausted and demonstrating diminishing ability to push. Spontaneous uterine contractions continue every 3 minutes, lasting 45 seconds, measuring 65 mm Hg on the average. Pelvic examination shows a cephalic presentation in left occiput posterior (LOP) presentation at –3 station with moderate molding of the head and a marked caput succedaneum.

Question Case 6B

Your best management is

A. Continued labor
B. Augmented labor
C. Forceps delivery
D. Cesarean delivery
E. External version

Answer: D

Assuming reassuring fetal status, the old rule of limiting the second stage of labor to 2 hours is now outdated. The information here, however, suggests molding of the head at a high station and a very tired mother. The forceps would be above the midforceps definition and, therefore, unsafe. Cesarean birth is the safest routine for mother and fetus.

ABNORMAL LABOR

This chapter deals primarily with APGO Objective(s):

OBJECTIVE 23   Abnormal Labor

A. Describe the causes, labor patterns, evaluation, and management of the abnormal labors, fetopelvic disproportion, and abnormal fetal presentations.

B. Describe the indications, contraindications and management of oxytocin (Pitocin) augmentation and induction of labor; for vaginal birth after cesarean delivery.

C. Describe the maternal and fetal complications resulting from abnormal labor and presentations.

(Continued)

D. Describe the management of labor emergencies, including breech presentation, shoulder dystocia, and umbilical cord prolapse.

Abnormal labor, or *dystocia* (literally, "difficult labor or childbirth"), results when anatomic or functional abnormalities of the fetus, the maternal bony pelvis, the uterus and cervix, and/or a combination of these interfere with the normal course of labor and delivery. The diagnosis and management of dystocia is a major health care issue, because more than one fourth of all cesarean deliveries are performed for this indication.

Abnormal labor describes complications of the normal labor process: *slower-than-normal progress (protraction disorder)* or a *cessation of progress (arrest disorder).* The patterns of abnormal labor are summarized in Table 7.1. Less specific terms have also been applied to abnormal labor patterns and remain in common usage. "*Failure to progress*" describes lack of progressive cervical dilation and/or descent of the fetus and is similar to both protraction and arrest disorders. "*Cephalopelvic disproportion*" is a disparity between the size or shape of the maternal pelvis and the fetal head, preventing vaginal delivery, and is similar to an arrest disorder. This may be caused by the size or shape of the pelvis and/or the fetal head, or a relative disparity as a result of malpresentation of the fetal head.

TABLE 7.1. Abnormal Labor Patterns

Prolonged latent phase
  No progress from latent to active phase of labor
    > 20 hr for nulliparas
    > 14 hr for multiparas
Protraction disorders
  Prolonged active phase of labor such that
    Cervical dilation proceeds at
      < 1.2 cm/hr for nulliparas
      < 1.5 cm/hr for multiparas
    Descent of the presenting part proceeds at
      < 1 cm/hr for nulliparas
      < 1.5 cm/hr for multiparas
Arrest disorders
  Secondary arrest of dilation: no cervical dilation for > 2 hr for nullipara or multipara in the active phase of labor
  Arrest of descent: no descent of the presenting part in > 1 hr in second stage of labor

CAUSES OF ABNORMAL LABOR

Correct diagnosis and management of abnormal labor requires evaluation of the mechanisms of labor: in classic terms, the "power," the "passenger," and the "passage," otherwise referred to as the uterine contractions, fetal factors (e.g., presentation and size), and the dimensions of the maternal pelvis, respectively.

Evaluation of the "Power"

The power, or *strength, duration, and frequency of uterine contractions,* may be evaluated both qualitatively and quantitatively. Frequency and duration of contractions can be subjectively evaluated by *manual palpation of the maternal abdomen during a contraction.* Strength of uterine contractions is often judged by how much the uterine wall can be "indented" by an examiner's finger during a contraction: strong contraction, no indentation; moderate contraction, some indentation; mild contraction, considerable indentation.

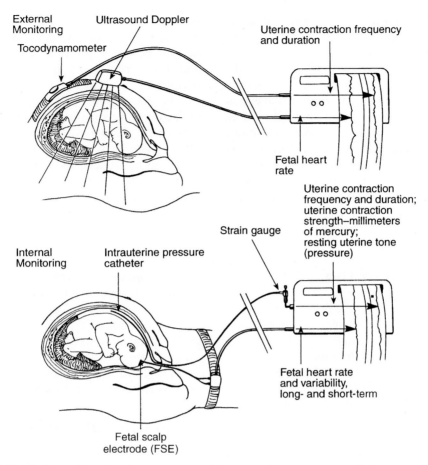

External Monitoring
Tocodynamometer
Ultrasound Doppler
Uterine contraction frequency and duration
Fetal heart rate
Uterine contraction frequency and duration; uterine contraction strength–millimeters of mercury; resting uterine tone (pressure)
Strain gauge
Internal Monitoring
Intrauterine pressure catheter
Fetal heart rate and variability, long- and short-term
Fetal scalp electrode (FSE)

FIGURE 7.1. Tocodynamometers and intrauterine pressure catheters.

Although subjective, such determinations by an experienced examiner are of some value. The frequency and duration of uterine contractions may be measured more accurately by using a *tocodynamometer* while performing external electronic fetal monitoring. A tocodynamometer is an external strain gauge, which is placed on the maternal abdomen; it records when the uterus tightens and relaxes, and for how long, but does not directly measure how much force the uterus is generating (i.e., strength) for a given contraction.

The actual pressure generated within the uterus cannot be directly measured without the use of an *internal* or *intrauterine pressure catheter* (IUPC). To use an IUPC, the physician introduces into the uterine cavity a narrow flexible tube that is attached to a strain gauge. The actual intrauterine pressure is transmitted through the tubing to the strain gauge, which then records the duration and frequency, as well as the strength, of the contractions in millimeters of mercury (Figure 7.1).

For cervical dilation to occur, each contraction must generate at least 25 mm Hg of peak pressure, with 50 to 60 mm Hg being considered the optimal intrauterine contractile pressure. The frequency of contractions is also important in generating a normal labor pattern; a minimum of three contractions in a 10-minute period is usually considered adequate. The expression "Montivedeo units" refers to the product of the number of contractions per 10 minutes times the average intensity (above baseline) of contractions as measured by the IUPC. Normal progress of labor is usually associated with 200 or more Montivedeo units. During the first stage of labor, arrest of labor should not be diagnosed until the cervix is at least 4 cm dilated (i.e., the latent phase of labor has been completed) and a pattern of uterine contractions adequate both in frequency and intensity has been established.

During the *second stage of labor,* the "powers" include both the uterine contractile forces and the voluntary maternal expulsive efforts (pushing). Maternal exhaustion, excessive anesthesia, or other conditions such as cardiac disease or neuromuscular disease may affect these combined forces so that they are insufficient to result in unassisted vaginal delivery. Forceps or vacuum-assisted vaginal delivery or cesarean delivery may then be required.

Evaluation of the "Passenger"

Evaluation of the passenger includes *clinical estimation of fetal weight and clinical evaluation of fetal lie, presentation, position, and attitude.* If a fetus has an estimated weight > 4000 to 4500 g, the incidence of dystocia, including shoulder dystocia or fetopelvic disproportion, is greater. Because ultrasound estimations of fetal weight are often inaccurate by as much as 500 to 1000 g, care must be taken to use such information in conjunction with the entire clinical assessment.

If the fetal head is asynclitic (turned to one side) or if the fetal head is extended, a larger cephalic diameter is presented to the pelvis, thereby increasing the possibility of dystocia. A *brow presentation* (occurring about 1 in 3000 deliveries) typically converts to either a vertex or face presentation, but, if persistent, causes dystocia requiring cesarean delivery. Likewise, a *face presentation* (about 1 in 600 to 1000 deliveries) requires cesarean delivery in most cases, although a mentum anterior presentation (chin toward mother's abdomen) may be delivered vaginally. In such cases with the chin beneath the pubis, the head may undergo flexion, rather than the normal extension, with subsequent delivery of the occiput over the perineum.

Persistent occiput posterior positions are also associated with longer labors (approximately 1 hour in multiparous patients and 2 hours in nulliparous patients). Occasionally, delivery from the occiput posterior position is not possible, and the vertex must be rotated to the occiput anterior position. The fetal head can be rotated manually or, if necessary, with forceps or vacuum. *In compound presentations, when one or more limbs prolapse alongside the presenting part* (about 1 in 700 deliveries), the extremity usually retracts (either spontaneously or with manual assistance) as labor continues. When it does not, or in the 15% to 20% of compound presentations associated with umbilical cord prolapse, cesarean delivery is required. When dystocia caused by the fetal position cannot be corrected either manually or with instruments, cesarean delivery is appropriate (Figure 7.2).

Fetal anomalies, including hydrocephaly and soft tissue tumors, may also cause dystocia. The use of prenatal ultrasound significantly reduces the incidence of unexpected dystocia for these reasons.

Evaluation of the "Passage"

Unfortunately, measurements of the bony pelvis are relatively poor predictors of successful vaginal delivery. This is because of the inaccuracy of measurements, as well as case-by-case differences, in fetal accommodation and mechanisms of labor. *Clinical pelvimetry* (i.e., manual evaluation of the diameters of the pelvis) cannot predict whether a fetus can successfully negotiate the birth canal, except in rare circumstances when the pelvic diameters are so small as to render the pelvis "completely contracted." X-ray or computed tomographic (CT) pelvimetry can be helpful in some cases, although the progress (or lack of progress) of descent of the presenting part in labor is the best test of pelvic adequacy. Before assuming that the bony pelvis is preventing vaginal delivery, adequate contractions must be ensured (see Table 3.1 and Figure 3.5). In addition to the bony pelvis, there are soft tissue etiologies of dystocia, such as a distended bladder or colon, an adnexal mass, a uterine fibroid, or an accessory uterine horn. In some instances,

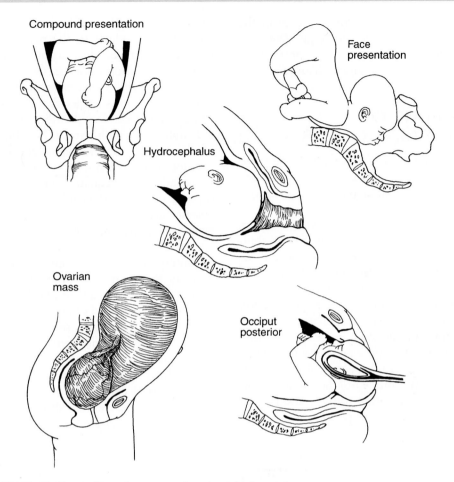

FIGURE 7.2.   Situations associated with dystocia.

epidural anesthesia may contribute to dystocia by decreasing the tone of the pelvic floor musculature.

EVALUATION OF ABNORMAL LABOR

Graphic documentation of progressive cervical dilation and effacement facilitates assessing a patient's progress in labor and identifying any type of abnormal labor pattern that may develop. Throughout labor, maternal and fetal well-being are continuously assessed along with the progress in labor. The mother, and all others present, should be provided emotional support and encouragement as the possibility of prolonged labor is faced and the various interventions are considered. Keeping the patient

and support person fully apprised of the situation is an important aspect of the management of potentially abnormal labor.

Each *pelvic examination* should provide the following information: dilation of the cervix in centimeters, percentage effacement of cervix, station of the presenting part, presence or absence of caput (molding of the fetal head), and position of the presenting part. The results of each examination are compared with previous examinations and any changes noted. In cases of failure of descent of the fetus, clinical reevaluation of the bony pelvis and its relationships to the fetus helps to identify the potential need for operative vaginal or cesarean delivery.

Uterine contractions can be assessed by manual palpation or by electronic tocomonitoring, as previously discussed. The uterine contraction pattern and/or the force of the contractions may be inadequate, either causing the abnormal labor pattern or resulting from a mechanical disorder.

PATTERNS OF ABNORMAL LABOR

Abnormal labor, or dystocia, is divided into prolongation disorders and arrest disorders. These abnormal labor patterns are demonstrated graphically in Figure 7.3.

A latent phase of labor exceeding 20 hours in a nulliparous patient or 14 hours in a multiparous patient is abnormal. The causes of such a *prolonged latent phase* of labor include abnormal fetal position, "unripe" cervix when labor commences, administration of excess anesthesia, fetopelvic disproportion, and dysfunctional/ineffective uterine contractions. The presence of a prolonged latent phase does not necessarily herald an abnormal active phase of labor. In addition, some patients who are initially thought to have a prolonged latent phase turn out only to have false labor. Although certainly of concern, particularly to the patient, a prolonged latent phase does not in itself pose a danger to the mother or fetus.

A *prolonged active phase* in the primigravid patient lasts longer than 12 hours or has a rate of cervical dilation of less than 1.2 cm/hr; for a multipara, 1.5 cm/hr. Causes of a prolonged active phase include fetal malposition, fetopelvic disproportion, excess use of sedation, inadequate contractions, and rupture of the fetal membranes before the onset of active labor. Risks associated with a prolonged active phase include an increase in operative vaginal deliveries or cesarean delivery, intrauterine infection, and fetal compromise. In the absence of nonreassuring fetal status, slow cervical dilation poses no threat to mother or fetus and can be allowed to progress. On the other hand, secondary arrest of dilation should be assessed promptly and acted upon appropriately.

In the multiparous patient, a prolonged active phase is defined as lasting more than 6 hours. Cervical dilation should occur at a rate of at least 1.5 cm/hr. Although a prolonged active phase is much less common in multiparous patients, the physician cannot be lulled into a false sense of security by the history of previous successful vaginal birth. Careful evaluation of all the factors is no less important in the multiparous patient than in the nulliparous patient.

Secondary arrest of dilation occurs when cervical dilation during the active phase of labor stops for 2 hours or more and is demonstrated by a flattening of the labor curve. Either dilation ceases because uterine contractions are no longer sufficient to maintain the progress of labor or labor arrests in spite of adequate uterine contractions, usually associated with too large a fetus, a fetal lie/position/attitude that prevents progress in labor, or a too small or abnormally shaped pelvis. Because ineffective contractions can be associated with mechanical factors such as disproportion and malpresentation, careful evaluation of all factors is necessary.

Active descent of the presenting part should occur progressively, beginning late in the first stage and throughout the second stage of labor. An "arrest of descent" over a

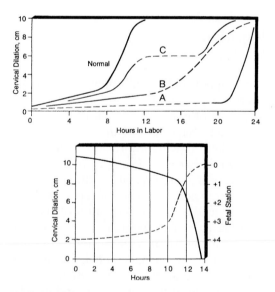

FIGURE 7.3. Abnormal labor. **Top,** Examples of labor patterns: *A,* prolonged latent phase; *B,* prolonged active phase; *C,* arrest of active phase. **Bottom,** Relation between descent of presenting part of fetus (*solid line*) and progressive dilation of cervix (*broken line*).

2-hour period is suggestive of either cephalopelvic disproportion or ineffective uterine contractions.

MANAGEMENT OF ABNORMAL LABOR

Induction of labor is the stimulation of uterine contractions before the spontaneous onset of labor, with the goal of achieving delivery. *Augmentation of labor* is the stimulation of uterine contractions that began spontaneously but are either too infrequent or too weak, or both. Stimulation of labor is usually carried out with intravenous oxytocin (Pitocin) administered as an intravenous piggyback solution by means of a metered pump. In this way, exact amounts of oxytocin may be given per minute. There are several regimens for oxytocin administration; two examples are presented in Table 7.2: a regular-dose oxytocin program and a low-oxytocin program. The use of an IUPC to document actual strength as well as frequency and duration of uterine contractions stimulated by oxytocin is often recommended once a regular contraction pattern has been established.

Prolongation of the first stage of labor can be minimized by avoiding unnecessary intervention; i.e., labor should not be induced when the cervix is not well prepared, or "ripe" (i.e., softened, anteriorly rotated, partially effaced). The degree of cervical ripening or readiness for labor is estimated by digital examination of the cervix.

The Bishop score has been used to try to quantify this determination (Table 7.3), and although not especially precise, it provides an excellent schema for cervical evaluation and a rough approximation of the likelihood of successful induction of labor and vaginal delivery.

Induction of labor is indicated if the anticipated benefits of delivery exceed the risks of allowing the pregnancy to continue. Therefore, careful evaluation of both mother and fetus is needed to make this decision. Currently, "elective" induction solely for convenience is controversial. Table 7.4 summarizes commonly cited indications and contraindications to labor induction.

When a cervix is not favorable, intravaginal *prostaglandin E$_2$ gel (dinoprostone)* has been used to ripen the cervix and, indeed, labor often ensues without the need of oxytocin stimulation. Dinoprostone is available in a retrievable polyester tape (Cervidil) or as a gel (Prepidil) with an insertion applicator. The former contains 10 mg dinoprostone, designed to release approximately 0.3 mg/hr over a 12 hour application. The tape can be removed if active labor ensues or if nonreassuring fetal or maternal events occur. The latter is designed for a 0.5 mg dose of gel that is given in shorter intervals, usually 4–6 hours. The main concern in the use of prostaglandin is uterine hyperstimulation, which in turn may cause uteroplacental insufficiency and, rarely, uterine rupture. Prostaglandins are relatively contraindicated in patients with

TABLE 7.2.	Oxytocin Administration for Induction and Augmentation of Labor		
Infusion	**Low Dose**	**Regular Dose**	
Initial IV infusion	1000 ml D$_5$LR	1000 ml D$_5$LR	
Piggyback infusion	20 U oxytocin in 1000 ml 0.9 N/S	20 U oxytocin in 1000 ml 0.9 N/S	
Initial infusion rate	1 mU/min	1 mU/min	
Interval and increment for increasing infusion rate	**1 mU q 30 min**	**1–2 mU q 15–30 min**	
Maximum infusion rate	**15–20 mU/min**	**Three contractions/10 min; no upper limit on infusion rate**	

TABLE 7.3. The Bishop Score for Cervical Status*

Factor	Points			
	0	1	2	3
Dilation	Closed	1–2 cm	3–4 cm	5+ cm
Effacement	0%–30%	40%–50%	60%–70%	80+%
Station	−3	−2, −1	0	+1, +2
Consistency	Firm	Medium	Soft	
Position	Posterior	Mid	Anterior	

*A score of 0 to 4 points is associated with the highest likelihood of failed induction; a score of 9 to 13 points is associated with the highest likelihood of successful induction.

TABLE 7.4. Induction of Labor: Common Indications and Contraindications

Indications	Contraindications
Post-term pregnancy	Placenta or vasa previa
Major maternal medical illnesses	Cord presentation
Fetal demise	Abnormal/unstable fetal lie
Suspected fetal compromise	Presenting part above inlet
Severe pregnancy-induced hypertension	Prior classical uterine incision
Premature rupture of membranes (at term)	Prior uterine incision of unknown type
Chorioamnionitis	Active genital herpes

concurrent asthma. Misoprostol is another cervical ripening agent as is insertion of *laminaria,* made from the stems of the seaweed *Laminaria japonica;* a synthetic form is also available. They are hygroscopic rods that are inserted into the internal cervical os. As the rods absorb moisture and expand, the cervix is slowly dilated (Figure 7.4). The risks associated with laminaria use include failure to dilate the cervix, cervical laceration, inadvertent rupture of the membranes, and infection.

A prolonged first stage of labor can be correctly diagnosed by accurately differentiating true labor from *false labor,* the latter being best treated with rest and sedation (Table 7.5).

A *prolonged latent phase* can be managed by either *rest* or *augmentation of labor* with intravenous oxytocin in a term pregnancy once mechanical factors have been ruled out. If the patient is allowed to rest, at times with the addition of intra-

muscular morphine sulfate, one of the following will occur: She will cease having contractions, in which case she is not in labor; she will go into active labor; or she will continue as before, in which case oxytocin may be administered to augment the uterine contractions. The use of *amniotomy,* or *artificial rupture of membranes,* is also advocated for patients with prolonged latent phase. It is believed that, after amniotomy, the fetal head will provide a better dilating force than would the intact bag of waters. In addition, there may be a release of prostaglandins, which could aid in augmenting the force of contractions. Before amniotomy is performed, the presenting part should generally be firmly applied to the cervix so as to minimize the risk of causing an umbilical cord prolapse. Amniotomy is usually performed with a thin, plastic rod with a sharp hook on the end. The end is guided to the open cervical os with the examiner's fingers, and the

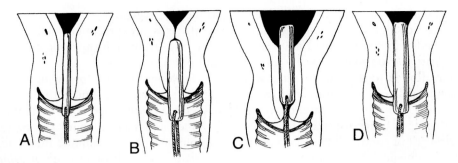

FIGURE 7.4. Use of laminaria. (*A*) Laminaria inserted properly just beyond the internal os. (*B* and *C*) Laminaria improperly inserted not far enough and too far, increasing the risk, respectively, of failure to dilate the cervix and inadvertent rupture of the membranes. (*D*) Properly placed laminaria that has expanded, causing cervical dilation.

TABLE 7.5. Differentiating Contractions of True and False Labor (Braxton Hicks Contractions)

True Labor	False Labor
Regular intervals, gradually increasing in frequency	Irregular intervals and duration
Increasing intensity	Intensity unchanged
Cervical dilation occurs	No cervical dilation
Back and abdominal discomfort	Lower abdominal discomfort
No relief from sedation	Relief from sedation

hook is used to snag and disrupt the amniotic sac. The clarity of the fluid should be noted and recorded, as well as the presence of meconium. The fetal heart rate (FHR) should be evaluated both before and immediately after rupture of the membranes.

During the *active phase of labor,* mechanical factors such as fetal malposition and malpresentation as well as fetopelvic disproportion must be considered before augmentation of uterine contractions with oxytocin. In cases in which the fetus fails to descend in the face of adequate contractions, disproportion is likely and cesarean delivery warranted. If no disproportion is present, oxytocin can be used if uterine contractions are judged to be inadequate. In cases of maternal exhaustion resulting in secondary arrest of dilation, rest followed by augmentation with oxytocin is often effective. If not already ruptured, artificial rupture of the membranes is also recommended.

Should fetal or maternal distress occur, prompt intervention is warranted. If this happens during the second stage of labor with the vertex low in the pelvis, forceps or a vacuum extractor can be used to effect a prompt vaginal delivery. In all other cases, cesarean delivery may be necessary. True nonreassuring status of either mother or fetus in the first stage of labor usually mandates cesarean delivery.

MANAGEMENT OF PROLONGED SECOND STAGE

In the past, a 2-hour second stage was considered an indication for cesarean delivery or operative vaginal delivery. Data now show that if the FHR is reassuring, it is safe to allow the mother to continue pushing in an attempt to accomplish vaginal delivery.

As long as both mother and fetus are doing well, the second stage of labor does not have to be concluded in any specific time frame. Should disproportion exist, no amount of extra time allotted to the second stage will allow vaginal delivery and cesarean delivery is necessary. If this is not the case, oxytocin may be used to improve the frequency and/or strength of contractions, especially if they are documented by intrauterine pressure catheter as being inadequate.

Bearing down efforts by the patient in conjunction with the uterine contractions help bring about delivery. Because this is the one phase of labor over which the patient has some control, emotional support and encouragement are of great importance. Labor positions other than the dorsal lithotomy, where the mother is to some extent pushing against gravity, may facilitate delivery. In addition, alternate positions may allow subtle changes in fetal presentation relative to the birth canal and bony pelvis, facilitating better accommodation to the birth canal and thereby vaginal delivery. The use of such positions (e.g., knee-chest, sitting, squatting, or birth-chair) requires the ability to continue needed fetal and maternal well-being monitoring, and the guidance of a physician or other clinician well versed in their use. Fetal accommodation may also be facilitated by allowing an epidural analgesia to "wear off," presumably associated with an increased tone of the pelvic floor muscles or an increased desire of the mother to push. In some cases, the use of an episiotomy may provide relief from the perineum that has resisted delivery. Similarly, forceps or vacuum extraction may be used to assist the necessary descent and rotation of the fetus, resulting in vaginal delivery.

RISKS OF PROLONGED LABOR

Prolonged labor can have deleterious effects on both fetus and mother. Maternal risks include infection, maternal exhaustion, lacerations, and uterine atony with possible hemorrhage. In addition, there are the attendant risks of any operative delivery, most especially maternal soft tissue injury to the lower genital tract and fetal trauma. Fetal risks of prolonged labor include asphyxia, trauma from difficult deliveries, and infection.

Prolonged labor (along with postdatism, growth restriction, and other situations associated with decreased amniotic fluid volume) is associated with the passage of meconium into the amniotic fluid and, subsequently, the risk of *meconium aspiration syndrome*. Fetuses who inhale meconium-stained fluid during labor or from the nasopharynx just after birth may suffer this syndrome, which includes both mechanical obstruction and chemical pneumonitis from the meconium material. Pathologic factors include atelectasis, consolidation, and barotrauma as well as some degree of direct removal of pulmonary surfactant by free fatty acids in meconium. In utero aspiration of meconium can also occur.

Intrapartum management of a patient with meconium-stained amniotic fluid may include *amnioinfusion*, by which a normal saline solution is slowly infused through a tube inserted into the uterine cavity, washing meconium-stained fluid out and replacing it with the saline solution. As the head is delivered, but before delivery of the fetal chest, careful suctioning of the nasopharynx and oropharynx should be performed. Postpartum examination of the area below the vocal cords of the neonate with a laryngoscope and suctioning out of meconium below the newborn's vocal cords, using an endotracheal tube, are also recommended procedures.

BREECH PRESENTATION

Breech presentation occurs in about 2% of singleton deliveries at term and more frequently in the early third and second trimesters. In addition to prematurity, other conditions associated with breech presentation include multiple pregnancy, polyhydramnios, hydrocephaly, anencephaly, uterine anomalies, and uterine tumors. The three kinds of breech presentation—*frank, complete, and incomplete breech* (Figure 7.5)—are diagnosed by a combination of Leopold maneuvers, pelvic examination,

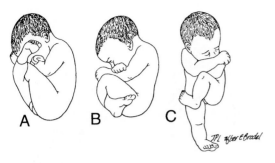

FIGURE 7.5. Breech presentations. (*A*) Frank breech. (*B*) Complete breech. (*C*) Incomplete breech, single footling.

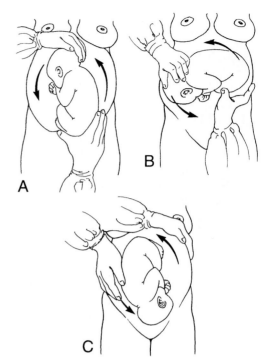

FIGURE 7.6. External cephalic version.

ultrasonography, and at times, other imaging techniques.

The morbidity and mortality rates for mother and fetus, regardless of gestational age or mode of delivery, are higher in the breech than in the cephalic presentation. This increased risk to the fetus comes from associated factors such as fetal anomalies, prematurity, and umbilical cord prolapse, as well as birth trauma.

Vaginal delivery of the preterm breech fetus weighing < 2000 g is avoided by many obstetricians because of concern about an increased risk of birth injury. Although the data to support this concern are contradictory, the practice of cesarean delivery for these smaller breech infants is common. At the other end of the spectrum, vaginal delivery of the term breech weighing > 4000 g is usually avoided, primarily because of concern about entrapment of the head after the vaginal delivery of the smaller body. Because of the wide margin of error in the estimated fetal weight (EFW) both by clinical estimation and by obstetrical ultrasonography, most recommend a cesarean delivery if the EFW is > 3800 g.

The risks of vaginal delivery of the breech at term or cesarean delivery for the breech are avoided in approximately half of appropriately selected cases by use of external cephalic version (Figure 7.6). Selection criteria include a normal fetus with reassuring fetal heart tracing, adequate amniotic fluid, presenting part not in the pelvis, no uterine operative scars, and no labor. The risks include placental abruption, cord accident, and uterine rupture. External version is more often successful in parous women. Whether to use tocolytics at the time of attempted version is controversial, but the use of anti-D immune globulin in D – women is recommended.

There are three types of vaginal delivery of the breech (Table 7.6). The keys to successful vaginal delivery of the term breech are appropriate selection of cases and patience during the delivery, allowing as much of the delivery as possible to be spontaneous.

The suggested criteria for a vaginal breech delivery include (*a*) a normal labor curve, (*b*) an estimated fetal weight between 2000 and 3800 g in the frank breech presentation, (*c*) a reassuring fetal heart tracing, (*d*) an adequate maternal pelvis by clinical pelvimetry (CT pelivmetry may also be employed), and (*e*) a normally flexed fetal head. Hyperextension of the fetal head occurs in about 5% of term breech fetuses, requiring cesarean delivery to avoid head entrapment. Because of the risk of umbilical cord prolapse, vaginal delivery of the footling breech is usually avoided. In the event of *cord*

TABLE 7.6.   Types of Vaginal Breech Deliveries

Total breech extraction
   Entire body extracted
Partial breech extraction
   Spontaneous delivery to umbilicus,
      remainder of body extracted
Spontaneous breech delivery
   No traction or manipulation of the
   fetus, which delivers
   spontaneously

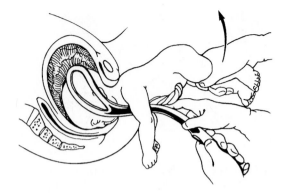

FIGURE 7.7.   Application of Piper forceps to the aftercoming head.

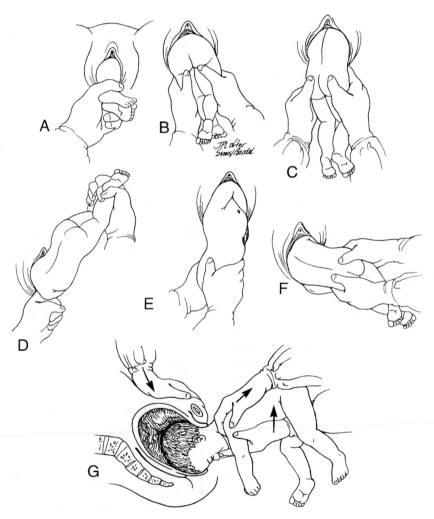

FIGURE 7.8.   Breech extraction. (*A–C*) Gentle traction on the feet and ankles, thighs, and pelvis. Note that traction is not applied above the pelvis. (*D*) Gentle traction and rotation as the scapulae become visible, sweeping the posterior and then anterior arm free in the process. (*E–G*) Mauriceau maneuver to deliver the head.

prolapse, the following steps should be taken: Place the mother in Trendelenburg position (head down); relieve pressure on the cord by pushing the fetal presenting part off of the umbilical cord; commence immediate plans for cesarean delivery.

The delivery of the aftercoming fetal head assisted with Piper forceps is shown in Figure 7.7, and the technique of breech extraction is presented in Figure 7.8.

INDICATIONS FOR OPERATIVE DELIVERY

Techniques of operative delivery include obstetric forceps, vacuum extraction, and cesarean delivery. Forceps are primarily used to supply traction to the fetal head to augment the forces expelling the fetus when the mother's voluntary efforts in conjunc-

tion with uterine contractions are insufficient to deliver the infant. Occasionally, forceps are used to rotate the fetal head before traction to complete the vaginal delivery. Forceps may also be used to control delivery of the fetal head, thereby avoiding any potentially precipitous delivery of the fetal head. Proper application of obstetric forceps by an experienced clinician is necessary to avoid the potential risk of trauma to both the maternal birth canal and the fetal head. Table 7.7 is a list of conditions necessary to apply forceps, and Table 7.8 is a classification of different types of forceps deliveries. Different types of forceps are available for different obstetric indications (i.e., rotations versus traction) and for different degrees of molding of the fetal head. Vacuum cups applied to the fetal head are sometimes used instead of forceps.

TABLE 7.7. Conditions for Operative Application

Cervix	Fully dilated
Membranes	Ruptured
Position and station of fetal head	Known and engaged
Anesthesia	Adequate for maternal comfort
Maternal pelvis	Evaluated and found adequate

TABLE 7.8. Forceps Classification*

Outlet forceps	The fetal skull has reached the perineal floor, the scalp is visible between contractions, the sagittal suture is in the anteroposterior diameter or in the right or left occiput anterior or posterior position, but not more than 45° from the midline
Low forceps	The leading edge of the skull is +2 station or more, rotation ≤ 45°
Midforceps	The head is engaged (0 station) but the leading edge of the skull is above +2 station

*The main controversy that has surrounded forceps delivery classification has been the definition of station used. Recently the American College of Obstetricians and Gynecologists (ACOG) redefined station for the purpose of forceps delivery classification, describing the leading bony point of the fetal head in centimeters at or below the level of the maternal ischial spines (0–+5) rather than the previously used system of thirds (0–+3).

CASE STUDIES

Case 7A

A 5-foot, 8-inch, 145-pound, 19-year-old G1 at 41 weeks' gestational age presents complaining of uterine contractions. Her antepartum course has been unremarkable; her fetus is active. Her fundal height is 40 cm, and her uterine contractions are occurring every 6 minutes and judged to be mild in intensity. Her estimated fetal weight is 8 lbs. Fetal heart tones are normal without abnormal decelerations. Pelvic examination shows the cervix to be 30% effaced and 1 cm dilated, with a cephalic part at −2 station, and membranes intact. Clinical pelvimetry is judged adequate.

Questions Case 7A

Which of the following are appropriate managements at this time?

A. Monitored labor
B. Ultrasound for fetal weight determination
C. Amniotomy
D. Cesarean delivery for fetopelvic disproportion
E. Patient discharged home with reassurance

Answer: A

The patient may or may not be in labor. Monitoring will help evaluate the pattern of uterine activity and the FHR. Because she is 41 weeks, there is more risk of uteroplacental insufficiency than there would have been 1 or 2 weeks earlier. Amniotomy is not advisable with a high presenting part. There is no indication for operative delivery, nor is it appropriate to send the patient home until it is known whether she is in labor and whether her

fetus demonstrates heart rate evidence suggestive of fetal compromise.

The patient develops regular, more intense uterine contractions and progresses to 6 cm dilation and 100% effacement with the vertex descending to −1 station. The head is felt to be right occiput transverse (ROT). Thereafter, uterine contractions become somewhat less intense and there is no further dilation for 2.5 hours. FHR monitoring continues to demonstrate a reassuring pattern. Your diagnosis at this time is

A. Prolonged latent phase
B. Prolonged active phase
C. Secondary arrest of labor
D. Cephalopelvic disproportion
E. Failure to progress

Answer: C

Components of your management should now include artificial rupture of membranes, along with

A. Fetal scalp electrode (FSE) application
B. Intrauterine pressure catheter insertion
C. X-ray pelvimetry
D. Pelvic ultrasonography

Answer: B

The passage and passenger are thought to be large enough and not too large, respectively. You must now assess the power (i.e., the strength as well as frequency and duration of uterine contractions). An FSE is commonly applied concurrent with rupture of the membranes and placement of an IUPC.

Artificial rupture of membranes is performed with appreciation of clear amniotic fluid. The cervix remains 6 cm dilated and the ROT vertex is at –1/–2. An IUPC and FSE are placed. Uterine contractions are found to be occurring every 4 to 5 minutes, lasting 30 seconds and generating 25 to 35 mm Hg of peak pressure. The FHR remains reassuring. Your best management now is

A. Fetal scalp blood sampling
B. Forceps delivery
C. Cesarean birth
D. Induction of labor
E. Augmentation of labor

Answer: E

Without a nonreassuring FHR pattern, fetal scalp sampling is unnecessary. Likewise, without evidence of fetal distress, operative delivery—transabdominal or transvaginal—is not indicated. You cannot induce labor because it is spontaneously begun. Augmentation is appropriate.

Pitocin augmentation is begun and continued for 5 hours; for the last 3 hours the IUPC shows 60 to 80 mm Hg uterine contractions that are occurring every 3 to 4 minutes and lasting 60 to 75 seconds. The resting uterine pressure is 15 mm Hg. The FHR remains reassuring. Over this 5-hour period, pelvic examination shows no change in cervical dilatation and that a large caput developed in the 4th to 5th hours. Your best management now is

A. Fetal scalp blood sampling
B. Forceps delivery
C. Cesarean birth
D. Induction of labor
E. Augmentation of labor

Answer: C

Operative vaginal delivery is contraindicated by dilation and station. Augmenta-tion has been successful in that an adequate mechanism of labor has been demonstrated for 4+ hours without progress.

Case 7B

A 31-year-old G2 P1001, who delivered an 8.5-lb son vaginally 8 years ago, presents at term in active labor and progresses rapidly to complete dilation. She then begins to push. After 2 hours of monitored labor, the vertex has progressed from –1 station to +1 station but with a prominent caput succedaneum noted. The FHR pattern is reassuring.

Question Case 7B

Which of the following are appropriate next steps in this patient's management?

A. Forceps delivery
B. Cesarean delivery
C. Continued monitored labor
D. Augmentation with oxytocin

Answer: C

After this patient has had a second stage of labor prolonged beyond the traditional 2-hour limit, there has been some descent from –1 to +1 station. Continued monitored labor is appropriate if clinical evaluation indicates that the fetus is not macrosomic or malformed or there is no obvious fetopelvic disproportion. If either is the case, cesarean delivery would be appropriate. Augmentation of the contractions would be appropriate if they were inadequate in frequency or intensity. Forceps delivery would be appropriate if either maternal or fetal condition warranted delivery and the fetus was in a position to be so delivered. In this case, at +1 station with caput succedaneum present, it is unlikely to be deliverable with forceps.

(Continued)

Case 7C

A 38-year-old G5 P4004 at term arrives in active labor, 5 to 6 cm dilated and 90% effaced with a presenting part at −1 station, and intact membranes. She has had no prenatal care and four previous vaginal deliveries of four boys all weighing 8.5 to 9 lb.

Because there are variable decelerations and a questionable loss of long-term variability, artificial rupture of membranes is performed, at which time the patient is found to have a frank breech presentation, now 7 cm dilated with the breech at −1 station. The FHR is now reassuring. Contractions are strong, occurring every 3 minutes.

Question Case 7C

Your best management would be

A. External version
B. Internal version
C. Piper forceps delivery
D. Cesarean birth
E. Monitored labor

Answer: E

There is debate of the propriety of vaginal breech delivery. Some physicians believe that the morbidity is too great for this procedure and opt for cesarean birth for all breech deliveries. Others will allow vaginal delivery of the breech in selected cases.

CHAPTER

INTRAPARTUM FETAL SURVEILLANCE

TABLE 8.1. Criteria for Diagnosis of Fetal Asphyxia

Any neonate who had hypoxia proximate to delivery severe enough to result in hypoxic encephalopathy will show other evidence of hypoxic damage, specifically including *all* of the following. The diagnosis of fetal asphyxia is unlikely unless all four criteria are met.

1. Metabolic or mixed acidemia (pH < 7.00) on an umbilical cord arterial sample, if obtained
2. Persistent Apgar scores of 0–3 for longer than 5 min
3. Evidence of neonatal neurologic sequelae such as seizures, coma and hypotonia
4. One or more of the following: cardiovascular, gastrointestinal, hematologic, pulmonary, or renal system dysfunction

Evidence suggesting a *nonreassuring fetal status* occurs in 5% to 10% of pregnancies, when there is concern that the function of the maternal-fetal physiologic unit is so altered that fetal death or serious injury may occur. The term *fetal distress* is also often used for this situation, but the term is imprecise and nonspecific, having a low positive predictive value even in high-risk situations and often being associated with a neonate that shows no evidence of intrauterine compromise as measured by Apgar scores and blood gas studies. Furthermore, when delivery is facilitated because of a nonreassuring fetal status, the delivery of a vigorous infant is not inconsistent. When, however, an infant is born with clinical evidence of intrauterine fetal compromise, the term *fetal asphyxia* should be used to describe the infant's status only when the situation fits the criteria suggested in the *Guidelines for Prenatal Care* of the American College of Obstetricians and Gynecologists (Table 8.1), although the presence of these criteria does not alone make the diagnosis of neonatal asphyxia. Thus, when this concern arises, the term *nonreassuring fetal status* associated with whatever findings elicit the comment should be used rather than *fetal distress*.

It is the task of the obstetric team to recognize this situation and to intervene as needed to avoid or minimize injury to the fetus. The decision to intervene is often difficult, because fetal heart rate (FHR) monitoring and fetal acid-base measurement are sometimes difficult to interpret. To help interpret these indirect measures of nonreassuring fetal status, the obstetric team correlates the intrapartum status with the patient's antepartum information, including historical risk factors (e.g., hypertension, maternal smoking), physical examination information (e.g., hypertension, fetal size), laboratory information (e.g., glucose tolerance data, ultrasound examinations), and dynamic testing information [e.g., biophysical profile determinations, nonstress test (NST), oxytocin challenge (OCT) testing]. When interpreting this information, the obstetric team is especially alert for items that are known to predispose to the *three categories of causes of nonreassuring fetal status:* uteroplacental insufficiency, umbilical cord compression, and fetal conditions/anomalies (Table 8.2).

The *uteroplacental unit* provides oxygen and nutrients to the fetus while receiving carbon dioxide and wastes, the products of the normal aerobic fetal and placental metabolisms. *Uteroplacental insufficiency* occurs when the uteroplacental unit starts to fail at this task. Initial fetal responses include fetal hypoxia; shunting of blood flow to the fetal brain, heart, and adrenal glands; and transient, repetitive late decelerations of the FHR. *If the cause of the fetal hypoxia is progressive and is not recognized and corrected, fetal respiratory and then metabolic acidosis can ensue. These patterns of nonreassuring fetal status are usually reversible either by altering the conditions of uteroplacental function or by rapid delivery of the infant.*

TABLE 8.2. Causes of Nonreassuring Fetal Status

Uteroplacental insufficiency	Placental edema
	Maternal diabetes
	Hydrops fetalis
	Rh isoimmunization
	Placental "accidents"
	Abruptio placentae
	Placenta previa ± accreta
	Postdatism
	Intrauterine growth restriction
	Uterine hyperstimulation
Umbilical cord compression	Umbilical cord accidents
	Umbilical cord prolapse or entanglement (gross, occult)
	Umbilical cord knot
	Abnormal umbilical cord insertion
	Anomalous umbilical cord
	Oligohydramnios (from any cause) with cord compression
Fetal conditions/anomalies	Sepsis (maternal/fetal; chorioamnionitis)
	Fetal congenital anomalies
	Intrauterine growth restriction
	Prematurity
	Postdatism

TABLE 8.3. Factors Determining the Apgar Score at 1 and 5 Minutes After Delivery

	Factors				
Score Assigned	Heart Rate	Respiratory Effort	Muscle Tone	Reflex Irritability	Color
0	Absent	Absent	Flaccid	No response	Blue, pale
1	< 100	Slow, irregular	Some flexion of extremities	Grimace	Pale body, blue extremities
2	> 100	Good, crying	Active motion	Vigorous crying	Completely pink

Interpretation: 7–10 normal; 4–7 mild to moderate neonatal depression; 0–4 severe neonatal depression.

Devised in 1952 by Dr. Virginia Apgar, an anesthesiologist, Apgar scores are a widely used measure of fetal status immediately after delivery. Their intended and main value is to determine the need for resuscitation. Five factors are rated on a three-point scale and the scores added, producing a final "Apgar" of 0 to 10 (Table 8.3). If delivery occurs promptly, the 1-minute Apgar score may be low, but the 5-minute score is usually high. If, however, the fetus continues to experience hypoxia, the time will come when the fetus will progressively switch over to anaerobic glycolysis, shunt more blood flow to vital organs, and progressively develop a metabolic acidosis superimposed on the respiratory one. Lactic acid accumulates as this process continues and progressive damage to vital organs occurs, especially the fetal brain and myocardium. At delivery, both the 1- and the 5-minute Apgar scores are often depressed, and if the intervention was not timely, serious and possibly permanent damage (and sometimes even death) results.

Fortunately, deleterious fetal acid-base changes are usually preceded by hypoxia manifest in FHR changes, which can be recognized by electronic monitoring or intermittent auscultation. Timely intervention is then usually possible once nonreassuring fetal status has been identified. The techniques of intrapartum monitoring are designed to discover this process as early as possible.

INTRAPARTUM MONITORING
Fetal Heart Rate Monitoring
METHODS OF FETAL HEART RATE EVALUATION

Before the popular use of electronic fetal monitoring (EFM), intermittent auscultation of the FHR after contractions was the technique used to assess intrapartum fetal well-being. With the use of EFM, FHR patterns have been identified and associated with various fetal conditions and prognoses. In the last few years, the now generalized use of these monitors has undergone re-evaluation. Continuous EFM of "high-risk patients" who have a predictable increased risk of intrapartum nonreassuring fetal status is usually not questioned. The value of EFM is questioned in "low-risk patients" whose risk of intrapartum nonreassuring fetal status is known to be small. Intermittent fetal heart rate auscultation, according to established guidelines for frequency of auscultation, is considered equally effective for these patients, although it is interesting that it is in this group of patients that the risk of unexpected nonreassuring fetal status is highest. During the

active phase of labor, the FHR should be evaluated at least every 15 minutes after a uterine contraction, with the frequency increasing to at least every 5 minutes in the second stage of labor.

FETAL HEART RATE

Fetal heart rates by EFM are described by rate and by pattern of variability. The techniques are described in Chapter 6. *The baseline FHR* ("normal FHR") at term is defined as 120 to 160 beats per minute (bpm), with slightly higher rates in preterm fetuses. *Baseline fetal tachycardia* is defined as >160 bpm for 10 or more minutes, and may be classified as mild if the baseline is between 161 and 180 bpm and severe if more than 181 bpm. Fetal tachycardia may be transient (usually <10 minutes) and without significance, although it is sometimes associated with situations that may require various interventions to avoid permanent fetal damage.

The most common cause of fetal tachycardia is elevated maternal temperature, which is often the first evidence of developing chorioamnionitis. Because the fetal oxygen-hemoglobin dissociation curve is adversely affected by increased temperature, a fetal tachycardia coupled with increased maternal temperature should prompt administration of antipyretics to the mother. If there is evidence of chorioamnionitis, antibiotic therapy is indicated.

Baseline fetal bradycardia is defined as less than 120 bpm for 10 or more minutes, and may be classified as moderate between 80 and 100 bpm and severe at less than 80 bpm. Heart rates between 100 and 119 bpm, although classified as a bradycardia, are rarely associated with fetal compromise unless accompanied by other evidence of nonreassuring fetal status. Fetal bradycardias may be associated with congenital heart block and with situations associated with severe fetal compromise such as placental abruption (Figure 8.1 and Table 8.4).

A *sinusoidal heart rate pattern* is when the rate is 120 to 160 bpm, but there is a smooth, undulating pattern of 5 to 10 bpm

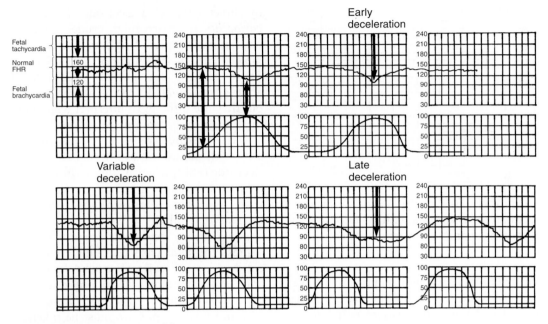

FIGURE 8.1.   Fetal heart rate patterns.

TABLE 8.4.   Baseline Fetal Heart Rates

Fetal Heart Rate (bpm)	Description	Associated Causes
> 160 for > 10 min	Fetal tachycardia	Maternal fever and infection Fetal infection Fetal anemia Maternal thyrotoxicosis Fetal tachyarrhythmias Maternal treatment with sympathomimetic or parasympatholytic (e.g., atropine) drugs Fetal immaturity Fetal hypoxia
120–160	Normal FHR	Normal function of maternal–fetal unit
< 120 for > 10 min	Fetal bradycardia	Maternal treatment with β-blockers (e.g., propranolol) Fetal congenital heart block (as in systemic lupus erythematosus, where an antibody may be produced that crosses the placenta and damages the conduction system of the fetus) Fetal anoxia

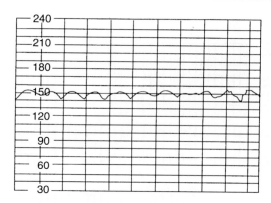

FIGURE 8.2. Sinusoidal fetal heart rate pattern associated with a fetal-maternal hemorrhage and severe fetal anemia.

in amplitude (very reminiscent of a sine wave) and shortened short-term variability (Figure 8.2). The cause of this pattern is unknown, although it has been associated with fetal anemia, Rh isoimmunization, and newborns with significant compromise. Sinusoidal-like patterns are sometimes seen after analgesic administration, so that the evaluation and treatment of this pattern are difficult. *Fetal arrhythmias* are seen in < 1% of monitored labors, are usually transient, and are diagnosed by fetal electrocardiography (ECG). If they persist, evaluation of the fetus for inherent pathology (especially hydrops and congenital anomalies) is indicated because some treatment may be needed with delivery or during the intrapartum period.

Fetal Heart Rate Variability

Fetal heart rate variability is the most reliable single EFM indicator of fetal status (fetal well-being). FHR variability results from a complex interplay of cardioinhibitory and cardioaccelerator centers in the fetal brain, which, in turn, are extremely sensitive to the fetal biochemical status (oxygenation and acid-base status). *The presence of good variability is highly suggestive of adequate fetal central nervous system (CNS) oxygenation.* Two types of variability are described (Figure 8.3). *Short-term variability* is the variation in amplitude seen on a beat-to-beat basis, normally 3 to 8 bpm, measured from R wave to R wave

by direct fetal scalp electrode. *Long-term variability* is an irregular, crude, wavelike pattern with a period of 3 to 5 cycles per minute and an amplitude of 5 to 15 bpm. These patterns are normally encountered after approximately 28 weeks' gestation, but they are difficult to interpret (especially their absence) before this gestational age.

Short-term variability is measurable only with the use of an internal fetal scalp electrode (FSE), whereas long-term variability may be measured, albeit not as well as with FSE, by Doppler measurement. Decreased variability is associated with fetal hypoxia and/or acidemia, drugs that may depress the fetal CNS (e.g., maternal narcotic analgesia), fetal tachycardia, fetal CNS and cardiac anomalies, prolonged uterine contractions (uterine hypertonus), prematurity, and fetal sleep. Care must be taken in the interpretation of decreased variability when a transient cause such as fetal sleep may be involved, lest an unnecessary intervention be considered.

Periodic Fetal Heart Rate Changes

The FHR may vary with uterine contractions by slowing or accelerating in periodic patterns. These changes in FHR are in response to two mechanisms: (*a*) intrinsic reflex FHR control, especially responses to hypoxia and acidemia as well as normal reflex responses; and (*b*) fetal myocardial hypoxia. Periodic FHR changes are classified into patterns based on their shape, magnitude (in beats per minute), and relationship to the same parameters of the uterine contractions with which they are associated. As indirect measures of fetal well-being, these patterns have some prognostic value in the antepartum and intrapartum evaluation of the fetus and in developing management plans (see Figure 8.1).

Accelerations of the FHR are defined as an increase in the FHR above the baseline of at least 15 bpm, usually of 15- to 20-second duration, and are associated with an intact fetal mechanism unstressed by hypoxia and acidemia. *FHR accelerations are, therefore, reassuring and usually indicative of fetal well-being.* Stimulation of the fetal scalp by

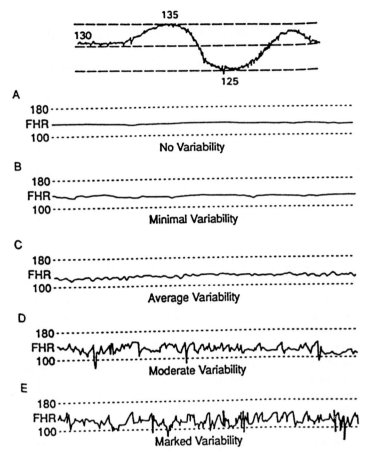

FIGURE 8.3.   Fetal heart rate variability. (*A*) Long-term variability. (*B–E*) Short-term variability.

digital examination usually engenders a heart rate acceleration in the uncompromised, nonacidotic fetus and is used by some obstetricians as a test of fetal well-being. External sound/vibration stimulation, also termed *acoustic stimulation,* elicits the same response and is also used for this purpose.

Early FHR decelerations are slowings of the FHR (never below 100 bpm) that begin as the uterine contraction begins, reach their nadir at the peak of the uterine contraction, and return to the baseline FHR with the end of the uterine contraction (i.e., mirror images of the uterine contraction). These early decelerations are the result of *pressure on the fetal head* (from the birth canal, digital examination, forceps application), causing a reflex response through the vagus nerve with acetylcholine release at the fetal sinoatrial node. This response may be

blocked with vagolytics such as atropine. *Early FHR decelerations are considered physiologic and are not a cause of concern.*

Variable FHR decelerations are slowings of the FHR that may start before, during, or after uterine contraction starts (hence, variable), but are characterized by a rapid fall in the FHR, often to below 100 bpm, and then a rapid return to baseline. These variable decelerations are also reflex mediated, usually associated with *umbilical cord compression* and mediated through the vagus nerve with sudden and often erratic release of acetylcholine at the fetal sinoatrial node, resulting in the characteristic sharp deceleration slope of these decelerations. Umbilical cord compression may result from wrapping of the cord around parts of the fetus, anomalies, or even knots in the umbilical cord, and is

TABLE 8.5.   Grading of Periodic Fetal Heart Rate Patterns

Pattern/Grade	Fall (bpm)	Duration (sec)
Variable		
Mild	Any value	< 30
Moderate	< 70	> 30, < 60
Severe	< 70	> 60
Late		
Mild	< 15	Any duration
Moderate	15–45	Any duration
Severe	> 45	Any duration

especially associated with oligohydramnios, in which the buffering space for the umbilical cord created by the amniotic fluid is lost. These variable decelerations are the most common periodic FHR pattern. They are often correctable by changes in the maternal position to relieve pressure on the umbilical cord. Infusion of fluid into the amniotic cavity (amnioinfusion) has also been used effectively to relieve pressure on the umbilical cord in cases of oligohydramnios or when rupture of membranes has occurred.

If the FHR falls below 100 bpm, a sterile vaginal examination is indicated to check for a prolapsed umbilical cord, a rare but emergent cause of the sudden development of this usually benign periodic FHR pattern. If the FHR falls below 60 to 70 bpm for more than 30 seconds, repetitive variable decelerations will often have a cumulative effect on fetal well-being, with the development of hypoxia, acidemia, and distress. If the FHR falls below 60 bpm, transient loss of fetal sinoatrial node function has been noted with transient "fetal cardiac arrest." These decelerations below 60 to 70 bpm require careful evaluation of cause. Both variable and late decelerations have been classified as mild, moderate, and severe, with the assertion that the risk of fetal hypoxia and acidosis increases with the degree of deceleration (Table 8.5).

Late FHR decelerations are slowings of the FHR that begin after the uterine contraction starts, *reach their nadir after the peak of the uterine contraction, and resolve to baseline after the uterine contraction is over* (i.e., also a mirror image of the contraction, but "late" relative to it). These late decelerations are viewed as significantly nonreassuring, especially if repetitive and most especially if associated with decreased variability. *Late decelerations are sometimes associated with uteroplacental insufficiency,* as a result of either decreased uterine perfusion or decreased placental function, and thus with decreased intervillous exchange of oxygen and carbon dioxide and *progressive fetal hypoxia and acidemia.* Therefore, they are associated with causes of uteroplacental insufficiency, including postdatism, placental abruption, maternal hypertension, maternal diabetes, maternal anemia, maternal sepsis, and problems with uterine contractions such as hyperstimulation or hypertonia.

Two mechanisms are postulated to associate late decelerations with fetal hypoxia and acidemia: chemoreceptor-mediated vagal reflex and hypoxic myocardial depression, or both. Intervention is usually required, the nature and timing depending on full evaluation of the maternal and fetal status. Certainly, the need to intervene increases with the progression of nonreassuring fetal status. One evaluation that is often used to help guide interventions is direct measurement of fetal acid-base status.

TABLE 8.6.	Normal Umbilical Cord and Fetal Scalp Blood Gas Values			
Umbilical Cord				
Venous	**Arterial**	**Values**		**Fetal Scalp**
7.34 ± 0.15	7.34 ± 0.15	pH		7.25–7.40
30 ± 15	15 ± 10	Po_2		15 ± 10
35 ± 8	45 ± 15	Pco_2		45 ± 15
5 ± 4	7 ± 4	Base deficit		7 ± 4

Measurement of Fetal Acid-Base Status

When the uteroplacental unit is functioning normally, even with the stress of uterine contractions, which cause a transient decrease in placental intervillous perfusion, fetal acid-base status is easily maintained in normal ranges. *Normal fetal acid-base status* is mirrored in the normal umbilical cord blood gas values at term (Table 8.6). When there is *uteroplacental insufficiency,* inadequate fetal oxygenation causes a switch from fetal aerobic to fetal anaerobic metabolism, resulting in the production of lactate and progressive fetal acidosis, compounding the deleterious effects of fetal hypoxia. Initially, the fetus responds by shunting blood flow to the brain and heart from other organs. With progressive hypoxia, late decelerations develop and, with the addition of acidosis, there is loss of beat-to-beat variability. Brain and myocardial damage follow, with subsequent high risk of other end-organ damage. When there are indicators of such an ominous situation (e.g., persistent late decelerations on EFM and decreased beat-to-beat variability), direct measurement of the fetal acid-base status is an option. The most common method is fetal scalp capillary blood gas or blood pH measurement.

FETAL SCALP pH/BLOOD GAS EVALUATION

The chorioamnion must be ruptured and the presenting part descended to allow access to the presenting fetal part through the cervical

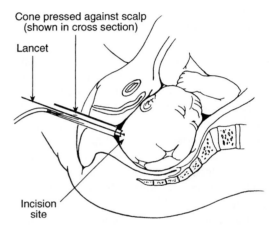

FIGURE 8.4. Fetal scalp blood sampling.

os, which must be dilated at least 2 to 3 cm. Given access to the fetal part, either head or breech, a plastic or metallic cone is inserted through the os and pressed against the fetal scalp. The scalp surface is thoroughly cleaned and the cone held with enough pressure to avoid dilution of the blood with amniotic fluid. A thin layer of silicone gel is often applied to the surface, serving to provide a smooth, uniform surface on which the blood droplet may form. A small incision is then made in the fetal scalp with a specialized lancet, and the drops of blood that form are collected in a heparinized capillary tube and analyzed. Pressure is applied to the incision site through one or two uterine contractions, until bleeding stops. Care must be taken not to make the incision over a fontanel or suture line. A caput succedaneum does not alter the pH information obtained (Figure 8.4).

TABLE 8.7. Classification of Neonatal Acidemia When Umbilical Cord pH is < 7.20

Type of Acidemia	P_{CO_2} (mm Hg)	HCO_3 (mEq/liter)	Base Deficit (mEq/liter)
Respiratory	≥ 65 (high)	> 17 (normal)	< 9 (normal)
Metabolic	< 65 (normal)	≤ 17 (low)	> 9 (high)
Mixed	≥ 65 (high)	≤ 17 (low)	> 9 (high)

Scalp blood samples are often difficult to interpret because absolute parameters that mandate specific interventions do not exist. Instead, as with other measures of fetal well-being, the information obtained must be correlated with the aggregate understanding of the status of the maternal-fetal unit at the time of the measure. Some general guidelines for the use of scalp pH include (a) a scalp pH greater than 7.25 is usually considered reassuring, requiring no further scalp sampling unless other measures of fetal well-being worsen; (b) a scalp pH between 7.20 and 7.24 raises concern about the possible development of fetal hypoxia/acidemia, and repeat scalp measurements usually are made within 15 to 30 minutes; (c) a scalp pH less than 7.20 means that fetal compromise is strongly expected, and interventions usually are required on an immediate basis to ameliorate the cause of the nonreassuring fetal status or to effect delivery. Determining whether the acidosis is respiratory, metabolic, or mixed in origin is often useful for management decisions (Table 8.7). Although a rare situation, maternal acidosis may complicate the evaluation of scalp pH results. For comparison, a free-flowing maternal venous sample may be evaluated for pH, with the fetal sample usually being approximately 0.1 pH unit below the maternal value.

FETAL OXYGEN SATURATION (FS$_p$O$_2$) MONITORING

Recently a modification of pulse oximetry technology has been introduced to intrapartum evaluation of fetal well being. A reflectance sensor is placed against the cheek (or forehead) of the fetus as an adjunct to fetal heart rate monitoring. The sensor contains LEDs emitting red and infrared light. Oxyhemoglobin weakly absorbs red light and strongly absorbs infrared light, and deoxyhemoglobin the opposite. A photodetector within the sensor captures reflected light and measures the absorption of each color. The data is used to determine the fraction of hemoglobin that is carrying oxygen, displayed as a percentage called *the fetal arterial oxygen saturation as determined by pulse oximetry (FS$_p$O$_2$)*. This information is displayed on the electronic fetal heart rate monitoring tracing (Figure 8.5). At present the normal range for FS$_p$O$_2$ in the term fetus in labor is thought to be 30% to 70%, with the critical threshold for a term infant believed to be 30% during labor. Values below 30% for more than ten minutes are thought to be associated with a predicted fetal scalp pH value of less than 7.20, decreasing by 0.02 pH units for each additional ten minutes below the threshold value. This technology is not presently recommended for routine intrapartum use, but rather, as an adjunct in term fetuses with nonreassuring FHR patterns. In this context FS$_p$O$_2$ data may be useful to determine which situation warrants expedited delivery (nonreassuring FHR tracing and FS$_p$O$_2$ value trending below 30%) and which (nonreassuring FHR tracing and FS$_p$O$_2$ value trending above 30%) may allow further monitored labor. As experience with this technology increases and data is accumulated to allow its use in fetuses of less than 36 weeks gestational age, its value and scope of uses may increase.

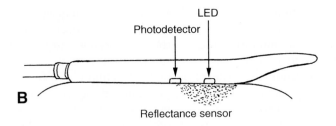

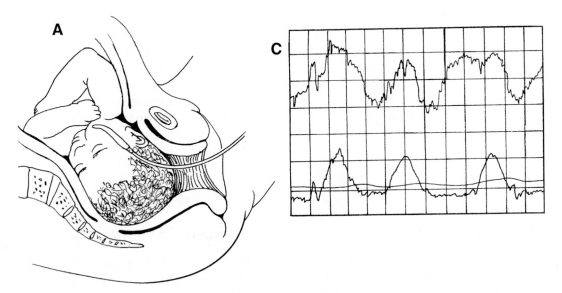

FIGURE 8.5.   Fetal oxygen saturation (FS_pO_2) monitoring. (*A*) Sensor in place against fetal cheek. (*B*) Reflectance sensor. (*C*) Electronic fetal heart rate monitor tracing with display of FS_pO_2 as a percentage.

MANAGEMENT

Interpretation of intrapartum fetal well-being measurements are made within the context of the entire obstetric situation, including maternal and fetal factors and the course and anticipated duration and outcome of labor. The number of variables to consider and the often imprecise nature of the information make these among the most difficult of medical decisions. In-depth training and experience in obstetrics are required to perform these complex tasks adequately.

Sometimes the FHR pattern demonstrates a single pattern. If it is reassuring, no intervention is needed; if it is not reassuring, the appropriate intervention is often clear. More often, however, the observed FHR pattern is a mixture of two more patterns and variations of baseline values. In these cases, it is usually prudent to manage the obstetric situation based on the most substantially nonreassuring of the patterns present.

In general, if there is evidence of progressive fetal hypoxia and acidosis in a situation where the time of vaginal delivery is remote, operative delivery by cesarean section is indicated for fetal reasons. Awaiting vaginal delivery is appropriate if, in the judgment of the obstetric team, vaginal delivery will occur soon enough that the progression of nonreassuring fetal status will not result in serious fetal injury and/or death, or when effective interventions to ameliorate the nonreassuring fetal status may be taken. In general, a scalp pH greater than 7.24 is reassuring; certainly, good variability on EFM is a reassuring factor. If meconium is present in the amniotic fluid, perinatal morbidity is increased by 5% to 10%, a condition that tends to dissuade continued labor when other evidence of nonreassuring fetal status is also present.

While awaiting vaginal delivery or while preparing for cesarean delivery, one or more of the following steps is appropriate: (a) discontinue oxytocin infusion that may have been started for induction or augmentation; (b) administer oxygen to the mother, usually 5 to 6 L/min by face mask; (c) check the maternal blood pressure, treating any hypotension with intravenous fluids and, if needed, pressors such as ephedrine;

(d) change the maternal position to left lateral position to decrease uterine pressure on the great vessels and thereby increase blood return to the heart, cardiac output, and uteroplacental blood flow; and (e) consider "intrauterine resuscitation," using an intravenous tocolytic (such as the β_2-sympathomimetic terbutaline, 0.25 mg I.V.P. or S.C.) to relax the uterine tone and slow the contraction rate, thereby increasing uteroplacental blood flow. Umbilical arterial and venous blood gases should be drawn immediately after the delivery from the cord attached to the placenta before placental separation. The data will help in the management of the newborn and shed light on the results of intrapartum interventions.

CASE STUDIES

Case 8A

Your patient is a 24-year-old G3 P2002 with an unremarkable antepartum course who presents at 41 weeks' gestational age having uterine contractions of increasing severity for 8 hours before being seen. On examination, the cervix is 3 to 4 cm, 80% effaced, −2 station; the fetus is in cephalic presentation with intact membranes. She is admitted, an intravenous line and appropriate laboratory studies are initiated, and external EFM is begun. After 30 minutes, the sample of EFM tracing seen in Figure 8A.1 is representative of her tracing.

Questions Case 8A

Which statement best describes the patient's intrapartum clinical situation?

A. FHR bradycardia and poor variability

B. FHR tachycardia and good variability

C. Normal FHR and good variability

D. Normal FHR and intermittent late decelerations

Answer: C

The baseline FHR is 120 to 125 bpm, within the normal range, and there is

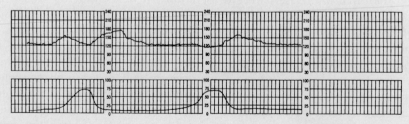

FIGURE 8A.1.

short- and long-term variability. There are no decelerations. This is a completely reassuring FHR tracing.

Labor continues for 4 hours and the patient's pelvic examination then shows 6 to 7 cm, 100%, 0 station. Membranes are artificially ruptured, an FSE and an intrauterine pressure catheter (IUPC) are placed, and after 15 minutes the patient is given 25 mg of meperidine intravenously for pain; 30 minutes later, the sample of EFM tracing seen in Figure 8A.2 is representative of her tracing. Which statement best describes the patient's intrapartum clinical situation?

A. FHR bradycardia and poor variability
B. Normal FHR and poor variability
C. Normal FHR, poor variability, and occasional variable decelerations
D. Normal FHR, poor variability, and occasional late decelerations

Answer: B

Apart from being 41 weeks' gestational age, there is no further historical information suggesting reasons for fetal distress. The patient's FHR tracing before the intra-

venous narcotic administration was normal, and the loss of variability after narcotic administration is consistent with narcotic effect. The single variable deceleration may be explained by pressure on the fetal head, which is at 0 station.

Labor continues for 3 hours, and the patient's pelvic examination then shows 9 to 10 cm, 100%, + 1 station. A representative sample of her EFM tracing at this time is seen in Figure 8A.3. Which statement best describes the patient's intrapartum clinical situation?

A. FHR tachycardia and poor variability
B. Normal FHR and poor variability
C. Normal FHR, poor variability, and occasional variable decelerations
D. Normal FHR, poor variability, and occasional late decelerations

Answer: D

This is a mixed pattern, with reassuring return of variability now that the narcotic effect is gone, but occasional late decelerations are noted. There is no indication for operative delivery because vaginal delivery may be expected in the near future in this multipara. Conservative interventions such as

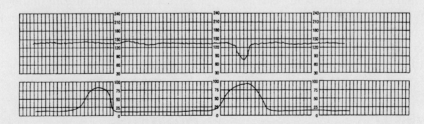

FIGURE 8A.2.

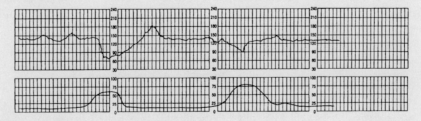

FIGURE 8A.3.

(Continued)

oxygen administration are indicated. Because she has had a previous cesarean section, and because of the intermittent late decelerations, close observation is indicated.

Case 8B

Your patient is a 17-year-old G1 at 39 weeks' gestation who presents with premature spontaneous rupture of membranes (clear fluid) after an antepartum course remarkable only for an iron deficiency anemia, which responded to hematemic therapy. After waiting 6 hours, you begin a Pitocin (oxytocin) induction of labor. The tracing seen in Figure 8B.1 is representative of her EFM trace 3 hours later, when the pelvic examination reveals a cervix dilated to 5 cm, 100%, vertex at 0/+1 station with a caput succedaneum, left occiput anterior (LOA), and the presence of the FSE and IUPC, which you placed before starting the induction.

Questions Case 8B

Which statement best describes the patient's intrapartum clinical situation?

A. Normal FHR baseline and variability without decelerations
B. Normal FHR baseline and variability with variable decelerations
C. Normal FHR baseline and decreased variability without decelerations
D. Normal FHR baseline and decreased variability with variable decelerations
E. Normal FHR baseline and decreased variability with late decelerations

Answer: D

Although there is a normal FHR, there is poor variability and severe variable decel-

erations. In a primigravida delivery, this loss of variability is not reassuring and intervention is indicated.

What is your best management now?

A. Continued monitoring, induced labor
B. Continued monitoring of labor, but discontinued induction
C. Fetal scalp blood sample
D. Forceps delivery
E. Cesarean birth

Answer: C

Continued labor without further evaluation of fetal well-being is inappropriate because the tracing is not reassuring. Repetitive late decelerations, and especially decreased variability, are associated with fetal compromise. Forceps delivery is impossible because the patient is not fully dilated. A case could be made for cesarean delivery in this patient remote from delivery, but the evidence of fetal compromise would not be sufficient for most obstetricians to proceed with cesarean birth. Fetal scalp sampling would provide more information on which to base a discussion.

A fetal scalp blood sample is performed. The pH is 7.13. The patient is still 5 cm dilated. What is your best management now?

A. Continued monitoring, induced labor
B. Continued monitoring of labor, but discontinue induction
C. Fetal scalp blood sample
D. Forceps delivery
E. Cesarean birth

Answer: E

There is now sufficient evidence of fetal compromise to warrant cesarean birth.

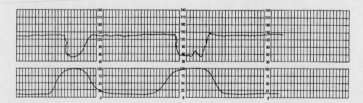

FIGURE 8B.1.

CHAPTER

IMMEDIATE CARE OF THE NEWBORN

CHAPTER OBJECTIVES

This chapter deals primarily with APGO Objective(s):

OBJECTIVE 13 Immediate Care of the Newborn

Explain the assessment of newborn status and immediate postpartum care of the newborn, including situations requiring immediate intervention.

Ninety percent of the over 4 million deliveries in the United States each year occur in hospitals equipped with sophisticated nurseries that include neonatologists. The delivering physician should be familiar with the initial assessment and immediate care of the newborn. Resuscitative efforts may be necessary in up to 5% of all cases of cesarean delivery and 2% of vaginal deliveries. The frequency of the need for these efforts increases in circumstances such as low-birth-weight infants and meconium staining. It is optimal to have highly trained personnel available in circumstances in which neonatal resuscitation is anticipated. Transport of the newborn in utero (i.e., maternal transport to a facility with more highly skilled clinicians and equipment) is appropriate in some cases. In other situations, personnel may be called to the delivery site on a stand-by basis. Table 9.1 lists some of these clinical situations.

TABLE 9.1. Examples of Cases That May Require Neonatal Resuscitation

Cesarean delivery
Non-reassuring fetal heart rate tracing
$FS_pO_2 < 30\%$ for more than 10 minutes in a term fetus
Moderate or thick meconium-stained amniotic fluid
Known or suspected fetal anomaly
Delivery of low-birth-weight infant
Maternal fever
"Difficult" delivery (e.g., breech delivery, shoulder dystocia)
Multiple gestation
Maternal diabetes

INITIAL ASSESSMENT

Once the newborn has been delivered, it is transported to the warming unit, which is equipped with a radiant heat source. The neonate is dried well to minimize evaporation and drop in core temperature. The nose and oropharynx are suctioned once again as the infant is placed in the supine position with the head lowered and turned to one side. The newborn is expected to both breathe and cry within the first 30 seconds of life. Suctioning as well as mild stimulation of the infant by rubbing the back or rubbing the sole of the feet help to stimulate the infant.

The initial evaluation of the infant is carried out at 1 and 5 minutes, using the Apgar scoring system (Table 9.2). The Apgar score is designed as a quick assessment of the newborn and should not be used to define birth asphyxia. These scores should not be used to identify the cause of the newborn's depression, nor can they be used to predict long-term neurologic outcome. In general, a low 1-minute Apgar identifies the newborn that requires particu-

TABLE 9.2. Apgar Scoring System

Sign	Score		
	0	1	2
Heart rate	Absent	< 100	> 100
Muscle tone	Limp	Some flexion of extremities	Active motion
Respiratory effort	Absent	Slow, irregular	Good cry
Reflex activity response to stimulation	No response	Grimace	Cough, sneeze, or crying
Color	Blue or pale	Body pink and extremities blue	Completely pink

lar attention. The 5-minute Apgar can be used to evaluate the effectiveness of any resuscitative efforts that have been undertaken. Apgar scores at 10, 15, and multiples thereof in minutes are also often recorded. The Neonatal Resuscitation Program (NRP) of the American Academy of Pediatrics and the American Heart Association recommend the assignment of Apgar scores every 5 minutes until 20 minutes or until two scores of 8 or greater are obtained. While not part of the original Apgar scoring system, many clinicians find these continued assessments of the newborn to be of value in ongoing clinical management.

Apgar scores of 7 to 10 are indicative of an infant who requires no active resuscitative intervention; scores of 4 to 7 are considered indicators of mildly to moderately depressed infants. Severely depressed infants with Apgar scores of less than 4 rarely require a full evaluation using the Apgar score. Instead, immediate resuscitative efforts are started, which may include endotracheal intubation and suctioning with the possible use of positive pressure oxygen.

The assessment of newborn metabolic well-being may also be done by an analysis of the umbilical cord blood gases. A 10- to 15-cm segment of umbilical cord is doubly clamped and cut so that it may be taken for assessment of pH, PO_2, PCO_2, and bicarbonate. It should be remembered that in the fetus freshly oxygenated blood from the placenta travels to the fetus through the umbilical vein while blood metabolized by the fetus travels back to the placenta through two umbilical arteries. Accordingly, the most meaningful assessment of metabolic status of the baby at the time of delivery is through analysis of umbilical artery blood gases. Normal values for umbilical arterial and venous samples are given in Table 9.3.

Acidemia is generally accepted as an increase in hydrogen ion concentration in an umbilical arterial sample resulting in a pH of less than 7.20. Further, asphyxia is usually defined as a combination of hypoxia and/or hypercarbia of sufficient level to produce metabolic acidosis. The terms acidemia, acidosis, and asphyxia should be used carefully when applied to the newborn condition because each term defines a series of changes that may or may not represent true metabolic compromise.

Meconium Staining of the Amniotic Fluid

Ten to fifteen percent of all fetuses and over twenty-five percent of postterm fetuses pass meconium (fecal material) in utero, in some cases in association with fetal stress albeit in others simply as a natural process. The amniotic fluid is then termed "meconium stained," and is often graded from thin to thick and particulate. About one third of infants born with meconium in the amniotic fluid will have meconium in the lungs, about one half will have abnormal chest x-rays, and about one tenth will develop significant respiratory distress. The latter situation is called "*meconium aspiration syndrome.*" Meconium aspiration syndrome may include mechanical obstruction and/or severe chemical pneumonitis associated with atelectasis, consolidation, and barotrauma, some degree of direct removal of pulmonary surfactant by free fatty acids in meconium, and/or persistent pulmonary hypertension. Ventilatory support and intensive medical management are often required, and the syndrome is associated with significant morbidity and mortality, the latter approaching 10%–20% in some series.

TABLE 9.3. Normal Umbilical Cord Blood Gas Values

	Arterial	Venous
pH	7.25–7.30	7.30–7.40
PCO_2 mm Hg	50	40
PO_2 mm Hg	20	30
Bicarbonate mEq/h	25	20

PCO_2 = carbon dioxide partial pressure;
PO_2 = oxygen partial pressure.

Meconium aspiration syndrome was thought to be caused primarily by the aspiration of meconium material, especially when the meconium was the thick, particulate variety. Nowadays, some degree of hypoxic antepartum or intrapartum stress is felt by many clinicians to be associated as well. In any event, two kinds of intervention are commonly used in an attempt to prevent meconium aspiration. The first is *amnioinfusion*, the slow infusion of normal saline into the uterus through a tube inserted through the open cervix during labor. The basic idea of the procedure is to "wash out" meconium from the amniotic fluid, replacing it with the saline fluid so as to decrease the amount and quality of meconium available for in utero and/or newborn aspiration. Further, in many situations the presence of meconium is associated with oligohydramnios, which is in turn associated with intermittent umbilical cord compression, decreased uteroplacental perfusion and progressive hypoxia, and fetal gasping in utero. Amnioinfusion may reverse this series of events. The second involves management of the airway immediately after birth, including immediate examination of the area below the vocal cords after birth and aspiration of any meconium material with an endotracheal tube. This procedure is generally recommended when the meconium is thick and particulate or in any situation where the infant is depressed, requiring positive pressure ventilation. In cases where the meconium is thin and light, clinical judgment is required, but many clinicians limit intervention to careful suctioning of the oropharynx.

Neonatal Asphyxia

The neonate for whom the diagnosis of neonatal asphyxia applies is characterized by significant newborn depression associated with severe hypoxia and a mixed respiratory and metabolic acidosis. Those who survive may have damage to one or more organ systems. Causes of neonatal asphyxia may include such situations as severe maternal disease, decreased uteroplacental blood flow, and trauma. Most neonates developing multiorgan failure have had neonatal asphyxia, but not all neonates having neonatal asphyxia proceed to permanent multiorgan damage.

The American College of Obstetricians and Gynecologists has suggested that the diagnosis of neonatal asphyxia is extremely unlikely unless four criteria are met: (1) Apgar scores less than 4 at 5 minutes of life, (2) umbilical artery pH less than 7.00, (3) neuromuscular signs and symptoms soon after birth (including seizures, coma, hypotonia), and (4) multiorgan system failure. The presence of these criteria does not alone make the diagnosis of neonatal asphyxia. When these criteria are present, the long-term prognosis of the neonate is uncertain, with long-term follow-up requisite to make a final determination.

ROUTINE CARE OF THE NEWBORN
Estimation of Gestational Age

A rapid overview of the gestational age of the newborn helps facilitate more highly skilled care if the newborn is felt to be premature. Table 9.4 provides guidelines for a rapid assessment using five measurements.

Umbilical Cord

The umbilical cord loses its bluish-white appearance within the first 24 hours after delivery. After clamping, the cord is normally not covered so that it may be exposed to air, thereby drying and separating more quickly. After a few days, the blackened, dried stump sloughs, leaving the granulating wound.

Urine and Stool

Over 90% of newborns pass stool within the first 24 hours. A congenital abnormality such as imperforate anus may be suspected if a stool has not been passed during the

TABLE 9.4. Estimation of Newborn Gestational Age			
	Estimated Gestational Age		
Anatomic Site	**≤ 36 weeks**	**37–38 weeks**	**≥ 39 weeks**
Scalp hair	Fine/fuzzy	Fine/fuzzy	Coarse
Ear lobe	No cartilage	Some cartilage	Thick cartilage
Breast nodule	2 mm	4 mm	6 mm
Sole creases	Anterior transverse crease	Creases across anterior 2/3s	Extensive creases covering the sole
Scrotum	Few rugae	Intermediate rugae	Extensive rugae

first 36 hours of life. Voiding typically occurs shortly after birth. Concern about a congenital defect of the urinary tract is appropriate if voiding has not occurred within the first day of life.

For the first two or three days of life, the stool is greenish-brown. Initially, the stools are sterile, but after the first few hours of life, bacteria can be found. With the ingestion of milk, the stool becomes more light/yellow and semi-solid.

Nutrition

It is recommended that nursing begin within the first 12 hours of delivery. Although growth-restricted or preterm infants require more frequent feedings, most term infants do well with feedings at 4-hour intervals. It is recommended that the infant be allowed to attempt to breast-feed at least five to ten minutes initially, with more time required, depending on various circumstances. Encouraging breast-feeding should be one of the focuses of prenatal education because of the biologic and emotional benefits that may be derived for both mother and newborn. Support for breast-feeding can be provided both through health clinicians in the hospital and outpatient facilities as well as support groups such as the LaLeche League.

As a result of the newborn's initial loss of urine, feces, and sweat, and because of the relative lack of nutrition in the first few days of life, newborn weight loss of less than 10% of birth weight should be anticipated. Of note, preterm newborns lose relatively more weight while regaining it at a slower rate than their term counterparts. Weight loss is usually regained in the first one to two weeks of life.

Conjunctivitis

Organisms such as N. gonorrhea, *Chlamydia*, and other bacteria may cause conjunctivitis in the newborn. In most states, application of silver nitrate as a prophylactic measure is required. In addition, various antibiotics have been used to manage the emerging resistant bacterial strains encountered.

Jaundice

Physiologic jaundice of the newborn (icterus neonatorum) occurs in up to one third of all newborns. Bilirubin levels of term infants may double to 5 mg/dl by the third or fourth day of life. It is at this level that jaundice becomes clinically apparent.

CASE STUDIES

Case 9A

A term infant is born by spontaneous vaginal delivery almost immediately on arrival in the labor unit. The infant is covered with meconium fluid, is limp, has a heart rate of 100, and only a grimace with stimulation.

Question Case 9A

Your management of the newborn will include

A. Oxygen by face mask
B. Intubation
C. Warming
D. External cardiac massage
E. Blood gas sampling
F. Stimulation

Answer: B, C, F

Intubation and removal of any meconium in the nasopharynx and below the cords is important to avoid meconium aspiration syndrome, especially in this situation where it is highly likely that positive pressure ventilation will be required. In this situation, such ventilation might drive meconium material deeper into the newborn respiratory tree worsening the risk and/or course of a subsequent meconium aspiration syndrome. Stimulation, warming, and oxygen in the interval immediately after birth as needed after aspiration of meconium are the first appropriate steps.

Case 9B

A term newborn is evaluated and found to have a heart rate of 110, irregular respirations, some flexion of its extremities, no reflexes, and a pale color.

Questions Case 9B

The newborn's Apgar score is

A. 2
B. 4
C. 6
D. 8

Answer: B

In assessing a newborn, the Apgar score is given for each of the five criteria. In this case, because the heart rate is greater than 100, 2 points are given. Slow, irregular respirations and some flexion of the extremities provide 1 point each. A lack of reflexes and a pale color each provide no points, for a total of 4.

Neonatal resuscitative efforts are provided to this infant. At the 5-minute assessment, the heart rate is now 120, respirations are strong, and the baby is crying loudly. There is active motion of all four extremities. The newborn is pink, with only bluishness of the extremities. It is sneezing and coughing. What is its 5-minute Apgar?

A. 6
B. 7
C. 8
D. 9

Answer: D

All of the parameters suggest 2 points for each category except color. In this case, 1 point is taken away for cyanotic extremities. The Apgar score is 9 at 5 minutes.

10

POSTPARTUM CARE

This chapter deals primarily with APGO Objective(s):

OBJECTIVE 14   Postpartum Care

A. Explain normal physiologic changes of the postpartum period.

B. Describe normal postpartum care and patient counseling.

OBJECTIVE 15   Lactation

A. Describe the normal anatomic/physiologic changes of the breast during pregnancy and the postpartum period.

B. Describe how to counsel a woman about the advantages of breast-feeding, and the lactating woman about issues such as frequency and duration of feeding and milk production.

(Continued)

C. Describe medications that are appropriate and inappropriate while breast-feeding.

D. Describe and explain the diagnosis and treatment of common postpartum breast abnormalities.

OBJECTIVE 22   Fetal Death

A. Describe the differential diagnosis, symptoms, physical findings, and diagnostic methods, and management for the causes of fetal death in each trimester.

B. Describe the emotional reactions to fetal death and their effect on its management.

C. Describe the maternal complications of fetal death, including disseminated intravascular coagulopathy.

OBJECTIVE 30   Anxiety and Depression

A. Describe the normal emotional responses to pregnancy.

B. Describe the signs and symptoms and management of postpartum depression and psychosis.

C. Describe the management of patients with psychiatric illness.

The *puerperium* is the 6- to 8-week period after birth during which the reproductive tract returns to its normal, nonpregnant state. Many of the physiologic changes of pregnancy have returned to normal within 1 to 2 weeks after delivery, whereas others may take much longer. The initial postpartum examination, traditionally scheduled at the end of this 6-week interval, is now often scheduled sooner. This is because many patients return to full nonpregnant activity in less than 6 weeks.

PHYSIOLOGY OF THE PUERPERIUM
Involution of the Uterus

The *uterus* weighs approximately 1000 g and has a volume of 5000 ml immediately after delivery compared with its nonpregnant weight of approximately 70 g and capacity of 5 ml. Immediately after delivery, the fundus of the uterus is easily palpable halfway between the pubic symphysis and the umbilicus. The immediate reduction in uterine size is a result of delivery of the fetus, placenta, and amniotic fluid as well as the loss of hormonal stimulation. Further uterine involution is caused by autolysis of intracellular myometrial protein, resulting in a decrease in cell size but not cell number. Through these changes, the uterus returns to the pelvis by 2 weeks postpartum, and is at its normal size by 6 weeks postpartum. Immediately after birth, uterine hemostasis is maintained by contraction of the smooth muscle of the arterial walls and compression of the vasculature by the uterine musculature.

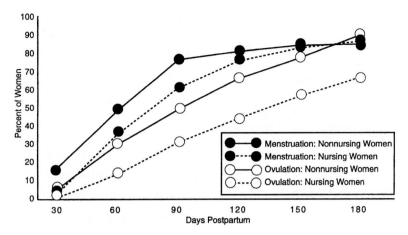

FIGURE 10.1.   Postpartum return of menstruation and ovulation.

Lochia

As the myometrial fibers contract, the blood clots from the uterus are expelled and the thrombi in the large vessels of the placental bed undergo organization. Within the first 3 days, the remaining decidua differentiates into a superficial layer, which becomes necrotic and sloughs, and a basal layer adjacent to the myometrium, which contained the fundi of the endometrial glands and is the source of the new endometrium.

This discharge is fairly heavy at first and rapidly decreases in amount over the first 2 to 3 days postpartum, although it may last for several weeks. In women who breast-feed, the lochia seems to resolve more rapidly, possibly because of a more rapid involution of the uterus caused by uterine contractions associated with breast-feeding. In some patients, there is an increased amount of lochia 1 to 2 weeks after delivery because the eschar that developed over the site of placental attachment has been sloughed. By the end of the third week postpartum, the endometrium is reestablished in most patients.

Cervix and Vagina

Within several hours of delivery, the cervix has reformed, and by 1 week, it usually admits only one finger (i.e., it is approximately 1 cm in diameter). The round shape of the nulliparous cervix is usually permanently replaced by a transverse, fish-mouth-shaped external os, the result of laceration during delivery. *Vulvar* and *vaginal tissues* return to normal over the first several days, although the *vaginal mucosa* reflects a hypoestrogenic state if the woman breast-feeds because ovarian function is suppressed during breast-feeding. The muscles of the pelvic floor gradually regain their tone. This may be aided by the use of Kegal exercises, consisting of repetitive contractions of these muscles. The hymen is now represented by several tags of tissue, the *myrtiform caruncles*.

Return of Ovarian Function

Ovulation can occur as early as 4 to 5 weeks postpartum if the woman chooses not to breast-feed. The mean time to ovulation in nonlactating women is approximately 10 weeks, with 50% of women ovulating by 90 days postpartum (Figure 10.1). Among breast-feeding women, the time to first ovulation depends on how long the woman breast-feeds. Ovulation is suppressed in the lactating woman in association with elevated prolactin levels. In these patients, prolactin remains elevated for 6 weeks, whereas in nonlactating women, prolactin levels return to normal by 3 weeks postpartum. Estrogen levels fall immediately after delivery in all patients, but begin to rise approximately 2 weeks after delivery if breast-feeding is not undertaken.

Abdominal Wall

Return of the elastic fibers of the skin and the stretched rectus muscles to normal configuration occurs slowly and is aided by exercise. The silvery *striae* seen on the skin usually slowly resolve. *Diastasis recti*, separation of the rectus muscles and fascia, usually also resolves over time.

Cardiovascular System

Pregnancy-related cardiovascular changes return to normal 2 to 3 weeks after delivery. Immediately postpartum, plasma volume is reduced by approximately 1000 ml, caused primarily by blood loss at the time of delivery. During the immediate postpartum period, there is also a significant shift of extracellular fluid into the intravascular space. The increased cardiac output seen during pregnancy also persists into the first several hours of the postpartum period. The elevated pulse rate seen during pregnancy persists for approximately 1 hour after delivery but then decreases. These conditions may contribute to decompensation sometimes seen in the early postpartum period in patients with heart disease. Immediately after delivery, approximately 5 kg of weight are lost as a result of diuresis and the loss of extravascular fluid. Further weight loss varies in rate and amount from patient to patient.

Hematopoietic System

The leukocytosis seen during labor persists into the early puerperium, thus minimizing the usefulness of identifying early postpartum infection by laboratory evidence of a mild to moderate elevation in the white cell count. There is some degree of autotransfusion of red cells to the intravascular space after delivery as the uterus contracts.

Renal System

GFR represents renal function and remains elevated in the first few weeks postpartum then returns to normal. Therefore, drugs with renal excretion should be given in decreased doses during this time. There may be considerable edema around the urethra after vaginal delivery, resulting in transitory urinary retention.

MANAGEMENT OF THE IMMEDIATE POSTPARTUM PERIOD

Hospital Stay

The amount of time a patient remains in the hospital after delivery continues to decrease. In the past, patients were kept in the hospital for 3 days after the birth of their first child, and 2 days after subsequent deliveries. Postpartum hospital stays for cesarean section patients were routinely 4 to 5 days. The period of hospitalization for many patients has been significantly reduced, primarily as a result of financial issues involving third-party payers. Concerns in these regards include the preparation of the mother for newborn care, infant feeding including the special issues involved with breast-feeding, and required newborn laboratory testing. Mandatory early discharge is considered inappropriate.

Maternal—Infant Bonding

It is recognized that shortly after delivery, the parents become totally engrossed in the events surrounding the newborn infant. Any significant separation of the mother from her infant that reduces activity such as cuddling, fondling, kissing, or gazing at the infant may have a negative impact on the involvement of maternal behaviors on a long-term basis. Contemporary obstetric units have enhanced these interactions by minimizing unnecessary medical interventions while increasing participation by the father and other family members. Rooming-in (mother and newborn are cared for in the same room rather than the newborn taken to a nursery) and an environment that facilitates breast-feeding also contribute to this atmosphere. Interaction between the infant and the new parents is also observed by the nursing staff with the resultant ability to identify any problems such as negative or even abusive actions toward the newborn.

Uterine Complications

The likelihood of serious *postpartum complications* is greatest immediately after delivery. Significant immediate postpartum hemorrhage occurs in approximately 1% of patients (see Chapter 12); infection is seen in approximately 5% of patients. Immediately after the delivery of the placenta, the uterus is palpated bimanually to ascertain that it is firm. Uterine palpation through the abdominal wall is repeated at frequent intervals during the immediate postpartum period to prevent and/or identify uterine atony. Perineal pads are applied, and the amount of blood on these pads as well as pulse and pressure are monitored closely for the first several hours after delivery to identify excessive blood loss.

Some patients will experience an episode of increased, "heavy" vaginal bleeding between days 8 and 14 postpartum, most likely associated with the separation and passage of the placental escar. This is self-limited and needs no therapy other than reassurance. In approximately 1% of cases, this bleeding persists or is excessive, *delayed postpartum hemorrhage,* in which case oxytocic therapy and/or suction evacuation of the uterus should be considered. Suction is successful in most cases, whether or not there is retained placental tissues as is found in one third of cases.

Analgesia

Postpartum analgesia is primarily indicated for perineal discomfort resulting from lacerations, episiotomy, and hemorrhoids or for postoperative pain from cesarean delivery or postpartum tubal ligation. Patients may also require pain medication for "afterbirth pains," the painful uterine contractions after delivery. This degree of discomfort from postpartum uterine contractions is seen more prominently in breast-feeding women because of the increased release of oxytocin during suckling. Common medications for this include acetaminophen (in cases of severe pain, combined with codeine), aspirin, and nonsteroidal anti-inflammatory drugs. Because hemorrhoids are varicosities of the hemorrhoidal veins, surgical treatment should not be considered for at least 6 months postpartum to allow for natural involution. Sitz baths, bowel softeners, and local preparations are useful, combined with reassurance that resolution is the most common outcome.

Breast Care

Breast engorgement in women who are not breast-feeding typically occurs 3 days postpartum and may be treated with techniques such as breast binders, ice packs, and avoidance of nipple stimulation. *Bromocriptine* (Parlodel), a dopamine receptor agonist that acts to suppress prolactin release by the anterior pituitary, was previously used for lactation suppression but is no longer recommended. Oral analgesics, such as codeine, are also useful adjuncts.

Occasionally, the breast-feeding mother may contract a *postpartum mastitis* manifest by high fever and usually chills, pain, and localized erythema and firmness of the breast. This is usually caused by infection with *Staphylococcus aureus* arising from the nursing infant's throat and nose and transmitted during nursing. Treatment includes penicillin G or a penicillinase-resistant drug such as dicloxacillin for penicillinase-reducing strains. For patients who are allergic to penicillin, erythromycin would be an appropriate alternative. Nursing from the affected side may be continued without danger to the infant. If an abscess develops, surgical drainage of the abscess in addition to antibiotic therapy is necessary.

Immunizations

Women who do not have anti-rubella antibody should be immunized for *rubella* during the immediate postpartum period. Breast-feeding is not a contraindication to this immunization. In some locations, a *tetanus toxoid booster* injection is also given at this time if needed. If the woman is D–, is not isoimmunized, and has given birth to a D+ infant, 300 mg of anti-D immune globulin (RhoGAM) should be administered before discharge. If the mother is positive for the *hepatitis B* surface antigen (HbSAg+), the newborn must be immunized before discharge.

Bowel Movement and Urination

It is common for a patient not to have a *bowel movement* for the first 1 to 2 days after delivery because patients have often not eaten for a long period of time. Stool softener (e.g., Colace, 100 mg orally twice daily, or Peri-Colace, 100 mg orally twice daily) is routinely prescribed in many institutions, especially if the patient has had a fourth-degree episiotomy repair or a laceration involving the rectal mucosa. Periurethral edema after vaginal delivery may cause *transitory urinary retention*. Patients should be monitored for urination after delivery, and if catheterization is required more than twice in the first 24 hours, placement of an indwelling catheter for 1 to 2 days is advisable as well as prophylactic administration of an antibiotic such as ampicillin.

Care of the Perineum

Perineal pain is minimized using oral analgesics, the application of an ice bag to minimize swelling, and/or a local anesthetic spray. Severe perineal pain unresponsive to the usual analgesics may signify the development of a hematoma, which requires evacuation if it continues to grow in size or becomes infected. *Infection of the episiotomy* is rare (< 0.1%) and usually is limited to the skin and responsive to broad-spectrum antibiotics. *Necrotizing fasciitis* is a rare but extremely serious infection requiring extensive resection and debridement of the perineum, cardiovascular support, and broad-spectrum antibiotic therapy. *Dehiscence*, like infection, is uncommon, with repair individualized on the basis of the nature and extent of the wound.

Contraception

Postpartum care in the hospital should always include discussion of *contraception*. As Figure 10.1 demonstrates, approximately 15% of nonnursing women are fertile at 6 weeks postpartum. All forms of contraception should be considered, although natural family planning methods (basal body temperature and cervical mucus evaluation) are not reliable until regular menses have been reestablished. Combined estrogen-progestin oral contraceptive preparations are not contraindicated by breast-feeding, although they may inhibit lactation slightly. Progestin preparations (oral northindrone or depo medroxyprogesterone acetate) have no effect or may slightly facilitate lactation. Once lactation is established, neither the volume nor the composition of breast milk is adversely affected by the administration of hormonal contraceptives, and there is no effect on the growth of breast-fed infants. Intrauterine device (IUD) insertion in the immediate postpartum interval is acceptable in the appropriately selected patient, but it must be remembered that the expulsion rate rises in this group to 10%–20% compared to an expulsion rate of 10% in the first year in the gynecologic patient (see Chapter 25).

Postpartum sterilization by tubal ligation is a popular method of permanent contraception, but usually the decision for this procedure should be made during the antepartum period and well documented in the chart. Then, if after delivery the patient still wishes sterilization, it may be performed without concern about the decision process (see Chapter 26). Because postpartum sterilization is associated with an increased incidence of guilt and regret when compared to "interval sterilization," consideration may be given to the advantages of laparoscopic sterilization 6–12 weeks postpartum, allowing time for further consideration of the permanence of the procedure in a time removed from childbirth and allowing time to ensure that the newborn is healthy. Finally, vasectomy should be considered as an alternative method of family planning for the couple.

Sexual Activity

Coitus may be resumed when the patient is comfortable. She should be counseled, especially if breast-feeding, that coitus may initially be uncomfortable because of a lack of lubrication and that the use of exogenous, water-soluble lubrication is helpful. The female superior position may be recommended, as the woman is thereby able to control the depth of penile penetration. The lactating patient may also be counseled to apply topical estrogen or a lubricant to the vaginal mucosa to minimize the dyspareunia caused by coital trauma to the hypoestrogenic tissue.

Patient Education

Patient education at the time of discharge should not be solely focused on postpartum and contraceptive issues. This is a good opportunity to reinforce the value and need for preventive health care and health care maintenance for both mother and infant. This should include a review of follow-up that has been arranged for the newborn and frequency and scope of health care for the new mother. Previously identified high-risk behaviors such as alcohol, tobacco, and drug abuse should once again be addressed. Infant safety concerns (e.g., automobile child restraints) are also appropriate topics of discussion. Postpartum follow-up of any preexisting medical conditions should also be reviewed.

Lactation and Breast-Feeding

An increasing belief in the advantages of breast-feeding has led many physicians to recommend this form of infant nutrition. As a result, more patients breast-feed and do so for a longer period of time. Benefits of breast-feeding include increased convenience for some mothers, decreased cost, improved infant nutrition for a variable period of time, and some protection against infection and allergic reaction. Successful breast-feeding depends on several factors, particularly the motivation of the mother and her ability to include breast-feeding in her daily activities. For some women, breast-feeding may be impossible, even if desired, because of restrictions on time caused by work. *Support by family and health care providers for the decision that best fits the total needs of the mother and baby is very important.* If breast-feeding is chosen, rooming-in during the hospital stay allows the mother to begin the process in a less pressured setting while allowing the hospital staff to provide helpful recommendations and support. *The decision to breast-feed or bottle feed is best made before delivery and is facilitated by balanced discussion during the antepartum visits.*

At the time of delivery, the drop of estrogen and other placental hormones is a major factor in removing the inhibition of the action of prolactin. Also, suckling by the infant stimulates release of oxytocin from the neurohypophysis. The increased levels of oxytocin in the blood result in contraction of the myoepithelial cells and emptying of the alveolar lumen of the breast. The oxytocin also increases uterine contractions thereby accelerating involution of the postpartum uterus. Prolactin release is also stimulated by suckling, with resultant secretion of fatty acids, lactose, and casein. *Colostrum* is produced in the first 5 days postpartum and is slowly replaced by maternal milk. Colostrum contains more minerals and protein but less fat and sugar than maternal milk, although it does contain large fat globules, the so-called colostrum corpuscles, which are probably epithelial cells that have undergone fatty degeneration. Colostrum also contains immunoglobulin A, which may offer the newborn some protection from enteric pathogens. Subsequently, on approximately the third to sixth day postpartum, milk is produced.

For milk to be produced on an ongoing basis, there must be adequate insulin, cortisol, and thyroid hormone, and adequate nutrients and fluids in the diet. Nutrients and fluids are especially important because maternal fat stores deposited during pregnancy provide only one third of the fat and calories needed to produce 850 ml of milk each day. The remainder must be supplied

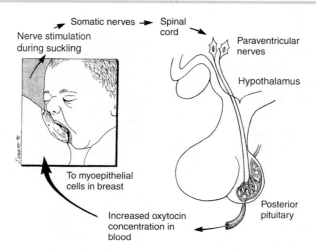

FIGURE 10.2. The somatosensory pathways for the suckling-induced reduced reflex release of oxytocin.

TABLE 10.1. Differential Diagnosis of Enlarged, Tender Breast Postpartum

Finding	Engorgement	Mastitis	Plugged Duct
Onset	Gradual	Sudden	Gradual
Location	Bilateral	Unilateral	Unilateral
Swelling	Generalized	Localized	Localized
Pain	Generalized	Intense, localized	Localized
Systemic symptoms	Feels well	Feels ill	Feels well
Fever	No	Yes	No

by an appropriate diet and fluid intake. All vitamins except K are found in human milk, but because they are present in varying amounts, maternal vitamin supplementation is recommended. Vitamin K may be administered to the infant to prevent hemorrhagic disease of the newborn. To maintain breast-feeding, the alveolar lumen must be emptied on a regular basis (Figure 10.2).

Nipple care is also important during breast-feeding. The nipples should be washed with water and exposed to the air for 15 to 20 minutes after each feeding. A water-based cream such as lanolin or A and D ointment may be applied if the nipples are tender. Fissuring of the nipple may make breast-feeding extremely difficult. Temporary cessation of breast-feeding, manual expression of milk, and use of a nipple shield will aid in recovery.

Engorgement, mastitis, and plugged duct (galactocele) are the three causes of enlarged, tender breast postpartum. They may be differentiated according to their signs and symptoms, presented in Table 10.1. Engorgement is treated by continued nursing or expression of milk by breast pump as well as application of heat and oral analgesics, and usually resolves spontaneously in 72 hours if not breast-feeding. Mastitis is associated with infection by *S. aureus β-hemolytic streptococci,* and *Haemophilus influenzae* and is treated with antibiotics

TABLE 10.2.   Medications and Breast-Feeding

Medication or Substance	Reason for Concern/Effect on Lactation
Contraindicated During Breast-Feeding	
Bromocriptine (Parlodel)	Suppresses lactation
Cyclophosphamide (Cytoxan)	Possible immune suppression; neutropenia; unknown effect on growth
Cyclosporine	Possible immune suppression; unknown effect on growth
Doxorubicin (Adriamycin)	Concentrated in milk; possible immune suppression; unknown effect on growth
Ergotamine (Ergotrate)	In dosages for migraine, emesis, diarrhea, convulsions
Lithium	50% therapeutic level in infant
Methotrexate	Possible immune suppression; unknown effect on growth
Substances of abuse (amphetamines, cocaine, heroin, marijuana, nicotine, and phencyclidine)	Growth restriction; neurologic damage; obstetric accidents
Uncertain Effects but of Concern When Breast-Feeding	
Antianxiety medications, antidepressants, and antipsychotics	No reported effects, but may be of special concern because of primary drug effect when given to nursing mothers for long periods of time
Chloramphenicol	Idiosyncratic bone marrow suppressions
Metoclopramide (Reglan)	Concentrated in milk; dopaminergic blockade
Metronidazole (Flagyl)	In vitro mutagen; consider discontinuing breast-feeding for 12–14 hr to allow secretion of single-dose regimens

(dicloxacillin, 500 mg orally four times a day) for at least 1 week. Nursing may be continued during treatment. A plugged duct is treated with warm packs and a breast pump. Rarely, incision and drainage may be required.

Drugs in the breast milk are a common concern for the breast-feeding mother. Less than 1% of the total dosage of any medication is seen in breast milk. This should be considered when any medication is prescribed by a physician or when any over-the-counter medications are contemplated by the patient (Table 10.2). Specific medications that would contraindicate breast-feeding include lithium carbonate, tetracycline, bromocriptine, methotrexate, and any radioactive substance, as well as all substances of abuse such as amphetamine, cocaine, heroin, marijuana, nicotine, and phencyclidine (PCP).

ANXIETY, DEPRESSION, AND THE POSTPARTUM PERIOD

Although pregnancy and childbirth are usually joyous times, for some patients the experience is followed by significant emotional distress. Identification of specific risk factors for postpartum and antepartum anxiety and depression is an important first step in identifying and dealing with these problems. Of patients with previous postpartum mental disease, approximately 25% have a recurrence after their next pregnancy. One third of patients with psychiatric illness during the postpartum period have a history of psychiatric disease. The exact cause of most of the postpartum emotional changes is unknown, although suggested etiologies

TABLE 10.3. Three Categories of Postpartum Mood Disorders

	Postpartum Psychosis	Postpartum Depression	Maternity Blues
Incidence	0.1%–0.2%	≥ 10%	50%–80%
Average time	2–3 days PP	2 weeks to 12 months PP	1–5 days PP
Average duration	Variable	3–14 months	2–3 days, resolution within 10 days
Symptoms	Similar to organic brain syndrome: confusion, attention deficit, distractibility, clouded sensorium	Irritability, labile mood, difficulty falling asleep, phobias, anxiety; symptoms worsen in evening	Mild insomnia, tearfulness, fatigue, irritability, poor concentration, depressed affect
Treatment	Apsychotic pharmacotherapy, antidepressant, 50% of patients also meet depression criteria	Antidepressant, pharmacotherapy, psychotherapy	Time, reassurance, watchful waiting; leads to PPD in 20% of patients

PP = postpartum; PPD = postpartum depression.

include changing hormone levels (as is seen with premenstrual changes), difficulty adjusting to a new life-style, and the stresses of parenthood.

There is a wide spectrum of response to pregnancy and delivery, ranging from mild depression ("maternity blues") to postpartum depression to the extreme response of postpartum psychosis (Table 10.3). The overall incidence of depression during the postpartum period appears not to be significantly greater than at other times of a woman's life. Early symptoms of depression include sleeplessness, loss of self-esteem, irritability, and mood swings. More serious symptoms include anorexia, obsessive behavior, panic, and delusions. A most disturbing symptom is the patient's estrangement from the newborn.

Both internal and external forces may result in postpartum psychiatric illness. A patient who does not cope well with stress is particularly susceptible to such poten-

tially traumatic stimuli as previous infertility, complications of the antepartum, intrapartum, or postpartum course, or conflicts in the roles of mother and wife. A supportive spouse and family can minimize the severity of any symptom complex.

Anxiety is very common during the antepartum and intrapartum periods, but can be minimized by having the patient as an active participant in the planning of and carrying out of the birthing process plan. Prepared childbirth and the rational use of minimal anesthesia at the patient's discretion may help the patient feel a sense of control. Active involvement of nursing personnel in the identification of significant anxiety and depression is also critical, because they observe the patient on a more ongoing basis than do physicians.

Treatment must be tailored to the patient's individual situation, with most cases of mild postpartum depression being managed by the attending physician in conjunction with the support of hospital staff such as nursing personnel and social workers. The mother who is fearful of, or is averse to, contact with the newborn should not be forced into contact. Both psychotherapy and medication such as antidepressants or lithium carbonate may be provided, usually in consultation with a clinical psychologist or psychiatrist. If conditions worsen despite outpatient efforts, inpatient therapy is warranted.

Whether during the antepartum, intrapartum, or postpartum period, depression and anxiety should be viewed as significant problems. It should be noted, however, that they are not necessarily solely related to pregnancy or its complications. Specifically, women are clinically depressed twice as frequently as men. Anxiety accompanies depression in three fourths of cases. The earliest clinical clue to the diagnosis of depression may be the inability to experience pleasure or happiness (anhedonia). Women particularly susceptible to depression are those with young children, those who are living in poverty, those who are abused, and those who have professional careers.

There appears to be some evidence for a hereditary factor that predisposes some patients to development of anxiety disorders. This may occur in as many as 10% to 15% of the population. Because every patient is subjected to some degree of stress, anxiety is usually seen in all patients, resulting in some shifts in mood as part of the normal life experience. As with depression, however, anxiety can become dysfunctional, with the patient seeing the world as a hostile or unsafe environment. Nonspecific nervousness, panic, irritability, and fear of losing control suggest significant anxiety disorder requiring treatment.

PERINATAL GRIEF

The loss of a child results in grief in the patient and the family. Grief occurs as the result of any significant loss, whether it be the death of an infant, the loss of the fetus before birth, or the loss of the "ideal child," as in the case of the birth of a handicapped infant. Perinatal grief is typically more severe the closer the loss is to term (i.e., third-trimester loss brings about a more extensive grief reaction than a first-trimester pregnancy loss). Health care providers should be sensitive to the patient's sense of guilt and failure in these circumstances. Postpartum depression is both more common and more severe in cases of perinatal loss.

Management of grief must occur not only in the postpartum period, but also during the prenatal period in the case of fetal death or diagnosis of abnormality before birth. Management of perinatal grief includes:

1. Anticipate the grief response.
2. Provide accurate information.
3. Encourage open expression of feelings.
4. Encourage photographing of the newborn and/or seeing and touching the infant.
5. Encourage active participation of the support person.
6. Assist the patient in disseminating information to family and friends.
7. Provide information regarding future pregnancies.
8. Arrange for appropriate consultations.

THE POSTPARTUM VISIT

At the time of the first postpartum visit, inquiries should be made into the following: status of breast-feeding, return of menstruation, resumption of coital activity, use of contraception, interaction of the newborn with the family, and resumption of other physical activities such as return to work. Involutional changes will have occurred in most instances. Inflammatory changes because of the healing of the cervix may result in minor atypia on a Papanicolaou smear performed at this time. Unless there is a past history of significant cervical dysplasia, repeating the Pap smear in 3 months is appropriate.

CASE STUDIES

Case 10A

A 24-year-old married woman has just delivered her first child, a healthy boy weighing 7 lb. Her antepartum and intrapartum courses were unremarkable. On the first day postpartum, she is noted to cry easily and to have slept poorly.

Question Case 10A

Which of the following are appropriate management steps at this time?

A. Reassure the patient that everything is okay and that feeling sad after a delivery is normal
B. Ask the nursing staff to ask the patient why she is crying
C. Ask a psychiatrist to evaluate the patient's apparent sadness
D. Ask a social worker to evaluate the patient's apparent sadness

Answer: A

Reassuring the patient is not inappropriate as a general measure, but it must be combined with some assessment of the apparent sadness. In general, this is best done at this level of distress by the physician or nursing staff; consultation to psychiatry or social services usually is not indicated.

Case 10B

A 23-year-old G1 delivers a healthy term boy by normal vaginal delivery after an unremarkable antepartum course and spontaneous labor. She decides to breast-feed, which is begun satisfactorily during her stay in the hospital. She and her new son are well at the time of discharge. Three days later, she calls complaining of the worst pain she has ever had in her breasts.

Questions Case 10B

On questioning, you learn that the pain is in the left side of her left breast, which is tender and swollen but does not feel especially warm to touch. Her temperature is 99° F and she feels generally well except for the pain. The most likely diagnosis is

A. Breast engorgement
B. Mastitis
C. Blocked duct
D. Neoplasm

Answer: C

Appropriate initial management includes

A. Incision and drainage
B. Antibiotic therapy
C. Warm packs and analgesics
D. Needle aspiration

Answer: C

Case 10C

A 28-year-old primigravida had a normal spontaneous delivery at term following an uncomplicated labor. Delivery anesthesia consisted of a pudendal block, there were no obstetric lacerations or episiotomy, and the placenta appeared normal and intact. Estimated blood loss was 400 cc.

Ten days after delivery she calls complaining of the onset of bleeding that is "as heavy as my period and very crampy." She says she has no fever and feels well otherwise. She is bottle-feeding and is using a nonhormonal method of contraception.

Questions Case 10C

The best management consists of

A. Reassuring the patient that the bleeding most likely will be self-

limited, and to use the analgesics provided and call back if the bleeding continues more than 3 days or becomes heavier or significantly more painful
B. Prescribing methergine 0.2 mg orally every 8 hours for two days and doxycycline 100 mg orally twice a day for 10 days
C. Advising the patient to go to the emergency room for evaluation for retained placental tissue
D. Advising the patient to come to the office the following day for evaluation

Answer: A

The patient calls back the next evening saying that the bleeding is significantly

heavier, with the passage of "lots" of clots, and is more painful. The best management at this time is to

A. Advise the patient to go to the emergency room for evaluation
B. Prescribe methergine 0.2 mg orally every 8 hours for two days and doxycycline 100 mg orally twice a day for 10 days
C. Advise the patient to go to the emergency room for evaluation for retained placental tissue
D. Advise the patient to come to the office the following day for evaluation

Answer: A

ABNORMAL OBSTETRICS

C H A P T E R

11

ISOIMMUNIZATION

CHAPTER OBJECTIVES

This chapter deals primarily with APGO Objective(s):

OBJECTIVE 20   D Isoimmunization

Describe the circumstances leading to Rh isoimmunization and the techniques used to determine its presence in the mother, the methods used to assess the severity of the disease in the fetus and newborn, and the appropriate use of immunoglobulin prophylaxis.

Isoimmunization refers to the development of antibodies to red blood cell antigens following exposure to such antigens from another individual. Transfusion is a source of such antigens, or in pregnancy, the "other individual" may be the fetus, 50% of whose genetic makeup is derived from the father. If the mother is exposed to fetal red cells during pregnancy or at delivery, she may develop antibodies to fetal cell antigens. Later in that pregnancy, or more commonly with the subsequent pregnancy, the antibodies can cross the placenta and hemolyze fetal red cells, leading to fetal anemia. In a pregnancy complicated by isoimmunization, the manufacture of maternal antibody that destroys fetal red cells is countered by the ability of the fetus to manufacture sufficient red cells to permit survival and growth.

NATURAL HISTORY

Isoimmunization can involve many of the *several hundred blood group systems.* This disorder is frequently referred to as Rh isoimmunization, because the Rhesus (Rh) system is most frequently involved. For the sake of this discussion, the Rh system will be used as an example, although it should be remembered that isoimmunization can and does develop with many other blood systems such as Kell, Duffy, Kidd, and others.

Within the Rh system, there are several specific antigens, the one most commonly associated with hemolytic disease being the D antigen. If a fetus is Rh+, having received the genes for the Rh D antigen from its father, and the mother lacks the Rh antigen (i.e., she is Rh–), the conditions exist for the development of isoimmunization. In the woman's first such pregnancy, the infant typically has no complications. If, however, the mother's blood is exposed to fetal red cells, even minuscule amounts, the woman can develop antibodies to the Rh D antigen. This can occur at the time of childbirth, or in other situations where fetomaternal hemorrhage may occur. These situations include amniocentesis; threatened, spontaneous, or elective/therapeutic abortion; ectopic pregnancy; bleeding associated with placenta previa and placental abruption; abdominal trauma; and external version. Antibody development occurs in approximately 15% of cases of an Rh– mother and Rh+ fetus. In a subsequent pregnancy, passage of minute amounts of fetal blood across the placenta, which occurs quite frequently, can lead to an *anamnestic response* of maternal antibody production. If the mother produces immunoglobulin M (IgM)-type antibodies, the molecules do not cross the placenta, because they are too large. In the case of Rh factor, however, the maternal antibody is predominantly the smaller IgG-type, which can freely cross the placenta and enter the fetal circulation. Once in the fetal vascular system, the antibody attaches to the Rh+ red blood cells and hemolyzes them. The bilirubin produced in this hemolytic process is transferred back across the placenta to the mother and metabolized. *The condition of the fetus is determined by the amount of maternal antibody transferred across the placenta and the ability of the fetus to replace the red blood cells that have been destroyed.*

In the first affected pregnancy, the infant may be anemic at delivery and may soon develop elevated levels of bilirubin, because hemolysis continues after birth and the newborn must now rely on its own, somewhat immature liver to metabolize the bilirubin. *In subsequent pregnancies,* with an Rh+ fetus, the process of antibody production and transfer may be accelerated, leading to the development of more significant anemia. In such cases, the fetal liver can manufacture additional red cells. However, this activity reduces the amount of proteins manufactured by the fetal liver. In turn, the reduced protein production can lead to a decreased oncotic pressure within the fetal vascular system, resulting in fetal ascites and subcutaneous edema. At the same time, the severe fetal anemia can lead to high output cardiac failure. This combination of findings is referred to as *hydrops fetalis.*

The tendency is for each subsequent baby to be more severely affected, but this is not always the case. The level of fetal dis-

TABLE 11.1. Risk of Rh Sensitization	
Obstetric/Medical Event	**Chance of Sensitization (percent)**
Ectopic pregnancy	< 1
Full-term pregnancy	1–2
Amniocentesis	1–3
Spontaneous abortion	3–4
Induced abortion	5–6
Full-term delivery, ABO compatible or incompatible	14–17
Mismatched blood transfusion	90–95

turbance may remain the same or, occasionally, may even be less than in the previous pregnancy. If subsequent fetuses are Rh–, which is commonly the case if the father is a heterozygote, the fetus is not affected at all (Table 11.1).

DIAGNOSIS

Isoimmunization can often be diagnosed on the basis of *history.* A woman with a previous diagnosis of isoimmunization or with a previous birth in which the neonatal course was consistent with this disorder is at risk for recurrence. As part of routine antenatal *laboratory evaluation,* maternal blood is tested for the presence of a variety of antibodies that may cause significant disturbances in the fetus. Any significant antibodies are further evaluated for the strength of antibody response, which is reported in a titer format (1:4, 1:16, and so on). During this testing process, other antibodies may be discovered that do not cause significant fetal/neonatal problems. The two most common of these are the anti-Lewis and anti-I. When these antibodies are found, titers are not reported because of their lack of clinical importance.

Determination of the father's Rh status is extremely helpful. If he is Rh–, the fetus is not affected. If he is Rh+, genotype testing can determine whether he is homozygous or heterozygous. Recently, direct Rh testing of the fetus has become possible, using cells floating within the amniotic cavity.

MANAGEMENT

Antibody titers would seem to be good markers of maternal antibody production, but in fact, such titers are of limited usefulness. In the first sensitized pregnancy, titers do seem to be helpful, but thereafter, they are of virtually no value because they do not reflect the current fetal condition. Even in the initial sensitized pregnancy, the greatest value is in distinguishing those pregnancies for which antibody production is so low as to be nonthreatening to the fetus from those for which there are likely to be significant consequence. *A titer of 1:16 or greater is generally considered the critical point* at which there is sufficient risk of fetal jeopardy to warrant additional evaluation.

Amniotic fluid assessment is of great value in managing the isoimmunized patient. Practical use of amniotic fluid analysis became a reality in about 1960, when Liley found that *the level of bilirubin in the amniotic fluid accurately reflects the condition of the fetus.* The mechanism by which bilirubin enters the amniotic fluid from the fetal compartment is still not understood. However, in the second half of normal pregnancy, the level of bilirubin normally decreases progressively. The level of bilirubin in an affected, isoimmunized patient can be evaluated in relation to natural decline. The level of bilirubin in the amniotic fluid is determined using a spectrophotometer. Normal amniotic fluid subjected to spectrophotometric analysis has a

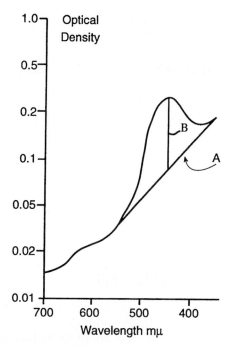

FIGURE 11.1.   Absorption curve of amniotic fluid by spectrophotometer in a patient with isoimmunization. (*A*) Anticipated curve for normal amniotic fluid. (*B*) Deviation of curve as a result of bilirubin in the amniotic fluid, expressed as ΔOD_{450}.

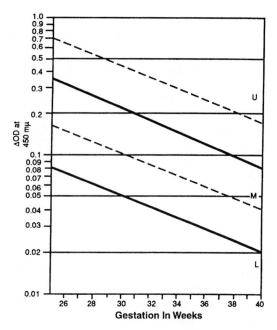

FIGURE 11.2.   Liley curve. The ΔOD_{450} was obtained as shown in Figure 11.1 and is plotted by gestational age. The condition of the fetus can be estimated by the zone in which the ΔOD_{450} decreases. In the upper (*U*) zone, the fetus is severely affected; in the middle (*M*) zone, moderately affected; and in the lower (*L*) zone, minimally affected or not affected.

characteristic curve, based on optical density (OD), as shown in Figure 11.1. The presence of bilirubin causes a characteristic deviation in this curve, at 450 nm. This degree of deviation is referred to as the ΔOD_{450}. Following the pioneering work of Liley and others, normal ΔOD_{450} values have been determined (Figure 11. 2). Experience has shown how optical density relates to the severity of fetal problems, as shown in the figure.

Amniotic fluid is obtained from the patient by amniocentesis at periodic intervals between the twentieth and thirtieth weeks of pregnancy, depending on the history of previous pregnancies. OD values are then plotted on a curve (as shown in Figure 11.2), which allows estimation of the degree of severity of the anemia in the fetus. Based on this level of severity, in conjunction with

the gestational age, a decision about expected management, transfusion of the fetus, or delivery can be made. *Markedly elevated ΔOD_{450} values indicate a severely affected fetus, intermediate values indicate a moderately affected fetus, and low values represent a fetus not or only mildly affected.*

Assessment of the affected fetus by *periodic ultrasonography* can be very helpful in detecting severe signs of the hemolytic process, namely subcutaneous edema and ascites. Under ultrasound guidance, the umbilical cord can be sampled directly [percutaneous umbilical blood sampling (PUBS)] and fetal blood can be taken for hematocrit determination to assess the severity of anemia. Later in pregnancy, general tests of fetal well-being are used in the isoimmunized patient, because the ability of an affected fetus to withstand the stresses of pregnancy and labor may be compromised.

TRANSFUSIONS

Transfusion of Rh– red blood cells to the fetus is indicated when, on the basis of the previous assessment, it is determined that the fetus *is in significant jeopardy* for hydrops or fetal death. Traditionally, blood was transfused into the fetal abdominal cavity where absorption of the transfused cells takes place over subsequent days. More recently, direct fetal transfusions into the umbilical cord (PUBS) under ultrasonography guidance are being used more frequently, with positive results. Physicians experienced and skilled in this technique are critical to its success. The procedure carries with it a risk of fetal death of up to 3%, a risk that must be weighed against the predicted future course for the fetus in utero and the potential adverse consequences of preterm delivery. The quantity of red blood cells to be transferred can be calculated using the gestational age and size of the fetus and the fetal hematocrit. Because the transferred cells are Rh–, they are not affected by the transplacental maternal antibody. Timing of subsequent transfusions can be determined based on the severity of disease and the predicted life span of the transfused cells.

PREVENTION

Maternal exposure and subsequent sensitization to fetal blood usually occurs at delivery and much less commonly during pregnancy. In the late 1960s, it was determined that the antibody to the D antigen of the Rh system could be prepared from donors previously sensitized to the antigen. Subsequently, it was found that *administration of this antibody (Rh immune globulin) soon after delivery could, by passive immunization, prevent an active antibody response by the mother in most cases.* Rh immune globulin is effective for only the D antigen of the Rh system. No similar preparations are available for patients sensitized with the many other possible antigens. It is now standard practice for Rh– patients who deliver Rh+ infants to receive an intramuscular dose of 300 mg of Rh immune globulin (i.e., RhoGAM) within 72 hours of delivery. With this practice, the risk of subsequent sensitization decreases from approximately 15% to approximately 2%. This residual 2% was determined to be the result of sensitization occurring *during the course of pregnancy* (as opposed to at delivery), usually in the third trimester. Administration of a 300-mg dose of Rh immune globulin to Rh– patients at 28 weeks was found to reduce the risk of sensitization to approximately 0.2%.

Prophylaxis with Rh immune globulin in Rh– women is not necessary if the father of the pregnancy is *known with certainty* to be Rh–. Although testing of the father can be done, *if there is any question as to the paternity, prophylactic administration of Rh immune globulin should be given as described,* because the risk is negligible and the potential benefits are considerable.

In summary, Rh– pregnant patients who have no antibody on initial screening are retested at 28 weeks (to detect the rare patient sensitized earlier in pregnancy). If no sensitization has occurred, they are given Rh immune globulin to protect them from antibody formation for the remainder of the pregnancy. If the father is known to be Rh–, this practice is not necessary. After delivery, the child's blood type and Rh status are determined, and if the child is Rh+, a second dose of Rh immune globulin is given to the new mother.

There are other situations when Rh immune globulin should be administered (Table 11.2). Because the amount of fetal red cells required to elicit an antibody response is minute, approximately 0.01 ml, *any circumstance in pregnancy in which fetomaternal hemorrhage can occur warrants Rh immune globulin administration.* Furthermore, because fetal red cell production begins with 6 weeks of conception,

TABLE 11.2. Indications for Rh Immune Globulin Administration in an Unsensitized Rh-negative Patient*

At approximately 28 weeks' pregnancy
Within 3 days of delivery of an
    Rh-positive infant
At the time of amniocentesis
After positive Kleihauer-Betke test
After an ectopic pregnancy
After a spontaneous or induced abortion

*Unless the father of the infant is known to be Rh–.

sensitization can occur in patients who have a spontaneous or scheduled pregnancy termination. Because the dose of antigen in such situations is low, a reduced dose of 50 mg of Rh immune globulin can be used to prevent sensitization. Amniocentesis and other trauma (e.g., from an auto accident) during pregnancy are also indications for the standard 300-mg dose of Rh immune globulin. In cases of trauma or bleeding during pregnancy, the extent, if any, to which fetomaternal hemorrhage has occurred can be evaluated using the Kleihauer-Betke test or similar test that allows the identification of fetal cells in maternal circulation. In the test, a sample of maternal blood is subjected to a strong base such as potassium hydroxide (KOH). Maternal cells are very sensitive to changes in pH and, therefore, promptly lyse and become "ghost" cells. Fetal cells are much more resistant to such agents and remain intact. The ratio of fetal to maternal cells can be assessed by counting 1000 or more total cells under the microscope and determining how many cells retain the dark appearance (representing fetal cells). Then the maternal blood volume is calculated and, using the ratio just described, the total amount of fetomaternal hemorrhage is derived. Because a standard 300-mg dose of Rh immune globulin effectively neutralizes 15 ml of fetal red blood cells, the appropriate dose can then be administered.

MANAGEMENT OF OTHER IRREGULAR ANTIBODIES

An increasing number of isoimmunizations are associated with other irregular antibodies as Rh-D isoimmunizations are less frequently encountered due to immunization. Differences in the frequencies of these antibodies and the likelihood that their presence will cause hemolytic disease of the newborn (HDN) depends on several factors, including the size and frequency of the antigenic stimulus, the relative potency of the antigen, and the type of antibody response (IgG or IgM).

Both Rh+ and Rh– mothers can produce these antibodies. When at risk for fetomaternal or exogenous antibody exposure, a positive antibody screen should be managed (Figure 11.3). Anti-Kell is the most important non-Rh cause of HDN and is usually associated with previous blood transfusion. When the mother is anti-Kell antibody positive, paternal Kell genotyping should be carried out. Ninety percent of fathers and their fetuses are Kell negative, and no further work-up is required as long as paternity is certain.

NONRHESUS BLOOD GROUP ISOIMMUNIZATION

With a decreasing prevalence of Rhesus-isoimmunization because of Rh prevention programs, ABO hemolytic disease and non-Rh D/non-ABO hemolytic disease are relatively more common.

ABO hemolytic disease is associated with milder fetal kernicterus and, rarely, hydrops, probably because of the relatively smaller number of A and B antigenic sites on fetal red blood cells and because anti-A and -B are IgM and thus do not traverse the placenta well; that which does cross has a high propensity for other binding sites besides fetal red blood cells. This disease usually occurs in the first pregnancy, and amniocentesis and early delivery are rarely indicated.

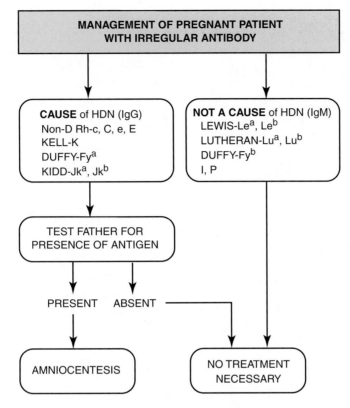

FIGURE 11.3. Management of other irregular antibodies. The more common irregular antibodies may be managed according to this flow sheet. It is important to determine paternity and paternal genotype before deciding against amniocentesis.

Non-Rh D/non-ABO hemolytic disease is frequently associated with blood transfusion, because "compatible" blood transfusion is matched only to the *ABO* and *Dd* antigens. Pregnant women who are affected by the common and uncommon antibodies that can cause hemolytic disease of the newborn are managed in the same way as those who are Rh–. Those women with antibodies that are very rarely associated with or unassociated with hemolytic disease of the newborn need not be treated.

CASE STUDIES

Case 11A

A 22-year-old G1 P0 presents for prenatal care at 28 weeks by dates and size. Her medical and family history is negative, and her physical examination is normal and consistent with her stated gestational age.

On review of her initial laboratory work you note that her blood type is O–. You ask her about the blood type of the father, but he has left town and she does not know what it is.

(Continued)

Questions Case 11A

What should your management be?

A. Offer RhoGAM on the possibility that the father is Rh+
B. Do not offer RhoGAM because the father's Rh status is unknown
C. Do not bring up the issue unless the patient asks

Answer: A

Because of the risk of isoimmunization and the low risk of administration of RhoGAM, it should be offered and given.

The patient declines because she does not want a medication unless she knows it is necessary. When she is 38 weeks, the patient learns that the father of the child is blood type O+. She asks if her baby will be damaged as a result. You respond

A. Certainly, because you failed to be treated appropriately
B. Probably, because you failed to be treated appropriately
C. Probably not, because it is the second or subsequent pregnancies that are usually affected
D. Certainly not, because it is always the second or subsequent pregnancies that are affected

Answer: C

You may reasonably reassure her and test for antibody to ascertain if any sensitization has occurred.

Case 11B

A 28-year-old gravida presents at 7 weeks' gestational age for prenatal care. Her antibody screen is positive for anti-Kell.

Question Case 11B

What is the first step in management of this situation?

A. Level II obstetric ultrasound
B. Amniocentesis
C. Cordocentesis
D. Determination of paternity

Answer: D

If the actual father is Kell-negative, no further evaluation is required. If not, or if paternity cannot be established, the mother must consider further evaluation, which may include invasive procedures that carry significant risk for the fetus.

12

POSTPARTUM HEMORRHAGE

This chapter deals primarily with APGO Objective(s):

OBJECTIVE 28   Postpartum Hemorrhage

Describe the differential diagnosis and risk factors of postpartum hemorrhage and the approach to its diagnosis and management, including identification of lacerations, the use of contractile agents, the management of volume loss, and the management of coagulopathy.

Excessive bleeding in the minutes and hours after delivery is a serious and potentially fatal complication. Hemorrhage can be sudden and profuse, or blood loss can occur more slowly but be prolonged and persistent. Postpartum hemorrhage is usually defined as a blood loss in excess of 500 ml of blood associated with delivery. Many patients lose considerably more blood than this, and the figure of 500 ml may actually represent the average amount of blood loss after vaginal delivery, with twice this amount lost at cesarean delivery. This problem with the definition of postpartum hemorrhage may affect some of the clinical statistics or cause clinicians to underestimate blood loss in order to avoid the classification of a normal delivery as one complicated by postpartum hemorrhage, but it probably has little if any effect on the recognition or treatment of true postpartum hemorrhage. This chapter discusses the causes of postpartum hemorrhage, followed by a general approach to the patient who bleeds excessively after giving birth.

MAJOR CAUSES OF POSTPARTUM HEMORRHAGE
Uterine Atony

Uterine atony is by far the most common cause of postpartum hemorrhage. Ordinarily, the uterine corpus (or body) contracts promptly after delivery of the placenta, constricting the spiral arteries in the newly created placental bed and preventing excessive bleeding from them. This muscular contraction, rather than coagulation, prevents excessive bleeding from the placental implantation site. When contraction does not occur as expected, the resulting uterine atony gives rise to postpartum hemorrhage.

A number of *factors predispose to uterine atony* (Table 12.1). These include conditions in which there is extraordinary enlargement of the uterus, such as hydramnios or twins; abnormal labor (both precipitous, prolonged, or augmented by oxytocin); and conditions that interfere with contraction of the uterus, such as uterine leiomyomas or use of magnesium sulfate. The clinical diagnosis of atony is based largely on the tone of the uterine muscle on palpation. Instead of the normally firm, contracted uterine corpus, a softer, more pliable—often called "boggy"—uterus is found. The cervix is usually open. Frequently, the uterus contracts briefly when massaged, only to become more relaxed when the manipulation ceases.

Management of uterine atony is both preventive and therapeutic. In the management of a normal delivery, it is customary to infuse oxytocin diluted in intravenous fluids (usually 20 units in 1 liter of fluid run at 125 to 165 ml/hr) starting soon after the placenta has been delivered. Oxytocin promotes contraction of the uterine corpus and decreases the likelihood of uterine atony. It is given in dilute solution because the intravenous administration of undiluted oxytocin can cause significant hypotension. Gentle bimanual massage of the uterus is also commonly performed in the belief that this will hasten uterine contraction and decrease blood loss as well as prevent uterine atony. Immediate breast-feeding also causes uterine contractions, and when performed probably also has similar effects.

TABLE 12.1. Factors Predisposing to Uterine Atony

Precipitous labor	Amnionitis (sepsis)
General anesthesia	Multiparity
Prolonged labor	Oxytocin use in labor
Uterine leiomyomas	History of postpartum hemorrhage
Macrosomia	Amniotic fluid embolus
Hydramnios	Magnesium sulfate in laboring patient
Twins	

Once uterine atony occurs and is diagnosed, management can be categorized as manipulative, medical, and surgical. Uterine massage alone is often successful in causing uterine contraction, and this should be done while preparations for other treatments are under way (Figure 12.1). Another manipulation, which is rarely used today, is packing of the uterine cavity with gauze, which serves as a temporizing measure while awaiting definitive therapy. Medical treatments include oxytocin, *Methergine* (methylergonovine maleate), and several prostaglandin preparations, administered separately or in combination. Methergine is a potent constrictor that can cause uterine contractions within several minutes. It is always given intramuscularly because rapid intravenous administration can lead to dangerous hypertension. Prostaglandin $F_{2\alpha}$ may be given intramuscularly or directly into the myometrium, and prostaglandin E_2 may be given by vaginal suppository. Both result in very strong uterine contractions. Typically, oxytocin is given prophylactically, as noted previously; if uterine atony occurs, the infusion rate is increased, and Methergine, prostaglandin, or both are given sequentially.

Occasionally, uterine massage and oxytocics are unsuccessful in bringing about appropriate uterine contraction, and surgical measures must be used. Surgical management of uterine atony may include ligation of the uterine arteries or hypogastric arteries, selective arterial embolization, and hysterectomy (Figure 12.2). At times, these procedures may be lifesaving. Management must

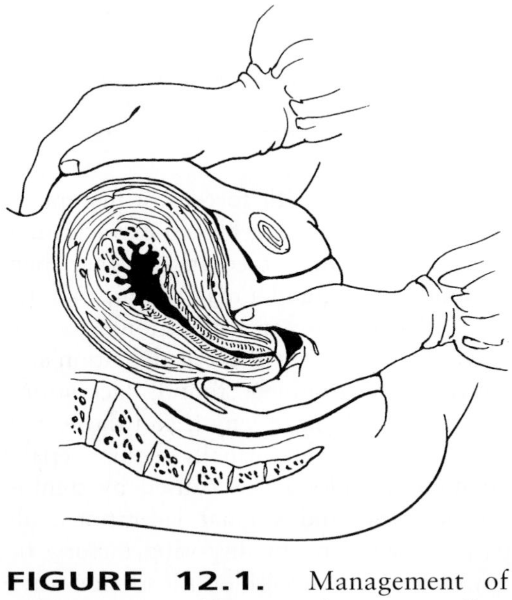

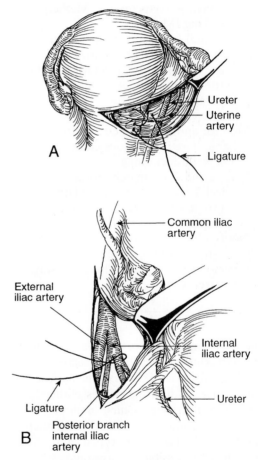

FIGURE 12.2. Surgical treatment of atonic uterine hemorrhage. (*A*) Ligation of the uterine artery. The artery crosses over the ureter and is ligated beyond this point at the uterine corpus. (*B*) Hypogastric artery ligation. Ligation of the anterior division of the internal iliac artery is performed after careful identification and retraction of the ureter, which usually overlies the bifurcation of the iliac artery into the external and internal iliac branches.

FIGURE 12.1. Management of uterine atony with manual massage. One hand gently massages the uterus from the abdomen while the other is inserted so that the cervix is cradled in the fingers and thumb to allow maximal compression and massage.

TABLE 12.2.   Management of the Patient with Postpartum Hemorrhage

Evaluate promptly once excessive bleeding is detected.

Review clinical course for probable cause.
- Any difficulty removing placenta?
- Were forceps used?
- Other predisposing factors?

Perform bimanual examination in recovery area/delivery room.
- Uterus boggy? Massage. Initiate or increase oxytocin; give Methergine, 0.2 mg IM.
- Placental fragments within uterus on exploration or on ultrasound examination? If so, return to delivery room for curettage.
- Laceration or hematoma? Repair in delivery room.

Monitor and maintain circulation.
- Large-bore intravenous catheters: 1 or 2 well functioning lines.
- Type and cross-match blood.
- Check hematocrit and coagulation profile with platelet count for baseline.

Notify obstetric physicians, nurses, and anesthesia and operating room personnel of potential need for surgical intervention.

Visualize cervix and vagina in search of lacerations.
- Repair if present.

Remember that postpartum hemorrhage may be from multiple causes (e.g., atony plus lacerations).

Observe patient constantly. Repeated bimanual examination. If bleeding persists, is the blood clotting? If not, consider disseminated intravascular coagulopathy.

Inform patient of the problem and what measures are being taken to correct it.
- Get an appreciation of her desires regarding further childbearing and hysterectomy.

Preoperative management options.
- Uterine packing.
- Prostaglandin administration.

Operative measures.
- Ligation of vessels.
  - Hypogastric artery ligation.
  - Uterine artery ligation.
- Selective arterial embolization.
- Hysterectomy is treatment of last resort in patient who wants to retain her uterus.

Intensive care measures.
- Hemodynamic, renal, and coagulation surveillance measures.

be individualized in cases of severe uterine atony, taking into account the degree of hemorrhage, the overall status of the patient, and her future childbearing desires (Table 12.2). When hemorrhage occurs, multiple large-bore intravenous access should be obtained, and blood should be typed and cross-matched for possible transfusion.

Lacerations of the Lower Genital Tract

Lacerations of the lower genital tract are far less common than uterine atony as a cause of postpartum hemorrhage, but they can be serious and require prompt surgical repair. *Predisposing factors* include an instru-mented delivery with forceps, a manipulative delivery such as a breech extraction, a precipitous labor, presentations other than occiput anterior, and a macrosomic infant.

Although minor lacerations to the cervix in the process of cervical dilation and delivery are routinely found, lacerations greater than 2 cm in length and those that are actively bleeding usually require repair. To minimize blood loss caused by significant cervical and vaginal lacerations, all patients with any predisposing factors, or any patient in whom blood loss soon after delivery appears to be excessive despite a firm and contracted uterus, should have a careful repeat inspection of the lower genital tract. This vaginal examination may require assistance to allow adequate visual-

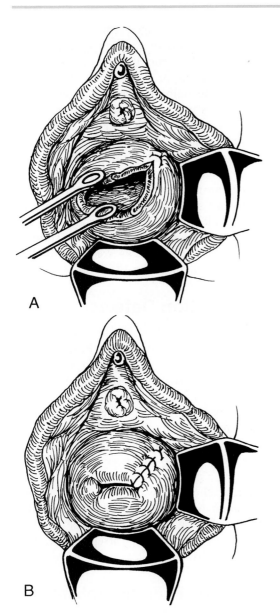

A

B

FIGURE 12.3. Repair of a cervical laceration. (*A*) After careful demonstration of the entire extent of the laceration, the first suture is placed above the apex of the laceration to prevent extension after the repair. (*B*) The laceration is then repaired, whether with interrupted sutures, as shown, or with figure-of-eight or running sutures.

ization. As a rule, repair of these lacerations is usually not difficult if adequate exposure is provided (Figure 12.3). Occasionally, however, extensive repair is required, necessitating general anesthesia.

Lacerations of the vagina and perineum (1st through 4th degree vaginal and peri-urethral lacerations) are not commonly causes of substantial blood loss, although the steady loss of blood, which may come from deeper lacerations, may be significant such that their repair when bleeding is requisite. Periurethral lacerations may be associated with sufficient edema to occlude the urethra causing urinary retention; a Foley catheter for 12 to 24 hours usually prevents this problem.

Retained Placenta

Separation of the placenta from the uterus occurs because of cleavage between the *zona basalis* and the *zona spongiosa*. Once separation occurs, expulsion is caused by strong uterine contractions. Retained placenta can occur when either the process of separation or the process of expulsion is incomplete. Predisposing factors to retained placenta include a previous cesarean delivery, uterine leiomyomas, prior uterine curettage, and succenturiate placental lobe.

Placental tissue remaining in the uterus can prevent adequate contractions and predispose to excessive bleeding. After expulsion, every placenta should be inspected to detect missing cotyledons, which may remain in the uterus. If retained placenta is suspected, either because of apparent absent cotyledons or because of excessive bleeding, it can often be removed by inserting two fingers through the cervix into the uterus and manipulating the retained tissue downward into the vagina. If this is unsuccessful or if there is uncertainty regarding the cause of hemorrhage, an ultrasound examination of the uterus is very helpful. A firmly contracted uterus exhibits a characteristic "stripe" on the ultrasound imaging, representing the newly contracted endometrial cavity. Absence of such a stripe implies placental tissue and/or blood clots remaining within the uterine cavity. Curettage with a suction apparatus and/or a large sharp curette may remove the retained tissue. Care must be exercised to avoid perforation through the uterine fundus.

Placental tissue may also remain in the uterus because separation of the placenta from the uterus may not occur normally. At times, placental villi penetrate the uterine wall to form what is generally called *placenta accreta*. More specifically, abnormal adherence of the placenta to the superficial lining of the uterus is termed placenta accreta, penetration into the uterine muscle itself is called *placenta increta*, and complete invasion through the thickness of the uterine muscle is termed *placenta percreta*. If this abnormal attachment involves the entire placenta, no part of the placenta separates. Much more commonly, however, attachment is not complete and a portion of the placenta separates while the remainder remains attached. Major, life-threatening hemorrhage can ensue. Hysterectomy is often required, although in a woman who desires more children, an attempt to separate the placenta by curettage, or other means of controlling the bleeding (such as uterine artery ligation or hypogastric artery ligation), is usually appropriate in trying to avoid a hysterectomy.

OTHER CAUSES OF POSTPARTUM HEMORRHAGE
Hematomas

Hematomas can occur anywhere from the vulva to the upper vagina as a result of delivery trauma. The frequency of hematoma formation is higher for the vulva and lower vagina than the upper vagina, whereas, conversely, the morbidity is higher with hematomas in the less accessible upper vagina. Hematomas may also develop at the site of episiotomy or perineal laceration. Hematomas may occur without disruption of the vaginal mucosa, when the fetus or forceps causes shearing of the submucosal tissues without mucosal tearing.

Vulvar or vaginal hematomas are characterized by exquisite pain with or without signs of shock. Hematomas that are less than 5 cm in diameter and are not enlarging

can usually be managed expectantly by frequent evaluation of the size of the hematoma and close monitoring of vital signs and urinary output. Application of ice packs can also be helpful. Larger and enlarging hematomas must be managed surgically. If the hematoma is at the site of episiotomy, the sutures should be removed and a search made for the actual bleeding site, which is then ligated. If not at the episiotomy site, the hematoma should be opened at its most dependent portion and drained, the bleeding site identified, if possible, and the site closed with interlocking hemostatic sutures. Drains and vaginal packs are often used to prevent reaccumulation of blood.

Coagulation Defects

Virtually any congenital or acquired abnormality in blood clotting can lead to postpartum hemorrhage. Abruptio placentae, amniotic fluid embolism, and severe preeclampsia are obstetric conditions commonly associated with disseminated intravascular coagulopathy (DIC). The treatment of coagulation defects is aimed at correcting the coagulation defect. When assessing a patient with postpartum hemorrhage, it should always be noted whether the blood that is passing from the genital tract is clotting. It also should be recalled that profuse hemorrhage itself can lead to coagulopathy.

Amniotic Fluid Embolism

Amniotic fluid embolism is a rare, sudden, and often fatal obstetric complication presumably caused primarily by entry of amniotic fluid into the maternal circulation, although there are probably significant biochemical as well as physical mediators of the syndrome. The diagnosis is classically based on the identification of fetal squames and lanugo in the maternal pulmonary system, although these findings are absent in perhaps one third of cases. The clinical diagnosis is based on five findings that occur in sequence: respiratory distress, cyanosis, cardiovascular collapse, hemor-

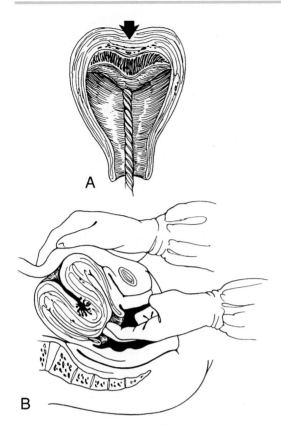

FIGURE 12.4. Uterine inversion. (*A*) Uterine inversion occurring with fundally implanted placenta. (*B*) Manual replacement of a partially inverted uterus.

rhage, and coma. The syndrome also often results in severe coagulopathy. Treatment is directed toward total support of the cardiovascular and coagulation systems, although maternal mortality still approaches 30%–50% in most series.

Uterine Inversion

Uterine inversion is a rare condition; the uterus literally turns inside out, with the top of the uterine fundus extending through the cervix into the vagina and sometimes even past the introitus. Hemorrhage with uterine inversion is characteristically severe and sudden. Treatment includes administration of an anesthetic that causes uterine relaxation (such as halothane) or another agent

with uterus-relaxing properties (such as terbutaline), followed by replacement of the uterine corpus. If this fails, surgical treatment, possibly including hysterectomy, may be needed (Figure 12.4).

GENERAL MANAGEMENT OF PATIENTS WITH POSTPARTUM HEMORRHAGE

Once excessive blood loss is identified, prompt assessment is mandatory. A general approach to management is outlined in Table 12.2. Because most cases of postpartum hemorrhage are caused by uterine atony, the uterus should be palpated abdominally, seeking the soft, boggy consistency of the relaxed uterus. If this is found, oxytocin infusion should be increased and either Methergine or prostaglandins given if the excessive bleeding continues.

Other questions help direct assessment:

Was expulsion of the placenta spontaneous and apparently complete?

Were forceps or other instrumentation used in delivery?

Was the baby large or the delivery difficult or precipitous?

Were the cervix and vagina inspected for lacerations?

Is the blood clotting?

As the cause of the hemorrhage is being identified, general supportive measures for patients with hemorrhage of any cause are initiated. Large-bore intravenous access; crystalloid infusions; type, cross-match, and administration of blood or blood components as needed; periodic assessment of hematocrit and coagulation profile; and monitoring of urinary output are all important.

The management of postpartum hemorrhage is greatly facilitated if patients at high risk are identified and preliminary preparations made before the bleeding episode. Table 12.3 reviews such precautionary measures.

TABLE 12.3. Precautionary Measures to Prevent or Minimize Postpartum Hemorrhage

Before delivery
   Identify any predisposing factors
   Determine baseline hematocrit
   Send blood specimen to blood bank for group and screen
   Establish well-functioning intravenous line with large-bore catheter
   Obtain baseline coagulation studies and platelet count if indicated
In delivery room
   Avoid excessive traction on umbilical cord

Inspect placenta for complete removal
Perform digital exploration of uterus
Massage uterus
Visualize cervix and vagina
Remove all clots in uterus and vagina before transfer to recovery area
In recovery area
   Closely observe patient for excessive bleeding
   Frequently palpate uterus with massage
   Determine vital signs frequently

CASE STUDIES

Case 12A

A 25-year-old G1 P0 has labor induced at 42 weeks' gestational age. Her induction is prolonged but finally results in a forceps-assisted delivery of a healthy, 9.5-lb boy. The placenta is expelled 9 minutes after delivery and appears to be intact. Inspection of the vagina and cervix reveals no lesions except the midline episiotomy. Intravenous oxytocin is begun in dilute solution at the time of placental delivery. During the repair of the midline episiotomy, excessive vaginal bleeding is noted. The patient is becoming tachycardic but her blood pressure is consistent with her intrapartum blood pressures.

Questions Case 12A

Which of the following causes of postpartum hemorrhage may be excluded from consideration at this time based on the information provided?

A. Coagulation defect
B. Uterine atony
C. Retained placental tissue
D. Vaginal laceration
E. None of the above

Answer: E

None can be excluded. Lacerations are sometimes missed on inspection, and placental tissue may be left behind with a placenta that appears to be intact.

Based on the information provided, which of the following is the most likely cause of this patient's postpartum hemorrhage?

A. Coagulation defect
B. Uterine atony
C. Retained placental tissue
D. Vaginal laceration
E. None of the above

Answer: B

Uterine atony is likely in this clinical situation, which includes prolonged pregnancy, Pitocin induction, prolonged labor, difficult delivery, and large infant. However, forceps delivery of a large baby is associated with lacerations of cervix and vagina, which are sometimes difficult to recognize without careful, complete inspection.

Your initial management should include all EXCEPT

A. Careful but rapid reexamination for lacerations
B. Administration of oxytocin
C. Administration of prostaglandin
D. Uterine artery ligation
E. Uterine massage

Answer: D

Initial measures are intended to facilitate uterine contraction and hemostasis. Operative interventions are indicated only if these maneuvers fail.

Case 12B

A 32-year-old G2 P0001 undergoes a spontaneous vaginal delivery of a healthy, 8-lb girl after an unremarkable spontaneous labor. After 10 minutes without spontaneous placental delivery, traction is applied to the umbilical cord. Placental tissue is expelled with the umbilical cord, but vaginal hemorrhage ensues immediately thereafter. The placenta is clearly not intact.

Questions Case 12B

All of the following are appropriate immediate interventions EXCEPT

A. Fluid resuscitation and cardiovascular support
B. Oxytocin administration
C. Manual exploration of the uterine cavity

D. Uterine massage
E. Notification of the operating room and anesthesia of a possible surgical emergency

Answer: E

All of these maneuvers are important for diagnostic and/or therapeutic reasons. Retained placental tissue can be assumed and treatment of an associated uterine atony should be undertaken immediately while attempts to remove the placental tissue proceed. The careful clinician should remember that lacerations are still a possible additional cause of bleeding, albeit unlikely. The need for possible surgical intervention is still remote, so that notification of the operating room is not necessary at this time.

Oxytocin administration, prostaglandin administration, and uterine massage reduce but do not stop the bleeding. Vaginal examination reveals placental tissue in the uterus, but repeated attempts to dislodge it are not successful. Indeed, careful examination between the retained placental tissue and the uterine wall does not reveal a "cleavage plane." What is the most likely diagnosis?

A. Placenta previa
B. Placental abruption
C. Placenta accreta
D. Uterine inversion
E. Endometrial carcinoma

Answer: C

The description is of placenta accreta, causing vaginal hemorrhage unresponsive to oxytocic and uterine atony. Uterine inversion is unlikely given the examination results. Endometrial carcinoma is exceedingly unlikely in this situation.

CHAPTER

13

POSTPARTUM INFECTION

CHAPTER OBJECTIVES

This chapter deals primarily with APGO Objective(s):

OBJECTIVE 29   Postpartum Infection

A. Describe the risk factors, differential diagnosis of infectious agents, and use of antibiotic prophylaxis for postpartum infection.

B. Describe the evaluation and management of presumed/actual postpartum infection.

Infections occurring during the puerperium are a relatively frequent cause of morbidity and, rarely, even mortality in obstetric practice. This chapter addresses common causes of infections in the days and weeks after delivery.

Many factors predispose to postpartum infection, including general health and concurrent medical problems, immune status, and of course concurrent infections (Table 13.1). Even the mode of delivery is itself a determinant of infection. After vaginal delivery, infection occurs much less frequently than after cesarean birth. The incidence of infection varies from 10% to as high as 50% in some populations, depending on the mode of delivery and presence of factors that predispose to postpartum infection (see Table 13.1).

PUERPERAL FEBRILE MORBIDITY

The definition of puerperal *febrile morbidity* is a *temperature of 38.0° C (100.4° F) or*

higher, the temperature to occur on any 2 of the first 10 days postpartum, exclusive of the first 24 hours. This guideline was written in the context of an oral temperature taken four times a day for the first ten postpartum days and is intended to help distinguish true infection from minor temperature elevations commonly seen in the early puerperium and presumed to be the result of breast engorgement. *Practically speaking, significant elevations in maternal temperature even within the first 24 hours postpartum, especially when accompanied by other evidence of infection, are usually thought to represent frank infection, and treatment is often instituted.* However, this "official" definition of puerperal morbidity does serve as a reminder that *not every postpartum temperature elevation reflects infection, and that, in borderline cases, expectant management is warranted.* After an overview of the evaluation of a patient with fever in the early puerperium, discussions of severe, common types of puerperal infection are provided.

TABLE 13.1. Factors That Predispose to Postpartum Infections

Maternal
  Obesity
  Low socioeconomic status
  Anemia
  Immunosuppression
  Chronic disease (e.g., diabetes
    mellitus)
  Vaginal infection, especially bacterial
    vaginosis
Associated with labor and delivery
  Rupture of fetal membranes
  Intra-amniotic infection
  Prolonged labor
  Multiple pelvic examinations during
    labor
  Internal electronic fetal monitoring,
    fetal scalp electrode (FSE), and/or
    intrauterine pressure catheter (IUPC)
  Cesarean birth, especially if prolonged
    operating time

EVALUATION OF THE FEBRILE POSTPARTUM PATIENT

The "sequence" of infection sites is somewhat predictable after vaginal or surgical delivery. On the first postoperative day, the lungs are the common cause of fever (atelectasis, pneumonia); on the second day, the urinary tract (cystitis, pyelonephritis); on the third day, the wound (superficial infection, necrotizing fasciitis); and on the fourth day, the extremities (thrombophlebitis). The common mnemonic phrase is *Wind, Water, Wound, and Walking.* The most common infection is metritis (infection of the uterine cavity and adjacent tissue), which is usually associated with the development of fever on the first or second days postpartum. Finally, infection of the breast (mastitis) is seen in the first few weeks postpartum, usually in patients who are breast-feeding.

When evaluating a febrile patient, a *history* of the labor and delivery can be helpful. If, for example, the patient had amnionitis and was febrile through labor, one would suspect metritis as the cause of fever. A careful history regarding pulmonary symptoms, urinary tract disturbance, and abdominopelvic pain and tenderness is of paramount importance. Pertinent information from the prenatal course of care is also often useful, such as medical problems that predispose to infection, a history of sexually transmitted diseases, or bacterial vaginosis. *Examination* should include the lungs, the back (for costovertebral tenderness), palpation of the abdomen, careful inspection of the incision site, a check for the presence of bowel sounds, examination of the perineum (if an episiotomy was performed or if a laceration occurred), a pelvic examination, assessment for calf tenderness, and inspection of any intravenous site. Although a pelvic examination may not elicit any findings other than uterine tenderness, one can confirm that lochia drainage is, in fact, occurring, and baseline information can be obtained concerning adnexal masses that may be important if the fever persists and an abscess develops. Blood cultures are not usually obtained unless the infection appears severe, sepsis is suspected, fever is especially high, or the response to limited therapy is delayed.

METRITIS

The most common infection after cesarean delivery is infection of the uterus. Often, such infection is improperly termed *endometritis* but, in fact, these infections usually extend well beyond the thin endometrial lining into the adjacent myometrium, the loose fibroareolar tissues within the parametrium, and sometimes beyond, with pelvic abscess formation. Hence, the *preferred term is metritis* for the initial "limited infection." An unusual condition is the *postcesarean phlegmon,* when infection proceeds from the lateral aspect of the uterus laterally to the pelvic sidewall, forming a pseudomass (Figure 13.1). The duration of labor, duration of rupture of membranes, and the presence of amnionitis

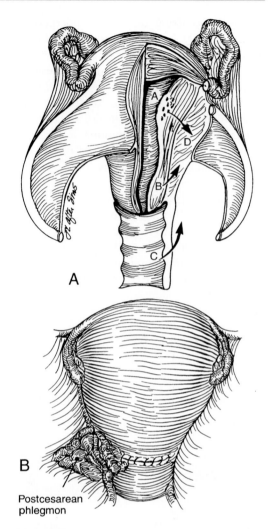

FIGURE 13.1. **A,** Metritis. Infection may extend from a placental site (*A*) or cervical/vaginal lacerations (*B, C*) into the loose parametrial tissues (*D*). **B,** Postcesarean phlegmon. Infection extends from the incision site laterally to the pelvic sidewall, seeming on pelvic examination to be a firm, three-dimensional mass next to the uterus.

during labor are the major factors leading to the development of metritis.

Fever is the characteristic feature in the diagnosis of metritis, and it may be accompanied by *uterine tenderness.* If the infection has spread to the parametrium and adnexa, tenderness may be present there as well. Signs of peritoneal irritation and diminished or absent bowel sounds, especially associ-

TABLE 13.2. Common Organisms Associated with Pelvic Infections

Aerobes		Anaerobes	
Gram-positive	**Gram-negative**	**Gram-positive**	**Gram-negative**
Staphylococcus	*Escherichia coli*	*Peptococcus*	*Bacteroides*
Streptococcus (A,B)	*Proteus*	*Peptostreptococcus*	
Enterococci (group D	*Klebsiella*	*Clostridium*	
Streptococcus)			

ated with ileus, indicate more serious infection, including the possibility of abscess formation. A leukocytosis in the range of 15,000 to 30,000 cells/ml^3 is common but difficult to interpret in the presence of the normal, early puerperium leukocytosis.

As with virtually all pelvic infections, metritis is polymicrobial in origin. Both aerobic and anaerobic organisms are commonly isolated, with anaerobic organisms predominating. The most common of these organisms are listed in Table 13.2. Because bacteria are normally found in the vagina and endocervix, it is difficult to culture the endometrial cavity properly because sampling devices are contaminated on transcervical sampling. On a practical basis, treatment using broad antibiotic coverage against a variety of common microorganisms is usually prescribed without cultures.

Various choices of *initial antibiotic therapy* are used, most of which are successful. Single-agent therapy has the benefit of ease of administration and is often cost saving; cephalosporins such as cefotetan and cefoxitin are commonly used. A combination of ampicillin and an aminoglycoside is also popular, as is the combination of clindamycin with gentamicin. Many such initial therapies have "gaps" in their total coverage—that is, one or more major pathogens are not sensitive to the antibiotic treatment. Therefore, *it is customary to provide additional antibiotic coverage if there has been no response within 48 to 72 hours.* Intravenous antibiotic administration while the patient is hospitalized is preferred for initial treatment. *Intravenous antibiotic therapy is continued until the patient is asymptomatic, has normal bowel function, and has been afebrile for at least 24 hours.* Subsequent outpatient oral antibiotic treatment is usually unnecessary (Table 13.3).

Occasionally a *pelvic abscess* further complicates the patient's recovery. Evidence that suggests abscess formation includes persistent fever despite antibiotic therapy, protracted malaise, delayed return of gastrointestinal function, localization of pain and/or tenderness in the abdominal cavity, and detection of a mass on pelvic/abdominal examination. Ultrasonography or other imaging scans [i.e., computed tomography (CT), magnetic resonance imaging] may be helpful in diagnosing a pelvic abscess. Management of a persistent pelvic abscess includes drainage by either percutaneous techniques, colpotomy (Figure 13.2), or laparotomy. Intra-abdominal rupture of a pelvic abscess is a surgical emergency. Sepsis may occur in association with pelvic infection, with or without frank abscess formation.

Prophylactic antibiotic therapy at the time of cesarean delivery has been shown to reduce significantly the likelihood of postpartum infection. A single dose of a broad-spectrum antibiotic [for example, cefazolin sodium (Ancef), 1 g] is usually given at the time of clamping of the umbilical cord, a practice designed to avoid confounding of subsequent bacterial cultures of the infant should they be necessary. Additional doses of antibiotics given after surgery do not seem to provide added protection against infection.

TABLE 13.3. Antibiotic Therapy for Metritis

Single-drug regimens
Cefazolin (Ancef)	1 g IV q 8 h
Cefotetan (Cefotan)	2 g IV q 12 h
Cefoxitin (Mefoxin)	1–2 g q 8 h
Ampicillin w/sulbactam (Unasyn)	1.5–3.0 g q 6 h
Ticarcillin w/clavulanic acid (Timentin)	3.1 g q 6 h

Multiple-drug regimens
Clindamycin–gentamicin
Clindamycin (Cleocin)	900 mg IV q 8 h
Gentamicin (Garamycin)	70–100 mg IV q 8 h*

Clindamycin–aztreonam
Clindamycin (Cleocin)	900 mg IV q 8 h
Aztreonam (Azactam)	2 g IV q 8 h

Cefoxitin–doxycycline
Cefoxitin (Mefoxin)	1–2 g q 8 h
Doxycycline	100 mg IV q 8 h

Ampicillin–gentamicin–clindamycin
Ampicillin	2 g q 6 h
Gentamicin (Garamycin)	
Clindamycin (Cleocin)	

*Adjust for impaired renal function; check serum levels for therapeutic range on first day.

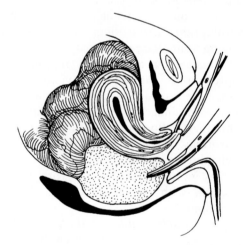

FIGURE 13.2. Drainage of abscess in posterior cul-de-sac of Douglas by colpotomy.

RESPIRATORY COMPLICATIONS/ INFECTION

Respiratory complications are especially common in the first 24 hours after delivery, particularly if general anesthesia was used. *Atelectasis* is also common if general anesthesia was used. Preoperative training in the use of an inspiratory inhaler and its postoperative use under supervision significantly reduces the incidence and severity of this complication. Atelectasis is arguably a cause of postoperative fever, but it is certainly associated with it, and its resolution often coincides with clinical defervescence. *Postoperative pneumonia* is uncommon and is usually seen in those with predelivery respiratory disease. *Aspiration pneumonia* is a feared complication of any surgery. However, it is especially likely to occur when general anesthesia is used in pregnancy, when there is relative gastric stasis, a greater likelihood of emesis, or a likely chance that anesthesia was used in an emergency situation.

URINARY TRACT INFECTIONS

Urinary tract infections are also commonly seen after cesarean delivery but may occur after vaginal delivery. Bladder catheterization, a practice common with both cesarean deliveries and epidural anesthesia, introduces bacteria into the lower urinary tract, which can lead to infection.

Dysuria (painful urination) is not as common in the puerperium as at other times because of a relative insensitivity of the bladder after delivery. *Frequency* of urination is also a normal occurrence postpartum, minimizing the value of this symptom during the postpartum period. *Costovertebral tenderness* may suggest an upper urinary tract infection. When a urinary tract infection is suspected, a clean-catch or catheterized urine sample should be obtained for urinalysis and for culture. Antibiotic treatment is begun with one of a variety of broad-spectrum agents, and if the patient is especially uncomfortable, urinary analgesia may be provided (phenazopyridine, 200 mg three times a day). The antibiotic can be changed if the culture results (usually available 24 to 48 hours later) indicate resistance of the bacteria to the initial antibiotic, especially if symptoms persist.

WOUND INFECTIONS, SEPARATIONS, AND DEHISCENCE

Infection of the *incision site* after cesarean delivery can occur, but is uncommon (3%–8% of cases in most series, reduced by 50% with prophylactic antibiotic use). Risk factors include obesity, diabetes, corticosteroid therapy, immunosuppression, anemia, and poor hemostasis from any cause with subsequent hematoma formation. Fever accompanied by pain, tenderness, and erythema around the incision are seen most frequently on the third and fourth days after delivery. Induration and drainage from the incision site may also be noted. As with any wound infection, the incision must be probed to determine the extent of infection, to ensure that the fascia is intact, and to permit adequate drainage of purulent or serosanguineous material. A culture of the site should be obtained, after which broad-spectrum antibiotic treatment is often initiated, although drainage alone may be adequate. Meticulous care of the open wound is also vital. If the infection disrupts the closure of the fascia, return to the operating room for debridement and reapproximation of the wound is necessary, with delayed closure of the skin being the usual management.

Infections of the episiotomy site are very uncommon (probably less than one fourth of 1% of cases), which is somewhat surprising given the bacterial milieu in that area. Infected episiotomy sites are tender and swollen. Poor tissue turgor often leads to breakdown of the sutures used in the initial repair. The sutures should be removed and drainage permitted, both to limit further spread of infection and to promote healing. Sitz baths also help in healing. Subsequent repair of the episiotomy site, if necessary, can be accomplished soon after the infection has cleared.

Necrotizing fasciitis is a rare infection that may be seen on the perineum or with abdominal incisions. It is caused by gas-forming organisms including *Clostridium*. This especially virulent and frequently fatal infectious process involves the subcutaneous tissue, muscle, and fascia. It may spread downward along the thighs or upward onto the abdomen and chest. This necrotic tissue must be immediately debrided until healthy tissue is reached. Antibiotics, cardiovascular system support, and subsequent skin grafting comprise the overall treatment. Without such vigorous care, fatality is virtually ensured; even with treatment, approximately 50% of the patients with necrotizing fasciitis do not survive. The key factor is early recognition of the possibility that a wound infection, whether perineal or abdominal, may represent this overwhelming infection.

SEPTIC PELVIC THROMBOPHLEBITIS

Septic pelvic thrombophlebitis is an uncommon infection and is a sequela of pelvic infection. The venous drainage of the pelvic organs tends to flow in a left-to-right fashion through the right ovarian vein. Venous stasis in these widely dilated veins, along with the presence of multiple bacteria if infection is present, can lead to septic thrombosis in these vessels; subsequent *microembolization* of the lungs or other organs by way of the inferior vena cava is possible.

Clinically, this infection is manifest as *residual fever and tachycardia* after several days of antibiotic treatment for presumed metritis. Usually the patient is asymptomatic with respect to uterine tenderness and bowel function. Although it is possible to diagnose this condition with CT scanning or other such imaging, it is customary to begin empiric treatment with *heparin.* Prompt resolution of the fever and tachycardia, usually within 24 hours, corroborates the diagnosis. Anticoagulation therapy is recommended for at least 7 and up to 30 days.

MASTITIS

In the lactating woman, breast infection occurs most commonly several weeks postpartum, but it can occur much later. Initially, symptoms can be misleading. Patients often complain of significant *fever* (often 103° F or more), *chills, malaise,* and *general body aching.* Breast symptoms may be somewhat vague, although breast tenderness is described if patients are asked specifically about this. Commonly, patients think they have a generalized viral infection and call their physician seeking information regarding medications to take for the flu while lactating.

After the onset of these signs and symptoms, evidence of infection becomes more localized to the breasts over the following days. Erythema and tenderness are present, often with a brawny and indurated area to palpation, which may be segmented in orientation. The infection is virtually always unilateral. Once the infection has progressed to produce fever and clinical findings, it may proceed to generalized sepsis very quickly, often in a matter of just a few hours. *Staphylococcus aureus* is cultured from the breast milk in about 50% of cases; no single predominant organism is identified in other cases. The origin of the infection is, in fact, the infant's pharynx; accordingly, there should be no concern on the part of the mother with respect to transmitting the infection to the infant.

It is no longer common practice to culture the breast milk. However, because of the prevalence of the *S. aureus* as the offender, an antibiotic that is penicillinase resistant, such as *dicloxacillin* (500 mg orally every 6 hours) is recommended. Resolution of symptoms is usually prompt, with marked improvement within 24 to 36 hours. Patients should be cautioned to complete the full antibiotic course to prevent recurrence. It is *not necessary to withhold nursing* on the infected breast, although some patients benefit greatly from uninterrupted rest for the first day or two of therapy.

Mastitis is usually distinguished from a blocked (inspissated) duct (see Chapter 10) on the basis of fever. At times, however, it may be difficult to distinguish these two entities, and antibiotic treatment is usually begun empirically.

CASE STUDIES

Case 13A

At 9 days postpartum, a new mother complains that she feels awful, is running a fever of 99° to 100° F, and "just aches all over." She is breast-feeding, but the baby *has been fretful the last 48 hours. She has no complaints of sore throat, dysuria, or pelvic pain (except the uterine cramps she has come to expect with breast-feeding),* and her breasts are not especially tender. On examination, the left breast is slightly warmer to touch and slightly more tender than the right.

Questions Case 13A

The most likely diagnosis is

A. Mastitis
B. Breast abscess
C. Fibrocystic disorder
D. Squamous cell carcinoma
E. Trauma and fat necrosis

Answer: A

Appropriate management includes

A. Surgical drainage of the infected breast
B. Cannulation of the breast ducts over the affected lobules
C. Administration of an oral penicillinase-resistant antibiotic
D. Instructions to cease breast-feeding until the infection clears
E. Mammography to rule out carcinoma

Answer: C

The presumptive diagnosis is early mastitis. Mastitis usually responds readily to oral antibiotic therapy. Surgical intervention for mastitis is not indicated, although drainage of an abscess may be. There is no risk to the baby or mother from continuing breast-feeding. The risk of carcinoma is exceedingly low.

Case 13B

A 27-year-old G1 P0 has induction of labor at 42 weeks for postdates pregnancy, undergoes induction with FSE and IUPC monitoring for 36 hours, and delivery is by cesarean section for fetal distress when she has dilated to 8 cm. The patient was afebrile before the surgery and was given

one dose of prophylactic antibiotics at the time of umbilical cord clamping.

Her immediate postpartum course is unremarkable. She is bottle feeding and lactation has not begun. On the third postpartum day, she develops a fever to 102.2° F with chills and lower quadrant abdominal pain. Examination reveals a tender uterine fundus and somewhat diminished but not absent bowel sounds. There is a slightly foul lochia, and the cervix is tender to manipulation. The breasts are nontender. A complete blood count reveals a hematocrit of 29 and a white blood cell (WBC) count of 14,500 with a left shift.

Questions Case 13B

The most likely diagnosis is

A. Mastitis
B. Metritis
C. Pelvic abscess
D. Septic pelvic thrombophlebitis
E. Atelectasis

Answer: B

Mastitis is unlikely in a bottle-feeding mother with normal breast findings. Metritis is highly likely given the prolonged labor with intrauterine catheter and scalp electrode and subsequent cesarean birth. Pelvic abscess is possible but it is somewhat early for this to develop. Septic pelvic thrombophlebitis is possible but likewise unlikely at this time. Atelectasis is unlikely to present 3 days after surgery with this temperature.

Your management at this time should include

A. Single-agent antibiotic therapy
B. Multiple-agent antibiotic therapy
C. Anticoagulation with heparin
D. Diagnostic laparoscopy or laparotomy
E. Observation

(Continued)

Answer: A

A single-agent antibiotic regimen suffices in most cases of simple metritis. Multiple-agent regimens are best left for situations in which the response to a single agent is unsatisfactory. Anticoagulation is not indicated at this time because the diagnosis of septic thrombophlebitis has not been made. Surgical evaluation is contraindicated with a diagnosis that is expected to respond to a simple antibiotic regimen. Observation to see if the fever continues is an option, but most clinicians proceed with therapy given a history that includes so many factors predisposing to metritis and these physical findings.

After 72 hours, the patient remains febrile and uncomfortable. Her WBC count is now 19,000. Your management at this time should include

A. Single-agent antibiotic therapy
B. Multiple-agent antibiotic therapy
C. Anticoagulation with heparin
D. Diagnostic laparoscopy or laparotomy as required
E. Observation

Answer: B

Multiple-agent antibiotic therapy is now indicated to cover the full range of aerobic and anaerobic organisms that may be expected in metritis.

Multiple-agent therapy is continued for 48 hours but the patient remains febrile. Examination of the abdomen reveals a less tender uterus and pelvic examination reveals a slightly tender uterus but no masses. Ultrasound examination does not reveal an abscess. The most likely diagnosis is

A. Mastitis
B. Metritis
C. Pelvic abscess
D. Septic pelvic thrombophlebitis
E. Atelectasis

Answer: D

Without evidence of abscess, the most likely diagnosis is metritis plus septic pelvic thrombophlebitis.

Your management at this time should include

A. Single-agent antibiotic therapy
B. Multiple-agent antibiotic therapy
C. Anticoagulation with heparin
D. Diagnostic laparoscopy or laparotomy as required
E. Observation

Answer: C

C H A P T E R

14

ABORTION

CHAPTER OBJECTIVES

This chapter deals primarily with APGO Objective(s):

OBJECTIVE 17   Spontaneous Abortion

Explain the differential diagnosis, diagnosis, and management of first trimester bleeding, including incomplete, missed, and threatened abortion, and also septic and recurrent abortion.

OBJECTIVE 37   Abortion

Describe the surgical and nonsurgical means of pregnancy termination and the evaluation and management of associated psychosocial considerations as well as complications such as hemorrhage and infection.

(Continued)

OBJECTIVE 22   Fetal Death

A. Describe the differential diagnosis, symptoms, physical findings, and diagnostic methods, and management for the causes of fetal death in each trimester.

B. Describe the emotional reactions to fetal death and their effect on its management.

C. Describe the maternal complications of fetal death, including disseminated intravascular coagulopathy.

Abortion is the termination of a pregnancy before viability, typically defined as 20 weeks from the first day of the last normal menstrual period or a fetus weighing less than 500 g. Whether spontaneous or induced, there are profound medical as well as emotional implications associated with abortion. Because the lay expression for spontaneous abortion is "miscarriage," care should be taken to explain the terminology to the patient.

SPONTANEOUS ABORTION

The *incidence of spontaneous abortion* is estimated at 50% of all pregnancies, an estimate based on the assumption that many pregnancies spontaneously terminate without clinical recognition. An incidence of recognized spontaneous abortion of 15% to 25% is commonly cited, with approximately 80% occurring during the first 12 weeks of pregnancy.

Approximately 50% of early spontaneous abortions are attributed to chromosomal abnormalities, of which trisomy accounts for 40% to 50%, monosomy C for 15% to 25%, triploidy for approximately 15%, and tetraploidy for approximately 5%. If the first abortus is chromosomally abnormal, a second abortus has an 80% chance of being abnormal as well. Risk factors associated with spontaneous abortion include increasing parity, increasing maternal age, increasing paternal age, and conception within 3 months of a live birth. Abnormal development of the early pregnancy (including the zygote, embryo, fetus, or placenta) is a common pathologic finding in spontaneous abortion. Expulsion of the pregnancy is typically preceded by death of the embryo or fetus.

The further that a pregnancy progresses before undergoing spontaneous abortion, the less likely that the fetus is chromosomally abnormal compared with first-trimester abortions. Second-trimester abortions are less likely to be chromosomal and more likely to be caused by maternal systemic disease, abnormal placentation, or other anatomic considerations. This difference is of great clinical significance, because these conditions can be treated and recurrent abortions can thereby potentially be prevented.

Maternal Factors

INFECTIOUS FACTORS

Maternal systemic conditions that have been associated with spontaneous abortion include infections such as *Listeria monocytogenes, Mycoplasma hominis, Ureaplasma urealyticum,* and toxoplasmosis as well as viral infections including rubella and cytomegalic inclusion disease.

SYSTEMIC FACTORS

Insufficient secretion of progesterone by the corpus luteum or the placenta may be associated with spontaneous abortion. *Luteal phase inadequacy* occurs in 3% of the general population but more frequently in those suffering spontaneous pregnancy loss. Luteal phase defect is diagnosed by appropriately timed endometrial biopsy, not serum progesterone assay. Treatment may include clomiphene, which acts by increasing follicle-stimulating hormone (FSH), and human chorionic gonadotropin (hCG), which is the physiologic luteotropic stimulus. Although uncommon, uncorrected medical conditions such as *hypothyroidism, systemic lupus erythematosus,* and *diabetes mellitus* are also associated with an increased incidence of spontaneous abortion.

The risk of spontaneous abortion also increases with maternal age. This may be related to an increased incidence of chromosomally abnormal pregnancies in older patients.

ENVIRONMENTAL FACTORS

Spontaneous abortion has also been related to environmental toxins, radiation, and immunologic factors. Both *smoking and alcohol consumption* have been linked to miscarriages. Women who smoke more than one pack of cigarettes per day have an almost twofold increase in their rate of spontaneous abortion. Women who drink more than 2 days per week experience twice the abortion rate of those who do not.

UTERINE FACTORS

Leiomyomata uteri, especially when located in a submucous position, have been associated with spontaneous abortion. It is uncommon for subserous or intramural leiomyomata of the uterus to be a causative factor of spontaneous abortion. Removal of the leiomyomata (myomectomy) is recommended only if it is determined that pregnancy wastage has been caused by this anatomic distortion.

Spontaneous abortion can also be caused by a *unicornuate* or *septate uterus,* with 20% to 30% of women with a unicornuate or septate uterus having reproductive difficulties, most frequently recurrent pregnancy loss. In utero exposure to *diethylstilbestrol (DES)* has been associated with abnormally shaped uteri as well as cervical incompetence.

Intrauterine synechiae (Asherman's syndrome) has been linked to spontaneous abortion, caused by an inadequate amount of endometrium to support implantation. This condition is typically a sequela of uterine curettage with subsequent destruction and scarring of the endometrium (Table 14.1).

Paternal Factors

Occasionally, a chromosomal abnormality in either parent may be a cause of spontaneous abortion. As a result, couples suffering recurrent abortions should have karyotyping of both parents. In addition, as with eggs, advanced age of sperm may also increase the rate of spontaneous abortion.

Fetal Factors

Genetic abnormalities of the conceptus are the most common cause of spontaneous abortion. More than 50% of abortions in the first trimester are caused by chromosomal anomalies, approximately half of which are autosomal trisomies. Whereas chromosomally abnormal pregnancies tend to terminate early, chromosomally normal pregnancies are usually lost later in gestation. Specifically, three fourths of aneuploid abortions occur before 8 weeks, whereas the incidence of euploid abortions is highest at 13 weeks.

Immunologic Factors

A successful pregnancy is dependent on an immunologic environment that permits the mother (host) to maintain the antigenically dissimilar fetus in the uterus. The exact mechanism for the success of the fetal allograft is yet undetermined. In patients who

TABLE 14.1.   Causes of Spontaneous Abortion

Genetic factors (10%–50%)
   Nondisjunction
   Balanced translocation/carrier state
Endocrine abnormalities (25%–50%)
   Luteal phase defect
   Thyroid disease
   Hyperandrogenism
   In utero DES exposure
Reproductive tract abnormalities
   (6%–12%)
   Leiomyomata uteri (submucous)
   Septate uterus
   Bicornuate or unicornuate uterus
   Incompetent cervix
   Intrauterine adhesions
   Abnormality of placentation
Infection
   Listeria monocytogenes
   Mycoplasma hominis
   Ureaplasma urealyticum
   Toxoplasmosis
   Syphilis
Systemic disease
   Diabetes mellitus
   Chronic renal disease
   Chronic cardiovascular disease
   Systemic lupus/lupus anticoagulant
Immunologic factor
   Hostile immunologic environment
      for fetal allograft
Environmental factors
   Toxins
   Radiation
   Smoking
   Alcohol
   Anesthetic gases

DES = diethylstilbestrol.

suffer from recurrent abortion, immunologic evaluation of both partners should be considered.

DIFFERENTIAL DIAGNOSIS OF ABORTION

Because the differential diagnosis of bleeding in the first trimester of pregnancy includes a wide range of possibilities such as ectopic pregnancy, hydatidiform mole, cervical polyps, and cervicitis, the patient should be examined whenever bleeding occurs. Any vaginal bleeding in the first half of an intrauterine pregnancy is presumptively called a *threatened abortion* unless another specific diagnosis can be made.

Threatened Abortion

Threatened abortion occurs in up to 25% of pregnancies with approximately half of these patients proceeding to spontaneous abortion. Those who carry a pregnancy complicated by threatened abortion to viability are at greater risk for preterm delivery, low-birth weight, and a higher incidence of perinatal mortality. There does not, however, appear to be a higher incidence of congenital malformations in these newborns. Some patients describe bleeding at the time of their expected menses, sometimes referred to as the *placental sign or implantation bleeding,* which may be the result of ruptured blood vessels in the endometrium. Low abdominal pain may accompany the bleeding. On examination the cervix is usually closed. Other sources of bleeding such as the cervix, urethra, and rectum should also be considered.

Ultrasonography is especially useful to determine if an early pregnancy is intact. Lack of a gestational sac does not, however, rule out a very early viable pregnancy. Ultrasonography, in conjunction with quantitative hCG, has been used to identify viable pregnancies at various stages of gestation. Transabdominal ultrasonography can identify an intact gestation if the quantitative β-hCG exceeds 5000 to 6000 mIU/ml, whereas transvaginal ultrasonography can typically identify an early intact pregnancy when the β-hCG level exceeds 1500 mIU/ml.

Inevitable Abortion

An *inevitable abortion* is defined as rupture of the membranes and/or cervical dilation during the first half of pregnancy such that pregnancy loss is unavoidable. It is unusual for a pregnancy to successfully reach viability in this circumstance. Uterine contractions typically follow and the products of conception are expelled. Conservative management of these patients significantly increases the risk of infection.

Complete Abortion

Complete abortion refers to a documented pregnancy that spontaneously passes all of the products of conception. Early in pregnancy, the fetus and placenta are often expelled in toto.

Incomplete Abortion

In those cases of spontaneous abortions in which partial expulsion of pregnancy tissue has occurred, bleeding and pain result. Suction curettage of the uterus is usually necessary to remove the remaining products of conception and prevent further bleeding and infection (see Chapter 24). Postevacuation treatment with an oxytocic (Methergine, 0.2 mg po q 4 h for 24 hours) and an antibiotic (doxycycline, 100 mg po bid for 3 days) reduces the risk of further bleeding and infection.

Missed Abortion

A *missed abortion* is the retention of a failed intrauterine pregnancy for an extended period, usually defined as more than two menstrual cycles. These patients present with an absence of uterine growth and may have lost some of the early symptoms of pregnancy. Although unusual, disseminated intravascular coagulopathy (DIC) can occur when an intrauterine fetal demise in the second trimester has been retained beyond 6 weeks after the death of the fetus. Evacuation of the uterus with suction curettage is recommended for pregnancy in the first trimester, whereas dilation and evacuation (D&E) or the use of prostaglandin suppositories is used for pregnancies that have advanced to the second trimester.

Recurrent Abortion

Recurrent abortion is a term used when a patient has had more than two consecutive or a total of three spontaneous abortions. In early abortions, there is a great likelihood of a chromosomal abnormality, whereas in later abortions, a maternal cause is more likely. Karyotyping is recommended for both parents when recurrent early abortion occurs, because there is a 3% chance of one parent being a symptomless carrier of a chromosomal abnormality after two fetal losses. The possibility of immunologic factors should also be explored. Correction of maternal medical conditions and/or anatomic deformities should be pursued for those patients with recurrent late abortions. These include surgical correction of uterine abnormalities, cerclage of the incompetent cervix, or lysis of intrauterine synechiae.

Recurrent abortion can be the result of *uterine anomalies,* such as septate uterus, with only approximately 25% of patients with septate uteri having problems with fetal wastage. Getting pregnant is usually not a problem, but maintaining pregnancy may require surgical management. Such management may include hysterography, hysteroscopy, and laparoscopy.

The *incompetent cervix* is diagnosed mainly by its classic history of sudden expulsion of a normal sac and fetus between the eighteenth and thirty-second week of pregnancy without prior pain or bleeding. Diagnosis is by history and observation of a lax, open cervical os. Increasingly, ultrasound visualization of shortening and funneling of the cervical canal during pregnancy is being used to make this diagnosis. Treatment is surgical by the *cerclage procedures,* which involve the placement of a "purse-string" suture about the cervix to close the incompetent cervix (Figure 14.1). Such sutures are commonly placed during pregnancy when the cervix is found to be dilating asymptomatically. The suture must be removed when labor ensues (or rupture of membranes occurs) or the patient must be delivered by cesarean birth. Allowing a patient to labor with a cerclage in place risks extensive laceration of the cervix and/or uterine rupture.

Intrauterine synechiae associated with *Asherman's syndrome* may occur after a vigorous curettage has denuded the

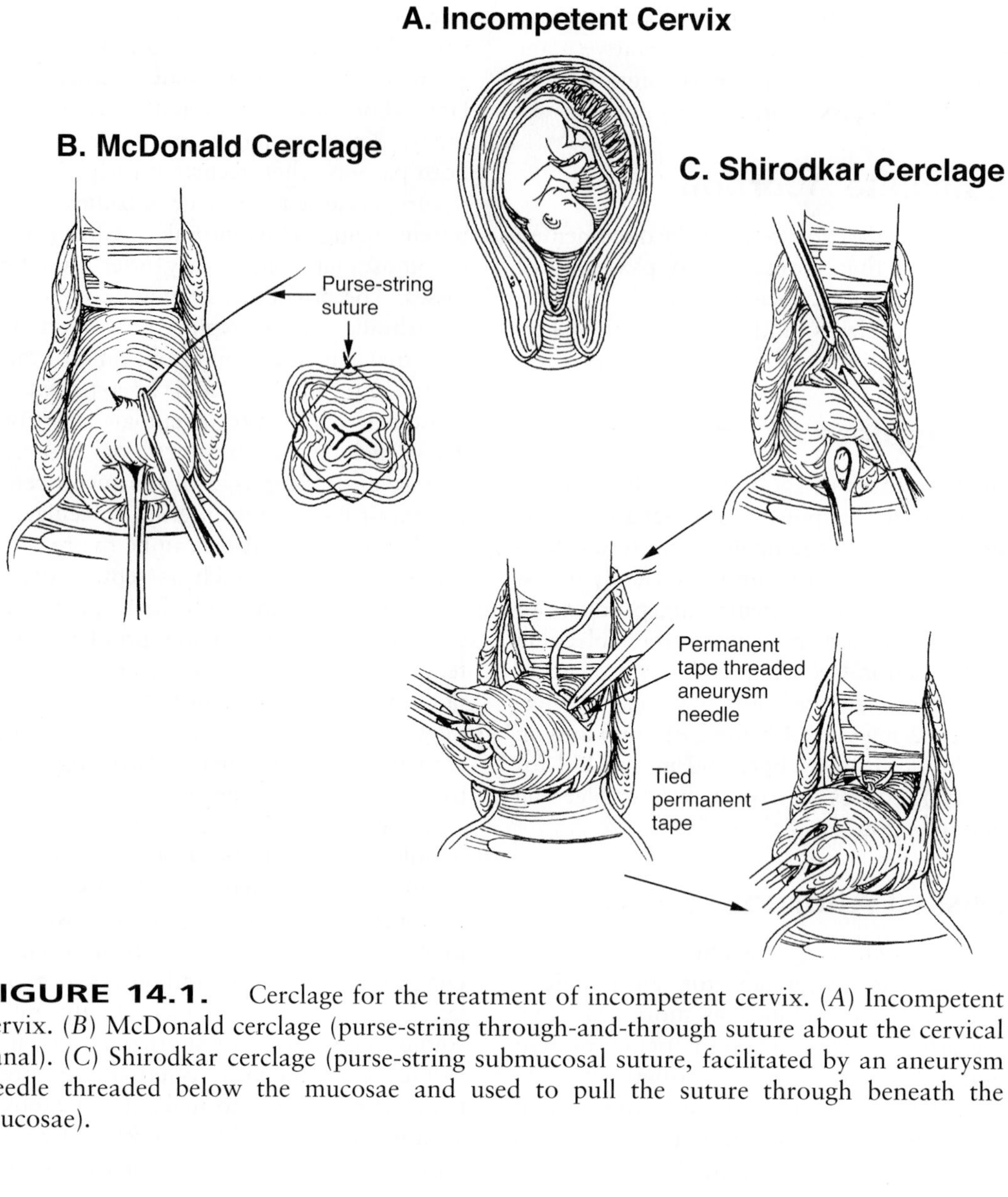

A. Incompetent Cervix

B. McDonald Cerclage

C. Shirodkar Cerclage

Purse-string suture

Permanent tape threaded aneurysm needle

Tied permanent tape

FIGURE 14.1. Cerclage for the treatment of incompetent cervix. (*A*) Incompetent cervix. (*B*) McDonald cerclage (purse-string through-and-through suture about the cervical canal). (*C*) Shirodkar cerclage (purse-string submucosal suture, facilitated by an aneurysm needle threaded below the mucosae and used to pull the suture through beneath the mucosae).

endometrium past the layer of the basalis so that webs of myometrium develop across the uterine cavity (the synechiae). Asherman's syndrome is associated with amenorrhea or irregular menses, infertility, and recurrent pregnancy loss. The diagnosis is confirmed by a hysterogram that shows the characteristic webbed pattern or by hysteroscopy. Treatment involves lysis of the synechiae and postoperative treatment with high doses of estrogen (conjugated estrogen, Premarin, 1.25 mg po two to four times per day for several weeks) to facilitate endome-

trial proliferation, leading to the reestablishment of a normal endometrial layer.

TREATMENT OF SPONTANEOUS ABORTION

No intervention is necessary for patients with threatened abortion even if the bleeding is accompanied by low abdominal pain and cramping. If there is no evidence of significant pathology on ultrasound evaluation, and the pregnancy is found to be intact, the patient can be reassured and allowed to continue normal activities. Intercourse is usually proscribed for 2 to 3 weeks, or longer, depending on the etiology of bleeding. Although commonly recommended, a short period of bed rest has no documented benefit.

If pain and bleeding persist, especially with significant hemodynamic alterations, or if ultrasound and hormonal evaluation identify a nonviable pregnancy, evacuation of the uterus should be carried out. Immediate considerations include control of bleeding, prevention of infection, pain relief, and emotional support.

Bleeding is controlled by ensuring that the products of conception have been expelled or removed from the uterus. In cases of complete abortion the uterus is small and firm, the cervix is closed, and ultrasound identifies an empty uterus. Evacuation of the uterus is accomplished via curettage in cases of incomplete, inevitable, missed, or septic abortions. Hemostasis is enhanced through uterine contraction stimulated by intravenous oxytocin or intramuscular Methergine (methylergonovine maleate). Removal of the products of conception also decreases the risk of infection, and this, combined with vaginal rest (no tampons, douches, or intercourse), provides adequate infection protection in most cases.

A mild analgesic may be required and should be offered. Rh—mothers should receive Rh immune globulin (RhoGAM). Chromosomal evaluation of spontaneous abortions is not recommended unless there is a history of recurrent abortion.

Emotional support is important for both the short- and long-term well-being of the patient as well as her partner. No matter how well prepared for the possibility of pregnancy loss a couple is, the event is a significant disappointment and cause of stress. When appropriate, the couple should be reassured that the loss was not precipitated by anything that they did or did not do and that there was nothing that they could have done to prevent the loss.

A follow-up office visit is generally scheduled for 2 to 6 weeks after the loss of a pregnancy. This is an appropriate time to evaluate uterine involution, assess the return of menses, and discuss reproductive plans. The causes (or lack of causes) of the pregnancy loss should also be reiterated. The impact of this loss on future childbearing should be discussed. A single pregnancy loss does not significantly increase the risk of future losses. Multiple pregnancy losses carry an increased risk for future pregnancies based, in part, on the higher likelihood of a continuing causative condition such as fibroids, immune diseases, or genetic disorders.

INDUCED ABORTION

Termination of an intact pregnancy before the time of viability can be done to safeguard the health of the mother or on a purely elective (i.e., voluntary) basis. Elective abortion has been legal since the Supreme Court decision of *Roe v. Wade*. Since that time, various local and state laws have been proposed to significantly limit access to elective abortion. These laws will continue to undergo many court challenges as our society struggles to define a consistent national policy.

Before undergoing an elective abortion, patients must be aware that choices are available. These include continuation of pregnancy with subsequent adoption, continuation of pregnancy and keeping the child, and elective abortion during either the first or second trimester. First-trimester pregnancies are typically terminated by means of suction curettage (i.e., vacuum aspiration performed through the cervix). Second-trimester abortions are most commonly performed through the cervix, using suction or destructive forceps, or by the use of prostaglandins, as in the form of intra-amniotic injections or vaginal suppositories.

Medical and/or surgical complications are associated with all choices, with the fewest complications related to elective abortion in the first trimester. Although there are complications associated with pregnancy termination, they are significantly fewer than those associated with carrying a pregnancy.

The most common complication following an induced abortion is infection. The patient usually presents with fever, pain, a tender uterus, and mild bleeding. Oral antibiotics and antipyretics are usually sufficient to manage these mild infections. If tissue remains in the uterus (incomplete abortion), suction curettage is also necessary. The second most common complication following induced abortion is bleeding. Risk of death from abortion during the first 2 months of pregnancy is less than 1 per 100,000 procedures, with increasing rates as pregnancy progresses. There is no apparent risk to future pregnancies if the first- or second-trimester abortion has been free of complications. There appears to be a slight increased risk of premature delivery if more than three first-trimester pregnancies are terminated by elective abortion.

Medical (i.e., nonsurgical) methods to induce first-trimester abortion include the antiprogesterone medication RU 486 (mifepristone), which is used in conjunction with a prostaglandin analog and methotrexate. Abortion is not always complete with this medical method, and suction and curettage to remove retained products of conception are required.

SEPTIC ABORTION

Occasionally, patients may present with a *septic abortion,* an infected complete or incomplete abortion in which the patient presents with sepsis, shock, hemorrhage, and possibly renal failure. It rarely occurs as a complication of a legal abortion but is more commonly associated with criminal abortions (i.e., those done illegally, under unsterile conditions, by persons who may have little or no knowledge of medicine or anatomy). Broad-spectrum parenteral antibiotics, fluid therapy, and prompt evacuation of the uterus are indicated. A careful evaluation for trauma, including perforation of the uterus or vagina, should also be carried out.

POSTABORTAL SYNDROME

Postabortal syndrome develops when the uterus fails to remain contracted after spontaneous abortion (with or without suction curettage) or elective/therapeutic abortion. The patient presents with crampy pain and/or bleeding, and is found to have an open cervix, bleeding, and a large, "softer-than-expected" uterus. The clinical situation is often indistinguishable from incomplete abortion, the question resolved only upon receipt of a pathology report of the tissue/material removed at suction curettage, the treatment for the condition. Treatment is completed by oxytocic and antibiotic therapy as in the treatment of incomplete abortion.

CASE STUDIES

Case 14A

A 20-year-old college student (G1 P1) presents with the complaint of 2 days of vaginal bleeding, 6 weeks after her last menstrual period. She has regular menstrual periods and uses condoms alone for contraception. She has had a positive home pregnancy test. The bleeding has been dark in color, painless, and began after intercourse.

Examination shows a small amount of dark blood in the vagina and at the cervical os. The cervix is closed and no tissue is visible. Bimanual examination reveals a slightly softened, normal size uterus and normal adnexa without masses or tenderness.

Questions Case 14A

Based on your assessment, your best course of management is

A. Perform a culdocentesis
B. Order a transvaginal ultrasound examination
C. Prescribe medroxyprogesterone (Provera) 10 mg/day
D. Recommend pelvic rest and light activity
E. Advise evacuation of the uterus by suction curettage
F. Order a serum quantitative β-hCG

Answer: F

Although a home pregnancy test is probably reliable, confirmation is indicated, which will also provide additional quantitative information. Therapeutic maneuvers are premature, although pelvic rest and light activity would probably be included in any situation. Invasive procedures and expensive imaging procedures are not indicated.

The quantitative β-hCG is reported as 846 mIU/ml. You indeed recommend pelvic rest and only light activity, with the likely diagnosis being threatened abortion. She returns in 48 hours; she still has bleeding, although now more like a menstrual period; and a repeat β-hCG is 146 mIU/ml. On examination her uterus is firm; the cervix closed; there is no uterine, cervical, or adnexal tenderness; and she is afebrile. Your working diagnosis is

A. Intrauterine pregnancy
B. Threatened abortion
C. Incomplete abortion
D. Complete abortion
E. Missed abortion
F. Ectopic pregnancy

Answer: D

The evidence suggests a failed pregnancy with expulsion of the intrauterine contents. There is no clinical evidence of ectopic pregnancy or infection.

Your best management is

A. Continued clinical observation for a few more days
B. Discussion of contraception
C. RhoGAM if she is Rh−
D. Transvaginal ultrasonography to rule out the life-threatening possibility of ectopic pregnancy

Answer: A, B, C

Case 14B

A 32-year-old (G2 P1001) presents with intense right lower-quadrant pain of 2 hours duration that is so severe she has difficulty walking. She tells you she had a positive urine pregnancy test in her doctor's office earlier in the week and that she was told she was approximately 6 weeks pregnant based on her last menstrual period and a pelvic examination.

In the last 2 weeks she has had some nausea and occasional emesis in the mornings and is not hungry. She has no history of sexually transmitted diseases. Her review of systems is negative.

On examination she has a temperature of 99.2° F, her blood pressure is 120/65, her pulse 90 and firm. Her abdomen is tender to palpation without masses or rebound, although bowel sounds are diminished. On pelvic examination, her cervix is slightly tender, her uterus is at a 6- to 8-week size and retroverted, and there is an indistinct tender fullness in the right adnexa.

(Continued)

Questions Case 14B

Your differential diagnosis includes

A. Intrauterine pregnancy
B. Threatened abortion
C. Incomplete abortion
D. Ectopic pregnancy
E. Corpus luteum cyst
F. Pelvic inflammatory disease (PID)
G. Appendicitis
H. Diverticulitis

Answer: A, D, E, G

Pregnancy inside and outside the uterus, a pregnancy-related corpus luteum cyst, and appendicitis are all consistent with the data. Incomplete abortion is not, as there is no bleeding. PID is unlikely, because she is pregnant and her fever is low, although this can be a presentation of *Chlamydia*-associated infection. Diverticulitis is uncommon in her age group.

Your best management is

A. Quantitative β-hCG
B. Quantitative serum progesterone
C. Transvaginal ultrasound
D. Culdocentesis
E. Diagnostic laparoscopy

Answer: A, B, C, D

The serum β-hCG will help define the pregnancy and assist in the interpretation of ultrasound findings. Serum progesterone is advocated by many to identify a pregnancy that is unlikely to be viable. Transvaginal ultrasound is indicated, because there is the question of an adnexal mass and the location of the pregnancy has not been determined. Invasive procedures are not indicated at this time.

The β-hCG is 2345 mIU/ml, and the serum progesterone is pending. Transvaginal ultrasound reveals a viable intrauterine pregnancy and a cystic right adnexal mass, $2 \times 3 \times 4$ cm. There is a small amount of fluid in the cul-de-sac of Douglas. Your most likely diagnosis is intrauterine pregnancy and a symptomatic corpus luteum cyst. You can reassure the patient and follow her clinically.

Case 14C

A 26-year-old (G3 P2002) presents in the emergency room, saying she had an abortion the previous day at a local clinic, complaining of central lower quadrant crampy pain and increasingly severe vaginal bleeding, but no fever or chills nor bowel or bladder symptoms. History reveals a last menstrual period, which would have made her about 12 weeks' gestational age at the time of the procedure, and this corresponds with the information given her at the clinic before and after the procedure. Upon discharge from the clinic, she was given a packet of oral contraceptives, told to contact her physician if she felt unwell, and return in 2 weeks for follow-up care.

On examination she is normotensive and afebrile, her abdomen is mildly tender suprapubically, but there is neither guarding nor rebound and bowel sounds are present and normal; her cervix is open 1 centimeter and clot and white material are present along with moderate bleeding; and her uterus is 12-week size, soft, slightly tender, and there are no adnexal masses.

Questions Case 14C

Your initial impression is

A. Incomplete abortion
B. Missed abortion
C. Uterine perforation
D. Appendicitis
E. Postabortal syndrome

Answer: A or E

From the information you have, the uterus is filled either with retained pregnancy tissue (incomplete abortion) or blood clot (postabortal syndrome). Missed abortion is a nonviable pregnancy retained in utero for more than 2 cycles; the "benign" nature of the history and physical findings argue against a surgical problem such as uterine perforation, although such remains in the differential diagnosis, or appendicitis.

Your management is

A. Send the patient home with instructions to follow-up within 24 hours with her private physician
B. Send the patient home with prescriptions for Methergine and doxycycline and an admonition to follow-up within 24 hours with her private physician
C. Suction-curettage followed by oxytocic and antibiotic therapy
D. Diagnostic laparoscopy and suction curettage

Answer: C

Whatever is in the uterus, pregnancy tissue or clot or both, it will not likely be expelled by intrinsic action of the uterus, even if stimulated by Methergine. Suction curettage is the treatment of choice fol-

lowed by oxytocics to avoid renewed uterine atony and prophylactic antibiotic therapy.

What laboratory tests are needed prior to discharge for discharge management?

A. Blood type and Rh
B. Rubella titer
C. CBC

Answer: A

Determination of blood type and Rh are important, because if the patient is Rh negative, RhoGAM administration is requisite unless it was given at the clinic where the pregnancy termination was performed. While not needed at the time of discharge, discovery that the patient is not rubella immune will allow vaccination at a follow-up visit, which will be beneficial in subsequent pregnancies. A complete blood cell (CBC) count is useful because it will detect an unexpected anemia allowing treatment, and an unexpectedly elevated white blood cell (WBC) count would warrant further evaluation for an early septic abortion or endomyometritis.

CHAPTER

15

ECTOPIC PREGNANCY

INCIDENCE

Implantation outside of the uterine cavity is termed *ectopic pregnancy,* a condition that significantly jeopardizes the mother and is incompatible with continuing the pregnancy. Catastrophic bleeding may occur when the implanting pregnancy erodes into blood vessels or ruptures through structures (typically the fallopian tubes) not suited to accommodate the growing conceptus. The effect of the ectopic pregnancy reaches beyond the incident pregnancy, reflected in decreased fertility and increased risk of recurrent ectopic pregnancy, depending on the amount of damage caused by the ectopic pregnancy, the treatment(s) used, and underlying causes.

Primarily because of an increasing prevalence of pelvic inflammatory disease (PID), the incidence of ectopic pregnancy has been increasing in the United States, from 4.5 per 1000 pregnancies in 1970 to an estimated 19.7 per 1000 pregnancies in 1992. Despite this nearly 2% incidence of ectopic pregnancy, maternal mortality rates have decreased markedly. In the 1970s,

there were 3.5 maternal deaths per 1000 cases of ectopic pregnancy; nowadays the rate is less than 1 per 1000. This improvement is primarily the result of earlier detection, allowing intervention before massive bleeding occurs and, in some cases, even prior to the development of any symptoms.

Pregnancies may implant in many locations in the genital tract and pelvis (Figure 15.1). The vast majority of ectopic gestations (95%) occur in the fallopian tube (*tubal pregnancy*). Four of five tubal pregnancies occur in the ampullary portion of the fallopian tube. Infrequent locations include the cervix, ovary, and peritoneal cavity (respectively, *cervical, ovarian, and abdominal pregnancy*). For women who have used assisted reproductive technology (ART) to achieve pregnancy, there is a significant increase in the incidence of nontubal ectopic pregnancies, especially the heretofore quite rare combined (or heterotropic) pregnancy, where one pregnancy is intrauterine and a second, ectopic.

Tubal pregnancy may result in any of three clinical scenarios: (1) tubal rupture with intraperitoneal hemorrhage; (2) tubal

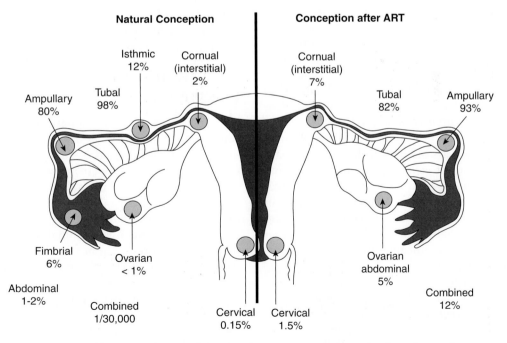

FIGURE 15.1. Incidence of types of ectopic pregnancy by location, after natural cycles and for women who have used assisted reproductive technology (ART).

abortion (i.e., expulsion of the pregnancy out the fimbriated end with or without hemorrhage); or rarely (3) tubal abortion with subsequent implantation on an intraperitoneal structure.

Patients with ectopic pregnancy not only are at risk for immediate morbidity and mortality from acute blood loss and risk of anatomic damage but also have a significantly reduced fertility rate, with fewer than one half of patients subsequently having a live full-term birth. As the *second leading cause of maternal mortality in the United States, ectopic pregnancy should be high in the differential diagnosis for any woman of reproductive age with acute pelvic or lower abdominal pain, with or without abnormal vaginal bleeding, and a positive pregnancy test.*

CAUSES OF ECTOPIC PREGNANCY

Knowing which patients are at higher risk can aid the physician in making an early diagnosis. The primary risk factor for ectopic pregnancy is a prior history of *salpingitis*. Damage from such infection may retard the passage of the fertilized ovum through the tube to the endometrial cavity, facilitating extrauterine implantation. Women with a history of salpingitis have a 6-fold increase in their risk of ectopic pregnancy. *A previous ectopic pregnancy also increases the risk of future ectopic implantations by approximately 10-fold.*

Age is an important risk factor. Women 35 to 44 years old have a threefold increase in the rate of ectopic pregnancy compared with women 15 to 24 years old. More than half of all ectopic pregnancies occur in women who have had *three or more pregnancies*. Finally, *black and Hispanic women* also have a significantly higher risk of ectopic pregnancy.

Contrary to some reports, *sterilization, contraception, and abortion do not increase ectopic pregnancy frequency.* Oral contraceptives prevent ovulation, thereby significantly reducing pregnancies in all locations. Intrauterine contraception devices (IUCDs)

prevent all types of pregnancies, although ectopic pregnancies may be reduced relatively less than intrauterine pregnancies, thereby giving the false impression that they are a risk factor. The higher prevalence of PID in IUCD users, however, may increase the patient's risk even after the removal of the IUCD.

In patients with previous sterilization, the chance of ectopic pregnancy is increased, but because sterilization failures are so uncommon, the net effect of sterilization is to protect against ectopic pregnancies. Although 85% of sterilization failures are associated with intrauterine pregnancies, the possibility of an ectopic pregnancy should always be considered in patients with sterilization failures. Abortion itself does not predispose to ectopic pregnancy, although associated infection may do so. There has been a reported effect of ovulation induction in increasing the risk of ectopic pregnancy. This has been difficult to determine, because there is the potential for subclinical tubal disease in some infertile patients, which may itself be the primary cause of the ectopic pregnancy.

CLINICAL EVALUATION OF POSSIBLE ECTOPIC PREGNANCY
Symptoms of Tubal Pregnancy

The classic presentation of a patient with an ectopic pregnancy includes *abdominal pain, amenorrhea, and vaginal bleeding.* The frequency of symptoms in patients with ectopic pregnancy is presented in Table 15.1.

Early ectopic pregnancies are asymptomatic. As the pregnancy grows, the most common symptom is abdominal or pelvic pain, which is present in nearly all patients. Pain is a result of the distended fallopian tube and/or irritation of the peritoneum by blood. The pain is generally described as colicky in character and may be unilateral (not necessarily on the same side as the ectopic) or bilateral, intermittent or constant, located in the lower or even upper

TABLE 15.1. Symptoms of Ectopic Pregnancy	
Symptoms	**Prevalence (%)**
Abdominal pain	95–100
Generalized	50
Unilateral	35
Shoulder	20
Back	5–10
Abnormal uterine bleeding	65–85
Amenorrhea	75–95
< 2 weeks	45
< 6 weeks	35
Syncope	10–18
Dizziness	20–35
Pregnancy symptoms	10–20
Nausea	15
Urge to defecate	5–15

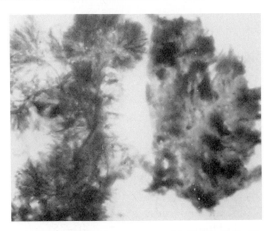

FIGURE 15.2. (*Left*) Typical fluffy villi of placenta. (*Right*) Shaggy decidua. (From Munsick RA. Clinical test for placenta in 300 consecutive menstrual aspirations. Obstet Gynecol 1982;60:738.)

abdomen. The proximal portions of the fallopian tube are not as able to adapt to the growing pregnancy, so an ectopic pregnancy in this area is likely to become symptomatic earlier in gestation.

In up to one fifth of patients with extensive intra-abdominal bleeding, irritation of the diaphragm causes referred pain to the shoulder. Irritation of the posterior cul-de-sac may cause an urge to defecate. Patients may present with a history of feeling faint or passing out while straining to have a bowel movement. Syncope occurs in one third of patients with ruptured tubal pregnancies, less frequently in unruptured cases.

Although patients with ectopic pregnancy typically have missed their normal menses, this history is often not given. By the time symptoms have developed, it has usually been 6 weeks since the last normal menstrual period. At this early stage, symptoms of pregnancy are not always present and cannot be used to rule in or rule out ectopic pregnancy.

As long as placental hormones are produced, there is usually no vaginal bleeding. Irregular vaginal bleeding results from the sloughing of the decidua from the endometrial lining. Vaginal bleeding in patients with an ectopic gestation may range from little or none to heavy, menstrual-like flow. In some patients, the entire "decidual cast" is passed intact, simulating a spontaneous abortion (Figure 15.2). Histologic evaluation of this tissue confirms whether placental villi are present. In any patient with a positive pregnancy test, whenever evaluation of tissue passed spontaneously or obtained by curettage does not demonstrate villi, an ectopic implantation should be assumed to be present until proved otherwise.

Physical Findings in Tubal Pregnancy

Physical examination findings range from a totally normal examination in early unruptured ectopic pregnancy to hypovolemic shock and an acute abdomen in cases of ruptured ectopic pregnancy. Most healthy reproductive-age women are able to compensate for mild to moderate degrees of blood loss so that extensive blood loss is usually required to cause a decrease in blood pressure and an increase in pulse. Five percent of patients present in hypovolemic shock, although blood loss is the major factor in 85% of ectopic pregnancy deaths. A summary of physical examination findings is presented in Table 15.2.

TABLE 15.2. Physical Examination in Ectopic Pregnancy

Finding	Prevalence (%)
Abdominal tenderness	80–90
Peritoneal signs	
Ruptured ectopic pregnancy cases	50
Unruptured ectopic pregnancy cases	5
Adnexal tenderness	75–90
Unilateral	40–75
Bilateral	50–75
Cervical motion tenderness	50–75
Adnexal mass	30–50
Contralateral	20
Uterus	
Normal size	70
Enlarged	15–30
Orthostatic changes	10–15
Temperature > 37°C	5–10
Vomiting	15

Fever is not expected, although a mild elevation in temperature in response to intraperitoneal blood may occur. A temperature of greater than 38° C may suggest an infectious etiology to a patient's symptoms. Abdominal distention and tenderness, with or without rebound, rigidity, or decreased bowel sounds, may be seen in cases of intra-abdominal bleeding. Abdominal tenderness is variable, present in 50% to 90% of patients with ectopic pregnancies. Cervical motion tenderness, caused by intraperitoneal irritation, and adnexal tenderness are commonly found. An adnexal mass is present in roughly one third of cases, but its absence does not rule out the possibility of an ectopic implantation. The uterus may enlarge and soften throughout the first trimester, thus simulating an intrauterine pregnancy. A slightly open cervix with blood or decidual tissue may be found and mistaken for a threatened and/or spontaneous abortion.

Differential Diagnosis

The rapid and accurate diagnosis of ectopic pregnancy is imperative to reduce the risk of serious complications or death. Up to one half of ectopic pregnancy-related maternal deaths have had a lag in treatment because of delayed or inaccurate diagnoses. *Any sexually active woman in the reproductive age group who presents with pain, irregular bleeding, and/or amenorrhea should have ectopic pregnancy as a part of the initial differential diagnosis.* Other elements of the differential diagnosis include complications of an intrauterine pregnancy (threatened, missed, completed, or incomplete abortion), nonpregnancy-related gynecologic conditions (acute and chronic salpingitis, follicular or corpus luteum cyst rupture, endometriosis, or adnexal torsion), and nongynecologic conditions (e.g., gastroenteritis and appendicitis).

Diagnostic Procedures

The initial assessment in the otherwise hemodynamically stable patient must include a *pregnancy test.* With the sensitive assays available today, a negative pregnancy test excludes the possibility of ectopic pregnancy. Urinary pregnancy tests, which detect human chorionic gonadotropin (hCG) levels to 50 mIU/ml, are now commonly available. They detect hCG as early as 14 days after conception and are positive in more than 90% of cases of ectopic pregnancy. Serum assays can detect the presence of hCG as early as 5 days after conception (i.e., before the missed menstrual cycle). However, because they require additional time and expertise to perform, they are often not used in a potentially emergent clinical setting.

If a positive pregnancy test is found when ectopic pregnancy is suspected, the remainder of the workup should focus on evaluation of the viability and location of the pregnancy. *Quantitative β-hCG levels* can be followed at 2-day intervals. Early in pregnancy, these levels should increase by at least 66% in 48 hours. Failure to meet this criterion suggests a pregnancy not growing appropriately, thus increasing the suspicion

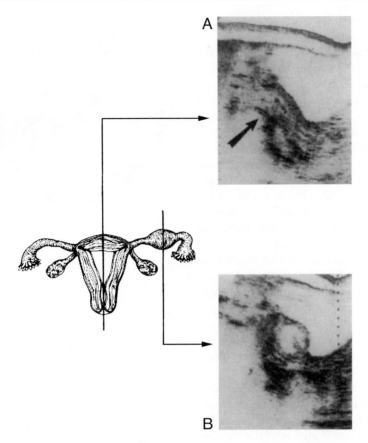

FIGURE 15.3.   Sonographic findings in tubal ectopic pregnancy. (*A*) Midline view through empty uterus (arrow pointing to empty uterus). (*B*) Paramidline view (arrow pointing to cystic mass in area of fallopian tube).

of ectopic pregnancy. An inappropriate increase in hCG identifies a potentially abnormal pregnancy but does not identify its location. No single hCG result can be used to rule in or rule out ectopic pregnancy, unless it is negative.

A useful adjunct to serial quantitative levels of hCG is pelvic *ultrasonography* (Figure 15.3). Ultrasonography cannot be relied on to routinely image a pregnancy outside the uterine cavity, but it can identify an intrauterine pregnancy with considerable accuracy, thus effectively ruling out ectopic pregnancy with the very rare possibility of coexistent intrauterine and extrauterine gestations (heterotopic pregnancy) as the exception. Transabdominal ultrasonography should be able to identify an intrauterine gestation by the time the hCG level reaches 5000–6000 mIU/ml. The more sen-

sitive transvaginal ultrasonography should show the pregnancy by the time the hCG level is 1500 mIU/ml. Failure to do so should further increase the suspicion that an ectopic pregnancy exists.

Although a low hematocrit is unusual, a complete blood count can document possible blood loss anemia and identify leukocytosis. If the white blood cell (WBC) count is greater than 20,000 (WBC/dl), infection may be more likely than an ectopic pregnancy.

Serum progesterone concentration has also been used as a screening test for ectopic pregnancy. A progesterone of less than 5.0 ng/ml strongly suggests a nonviable pregnancy, either intra- or extrauterine. Serum progesterone levels greater than 25 ng/ml help in cases of suspected ectopic gestation, because only 2.5% of all abnormal pregnancies (ectopic or intrauterine) have serum progesterone levels above this level.

Curettage of the uterine cavity can also help rule out ectopic pregnancy. Although intrauterine and ectopic pregnancy can exist simultaneously in rare cases, identification of chorionic villi in curettings identifies an intrauterine location of the pregnancy and essentially rules out ectopic pregnancy. The Arias-Stella reaction, a hypersecretory endometrium of pregnancy seen on histologic examination, is compatible not only with ectopic pregnancy but also with intrauterine pregnancy and is, therefore, not useful in identifying an ectopic pregnancy. Instrumentation of the uterine cavity should be undertaken only after thorough consideration of the likelihood that an ongoing pregnancy might be interrupted.

Culdocentesis can aid in the identification of a hemoperitoneum, which, in turn, may indicate a ruptured ectopic pregnancy, although other conditions such as a ruptured corpus luteum cyst can also cause a hemoperitoneum. An 18-gauge needle is inserted posterior to the cervix, between the uterosacral ligaments, and into the cul-de-sac of the peritoneal cavity (Figure 15.4). Aspiration of clear peritoneal fluid (*negative culdocentesis*) indicates no hemorrhage into the abdominal cavity but does not rule out an unruptured ectopic pregnancy. Aspiration of blood that clots can indicate either penetration of a vessel or such rapid blood loss into the peritoneal cavity that the blood clot has not had time to undergo fibrinolysis. Nonclotting blood is evidence of hemoperitoneum (*positive culdocentesis*) in which the blood clot has undergone fibrinolysis. If nothing is aspirated (*equivocal or nondiagnostic culdocentesis*), no information is obtained. Unfortunately, no finding on culdocentesis can definitively rule in or rule out ectopic pregnancy, although a positive culdocentesis identifies blood in the peritoneal cavity and confirms the need for further evaluation to identify the source of the bleeding.

The most accurate technique of identifying an ectopic pregnancy is by direct visualization, which is done most commonly via laparoscopy or laparotomy. Even laparo-

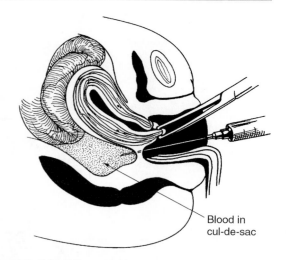

FIGURE 15.4.   Culdocentesis.

scopy, however, carries a 2% to 5% misdiagnosis rate, because an extremely early tubal gestation may not be identified because it may not distend the fallopian tube sufficiently to be recognized as an abnormality (false negative). False-positive diagnoses may also occur because a hematosalpinx may be misinterpreted as an unruptured ectopic pregnancy.

MANAGEMENT OF ECTOPIC PREGNANCY

The traditional management of a tubal pregnancy is surgical removal. Conservative surgical techniques have been developed that maximize preservation of reproductive organs. If done through the laparoscope, definitive diagnosis and treatment can be accomplished at the same operation with minimal morbidity, cost, and hospitalization. In a *linear salpingostomy* (Figure 15.5), the surgeon makes an incision on the fallopian tube over the site of implantation, removes the pregnancy, and allows the incision to heal by secondary intention. A *segmental resection* is the removal of a portion of the affected tube with the potential of reanastomosing the tube at the initial operation or at a later time (Figure 15.6). *Salpingectomy* is removal of the entire tube, a procedure reserved for those cases in which little or no normal tube remains.

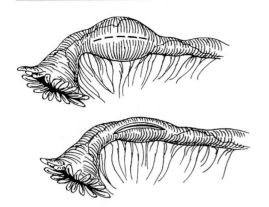

FIGURE 15.5. Surgical management of ectopic pregnancy: linear salpingostomy.

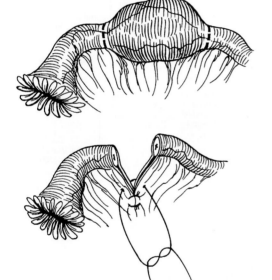

FIGURE 15.6. Surgical management of ectopic pregnancy: segmental resection and tubal reanastomosis.

TABLE 15.3. Single-dose Methotrexate Protocol for Ectopic Pregnancy Treatment	
Day	**Therapy**
0	hCG, D&C, CBC, SGOT, BUN, creatinine, blood type + Rh
1	MTX, hCG*
4	hCG†
7	hCG

BUN = blood urea nitrogen; CBC = complete blood count; D&C = dilation and curettage; hCG = quantitative β-human chorionic gonadotropin; MTX = intramuscular methotrexate, 50 mg/m²; SGOT = serum glutamic oxaloacetic transaminase.
*In those patients not requiring D&C before MTX initiation (hCG < 2000 mIU/ml and no gestational sac on transvaginal ultrasound), day 0 and day 1 are combined.
†With a 15% decline in hCG titer between days 4 and 7, follow weekly until hCG is < 10 mIU/ml.

In selected cases, nonsurgical therapy may be advocated for the early, unruptured ectopic pregnancy. Expectant management involves no surgery and no medical therapy but allows the pregnancy to spontaneously regress as documented by serial hCG levels. *Methotrexate,* a folic acid antagonist, has been successfully used to treat ectopic pregnancy via the oral or intramuscular routes, as well as by direct injection into the ectopic gestational sac. Table 15.3 shows a management protocol using methotrexate as a single-dose intramuscular treatment for unruptured ectopic gestations. This therapy is usually reserved for cases in which the ectopic gestation is less than 3.5 cm in diameter and no cardiac activity in the pregnancy is seen on ultrasound.

When conservative surgery or nonsurgical treatment is used, the patient must be followed post-therapy with serial quantitative β-hCG levels to monitor regression of the pregnancy. Subsequent surgery or methotrexate therapy is needed if trophoblastic function persists as evidenced by persistent or rising levels of hCG.

Rh-negative mothers with ectopic pregnancy should receive *Rh immune globulin (Rho-GAM)* to prevent Rh sensitization.

Although traditionally diagnosed at the time of surgery, ectopic pregnancies are increasingly suspected and treated without either laparoscopy or laparotomy, thereby avoiding the inherent morbidity and cost of surgery. The algorithm shown in Figure 15.7 is an example of the nonsurgical

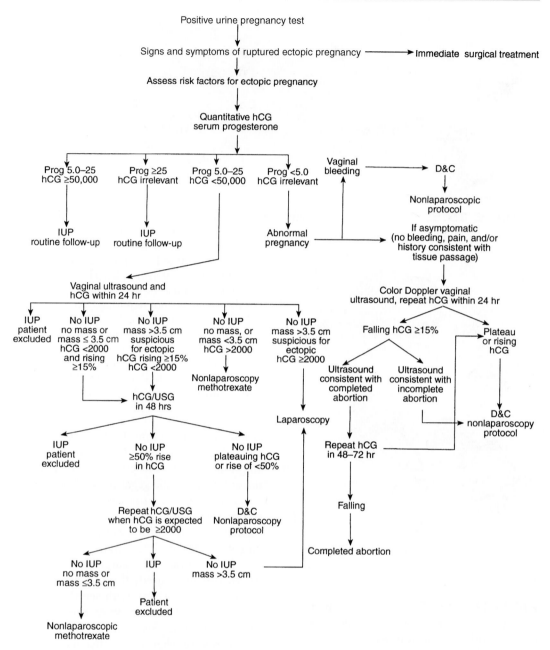

FIGURE 15.7. Nonsurgical diagnosis and treatment of ectopic pregnancy.

diagnosis and treatment of ectopic pregnancy. Figure 15.8 demonstrates how this may be accomplished with minimal use of surgery.

Combined Pregnancy

Combined pregnancy (coincident or heterotopic pregnancy) occurs in approximately 1 in 30,000 pregnancies with simultaneous intrauterine and extrauterine gestations. Associated with abnormal development of one twin or superfetation, the treatment of the intrauterine pregnancy is individualized depending on the maternal status and wishes as well as the gestational age and clinical status of the pregnancy. Management of the extrauterine pregnancy must

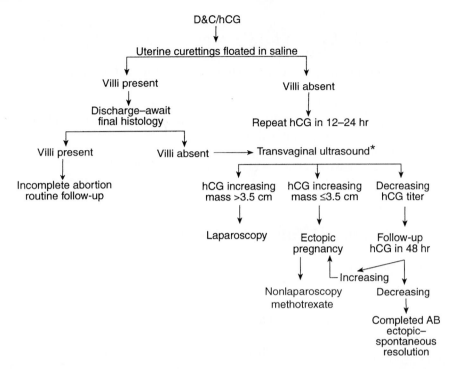

FIGURE 15.8. Diagnosis and treatment of ectopic pregnancy with minimal surgery (dilation and curettage). *Repeat transvaginal ultrasound if performed > 48 hours earlier. AB = abortion.

account for the possible effect on the intrauterine gestation. Approximately 1 in 3 of the intrauterine pregnancies are reported as surviving in the limited number of cases reported.

Nontubal Ectopic Pregnancy

Ectopic implantations outside of the fallopian tube may present in a variety of ways and at different times in gestation, primarily related to the site of implantation. All are uncommon, deriving part of their morbidity from their locations and the remainder from delayed diagnosis.

Abdominal pregnancy occurs in 1 in 3000 to 4000 pregnancies after normal menstrual cycles and more frequently after assisted reproductive technology, involving implantation on peritoneal surfaces—in order of frequency, on the adnexae, broad ligaments, sigmoid colon, uterine fundus, and elsewhere in the abdominopelvic cavity. There are two types of abdominal pregnancy. *Primary abdominal pregnancy* is pri-

mary implantation of the fertilized ovum, occurring in association with müllerian tract anomalies, delayed ovulation, endometriosis, PID, and fallopian tube dysfunction. *Secondary abdominal pregnancy,* which is more common, involves reimplantation somewhere in the abdominal cavity after the pregnancy has been separated from its primary site of implantation such as in tubal abortion (expulsion of a tubal pregnancy out the fimbriated end), tubal pregnancy rupture, or uterine rupture. Physical findings and symptoms are widely variable, depending on gestational age and site of implantation. Diagnosis is confirmed primarily by ultrasonography.

Abdominal pregnancy is usually discovered long before fetal viability, with treatment being removal of the pregnancy, but not the placenta if it is well developed and attached to vascular, vital structures because of the often uncontrollable hemorrhage that frequently ensues. The management of abdominal pregnancy with a near viable pregnancy is extremely uncommon. Survival

TABLE 15.4.	Rubin's Criteria for Cervical Pregnancy

Cervical glands opposite placental attachment, chorionic villi in cervical canal, no chorionic villi in corpus
Intimate attachment of placenta to cervix
All or part of placenta must be situated below entrance of uterine vessels and anterior/posterior uteroperitoneal reflections
No fetal elements in corpus uteri
Internal cervical os closed, external cervical os open or closed

TABLE 15.5.	Spiegelberg's Criteria for Ovarian Pregnancy

Fallopian tube:	1. Intact, including fimbria
	2. Clearly separate from ovary
	3. Microscopically free of gestational tissue
Ovary:	1. Occupies normal position
	2. Connected to uterus by ovarian ligament
	3. Ovarian tissue in wall of gestational sac

of the fetus occurs in only 10% to 20% of cases, with up to one half having significant deformity. The patient is given the option of continuing the pregnancy to fetal viability with operative delivery or operative termination of the pregnancy at the time of diagnosis. In either case, removal of the placenta is usually not attempted because of the risk of uncontrollable hemorrhage. Treatment with methotrexate is commonly used to induce regression of the retained placenta.

Cervical pregnancy occurs in 1 in 10,000 to 20,000 pregnancies, when the ovum implants in the cervical mucosa below the level of the histologic cervical internal os (Table 15.4). Cervical pregnancy often presents as an incomplete or threatened abortion, with uncontrollable hemorrhage as removal of the pregnancy tissue is attempted. Surgical treatment that avoids hysterectomy, such as conization, and arterial embolization have been described for definitive management of cervical pregnancy. However, hysterectomy is often needed to control the significant vaginal bleeding that may ensue when the cervical pregnancy is disrupted, especially common when the pregnancy is 12 weeks' gestational age or more. Methotrexate has been used when the diagnosis is made earlier, thereby avoiding the need for surgical intervention.

Ovarian pregnancy occurs uncommonly as well, with an incidence estimated from 1 in 7000 to 1 in 50,000 pregnancies after normal menstrual cycles. The types of ovarian pregnancy are primary and reimplantation, or secondary, as with abdominal pregnancy. The criteria of Spiegelberg define the requirements for ovarian pregnancy (Table 15.5), which has a low morbidity rate, because it is often diagnosed as a tubal pregnancy and successfully treated by surgery, either wedge resection of the pregnancy or oophorectomy, depending on the extent of ovarian damage.

CASE STUDIES

Case 15A

A 20-year-old college student (G1 P0) presents with the complaint of 2 days of vaginal bleeding, 6 weeks after her last menstrual period. She has had a positive urinary pregnancy test. The bleeding has been dark in color, painless, and began after intercourse. She has had no prior surgeries. She has had one episode of "a pelvic infection" in the past.

Examination shows a small amount of dark blood in the vagina and at the cervical os. The cervix is closed and no tissue is visible. Bimanual examination reveals a slightly softened uterus and an unremarkable adnexal examination.

Questions Case 15A

Your best course of management is

A. Advise an immediate culdocentesis
B. Request a transvaginal ultrasound examination
C. Prescribe medroxyprogesterone (Provera), 10 mg/day
D. Recommend pelvic rest and light activity
E. Advise evacuation of the uterus by suction curettage

Answer: D

A likely diagnosis in this situation is a threatened abortion, but a history of a "pelvic infection" is present in up to 70% of patients with ectopic pregnancies and should increase the clinician's suspicion that an unruptured ectopic pregnancy may be present. A transvaginal ultrasound examination may help to identify the presence of an intrauterine pregnancy, making the diagnosis of threatened abortion more probable. However, a β-hCG of greater than 1500 mIU/ml is generally required

before an intrauterine pregnancy is routinely visualized on transvaginal sonogram. Culdocentesis is a useful test to identify intra-abdominal bleeding, but the patient's history is not suggestive of rupture or leakage from an ectopic implantation site. Because culdocentesis is invasive, it should be reserved for those cases in which the possibility of intra-abdominal bleeding is greater and the need for diagnostic information is more acute. Recommendations of therapy must be reserved until the possibility of an ectopic pregnancy has been addressed. If there is a delay before obtaining the ultrasound, treating the condition as a presumed threatened abortion is appropriate.

The patient returns the following day with continued spotting and the passage of a "glob of tissue," which she has brought in a jar. She is still without pain, although vaguely uncomfortable. The rush pathology report on the tissue is "necrotic debris and blood clot, unable to make histologic diagnosis, specifically, cannot discern whether or not there are chorionic villi present." Your best course of management is

A. Advise an immediate culdocentesis
B. Request a transvaginal ultrasound examination
C. Obtain serum quantitative β-hCG
D. Recommend pelvic rest and light activity
E. Advise evacuation of the uterus by suction curettage

Answer: B, C

Now the concern of passage of a decidual cast and an associated ectopic pregnancy is raised. β-hCG level will help in the

(Continued)

interpretation of the transvaginal ultrasound examination.

The β-hCG is reported as 3100 mIU/ml. The transvaginal ultrasound is reported as a uterine cavity with indistinct, disorganized echoes and a cystic left adnexal mass, distinct from the ovary, which contains a cyst as well. There is some fluid in the cul-de-sac of Douglas. Your working diagnosis is now

A. Intrauterine pregnancy
B. Threatened abortion
C. Incomplete abortion
D. Completed abortion
E. Ectopic pregnancy

Answer: D or E

Intrauterine pregnancy and threatened abortion have been effectively eliminated by the transvaginal sonogram. Incomplete abortion is likewise unlikely given the scant tissue seen on ultrasound. The tissue passed may have been a decidual cast and the cystic mass on the left, an ectopic pregnancy; or the patient may have a benign cyst and passed her pregnancy completely.

Your best course of management is

A. Advise an immediate culdocentesis
B. Request a transvaginal ultrasound examination in 48 hours
C. Obtain serum quantitative β-hCG in 48 hours
D. Recommend pelvic rest and light activity
E. Advise evacuation of the uterus by suction curettage and diagnostic laparoscopy

Answer: B, C, D, or E

Given the lack of symptoms, observation with careful patient instruction and a repeat evaluation would be an acceptable management in a cooperative patient. Given the history of PID and the presence of a cyst consistent with a corpus luteum and another extrauterine and extraovarian

cystic structure, ectopic pregnancy is a distinct possibility so that surgical evaluation at this time would also be an acceptable management. What would be unacceptable would be to assume a completed abortion and dismiss the patient from follow-up.

Case 15B

A 25-year-old G1 P0 patient begins to cramp and passes a clump of spongy tissue, which she brings to the office. A transvaginal ultrasound examination 1 week ago revealed an intrauterine gestational sac. On examination, her uterus is small and firm and her cervical os is closed with minimal bleeding.

Questions Case 15B

The best course of management is

A. Observe only
B. Observe and send specimen for pathologic evaluation
C. D&C
D. Diagnostic laparoscopy
E. Methotrexate therapy

Answer: B

The specimen may represent a completed abortion or it may be a decidual cast associated with an ectopic pregnancy. The latter is much less likely in this case, because of the ultrasound documented intrauterine pregnancy 1 week ago. In general, any tissue must be sent for histologic evaluation. A D&C would be appropriate if bleeding is persistent and incomplete abortion was suspected. Diagnostic laparoscopy would be used only if ectopic pregnancy was more likely, and treatment such as methotrexate is inappropriate unless ectopic pregnancy is diagnosed.

The specimen is reported as "products of conception." You continue to follow the patient who continues to complain of lower abdominal pain. Her initial β-hCG was 4700 mIU/ml, and now, 4 days later, it is 4000 mIU/ml. Your most likely diagnoses include

A. Missed abortion
B. Molar pregnancy
C. Choriocarcinoma
D. Combined pregnancy
E. Retained placental tissue

Answer: E then D, in order of likelihood

Retained placental tissue is the most common cause of this situation, and suction curettage is indicated. A transvaginal ultrasound will help in evaluation of the differential diagnoses, which should include the rare combined pregnancy. Gestational trophoblastic disease is unlikely given the relatively low β-hCG level.

Case 15C

A 32-year-old G2 P2002 who has had tubal ligation presents with 7 weeks of amenorrhea and vaginal spotting. Pelvic examination reveals a 6-week-size anteverted uterus, a closed cervical os with minimal dark blood in the vaginal vault, and no palpable findings on adnexal examination. A urine pregnancy test is positive.

Questions Case 15C

Appropriate next steps in this patient's management include

A. Quantitative serum β-hCG
B. Quantitative serum progesterone
C. Transvaginal pelvic ultrasound
D. D&C
E. Diagnostic laparoscopy

Answer: C; possibly A and/or B

At 6 weeks' gestational age with a positive urinary pregnancy test, transvaginal ultra-sound should be able to identify an intrauterine pregnancy in virtually all cases. However, serum progesterone and β-hCG measurement would be helpful if no gestational sac were seen. Serum progesterone may help identify the viability of the pregnancy. Invasive procedures are not indicated in the absence of a diagnosis.

The serum β-hCG is 3650 mIU/ml; the progesterone is 12 ng/ml. The transvaginal ultrasound is reported as no definite intrauterine pregnancy and no definitive extrauterine gestation or fluid in the cul-de-sac of Douglas. The patient's spotting has subsided somewhat, but she now complains of left lower quadrant crampy pain. Your most likely diagnosis is

A. Intrauterine pregnancy
B. Threatened abortion
C. Incomplete abortion
D. Completed abortion
E. Ectopic pregnancy

Answer: E

Your best course(s) of management is

A. Observation
B. D&C
C. Operative laparoscopy
D. Exploratory laparotomy
E. Methotrexate therapy

Answer: C or D, or B with E

Operative evaluation, either by operative laparoscopy or open laparotomy, is appropriate. Alternatively, a D&C would exclude the diagnosis of intrauterine pregnancy, thereby confirming the diagnosis of an extrauterine pregnancy allowing medical management, with methotrexate.

CHAPTER

16

MEDICAL AND SURGICAL CONDITIONS OF PREGNANCY

CHAPTER OBJECTIVES

This chapter deals primarily with APGO Objective(s):

OBJECTIVE 18 Medical and Surgical
Conditions in Pregnancy

Describe the diagnosis and
management of the common medical
and surgical complications in the
pregnant patient, including their
effects on the pregnancy and the
effects of pregnancy on the condition;
include consideration of anemia,
diabetes mellitus, urinary tract
disorders, infections including herpes,
rubella, streptococcus, hepatitis B,
human immunodeficiency virus,
human papilloma virus, and other

sexually transmitted diseases, cytomegalovirus and varicella infection, cardiac disease, asthma, the abuse of alcohol, tobacco, and other substances, and the causes of the acute ("surgical") abdomen.

Virtually any maternal medical or surgical condition can complicate the course of a pregnancy and/or be affected by pregnancy. Physicians providing obstetric care must have a thorough understanding of the effect of pregnancy on the natural course of a disorder, the effect of the disorder on a pregnancy, and the change in management of the pregnancy and/or disorder caused by their coincidence. In this chapter, selected common medical and surgical complications that may be encountered during the course of obstetric care are discussed. Only a small portion of possible medical-surgical disorders are included here; more detailed coverage is the province of textbooks of maternal-fetal medicine, internal medicine, and surgery.

The following 17 disorders or groups of disorders in pregnancy are discussed in this chapter.

1. Anemias
2. Urinary tract infection
3. Renal disease
4. Respiratory disease
5. Cardiac disease
6. Glucose intolerance and diabetes mellitus
7. Thyroid disease
8. Infectious diseases
9. Thromboembolic disorder
10. Neurologic disease
11. Gastrointestinal disease
12. Dental disease
13. Hepatobiliary diseases
14. Abdominal surgical conditions and abdominal trauma
15. Substance abuse
16. Coagulation disorders
17. Cancer

1. ANEMIAS IN PREGNANCY

The plasma and cellular composition of blood changes significantly during the course of pregnancy because of an expansion of plasma volume proportionally greater than that of the red blood cell (RBC) mass (Table 16.1). On the average, there is a 1000 ml increase in plasma volume and a 300 ml increase in red cell volume (a 3:1 ratio). Because the hematocrit (Hct) reflects the proportion of blood made up primarily of red blood cells, Hct demonstrates a "physiologic" decrease during pregnancy (the so-called *physiologic anemia of pregnancy*). This decrease in Hct is not actually an anemia. *Anemia in pregnancy is generally defined as an Hct less than 30% or a hemoglobin of less than 10 g/dl.* Because of monthly blood loss with menstrual flow and contemporary dietary practices, which may lack sufficient iron and protein, women often enter pregnancy with a lowered iron store and sometimes a lowered Hct. When faced with the expansion of the maternal red cell mass and fetal iron needs, additional demands on the mother for iron outstrip the stores that are available; the result is *iron-deficiency anemia*. It is for these reasons that supplemental iron is appropriately prescribed for pregnant women. Iron-deficiency anemia is by far the most frequent type of anemia seen in

| TABLE 16.1. | Hematologic Laboratory Values in Pregnancy | | |

Test	Nonpregnant	Pregnant
Hb (g/dl)	12–16	10–13
Hct (%)	37–45	30–39
RBC (ml/mm³)	4.2–5.4	3.8–4.4
WBC (1000/mm³)	4.7–5.4	6–16
MCV (f/L)	80–100	70–90
MCH (pg/cell)	27–37	23–31
MCHC (d/dl/RBC)	32–35	32–35
Reticulocyte count (%)	0.5–1.0	1.0–2.0
Serum iron (μg/dl)	50–110	30–100
TIBC (μg/dl)	250–300	280–400
Transferrin saturation (%)	25–35	15–30
Serum folate (ng/ml)	4–16	4–10
Serum vitamin B_{12} (ng/ml)	70–85	70–500

Hb = hemoglobin; Hct = hematocrit; MCH = mean corpuscular hemoglobin; MCHC = mean corpuscular hemoglobin concentration; MCV = mean corpuscular volume; RBC = red blood cell; TIBC = total iron-binding capacity; WBC = white blood cell.

pregnancy, accounting for more than 90% of cases.

Because iron deficiency is the most common form of anemia in pregnancy, extensive evaluation of anemic pregnant patients should be delayed until an empiric trial of iron therapy is given and the effect observed. If the presumed iron-deficiency anemia is severe, the classic findings are small, pale erythrocytes manifest on peripheral blood smears (microcytic, hypochromic anemia) and red cell indices that indicate a low mean corpuscular volume (MCV)—generally < 80 f/L—and low mean corpuscular hemoglobin concentration (MCHC)—generally < 30%. Further laboratory studies usually demonstrate a decreased serum iron (generally < 50 mg/dl), an increased total iron-binding capacity, and a decrease in serum ferritin. A recent dietary history is also highly suggestive, especially if *pica* exists (the consumption of non-nutrient substances such as starch, ice, or dirt). Such dietary compulsions may contribute to iron deficiency by decreasing the amount of nutritious food and iron consumed.

Iron therapy is generally given in the form of ferrous sulfate or ferrous fumarate taken two times a day, a 325-mg tablet that contains approximately 60 mg and 100 mg of elemental iron, respectively. The uptake of iron is increasingly efficient as pregnancy progresses, 10% initially, increasing to nearly 30% in the last trimester. A response to therapy is first seen as an increase in the reticulocyte count approximately 1 week after the institution of iron therapy. Because of the plasma expansion associated with pregnancy, the Hct may not increase significantly but rather stabilizes or increases only slightly.

The second most common form of anemia seen in pregnancy is *folate deficiency* (or *megaloblastic anemia*). Although folate is found in green leafy vegetables, the demands of fetal and maternal growth during pregnancy (800 mg/day) outstrip the usual adult intake of 50 to 100 mg/day, requiring folate supplementation. Folate deficiency is especially likely in multiple gestation or when patients are taking medications such as phenytoin (Dilantin), nitrofurantoin, pyrimethamine, or trimethoprim or drinking ethanol in large quantities. Folate deficiency on blood smear is characterized by hypersegmented neutrophils and indices that suggest large cell volume (macrocytic anemia). Serum folate levels < 4 ng/ml and erythrocyte folate activity < 20 ng/ml are diagnostic. Treatment of folate deficiency anemia is 1 mg of folate orally on a daily basis, the amount generally found in most prenatal vitamin supplements. Because gastrointestinal absorption of folate is low (only 10 to 20 mg every 8 hours), divided doses may increase absorption in severe cases. With especially severe disease or in the case of malabsorption (malabsorption syndrome or surgical resection of the upper bowel), parenteral administration may be indicated.

With a *mixed iron and folate deficiency anemia,* the microcytic changes of iron deficiency negate the megaloblastic changes of folate deficiency, resulting in a normocytic and normochromic anemia. In such cases, treatment with either iron or folate alone will not be followed by an increase in red cell production; both therapies must be instituted simultaneously.

Vitamin B_{12} deficiency also causes a *macrocytic megaloblastic anemia,* although it is quite rare (1/6000 to 1/8000 pregnancies). Because the normal adult female has a multiple-year store of vitamin B_{12}, this disease is usually seen in women with chronic malabsorption from disease (such as sprue, pancreatic disease, Crohn's disease, or ulcerative colitis) or surgical resection. Parenteral vitamin B_{12} is a rapid and effective treatment.

The hereditary hemolytic anemias are also rare causes of anemia in pregnancy. Some examples are hereditary spherocytosis, an autosomal dominant defect of the erythrocyte membrane; glucose 6-phosphate dehydrogenase deficiency; and pyruvate kinase deficiency.

Thalassemia trait may also present as microcytic, hypochromic anemia, but unlike iron-deficiency anemia, the serum iron and total iron-binding capacity are normal. In addition, hemoglobin A_2 (HbA_2) is elevated.

The direct fetal consequences of anemia are minimal, although infants born to mothers with iron deficiency may have diminished iron stores as neonates. The maternal consequences of anemia are those associated with any adult anemia. If the anemia is corrected, the woman with an adequate red cell mass enters the labor and delivery process with additional protection against the need for transfusion.

The *hemoglobinopathies,* including the sickle-cell diseases and the thalassemias, are disorders of polypeptide chains that comprise the oxygen-carrying hemoglobin molecule found in the blood cells (Table 16.2). These disorders usually involve abnormalities of the β-globulins; the oxygen-carrying capacity of the hemoglobin molecule, including its structural integrity under conditions of low oxygen tension, is impaired. When this results in deformity of the normal spheroid shape of the RBC, vaso-occlusive "crisis" ensues.

These disorders may be grouped into those with minimal maternal and fetal morbidity (sickle-cell trait, HbSA; sickle-cell β-thalassemia disease, HbS-β-thal) and those with considerable maternal morbidity and occasional mortality (sickle-cell disease, HbSS; sickle-cell-hemoglobin C, HbSC). Patients with sickle-cell disease (defined as less than 40% HbS on quantitative hemoglobin electrophoresis) are inclined to develop maternal urinary tract infections, particularly asymptomatic bacteriuria and renal and gallbladder stones. Otherwise the pregnancies of patients with HbSA and HbS-β-thal are generally unaffected. Patients who are HbSS or HbSC, in contrast, may suffer vaso-occlusive episodes ("crises") with acute episodes of uteroplacental insufficiency and morbidity, such as prematurity and intrauterine growth restriction.

Although prophylactic maternal red cell transfusions have been popular, the risks of multiple blood transfusions and the general improvement in outcome in patients with hemoglobinopathies without transfusion have shifted the therapeutic emphasis to conservative management. Transfusions are, for the most part, reserved for complications of hemoglobinopathies such as congestive heart failure, sickle-cell disease crises, and severely low levels of hemoglobin. Careful antenatal assessment of fetal well-being and growth using standard techniques is an important part of managing patients with hemoglobinopathies.

TABLE 16.2. The Hemoglobinopathies

Characteristic	Sickle-Cell	HbSC Disease	Sickle-Cell β-Thalassemia	α-Thalassemia	β-Thalassemia
Globin abnormality	HbS (valine substituted for glutamic acid at the sixth position) in one or both chains	One globin is HbS and the other is HbC (lysine substituted for valine at the position)	One globin is HbS and one globin allele codes for β-thalassemia; decreased synthesis of HbA	Normal hemoglobins; decreased production of globin chains	Normal hemoglobin; decreased production of β globin chains
Genetics	Autosomal recessive Sickle-cell trait: heterozygous (one chain affected); < 40% HbS; 1 in 12 black Americans Sickle-cell disease: homozygous (both chains affected); 1 in 500 pregnancies in black Americans	Autosomal recessive; 1 in 700 patients at risk	Autosomal recessive; 1 in 1700 pregnancies; severity of disease depends on β allele—from no HbA production (severe disease) to moderate production (milder disease)	Autosomal recessive; severity of disease (microcytic, hypochromic anemia) depends on expression and amount of globin produced—from none (homozygous) to 25%–75% (heterozygous)	Autosomal recessive; point mutations cause decreased β chain synthesis Homozygous: β-thalassemia major (Cooley's anemia); no HbA produced; most is HbF or HbA$_2$; severe disease Heterozygous: β-thalassemia or β-thalassemia minor; one normal and one abnormal β globin allele; usually mild to moderate disease
Risk groups	African, Mediterranean, Turkish, Arabian, and East Indian heritage			Asian, African, East Indian, and Mediterranean heritage	Mediterranean, Middle Eastern, African, East Indian, and Asian heritage

2. URINARY TRACT INFECTION IN PREGNANCY

Urinary tract infections (UTIs) are common in pregnancy. Approximately 8% of all women (pregnant and nonpregnant) have greater than 10^5 colonies of a single bacteria on a midstream culture. Approximately 25% of the pregnant portion of this group develop an acute, symptomatic UTI. Compared with nonpregnant women with similar colony counts on urine culture, *asymptomatic bacteriuria* in pregnancy is more likely to lead to cystitis and pyelonephritis. The increased incidence of symptomatic infection during pregnancy is thought to be caused by pregnancy-associated urinary stasis and glucosuria. This relative urinary stasis in pregnancy is a result of progesterone-induced decreased ureteral tone and motility, mechanical compression of the ureters at the pelvic brim, and compression of the bladder and ureteral orifices. In addition, the pH of the urine is increased because of increased bicarbonate excretion, which enhances bacterial growth, as does the mild glycosuria common in pregnancy.

It is standard to obtain a urine culture at the onset of prenatal care and to treat patients with asymptomatic bacteriuria. Ampicillin (500 mg po qid), sulfisoxazole (Gantrisin; 1 g po qid), or nitrofurantoin (Macrodantin; 50 mg po qid) for 7 to 10 days is usually quite effective, because the most common organism is *Escherichia coli*. In the third trimester, sulfas should be avoided because they compete with bilirubin for albumin-binding sites in the fetus and theoretically may produce hyperbilirubinemia of the newborn. Nitrofurantoin should be avoided in late pregnancy because of the risk of hemolysis as a result of deficiency of erythrocyte phosphate dehydrogenase in the newborn.

Approximately 25% to 30% of patients not treated for asymptomatic bacteriuria proceed to symptomatic UTI; hence, this treatment should prevent approximately 70% of symptomatic UTIs in pregnancy. However, 1.5% of patients with initial negative cultures also develop symptomatic UTIs in pregnancy. Suppressive antimicrobial therapy (nitrofurantoin, 50 to 100 mg po qd) is indicated if there are repetitive UTIs during pregnancy or following pyelonephritis during pregnancy. Consideration should be given to postpartum radiology evaluation of these patients to identify renal parenchymal and urinary collecting duct abnormalities.

Acute cystitis occurs in approximately 1% of pregnancies. Patients complain of urinary frequency, urgency, dysuria, and bladder discomfort. Occasionally, hematuria is also seen. Fever is unlikely, and its presence should suggest upper UTI. The treatment of cystitis is the same as that of asymptomatic bacteriuria.

Patients with *pyelonephritis* are acutely ill, with fever, costovertebral tenderness, general malaise, and often dehydration. Approximately 20% of these ill patients demonstrate increased uterine activity and preterm labor, and approximately 10% have positive blood cultures if they are obtained in the acute febrile phase of the disease. Pyelonephritis occurs in 2% of all pregnant patients and is one of the most common medical complications of pregnancy requiring hospitalization.

After a urinalysis and urine culture are obtained, patients are treated with intravenous hydration and antibiotics, commonly a first-generation cephalosporin or ampicillin. Uterine contractions may accompany these symptoms; if they are uncontrolled, preterm labor may ensue. Contractions usually cease but specific tocolytic therapy may be required. It is known that *E. coli* can produce phospholipase A, which in turn can promote prostaglandin synthesis, resulting in an increase in uterine activity. Fever is also known to induce contractions so that antipyretics are required for a temperature greater than 100° F. Attention must be paid to the patient's response to therapy and her general condition; sepsis occurs in 2% to 3% of patients with pyelonephritis. If improvement does not occur within 48 to 72 hours, urinary tract obstruction or urinary calculus should be considered along with a reevaluation of antibiotic coverage. A "single-shot" intravenous pyelogram and/or ultrasonography with attention to the ureters and kidneys is an integral part of the evaluation.

The organisms most commonly cultured from the urine of symptomatic pregnant patients are *E. coli* and other gram-negative aerobes. Follow-up can be with either frequent urine cultures or empiric antibiotic suppression with an agent such as nitrofurantoin.

Recurrent symptoms or failure to respond to usual therapy suggests another etiology for the findings. In these patients, a complete urologic evaluation 6 weeks after pregnancy may be warranted.

Urinary calculi are identified in approximately 1 in 1500 patients during pregnancy, although pregnancy per se does not promote stone development. Persistently alkaline urine is frequently associated with patients with urinary calculi, as is UTI with *Proteus* species. Symptoms similar to those of pyelonephritis but without fever are suggestive of urinary calculi. Microhematuria is more common with this condition than in uncomplicated UTI. Although typically renal colic pain may be found, it is seen less frequently in pregnancy than in the non-pregnant state due to the hormone-induced relaxation of ureteral tone. Usually, hydration and expectant management, along with straining of urine in search of stones, suffice as management. Occasionally, however, the presence of a stone can lead to infection and/or complete obstruction, which may require drainage by either ureteral stent or percutaneous nephrostomy. When the diagnosis of urinary calculi is uncertain, a limited-exposure intravenous pyelogram may be obtained.

3. RENAL DISEASE IN PREGNANCY

Pregnancy has profound effects on renal function, including a nearly 50% increase in glomerular filtration. The normal nonpregnant values for serum creatinine (Cr) and urea nitrogen decrease from a mean of 0.8 and 13 mg/100 ml, respectively, to mean values of 0.6 and 9 mg/100 ml.

Pregnancy in patients with preexisting renal disease is encountered frequently, because treatments such as dialysis and transplantation allow these patients health sufficient to support ovulation and pregnancy. *During preconception counseling,* these patients should be advised of the significant risks involved in a pregnancy and that pregnancy should be avoided unless their blood Cr levels are < 2 mg/100 ml and their diastolic blood pressure is < 90 mm Hg.

Pregnancy often has no adverse effect on patients with chronic renal disease. In general, patients with mild renal impairment (serum Cr < 1.4 mg/dl) have relatively uneventful pregnancies provided other complications are absent. Patients with moderate renal impairment (serum Cr > 1.4 to < 2.5 mg/dl) have a more guarded prognosis with an increased incidence of deterioration of renal function. In approximately 50% of patients with renal disease, proteinuria manifests. An increase in proteinuria during pregnancy is not, by itself, a serious consequence. *The presence of hypertension before pregnancy or the development of hypertension during pregnancy is a more worrisome finding with respect to both the course of the patient's renal disease and the pregnancy.*

Chronic renal disease is associated with an increased risk of first trimester spontaneous abortion. When pregnancy continues, there is an increased incidence of intrauterine growth restriction, so that serial assessment of fetal well-being and growth is recommended in most cases. Pregnancy following renal transplantation is generally associated with a good prognosis if at least 2 years have lapsed since the transplant was performed and thorough renal assessment reveals no evidence of active disease or rejection.

4. RESPIRATORY DISEASE IN PREGNANCY

The mechanical and hormonal changes associated with pregnancy alter the functional characteristics of the respiratory system (Figure 16.1). Most women experience

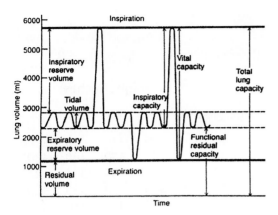

FIGURE 16.1.   Respiratory changes in pregnancy.

dyspnea of pregnancy in the latter half of pregnancy because of changes such as increased abdominal pressure associated with the expanding uterus, which cause decreased diaphragmatic excursion. Reassurance and advice to sleep in a semisitting position usually suffice for this problem.

Upper Respiratory Infections and Pneumonia in Pregnancy

Associated with the rhinovirus, adenovirus, picornavirus, parainfluenza virus, and respiratory syncytial virus, the incidence and severity of the viral common cold [*upper respiratory infection* (URI)] is unchanged in pregnancy. After appropriate evaluation excludes more serious problems such as influenza, mycoplasma pneumonia, and streptococcal pharyngitis, supportive care emphasizing hydration, rest, good diet, and antipyretics (e.g., acetaminophen) usually suffices. Decongestants such as pseudoephedrine may be used sparingly if needed for symptomatic relief. Fetal involvement is extremely uncommon because these mild viral respiratory illnesses do not have a viremic phase.

Pneumonia is an uncommon but serious complication in pregnancy, occurring in 0.1%–1.0% of pregnancies. It is a major cause of nonobstetric maternal death, with a reported overall mortality rate of 3% to 4%. *Bacterial pneumonia* presents as an acute febrile illness with chills and productive cough, leukocytosis, and lobar pattern infiltrate on chest x-ray. *Streptococcus pneumoniae* accounts for 30%–50% of these infections; others are caused by *Haemophilis influenzae, Klebsiella pneumoniae,* and *Staphylococcus aureus.* Conversely, *Mycoplasma pneumoniae* presents atypically as a slowly progressive headache, low-grade fever, myalgia, and nonproductive cough. Gram staining of the sputum, complete blood count (CBC), electrolytes, urinalysis, and blood gas determinations are important to exclude maternal hypoxia that may adversely affect the fetus. Management includes hydration, antipyretics (on a regular schedule when the maternal temperature is above 100° F), antibiotic therapy, respiratory toilet and oxygen supplementation if needed (as with low maternal PO_2, fetal tachycardia, and/or maternal respiratory distress), and evaluation of fetal well-being. Uncomplicated pneumococcal pneumonia is treated with penicillin G (600,000 units q 12 h for 7 to 10 days); mycoplasma and legionella pneumonia, with erythromycin (500 mg po qid for 14 days).

Influenza pneumonia presents as fever, malaise, headache, and a nonproductive cough, with a negative chest x-ray. Spontaneous resolution usually occurs within 3–4 days and care is supportive. *Varicella pneumoniae,* conversely, occurs in up to 20% of women with varicella infection (chicken pox) and has a maternal mortality rate of 25%–35%. Presenting as pleuritic chest pain, dyspnea, cough, and hemoptysis 2–6 days after the rash, this serious complication of pregnancy requires hospitalization with immediate acyclovir therapy (8–10 mg/kg every 8 hours) and vigorous supportive therapy for mother and fetus.

ASTHMA

Bronchial asthma is encountered in approximately 1% of pregnant patients, about 15% of whom have one or more severe asthma attacks during pregnancy. The overall course of asthma tends to be the same from pregnancy to pregnancy, with approximately 40% of women experiencing no change in their asthma, about 20% noting improvement, and the remaining 40% worsening of symptoms. Because of these associations, the modern management of asthma in pregnancy rests on four key components. First, serial objective measurement of pulmonary function during pregnancy, usually with peak flow measurements. Second, identify situations or substances that trigger asthma and develop plans to avoid them. This aspect of care is often given insufficient attention compared to medical therapy, but is the aspect of care that may greatly decrease the frequency of exacerbations and severity of illness. Third, appropriate pharmacologic management. Fourth, patient education with respect to the first three components and reassurance that such management is not harmful, indeed is beneficial, to the fetus. The management of asthma in pregnancy also includes evaluation of fetal growth and well-being as indicated.

Asthma is a chronic disease characterized by hyper-responsivity to allergens, air pollutants, exercise, viral infections, and cold air. Bronchospasm, mucosal edema, and mucous plugging of the airways result in air trapping and hyperinflation of the lungs, clinically manifest as wheezing, dyspnea, respiratory distress, and in the worse case, respiratory failure. Measurement of the peak flow (peak expiratory flow rate, or PEFR) provides objective measurement of the degree of obstruction, as this pulmonary function is unchanged by pregnancy, and is used for diagnosis and to monitor the response to therapy (Table 16.3). Hypoxia may also ensue, and with severe exacerbations, carbon dioxide (CO_2) retention associated with alveolar hypoventilation may follow. Arterial blood gas determination is the cornerstone of evaluation of these parameters. Pulse oximetry is limited in value in that it does not provide data on the clearing of CO_2. Chest x-ray is useful to evaluate for infiltrate and infection, noting that infiltrates may not be apparent on x-ray until after a dehydrated patient is sufficiently rehydrated. Eosinophils on sputum Gram stain may suggest an allergic etiology, whereas neutrophils, an infectious cause.

TABLE 16.3. Predicted Peak Expiratory Flow Rates (PEFR)

Age (years)	Height (inches)			
	58	60	64	68
15	370	380	410	440
20	360	370	400	430
25	350	365	395	425
30	340	360	390	420
35	335	350	380	410
40	300	340	370	400

Adapted with permission from Knudson RJ, et al. Changes in the normal maximal expiratory volume curve with growth and aging. Am Rev Respir Dis, 1983; 127; 725–734.

ACUTE EXACERBATIONS OF ASTHMA IN PREGNANCY

An exacerbation of known asthma, or on occasion the first diagnostic episode, during pregnancy requires evaluation consisting of careful history to determine if there is an identifiable allergen or other inciting cause (so that it can be eliminated, avoiding repeat exacerbation), physical examination, and peak flow measurement. A peak flow less than approximately 60%–70% of the predicted value should engender therapy, although therapy may be required at higher peak flow values depending on the clinical presentation and asthmatic history. Arterial blood gas and chest x-ray should be considered and usually performed except in mild cases. A productive cough warrants sputum evaluation. Medical therapy is centered in beta$_2$-agonist therapy (Table 16.4). Bronchodilation starts within 5–10 minutes with therapy repeated as often as every 20–30 minutes. Subcutaneous terbutaline (0.25 mg subcutaneous every 20–30 minutes for up to 3 doses) may be substituted for inhaled agents. A rapid response allows continued therapy on an outpatient basis. The use of a methylxanthine preparation such as theophylline or aminophylline [which inhibits

TABLE 16.4.	Medications for Asthma in Pregnancy	
Medication		**Dosage**
Beta-agonists	Albuterol	1–2 puffs q 3–4 hr to bid from inhaler
		1.5 mg in nebulizer administration
	Terbutaline	0.25 mg subcutaneous
Corticosteroid	Hydrocortisone	2 mg/kg as an intravenous bolus, followed by maintenance if needed 0.5 mg/kg/hr OR
		60 mg po initial dose, then 60–120 mg/day po in divided doses; with improvement, corticosteroids are usually tapered to a single dose daily gradually reduced over 7–14 days
Anti-inflammatory	Cromolyn sodium	2 puffs qid by inhaler or 2 sprays in each nostril bid-qid

phosphodiesterase, increasing cyclic adenosine monophosphate (cAMP) and controlling bronchospasm] is controversial in the treatment of acute exacerbation. One advantage cited is that methylxanthine use is often helpful to reduce the frequency and severity of exacerbations. Theophylline may be conveniently given intravenously as a loading dose of 6 mg/kg over 20 to 30 minutes, followed by a maintenance dose of 0.9 mg/kg/hr, pending transition to oral therapy. Therapeutic serum theophylline levels range from 10 to 20 mg/ml. If the response is not rapid or of sufficient magnitude (a severe exacerbation), corticosteroids should be given. If an incomplete response after 1–2 hours of therapy or peak flows remain below 60%, an agent such as hydrocortisone should be given (see Table 16.4). Remember that glucocorticosteroids cross the placental barrier and are associated with intrauterine growth restriction, a risk already present as a result of the asthma. Antibiotic therapy is reserved for clearly identified pulmonary infection. Careful attention to full hydration is also important. Electronic fetal heart monitoring and oxygen administration to maintain a PO_2 over 70 mm Hg or O_2 saturation over 95% completes the management of acute asthmatic exacerbation in pregnancy.

CHRONIC ASTHMA IN PREGNANCY

Chronic *mild* asthma is brief intermittent symptoms occurring once to twice a week. The peak flows remain over 80%–90% of expected values on serial measurement, and maintenance therapy usually consists of an inhaled beta$_2$-agonist used 1–2 puffs once or twice daily. Chronic *moderate* asthma is characterized by symptoms more frequent than twice a week or which last for several days or interfere with sleep. Peak flows of 60%–80% are common. Therapy consists of relatively short-acting "rescue medication regimens," including inhaled beta$_2$-agonists and, to reduce inflammation, either inhaled corticosteroids or cromolyn. Sustained-release theophylline may be useful for those with sleep disruption. *Severe* asthmatic patients have continuous symptoms that limit their activity and interfere with sleep, often with repeated emergency room visits. Their medical therapy involves the same medications on a more vigorous basis. Serial fetal evaluation for growth and acute monitoring for fetal well-being during exacerbations are essential. Finally, constant attention to allergens and other environmental factors, especially those that may be new, must be a regular part of care, as their elimination can greatly decrease the frequency and severity of the disease.

TABLE 16.5. Medical Management of Tuberculosis in Pregnancy

Recent PPD conversion (within 2 years) and no evidence of active disease (negative chest x-ray)	Isoniazid* 300 mg/day, starting after 1st trimester and continuing for 6–9 months
PPD conversion of unknown duration (> 2 years) and under 35 years of age†	Isoniazid 300 mg/day for 6–9 months postpartum
Active tuberculosis in pregnancy	Dual agent therapy (isoniazid and rifampin) for 9 months; ethambutol replaces rifampin if there is isoniazid resistance

*Pyridoxine (vitamin B_6) supplementation (50 mg/day) for all patients taking isoniazid is requisite to combat the neuropathy often associated with isoniazid therapy.
†Not recommended for women over 35 because of concerns about hepatotoxicity.
PPD = purified protein derivative.

LABOR AND DELIVERY FOR ASTHMATIC PATIENTS

The existing asthmatic care regimen is maintained in labor for the stable asthmatic patient. Intravenous hydrocortisone (100 mg every 8 hours) is indicated for those who have or are receiving steroids during pregnancy. Analgesia with morphine or meperidine may not be wise whereas fentanyl may be used. Lumbar epidural analgesia is an excellent choice for asthmatic women. Induction of labor with oxytocin or prostaglandin E_2 is permissible, while the use of 15-methyl prostaglandin $F_{2\alpha}$ may exacerbate asthma and should be avoided.

Tuberculosis in Pregnancy

While still an uncommon problem in pregnancy, the incidence of tuberculosis has increased recently, approaching 0.1% in endemic areas of the United States. Risk factors include exposure to persons known or suspected to be infected, human immunodeficiency virus (HIV) infection, birth/past residence in a country with a high tuberculosis prevalence, medically underserved status, substance (alcohol or drug) abuse, and being a health professional. Symptomatic pregnant patients (cough, fever, malaise, weight loss, night sweats, hemoptysis) may be encountered from time to time, but most pregnant patients with tuberculosis are asymptomatic. As a result, initial prenatal care should include screening with a purified protein derivative (PPD) skin test. Medical management depends on the duration of PPD-positive status (conversion) and the presence or absence of active disease (Table 16.5). Breast-feeding is safe (a multivitamin containing pyridoxine should be taken) as long as the infant is not taking concurrent oral TB therapy. Newborns of women taking TB therapy should receive a PPD at birth and at 3 months of age.

Smoking in Pregnancy

It is estimated that 33% of pregnant women smoke, despite vigorous public education programs that explain the risks to the smoker (cancer, heart disease, and so on) and fetus. Pregnant smokers also place their infants at increased risk of decreased birth weight, intrauterine growth restriction, abruptio placentae, and perhaps long-term neurologic abnormalities (Table 16.6). *Patients should be counseled to stop or at least significantly reduce smoking during pregnancy.*

5. CARDIAC DISEASE IN PREGNANCY

In the past, most pregnant patients with cardiac disease had rheumatic heart disease;

TABLE 16.6.   Reproductive Effects of Smoking

Decreased fertility
Increased risk of spontaneous abortion
Increased risk of ectopic pregnancy
Decreased birth weight (average =
    1 pound)
Increased risk of preterm delivery
    (preterm labor, premature rupture of
    membranes)
Increased risk of abruptio placentae and
    placenta previa
Increased risk of sudden infant death
    syndrome
Increased risk of developmental problems

TABLE 16.7.   New York Heart Association Functional Classification of Heart Disease

Class I	No cardiac decompensation
Class II	No symptoms of cardiac decompensation at rest
	Minor limitations of physical activity
Class III	No symptoms of cardiac decompensation at rest
	Marked limitations of physical activity
Class IV	Symptoms of cardiac decompensation at rest
	Increased discomfort with any physical activity

patients with congenital heart disease usually died before reaching reproductive age. Modern treatment of congenital and acquired heart disease allows many patients to reach their reproductive years and become pregnant. As a result, patients with rheumatic heart disease and acquired infectious valvular heart disease (often associated with drug use) comprise only 50% of pregnant cardiac patients. Considering that pregnancy is associated with a cardiac output increase of 40%, the risks to mother and fetus are often profound for patients with preexisting cardiac disease. Ideally, cardiac patients should have preconceptional care directed at maximizing cardiac function. They should also be counseled about the risks their particular heart disease poses in pregnancy. Some patients may choose to avoid pregnancy; others may choose to terminate a pregnancy rather than assume the risks to themselves and/or their fetus; still others may choose to continue pregnancy under intense medical and obstetric management.

The *classification of heart disease* of the New York Heart Association is useful to evaluate all types of cardiac patients with respect to pregnancy (Table 16.7). It is a functional classification, which is independent of type of heart disease. Patients with

septal defects, patent ductus arteriosus, and mild mitral and aortic valvular disorders often are in classes I or II and do well throughout pregnancy. Primary pulmonary hypertension, uncorrected tetralogy of Fallot, Eisenmenger syndrome, and certain other conditions are associated with a much worse prognosis (frequently death) through the course of pregnancy. For this reason, patients with such disorders are strongly advised not to become pregnant.

General management of the pregnant cardiac patient consists of avoiding conditions that add additional stress to the workload of the heart beyond that already imposed by pregnancy, including prevention and/or correction of anemia, prompt recognition and treatment of any infections, a decrease in physical activity and strenuous work, and proper weight gain. A low sodium diet and resting in the lateral decubitus position to promote diuresis are especially helpful interventions. Adequate rest is essential. For patients with class I or II heart disease, increased rest at home is advised. In more severe classes, hospitalization and treatment of cardiac failure are often required. Coordinated management between obstetrician, cardiologist, and anesthesiologist is necessary for patients with significant cardiac dysfunction.

TABLE 16.8. American Heart Association (AHA) Recommendations for Prevention of Bacterial Endocarditis in Patients Undergoing Genitourinary Procedures

Drug	Regimen
Standard Regimen	
Ampicillin, gentamicin, and amoxicillin	Ampicillin 2 g IV or IM; gentamicin 1.5 mg/hr IV 30 minutes before procedure, not to exceed 80 mg, followed by amoxicillin, 1.5 g po 6 hours later, or repeat parenteral regimen 8 hours later
Penicillin Allergic Regimen	
Vancomycin, gentamicin	Vancomycin 1.0 g over 1 hour IV plus gentamicin 1.5 mg/hr 1 hour before procedure, not to exceed 80 mg; repeat 8 hours after initial regimen

TABLE 16.9. Anticoagulation with Heparin

Loading dose	5000 U IV by rapid administration
Continuous infusion	Hourly rate to achieve 30,000–35,000 U/24 hours; adjust rate to achieve aPTT 1.5–2.5 times control
Long-term anticoagulation	17,500 U every 12 hours; adjust dose to achieve aPTT 1.5–2.5 times control at 6 hours

aPTT = activated partial thromboplastin time.

The fetuses of patients with functionally significant cardiac disease are at increased risk for low-birth weight and prematurity. A patient with congenital heart disease is more likely (1% to 5%) to have a fetus with congenital heart disease; antepartum fetal cardiac assessment using ultrasound is recommended.

The antepartum management of pregnant cardiac patients includes serial evaluation of maternal cardiac status as well as fetal well-being and growth. Anticoagulation, antibiotic prophylaxis for subacute bacterial endocarditis (SBE), invasive cardiac monitoring, and even surgical correction of certain cardiac lesions during pregnancy can be all accomplished if necessary (Tables 16.8 to 16.10). The *intrapartum and postpartum management of pregnant cardiac patients* includes consideration of the increased stress of delivery and postpartum physiologic adjustment. Labor in the lateral position to facilitate cardiac function is often desirable. Every attempt is made to facilitate vaginal delivery, given the increased cardiac stress of cesarean section. Because cardiac output increases by 40% to 50% during the second stage of labor, shortening this stage by the use of forceps is often advisable. Conduction anesthesia to reduce the stress of labor is also recommended. Even with patients who are stable at the time of delivery, it must be remembered that an additional increase in cardiac output is manifest in the puerperium because of the additional 500 ml added to the maternal blood volume as the uterus contracts to a nonpregnant configuration. Indeed, the majority of obstetric patients who die with cardiac disease do so following delivery.

TABLE 16.10. Commonly Prescribed Cardioactive Drugs in Pregnancy

Drug	Indication	Adverse Fetal Effects	FDA Pregnancy Category*	Adverse Maternal Effects
Digitalis (digoxin)	Heart failure; arrhythmias, especially atrial fibrillation	Toxicity; neonatal death with overdosage	C	Arrhythmias; conduction disturbances; anorexia; emesis
Loop diuretics (furosemide, bumetanide)	Heart failure; hypertension; constrictive pericarditis	Growth restriction	C	Electrolyte disturbances
Thiazides (hydrochlorothiazide, direct acting)	Hypertension, heart failure, pulmonary	Neonatal jaundice; thrombocytopenia; hemolytic anemia; hypoglycemia	C	Electrolyte disturbances
Vasodilators (hydralazine, isosorbide)	Hypertension; angina	Teratogenic in animals; thrombocytopenia; leukopenia reported in newborn	C	Hypotension; nausea; diarrhea; headache
β-Adrenergic blockers (propranolol, metropolol)	Angina; hypertrophic cardiomyopathy; hypertension; mitral valve prolapse; arrhythmia	During delivery: bradycardia; hypotension; oliguria; hypoglycemia	C	Uterine contraction; bradycardia; hypotension; bronchospasm
Calcium-channel blockers (nifedipine, verapamil)	Angina; hypertension; arrhythmia (verapamil)	Teratogenicity in small animals; no controlled human studies	C	Constipation (verapamil); bradycardia; conduction disturbances; hypotension

*B = negative animal studies; no human studies showing risk; should be used in pregnancy only if clearly indicated; C = animal studies show teratogenic effects; no human studies; should be used in pregnancy only if the potential benefit justifies the potential risk to the fetus.
FDA = Food and Drug Administration.

Mitral valve prolapse may occur in as many as 5% of pregnancies. Occurring when the mitral valve prolapses into the left atrium during systole, this condition is usually asymptomatic except for a late systolic murmur sometimes associated with a late systolic click. Pregnancy is unaffected in this situation, with SBE prophylaxis being of questionable value. In a minority of patients, regurgitation is severe with left atrial and ventricular enlargement and dysfunction. Echocardiography helps determine the severity of disease. Blockage of β-adrenergic receptors with propranolol may aid in management of associated symptoms such as chest pain, palpitations, tachycardia, dysrhythmia, and anxiety.

Rheumatic heart disease remains a common cardiac disease in pregnancy. As the severity of the associated valvular lesion increases, these patients are at higher risk for thromboembolic disease, SBE, cardiac failure, and pulmonary edema. A high rate of fetal loss is also seen in women with rheumatic heart disease. Approximately 90% of these patients have mitral stenosis, whose associated mechanical obstruction worsens as cardiac output increases during pregnancy. Mitral stenosis associated with atrial fibrillation has an especially high likelihood of congestive failure.

Maternal cardiac arrhythmias are occasionally encountered during pregnancy. Paroxysmal atrial tachycardia is the most commonly encountered maternal arrhythmia and is usually associated with too strenuous exercise. Underlying cardiac disease such as mitral stenosis should be suspected when atrial fibrillation and flutter are encountered.

Peripartum cardiomyopathy is a rare but especially severe pregnancy-associated cardiac condition. It occurs in the last month of pregnancy or the first 6 months following delivery and is difficult to distinguish from other cardiomyopathies except for its association with pregnancy. A myocarditis is responsible for some of these cases, whereas in other cases no apparent etiology can be determined.

A classic patient at increased risk for peripartum cardiomyopathy is one who is black, multiparous, and over 30 years of age and who has a history of twins or preeclampsia. Management includes bed rest, digoxin, diuretics, and in some cases, anticoagulation. The mortality rate is high. The best clinical sign related to prognosis is cardiac size 6 months after diagnosis. In patients with persistent cardiomegaly, the risk of death in the near future is great. In patients in whom the heart size has returned to normal, the prognosis is better, although recurrence in a subsequent pregnancy is likely. Counseling the patient about the benefits of sterilization is warranted.

There are several uncommon cardiac conditions seen in pregnancy that warrant discussion. *Marfan's syndrome* is inherited as an autosomal dominant trait and is manifest by abnormality of the connective tissue. It is characterized by aortic aneurysm, ectopia lentis, and long extremities. Patients suffer dyspnea and chest pain and demonstrate an aortic diastolic murmur and midsystolic click. Rupture of the aneurysm makes pregnancy especially dangerous for these patients, because there is a 25% to 50% risk of maternal mortality and a 50% chance that the offspring will inherit the disease.

6. GLUCOSE INTOLERANCE AND DIABETES MELLITUS IN PREGNANCY

Approximately 2% of pregnancies are complicated by diabetes that either develops during pregnancy or was antecedent to pregnancy. In either case, diabetes has significant implications for pregnancy, and conversely, pregnancy significantly affects diabetes.

Classification of Diabetes Mellitus

The White classification was used for many years to group cases of diabetes during pregnancy on the basis of age at onset of diabetes, duration of diabetes, and complications such as vascular disease. In recent years, the simpler *classification of the American Diabetic Association* (ADA) has become more commonly used (Table 16.11).

TABLE 16.11. Classifications of Diabetes in Pregnancy			

ADA Classification

Type I diabetes	Diagnosed in childhood, often brittle and difficult to control
Type II diabetes	Adult-onset glucose intolerance
Gestational diabetes	Glucose intolerance identified during pregnancy

The diabetic status is then described, for example, type II diabetes
with mild vascular disease

White Classification

A	Gestational diabetes; onset in pregnancy	D	Onset under age 10
			Duration > 20 years
B	Onset after age 20		Some vascular disease; retina, legs
	Duration less than 10 years	E	Pelvic arteriosclerosis by x-ray
	No vascular disease	F	Vascular nephritis
C	Onset between ages 10 and 19	R	Proliferative retinopathy
	Duration 10–19 years	T	Transplantation
	No vascular disease		

In the ADA classification, three forms of glucose intolerance are identified. *Type I diabetes* refers to diabetes diagnosed in childhood and is often brittle and difficult to control. It is thought to result from an immunologic destruction of cells of the pancreas. Diabetic ketoacidosis (DKA) is common in patients with this type of diabetes. *Type II diabetes* refers to the patient who has adult-onset glucose intolerance. These patients are frequently overweight and can often be controlled with a carefully followed diet. This type of diabetes is thought to result from exhaustion of the cells rather than their destruction. *Gestational diabetes* refers to a new glucose intolerance identified during pregnancy. In most patients, it is a reversible condition, although glucose intolerance in subsequent years occurs more frequently in this group of patients.

Interrelations between Pregnancy and Diabetes Mellitus

EFFECTS OF PREGNANCY ON GLUCOSE METABOLISM/DIABETES

Dietary habits are frequently changed during pregnancy, most notably with a decrease in food intake early in pregnancy because of nausea and vomiting and altered food choices. Several pregnancy-associated hormones also have a major effect on glucose metabolism. Most notable of these is *human placental lactogen* (HPL), which is produced in abundance by the enlarging placenta. HPL affects both fatty acid and glucose metabolism. It promotes lipolysis with increased levels of circulating free fatty acids and causes a decrease in glucose uptake and gluconeogenesis. In this manner, HPL can be thought of as an anti-insulin. The increasing production of this hormone as pregnancy advances generally requires ongoing changes to be made in insulin therapy to adjust for this effect.

Other hormones that have demonstrated lesser effects include *estrogen and progesterone*, which interfere with the insulin-glucose relation, and *insulinase*, which is produced by the placenta and degrades insulin to a limited extent. These effects of pregnancy on glucose metabolism make the management of pregnancy-associated diabetes difficult. DKA, for example, is more common in pregnant patients.

EFFECTS OF GLUCOSE METABOLISM/DIABETES ON THE MOTHER

With increased renal blood flow, the simple diffusion of glucose in the glomerulus

TABLE 16.12. Maternal and Fetal Complications of Pregnancy Associated with Maternal Diabetes

Maternal effects
  Hyperglycemia and glucosuria
  Diabetes ketoacidosis
  Increased incidence of urinary tract
    infection
  PIH/preeclampsia
  Retinopathy
Fetal/neonatal effects
  Congenital anomalies
  Macrosomia
  Hypoglycemia
  Hyperbilirubinemia
  Hypocalcemia
  Polycythemia
  Hydramnios
  Intrauterine fetal demise/spontaneous
    abortion

PIH = pregnancy-induced hypertension.

increases beyond the ability of tubular reabsorption, resulting in a normal *glucosuria* of pregnancy, commonly of approximately 300 mg/day. With diabetic patients this may be much higher, but because of poor correlation with blood glucose concentrations, using urinary glucose is of little value in glucose management during pregnancy. This glucose-rich urine is also an excellent environment for bacterial growth so that pregnant diabetic mothers have twice the incidence of *UTI* that nondiabetics have.

In addition to the added difficulties of glucose management and the increased risk of DKA during pregnancy, diabetic mothers have a twofold increase in the incidence of *pregnancy-induced hypertension* (PIH), or *preeclampsia,* over nondiabetic patients. Diabetic retinopathy worsens in approximately 15% of pregnant diabetic patients, some proceeding to proliferative retinopathy and loss of vision if the process remains untreated by laser coagulation (Table 16.12).

EFFECTS OF GLUCOSE METABOLISM/DIABETES ON THE NEONATE

Infants of diabetic mothers are at a three-fold increased risk of congenital anomalies over the 1% to 2% baseline risk of all patients. The most commonly encountered anomalies are cardiac and limb deformities. Sacral agenesis is a unique but rare anomaly for this group. *Excessive fetal growth, or macrosomia* (usually defined as a fetal weight in excess of 4500 g), is more common in diabetic pregnant patients because of the fetal metabolic effects of increased glucose transfer across the placenta. This excessive neonatal size can lead to problems with fetopelvic disproportion, requiring cesarean section or causing shoulder dystocia at the time of attempted vaginal delivery.

The *neonatal hypoglycemia* often encountered in these infants is thought to result from the sudden change in the steady-state arrangement, wherein increased glucose crossing the placenta was countered in the fetus by an increase in insulin levels. Once separated from the maternal supply of glucose, the higher level of insulin causes a significant neonatal hypoglycemia. In addition, these newborns are subject to an increased incidence of *neonatal hyperbilirubinemia, hypocalcemia, and polycythemia.*

Another complication of pregnancy in diabetic patients is an amniotic fluid volume increased above 2000 ml, a condition known as *hydramnios, or polyhydramnios.* Encountered in approximately 10% of diabetics, the increases in amniotic fluid volume and uterine size are associated with an increased risk of abruptio placentae and preterm labor. This condition is also a predisposing factor for *postpartum uterine atony.*

The risk of *spontaneous abortion* is similar in well-controlled diabetic and nondiabetic patients, but the risk is significantly increased if glucose control is poor. There is also an increased risk of *intrauterine fetal demise* and *stillbirth,* especially when diabetic control is inadequate (see Table 16.12).

Infants of diabetic mothers also tend to have a fivefold to sixfold increased fre-

| TABLE 16.13. | Glucose Tolerance Tests in Pregnancy |

1-hour Glucola screening test
   50-g glucose challenge with no glucose preparation and with sampling at 1-hour postchallenge
   Normal value: < 140 mg/100 ml (< 7.8 mM/L) plasma glucose
3-hour glucose tolerance test
   100-g glucose challenge after 3 days glucose preparation with sampling as shown
   Normal values:

| | *Less than stated mg/100 ml (mM/L) at:* | | | |
Time (hour)	Fasting	1	2	3
Plasma glucose	105	190	165	145
	(5.8)	(10.6)	(9.2)	(8.1)
Blood glucose	90	165	145	125
	(5.0)	(9.2)	(8.1)	(6.9)

quency of *respiratory distress syndrome.* The usual tests of lung maturity are often poorly predictive for these infants.

Laboratory Diagnosis of Glucose Intolerance/Diabetes in Pregnancy

Approximately 1% of all pregnant patients are known to have been diabetic before pregnancy. For these patients, management ideally begins before conception with the goal of optimal glucose control before and during pregnancy. Although there is controversy as to whether this causes a reduction in the risk of congenital anomalies, other maternal and neonatal benefits make it clear that a diabetic woman entering pregnancy should be at optimum glucose control if at all possible.

Gestational diabetes is usually identified by prenatal screening of all pregnancy patients, although it may be suspected in patients with known risk factors for gestational diabetes, including a history of giving birth to an infant weighing > 4000 g, a history of repeated spontaneous abortions, a history of unexplained stillbirth, a strong family history of diabetes, obesity, and/or persistent glucosuria. *Of patients identified*

as having gestational diabetes, however, 50% do not have such risk factors. This is the rationale for universal glucose screening in pregnancy.

The most commonly used screening test for glucose intolerance during pregnancy does not require the patient to be in a fasting state: 1 hour after consuming 50 g of glucose solution (Glucola), blood is drawn for plasma glucose determination. Patients whose glucose value exceeds 140 mg/mL require a 3-hour glucose tolerance test. Two or more abnormal values on the 3-hour test make the diagnosis of gestational diabetes. One abnormal value is considered suspicious, and testing is repeated in 4 to 6 weeks, depending on the gestational age at the time of the initial test. The standards are summarized in Table 16.13, which includes values in the more common international notation of millimoles per liter (equal to milligrams per 100 milliliters divided by 18).

In patients lacking any risk factors, the *1-hour glucose screening is usually performed between 24 and 28 weeks' gestation,* because glucose intolerance is generally manifest after that time. In patients with factors suggesting possible glucose intolerance, the testing is performed at the onset of prenatal care and, if normal at that time, repeated as the third trimester commences. Using this screening method, approximately 15% of patients have an abnormal screening test. Of those patients who then proceed to have the standard 3-hour oral glucose tolerance test, approximately 15% are diagnosed as having gestational diabetes.

Management of Diabetes during Pregnancy

Often overlooked in the overall management of a patient whose pregnancy is complicated by diabetes mellitus is the importance of *patient education*. The long-standing diabetic patient should realize that much tighter control of her glucose levels is advised during pregnancy, with greater attention and more frequent glucose monitoring. The impact of pregnancy on diabetes and vice versa must also be emphasized to the pregnant diabetic patient. The newly diagnosed diabetic patient should receive general diabetic counseling along with information about the unique features of the combination of diabetes and pregnancy. With either type of patient, intense management may be quite stressful, and all those involved with obstetric care should be mindful of the need for extra attention that many of these patients need.

The overall goal of management is to control glucose values within fairly circumscribed limits, to serially evaluate fetal well-being, and to time delivery to maximize outcome for both mother and fetus/neonate. *The mainstay of diabetes management is nutritional counseling about an appropriate diet.* Although the recommended increase in daily caloric intake has been proposed as 30 kcal/kg of ideal body weight, most pregnant diabetic patients end up on a daily caloric recommendation of 2300 to 2400 calories, comprised of approximately 25% fat, 25% protein, and 50% complex carbohydrates. With careful attention to diet, most gestational diabetic mothers do not require insulin.

Patients are generally followed with morning fasting and 2-hour postbreakfast plasma glucose determinations, optimally obtained the morning of their office visit. For "ideal" control, the fasting plasma glucose should be maintained in the 90 to 100 mg/100 ml range and the 2-hour post-breakfast plasma glucose maintained at less than 120 mg/100 ml, although values up to 140 mg/100 ml may be acceptable in selected circumstances. Home glucose monitoring is now widely available in convenient kits that require a level of sophistication that most patients can achieve.

For patients who do not need exogenous insulin, the perinatal outcome is good. Pregnancy is allowed to continue to term with delivery planned at that time. Careful evaluation of fetal weight by ultrasonography is important, because the incidence of macrosomia remains increased in these patients.

Insulin therapy is required for the patient whose plasma glucose values exceed the limits noted for glucose tolerance testing or exceed the "ideal" levels for dietary management. Insulin does not cross the placenta and, therefore, does not directly affect the fetus. Instead, enough insulin is given to maintain normal blood glucose levels, because glucose does cross the placenta and in excessive concentration can harm the fetus. A mixture of short- and long-acting insulin is given in morning and evening injections so that there is insulin activity at all times, thus maintaining a uniform blood glucose level. A common method is to administer two thirds of the dose in the morning and one third in the evening. The insulin requirements of a pregnant patient are expected to increase because of increased "insulin resistance" as pregnancy progresses.

Once the patient has begun insulin therapy, plasma glucose values are obtained four times a day, typically at 7:00 A.M., 11:00 A.M., 4:00 P.M., and 10:00 P.M. Insulin doses are adjusted to maintain a fasting level under 100 mg/100 ml and other levels under 120 mg/100 ml. Understanding the duration of action of each type of insulin provides a logical framework for adjusting insulin doses if needed. The fasting glucose reflects the dose of NPH insulin given before dinner on the previous evening. The

11:00 A.M. plasma glucose value reflects the morning regular insulin received 3 to 4 hours earlier. The 4:00 P.M. plasma glucose value reflects the morning NPH, and the 10:00 P.M. plasma glucose value reflects the evening doses of regular insulin. Incremental changes in glucose administration should be approximately 1 to 3 units at a time to avoid rapid changes in glucose values. A flow sheet is kept by the patient showing time and dosage of insulin and self-blood-sugar determinations as well as any comments about reactions, and so on.

A fraction of hemoglobin known as hemoglobin A_{1c} reflects glucose values over the preceding 6 to 8 weeks. This test has been used to monitor glucose control and to predict the likelihood of congenital anomalies in diabetics early in pregnancy. Overall, the value of this test has been disappointing in clinical use. Fructosamine, which reflects glucose values over the shorter interval of 2 to 3 weeks, also has limited clinical value.

Pregnant diabetic patients, especially type I diabetics, are prone to DKA. This serious complication can usually be avoided with frequent monitoring of blood glucose levels, attention to diet, careful insulin administration, and the avoidance of infections. Management of DKA is not different from management of DKA in nonpregnant patients and consists of adequate fluids, insulin, glucose, and electrolyte stabilization. Fetal death can accompany DKA, so electronic fetal monitoring of the fetus is essential until the maternal metabolic status is stabilized. At the other end of the spectrum, hypoglycemia is encountered at times, especially early in pregnancy, when nausea and vomiting interfere with caloric intake. Although hypoglycemia does not have untoward effects on the fetus, the symptoms and potential trauma that the patient may experience should be avoided.

Infections are more frequently encountered in diabetic mothers. Periodic urine cultures should be obtained to detect asymptomatic bacteriuria, because the risk of UTI and pyelonephritis is twice that of the nondiabetic gravida. Patients should also be told to promptly report any other symptoms that suggest infection, so that aggressive treatment can be initiated.

Because of the risk of progressive retinopathy, diabetic patients should have an initial ophthalmologic evaluation and serial examinations during their pregnancies.

Fetal Assessment in Diabetic Pregnancy

Beginning at approximately 30 to 32 weeks of gestation, various measures to evaluate the fetal growth and well-being are undertaken. *Daily fetal kick counts* are an inexpensive and reliable screening test. Serial *nonstress testing and/or biophysical profile* measurements are also initiated, usually on a once or twice weekly schedule, but more frequently if clinical indicators warrant. Serial ultrasonography is performed to detect fetal anomalies and developing polyhydramnios and to follow fetal growth. Both intrauterine growth restriction and macrosomia are seen in infants of diabetic mothers. When the estimated fetal weight by ultrasound is > 4500 g, *macrosomia* is diagnosed; when > 5000 g, cesarean section for delivery is often recommended to avoid the risk of shoulder dystocia and similar birth trauma.

Delivery in Diabetic Pregnancy

In general, the goal is for the pregnant diabetic to deliver a healthy child vaginally. The adequacy of glucose control, the well-being of the infant, estimated fetal weight by ultrasound, the presence of hypertension or other complications of pregnancy, the gestational age, the presentation of the fetus, and the status of the cervix are all factors involved in decisions regarding delivery. In the *well-controlled diabetic with no complications, induction at term (38 to 40 weeks) is often undertaken.*

If an *earlier delivery* is deemed necessary for either fetal or maternal indications, fetal maturity studies are performed before effecting delivery. To avoid the potential delivery of an infant who might suffer respiratory distress syndrome, some clinicians require that two or more tests indicate fetal lung maturity, instead of a single test used for nondiabetic patients. Ideally, the presence of phosphatidylglycerol confirms the presence of fetal lung maturity, but this phospholipid might not be present in detectable amounts even late in pregnancy.

The route of delivery is influenced by the estimated fetal weight. If the estimated fetal weight is > 4500 g, cesarean section rather than attempted vaginal delivery may be considered, depending on maternal factors such as pelvic size. When the estimated fetal weight is > 5000 g, the risk of birth trauma is significantly increased and cesarean delivery is usually recommended.

Whether the patient's labor begins spontaneously or is induced, *intrapartum glucose control* is generally managed by a constant glucose infusion of a 5% dextrose solution at 100 ml/hr with frequent plasma glucose assessments. Short-acting insulin may be administered if needed, either by constant infusion or by intermittent injection. Somewhat surprisingly, patients whose glucose has been difficult to control through pregnancy often have very satisfactory levels of glucose in labor when so managed.

Postpartum Management in Diabetic Pregnancy

With delivery of the placenta, the source of the "anti-insulin" factors is removed. HPL has a short half-life, and its effect on plasma glucose is evident within hours. Many patients do not require any insulin whatsoever in the first several days postpartum, and routine management generally consists of frequent glucose determinations using a sliding-scale approach with minimal insulin injections. For patients with gestational diabetes, no further insulin is required postpartum. In patients with preexisting diabetes, insulin is generally resumed at 50% of the prepregnant dose once a patient is taking a normal diet. Thereafter, insulin can be adjusted over the ensuing weeks, with requirements usually reaching the prepregnancy level.

Over 95% of gestational diabetic mothers return to a completely normal glucose status postpartum. Glucose tolerance screening is advocated 2 to 4 months postpartum for these patients to detect the 3% to 5% who remain diabetic and require treatment. A fasting plasma glucose of ≥ 140 mg/dl or a 2-hour post-75 g glucose load of > 200 mg/dl requires close follow-up.

Diabetic women are best advised to have their pregnancies early in their reproductive lives, before the development of serious vascular complications. Contraception is best accomplished by barrier methods or intrauterine devices, because oral contraceptives may adversely affect maternal blood vessels.

7. ENDOCRINE DISEASE IN PREGNANCY
Thyroid Disease in Pregnancy

Thyroid function in pregnancy remains normal, although some clinical manifestations of pregnancy (e.g., warm skin, palpitations) may mimic thyroid dysfunction. The diagnosis of thyroid disease in pregnancy depends on the interpretation of laboratory tests. Total thyroxine (T_4) and 3,5,3'-triiodothyronine (T_3) serum concentrations are elevated, and the T_3 resin uptake (T_3RU) is lowered during pregnancy because of estrogen-induced increases in thyroxine-binding globulin (TBG). Free T_4 (FT_4) and free T_3 (FT_3) concentrations are unchanged, however. Calculation of the index for FT_3 (FT_3I) and FT_4 (FT_4I) aids in the diagnosis of hyperthyroidism and hypothyroidism, because a high value is consistent with hyperthyroidism and a low value, with hypothyroidism. Thyroid-stimulating hormone (TSH) concentration is unchanged in pregnancy. The availability of new sensitive TSH (sTSH) tests may help to clarify the situation even more than traditional thyroid function testing (Table 16.14).

Hyperthyroidism complicates approximately 0.2% of pregnancies, and in 85% of cases it is associated with Graves disease,

TABLE 16.14. Thyroid Function Studies during Pregnancy

	Nonpregnant	Pregnant		
Test	Normal	Normal	Hyperthyroid	Hypothyroid
Total T$_4$	Normal	Increased	Increased	Decreased
FT$_4$	Normal	Normal	Increased	Decreased
FT$_4$I	Normal	Normal	Increased	Decreased
Total T$_3$	Normal	Slightly increased	Normal to slightly increased	Normal to slightly decreased
FT$_3$I	Normal	Normal	Normal to increased	Normal to increased
T$_3$RU	Normal	Decreased	Increased	Decreased
TSH	Normal	Normal	Normal to decreased	High
TSAb	Negative	Negative	Often positive	Negative

FT$_3$I = index for free 3,5,3'-triiodothyronine; FT$_4$ = free thyroxine; FT$_4$I = index for FT$_4$; T$_3$RU = T$_3$ resin uptake; TSAb = thyroid-stimulating antibody; TSH = thyroid-stimulating hormone.

with the remainder of cases associated with acute and subacute thyroiditis, chronic lymphocytic thyroiditis (Hashimoto's disease), toxic nodular goiter, and hydatidiform mole and choriocarcinoma. The diagnosis is suspected with the classic stigmata of hyperthyroidism (nervousness, palpitations, heat intolerance, weakness, diarrhea, tachycardia, hyperreflexia, tremor, exophthalmos, and skin and hair changes), with or without goiter and confirmed by elevated thyroid function studies and reduced levels of sTSH. Infants of hyperthyroid mothers are at increased risk for low birth weight.

Treatment with propylthiouracil (PTU) blocks intrathyroid synthesis of T$_4$ as well as peripheral conversion of T$_4$ to T$_3$ and has the additional advantage of less placental transfer to the fetus than the other common medicine methimazole (Tapazole). Hyperthyroidism is usually brought under control in 3 to 4 weeks via the usual regimen of PTU: an initial dose of PTU of 300 to 400 mg/day in oral divided doses. After the patient is clinically euthyroid, the dosage may be tapered and the patient followed for evidence of relapse. PTU should be tapered to < 100 mg/day at term. Skin rash, pruritus, fever, and nausea are complications in approximately 3% of patients, and if severe, methimazole may be substituted

(30 to 40 mg/day in divided doses as initial therapy and 10 mg/day as the tapering target for the time of term pregnancy).

Fortunately, the dangerous complications of PTU therapy—granulocytopenia and agranulocytosis—are rare (0.2% of cases) and usually resolve with alternate therapy. The FT$_4$ is the first thyroid function parameter to decrease, followed in a few weeks by FT$_3$I. Because the plasma half-life of T$_4$ is 7 days, laboratory testing at intervals of less than 1 week is not rewarding. Although *neonatal hypothyroidism* may result from suppression of the fetal thyroid with PTU, PTU has minimal transfer to breast milk and may be safely used while nursing. On the contrary, methimazole is secreted in breast milk and is not recommended during nursing.

Radioactive iodine is contraindicated during pregnancy because of its effect on the fetal thyroid. Surgical therapy is rarely warranted during pregnancy.

Hypothyroidism is rarely encountered in pregnancy, because it is associated with anovulation and infertility. The diagnosis is suspected with the classic stigmata of hypothyroidism (tiredness, lethargy, weakness, cold intolerance, and constipation), with or without goiter, and confirmed by lowered thyroid function studies. Management with replacement thyroxine (Synthroid) is indicated (0.1 to 0.2 mg/day in a single oral dose to achieve clinical euthyroidism). TSH levels take 8 weeks to return to normal after initiation of therapy and hence have limited clinical value.

8. INFECTIOUS DISEASES IN PREGNANCY
Group B Streptococcus

The group B β-hemolytic streptococcus is an important cause of perinatal infections. Asymptomatic cervical colonization occurs in up to 30% of pregnant women, but cultures may be positive only intermittently even in the same patient. Approximately 50% of infants exposed to the organism in the lower genital tract will become colonized. For most of these infants, such colonization is of no consequence, but for approximately 2 to 3 infants per 1000 live births, significant clinical infection occurs.

There are two manifestations of clinical infection of the newborn. *Early-onset infection* is manifest as septicemia and septic shock, pneumonia, and/or meningitis. Such an infection is much more likely in premature infants than in term gestations. The mortality rate exceeds 50%. *Late-onset infection* occurs up to 4 weeks after delivery. Meningitis is the most common specific infection and the mortality rate in these cases is approximately 25%. Prematurity is not a factor for late-onset infection.

Current recommendations include treatment of patients at high risk for perinatal infection (e.g., preterm labor, ruptured membranes) and screening of all patients late in pregnancy. Neither approach is ideal.

In the mother, postpartum endometritis may be caused by infection with group B streptococcus. The onset is often sudden and within 24 hours of delivery. Significant fever and tachycardia are present; sepsis may follow.

Syphilis

Syphilis is caused by the motile spirochete *Treponema pallidum,* which survives only in vivo. The spirochete is transmitted by direct contact, invading intact mucous membranes or areas of abraded skin. *T. pallidum* is generally considered to cross the placenta to the fetus after 16 weeks of gestation, although transmission has been documented at as early as 6 weeks of gestation.

Abortion, stillbirth, and neonatal death are more frequent in any untreated patient, whereas neonatal infection is more likely in primary or secondary rather than latent syphilis. Infants with congenital syphilis may be asymptomatic or have the classic stigmata of the syndrome, although most infants do not develop evidence of disease for 10 to 14 days after delivery. Early evidence of disease includes a maculopapular rash, snuffles, mucous patches on the oropharynx, hepatosplenomegaly, jaundice, lymphadenopathy, and chorioretinitis. Later signs include Hutchinson's teeth, mulberry molars, saddle nose, and saber shins.

Serologic testing is the mainstay of diagnosis. Nontreponemal tests identify antibodies developed in response to nonspecific antigens from the immunologic inflammatory response to the spirochete. Test results are reported in quantitative titers (e.g., 1:8); the higher the titer, the greater the inflammatory response. Because false-positive Venereal Disease Research Laboratory (VDRL) and rapid plasma reagin (RPR) tests can be seen in chronic diseases such as leprosy, autoimmune diseases (e.g., lupus), and in drug addiction, treponemal-specific tests are used to confirm infection and identify antibody specific against *T. pallidum.* A positive result indicates either active disease or previous exposure. Dark-field microscopy can be used to identify the spirochete directly (Table 16.15).

Treatment consists of a single 2.4-million-unit intramuscular benzathine penicillin injection for primary and secondary infection or latent disease of < 1-year duration. For latent disease of > 1-year duration, three injections are given at weekly intervals. Patients with known penicillin sensitivity generally require desensitization, because penicillin is the only antibiotic that can cross the placenta in adequate amounts to treat the fetus. Posttreatment titers

TABLE 16.15. Sensitivity and Specificity of Serologic Test for Syphilis

Test	Sensitivity			
	1°	2°	Early	Latent
VDRL	78	100	96	71
RPR	86	100	98	73
FTA-ABS	84	100	100	96
MHA-TP	76	100	97	94

FTA-ABS = fluorescent treponemal antibody, absorbed; MHA-TP = microhemagglutination-*Treponema pallidum;* RPR = rapid plasma reagin; VDRL = Venereal Disease Research Laboratory. (After Larsen S, Hunter E, Kraus S, eds. A Manual of Tests for Syphilis. Washington, DC: American Public Health Association, 1990.)

should be followed serially for 2 years. A fourfold increase in serologic titer or persistent or recurrent signs or symptoms indicates inadequate treatment or reinfection, and retreatment is indicated in either case. Response to therapy is again evaluated by following serologic titers.

Gonorrhea

Routine antepartum screening for *Neisseria gonorrhoeae* is universal. Recovery rates vary from 1% to 8%, depending on the population screened. Infection above the cervix (i.e., of the uterus, including the fetus, and the fallopian tubes) is rare after the first weeks of pregnancy. At delivery, however, infected mothers may transmit the organism, causing gonococcal ophthalmia in the neonate. In the past, such infection was a prominent cause of blindness, but currently used routine prophylactic treatment of the newborn's eyes with silver nitrate or tetracycline is very effective in preventing neonatal gonorrhea.

Bacterial Vaginosis

Bacterial vaginosis (BV) is the current term for vaginitis previously called *nonspecific* vaginitis, *Haemophilus vaginalis vaginitis, Corynebacterium vaginalis vaginitis,* and *Gardnerella vaginalis vaginitis.* The multiple names demonstrate the present understanding that bacterial vaginosis is a syndrome that involves a marked change in the vaginal flora, resulting in a loss of lactobacilli, an elevated pH, and an increase in other flora—particularly *G. vaginalis, Mycoplasma hominis,* and various anaerobic bacteria such as *Bacteroides, Peptostreptococcus,* and *Mobiluncus* species. Because this is not an inflammatory vaginitis, increased numbers of white blood cells (WBCs) are not seen on wet preparation of the discharge (Table 16.16). Predisposing factors include but are not limited to multiple sexual partners, longer history of coital experience, and the presence of other sexually transmitted diseases, especially *Trichomonas vaginalis.* The evidence for the sexual transmission of bacterial vaginosis is unclear, because the treatment of male partners has not affected the incidence in their partners.

Approximately 50% of women with bacterial vaginosis are asymptomatic. The others have variable complaints, including an increase in the amount of discharge and a "fishy" or "musty" vaginal odor and sometimes a thin gray to white discharge that stains the undergarments. Vulvar and vaginal pruritus are uncommon, because bacterial vaginosis is not an inflammatory condition. The diagnosis is made by finding three of four signs: (*1*) a thin homogeneous discharge that tends to adhere to the vaginal walls, (*2*) a vaginal pH elevated above 4.5, (*3*) a positive potassium hydroxide (KOH) "amine" or "whiff" test, and (*4*) the presence of *clue cells* on microscopic examination. A whiff test is performed by mixing a few drops of 10% KOH with the vaginal secretions; if positive, the characteristic fishy odor is easily discovered. Clue cells, which are epithelial cells studded with large numbers of bacteria that obscure the cell border, are the single most reliable diagnostic criterion when they account for greater than 20% of the cells seen (Figure 16.2).

Bacterial vaginosis has been associated with an increased incidence of pelvic

TABLE 16.16. Common Vaginal Infections

Characteristic	Normal	Infection		
		Bacterial Vaginosis	*Candida* **Vulvovaginitis**	*Trichomonas* **Vaginitis**
Common patient complaint	None	Discharge; fishy odor, possibly worse after intercourse	Itching, burning, discharge	Frothy discharge, bad odor, vulvar pruritus, dysuria
Vaginal pH	3.8–4.2	> 4.5	< 4.5 (usually)	> 4.5
Discharge appearance	White, flocculent	Thin, homogeneous, white, gray, adherent, often increased amount over normal	White, curdy ("cottage cheese"), sometimes increased amount over normal	Yellow, green, frothy, adherent, increased amount over normal
Amine odor (KOH whiff test)	Absent	Present (fishy)	Absent	Often present (fishy)
Microscopic	Lactobacilli	Clue cells, coccobacillary bacteria, no WBCs	Mycelia budding, yeast, pseudohyphae with KOH preparation	Trichomonads, WBCs > 10 pf

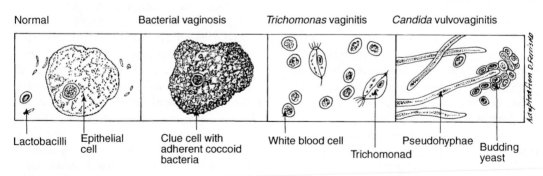

Normal   Bacterial vaginosis   *Trichomonas* vaginitis   *Candida* vulvovaginitis

Lactobacilli   Epithelial cell   Clue cell with adherent coccoid bacteria   White blood cell   Pseudohyphae   Budding yeast   Trichomonad

FIGURE 16.2. Wet mount of normal vaginal secretion and secretion from patient with bacterial vaginosis.

inflammatory disease, posthysterectomy infection, postabortal pelvic inflammatory disease, preterm labor and delivery, premature rupture of membranes, amniotic fluid infection, and postpartum endometritis. Treatment with intravaginal or oral metronidazole (Flagyl, 500 mg po bid for 7 days; Metrogel 0.75%, 5 g intravaginally once or twice for 5 days; Clindamycin cream 2%, 5 g for 7 days) is effective therapy, although recurrence is common. Oral therapy with other broad spectrum antibiotics may also be effective.

Genital Herpes

Herpes simplex virus (HSV) is a DNA virus that poses significant risk to the fetus/neonate. Herpes infections are categorized as either primary or recurrent; it is the primary form that poses the greatest risk to the fetus. Delivery through a lower genital tract with primary herpes virus infection is associated with neonatal infection in 50% or more of cases, a neonatal mortality rate of approximately 50% of those infected, and serious neurologic sequelae in nearly 75% of survivors. The risk of neonatal infection is much lower with recurrent infections, presumably because of a decreased inoculum size.

The diagnosis of HSV infection is suspected when clinical examination shows the characteristic tender vesicles with ulceration followed by crusting. Confirmation is by cell culture, with most positive results reported within 72 hours. Multinucleated giant cells can be seen on Pap smears or with the use of a Tzanck test in roughly 50% of cases.

If infection with herpes virus is suspected during the course of pregnancy, a culture from a lesion is generally obtained to confirm the diagnosis. In such patients, or any patient with a history of herpes virus infection, careful visualization of the lower genital tract is important at the onset of labor or when rupture of membranes occurs. If no lesions are identified, vaginal delivery is deemed safe. Cesarean delivery is recommended if herpes lesions are identified on the cervix, in the vagina, or on the vulva at the time of labor or spontaneous rupture of membrane (SROM). This is true whether or not the lesions are associated with primary or recurrent infection. Recent evidence suggests that the risk of neonatal infection may be much higher in first episode primary infection (30% to 50%) as compared to recurrent disease (3% to 5%), although this information does not alter the recommendation for cesarean birth when lesions are present. Serial culturing for HSV near term does not predict if a patient will be shedding virus at delivery and hence should be abandoned as a routine antenatal test. Despite this, 1 of 20 infants delivered by cesarean section for this reason develop HSV infection. Acyclovir is used if symptoms are serious, although its safety in pregnancy has not been fully ensured.

Cytomegalovirus

Cytomegalovirus (CMV) infection affects 1% of births in the United States and is the most common congenital infection. CMV is a DNA virus that may be transmitted in saliva, semen, cervical secretions, breast milk, blood, or urine; CMV infection is often asymptomatic, although it can cause a short febrile illness. Like the herpes virus to which it is related, CMV may have a latency period, only to reactivate at a later time. Maternal seronegativity, and hence susceptibility, is inversely proportional to socioeconomic status.

Either primary or recurrent maternal infection is associated with a 0.5% to 1.5% risk of intrauterine infection, although severely affected infants are more often associated with primary seroconversion during pregnancy. Approximately 10% of infected infants demonstrate congenital defects of varying severity, including microcephaly with or without intracranial calcifications, intrauterine growth restriction, or hepatosplenomegaly. Approximately 10% of asymptomatic CMV-infected infants subsequently develop sensoneural hearing loss, chorioretinitis, mild neurologic effects, and dental defects.

The diagnosis is clinical and by exclusion. There is no reliable serologic testing presently available.

There is no treatment of maternal or neonatal CMV infection. Prevention of infection by habits emphasizing personal cleanliness and selectivity of personal contacts is important. Unlike herpes, active lower genital tract infection is not associated with increased risk to the neonate and is not an indication for cesarean section.

Rubella

Rubella (German or 3-day measles) is an RNA virus with important perinatal impact if infection occurs during pregnancy. Approximately 15% of reproductive-age women lack immunity to this virus and are susceptible to infection. A history of prior infection is unreliable in 50% of cases. The virus is spread by airborne droplets, with an incubation period of 14 to 21 days postexposure. Clinical disease is associated with communicability from approximately 7 days before rash development through 4 days after the onset of rash. Once infection occurs, immunity is lifelong.

If a woman develops rubella infection in the first trimester, there is an increased risk of both spontaneous abortion and congenital rubella syndrome. Although 50% to 70% of infants with congenital rubella appear normal at birth, many subsequently develop signs of infection. Common defects associated with the syndrome include congenital heart disease (e.g., patent ductus arteriosus), mental retardation, deafness, and cataracts. The risk of congenital rubella is related to the gestational age at the time of infection such that up to 90% of infants acquire the syndrome if infection occurs at less than 11 weeks; 33% at 11 to 12 weeks; 25% at 13 to 14 weeks; 10% at 15 to 16 weeks; and 5% in the third trimester. Primary infection can be diagnosed using acute and convalescent sera for immunoglobulin (Ig)-M and IgG antibodies.

Because of the fetal implications, prenatal screening for IgG rubella antibody is routine. Young women should be vaccinated remote from pregnancy if they are found to be susceptible. The vaccine uses a live attenuated rubella virus that induces antibodies in more than 95% of vaccinations. Because there is a 5% failure rate, the patient should be rechecked 6 weeks after vaccination to ensure antibody response. It is recommended that pregnancy be delayed 3 months following immunization although congenital rubella syndrome following vaccination during an undiagnosed pregnancy has not been reported. In women whose prenatal screen identifies a lack of rubella antibody, vaccination at the time of hospital discharge postpartum is recommended. Such management poses no risk to the new-

born or other children; breast-feeding is not contraindicated.

Because there is no effective treatment for a pregnant patient infected with rubella, patients who do not have immunity are advised to avoid potential exposure. Human immune γ-globulin does not prevent or lessen the effect of infection; no antiviral therapy is available. Maternal treatment is supportive.

Toxoplasmosis

Infection with the intracellular parasite *Toxoplasma gondii* occurs primarily through ingestion of the infectious tissue cysts in raw or poorly cooked meat or through contact with feces from infected cats, which contain infectious sporulated oocytes. The latter may remain infectious in moist soil for more than 1 year. Only cats who hunt and kill their prey are reservoirs for infection, not those who exclusively eat prepared foods. Asymptomatic infection is common. Approximately 33% of reproductive-age women have antibodies to toxoplasmosis.

Infection in the first trimester causes more severe fetal disease than infection in the third trimester, but conversely, the rates of infection are less in the first than in the third trimester.

Approximately 60% of infants whose mothers are infected during pregnancy have serologic evidence of infection. Of these, 75% show no gross evidence of infection at birth. However, congenital disease can cause severe mental retardation with chorioretinitis, blindness, epilepsy, intracranial calcifications, and hydrocephalus.

Because infection is usually asymptomatic, diagnosis depends on serologic testing. Unfortunately, these tests cannot predict the time of infection with accuracy, so that the routine screening of patients is not recommended. Furthermore, such testing is of limited value in specific clinical situations. Fetal blood testing is possible if infection is likely to have occurred.

Treatment of suspected first trimester infection focuses on counseling about the risks of serious congenital infection and the potential option of therapeutic pregnancy termination. Treatment for patients for whom pregnancy termination is not an option or for those suspected of being infected later in pregnancy is a combination of sulfadiazine and pyrimethamine. However, pyrimethamine is teratogenic in laboratory animals in the first trimester so that its use is not recommended during this time.

Prevention of infection should be an important part of prenatal care, including the suggestion that all meats be thoroughly cooked and that cats be kept indoors and fed only store-bought foods. If a cat is kept outside, others should feed and care for the cat and its wastes.

AIDS

Approximately 18% of Americans infected with human immunodeficiency virus (HIV) are women, the group whose infection rate is rising most rapidly. Over 85% of these women are of childbearing age. The primary acquisition routes for women are sexual contact and intravenous drug abuse. More than 80% of pediatric HIV infection is the result of vertical transmission from mother to fetus.

HIV is a single-stranded RNA-enveloped human retrovirus that has the ability to become incorporated into cellular DNA. The virus attaches to cells with high CD4 surface receptor concentrations such as lymphocytes, monocytes, and some neural cells. Via a reverse transcriptase, the virus encodes for DNA production, hence viral replication.

A few weeks after infection, most individuals have an acute seroconversion reaction. Antigen appears in a few weeks, followed quickly by antibody in most cases. Thereafter, the usual estimated latency period is almost 11 years. HIV infection becomes acquired immune deficiency syndrome (AIDS) as the helper (CD4) lymphocyte count decreases and the host becomes more susceptible. The presence of a defining opportunistic infection or a CD4 count < 200 mm^3 is diagnostic of AIDS, after

which the prognosis is poor, with survival more than 2 years uncommon.

The diagnosis of HIV infection is suspected with the receipt of a positive enzyme-linked immunosorbent assay (ELISA), based on an antigen-antibody reaction. The Western blot test, which identifies antibodies to specific portions of the virus, is performed to confirm the ELISA. Approximately 10% of patients have an indeterminate Western blot, but when repeated in 4 to 6 months, the test is usually positive. The sensitivity and specificity of the combined tests are approximately 99%. Pretest counseling is important given the health, social, and financial ramifications of a positive test. Testing should be offered to women at high risk, especially those with multiple sexual partners and those who abuse drugs or consort with those who do. Given the reluctance of some women to reveal such behaviors, it may be prudent to offer all women testing in areas of low HIV infection prevalence and to recommend routine testing in areas with high prevalence.

Independent of other problems such as drug abuse, HIV infection appears to have no direct effect on pregnancy, including birth weight, gestational age at delivery, or abortion rates. Conversely, pregnancy does affect the immune system and may affect the course of HIV infection, although the effect is probably small.

Transplacental intrauterine transmission of HIV infection is the most significant means of fetal transmission. Between 25% and 33% of infants born to an HIV infected mother become HIV infected. There is no advantage of cesarean section over vaginal birth, although the use of fetal scalp electrodes, fetal scalp blood sampling, and the like should be avoided in labor. The administration of zidovudine (SDV or AZT) to the mother during the antepartum and intrapartum periods and to the infant postpartum has been associated with a decrease in the rate of transmission of HIV from mother to infant, to under 8% (Table 16.17). Likewise, breast-feeding should be discouraged when the mother is infected, although the risk of breast-feeding is unclear.

TABLE 16.17.	Zidovudine Therapy to Reduce Vertical HIV Transmission

Regimen	Administration
Antepartum	500 mg po daily from 14 to 34 weeks of gestation until labor
Intrapartum	IV administration during labor: 2 mg/kg loading dose followed by a continuous infusion at 1 mg/kg/hr until delivery
Postpartum	Oral administration of zidovudine syrup, 2 mg/kg, every 6 hours for 6 weeks

HIV= human immunodeficiency virus.

9. THROMBOEMBOLIC DISORDERS IN PREGNANCY

An increase in key coagulation factors and venous stasis as a result of relaxed vasculature increases the risk of thromboembolic disorders during pregnancy and the puerperium. This group of disorders includes phlebitis, both superficial and deep vein, and pulmonary embolism.

Superficial thrombophlebitis is the most common thromboembolic disorder in pregnancy, occurring in 1/500 to 1/750 pregnancies; three fourths of cases occur in the initial 72 hours following delivery. With superficial phlebitis, redness and tenderness are accompanied by palpable veins in the involved area, usually the calves. Superficial phlebitis offers little maternal risk beyond discomfort and is treated with elevation of the legs, rest, heat, and mild analgesics.

The risk of *deep venous thrombosis* is probably increased in pregnancy and is also increased in the postpartum period from 0.15% to 3%. The clinical presentation may be varied, depending on the level of involvement in the lower extremities. Calf pain with tenderness to manipulation and edema can be present in differing degrees. Popliteal tenderness may be noted. Various techniques of diagnosis are available, none of which is entirely satisfactory. The gold standard is venography, but Doppler examination and impedance plethysmography can be helpful. The differential diagnosis includes rupture of a Baker cyst, muscle strain or hematoma, arterial insufficiency, arthritis, lymphangitis, myositis, bone disease, varicose veins, and superficial thrombophlebitis.

Treatment of deep venous thrombosis is with heparin anticoagulation (Table 16.18). Coumadin is reserved for the postpartum state, because it can be teratogenic in early pregnancy and may cause fetal bleeding in later pregnancy. With heparin, rest, and analgesia, symptoms of deep venous thrombosis subside in approximately 1 week, but heparin is continued well into the postpartum period.

Deep venous thrombosis is often a forerunner of *pulmonary embolism* (PE), although the initial presentation can be pulmonary. Unfortunately, clinical findings of tachypnea, shortness of breath, electrocardiogram (ECG) changes, and other so-called classic signs may be misleading. The differential diagnosis includes muscle strain, acute anxiety attack, acute pulmonary edema, and atelectasis.

When a pulmonary embolus is suspected, arterial blood gases should be obtained. $PaO_2 < 80$ mm Hg suggests PE. Regardless of cause, patients with a diminished PaO_2 need oxygen therapy. The ventilation/perfusion lung scan is helpful in diagnosing PE. Results are often given as "low" or "high" probability for PE; at times, pulmonary angiography is necessary to confirm the diagnosis.

Two thirds of patients who die from a PE do so within 30 minutes of the acute event. The mortality rate of PE in pregnancy may be reduced to < 1% with prompt anticoagulation. Initial anticoagulation is by intravenously administered heparin [100 to

TABLE 16.18. Heparin Anticoagulation for Deep Vein Thrombophlebitis during Pregnancy			
Route	**Loading Dose**	**Maintenance**	**Subcutaneous Continuation of Therapy**
Intravenous	100 U/kg	Continuous infusion: 1000 U/hr to maintain a PTT that is prolonged 1.5–2 times the baseline for 7–10 days	Maintenance during remainder of the pregnancy (after acute therapy; 10,000–20,000 U) every 12 hours sc and for first 6 weeks postpartum
Subcutaneous	150 U/kg	15,000–20,000 U sc every 12 hours to maintain a midinterval PTT of 1.5 times the baseline	Same as above

PTT = partial thromboplastin time.

120 U/kg loading dose, followed by a continuous infusion to maintain the partial thromboplastin time (PTT) at twice its normal value]. Coumadin may be used postpartum to maintain a therapeutic prothrombin time (PT) of 1.5 to 2.5 times the normal (e.g., 21 to 35 seconds when the control is 14 seconds). If the patient develops recurrent embolus despite anticoagulation therapy, vena cava ligation or insertion of a balloon/filter distal to the renal veins may be considered postpartum.

Septic pelvic thrombophlebitis occurs postpartum, the result of bacterial infection in the uterus, with spread to the ovarian veins, typically on the right. Patients under treatment for pelvic infection may have persistent fever spikes despite improvement in other aspects of infection, such as uterine tenderness. In some cases, a palpable and tender mass representing the right uterine vein can be identified. Response to heparinization is prompt, although spontaneous resolution can also occur.

10. NEUROLOGIC DISEASE IN PREGNANCY

Epilepsy in Pregnancy

Epilepsy occurs in approximately 0.5% of pregnant women and is characterized by paroxysmal changes in sensory, cognitive, emotional, or psychomotor function as a result of disordered brain function. Epilepsy may be caused by neurologic injury, brain lesions, or idiopathic dysfunction. During pregnancy, elevated estrogen levels excite seizure foci, whereas elevated progesterone levels counteract this effect. As a result, epileptic activity is unchanged in 50% of patients, increased in 40% of patients, and decreased in 10% of patients. Prepregnancy frequency of seizures is the best predictor of seizure activity during pregnancy. Only 25% of patients who have been seizure-free in the 9 months before pregnancy may expect a worsening of their condition.

Patients with epilepsy appear to have a threefold to fourfold increased risk (6% to 10%) of bearing children with congenital anomalies. However, because many standard anticonvulsants also have teratogenic effects, the cause-and-effect relationships are uncertain. There is also an increased incidence of seizure disorders in the offspring of epileptic mothers (1/30). During a seizure, there is the additional risk of acute uteroplacental insufficiency and abruptio placentae.

Phenytoin (Dilantin) has been the standard anticonvulsant for the management of epilepsy. Its use during pregnancy is associated with the *fetal hydantoin syndrome*, which includes microcephaly, facial clefts and dysmorphism, limb malformations, and distal phalangeal and nail hypoplasia. Phenobarbital is also associated with cleft lip and palate, albeit at a reduced frequency. Because of these concerns for teratogenesis, the *most commonly used anticonvulsant in pregnancy is now carbamazepine* (Tegretol), which appears to be relatively safe with respect to congenital anomalies. Most anticonvulsants also cause bone marrow suppression and depression of vitamin K-dependent clotting factors so that there is a higher risk of fetal and neonatal hemorrhage. Supplemental folate and neonatal administration of vitamin K are indicated.

11. GASTROINTESTINAL DISEASE IN PREGNANCY

In response to incursion of the enlarging uterus into the abdominal cavity as pregnancy advances, the hormonal milieu of pregnancy, and increased nutritional needs, gastrointestinal (GI) function is markedly altered during pregnancy. Symptoms and findings may be associated with these physiologic changes or may be related to disease.

Alterations of GI function and their clinical manifestations are reviewed in Table 16.19.

Nausea and Vomiting in Pregnancy and Hyperemesis Gravidarum

The majority of women experience some degree of nausea and vomiting during pregnancy. At least 66% of women experience nausea and 50% emesis in the first trimester, with the frequency of these symptoms lessening as the second and third trimesters ensue. Classically, symptoms are predominantly present in the morning ("morning sickness"), but they may occur throughout the day and evening. A variety of causes have been suggested for these symptoms, although none has been clearly determined. Frequent small feedings and avoidance of foods that are unpleasant to the patient usually relieve symptoms to a manageable level. Prenatal vitamin supplements may aggravate these GI symptoms and can be withheld until symptoms abate.

TABLE 16.19. Alterations of Gastrointestinal Function in Pregnancy and Their Clinical Manifestations

Alteration of GI Function	Characteristics	Clinical Manifestation
Esophageal	Reduced resting LES pressure Altered esophageal motility	Gastroesophageal reflux Heartburn Erosive esophagitis
Gastric	Decreased gastric emptying Increased residual volume	Increased risk of anesthesia-associated aspiration Decreased incidence of duodenal ulcer
Small bowel	Altered propulsive motility Increased transit time Increased activity/efficiency of brush borders	Stasis/bacterial overgrowth Pseudo-obstruction Sequestration of bile salts Increased absorption of some nutrients
Large bowel/colon	Reduced contractility Increased water and sodium absorption	Constipation Pseudo-obstruction

GI = gastrointestinal; LES = lower esophageal sphincter.

Symptoms of nausea and vomiting in early pregnancy should not be presumed to be morning sickness. It is necessary to rule out other more serious causes of such symptoms. Fortunately, nausea and vomiting in pregnancy are short lived and most patients can look forward to cessation of symptoms as the second trimester begins.

A variety of antiemetics can be prescribed if the above measures fail to provide adequate relief, but unfortunately, none is completely effective and all carry risks (Table 16.20). Of historical interest is the compound medication Bendectin, a combination of the antihistamine doxylamine and vitamin B_6 (pyridoxine), which was reasonably effective as an antiemetic in pregnancy. Although there is no evidence to support an increased teratogenic risk for the compound, medicolegal concerns led the manufacturer to withdraw the medication from the market. Recently similar formulations have been reintroduced into the marketplace, but their acceptance has yet to be determined.

Hyperemesis gravidarum (intractable emesis during pregnancy) is a more severe form of nausea and vomiting, occurring in approximately 4 out of 1000 pregnancies; it is associated with severe symptoms as well as weight loss, dehydration, ketosis, and electrolyte disturbances. Hospitalization and treatment with balanced crystalloid solutions and necessary electrolytes and "NPO status" generally eliminate symptoms and correct metabolic disturbances in a short time. Diet can then be reinstituted slowly and progressively. Recurrences sometimes necessitate repeat hospitalizations.

Gastroesophageal Reflux in Pregnancy

At least 50% of patients experience gastroesophageal reflux in the third trimester of pregnancy. It does not alter the course of pregnancy, nor is it detrimental to the fetus; it is, however, uncomfortable for the patient and may lead to long-term esophageal

TABLE 16.20. Antiemetics in Pregnancy

Antiemetic	Action	Regimen	FDA Pregnancy Category*
Metoclopramide (Reglan)	Stimulates motility of upper GI tract and increases LES	10 mg po qid, pc and hs	B
Meclizine (Antivert)	Antihistamine; inhibits spasmogenic effects of histamine	12.5–25 mg po qid	B
Promethazine (Phenergan)	A phenothiazine derivative with lessened psychoactive action; an H_1-receptor blocker; also has sedative and antiemetic effect	25 mg q 4–6 h po or pr	C

*B = negative animal studies; no human studies showing risk; should be used in pregnancy only if clearly indicated; C = animal studies show teratogenic effects; no human studies; should be used in pregnancy only if the potential benefit justifies the potential risk to the fetus.
FDA = Food and Drug Administration; GI = gastrointestinal; LES = lower esophageal sphincter.

changes. The cause is a combination of decreased intra-abdominal space and increased pressure from the enlarging uterus as well as the effect of progesterone to decrease lower esophageal sphincter (LES) tone.

Treatment includes reassurance, elevating the head of the patient's bed, small more frequent meals, and liberal use of antacids at bedtime and after meals. Metoclopramide (Reglan) is especially useful because it increases LES tone and is an antiemetic (see Table 16.20). Antacids such as magnesium and aluminum hydroxide preparations (15 to 30 ml po qhs and pc) are also helpful.

Peptic Ulcer Disease in Pregnancy

GI hemorrhage resulting from peptic ulcer is managed by nasogastric suction and ice water lavage, blood replacement as needed, monitoring of fetal well-being as appropriate by gestational age, and surgery if the bleeding is unresponsive to these medical managements.

Ptyalism in Pregnancy

Ptyalism, or excessive salivation, is especially annoying for a small number of patients, sometimes approaching 1 liter per day. Medical treatment with tincture of belladonna or atropine alters ptyalism only slightly, so reassurance of the time-limited nature of the problem is a mainstay of management.

Pica

Pica, a craving for nonfoodstuffs such as laundry starch, ice, dirt, or clay, is common in pregnancy. It is attributed to certain ethnic groups but its true incidence is hidden in denial. Pica can be deleterious when ingestion of the materials interferes with needed food and mineral intake, resulting in anemia and/or sequelae of poor nutrition. Treatment consists of detection, counseling, encouragement to control pica, and replacement therapy, including iron, folic acid, and prenatal vitamins.

Appendicitis in Pregnancy

Appendicitis complicates approximately 0.1% of pregnancies and is the most common surgical emergency in pregnancy. Maternal mortality rate is 2% in the first and second trimesters and approaches 10% in the third trimester compared with 0.25% in nonpregnant patients. The increased mortality rate is due primarily to delay in diagnosis and to a doubling in the rate of perforation during pregnancy. Premature labor is the most common perinatal complication.

The diagnosis is suspected when nausea and vomiting are preceded by anorexia and associated with periumbilical or right lower quadrant pain. The gravid uterus may mask the diagnosis by altering the position of the appendix and sequestering inflammatory exudate. The differential diagnosis in the first trimester includes ectopic pregnancy, salpingitis, ruptured corpus luteum cyst, dermoid cyst, and adnexal torsion. Late in pregnancy, round ligament pain, preterm labor, abruptio placentae, and degenerating leiomyoma of the uterus are more likely diagnostic possibilities.

Appendectomy with or without vigorous antibiotic therapy is necessary. Electronic fetal monitoring during and after surgery is essential with tocolysis if labor ensues in a preterm pregnancy. Whether to administer tocolytics prophylactically when operating on a preterm patient is controversial.

Inflammatory Bowel Disease in Pregnancy

Regional enteritis is seen in approximately 0.02% and ulcerative colitis in approximately 0.01% of childbearing-age women and is also seen on occasion in pregnancy. The morbidity of the former is related primarily to abdominal abscesses or intestinal obstruction and the latter to toxic megacolon, colonic perforation, and colonic stricture.

Regional enteritis is a chronic inflammatory condition of the bowel that causes diarrhea and pain and malabsorption of iron and vitamin B_{12} if the terminal ileum is involved. Regional enteritis appears to be unaffected by pregnancy and vice versa. Treatment consists of rest and a high-calorie, high-protein, low-fat diet. Antidiarrheals such as diphenoxylate (Lomotil; 10 ml q 6–8 h) help with that symptom. Prednisone can be used for acute exacerbations. Cesarean birth should be considered if there are perirectal abscesses and fistulae.

Ulcerative colitis is a more acute condition than regional enteritis and is associated with bloody, watery diarrhea. Pregnancy does not exacerbate the disease, whereas severe ulcerative colitis is associated with an increased risk of spontaneous abortion and premature labor. Treatment consists of a low residue diet, antidiarrheals such as diphenoxylate, steroids, and sulfasalazine (Azulfidine; starting with 1 mg/day po and increasing to 2 to 4 mg/day) for its anti-inflammatory and immunosuppressive effect.

12. DENTAL DISEASE IN PREGNANCY

Pregnancy-associated gingivitis is encountered in approximately 50% of pregnancies. The gums are hypertrophied, red, and inflamed because of the hormonal changes of pregnancy. They are uncomfortable, bleed easily, and are more susceptible to poor dental hygiene. Pregnancy-associated gingivitis is related to poor dental hygiene combined with the hormonal changes of pregnancy. Occasionally an inflammatory growth appears in the papilla area between the teeth. Misnamed "pregnancy tumor," this is simply a pyogenic granuloma that exacerbates the pregnancy-associated gingivitis. Good dental hygiene and astringent mouthwashes offer some relief of this problem, which regresses with the end of pregnancy.

Emergency and routine dental care can be provided as usual, although many dentists try to minimize intervention during pregnancy. *Local anesthetics without epinephrine offer little risk.* Other modalities such as nitrous oxide are best avoided during pregnancy.

13. HEPATOBILIARY DISEASES IN PREGNANCY
Hepatitis

Hepatitis is the major cause of jaundice (bilirubin > 4 mg/dl) during pregnancy. Viral hepatitis takes several forms, including the more common hepatitis A (HAV), hepatitis B (HBV), and hepatitis C (HCV; parenterally transmitted non-A, non-B hepatitis) and the less common hepatitis D (HDV; also called the d agent) and hepatitis E (HEV; formerly known as epidemic or waterborne non-A, non-B hepatitis). *Hepatitis A* is spread by ingestion of contaminated food or water and by fecal-oral transmission and accounts for approximately 10% of cases of hepatitis in pregnancy. It has an incubation period of 15 to 50 days, and the symptoms and signs are often vague. There is little, if any, effect on pregnancy. Pregnant women exposed to hepatitis A can be given γ-globulin, following the guidelines for nonpregnant adults.

Hepatitis C virus formerly followed transfusion with blood or blood components but screening for hepatitis C antibody in donor blood has virtually eliminated such transmission. Approximately 1% of the population has evidence of hepatitis C infection. HCV has an incubation period of approximately 50 days. It can also spread through sexual contact. Many cases of hepatitis C are mild; its effects on pregnancy are similar to but much less severe than those of hepatitis B. Hepatitis D is uncommon but often associated with a fulminant hepatitis. Hepatitis E is clinically similar to hepatitis A but milder, except in pregnancy when maternal mortality rate may be quite high. Hepatitis C, D, and E combined account for approximately 10% of cases of hepatitis in pregnancy.

Hepatitis B virus is the most common hepatitis in pregnancy, accounting for approximately 80% of cases. It is spread by infected blood or serous body products via percutaneous or permucosal routes and has an incubation period of 15 to 50 days. Groups at special risk for HBV include intravenous drug users, homosexuals, health care workers and others who come in contact with potentially infected materials on a regular basis, and individuals with multiple sexual partners or whose partners include high-risk individuals. Hemophiliacs and others receiving blood components regularly are also at risk.

The course of HBV infection is not significantly affected by pregnancy. There is a wide range of clinical presentations, from asymptomatic illness through a mild episode with low-grade fever and nausea to hepatic failure, coma, and death in unusual circumstances. Serum chemistry abnormalities include elevated serum transaminase levels, often above 1000 mU/ml, and an increased serum albumin. Most patients recover completely within 3 to 6 months, and fewer than 10% develop chronic infection with circulating HBV antigens.

Vertical transmission to the fetus at delivery is now recognized to pose significant danger to the neonate. Untreated, the majority of infants who are infected become chronic carriers capable of transmitting the infection to others. Hepatic carcinoma and cirrhosis are other unusual sequelae. These adverse outcomes have led to the recent institution of universal screening of all pregnant patients for the presence of the hepatitis B surface antigen (HBsAg). Women so identified should also undergo testing for antibodies and for the presence of the envelope (e) antigen, which is associated with an 80% risk of fetal transmission and of the infant becoming a chronic carrier.

If its mother is identified as a carrier or develops HBV during pregnancy, the neonate should receive both active immunization for hepatitis (hepatitis B vaccine) and passive immunization with hepatitis B immunoglobulin (HBIG). Hepatitis B recombinant vaccine is recommended for pregnant women who are at high risk for contracting HBV. HBIG should be given to susceptible pregnant women within 48 hours of exposure to HBV.

During pregnancy, the diagnosis of hepatitis is made on the basis of liver function studies as well as the presence or absence of antigens and corresponding antibodies. Treatment is supportive, with hospitalization usually being recommended until patients are capable of maintaining good nourishment.

Cholestasis in Pregnancy

Cholestasis of pregnancy (pruritus gravidarum) occurs in < 0.1% of pregnancies and is the second most common cause of jaundice in pregnancy. It usually occurs in the third trimester, although it is encountered throughout pregnancy. The etiology is unclear but probably involves an increased hepatic sensitivity to estrogen, resulting in cholestasis without the hepatocellular damage seen in cholecystitis or cholelithiasis.

Patients present with generalized, often intense, pruritus associated with fatigue, jaundice, and often dark urine. Laboratory evaluation reveals serum bile acid levels elevated to 10 to 100 times normal, elevated serum alkaline phosphatase to 10 times normal, and bilirubin levels elevated up to 5 mg/ml.

The main effect of cholestasis of pregnancy is the discomfort of intense pruritus. Occasional coagulation abnormalities as a result of decreased vitamin K absorption have been reported.

Treatment consists of antipruritics such as diphenhydramine hydrochloride (Benadryl) or hydroxyzine hydrochloride (Vistaril), topical skin preparations containing lanolin as a base, and reassurance. Cholestyramine may decrease the bile acid levels but is associated with GI disturbances (nausea and diarrhea). Phenobarbital may be tried if cholestyramine is not effective in inducing hepatic microsomal function. Recurrence in future pregnancies and with use of oral contraceptives is likely.

Cholelithiasis in Pregnancy

Cholelithiasis and *cholecystitis* complicate more than 3% of pregnancies. Properly treated, maternal and fetal outcomes are uncompromised, whereas failure to treat cholelithiasis effectively is associated with an increased fetal mortality rate. The pathogenesis and pathophysiology in pregnancy are also unchanged, with supersaturation of bile with cholesterol being followed by crystallization and formation of gallstones, uncomfortable distention of the gallbladder, and blockage of the cystic duct, which causes biliary colic and jaundice. An association with fatty food intake is noted. In pregnancy, increased estrogen/progesterone concentrations may increase the concentration of cholesterol and the rate of stone formation.

The clinical history of food-associated colic and laboratory evidence of elevated liver enzymes and bilirubin are confirmed by ultrasonography of the gallbladder.

Asymptomatic cholelithiasis in pregnancy requires no treatment except admonitions about fatty food intake. Biliary colic is treated with nasogastric suction, hydration, analgesia, and antibiotics if needed. Lack of improvement or the development of pancreatitis is usually indication for cholecystectomy. Cholecystectomy is second only to appendectomy as the most frequent nonobstetric surgical procedure performed during pregnancy. Cholecystectomy during pregnancy is associated with a 5% fetal loss rate, which rises to about 60% if pancreatitis is present at the time of surgery.

Acute Fatty Liver of Pregnancy

Acute fatty liver of pregnancy is a rare complication of pregnancy, but its severity and maternal mortality rate of 30%–75% and fetal mortality rate of 90% make its timely diagnosis and treatment of importance. Acute fatty liver usually occurs late in pregnancy in primigravidas and is characterized by vague gastrointestinal symptoms becoming worse over several days' time. Thereafter headache, mental confusion, and epigastric pain may ensue, and if untreated, there may be rapid development of coagulopathy, coma, multiple organ failure, and death. Laboratory findings include an initial modest elevation in bilirubin and an elevation of transaminase levels, but the magnitude of these elevations is not great and the disease may be misdiagnosed as being minor in nature. Treatment of this serious complication is correction of coagulopathy and electrolyte imbalances, cardiorespiratory support, and delivery as soon as feasible by the vaginal route, if possible.

14. ABDOMINAL SURGICAL CONDITIONS AND ABDOMINAL TRAUMA IN PREGNANCY

Abdominal Surgical Conditions in Pregnancy

Careful management of patients with surgical conditions should provide optimal care for the mother and consideration for optimal perinatal outcome. Any pregnant patient presenting with a potential surgical condition should be fully evaluated regardless of her pregnant status (i.e., necessary radiographic or other studies should not be avoided just because the patient is pregnant). For procedures such as x-rays of the chest, an abdominal shield may be used to avoid unnecessary exposure to the fetus. In general, exposure to low doses of radiation is considered safe for the fetus, especially when compared with the misdiagnosis of a serious surgical condition.

The fetus should be monitored as thoroughly as possible consistent with the stage of gestation and need for intervention. For a viable pregnancy this means electronic fetal monitoring for fetal heart tones and the possibility of uterine activity. The supine position should be avoided, if possible, to prevent the supine hypotensive syndrome. Oxygen administration may be helpful and is ordinarily not harmful. In general, those caring for these patients should be constantly aware of both maternal and fetal considerations. For example, in pregnancy the residual lung volume is diminished, providing less reserve for respiratory function. As another example, delayed gastric emptying makes aspiration of stomach contents more likely should surgery be necessary.

Abdominal Trauma in Pregnancy

Abdominal trauma, regularly encountered in pregnancy, is most commonly associated with automobile accidents, falls, and interpersonal violence. Prevention includes correct and consistent use of seat belts (both lap and shoulder harness) and avoiding situations and activities in which falls are likely.

A special type of trauma that must be kept in mind is physical abuse. This may occur in up to 10% of pregnant patients and may not be divulged by the patient. Frequently, a variety of somatic complaints, including abdominal symptoms, may be offered or excuses given for obvious signs of trauma.

From an obstetric viewpoint, the most important consideration about abdominal trauma is the possibility of abruptio placentae. Direct trauma to the uterus is not necessary for a shearing effect on the placenta to occur. Patients whose pregnancies have proceeded beyond the point of viability must be monitored for several hours following abdominal trauma to detect possible fetal heart rate abnormalities, resulting from diminished oxygenation because of the abruption. Because of this risk, these patients should be monitored while lying on their side so as to deflect the large uterus away from the great vessels where pressure may impede cardiac function and hence uteroplacental blood flow.

Monitoring for vaginal bleeding is important, although the bleeding may be concealed in some cases. Uterine tenderness may be a sign of abruption. Some degree of fetal-maternal hemorrhage may occur in 5% to 25% of cases; it is usually of insignificant volume. A test to detect fetal-maternal hemorrhage, such as the Kleihauer-Betke test, should be performed, and RhoGAM administered as appropriate. In some cases, coagulation studies are obtained to detect subtle changes associated with placental abruption. Tetanus toxoid should be administered to pregnant patients following the same guidelines as those for nonpregnant patients.

Uterine rupture is usually associated with only very severe direct abdominal trauma. Diagnosis and treatment are as described for uterine rupture associated with labor. Fetal injury from abdominal trauma is very rare, with fetal death usually being associated with impaired maternal status or abruptio placentae.

15. SUBSTANCE ABUSE IN PREGNANCY

The use of a variety of legal and illicit drugs and legal but potentially harmful substances during pregnancy has climbed at an alarming rate in recent years. Management of patients involved in the use and abuse of these materials is compounded by a variety of social problems, frequently inadequate prenatal care and poor nutrition. Despite these frustrations, help and encouragement to these patients must be given at every opportunity, because the consequences are so significant to the mother and her offspring.

Smoking

A decrease in the incidence of smoking has occurred more slowly in women than in men, and regrettably, young women now appear to be initiating smoking at an earlier age than in years past. It is estimated that 30% of reproductive-age women smoke, the incidence doubling if there is concurrent use of other substances of abuse. A variety of adverse pregnancy outcomes have been associated with cigarette smoking (see Table 16.6). These complications result from the effects of carbon monoxide and altered placental perfusion caused by vasoconstriction induced by nicotine. The pregnant woman who smokes endangers not only herself but also her unborn child. For some women, pregnancy provides a unique opportunity to cease or at least reduce smoking, an incentive that may be aided by the diminished appetite and nausea seen in pregnancy.

Alcohol

Ethyl alcohol is a potent central nervous depressant that has great potential for overuse and abuse. One beer, one glass of wine, or one standard mixed drink contains approximately 0.5 ounce of absolute ethyl alcohol. A total of 75% of Americans use alcohol to some extent, including an unknown percentage of pregnant women. With the ingestion of approximately

TABLE 16.21.	Fetal Alcohol Syndrome

Mental retardation
  Performance defects
  Lowered IQ
Growth
  Prenatal and postnatal growth restriction
Congenital anomalies
  Brain defects
  Cardiac defects (especially ventricular
    septal defects)
  Spinal defects
	Craniofacial anomalies
	  Flattened nasal bridge
	  Absent to hypoplastic philtrum
	  Broad upper lip
	  Hypoplastic upper lip vermillion
	  Micrognathia
	  Microphthalmia
	  Short nose
	  Short palpebral fissure

3 ounces of alcohol daily during pregnancy, *fetal alcohol syndrome* is observed (Table 16.21); effects consist of prenatal and postnatal growth deficiency, mental retardation, behavioral disturbances, and congenital defects such as craniofacial anomalies.

In theory, lesser consumption in pregnancy is associated with lesser effects—described as *fetal alcohol effects*—which include minor anomalies, moderate growth deficiency, "mild" mental retardation, and subtle behavioral changes. In fact, it is unknown what the lower threshold for safe use of alcohol in pregnancy is, if one exists, so that the best recommendation is abstinence during pregnancy. *Indeed, excluding genetic causes, alcohol use in pregnancy is the most common cause of mental retardation.* The performance defects associated with fetal alcohol syndrome include an average IQ of 60 to 70 for severely affected infants, fine motor dysfunction, infant irritability, and hyperactivity in later childhood. The risk of spontaneous abortion is also increased in patients consuming alcohol.

Ethanol freely crosses the placenta and fetal blood-brain barrier, presumably causing its deleterious effects by direct toxicity of ethanol and its metabolites such as acetaldehyde. Toxicity appears to be dose-related and is greatest in first trimester exposure.

Cocaine

Cocaine has become the drug of choice in the United States because of easy accessibility and relatively low cost. This effective local anesthetic also has profound sympathomimetic action by dopamine potentiation (it blocks the reception of dopamine and norepinephrine), making it a very potent central nervous stimulant, which has led directly to its great potential for addiction and abuse.

This highly addictive substance causes multiple medical problems, both directly and as a result of sequelae of the lifestyle associated with drug dependence. The former include acute myocardial infarction, cardiac arrhythmias, aortic rupture, stroke, seizures, bowel ischemia, hyperthermia, and sudden death syndrome. The latter includes poor diet and hygiene; chronic lack of health care; increased risk of physical and emotional violence; and for women, sexual promiscuity/prostitution with associated risks of sexually transmitted diseases.

Cocaine use is associated with an increased incidence of spontaneous abortion and in utero fetal demise. Cocaine abusers are at increased risk for premature rupture of membranes (20%), preterm labor and delivery (25%), intrauterine growth restriction (25% to 30%), meconium-stained amniotic fluid (30%), and placental abruption (6% to 10%). In utero cerebral infarction has been reported in cocaine-abusing women. Cocaine use is associated with congenital anomalies such as segmental intestinal atresia, limb-reduction defects, disruptive brain anomalies, congenital heart defects, prune-belly syndrome, and urinary tract anomalies. Surviving infants are at higher risk for sudden infant death syndrome (SIDS), poor learning performance, and behavioral problems.

Marijuana

Between 5% and 15% of pregnant women are thought to use marijuana or hashish during pregnancy. The active component, 9-tetrahydrocannabinol (THC), is a highly active psychotropic compound that is teratogenic in animal models but equivocally so in human studies. Its use should be avoided in pregnancy.

Opiates

Heroin abuse is associated with a threefold to sevenfold increase in the rates of stillbirth, fetal growth restriction, premature labor and delivery, and neonatal mortality, probably as a result of both drug effects and the dangers of the narcotic abuser's lifestyle. Methadone treatment in pregnancy is associated with improved outcomes.

Newborn narcotic withdrawal syndrome is seen in up to 66% of infants born to users and is potentially fatal. The syndrome is less frequently seen in the offspring of methadone-treated women, but its severity is the same as for neonates of untreated women. Neonatal withdrawal syndrome is characterized by high-pitched cry, poor feeding, hypertonicity, tremor, hyperirritability, sneezing, diarrhea, and seizures. Neonatal symptoms usually appear in 1 to 2 days, although the syndrome can appear up to 10 days after birth, when the infant has been discharged from direct patient care.

Hallucinogens

There is no good evidence of direct chromosomal damage or untoward pregnancy outcome from the use of lysergic acid diethylamide (LSD) or other hallucinogenic substances. However, there are very few studies of this type of drug abuse in pregnancy. The use of hallucinogenics, in or out of pregnancy, should be actively discouraged.

16. COAGULATION DISORDERS IN PREGNANCY

Thrombocytopenia in Pregnancy

Thrombocytopenia is generally diagnosed when the platelet count is less than 100,000/mm³, although thrombocytopenia-associated bleeding usually occurs at platelet concentrations of less than 20,000/mm³. Although leukemia and other neoplastic processes may be responsible for thrombocytopenia, these conditions are fortunately quite rare in obstetric patients. Drugs are common causes of thrombocytopenia. The list of drugs that cause thrombocytopenia is extensive and includes acetaminophen and a variety of antibiotics (Table 16.22). Because pregnant women consume various drugs, it may be difficult to assign the cause of thrombocytopenia to a specific drug, and an empiric withdrawal of medications may be required to make a diagnosis of drug-associated disease.

Immune thrombocytopenic purpura (ITP) is an autoimmune disorder characterized by the development of an IgG class antiplatelet antibody, occurring in 1 to 2 out of 1000 pregnancies. The diagnosis is suspected with thrombocytopenia and confirmed by direct assay of platelet-associated IgG and C3 with radioactively labeled IgG antisera. Bone marrow aspiration reveals megakaryocyte hyperplasia.

Maternal treatment of ITP is initially with corticosteroids (usually Prednisone, 1.0 to 1.5 mg/kg/day). If unsuccessful, γ-globulin may be administered instead of performing a splenectomy, which formerly was the second-line treatment of this disorder. Because transfused platelets have a half-life of minutes to 2 to 3 days, compared with the normal half-life for platelets of 7 to 12 days, transfusion is not a useful therapy.

Because the maternal IgG antiplatelet antibodies cross the placenta, the fetus is also at risk, especially from trauma associated with vaginal delivery. Controversy

TABLE 16.22. Drugs Associated with Thrombocytopenia or Abnormal Platelet Function

Anti-inflammatory agents	Destruction
Aspirin	Chlorothiazide
Ibuprofen (Motrin)	Diazepam (Valium)
Indomethacin	Diphenylhydantoin (Dilantin)
Mefenamic acid (Ponstel)	Quinidine
Antibiotics	Sulfisoxazole (erythromycin)
Ampicillin	Others
Penicillin G	Acetaminophen
Gentamicin	Chlorpromazine (Thorazine)
Nitrofurantoin	Cimetidine
Cardiovascular drugs	Furosemide (Lasix)
Dipyrimadole (Persantine)	Heparin
Propranolol	Phenylbutazone
Theophylline	Sulfonamides
	Tolbutamide

exists over when cesarean section is appropriate. One approach is to use percutaneous umbilical blood sampling, with cesarean section being used for fetuses with a platelet count of < 50,000/mm^3. Fetal scalp electrodes should not be used in the labor of patients with ITP. A variation of this theme is isoimmune thrombocytopenia, in which there is maternal production of platelet antibodies directed against fetal platelet antigens that the mother's platelets do not have. Occurring in approximately 1/1000 pregnancies, fetal morbidity is reduced by maternal corticosteroid therapy and liberal use of cesarean delivery.

Systemic lupus erythematosus (SLE) can have thrombocytopenia as one of its manifestations. Patients with low platelet counts should be evaluated for this autoimmune disorder. Thrombocytopenia is also seen in the *hypertensive-associated HELLP syndrome* (*h*emolysis, *e*levated *l*iver enzymes, and *l*ow *p*latelet count).

Disseminated intravascular coagulopathy (DIC) in obstetrics is associated with placental abruption, retention of a dead fetus, sepsis, preeclampsia, following massive transfusion, and amniotic fluid embolism. Patients with these conditions must be carefully monitored for evidence of DIC. Findings include prolonged bleeding, decreased clotting factors, and elevated fibrin degradation products. The possibility may be evaluated at the bedside by drawing a small amount of blood into a sample tube that lacks anticoagulants; failure to clot supports the working diagnosis of DIC.

Lupus anticoagulant refers to immunoglobulins that interfere with phospholipid-related coagulation tests that were initially discovered in patients with SLE. Subsequently, it has been found that some patients with this clotting inhibitor lack other evidence of the more commonly seen SLE. The problem in these patients is that abnormal intravascular clotting occurs in the arterial system. Paradoxically, the activated partial thromboplastin time (aPTT) is prolonged, owing to the interference in this test by the immunoglobulins.

Patients with lupus anticoagulant have a rate of reproductive wastage in excess of 90%. Spontaneous abortions and intrauterine growth restriction are commonly seen. Second or third trimester fetal loss without apparent etiology may be associated with this antiphospholipid syndrome. Screening of patients with poor reproductive histories includes the aPTT and a test for anticardi- olipin antibodies, which have been shown to be associated with this clinical picture. Treatment of patients with these disorders includes steroids and low-dose aspirin.

Hereditary Coagulation Defects

Hemophilia A and hemophilia B are X-linked recessive disorders caused by low factor VIII coagulant activity or deficiency of factor IX, respectively, exclusively affecting males. The importance of these disorders in obstetrics involves providing genetic counseling to women at risk for delivering an affected male fetus. *Von Willebrand's* disease is an inherited defect of coagulation in which the von Willebrand factor portion of the factor VIII complex is abnormal. Occurring in approximately 1/10,000 pregnancies, a bleeding diathesis and family history are confirmed by a prolonged bleeding time, low factor VIII level, and abnormal platelet adhesion. Factor VIII-rich cyropre- cipitate is given if the factor VIII level is not > 50% of normal at labor or delivery. *Antithrombin III deficiency* is an autosomal dominant deficit affecting the production of the regulatory protein that inhibits throm- bin, factor Xa, and other serine proteases. More than 50% of the 1/2000 who have this disease also develop a deep vein throm- bosis. Peripartal heparin anticoagulation is required for these patients.

17. CANCER IN PREGNANCY
Breast Cancer in Pregnancy

About 3 in 10,000 pregnancies are compli- cated by breast cancer. The relationship between breast cancer and pregnancy is uncertain. Diagnosis of breast cancer during pregnancy is made more difficult by the change of breast size and consistency. The diagnosis may, therefore, be delayed. To date, the stage-for-stage survival rates for breast cancer are unaffected by pregnancy.

Treatment of breast cancer must be individualized. Pregnancy termination has no recognized advantage in the treatment of localized breast cancer. Disseminated breast cancer is often responsive to hormonal abla- tion so that pregnancy termination in early pregnancy may be advisable, whereas in later pregnancy awaiting fetal lung maturity before delivery may pose an acceptable risk to the patient. Chemotherapeutic agents can be administered to the pregnant patient in the second and third trimesters in selected cases. There is no evidence that breast can- cer adversely affects the pregnancy.

Colorectal Cancer

Colorectal carcinoma is uncommon in women under 40 years of age and is encountered in an estimated 1 in 100,000 pregnancies. The prognosis is determined by the stage and grade of tumor; the cancer is unaffected by pregnancy and vice versa.

CASE STUDIES

Case 16A

A 23-year-old G1 is seen at 8 weeks' gestational age for obstetric care. Her mother is an insulin-dependent diabetic.

Questions Case 16A

Which, if any, of the following laboratory studies should be performed?

A. Fasting blood sugar (FBS) at initial prenatal testing
B. Fasting blood sugar at the 28-weeks laboratory testing
C. 1-hour Glucola at initial prenatal testing
D. 1-hour Glucola at the 28-weeks laboratory testing
E. 3-hour glucose tolerance test (GTT) at initial prenatal testing

Answer: C

Given the patient's family history of diabetes, testing before 28 weeks is indicated. The most commonly performed test would be a 1-hour Glucola. A fasting blood sugar would be less desirable, because it might miss an early glucose intolerance. Glucose tolerance testing is inappropriate as an initial screening test.

The 1-hour Glucola is reported as 181 mg/100 ml. Appropriate management steps include

A. A 2500-calorie ADA diet
B. 1-hour Glucola at the 28-weeks laboratory testing
C. 3-hour GTT
D. 3-hour GTT at the 28-weeks laboratory testing
E. Routine obstetric care

Answer: C

The 1-hour Glucola is above the 140 mg/100 ml screening limit, so glucose toler-

ance testing is required. Delay to 28 weeks is inappropriate, because the effects of glucose intolerance/diabetes are additive over time and, perhaps, more profound in early pregnancy.

A 3-hour GTT is performed, and the results are 150, 199, 256, and 199 mg/100 ml. The ADA diet was begun immediately after the GTT was performed, 3 days ago. What will your management plan include?

A. FBS and 2-hour post-prandial blood glucose in 1 to 2 weeks
B. FBS and 2-hour post-prandial blood glucose at 28-weeks laboratory testing
C. 3-hour GTT in 1 to 2 weeks
D. 3-hour GTT at 28-weeks laboratory testing

Answer: A

Further GTTs are not required because the diagnosis is made. The question is whether diet alone will control the patient's blood sugars or whether insulin therapy will be required. Thus testing in 1 or 2 weeks is required, because a wait to 28 weeks may expose the fetus to abnormal blood sugars for an excessive period of time.

Case 16B

A 19-year-old G2 P1001 at 35 weeks of gestational age complains of a backache following an automobile accident. While she was driving to work, her automobile was hit from behind, buffeting her against the restraints of her lap/shoulder harness. Her abdomen hit the steering wheel lightly. Her antepartum course has heretofore been unremarkable. She notes nothing amiss except a sore back and a bruise over the lower part of her abdomen.

(Continued)

Question Case 16B

Physical examination is entirely normal except for the bruise she has mentioned. Her cervix is closed and there is no vaginal bleeding. Ultrasound examination is normal. Appropriate management includes

A. Obstetric ultrasound in 1 week
B. Electronic fetal monitoring within 1 week
C. Electronic fetal monitoring at this time
D. Amniocentesis

Answer: C

Abruptio placentae and preterm labor may manifest some hours after trauma to the gravid abdomen. Monitoring for uterine and fetal status is necessary, perhaps for 24 hours, according to some authorities.

Case 16C

A 20-year-old G1 presents for prenatal care after missing her menstrual period the previous month. Her medical history and physical examination are all unremarkable except

1. She had a short episode of drug use in her midteens, but successfully completed a drug rehabilitation program 4 years ago. She reports being drug-free since.
2. She has frequent respiratory infections.
3. She has a friable cervix.

Questions Case 16C

Which of the following problems is a special concern in this case?

A. Gonorrhea
B. Syphilis
C. Hepatitis
D. HIV infection
E. Bacterial vaginosis

Answer: D

Her history of involvement with the drug culture puts her at higher risk for any sex-

ually transmitted disease (STD). Frequent infection also suggests immunocompromise. The friable cervix could be associated with cervicitis; however, cervical dysplasia is more frequent in patients with HIV infection.

On review of the prenatal laboratory evaluations, you note

1. ELISA and Western blot are both HIV+
2. Gonorrhea culture is positive
3. Urine toxicology positive for cocaine and THC
4. Pap smear reveals high-grade squamous intraepithelial lesion (HGSIL)

Immediate management includes discussion of all the following EXCEPT

A. Therapeutic termination of the pregnancy
B. Delay in treatment until after delivery
C. The risk of HIV transmission to the baby
D. HIV infection for the patient
E. The evaluation of the HGSIL positive Pap smear
F. Sexual practices, partners, and STDs

Answer: B

Vertical transmission of HIV to the fetus is approximately 10% with proper treatment, although the mother's ultimate prognosis is less comforting. Therapeutic abortion or plans for caring for a well or a sick infant must be discussed. The patient clearly needs further drug rehabilitation and treatment of infection.

Case 16D

An 18-year-old G2 P1001 at 30 weeks of gestation by dates and midtrimester ultrasound complains of a dull right lower quadrant and low back pain for 48 hours, associated with lack of appetite, mild nausea, no emesis, and frequent runny stools. Her pregnancy has so far been unremarkable, with the exception of hyperemesis in the first trimester (which resolved spontaneously) and a bout of the flu 1 week ago associated with nausea and diarrhea.

On physical examination, her temperature is 99.9° F, pulse 80, and blood pressure 110/75. Her fundal height is 31 cm and her uterus slightly tender. There are palpable fetal movements, the fetal heart rate (FHR) is 150 with a reactive NST, there is mild right CVA tenderness, and there are minimal bowel sounds and mild tenderness in both lower quadrants and the right upper quadrant. Her cervix is long and closed.

Question Case 16D

The more likely elements of your differential diagnosis include all of the following EXCEPT

A. Gastroenteritis
B. Pyelonephritis
C. Diverticulitis
D. Appendicitis

Answer: C

This patient's relatively generalized discomfort is consistent with a renewed flu-gastroenteritis, early appendicitis, and early pyelonephritis. Diverticulitis is extremely unlikely because of the patient's age and lack of previous symptoms.

Case 16E

A 22-year-old G2 P1001 at 29 weeks' gestational age complains of shortness of breath, fever and chills, and crampy abdominal pain. She has asthma, with stable peak flow measurements of 380–410 during this pregnancy, using an albuterol inhaler twice a day. On physical examination her temperature is 100.8° F, her pulse 90, her respiratory rate 28, her blood pressure 110/75, her weight 135 lb, and her height 63 inches. Her nasopharynx is injected, her chest examination reveals bilateral wheezes and scattered rhonchi,

her abdomen is soft, FH 30 cm, and FHT 150. Her cervix is long and closed.

Questions Case 16E

Your initial evaluation should consist of

A. Peak flow
B. Chest x-ray
C. Obstetric ultrasound
D. Sputum for Gram stain
E. Arterial blood gas

Answer: A,B,E

Objective measurement of respiratory status is requisite to determine the kind and place of care, hence peak flow and blood gas determinations. Given the fever and chest findings, a chest x-ray to evaluate for possible pneumonia is important.

Her peak flow measurements were 275, 285, 285; her blood gas shows mild hypoxia. Her chest x-ray demonstrates no infiltrate. Your management should consist of

A. Outpatient management consisting of the addition of an inhaled steroid and re-evaluation at the next prenatal visit
B. Outpatient management consisting of the addition of an inhaled steroid and a broad spectrum antibiotic and re-evaluation at the next prenatal visit
C. Inpatient management consisting of oxygen supplementation, hydration, and repeat of chest x-ray in 12–24 hours, respiratory toilet, and broad spectrum antibiotic therapy

Answer: C

Given the possibility of pneumonia, inpatient therapy is the best response with re-evaluation in 12–24 hours. With hydration, an underlying pneumonia may be discovered. Starting antibiotic therapy at the time of hospitalization or if further information confirms a pneumonic process is controversial.

CHAPTER

17

HYPERTENSION IN PREGNANCY

This chapter deals primarily with APGO Objective(s):

OBJECTIVE 19   Preeclampsia–Eclampsia
Syndrome

Define pregnancy-induced hypertension, preeclampsia, and eclampsia, and describe the pathophysiology, diagnosis, maternal and fetal managements, and potential maternal and fetal complications of these conditions.

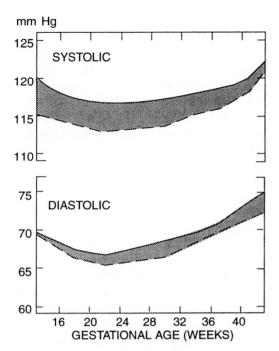

mm Hg

FIGURE 17.1. Range of blood pressures in normotensive pregnancy. Note the decrease in blood pressure in the second trimester.

Hypertensive disorders are among the most common and yet serious conditions seen in obstetrics. These disorders cause substantial morbidity and mortality for both mother and fetus, despite improved prenatal care. The etiology of hypertension unique to pregnancy remains unknown.

Hypertension in pregnancy is generally defined as a sustained systolic blood pressure at or above 140 mm Hg, or a diastolic blood pressure of 90 mm Hg or greater. This definition requires that the increased blood pressures be present on at least two separate occasions, 6 hours or more apart. Although this definition seems quite clear, its use in clinical practice is difficult because of various problems in obtaining a reliable assessment of blood pressure.

The position of the patient influences blood pressure. It is lowest with the patient lying in the lateral position, highest when the patient is standing, and at an intermediate level when she is sitting (Figure 17.1). The choice of the correct size blood pressure cuff also influences blood pressure readings,

with falsely high measurements noted when normal sized cuffs are used on large patients. Also, during the course of pregnancy, blood pressure typically declines slightly in the second trimester, increasing to prepregnant levels as gestation nears term. If a patient has not been seen previously, there is no baseline blood pressure against which to compare new blood pressure determinations, thereby making the diagnosis of pregnancy-related hypertension more difficult.

Pregnancy-induced hypertension (PIH) develops in 5% to 10% of pregnancies that proceed beyond the first trimester, with a 30% incidence in multiple gestation, regardless of parity. Maternal morbidity is directly related to the severity and duration of hypertension; with sound obstetric management, maternal mortality is rare, however, even when associated with such complications as abruptio placentae, hepatic rupture, or preeclampsia/eclampsia. Perinatal mortality increases progressively with each 5 mm Hg increase in mean arterial pressure, primarily associated with uteroplacental insufficiency and abruptio placentae.

HYPERTENSIVE DISEASE IN PREGNANCY
Classification

Various classifications of hypertensive disorders in pregnancy have been proposed. Table 17.1 presents a commonly used classification. Because hypertensive disorders in pregnancy represent a spectrum of disease, classification systems should not be considered as rigid markers on which all management decisions are made.

Hypertension in late pregnancy in the absence of other findings suggestive of preeclampsia has been termed *transient hypertension of pregnancy or gestational hypertension.* Although isolated hypertension is certainly seen in late pregnancy and in the first few days postpartum, caution should be taken in assuming that these patients have hypertension alone.

Preeclampsia is defined as *the development of hypertension with proteinuria or*

TABLE 17.1. Hypertensive Disorders in Pregnancy*

Pregnancy-induced hypertension
Transient hypertension
Preeclampsia
    Mild
    Severe
Eclampsia
Chronic hypertension preceding
    pregnancy (any etiology)
Chronic hypertension (any etiology)
    with superimposed pregnancy-induced
    hypertension
    Superimposed preeclampsia
    Superimposed eclampsia

*Classification of the American College of
  Obstetricians and Gynecologists (ACOG).

edema (or both) induced by pregnancy, generally in the second half of gestation. The high prevalence of edema in pregnancy renders this finding much less important than blood pressure recordings in making the diagnosis of preeclampsia. Preeclampsia is more common in women who have not carried a previous pregnancy beyond 20 weeks and is more frequent at the extremes of the reproductive years. Preeclampsia is classified as severe if there is a blood pressure greater than or equal to 160 mm Hg systolic or 110 mm Hg diastolic, marked proteinuria (generally > 1 g/24-hr urine collection, or 2+ or more on dipstick of a random urine), oliguria, cerebral or visual disturbances such as headache and scotomata, pulmonary edema or cyanosis, epigastric or right upper quadrant pain (probably caused by subcapsular hepatic hemorrhage or stretching of Glisson's capsule), evidence of hepatic dysfunction, or thrombocytopenia. These myriad changes illustrate the multisystem alterations associated with preeclampsia.

Eclampsia is the presence of convulsions, which are not caused by neurologic disease, in a woman whose condition also meets the criteria of preeclampsia. Eclampsia occurs in 0.5% to 4% of deliveries. Most cases of eclampsia occur within 24 hours of delivery, but about 3% of cases are diagnosed between 2–10 days postpartum.

Chronic hypertension is defined as hypertension present before the twentieth week of gestation or beyond 6 weeks postpartum. Chronic hypertension can be owing to a variety of causes, although the majority of cases are deemed essential hypertension. The greatest risk to a woman with chronic hypertension during pregnancy is the development of superimposed preeclampsia or eclampsia, which occurs in approximately 25% of cases. At times, it is difficult to distinguish between preeclampsia and chronic hypertension when a patient is seen late in pregnancy with an elevated blood pressure. In such cases, it is always wise to assume that the findings represent preeclampsia and treat accordingly. Finally, *preeclampsia or eclampsia superimposed on chronic hypertension* is defined as the development of preeclampsia or eclampsia in a patient with preexisting chronic hypertension.

Pathophysiology

Hypertension in pregnancy affects the mother and newborn to varying degrees, depending on the severity of disease. Given the characteristic multisystem effects, it is clear that several pathophysiologic mechanisms are involved. Unfortunately, present understanding of these mechanisms lags behind the ability to describe the clinical manifestations. One common pathophysiologic finding in hypertension in pregnancy, especially when there is progression to preeclampsia, is *vasospasm.* Although numerous theories—ranging from poor nutrition to climate changes—have been proposed to explain this vascular phenomenon, the etiology of the vasospasm remains unknown.

Interestingly, it has been shown that women with uncomplicated pregnancies are extraordinarily resistant to the effects of the potent pressor angiotensin II, whereas those patients destined to develop preeclampsia do not demonstrate the decreased peripheral resistance normally seen in pregnancies. Hepatocellular dysfunction, coagulopathy, and renal dysfunction are also encountered, usually in severe cases of the disease.

Presumably because of vasospastic changes, placental size and function are decreased. The results are progressive fetal hypoxia and malnutrition as well as an increase in the incidence of intrauterine growth restriction, oligohydramnios, and dysmaturity. With the stress of uterine contractions during labor, the placenta is often incapable of supporting the fetus, resulting in intrapartum uteroplacental insufficiency with progressive fetal hypoxia and acidosis.

Evaluation

The history and physical examination are directed toward detection of pregnancy-associated hypertensive disease and its stigmata. A review of current obstetric records, if available, is especially helpful to ascertain changes or progression in findings. *Visual disturbances,* especially scotomata (spots before the eyes), or unusually severe or persistent headaches are indicative of vasospasm. *Right upper quadrant* (RUQ) *pain* may indicate liver involvement, presumably involving distention of the liver capsule. Any history of *loss of consciousness or seizures,* even in the patient with a known seizure disorder, may be significant.

The patient's weight is compared with her pregravid weight and with previous weights during this pregnancy, with special attention to excessive or too rapid weight gain. Peripheral edema is common in pregnancy, especially in the lower extremities; however, persistent edema unresponsive to resting in the supine position is not normal, especially when it also involves the upper extremities and face. Indeed, the puffy-faced, edematous hypertensive pregnant woman is the classic picture of severe preeclampsia. Careful blood pressure determination in the sitting and supine positions is necessary. Fundoscopic examination may detect vasoconstriction of retinal blood vessels, presumably indicative of similar vasoconstriction of other small vessels. Tenderness over the liver attributed in part to hepatic capsule distention may be associated with complaints of RUQ pain. The patellar and Achilles deep tendon reflexes should be carefully elicited and hyperreflexia noted. The demonstration of clonus at the ankle is especially worrisome.

The maternal and fetal laboratory evaluations for pregnancy complicated by hypertension are presented in Table 17.2 and demonstrate, by the wide range of tests, the multisystem effects of hypertension in pregnancy. Maternal liver dysfunction, renal insufficiency, and coagulopathy are significant concerns and require serial evaluation. Evaluation of fetal well-being with ultrasonography, nonstress test (NST)/oxytocin challenge test (OCT), and/or biophysical profile is crucial.

Management

The goal of management of hypertension in pregnancy is to balance the management of both fetus and mother to optimize the outcome for each. In general, maternal blood pressure should be monitored and the mother should be observed for the sequelae of the hypertensive disease. Intervention for maternal indications should occur when the risk of permanent disability or death for the mother without intervention outweighs the risks to the fetus caused by intervention. For the fetus, there should be regular evaluation of fetal well-being and fetal growth, with intervention becoming necessary if the intrauterine environment provides more risks to the fetus than delivery with subsequent care in the newborn nursery.

MANAGEMENT OF PREECLAMPSIA

The severity of the preeclampsia and the maturity of the fetus are the primary considerations in the management of preeclampsia. Care must be individualized, but there are well-accepted general guidelines.

The mainstay of patients with *mild preeclampsia* and an immature fetus is *bed rest,* preferably with as much time as possible spent in a lateral decubitus position. In this position, cardiac function and uterine blood flow are maximized and maternal blood pressures in most cases are normalized.

TABLE 17.2.   Laboratory Assessment of Pregnant Hypertensive Patients

Test or Procedure	Rationale
Maternal studies	
Complete blood count	Increasing hematocrit may signify worsening vasoconstriction and decreased intravascular volume
Platelet count	Thrombocytopenia and coagulopathy are associated with worsening PIH
Coagulation profile (PT, PTT)	
Fibrin split products	
Liver function studies	Hepatocellular dysfunction is associated with worsening PIH
Serum creatinine	Decreased renal function is associated with worsening PIH
24-hour urine for	
Creatinine clearance	
Total urinary protein	
Uric acid	
Fetal studies	To assess for pregnancy-associated
Ultrasound examination	hypertension effects on the fetus
	IUGR
Fetal weight and growth	Oligohydramnios
Amniotic fluid volume	Chronic fetal stress/distress
Placental status	
NST/OCT	
Biophysical profile	

IUGR = intrauterine growth restriction; NST/OCT = nonstress test/oxytocin challenge test; PIH = pregnancy-induced hypertension; PT = prothrombin time; PTT = partial thromboplastin time.

This improves uteroplacental function, allowing normal fetal growth and metabolism. For a patient with mild preeclampsia who has access to medical care and is motivated to care for herself, bed rest at home with daily weighing (if possible), fetal movement count records, and home blood pressure determinations (if available) usually suffice. The patient is instructed to recognize the signs and symptoms that indicate worsening of the preeclampsia and to notify her physician in such an event. In the absence of significant changes in her condition, such care allows the fetus to grow and become more functionally mature. In addition, induction of labor, if needed, is more likely to be successful as gestational age approaches term.

Hospitalization is recommended if the patient lacks either transportation for frequent prenatal visits or motivation to maintain bed rest, or for the patient in whom expectant management at home does not result in normalization of blood pressure. The same regimen is used in the hospital, but better compliance is ensured in this more controlled environment.

For the patient with *worsening preeclampsia* or the patient who has *severe preeclampsia or eclampsia,* stabilization with magnesium sulfate, antihypertensive therapy (as indicated), monitoring for maternal and fetal well-being, and delivery by either induction or cesarean delivery are required. A 24-hour delay in delivery to allow for steroid administration to enhance

TABLE 17.3.	Magnesium Toxicity

Serum Concentration (mg/dl)	Manifestation
1.5–3	Normal concentration
4–7	Therapeutic levels
5–10	ECG changes
8–12	Loss of patellar reflex
9–12	Feeling of warmth, flushing
10–12	Somnolence; slurred speech
15–17	Muscle paralysis; respiratory difficulty
> 30	Cardiac arrest

ECG = electrocardiogram.

fetal pulmonary maturity may be indicated in some cases.

For more than half a century, *magnesium sulfate* has been used to prevent eclamptic convulsions. It has virtually no effect on blood pressure. Other anticonvulsants such as diazepam and phenytoin are infrequently used in obstetrics. Magnesium sulfate may be administered by intramuscular or intravenous routes, although the latter is far more common. An initial 4-g loading dose is given intravenously over 20 to 30 minutes, followed by a constant infusion of 1 to 3 g/hr. In 98% of cases, convulsions will be prevented. Therapeutic levels are 4 to 7 mEq/L, with toxic concentrations having predictable consequences (Table 17.3). Frequent evaluations of the patient's patellar reflex and respirations are necessary to monitor for manifestations of rising serum magnesium concentrations. In addition, because magnesium sulfate is excreted solely from the kidney, maintenance of urine output at ≥ 25 ml/hr will help avoid accumulation of the drug. Reversal of the effects of excessive magnesium concentrations is accomplished by the slow intravenous administration of 10% calcium gluconate along with oxygen supplementation and cardiorespiratory support if needed.

Antihypertensive therapy is indicated if the diastolic blood pressure is repeatedly above 110 mm Hg. Hydralazine (Apresoline) is often the initial antihypertensive medication of choice, given in 5-mg increments intravenously until an acceptable blood pressure response is obtained. A 10- to 15-minute response time is usual. The goal of such therapy is to reduce the diastolic pressure to the 90 to 100 mm Hg range. Further reduction of the blood pressure may impair uterine blood flow to rates dangerous to the fetus. Other antihypertensive agents may be used (Tables 17.4 and 17.5).

Once anticonvulsant and antihypertensive therapies are established, attention is directed toward *delivery*. Induction of labor is often attempted, although cesarean delivery may be needed either if induction is unsuccessful, or not possible, or if maternal or fetal status is worsening. At delivery, blood loss must be closely monitored, because patients with preeclampsia or eclampsia have significantly reduced blood volumes. *After delivery,* patients are kept in the labor and delivery area for 24 hours, or longer if the clinical situation warrants, for close observation of their clinical progress and further administration of magnesium sulfate to prevent postpartum eclamptic seizures. Approximately 25% of all preeclamptic patients who have eclamptic seizures have them before labor, approximately 50% during labor, and approximately 25% after delivery. Usually, the vasospastic process begins to reverse itself in the first 24 to 48 hours after delivery, as manifest by a brisk diuresis.

The management of patients with *chronic hypertension in pregnancy* involves closely monitoring maternal blood pressure and watching for the superimposition of preeclampsia or eclampsia and following the fetus for appropriate growth and fetal well-being. Also, the patient should be encouraged to increase the amount of time she rests. Medical treatment of milder forms of chronic hypertension has been disappointing in that no significant improvement in pregnancy outcome has been

TABLE 17.4. Antihypertensive Medications Used in Pregnancy

Medication	Mechanism of Action	Effects
Thiazide	Decreased plasma volume and CO	CO decreased; RBF decreased; maternal electrolyte depletion; neonatal thrombocytopenia
Methyldopa	False neurotransmission, CNS effect	CO unchanged; RBF unchanged; maternal lethargy, fever, hepatitis, and hemolytic anemia
Hydralazine	Direct peripheral vasodilation	CO increased; RBF unchanged or increased; maternal flushing, headache, tachycardia, lupus-like syndrome
Propranolol	β-adrenergic blocker	CO decreased; RBF decreased; maternal increased uterine tone with possible decrease in placental perfusion; neonatal depressed respirations
Labetalol	α- and β-adrenergic blocker	CO unchanged; RBF unchanged; maternal tremulousness, flushing, headache; neonatal depressed respirations
Nifedipine	Calcium-channel blocker	CO unchanged; RBF unchanged; maternal orthostatic hypotension and headache (also a tocolytic); no neonatal effects known

CNS = central nervous system; CO = cardiac output; RBF = renal blood flow.

TABLE 17.5. Drug Therapy for Hypertensive Emergencies in Pregnancy

Drug	Regimen	Course of Action
Hydralazine (Apresoline)	10–50 mg IM q 3–6 h; 5–25 mg IV q 3–6 h	Onset, 10–20 minutes; maximum effect, 20–40 minutes; duration, 3–8 hours
Nifedipine	10 mg po q 4–8 h	Onset, 5–10 minutes; maximum effect, 10–20 minutes; duration, 4–8 hours
Labetalol	20–50mg IV q 3–6 h	Onset, 1–2 minutes; maximum effect, 10 minutes; duration, 6–16 hours

demonstrated. Antihypertensive medication is generally not given unless the diastolic blood pressure exceeds 110 mm Hg; the purpose of such medications is to reduce the likelihood of maternal stroke. Methyldopa is the most commonly used antihypertensive medication for this purpose. It was formerly taught that diuretics were contraindicated during pregnancy, but diuretic therapy is no longer discontinued in the patient who was already on such therapy before becoming pregnant.

MANAGEMENT OF THE ECLAMPTIC SEIZURE

The eclamptic seizure is life-threatening for mother and fetus. Maternal risks include musculoskeletal injury (including biting the tongue), hypoxia, and aspiration. Maternal therapy consists of inserting a padded tongue blade, restraining gently as needed, providing oxygen, and gaining an intravenous (IV) access. Eclamptic seizures are usually self-limited so that medical therapy should be directed to the initiation of magnesium therapy (4 g slowly IV) to prevent further seizures rather than to anticonvulsant therapy with diazepam or similar drugs. Transient uterine hyperactivity for 2 to 15 minutes is associated with fetal heart rate (FHR) changes, including bradycardia or compensatory tachycardia, decreased beat-to-beat activity, and late decelerations. These are self-limited and not dangerous to the fetus unless they continue for 20 minutes or more. Delivery during this time imposes unnecessary risk for mother and fetus and should be avoided. Arterial blood gases should be obtained, any metabolic disturbance should be corrected, and a Foley catheter should be placed to monitor urinary output. If the maternal blood pressure is very high, if maternal urinary output is low, or if there is evidence of cardiac disturbance, consideration of a central venous catheter and, perhaps, continuous electrocardiogram (ECG) monitoring are appropriate.

HELLP SYNDROME

HELLP is the acronym for a specific set of hypertensive patients who have *hemolysis (H), elevated liver (EL) enzymes, and low platelet (LP) count.* This syndrome is now appreciated as a distinct clinical entity, occurring in 4% to 12% of patients with severe preeclampsia or eclampsia. Patients with HELLP syndrome are often multiparous, somewhat older than the average obstetric patient, and somewhat less hypertensive than many preeclamptic patients. The liver dysfunction may be manifest as RUQ pain and is all too commonly misdiagnosed as gallbladder disease or indigestion. Major morbidity and mortality with unrecognized HELLP make accurate diagnosis imperative. Unfortunately, the first symptoms are often rather vague, including nausea and emesis and a nonspecific viral-like syndrome. Treatment of these gravely ill patients is best done in a high-risk obstetric center and consists of cardiovascular stabilization, correction of coagulation abnormalities, and delivery. Parenteral analgesia in labor is appropriate, but pudendal or epidural anesthesia is contraindicated because of the risk of bleeding. Platelet transfusion before or after delivery is indicated if the platelet count is fewer than 20,000/mm^3, and it may be advisable to transfuse patients with a platelet count below 50,000/mm^3 before proceeding with a cesarean birth.

CASE STUDIES

Case 17A

A 38-year-old G2 P1001 presents for prenatal care at 10 weeks of gestational age by good dates and initial pelvic examination. Her obstetric history includes a normal pregnancy and delivery at age 17. She was diagnosed as having essential hypertension 4 years ago and was placed on a *diuretic and methyldopa; she says her blood pressure "runs approximately 140/90 most of the time."*

On physical examination, the patient weighs 280 pounds. A blood pressure taken with a large cuff is 135/85 supine and 140/95 sitting. She has mild arteriolar

(Continued)

narrowing on fundoscopic examination, a normal cardiovascular examination, a 10-week-size uterus, normal deep tendon reflexes (DTRs), and 1+ lower extremity peripheral edema. Her urine sample dipstick shows 1+ protein and trace glucose.

Questions Case 17A

Your initial diagnosis is

A. PIH
B. Mild preeclampsia
C. Severe preeclampsia
D. Eclampsia
E. Chronic hypertension
F. Chronic hypertension with superimposed PIH

Answer: E

This patient's hypertension precedes her pregnancy. Although her status nears the definition of mild preeclampsia, which would give her the diagnosis of chronic hypertension with superimposed mild preeclampsia, her stable history precludes this diagnosis at her initial visit.

Your initial management should

A. Discontinue the diuretic and methyldopa
B. Recommend strict bed rest at home
C. Recommend therapeutic abortion
D. Hospitalize for the remainder of pregnancy
E. None of these

Answer: E

Initial management should be to maximize rest, but strict bed rest at home is too much restriction at this time. Modern obstetric practice is not to change the antihypertensive medications of chronic hypertensive patients who become pregnant. Instead, the regimen is continued while maternal and fetal evaluations commence. There is no indication for hospitalization or for therapeutic abortion.

Case 17B

A 19-year-old G1 has had an unremarkable antepartum course since her first prenatal visit at 8 weeks. At the start of her thirty-second week she complains of swollen hands and feet and "puffy eyes," which have been getting worse for the last 2 days. Her blood pressure is 150/95 compared with her usual blood pressure of 130/70. After resting for 30 minutes, her blood pressure is 145/85. Her dipstick urinary protein is 1–2+. She reports daily fetal movement that has not changed and denies headache, abdominal pain, or dizzy spells.

Questions Case 17B

Your initial diagnosis is

A. PIH
B. Mild preeclampsia
C. Severe preeclampsia
D. Eclampsia
E. Chronic hypertension
F. Chronic hypertension with superimposed PIH

Answer: B

This patient has mild preeclampsia. Her 1–2+ proteinuria is disconcerting, but her rapid improvement in blood pressure with 30 minutes of rest is reassuring, as is her history of an active fetus.

All of the following evaluations are indicated at the present time EXCEPT

A. Obstetric ultrasound
B. Amniocentesis for fetal lung maturity determination
C. Biophysical profile
D. Complete blood count (CBC), coagulation profile, and liver function studies
E. 24-hour urine collection for total protein and creatinine clearance

Answer: B

Because there is no need to deliver the fetus at this time, fetal lung maturity is not an issue. Ultrasound can evaluate amniotic fluid volume and provide the biophysical profile. The chemical evaluations of maternal status are indicated, if for no other reason than to serve as a baseline evaluation if the mother's condition deteriorates. A pelvic examination is a wise precaution at this time to evaluate the favorability of the cervix, because the potential for induction exists if the maternal or fetal status worsens.

Case 17C

A 26-year-old G1 at 39 weeks' gestational age presents to labor and delivery in early labor, contracting every 4 to 5 minutes, dilated to 5 centimeters, and effaced to 90% with the fetal head at zero station. She has been at bed rest at home for two weeks with a diagnosis of mild preeclampsia (blood pressures on office visits in the range of 140–150/80–90 after the start of bed rest). Because of her mild preeclampsia and concerns about the quality of her uteroplacental function, a fetal scalp clip is placed and the fetal heart rate pattern is reassuring. Two hours after admission, the patient suddenly becomes unresponsive and seizes.

Questions Case 17C

Initial management consists of

A. Immediate cesarean section
B. Diazepam, 10–20 mg IV push
C. Mg^{++}, 4 g IV over 15–20 minutes and then at a rate of 1–3 g/hr
D. Injury prevention, including tongue blade
E. Placement of Foley catheter

Answer: C, D, E

The patient is eclamptic, and eclamptic seizures are usually self-limited. Thus, management is directed toward injury prevention and the initiation of Mg sulfate therapy to prevent further seizure activity. Anticonvulsant therapy is rarely indicated.

The seizure lasts 3 minutes, but at 1½ minutes, the fetal heart rate changes, demonstrating a bradycardia of 80.

Management now consists of

A. Apresoline intravenous
B. Ephredrine intravenous
C. Immediate cesarean delivery
D. Continuation of present management
E. Immediate forceps delivery

Answer: D

Fetal heart rate alterations (bradycardia, decelerations, altered beat-to-beat variability) are common and usually transient. Urgent delivery by cesarean section is not needed for the fetus and may pose additional risks to the mother. If the non-reassuring fetal heart rate pattern persists for 20 minutes or more, however, consideration of urgent delivery should be entertained.

18

MULTIFETAL GESTATION

This chapter deals primarily with APGO Objective(s):

OBJECTIVE 21   Multifetal Pregnancy

A. Describe the mechanisms of and the altered maternal and fetal physiology associated with monozygotic, dizygotic, and multizygotic gestation.

B. Describe the diagnosis and the antepartum, intrapartum, and postpartum management of multifetal gestation.

At first glance, twin pregnancy is often considered a novelty, with pleasant images of identical children dressed alike. In fact, pregnancies with multiple fetuses pose significant medical risks for both the mother and her offspring. Special care is necessary to achieve an optimal outcome. Caring for two or more infants likewise challenges even the most devoted parents. This chapter provides an overview of twin pregnancy—its diagnosis and antepartum, intrapartum, and postpartum care—with reference to pregnancies with three or more fetuses when relevant. In general, all potential complications with twin pregnancies are somewhat more frequent and more serious as the number of fetuses increases.

INCIDENCE OF MULTIPLE GESTATION

The overall incidence of recognized twins in the United States is almost 3% with the rate rising due to an increase in older gravidas and the wider availability and use of assisted reproductive technologies. The natural rate of twinning is approximately 1 in 90 and is slightly higher in blacks than in whites. Twin gestations can be characterized as dizygotic (fraternal) or monozygotic (identical). *Dizygotic twins* occur when two separate ova are fertilized by two separate sperm, and in fact, represent two siblings who happen to be born at approximately the same time. *Monozygotic twins* represent division of the fertilized ovum at various times after conception. There is a marked difference in the incidence of twinning in various populations, almost exclusively due to the incidence of dizygotic twinning. The *incidence of monozygotic twinning* is fairly constant around the world at *approximately 1 in 250 pregnancies*, whereas *dizygotic twinning* occurs as frequently as *1 in 20 pregnancies* in certain African countries. Increasing age and increasing parity are independent factors for dizygotic twinning. A familial factor is present in twinning that follows the maternal lineage. Ultrasonography, which allows early detection and serial evaluations, has provided valuable information concerning the outcome of twin pregnancies. Only approximately 50% of twin pregnancies detected in the first trimester result in the delivery of viable twins, with the remaining associated with death and resorption of one embryo/fetus with eventual delivery of a single fetus. Both spontaneous abortions and congenital anomalies occur more frequently in multiple pregnancies than in singleton pregnancies.

The likelihood of twinning is increased significantly if *fertility agents or other assisted reproductive technologies* are used. With clomiphene citrate induction of ovulation, the twinning rate is approximately 6% to 8%. With the use of exogenous gonadotropin therapy, the rate increases to approximately 25% to 35%. Because in vitro fertilization programs typically insert several fertilized ova into the uterine cavity, multiple fetuses would be expected to occur in some instances; in fact, the rate of two or more fetuses is approximately 35% to 40%.

The incidence of three or more pregnancies may be approximated by 90 raised to the power of the number of fetuses minus one. Thus triplets are 1 in 90^2, or 1 in 8100; quadruplets, 1 in 90^3, or 1 in 729,000; and so forth.

NATURAL HISTORY

As the number of fetuses increases, the expected *duration of pregnancy* diminishes. Compared with singleton pregnancies, which deliver at 40 weeks, twins deliver at an average of 37 weeks, triplets at 33 weeks, and quadruplets at an average of 29 weeks. Thus with each additional fetus, the length of gestation is decreased by approximately 4 weeks. Although all twins face certain risks, *monozygotic twins face additional risks related to the time when twinning occurs*. The developmental sequence associated with the separation of the conceptus into twins explains the basis for these problems as well as the configuration of the fetal membranes at delivery. If division of the conceptus occurs within 3 days of fertilization, each fetus will be surrounded by an amnion and chorion, and the membranes are termed diamniotic dichorionic. If division occurs between the fourth and eighth day following fertilization, the chorion has already begun to develop, whereas the amnion has not. Therefore, each fetus will be surrounded by an amnion, but a single chorion will surround both twins, a condition termed diamniotic monochorionic. Division from day 9 to day 12 takes place after development of both the amnion and the chorion, and the twins will share a common sac, a condition termed monoamniotic/monochorionic (Figure 18.1). Division thereafter is incomplete, resulting in the development of conjoined twins, which may be fused in any of a multitude of ways, but usually at the chest and/or abdomen. This

rare condition is seen in approximately 1 in 70,000 deliveries.

Further development can result in various vascular anastomoses between the fetuses that, in turn, can lead to a condition known as *twin–twin transfusion syndrome*. In this circumstance, blood flow of the fetuses mixes such that there is net flow from one twin to another, at times with disastrous consequences. The so-called donor twin can have impaired growth, anemia, hypovolemia, and other problems. On the other hand, the recipient twin can develop hypervolemia, hypertension, polycythemia, and congestive heart failure as a result of this abnormal transfusion. A secondary manifestation involves the amniotic fluid dynam-

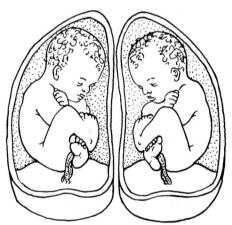

A Two placentas, two amnions, two chorions — dichorionic diamniotic

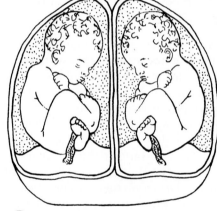

B One placenta, two amnions, two chorions — dichorionic diamniotic

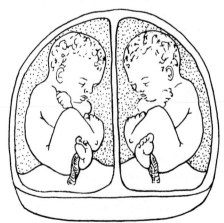

C One placenta, two amnions, one chorion — monochorionic diamniotic

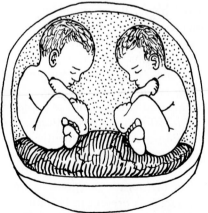

D One placenta, one amnion, one chorion—monochorionic monoamniotic

FIGURE 18.1. Development of the amnion and chorion in twin pregnancies.

ics. Because of transudate across the skin or, probably more important, increased urinary output owing to its hypervolemia, the recipient produces abundant amniotic fluid, whereas the donor twin may in fact have oligohydramnios. The hydramnios in one twin further compounds the risk of preterm labor in multifetal pregnancies. Recently, intrauterine laser ablation of the vascular anastomoses has met with some success in treating this difficult problem. Other vascular abnormalities include absence of an umbilical artery, which may be associated in 30% of cases with other congenital problems, especially renal agenesis. A single umbilical artery is seen in approximately 3% to 4% of twins, compared with 0.5% to 1% of singletons.

Multifetal pregnancy is associated with increased *perinatal morbidity,* three to four times that for a comparable singleton pregnancy in the case of twin gestation. The most significant cause of morbidity is preterm labor and delivery, followed by intrauterine growth restriction, polyhydramnios (in approximately 10% of multiple gestations, predominantly monochorionic gestations), maternal disease (especially preeclampsia), congenital anomalies, postpartum hemorrhage, and placental and umbilical cord accidents. The spontaneous abortion rate is higher in multiple gestation.

DIAGNOSIS OF MULTIPLE GESTATION

Twin pregnancy is usually *suspected when the uterine size is excessively large for the calculated gestational age.* Although there is a variation in fundal height measurements in singleton pregnancies, an increase of 4 cm between the week gestation and the carefully measured fundal height should prompt evaluation to detect twins, reassign gestational age, diagnose hydramnios, or provide other explanation for the discrepancy. In modern obstetrics, the diagnosis of twins or multiple gestation is *usually made by obstetric ultrasonography.* The differential diagnosis includes incorrect dates, leiomyoma uteri or other tumors, polyhydramnios of other etiology, and in early pregnancy, hydatidiform mole.

Once the diagnosis of twin pregnancy has been made, subsequent antenatal care addresses each of the *potential concerns* for mother and fetus as listed in Table 18.1. Although the maternal blood volume is greater with a twin gestation than with singleton pregnancy, the anticipated blood loss at delivery is also greater. Anemia is more common in these patients, and a balanced diet with iron, folate, and possibly other micronutrients is important. Although the value of bed rest in prolonging gestation is controversial, it is generally advised that a

TABLE 18.1. Antenatal Management of Twin Pregnancies	
Concern	**Action**
Adequate nutrition	Balanced diet; additional increase in daily caloric intake; multivitamin and mineral supplements (e.g., folate)
Increased blood loss at delivery	Prevent anemia (iron)
Fetal growth	Increasing rest beginning at 24–26 weeks—the value of this is unclear, but also may decrease preterm labor
Preterm labor	Educate patient on signs of labor; increase bed rest; cervical examinations every 1–2 weeks; home monitoring in select cases
Pregnancy-induced hypertension	Frequent blood pressure determinations; frequent urinary protein assessment
Fetal growth, discordant growth	Periodic ultrasonography examinations

woman limit her activity after 24 to 26 weeks to avoid *premature labor,* which is more common in twin gestations. Careful attention to detection of uterine contractions is important, and the patient should be cautioned about signs of preterm labor, such as low back pain, a thin vaginal discharge, and diarrhea. Cervical examinations to detect early effacement and dilation are usually done every 1 to 2 weeks beginning in the midtrimester. At these visits, evidence suggesting pregnancy-induced hypertension is also gathered, which includes careful measurement of blood pressure and testing for protein in the urine. Beginning at 30 to 32 weeks, daily fetal kick counts are usually begun to help assess *fetal well-being.* Although somewhat surprising, patients can almost always distinguish movements of different fetuses. Nonstress tests (NSTs) or other fetal monitor testing is begun as the pregnancy approaches term. Fortunately, fetal lung maturity is achieved somewhat earlier in twin pregnancies than in singleton pregnancies.

The chief antenatal assessment in twin pregnancy remains the periodic ultrasonography examination, which is done approximately every 4 weeks after 20 weeks' gestation. At each examination, growth of each fetus is assessed and an estimate of amniotic fluid volume made. If growth is discordant, usually defined as a 20% difference in weight (the difference in weight divided by the weight of the larger fetus is 20% or more), ultrasonography may be performed more often and tests of fetal well-being (such as an NST and kick counts) are begun at 30 to 32 weeks. Fetal breathing and body movements as well as body tone (elements of the biophysical profile) can also be determined with ultrasonography.

INTRAPARTUM MANAGEMENT

Intrapartum management is largely *determined by the presentation of the twins.* In general, if the first (presenting) twin is in the cephalic (vertex) presentation, labor is allowed to progress to vaginal delivery, whereas if the presenting twin is in a position other than cephalic, cesarean delivery is often performed. During labor, the heart rate of both fetuses is monitored separately. Approaches to the delivery of twins vary, depending on gestational age, presentation of the twins, and the experience of the attending physicians. Regardless of the delivery plan, access to full obstetric anesthetic and pediatric services is mandatory, in that cesarean delivery may be required on short notice.

If vaginal delivery of the first twin is accomplished and the second twin is also cephalic, delivery of the second twin generally proceeds smoothly. With proper monitoring of the second twin, there is no urgency in accomplishing the second delivery. If the second twin is presenting in any way other than cephalic, there are two primary manipulations that may effect vaginal delivery. The first is *external cephalic ver-*

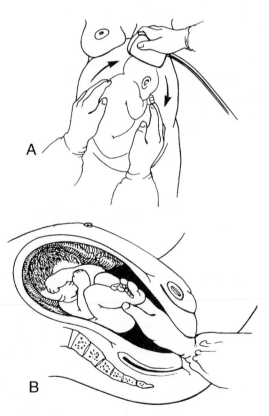

FIGURE 18.2. (*A*) External cephalic version. (*B*) Breech extraction (internal podalic version).

sion whereby, using ultrasonographic visualization, the fetus is gently guided into the cephalic presentation by abdominal massage and pressure. The second maneuver is *breech extraction,* in which the physician reaches a hand into the uterine cavity, identifies the lower extremities of the fetus, and gently delivers the infant via breech delivery. The possibility of a prolapsed umbilical cord must always be borne in mind when delivery of twins is to be accomplished (Figure 18.2). Postpartum, the overdistended uterus may not contract normally, leading to uterine atony and postpartum hemorrhage.

CASE STUDIES

Case 18A

At 32 weeks of gestation, a 35-year-old G1 P0 with known twins is noted to have a fundal height not commensurate with gestational age. Her weight gain and blood pressure are normal as are her antenatal laboratory studies. She says the babies are moving normally and that she feels well, although "rather large."

Questions Case 18A

Which of the following interventions, if any, are indicated?

A. Oxytocin challenge test (OCT)
B. Ultrasound
C. Induction of labor if cephalic/cephalic presentation
D. Cesarean birth

Answer: B

Intrauterine growth restriction and discordant growth are both common in twin pregnancies. Measurements of each fetus for comparison may reveal abnormal development. If found, further testing with possible delivery is indicated. Evaluation of fetal well-being at the time of obstetric ultrasound and NST are noninvasive tests that yield valuable information. Given the risk of premature labor, OCT is less commonly used and would best be reserved if the NST is not reassuring. Delivery should be contemplated only if one or both fetuses are compromised.

At ultrasound her twins are noted to be monochorionic/diamniotic, with both twins moving actively in adequate amounts of amniotic fluid. Comparison of twin A to twin B shows a 25% difference in weights, with Twin A being the larger. An NST is reactive for both twins so that the biophysical profile is 10/10 for each twin. Your best explanation and recommendations are

A. Cesarean birth now, because the discordant growth is a harbinger for intrauterine fetal death in the near future for Twin B
B. Induction of labor, because the discordant growth is a harbinger for intrauterine fetal death in the near future for Twin B
C. Biweekly NSTs and weekly biophysical profiles (BPPs) and evaluation for fetal growth
D. Amniocentesis

Answer: C

Without evidence of intrauterine compromise, delivery is not indicated. Evaluation of fetal well-being and growth is needed, however, on a biweekly basis, with delivery being considered if the disparity in growth widens or information consistent with a nonreassuring fetal status develops.

CHAPTER

19

FETAL GROWTH ABNORMALITIES

Intrauterine Growth Restriction and Fetal Macrosomia

CHAPTER OBJECTIVES

This chapter deals primarily with APGO Objective(s):

OBJECTIVE 33   Fetal Growth
 Abnormalities

Define macrosomia and intrauterine fetal growth restriction and for each, describe the associated risk factors, recognized causes, associated morbidity and mortality, and methods used in diagnosis and management of each.

INTRAUTERINE GROWTH RESTRICTION

The term *intrauterine growth restriction* (IUGR) is used to describe infants whose weights are much lower than expected for their gestational age. *A fetus/infant whose weight lies in the lowest 10% of the normal population for a specified gestational age is designated as having IUGR*, a determination based on standard weight/gestational age tables. By definition then, the prevalence of IUGR will be 10%. Unlike "low birth weight," IUGR is based on weight for a *specific gestational age*. Thus careful assessment of gestational age is crucial to diagnosing and, therefore, managing patients with IUGR.

The fetus with IUGR is best viewed as fragile, that is, potentially lacking adequate reserves for continued intrauterine life, the stress of labor, or neonatal adaptation. Such infants are at greater risk for intrauterine fetal death or neonatal death, asphyxia, and fetal distress before or during labor; and once delivered, they are at risk for meconium aspiration, hypoglycemia, hypothermia, respiratory distress, and many other problems. Indeed, the perinatal mortality rate is increased 7- to 10-fold with IUGR— about 120 per 1000 for all cases of growth restriction and about 100 per 1000 if anomalous infants are excluded. About one third of stillborns are growth restricted. The perinatal morbidity rate for growth-restricted infants is also exceedingly high. Because of these risks, it is important to identify such infants in utero, maximize the quality of their intrauterine environment, plan and implement their delivery using the safest means possible, and provide needed care in the neonatal period.

Etiology

For a fetus to thrive in utero, an adequate number of fetal cells must be present and differentiated properly. In addition, sufficient foodstuffs, other nutrients, and oxygen must be available via an adequately functioning uteroplacental unit to allow growth in number of cells and then in size. Early in pregnancy, fetal growth is primarily by cellular hyperplasia, or cell division, so that *early-onset IUGR* leads to an irreversible diminution of organ size and perhaps function. This type of IUGR is associated with heritable factors, immunologic abnormalities, chronic maternal disease, fetal infection, and multiple pregnancy. Later in pregnancy, fetal growth is more and more dependent on cellular hypertrophy rather than hyperplasia so that *delayed-onset IUGR* results in decreased cell size and is amenable to restoration of size with adequate nutrition. The normal fetus grows throughout pregnancy, but the rate of growth falls off after 37 weeks' gestational age as the fetus begins to use energy to deposit fat in addition to cellular growth. Uteroplacental insufficiency is the primary cause of this kind of IUGR. The placenta grows early and rapidly compared to the fetus, reaching a maximum surface area of about 11 m^2 and weight of 500 grams at about 37 weeks' gestational age. Thereafter, there is a slow but steady decline in placental surface area (and hence function), primarily because of microinfarctions of its vascular system. Because there is a close relationship between placental surface area and fetal weight, factors that act to decrease placental size (surface area, weight) are associated with decreased (restricted) growth.

Although a number of *causes of IUGR* have been recognized (Table 19.1), a definite cause of IUGR cannot be identified in approximately 50% of all cases. Therefore, surveillance for evidence of IUGR is an important part of every antepartum visit. Causes of IUGR can be conveniently grouped into maternal and fetal origins. Maternal smoking has been known for many years to be associated with decreased birth weight, to a magnitude of roughly 0.5 pound at term. Because maternal habits are important causes of growth restriction, modification of such behavior can improve outcome.

The recommended maternal *weight gain* during pregnancy is approximately 25–35 pounds (11.4–15.9 kg). If there are marked nutritional deficiencies, however, a decrease in fetal weight has been demonstrated.

TABLE 19.1. Causes/Risk Factors of Intrauterine Growth Restriction

Maternal		Fetal

Maternal

Cardiovascular
  Hypertension
  Cyanotic heart disease
  Cyanotic pulmonary
  disease
Metabolic
  Low maternal
  prepregnancy weight
  (< 90% ideal body
  weight)
  Poor nutrition, poor
  weight gain

Diabetes
Significant anemia;
  hemoglobinopathies
Behavioral
  Substance abuse (drugs,
  alcohol)
  Smoking

Obstetric

History of growth
  restriction in previous
  pregnancy
Elevated MSAFP/hCG

Antiphospholipid
  syndrome
Multifetal pregnancy
Abnormal placentation

Fetal

Infection: rubella,
  cytomegalovirus
Congenital anomalies

MSAFP/hCG = maternal serum alpha-fetoprotein/human chorionic gonadotropin.

In studies performed during World War II, severe famine and marked caloric restriction resulted in decreased birth weights of 0.5 to 1.0 pound, depending on the nutritional status of the women before the onset of nutritional deprivation. It is difficult to define the role of less severe forms of nutritional deficiencies on fetal growth. In pregnancies with multiple fetuses, even normal nutrition may not be enough to provide adequate nutrition for all fetuses, resulting in IUGR.

The most common known maternal factor associated with IUGR is *hypertensive disease* (either pre-existing hypertension or pregnancy-associated hypertensive disease such as preeclampsia). Vasospasm diminishes uteroplacental blood flow and hence the ability of the mother to provide adequate nutrition to the fetus through the placenta, which is often of smaller size and surface area. From 25% to 30% of all cases of IUGR are associated with maternal hypertensive disease. Other maternal disorders may likewise interfere with fetal growth, notably *cyanotic heart disease and hemoglobinopathies.*

Fetal causes of IUGR include congenital infections and anomalies. The most clearly understood *fetal infections* that interfere with growth are rubella and cytomegalovirus infections, especially at early gestational ages. These infections may

be manifest only as mild "flu-like" illnesses, but their occurrence should be noted. Damage to the fetus during organogenesis can result in a decreased cell number, which is manifest by diminished growth later in gestation. Probably 5% or less of all cases of IUGR are related to early infection with these or other viral agents. Bacterial infections have not been implicated in IUGR. *Congenital anomalies* account for up to 15% of all cases of IUGR. Chromosomal anomalies such as trisomy 21, 18, and 13 are typically associated with diminished fetal growth. Other genetic abnormalities, such as certain congenital heart defects and a variety of dysmorphic syndromes, likewise result in smaller than expected infants.

Evaluation and Management

The diagnosis of IUGR is based on a fetus whose weight falls behind the 10th percentile for a given age. Unfortunately, this definition requires two data whose intrauterine measurement is both difficult and imprecise. Late prenatal care, a common problem, further exacerbates this imprecision because dating is more difficult later in pregnancy. Some elements of maternal history are associated with IUGR, and the presence of these alerts the clinician to a higher possibility of the development of IUGR (see Table 19.1). A patient with a history of having a child with IUGR is at increased risk for a recurrence of this problem. Personal habits such as smoking and use of alcohol or other drugs of abuse such as cocaine should be part of the routine obstetric history obtained at the onset of prenatal care. Recognition of such elements in the history is important so every effort can be made to discourage such behavior. A medical history of disorders potentially interfering with fetal growth, primarily hypertension, should be obtained at the onset of prenatal care.

Physical examination is limited in usefulness in diagnosing IUGR, but it serves as an important screening test for abnormal fetal growth. Maternal size and weight gain throughout pregnancy have a limited use, but access to such information is readily available and a low maternal weight or little or no weight gain through pregnancy can suggest IUGR. Serial measurement of fundal height at every antepartum visit is perhaps the most useful initial evaluation for IUGR. Between approximately 15 and 36 weeks' gestation, *fundal height measurement* should advance in centimeter increments in close parallel with gestational age in weeks. Thus a patient at 28 weeks' gestation would be expected to have a fundal height of close to 28 cm. Serial measurements, especially by the same examiner, can serve as an effective screening test for IUGR, because an increase in fundal height less than expected may suggest the diagnosis of IUGR and raise the need for additional testing (Figure 19.1). Clinical estimations of fetal weight are not very helpful in diagnosing IUGR, except when fetal size is grossly diminished.

Ultrasonography has provided an important obstetric tool to diagnose and assess IUGR. Measurements of various fetal structures can be compared with standardized tables that reflect normal growth. The measurement of the biparietal diameter, head circumference, abdominal circumference, and femur length are among the measurements usually obtained. Ratios of these measurements and equations can provide useful information with respect to fetal size.

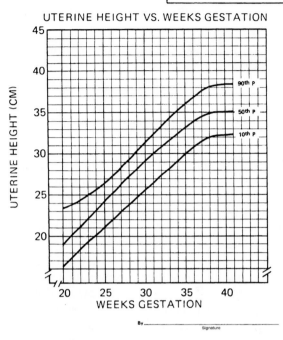

FIGURE 19.1. Fundal height evaluation as a screening test for intrauterine growth restriction. (From Scott JR, Di Saia PJ, Hammond CB, et al: *Danforth's Obstetrics and Gynecology,* 8th ed. Philadelphia, Lippincott Williams & Wilkins, 1999.)

The diameter of the cerebellum appears to be unaltered by a number of the factors that lead to growth restriction. Accordingly, in patients with uncertain gestational age, measurement of the diameter of this structure may prove helpful.

By the use of ultrasonography, IUGR can be distinguished as asymmetric or symmetric. *Asymmetric IUGR* refers to an unequal decrease in the size of structures. For example, the abdominal circumference may be low, but the biparietal diameter may be at or near normal. Such asymmetry can be seen with severe nutritional deficiencies and with hypertension, when fetal access to nutrients is compromised. In *symmetric IUGR,* all structures are approximately equally diminished in size with a relative sparing of fetal brain and heart compared

TABLE 19.2. Symmetric and Asymmetric Intrauterine Growth Restriction

Asymmetric	Ultrasound Measurement	Symmetric
Appropriate for dates	BPD	May be smaller than dates suggest
< 10th percentile for dates	EFW	< 10th percentile for dates
> 95th percentile for dates	HC/AC ratio	In "normal" range for dates
Low for dates	AFV	Normal or low for dates

AFV = amniotic fluid volume; BPD = biparietal diameter; EFW = estimated fetal weight; HC/AC = head to abdominal circumference.

with asymmetric IUGR. Congenital anomalies or early intrauterine infection can alter cell number and lead to this type of IUGR. This distinction is not always clear, but it does serve as a guide in seeking the etiology of IUGR (Table 19.2).

In patients at increased risk for IUGR, a *baseline ultrasonography* examination should be obtained early in prenatal care and usually repeated periodically. Because growth restriction is related to gestational age, all patients whose length of pregnancy is uncertain should be assessed with physical examination and ultrasonography to establish an accurate gestational age as early in pregnancy as possible. Ultrasonography also can identify the amount of amniotic fluid present. The combination of oligohydramnios (diminished amniotic fluid volume) and IUGR is especially worrisome because it is associated with severe disease and/or worsening outcome. The mechanism is thought to be decreased fetal blood volume, which diminishes renal blood flow, which in turn leads to a reduction of urine output, a primary source of amniotic fluid in the second half of pregnancy.

Direct studies of the fetus are useful in selected patients with IUGR. Fetal tissue can be obtained via amniocentesis (fetal fibroblasts floating in the amniotic fluid), chorionic villus sampling (CVS; or biopsy of placenta), direct blood sampling [percutaneous umbilical blood sampling (PUBS)], or removal of fetal plasma and cells. PUBS also permits immunoglobulin studies and viral cultures to be obtained in patients with suspected viral infections as a cause of IUGR.

Moreover, the level of oxygenation and the acid-base status can be assessed with this technique. PUBS and to some extent CVS are less widely available than ultrasound-directed amniocentesis.

Once IUGR has been diagnosed, *the goal is to deliver the healthiest possible infant at the optimal time.* This involves a balance between the degree of prematurity estimated at the time of diagnosis with the degree of suspected fetal compromise. Initial management consists of a comprehensive attempt to determine a cause for the IUGR. If a correctable etiology is found, corrective action should be taken. Management of the patient with IUGR can be categorized as antepartum, intrapartum, and postpartum (or neonatal) [Table 19.3]. Antepartum management consists of efforts to determine the cause of the IUGR, promote growth, and monitor carefully for fetal compromise. Ultrasonography by experienced personnel can usually identify congenital anomalies that may be associated with IUGR. Measurements of amniotic fluid volume and fetal structures can be made on a serial basis. The degree of IUGR can then be followed in the ensuing weeks. Ultrasound evaluation every three or four weeks to follow the extent of growth restriction, and whether it is improving or worsening, is an important part of the overall management plan for IUGR. Worsening IUGR, for example, may be a key factor in the timing of delivery in combination with gestational age and measurements of fetal well-being. Bed rest, or at least limited activity, is often prescribed for patients with IUGR, because

TABLE 19.3. Assessment and Management of Patient with Intrauterine Growth Restriction

Antepartum	Intrapartum	Postpartum (Neonatal)
Eliminate cause, if possible	Electronic fetal monitoring	Pharyngeal suction
Bed rest, frequent fetal movement counts	Preparation for cesarean delivery; amnioinfusion	Effective neonatal resuscitation as needed
Serial sonography	Oxygen therapy	Avoid hypoglycemia
NST; CST; BPP	Neonatal/anesthesia consultation	Avoid hypothermia; oxygen therapy, if needed
Doppler ultrasound		Avoid hyperviscosity syndrome
Amniocentesis for maturity studies		
PUBS		

BPP = biophysical profile; CST = contraction stress test; NST = nonstress test; PUBS = percutaneous umbilical blood sampling.

limitation of activity, especially with the patient lying in the left-lateral position, maximizes uterine blood flow. This has a salutary effect on fetal growth.

Determination of fetal activity by the so-called kick counts is a useful way of assessing *fetal well-being*. Various electronic fetal monitoring tests, such as the nonstress test (NST) or contraction stress test (CST), or electronic fetal monitoring combined with ultrasound [the biophysical profile (BPP)] can be used once or twice a week (or even more frequently) to assess the condition of the fetus. Although these tests can be helpful if the results are normal, the high false-positive rate must be considered when management decisions regarding delivery are made. Use of these tests in combination may reduce this false-positive rate. Examination of the blood flow through the umbilical cord with Doppler ultrasound may be useful in patients with IUGR. An umbilical artery systolic-end diastolic ratio of more than 3.0 may be associated with increased placental resistance. In selected patients with IUGR of uncertain cause, fetal blood aspirated directly through PUBS can be analyzed for viral antibody titer, chromosomes, and other parameters that reflect fetal oxygenation and acid-base status. Amniocentesis for tests of fetal lung maturity may provide information helpful in selecting the timing of delivery.

The decision regarding proper *time for delivery* is based on a combination of factors. The fetus who is thought to be in marked jeopardy may be delivered by scheduled cesarean section without a trial of labor if its ability to withstand labor is questionable and an induced labor is likely to be lengthy. If induction of labor is undertaken, however, constant electronic fetal monitoring to detect signs suggestive of fetal jeopardy is important. Preparations for cesarean delivery should be made, because rapid deterioration of the fetus may occur. Consultation with anesthesia and neonatology personnel is important for optimal care of the patient and her newborn. Amnioinfusion (instillation of warmed normal saline via transcervical catheter) may be helpful if fetal heart rate decelerations thought to be caused by diminished amniotic fluid volume are present. Maternal oxygen therapy may be beneficial throughout the course of labor.

Expert *neonatal care* is critical because of the reduced capacity of the fetus/infant to adapt and adjust to extrauterine life. Because of the frequent passage of meconium before delivery, the mouth and nasopharynx must be suctioned, usually with direct visualization of the vocal cords. These infants are prone to other complications such as respiratory distress, hyperviscosity syndrome, hypoglycemia, and hypothermia. Hyperviscosity syndrome results from the fetus' attempt to compensate for poor placental oxygen transfer by increasing the hematocrit to more than 65%. After birth, this marked polycythemia can cause multiorgan thrombosis, heart failure, and hyperbilirubinemia. Growth-restricted fetuses also have had less fat deposition in late pregnancy, so that newborn euglycemia cannot be maintained by the normal mechanism of mobilization of glucose by fat metabolism. Fortunately, infants who survive the neonatal period have a generally good prognosis.

FETAL MACROSOMIA

Fetal macrosomia is defined, depending on the definition used, as > 4000 or 4500 g or a fetal weight greater than the ninetieth percentile for a given gestational age. Identification of these fetuses is important, and when possible, the underlying cause must be treated. The physician must anticipate the potential problems of vaginal delivery of a large infant, including a prolonged second stage of labor, shoulder dystocia, and immediate neonatal injury.

Macrosomia is associated with maternal obesity, maternal diabetes, and excessive maternal weight gain during pregnancy. Diagnosis is suspected when the fundal height is > 4 cm above the expected height for a given gestational age (see Figure 19.1). The diagnosis is confirmed by ultrasonography. The differential diagnosis includes a large but normal fetus, multiple gestation, polyhydramnios, uterine leiomyoma or other gynecologic tumor, and in early pregnancy, molar pregnancy.

Antepartum care focuses on management of any treatable cause of macrosomia. Intrapartum management consists of choice of delivery route. Some advocate cesarean birth for macrosomic fetuses, whereas others argue that the perinatal outcome is the same so that the risk to the mother is not justified. When vaginal delivery is chosen, the physician must be prepared to deal with shoulder dystocia by using maneuvers such as hyperflexion of the thighs [McRoberts maneuver (see Figure 21.1)], as well as suprapubic pressure (see Figure 21.2).

CASE STUDIES

Case 19A

A 36-year-old G2 P0010 is seen for her first prenatal visit at 8 weeks. Her medical history includes essential hypertension, smoking, and poor dietary habits. She had three hospitalizations for pelvic inflammatory disease and one for a cone biopsy of the cervix. Her family history includes a sister with Down syndrome, a mother and grandmother with insulin-dependent diabetes, and a sister with carcinoma of the breast.

On physical examination, the patient's blood pressure is 160/95, and she has 1+

proteinuria. She weighs 200 pounds and is 5 feet 1 inch tall. Her general physical examination is normal with the following specific findings: (1) normal breast examination, (2) 2/6 holosystolic murmur without radiation or extra sounds, (3) obese abdomen without masses, (4) cervix consistent in appearance with her history, (5) retroverted 14-week-size uterus that is slightly irregular in shape, and (6) 2+ dependent edema and normal deep tendon reflexes (DTRs).

Question Case 19A

This patient is at increased risk for a growth-restricted infant. Of the several risk factors mentioned, which pose the least likely threat?

A. Poor nutrition
B. Hypertension
C. Smoking
D. Family history of diabetes

Answer: D

Poor nutrition is a risk, although the maternal–fetal unit is able to compensate for considerable dietary inadequacy. This patient's hypertension and smoking are major risk factors, both having great potential for diminution of placental function. Diabetes may be associated with abnormal fetal growth, both growth restriction and macrosomia.

Case 19B

A 28-year-old G2 P1001 at 32 weeks of gestational age has a fundal height of 26 cm. A late first trimester ultrasound had been consistent with her gestational age by dates. Her first baby was delivered by cesarean section for fetal distress. The baby was reportedly "too small" and had not "grown right." The child is well at home but is suffering some difficulty in school.

Questions Case 19B

Information from an ultrasound examination would provide all of the following information EXCEPT

A. Biophysical profile (BPP)
B. Evaluation of fetal growth
C. Evaluation for fetal anomalies
D. Evaluation of amniotic fluid volume
E. PUBS for genetic evaluation

Answer: E

The first four choices address the issues of fetal growth and fetal well-being, both of which require assessment at this time. PUBS has a place in the evaluation of the growth-restricted fetus, but only after the diagnosis of IUGR has been made and then under specific conditions when the risk of the procedure outweighs the risk of not obtaining the information from the test. It is not yet apparent that PUBS is indicated.

Ultrasonographic evaluation shows concordant growth of fetal head and trunk, but an overall growth in the twentieth percentile for the estimated gestational age. The biophysical profile is reassuring (10 of 10). How should this patient be managed? What tests should be used and how often are they to be done?

A. NST, BPP, and assessment of interval fetal growth weekly
B. NST, BPP, and assessment of interval fetal growth biweekly
C. NST, BPP, and assessment of interval fetal growth at 36 weeks
D. NST, BPP, and assessment of interval fetal growth when the patient goes into labor

Answer: A

Continued growth and evidence of fetal well-being are the main issues. If data suggest a nonreassuring fetal status, delivery by appropriate means is indicated.

At her 37-week evaluation, the NST is reactive, and the BPP is 10/10. The infant has grown but is still at the twentieth percentile. Your plan of management is

A. The same
B. Induction of labor
C. Cesarean birth

(Continued)

Answer: A

Maintain the same management because the fetus has grown, although still in the twentieth percentile, and the tests show evidence of fetal well-being.

At her 38-week evaluation, the NST is reactive, and BPP is 8/10 with markedly decreased amniotic fluid. The infant has grown but is in the eighteenth percentile. Your plan of management is

A. The same
B. Induction of labor
C. Cesarean birth

Answer: B

Oligohydramnios is an ominous sign in a growth-restricted fetus, and at 38 weeks delivery is indicated. A trial of labor is appropriate, but preparation for cesarean birth should be made because it is unknown what fetal reserves remain to deal with the stress of labor.

CHAPTER

20

THIRD-TRIMESTER BLEEDING

CHAPTER OBJECTIVES

This chapter deals primarily with APGO Objective(s):

OBJECTIVE 24   Third-Trimester Bleeding

A. Describe the approach to the patient with third trimester bleeding, including the methods to differentiate among its causes (such as placenta previa and abruptio placentae), the maternal and fetal complications associated with these causes, and the management of them.

B. Describe the management of shock secondary to obstetric hemorrhage, including the components of and indications for the use of the various blood products.

An estimated 5% of women describe bleeding of some extent during pregnancy. At times, the amount of bleeding is hardly more than "spotting," whereas at other times profuse hemorrhage can lead to maternal death in a very short time. In most cases, antepartum bleeding is minimal spotting, often following sexual intercourse, and is thought to be related to trauma to the friable ectocervix. Table 20.1 lists causes of bleeding in the second half of pregnancy.

TABLE 20.1. Causes of Bleeding in the Second Half of Pregnancy

> Vulva
> > Varicose veins
> > Tears or lacerations
> Vagina
> > Tears or lacerations
> Cervix
> > Polyp
> > Glandular tissue (normal)
> > Cervicitis
> > Carcinoma
> Intrauterine
> > Uterine rupture
> > Placenta previa
> > Abruptio placentae
> > Vasa previa

A previous Pap test and examination of the lower genital tract should eliminate the likelihood of lower genital tract neoplasms in most cases. At times, patients may mistake bleeding from hemorrhoids or even hematuria for vaginal bleeding, but the difference is easily distinguished by examination.

The two causes of hemorrhage in the second half of pregnancy that require greatest attention, because of the associated maternal and fetal morbidity and mortality rates, are *placenta previa* and *abruptio placentae*. Various characteristics of these entities are compared in Table 20.2.

PLACENTA PREVIA

Placenta previa refers to an *abnormal location of the placenta over, or in close proximity to, the internal cervical os.* Placenta previa can be categorized as *complete or total* if the entire cervical os is covered; *partial,* if the margin of the placenta extends across part but not all of the internal os; *marginal,* if the edge of the placenta lies adjacent to the internal os; and *low lying,* if the placenta is located near but not directly adjacent to the internal os (Figure 20.1). The etiology of placenta previa is not understood, but abnormal vascularization has long been proposed as a mechanism for this abnormal placement of the placenta. In

---

TABLE 20.2. Characteristics of Placenta Previa and Abruptio Placentae

Characteristic	Placenta Previa	Abruptio Placentae
Magnitude of blood loss	Variable	Variable
Duration	Often ceases within 1–2 hours	Usually continues
Abdominal discomfort	None	Can be severe
Fetal heart rate pattern on electronic monitoring	Normal	Tachycardia, then bradycardia; loss of variability; decelerations frequently present; intrauterine demise not rare
Coagulation defects	Rare	Associated, but infrequent; DIC often severe when present
Associated history	None	Cocaine use; abdominal trauma; maternal hypertension; multiple gestation; polyhydramnios

DIC = disseminated intravascular coagulation.

some cases, such as in twin pregnancy or if it is hydropic, the placenta may extend to the region of the internal cervical os because of its size alone. Increasing maternal age, increasing parity, and previous cesarean delivery are factors commonly associated with placenta previa, although recent evidence suggests that age alone is not an important factor.

The incidence of placenta previa varies with gestational age, usually reported overall as approximately 1 in 250 pregnancies. There is great variation in incidence, however, with parity. The incidence in nulliparas is only 1 in 1000 to 1500, whereas that in grandmultiparas is as high as 1 in 20. Women with the highest risk for placenta previa are grandmultiparas, those who have had a previous placenta previa (4% to 8%), and those who have had four or more cesarean sections. With common use of ultrasonography examinations, it has been shown repeatedly that the placenta may cover the internal cervical os in approximately 5% of pregnancies when examined at midpregnancy, a finding seen even more frequently earlier in gestation. Because of subsequent growth of both the upper and lower uterine segments, the placenta appears to "migrate" away from the internal os in the majority of cases. The likelihood of this apparent movement diminishes as the gestational age at first detection increases.

The average gestational age at the time of the first bleeding episode is 29 to 30 weeks. Although the bleeding may be substantial, it almost always ceases spontaneously, unless digital examination or other trauma occurs. The bleeding is caused by separation of part of the placenta from the lower uterine segment and cervix, possibly in response to mild uterine contractions. The blood that is lost is usually maternal in origin. The patient often describes a sudden onset of bleeding without any apparent antecedent signs. There is no pain associated with placenta previa in most cases, unless coincident with labor or with an abruptio placentae (approximately 5% to 10% of cases).

Ultrasonography has been of enormous benefit in localizing the placenta, especially when the placenta is anterior or lateral. If the placenta lies in the posterior portion of the lower uterine segment, its exact relation with the internal os may be more difficult to ascertain. In most cases, though, ultrasonography examination can accurately diagnose placenta previa (Figure 20.2) or, by illustrating the placenta location away from the cervix and lower uterine segment, exclude it as a cause for bleeding. In some instances, transvaginal ultrasonography may be a useful adjunct to the transabdominal approach, especially in the case of posterior placenta.

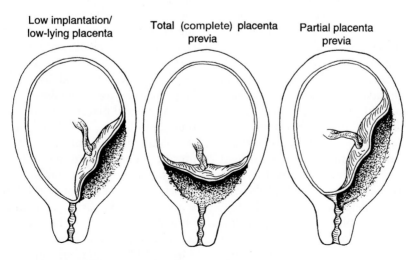

Low implantation/low-lying placenta   Total (complete) placenta previa   Partial placenta previa

FIGURE 20.1.   Placenta previa.

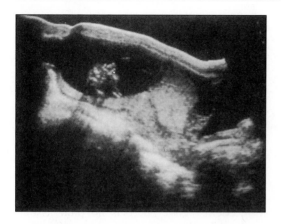

FIGURE 20.2.   Posterior placenta previa on transabdominal ultrasound.

The basic management of patients with placenta previa includes initial hospitalization with hemodynamic stabilization, followed by expectant management until fetal maturity has occurred. Ideal expectant management would be continuous hospitalization with enforced bed rest and immediate access to emergency care, but this is increasingly prohibited by cost issues. After initial hospital management, care as an outpatient may be considered if certain criteria are met. These include a highly motivated patient who clearly understands and will comply with instructions concerning restrictions of activity, the constant attendance of a responsible adult to assist in the event of an emergency situation, and the presence of ready transportation to the hospital.

The number of bleeding episodes is unrelated to the degree of placenta previa or to the prognosis for fetal survival. Such expectant management combined with appropriate use of blood transfusion and cesarean birth have resulted in the lowering of the maternal mortality rate from 25%–30% to < 1% and the perinatal mortality rate from 60%–70% to < 10%. If the fetus is thought to be mature by gestational age criteria or by amniocentesis for fetal lung maturity testing, there is little benefit to be gained by a delay in delivery. The further from term that bleeding from placenta previa occurs, the more important it is to delay delivery to allow for further fetal growth and maturation. The degree of

bleeding and the maturity of the fetus must be constantly weighed in managing these patients. Fetal maturity is usually assessed at approximately 36 weeks, with cesarean delivery performed once the fetus is deemed mature.

In some cases, when the location of the placenta cannot be accurately determined by ultrasound and delivery is required, the route of delivery is determined by a *double setup examination*. This procedure involves careful evaluation of the cervix in the operating room with full preparations for rapid cesarean delivery. If placental tissue is seen or palpated at the internal cervical os, prompt cesarean delivery is performed. If the placental margin is away from the internal os, artificial rupture of the membranes and oxytocin induction of labor may be performed in anticipation of vaginal delivery. Before the widespread use of ultrasound, this procedure was done more frequently than it is in modern obstetrics; nonetheless, it is still an important tool in selected cases.

An attempt at vaginal delivery of a patient with placenta previa may be indicated if the delivery can be accomplished with minimal blood loss and if the fetus is dead, has major fetal malformations, or is clearly previable. If making such an attempt is appropriate, ceasing the process and moving to cesarean delivery for a maternal indication must always be considered. Placenta previa is associated with a nearly doubling of the rate of congenital malformations, the most serious including major anomalies of the central nervous system, gastrointestinal tract, cardiovascular system, and respiratory tract. At the time of diagnosis of placenta previa, a detailed fetal survey should be performed for anomalies.

Abnormal placental location can be further complicated by abnormal growth of the placental mass into the substance of the uterus, a condition termed *placenta previa accreta*. In placenta previa accreta, the poorly formed decidua of the lower uterine segment offers little resistance to trophoblastic invasion. The incidence of this severe complication is variously reported as 5% to 10% of placenta previas, although the incidence is much higher in patients

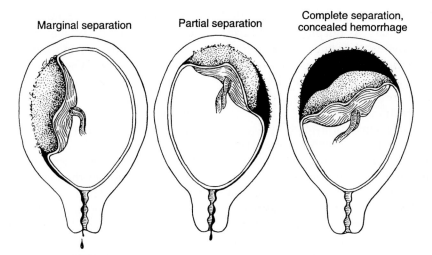

FIGURE 20.3.   The relation between vaginal bleeding and abruptio placentae.

with multiple previous cesarean sections. At the time of delivery, sustained and significant bleeding may ensue, often requiring hysterectomy.

ABRUPTIO PLACENTAE

Whereas placenta previa refers to the abnormal location of the placenta, abruptio placentae, often called placental abruption, refers to the *premature separation of the normally implanted placenta* from the uterine wall. Although it shares some clinical features with placenta previa, particularly vaginal bleeding, other characteristics serve to distinguish abruptio placentae from placenta previa, the most important of which are abdominal discomfort and painful uterine contractions (see Table 20.2).

Placental abruption occurs when there is hemorrhage into the decidua basalis, leading to premature placental separation and further bleeding. The cause for this bleeding is not known. Placental abruption is associated with maternal hypertension and sudden decompression of the uterus in cases of rupture of membranes in a patient with excessive amniotic fluid (hydramnios) or after delivery of the first of multiple fetuses. A more recent and serious association involves cocaine use by the mother,

which leads to intense vasoconstriction and, in some cases, sudden separation of the placenta from the uterine wall. Placental abruption can also occur following trauma, even when the extent of injury is not considered serious. For example, pregnant women involved in motor vehicle accidents can sustain placental abruption even though lap belts and shoulder strap restraints are used. Moreover, direct trauma to the abdomen is not required, because sudden force applied elsewhere to the body can result in coup and contrecoup injury.

The anatomic relation between vaginal bleeding and placental abruption is shown in Figure 20.3. If the bleeding and subsequent separation of a placenta permit access to the cervical os, vaginal bleeding will be apparent. If the placental location is higher in the uterus, or if the bleeding is more central and the margins of the placenta remain attached to the underlying uterus, blood may not escape into the vagina. Thus the amount of vaginal bleeding is extremely variable, from none to heavy. The bleeding into the basalis stimulates the uterine muscle to contract, and the uterus will be painful to the patient and tender to touch. Unusually painful uterine contractions are frequent and the uterus may feel constantly tense. At times, the bleeding can penetrate the uterine musculature to such an extent that, at the time of cesarean delivery, the entire uterus has a purplish or bluish appearance, owing to such extravasation of blood (*Couvelaire uterus*). Despite its unusual appearance, no treatment is required, because spontaneous resolution of the condition occurs postpartum.

Because the separation of the placenta from the uterus interferes with oxygenation of the fetus, a nonreassuring fetal status is quite common in cases of significant placental abruption. Thus, in any patient in whom placental abruption is suspected, electronic fetal monitoring should be included in the initial management. Fetal death caused by deprivation of oxygen is, unfortunately, not rare with placental abruption.

Coagulation abnormalities may also be found, thereby compounding the patient's already compromised status. Placental abruption is the most common cause of consumptive coagulopathy in pregnancy and is manifested by hypofibrinogenemia as well as by increased levels of fibrin degradation products. The platelet count can also be decreased, and prothrombin time and partial thromboplastin time can be increased as well. Such coagulopathy is a result of intravascular and retroplacental coagulation. The intravascular fibrinogen is converted to fibrin by way of the extrinsic clotting cascade. Thus not only is serum fibrinogen decreased but platelets and other clotting factors are thereby also depleted. Transfusion with crystalloid and whole blood should be implemented as soon as possible for those patients who require either volume replacement or oxygen-carrying capacity. Whole blood helps to replace not only volume but also oxygen-carrying capacity. Whole blood may also contain some clotting factors, including fibrinogen. Many experts recommend component therapy (e.g., packed red cells, platelets, fresh frozen plasma) rather than whole blood therapy (Table 20.3). The extent of placental abruption is generally categorized as the proportion of the maternal surface of the placenta on which a clot is detected at the time of delivery (e.g., 50% abruption).

Ultrasound is of little benefit in diagnosing placental abruption, except to exclude placenta previa as a cause for the hemorrhage. Relatively large retroplacental clots may be detected on ultrasound examination, but the absence of ultrasonographically identified retroplacental clots does not rule out the possibility of placental abruption, and conversely, a retroplacental echogenic area can be seen in patients without placental abruption. The diagnosis rests on the classic clinical presentation of vaginal bleeding, a tender uterus, and frequent uterine contractions with some evidence of fetal distress. The extravasation of blood into the uterine muscle causes contractions such that the resting intrauterine pressure, when measured with an intrauterine pressure catheter, is often elevated; this sign can be helpful in making the diagnosis.

Management of a patient with placental abruption when the fetus is mature is hemodynamic stabilization and delivery. Careful attention to blood component therapy is

TABLE 20.3. Blood Replacement Products

Component (volume/unit)	Factors Present	Discussion
Packed RBCs (200)	RBCs only	Replaces RBC cell mass only
Fresh-frozen plasma (200–400)	All procoagulants; no platelets	~1 g fibrinogen per unit
Cryoprecipitate (20–50)	Fibrinogen; factors VIII and XIII	Variable fibrinogen content; averages 0.25 mg/bag
Fresh whole blood (500)	RBCs and all procoagulants	Often difficult to obtain

RBCs = red blood cells.

critical, and the coagulation status must be followed closely. Unless there is evidence of fetal distress or hemodynamic instability, vaginal delivery by oxytocin induction of labor is preferable to a cesarean delivery, although the maternal or fetal status may require that abdominal delivery be performed. When the fetus is not mature and the placental abruption is limited and not associated with premature labor or fetal or maternal distress, observation with close monitoring of both fetal and maternal well-being may be considered while awaiting fetal maturity.

VASA PREVIA

Although rarely encountered, vasa previa presents significant risk to the fetus. In vasa previa, the umbilical cord inserts into the membranes of the placenta (rather than into the central mass of the placental tissue), and one such vessel lies below the presenting fetal part in the vicinity of the internal os. If this vessel ruptures, fetal bleeding occurs. Because of the low blood volume of the fetus, seemingly insignificant amounts of blood may place the fetus in jeopardy. A small amount of vaginal bleeding associated with fetal tachycardia may be the clinical presentation. A test to distinguish fetal blood from maternal blood, such as the Kleihauer-Betke or the Apt test, can be of value when such a condition is suspected. These tests distinguish between maternal and fetal blood on the basis of the marked resistance to pH changes in fetal red cells compared with the friable nature of adult red cells in the presence of strong bases. Immediate cesarean section is the only way to save the fetus in vasa previa.

UTERINE RUPTURE AS A CAUSE OF OBSTETRIC HEMORRHAGE

Separation of the muscular wall of the pregnant uterus occurs in a fraction of one percent of pregnancies, most commonly associated with labor in a patient who has had a cesarean section (vaginal birth after cesarean section, VBAC). The incidence approaches 0.5% for patients with an uncomplicated previous lower segment transverse cesarean section, but may approach one in four to one in three patients with previous incisions of the upper uterine segment or fundus (previous classical cesarean section, previous myomectomy, or repair of congenital uterine anomalie). Other conditions associated with such intrapartum rupture include uterine hyperstimulation (either endogenous, as in chorioamnionitis, or exogenous with pitocin induction or augmentation of labor), uterine anomalie, placenta increta or percreta, grandmultiparity, obstructed labor (fetal macrosomia, uterine myomas blocking the birth passage, fetopelvic disproportion), and previous perforation of the uterus associated with dilatation and curettage (D&C), hysteroscopy, or forceps delivery. Often such separation occurs slowly involving only the muscular wall without breach of the overlying peritonium. In this case, *uterine scar dehiscence or uterine window formation,* bleeding is minimal, the fetus remains in utero, uterine function continues, there is no disruption of placental function if the scar is not under the placenta, and delivery is unimpeded. The rent is discovered during the postpartum examination. Uterine rupture is when the rent is relatively more rapid with disruption of the peritoneum and uterine wall, bleeding, extrusion of the fetus from the uterus, separation of the placenta with nonreassuring fetal status, and/or shock, and on occasion disseminated intravascular disease (DIC).

Because uterine rupture may be difficult to recognize, close intrapartum surveillance with appreciation of the risk factors is requisite. The most common early finding is nonreassuring fetal status, with fetal heart rate decelerations, bradycardia, and/or failure to detect fetal heart activity in about one half to three fourths of cases. Bleeding, shock, pain, and altered uterine activity are also noted in varying numbers of patients. Management consists of immediate exploratory laparotomy, retrieval and hopefully resuscitation of the fetus, and repair of the uterine rent. In most cases, repair is possible, although in some cases damage is sufficiently severe that hysterectomy is required. The management of women with a previous uterine rupture confined to the lower uterine segment is controversial, as the repeat rupture rate is about 5%. If the uterine rupture involves the upper segment of the uterus, the repeat rate approaches one third and cesarean delivery at 36–37 weeks is recommended.

Antepartum uterine rupture is rarely spontaneous, but is rather associated with trauma in most situations. Auto accidents with improper seat belt placement and assault are the two most common situations encountered.

APPROACH TO A PATIENT WITH VAGINAL BLEEDING IN THE SECOND HALF OF GESTATION

In any woman with vaginal bleeding during the second half of pregnancy, fetal and maternal status should be evaluated promptly. At the same time that a search is undertaken for the cause of the bleeding, attention must be directed toward stabiliza-tion of the maternal hemodynamic state. The approach is not unlike that for any hemorrhaging patient and includes ready access for fluid replacement through one or more large-bore intravenous catheters, serial complete blood counts, type and cross-match of ample amounts of blood, and if the condition is unstable, intracardiac monitoring. Attention to urinary output is a simple and important reflection of the volume status of a patient. Because normal antepartum blood volume expansion is substantial, pregnant women may lose considerable amounts of blood before vital sign changes are apparent.

In more than half of the cases of significant vaginal bleeding in pregnancy, no specific cause can be discovered despite careful evaluation. In general, patients with significant bleeding should remain hospitalized until delivery, although in some cases minimal bleeding ceases, and the patient appears normal in every way. Caution is advised, however, because patients with bleeding of undetermined etiology can be at greater risk for preterm delivery, intrauterine growth restriction, and fetal distress than patients with bleeding of known cause.

CASE STUDIES

Case 20A

A 26-year-old G1 at 29 weeks of gestation by last menstrual period (LMP) has phoned the hospital, saying she had an episode of bright red vaginal bleeding without other symptoms approximately 2 hours ago. You have not seen her previously.

Questions Case 20A

Your best instruction to her is to

A. Call back if there is another episode of bleeding

B. Come in for evaluation
C. Make an office appointment
D. Make an appointment in radiology for ultrasound evaluation

Answer: B

Immediate evaluation of fetal and maternal status is required. Placenta previa may present in this manner; and although the first bleeding episode may have been self-limited, the second may be much more profuse. Although there are no reported symptoms, abruptio placentae is still a possibility with the associated need for prompt fetal evaluation.

The patient arrives at the hospital and is found to have stable vital signs. Further history includes a fall, in which she hit her abdomen, approximately 6 hours before the bleeding episode. The patient's physical examination reveals a very mildly tender uterus over the area of the fall and minimal vaginal spotting, and speculum examination shows no cervical dilation or evidence of rupture of membranes. Immediate management should include all EXCEPT

A. IV fluids
B. Electronic fetal monitoring
C. Ultrasound evaluation
D. Amniocentesis
E. Kleihauer-Betke test

Answer: D

Because the mother is hemodynamically stable, immediate evaluation of fetal status, using electronic fetal monitoring and ultrasound, is indicated because you have not established a cause of the bleeding. Ultrasound examination is often advised before any vaginal examination, although a careful speculum examination is advocated before ultrasound examination by some authorities. Venous access is indicated in the event of further bleeding. Amniocentesis may be indicated in the future, but at present it is too invasive for the information needed.

Evaluation reveals a normal 29-week fetus with normal movement and amniotic fluid volume and a partial placenta previa, which is posteriorly located. The Kleihauer-Betke test is negative. Over the next 12 hours, there is no more bleeding and no other symptoms. The best management at this time is

A. Cesarean birth to avoid further risk to mother and fetus

B. Amniocentesis for lecithin:sphingomyelin (L:S) ratio in preparation for cesarean birth
C. Resumption of normal activities, because it is only a marginal and not full placenta previa
D. Bed rest
E. Schedule a cesarean birth for 40 weeks of gestation

Answer: D

Bed rest and pelvic rest are the basics of management. A marginal placenta previa at 29 weeks may "resolve" by term, so cesarean section is not a certainty. With fetal well-being ensured for the time and no further bleeding, delivery is not indicated.

Case 20B

A 26-year-old G6 P5005 presents for her routine antepartum visit at 18 weeks' gestational age. She is distressed because at her ultrasound visit the day before she was told by the technician that her placenta was partly over the opening of her womb.

Question Case 20B

Which of the following would you tell the patient?

A. She has a placenta previa and will definitely require cesarean section
B. She has a vasa previa and will definitely require cesarean section
C. She has a placental abruption and will definitely require cesarean section
D. She has a placenta previa and may require cesarean section
E. She has a vasa previa and may require cesarean section
F. She has a placental abruption and may require cesarean section

(Continued)

Answer: D

The ultrasound is consistent with a partial placenta previa. Because the growth of the upper and lower uterine segments may result in the placenta "migrating away" from the cervical os, it is too early to be certain that cesarean section will be required.

Case 20C

A 31-year-old G3 P1011 who believes she is approximately 8 months pregnant calls complaining of bright red vaginal bleeding and some cramps for the last hour. On questioning, you learn she has had no pre-natal care, was in a drug rehabilitation program but left a few weeks ago, and is homeless.

Questions Case 20C

Your best action is which of the following?

A. Because she has had no prenatal care to this point, there is little you can do until she is in labor; thus you advise her to call again when she is in labor
B. Ask her to come in for evaluation
C. Ask her to come in for induction of labor
D. Ask her to call your office for an appointment sometime in the next 2 weeks
E. Tell her to return immediately to her drug program

Answer: B

She needs evaluation for antepartum bleeding, which may have several causes, including placenta previa, abruptio pla-centae, and labor. Neither induction nor any delay in evaluation is indicated.

She is evaluated, and you discover a nor-motensive, slightly disoriented woman with a fundal height of 30 cm and a slightly tender uterus. She has irregular

uterine contractions and a baseline fetal heart rate of 150 with good beat-to-beat variability. Ultrasound shows a 30-week gestation with adequate amniotic fluid and a fundal placenta without evidence of pla-centa previa or abruptio placentae. Urine drug screen is positive for cocaine and alcohol. Careful pelvic examination by speculum shows her cervix to be closed with minimal bleeding and no evidence of rupture of membranes. Your most likely diagnosis is

A. Labor
B. Abruptio placentae
C. Placenta previa
D. Cervicitis
E. Cervical carcinoma

Answer: B

There is no evidence of placenta previa or labor. Although there is no evidence of abruptio placentae on ultrasound, it occurs more frequently in patients who use cocaine.

Your best management is

A. Observation at home
B. Observation in the hospital
C. Induction of labor
D. Cesarean birth
E. Discharge to the drug rehabilitation program

Answer: B

There is no evidence of maternal or fetal compromise requiring delivery. Given her drug use, noncompliance, and homeless status, observation in the hospital is espe-cially appropriate, with serial evaluation of maternal and fetal status.

Case 20D

A 24-year-old G2 P1001 is in early spon-taneous labor. She had a lower segment cesarean section for "failure to progress" three years earlier. On physical examina-

tion her uterus appears normal in size and configuration and appropriate for a term singleton gestation. Her birth canal seems adequate in size and her spontaneous mechanism of labor normal.

Questions Case 20D

She asks about her risk of uterine rupture during labor. You suggest it is

A. 0.5%
B. 5.5%
C. 10.5%
D. 15.5%

Answer: A

After she reaches about 6 centimeters, she makes no progress for 3 hours. Pitocin augmentation is begun, and she again progresses in dilation. When she is about 8 centimeters, moderate bright red vaginal bleeding is noted, the patient's blood pressure falls markedly, and variable fetal heart rate decelerations are noted. The patient complains of increased uterine pain. Your management consists of

A. An epidural anesthesia
B. Fluid bolus and cessation of augmentation
C. Exploratory laparotomy
D. Reassurance and continued augmented labor

Answer: A

CHAPTER

21

POSTTERM PREGNANCY

CHAPTER OBJECTIVES

This chapter deals primarily with APGO Objective(s):

OBJECTIVE 32   Postterm Pregnancy

Describe normal, prolonged, and postterm pregnancy, and the complications, methods of fetal surveillance, and the maternal and fetal management associated with them.

Normal pregnancy lasts from 38 to 42 weeks, which is considered "term." Stated another way, term is the due date or estimated date of confinement (EDC) ± 2 weeks. *A patient who has not delivered by the completion of the forty-second week* (294 days from the first day of the last normal menstrual period) is said to be postterm (a common synonym is postdates). This condition occurs in approximately 8% to 10% of pregnancies and carries with it an increased risk of adverse outcome. The increased morbidity and mortality in a small percentage of cases, however, warrants careful evaluation of all postterm pregnancies. In addition, postterm pregnancies can create significant stress for the patient, her family, and those caring for her. Therefore, the physician should reassure the patient and discuss with her the options for management.

ETIOLOGY

The most common "cause" of postterm pregnancy is inaccurate estimation of gestational age (dating). Inaccurate dating is more likely in women with irregular menses, those who seek prenatal care later in pregnancy, those with delayed ovulation (for example, a woman who has just stopped using oral contraceptives), and those who simply do not remember their last menstrual period accurately. Inaccurate dating leading to the erroneous classification of a pregnancy as postterm has two important sequelae. First, these pregnancies are labeled "high-risk," costly increased evaluations are employed, and the likelihood of intervention increases. The latter leads to the second sequela—increased intervention usually means delivery by induction or cesarean section, both of which are associated with increased maternal and fetal morbidity. Other less common causes are listed in Table 21.1. Uterine contractility has also been shown to be diminished in some cases of postterm pregnancy, suggesting a cause intrinsic to the myometrium. Whatever the etiology, there is a tendency for recurrence of postterm pregnancy. *Approximately 50% of patients having one postterm pregnancy will experience prolonged pregnancy with the next gestation.*

TABLE 21.1. Factors Associated with "Postterm" Pregnancy

Factor	Discussion
Inaccurate or unknown dates	*Most common cause;* high association with and major risk factor of late or no prenatal care
Irregular ovulation; variation in length of follicular phase	Results in overestimation of gestational age
Altered estrogen:progesterone ratio Anencephaly	Decreased production of 16α-hydroxydehydroepiandrosterone sulfate, a precursor of estriol
Fetal adrenal hypoplasia	Decreased fetal production precursors of estriol
Placental sulfatase deficiency	X-linked disease prevents placenta conversion of sulfated estrogen precursors
Extrauterine pregnancy	Pregnancy not in uterus, no labor (see Chapter 15)

EFFECTS

The morbidity and mortality rates for the postterm fetus increase severalfold compared with term pregnancies because of several reasons. Approximately 20% of truly postterm newborns demonstrate some elements of *dysmaturity, or postmaturity syndrome.* Dysmature infants often are growth-restricted and have loss of subcutaneous fat, giving the child a wizened, elderly appearance. Integumentary changes are also seen, including long nails, scaling epidermis, and meconium staining of the nails, skin, and umbilical cord. These infants may demonstrate altered glucose and bilirubin metabolism and are at risk for hypoglycemia and hyperbilirubinemia.

Approximately 25% of prolonged pregnancies result in a *macrosomic infant* (i.e., birth weight > 4000 or 4500 g, depending on the definition used) and may occur in any prolonged pregnancy, although maternal obesity or diabetes mellitus raises the risk. These infants may demonstrate altered glucose and bilirubin metabolism and are at risk for hypoglycemia and hyperbilirubinemia. They have an increased incidence of birth trauma, especially shoulder dystocia, fracture of the clavicle, and associated brachial plexus injury (Erb, or Erb-Duchenne, palsy) during vaginal delivery as well as of the need for cesarean section as a result of fetopelvic disproportion. *Brachial plexus injury* is reported in approximately 1 in 500 term deliveries and is especially likely in the delivery of macrosomic infants, breech deliveries, or in difficult deliveries, although it may occur in the seemingly uneventful, easy delivery. In the *Erb (or Erb-Duchenne) palsy,* or paralysis, stretch or tear injury to the upper roots of the brachial plexus results in paralysis of the deltoid and infraspinatus muscles and flexor muscles of the forearm, causing the limb to hang limply close to the side, forearm extended and internally rotated; finger function is usually retained. Less frequently, damage is limited to the lower nerves of the brachial plexus, causing *Klumpke's paralysis,* or paralysis of the hand. As most injuries are mild, treatment is expectant, with splints and physical

therapy and the anticipation of complete or nearly complete recovery in three to six months. In fetal macrosomia, there can also be maternal trauma, with lacerations of the maternal perineum or, in the case of cesarean delivery, of the uterus and other pelvic organs.

The *diminished amniotic fluid volume, or oligohydramnios,* associated with postterm pregnancy is largely responsible for the *increased fetal stress and nonreassuring fetal status* seen late in pregnancy and in the intrapartum period. Amniotic fluid volume reaches its maximal amount of approximately 1 liter at 36 to 37 weeks' gestation and thereafter diminishes to an average of less than half that at 42 weeks. The umbilical cord normally floats freely in the amniotic fluid. The loss of significant fluid volume means a loss in protection for the umbilical cord so that impingement on the cord can occur, which may be manifest on electronic fetal heart rate monitoring as variable decelerations. *Cord accidents* (complete occlusion of the umbilical cord) are more common when there is oligohydramnios, and unfortunately, are not always preceded by fetal heart rate abnormalities.

Another special concern in postterm pregnancies is meconium passage and the possibility of aspiration of meconium (*meconium aspiration syndrome*), which can lead to severe respiratory distress from mechanical obstruction of both small and large airways as well as meconium chemical pneumonitis. Meconium passage is not limited to postterm pregnancies, although postterm pregnancy, especially if there is oligohydramnios, is a substantial risk factor; it is seen in 13% to 15% of all term pregnancies. The incidence of meconium passage increases as pregnancy becomes prolonged. Because diminished amniotic fluid volume is also present in postterm pregnancy, the neonate is more likely to aspirate more concentrated solutions of this potentially toxic, particulate meconium.

Increasingly severe *placental dysfunction* with decreased transfer of water, electrolytes, glucose, amino acids, and oxygen can occur in postterm pregnancy. In normal pregnancy, the placenta reaches its maximum size and surface area at about 37 weeks gestational age with functional peak at the same time. Thereafter, size, surface area, and function decrease. To compensate, especially in the postdates intervals, the fetus may decrease its energy requirements by decreasing growth and deposition of fat and glycogen. Second, it may slow movement. Lastly, it may experience degrees of hypoxia, during movement or with contractions, or at rest. Approximately 40% of placentas from postterm pregnancies demonstrate placental infarcts, calcification, and fibrosis consistent with decreased functional capability. This intrauterine nutritional and respiratory deprivation may contribute to fetal stress and to the development of postmaturity syndrome, and to fetuses who demonstrate nonreassuring fetal status, antepartum or in labor.

DIAGNOSIS

The diagnosis of postterm pregnancy rests on establishment of the correct gestational age. Every effort should be made to accurately assess gestational age as early as possible in pregnancy, when the parameters used for this purpose are most discriminating and reliable. With improved access to prenatal care and the greater importance placed on accurate gestational age assessment, the percentage of patients in whom postterm pregnancy is suspected but whose dates are uncertain has diminished. Nonetheless, a substantial number of patients do not seek prenatal care early in pregnancy or do not have an accurate gestational age determination. Physicians should be suspicious of the presumed due date of any patient who first appears for prenatal care late in pregnancy who might be "1 or 2 months overdue." Care should be taken to properly evaluate and monitor her fetus for these problems associated with postterm pregnancy.

MANAGEMENT

The first step in management of postterm pregnancy is a careful review of the information used to establish the gestational age to be as certain as possible that the estimate is correct. *Once a patient approaches 41 weeks' gestation (1 week past her due date), the management options are either to induce labor or to continue surveillance of fetal well-being until spontaneous labor occurs.*

If gestational age is felt to be firmly established, factors that influence the decision of whether to deliver or not rest with the patient's concerns and desires, the assessment of fetal well-being, and the status of the cervix. Induction of labor is appropriate if the cervix is favorable (see Chapter 7, Induction of Labor and the Bishop Score) and if the patient prefers labor induction.

If the cervix is not favorable or the patient does not wish induction of labor, fetal well-being is monitored while awaiting spontaneous labor or a change in the cervix so that induction is appropriate. A variety of management schemes have been devised for this "waiting period," none of which is clearly superior. Daily fetal movement counting is included in most management plans, with decreased perceived fetal movement an indication for further, timely evaluation of fetal well-being. Weekly monitoring of amniotic fluid volume is commonly employed, often employing an amniotic fluid index (AFI) measurement where the largest pocket of fluid is measured in each of the four quadrants of the uterus and summed; a value of more than 5 or so is considered within normal limits and less than that, oligohydramnios. This diagnosis is usually considered a sufficient indication for delivery. Antepartum fetal heart rate monitoring is also commonly used, either nonstress tests (NSTs) employed twice a week or oxytocin challenge tests employed once or twice a week. The biophysical profile (BPP) is a combination of ultrasound and fetal heart rate monitoring information and may be used once or twice a week. Doppler flow studies of the umbilical artery are also considered useful. These studies are discussed in Chapter 5. All of these tests are most useful when the data obtained are viewed in the context of the whole pregnancy, maternal and fetal factors.

If the gestational age is not well established, the clinician uses whatever information is available to determine the best date. Amniocentesis is not especially helpful, as fetal lung maturity is rarely a question in the postterm evaluation. When the best date is selected, a management plan similar to that for a postterm pregnancy with well-established dates is used.

Although there is no absolute time within which labor must be induced, many physicians believe that delivery should be effected by either 42 or 43 weeks. Induction of labor can be attempted using intravenous oxytocin (Pitocin) or prostaglandin vaginal suppositories (Prostin; carboprost tromethamine). In some patients, if the cervix is quite unfavorable, cervical "ripening" can be accelerated using an intracervical or intravaginal preparation of prostaglandin or laminaria, a hydrophilic device that dilates the cervix (see Chapter 7). Rarely, cesarean section without attempted induction may be performed. Proponents of such cutoff dates are said to favor *"aggressive management,"* citing increased morbidity and mortality after 42 or 43 completed weeks' gestation. Modern methods for surveillance of fetal well-being make it less logical to be dogmatic about mandatory induction at a given gestational age. Proponents of *"expectant management"* allow pregnancy to continue for some time as long as there is evidence of fetal well-being.

Because of the risk of macrosomia-associated birth trauma, ultrasonographic estimation of fetal weight should be obtained before any induction of labor in a postterm pregnancy. If the estimated fetal weight is > 4500 to 5000 g, cesarean section is often the appropriate mode of delivery.

Patients with postterm pregnancies should be advised to come promptly to the hospital when labor pains commence. Once the onset of regular contractions occurs, careful electronic fetal monitoring should be used throughout labor because of the risk of fetal stress/distress. Intrapartum management includes the artificial rupture of membranes, when possible, to allow detection of meconium and to allow the placement of a fetal scalp electrode and intrauterine pressure catheter (IUPC). If the decreased amniotic fluid is sufficient to permit undue pressure on the umbilical cord, deceleration of the fetal heart rate may occur. Infusion of normal saline through the IUPC (amnioinfusion) may provide a buffer for the cord and eliminate these decelerations. Because of the increased risk of cesarean delivery for fetal stress and because of the potential problems associated with meconium, both anesthesia and pediatric personnel should be alerted that a postterm patient is in labor.

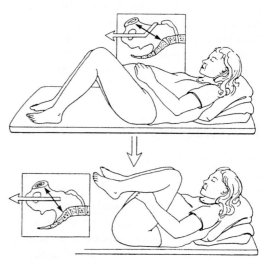

FIGURE 21.1.   McRoberts maneuver: hyperflexion of thighs to aid in management of shoulder dystocia.

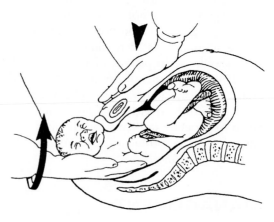

FIGURE 21.2.   Rotation plus suprapubic pressure to aid in management of shoulder dystocia.

At the time of delivery, special precautions are taken. If meconium passage has been noted, the infant's nasopharynx and oropharynx should be suctioned before delivery of the shoulders, since compression of the chest has forced fluid within the chest upward to the pharynx. Pediatric support should be in the delivery room to provide prompt visual examination of the infant's airway to a level beneath the larynx and to suction any meconium material. This infant management significantly decreases, but does not eliminate, the likelihood of meconium aspiration syndrome. Because of the risk of macrosomia, the physician performing the delivery should be familiar with the techniques used to treat shoulder dystocia such as exaggerated flexion of the thighs (Figure 21.1) and suprapubic pressure (Figure 21.2).

CASE STUDIES

Case 21A

A 35-year-old G1 P0 patient presents on June 6 for prenatal care, saying that her previous doctor said she was due "about now." The prenatal records she brings include the notation of a "light last menstrual period" (LMP) on September 20; a "period" on August 25; fetal movement "sometime just before Christmas"; a first pelvic examination on November 1, which showed an anteverted 10- to 11-week-size uterus; and an ultrasound on January 4 consistent with a 15-week gestation and another on May 15 consistent with a "term" pregnancy. The patient says the baby is moving as much this week as during the previous 2 weeks. The patient has no obstetric risk factors. Physical examination is completely normal. The fundal height is 38 cm and the cervix is closed and uneffaced with the vertex at −1 station. The patient asks to be induced and delivered now.

Questions Case 21A

She should be told that

A. Another ultrasound should be obtained to clarify her gestational age
B. No action by the physician is needed
C. Induction is appropriate at this time
D. Further evaluation is needed before a course of management can be recommended

Answer: D

The patient's gestational age requires clarification before a rational management can be formulated. In addition, induction without indication poses undue risks to mother and fetus, especially with an unfavorable cervix as depicted in this case. Ultrasound is most useful in determination of gestational age in late first and second trimesters but much less accurate (± 2 to 3 weeks) in the third trimester.

Based on the information given, the best estimate of this patient's gestational age is

A. 38 weeks
B. 39 weeks
C. 40 weeks
D. 41 weeks
E. 42 weeks
F. 43 weeks

Answer: D

The LMP of September 20 was "light," whereas that of August 25 was "normal."

(Continued)

Although this is insufficient to establish dates, the "normal" LMP of August 25 is consistent with the first pelvic examination and midtrimester ultrasound and not inconsistent with the late trimester ultrasound. Thus setting a gestational age of 41 weeks is appropriate.

All of the following studies are appropriate at this time EXCEPT

A. Ultrasound to establish gestational age
B. Ultrasound to evaluate amniotic fluid volume
C. Biophysical profile
D. Electronic fetal monitoring of the fetus (nonstress or stress test)

Answer: A

Ultrasound is relatively imprecise in the last trimester for gestational age measurement, although it is useful for evaluation of amniotic fluid volume and for biophysical profile measurement. Likewise, electronic fetal monitoring (e.g., nonstress test) to assess the fetal status is appropriate.

All the studies performed on this patient were reassuring as to maternal and fetal status. One week later, on June 13 the patient reports that the baby is still moving well, although she feels more pelvic pressure and has been having cramps. On physical examination, the fundal height is unchanged and the cervix is 90% effaced and 3 cm dilated, with the vertex at 0 station with intact membranes. The patient again requests induction of labor. She should now be told that

A. Another ultrasound to determine gestational age is necessary
B. She should not worry; she will deliver when she is ready
C. Induction of labor is appropriate
D. Further studies are necessary before a course of management can be recommended

Answer: C

The patient's cervical examination has now changed to one favorable for induction, which is now the least risky management for mother and fetus. If the cervical examination had been unchanged, continued evaluation of fetal well-being would have been appropriate. Delivery would be indicated if there were evidence of fetal distress or at 42 or 43 weeks, depending on the physician's attitude toward the maximum allowable duration of gestation.

Case 21B

A patient G1 P0 at 41 weeks confirmed by first trimester ultrasound has had an unremarkable pregnancy. Fetal well-being studies are normal. The fundal height is 45 cm. On pelvic examination, the cervix is uneffaced and closed and the cephalic part is at –3 station. After 1 week of expectant management, the patient reports good fetal movement and some mild, somewhat regular contractions. On examination, fundal height is 44 cm, fetal heart rate is 140 beats per minute, and pelvic examination shows the vertex at –3 station, intact membranes, and a cervix dilated to 4 cm and 100% effaced. The patient requests induction of labor.

Question Case 21B

The patient should be told that

A. Another ultrasound will be ordered for clarification of gestational age
B. She should not worry; she will deliver when she is ready
C. Labor will be induced now
D. She is in labor

Answer: D

The duration of pregnancy is clear and no further studies are needed. A patient in early labor at 42 weeks' gestation should be allowed to labor there being no contraindication to the contrary.

Case 21C

A 19-year-old obese G3 P2002 presents in labor and delivery at 42 2/7 weeks' gestational age based on dates on a first trimester ultrasound, which was congruent. Her first two pregnancies ended in spontaneous labor and vaginal delivery of a 4200 g girl and a 4800 g boy, respectively. Her antepartum care was complicated by episodic care, including failure to obtain a 1-hour glucose tolerance test and to adhere to recommendations for evaluation of fetal well-being in the last 3 weeks of pregnancy. On examination her fundal height is 48 cm, her clinical pelvimetry is considered adequate, and she is dilated 5 cm at 95% effacement, vertex presentation at −2 station, and membranes intact.

Questions Case 21C

Proper management would include

A. Monitored labor
B. Amniotomy to engage the vertex
C. Cesarean section
D. Ultrasound determination of fetal weight

Answer: D

The fundal height and history are suggestive of repetitive macrosomia and postdates pregnancy.

On ultrasound evaluation, a male infant with an estimated fetal weight of 4900 g is noted. Proper management would include

A. Monitored labor
B. Amniotomy to engage the cervix
C. Cesarean section

Answer: C

The successful vaginal delivery of one macrosomic infant does not guarantee that of this pregnancy. Macrosomic infants have substantial risks at delivery, including shoulder dystocia and Erb palsy.

C H A P T E R

22

PRETERM LABOR

CHAPTER OBJECTIVES

This chapter deals primarily with APGO Objective(s):

OBJECTIVE 25   Preterm Labor

Describe the predisposing factors and causes of preterm labor and preterm delivery and the approach to and management of the patient with preterm contractions/labor, including the use of tocolytics, antibiotics, and steroids.

Labor occurring prior to the completion of 37 weeks of gestation, or 259 days from the last menstrual period (LMP), is considered preterm labor. Because *preterm birth* resulting from *preterm labor* (PTL) is the most common cause of perinatal morbidity and mortality, its prevention and treatment are major concerns in obstetric care. The *consequences of PTL and preterm birth* occur with increasing severity and frequency the earlier the gestational age of the newborn. Seventy-five percent of neonatal deaths that are not due to congenital malformations are associated with premature labor and birth. Besides perinatal death in the very young fetus, common complications of PTL include respiratory distress syndrome (RDS; also called hyaline membrane disease), intraventricular hemorrhage, necrotizing enterocolitis, sepsis, neurologic impairment, and seizures. Long-term morbidity associated with PTL and delivery includes bronchopulmonary dysplasia and developmental abnormalities. The significant impact of preterm birth is best summarized by this fact: *The 8%–10% of babies born prematurely account for 60%–75% of all perinatal morbidity and mortality in the United States.*

In the consideration of the consequences of preterm delivery, it is important to *separate the concepts of low birth weight and prematurity.* Prematurity reflects gestational age, whereas low birth weight is based on the single parameter of weight, usually 2500 g or less. For example, a growth-restricted fetus of a hypertensive patient may weigh well under 2500 g at 40 weeks' gestation. Such an infant is a low-birth-weight infant but not preterm and will suffer the consequences associated with low birth weight and the effects of maternal hypertension, but not of premature birth. Likewise, an infant of a diabetic mother may be delivered before term, weigh in excess of 2500 g, and still have the significant perinatal morbidities of preterm birth and maternal diabetes.

Many preterm births are the result of deliberate intervention for a variety of pregnancy complications and hence have unavoidable perinatal complications (e.g.,

delivery of a preterm fetus because of maternal eclampsia). A major cause of preterm birth, however, is PTL. *PTL is functionally defined as the presence of regular uterine contractions, occurring with a frequency of 10 minutes or less between 20 and 36 weeks' gestation, with each contraction lasting at least 30 seconds. This uterine activity is accompanied by cervical effacement, cervical dilation, and/or descent of the fetus into the pelvis.* However, variations of this definition are commonly used, and much of the criteria rest with data whose subjective measurement is difficult, so it is often difficult to know when a patient is really in PTL. This presents a problem because treatment appears to be more effective when initiated early in the course of PTL; waiting for cervical changes to occur to establish a definitive diagnosis may limit successful therapy.

ETIOLOGY AND PREVENTION OF PRETERM LABOR

A number of causes and associated factors have been implicated in PTL (Table 22.1). About 10% of preterm births are in multiple gestations, although multiple gestation accounts for only about 1% of pregnancies. If a patient's first pregnancy ends in preterm labor and delivery, her risk in a subsequent pregnancy is increased two-fold, and if she has a second preterm labor and delivery, her risk increases still further to three-fold for the next pregnancy. However, an intervening term labor and delivery decrease the risk in similar proportion. Unfortunately, in most cases, PTL is idiopathic (i.e., no cause or risk factor can be identified).

Patient and physician education has focused on *recognition of the signs and symptoms* that suggest PTL (Table 22.2). Patients with such symptoms should be strongly advised to seek prompt medical attention, and physicians and nurses providing obstetric care must carefully evaluate all such patients. Patient education to help recognize these signs and symptoms is an important part of care, although maternal

TABLE 22.1. Factors Associated with Preterm Labor

Dehydration	Uterine distortion
Premature rupture of membranes (PROM)	Leiomyomas
Incompetent cervix	Septate uterus, uterine didelphis, and
Primary	other anomalies
Secondary to surgery (e.g., cone biopsy	Placental abnormalities
of cervix)	Abruptio placentae
Infections	Placenta previa
Urinary	Maternal smoking (strong implications)
Cervical	Substance abuse
Bacterial vaginosis	Iatrogenic: induction of labor
Intra-amniotic	
Excessive uterine enlargement	
Hydramnios	
Multiple gestation	

TABLE 22.2. Symptoms and Signs of Preterm Labor

Menstrual-like cramps
Low, dull backache
Abdominal pressure
Pelvic pressure
Abdominal cramping (with or without diarrhea)
Increase or change in vaginal discharge (mucous, watery, light bloody discharge)
Uterine contractions, often painless

recognition of uterine activity that leads to premature cervical changes is often inaccurate. There are indicators that often precede PTL. Patients destined to develop frank PTL may have increased uterine irritability and more frequent contractions in the weeks before the actual diagnosis of labor. At times they experience a sensation of pelvic pressure. Electronic fetal monitoring (periodic monitoring at home along with frequent contact with personnel trained in recognition of PTL) has been suggested as being beneficial for patients at high risk for PTL, but the value of this approach is dubious at best and infrequently used nowadays. Unfortunately, educational and risk scoring programs to identify patients likely to experience PTL have also been disappointing.

Early asymptomatic dilation and effacement of the cervix seem to be associated with an increased likelihood of PTL. For patients at higher risk for PTL, cervical examinations can be performed periodically through the second half of gestation.

EVALUATION OF A PATIENT IN SUSPECTED PRETERM LABOR

Once a patient describes symptoms and signs suggestive of PTL, evaluation should be prompt. Application of an *external electronic fetal monitor* may help to quantify the frequency and duration of contractions; the intensity of uterine contractions is assessed very poorly on an external monitor, but abdominal palpation by experienced personnel can prove helpful. The status of the cervix should be determined, either by visualization with a speculum or by gentle digital examination. Because digital examination is contraindicated if there is premature rupture of membranes, speculum evaluation should be performed first if there is indication of membrane rupture. If there is membrane rupture, cervical dilation and effacement are estimated by inspection rather than by digital examination. Changes in cervical effacement and dilation on subsequent examinations are important in the evaluation of both the diagnosis of PTL and the effectiveness of management. Subtle changes are often of great clinical importance so that serial examinations by the same examiner are optimal although not always practical. Ultrasound measurement of cervical length is being performed on patients with a history of preterm labor or signs and symptoms of same, and is felt by some to be of value. Further experience with this technique is needed.

Because urinary infections can predispose to uterine contractions, a urinalysis and urine culture should be obtained. At the time of speculum examination, a cervical culture should be taken for group B β-streptococcus. Empiric treatment for group B streptococcus with penicillin or ampicillin is generally given until culture results are available. When indicated by history or physical examination findings, cultures for *Chlamydia* and *Neisseria gonorrhoeae* should be obtained. *Chlamydia* has been implicated in some cases of PTL. A normal saline wet preparation is also useful to evaluate for bacterial vaginosis, which is associated with premature labor and premature rupture of the membranes.

An increase in the concentration of fetal fibronectin (fFN) has been associated with preterm labor. fFN is an extracellular glycoprotein normally found in the cervical mucus in early pregnancy and then again near term. A preterm rise in the concentration of fFN may be associated with the impending onset of preterm labor, and its absence from cervicovaginal secretions is uncommonly associated with a patient who delivers in the 7 days after the sample is taken. Experience with the use of the measurement of fFN in cervicovaginal secretions and its possible beneficial use is accumulating.

Ultrasound examination can be useful in assessing the gestational age of the fetus, estimation of the amniotic fluid volume (spontaneous rupture of membranes with fluid loss may precede PTL and may be unrecognized by the patient), fetal presentation, and placental location. The technique also can reveal the existence of fetal congenital anomalies. Because placenta previa and abruptio placentae may lead to preterm contractions, patients should also be monitored for bleeding.

Because either clinical or subclinical infection of the amniotic cavity is thought to be associated with PTL in some cases, *amniocentesis* may be performed. The presence of bacteria in amniotic fluid is correlated not only with PTL but also with the subsequent development of infection, which is less responsive to therapy. The presence of white cells in the amniotic fluid increases the likelihood of infection developing. Antibiotic therapy before delivery is instituted if infection is diagnosed or strongly suspected. At the time of amniocentesis, additional amniotic fluid may be obtained for pulmonary maturity studies, which could have bearing on subsequent management. Tocolysis, the suppression of uterine contractions by pharmacologic means, may not be appropriate if there is indication of fetal lung maturity.

MANAGEMENT OF PRETERM LABOR

The purpose in treating PTL is to delay delivery, if possible, until fetal maturity is attained. Management involves *two broad goals: (1)* the detection and treatment of disorders associated with PTL and *(2)* therapy for the PTL itself. Although it is fortunate that more than 50% of patients with preterm contractions have spontaneous resolution of abnormal uterine activity, this complicates the evaluation of treatment. One may not know whether there was actual PTL or simply normal preterm uterine activity. It may be difficult to know whether it was the treatment that stopped the PTL or whether it would have stopped without therapy.

Because dehydration has been known to lead to uterine irritability, *therapy often begins with intravenous hydration.* In a significant number of patients, this therapy alone causes cessation of uterine contractions, although its value in patients who are already well hydrated is controversial.

TABLE 22.3. Agents Used in Treating Preterm Labor

Class (Example)	Action	Comments
Magnesium sulfate	Competes with calcium for entry into cells	High degree of safety; often used as first agent; may cause flushing or headaches; at high levels may cause respiratory depression (12–15 mg/dl) or cardiac depression (> 15 mg/dl); contraindicated in patients with hypocalcemia or who have myasthenia gravis
β-adrenergic agents (ritodrine, terbutaline)	Increase cAMP in cell, which decreases free calcium	β-receptors are of two types: β_1-receptors predominate in the heart and intestines and β_2-receptors predominate in the uterus, lungs, and blood vessels; side effects include hypotension, tachycardia, anxiety, chest tightening or pain, ECG changes; increased pulmonary edema occurs very infrequently but is possible, especially with fluid overload; relatively contraindicated in patients with asthma or coronary artery disease and in those with renal failure
Prostaglandin synthetase inhibitors (indomethacin)	Decrease prostaglandin (PG) production by blocking conversion of free arachidonic acid to PG	Premature constriction of ductus arteriosus possible especially after 34 weeks; bradycardia and growth restriction hypoglycemia have been reported, but concern has decreased with broader experience
Calcium-channel blockers (nifedipine)	Prevent calcium entry into muscle cells	Problems include possible decrease in uteroplacental blood flow, fetal hypoxia, and hypercarbia

Various tocolytic therapies have been used in the management of PTL (Table 22.3); specific regimens are detailed in Tables 22.4 and 22.5. *Unfortunately, tocolytics have not been clearly shown to prolong pregnancy beyond several days.* Different treatment regimens address specific mechanisms involved in the maintenance of uterine contractions, and each, therefore, may be best suited for certain patients.

Typically, *patients diagnosed as having PTL receive one form of therapy, with the addition or substitution of other forms if the initial treatment is unsuccessful.* As noted in Table 22.3, adverse side effects, at times serious and even life-threatening to the mother, can occur. These possibilities must be taken into account in selecting a therapy. The maturity of the fetus is a consideration in deciding how aggressively to pursue therapy, and in general, the vigor

---

TABLE 22.4.   Administration of Magnesium Sulfate for Preterm Labor

- 6 g MgSO$_4$ are mixed in 100–150 ml of D$_5$W and infused over 15–20 minutes as a loading dose
- 40 g MgSO$_4$ are mixed in 1000 ml of D$_5$W, providing an MgSO$_4$ concentration of 1 g MgSO$_4$ in 25 ml of solution
- Using a piggyback infusion via an infusion pump, the physician usually begins infusion at 2 g/hr (50 ml/hr) and increases it in 0.5-g/hr increments as needed

---

TABLE 22.5.   Administration of Nifedipine for Preterm Labor

- Loading dose: 30 mg
- Immediate tocolysis: 20 mg po q 6–8 h; may increase to q 4 if blood pressure remains > 80/50
- Maintenance: 10–20 mg q 8 h if necessary
- Cautions: Contraindicated in patients with myasthenia gravis, renal failure, hypoglycemia or active hepatitis and/or hepatic failure; may potentiate the effect of magnesium sulfate, leading to hypotension and respiratory depression
- Pharmacology: Inhibits calcium transport through L-type or slow-type channels, causing significant reductions in systemic and pulmonary vascular resistance and tocolysis; specific uterine effects include inhibition of myometrial contractility and reduction of uterine vascular resistance; potentiates magnesium sulfate but may be used concurrently with β-blockers such as terbutaline
- Side effects: Flushing is common; headache in 5%–10% of patients; hypotension and tachycardia are rare; no known teratogenic effects
- Other uses: Treatment of hypertension in pregnancy

---

with which therapy is undertaken diminishes as the gestational age of the fetus increases. One might be more willing to accept potential adverse effects for a patient in PTL at 35 weeks as opposed to 26 weeks. It is customary to not initiate or to stop therapy at 35–36 weeks. Treatment sequences may vary from hospital to hospital, depending on the individual hospital experience and the success rate with various therapeutic regimens.

Contraindications to tocolysis include advanced labor, a mature fetus, a severely anomalous fetus, intrauterine infection, significant vaginal bleeding, conditions in which the adverse effects of tocolysis may be marked, and a variety of obstetric complications that contraindicate delay in delivery.

From 24 to 34 weeks, management generally includes administration of certain *steroids*, such as betamethasone, *to enhance pulmonary maturity.* Both the incidence and severity of RDS appear to be reduced with this therapy. The salutatory effect for the fetus appears to wane after 7 days, so the therapy may be repeated weekly. In addition, sequelae of RDS such as intracerebral hemorrhage and necrotizing enterocolitis occur less frequently in infants whose mother received betamethasone or a similar agent.

Because tocolytic therapy is often unsuccessful, maternal transfer of a woman in preterm labor (after stabilization) to a center with a neonatal intensive care unit (NICU) is highly advisable.

CASE STUDIES

Case 22A

A 26-year-old G2 P0101 presents with complaints of vaginal discharge, urinary frequency, and a sensation of pelvic pressure. She says she may be contracting sometimes, but she isn't sure. She is at 28 weeks' gestation by dates and early ultrasound examination. Her first child was delivered by ceasarean section at 29 weeks' gestation after tocolysis with magnesium sulfate and terbutaline had failed and the fetus was found to be breech. Her past medical history includes three episodes of Chlamydia infection, the last in the first trimester of this pregnancy. Her antenatal course during this pregnancy has been otherwise unremarkable.

Questions Case 22A

Based on this history, all of the following are indicated at this time EXCEPT

A. Urinalysis (UA), culture and sensitivity (C&S)
B. Obstetric ultrasound
C. Cervical evaluation
D. Amniocentesis
E. Cervical cultures for *Chlamydia, N. gonorrhoeae,* and group B β-streptococcus

Answer: D

With a history of urinary frequency and previous *Chlamydia* infection, urinalysis and appropriate cultures are important initial steps. Cervical evaluation is crucial in determining if this patient with a previous PTL and delivery is again in PTL, for which she is at high risk. Obstetric ultrasound is useful, but not immediately. Evaluation for uterine activity by electronic fetal monitor (EFM) is appropriate to assess for the presence of significant uterine contractions. Finally, amniocentesis is

not indicated in the initial evaluation, because at this time the patient is not known to be in PTL.

The patient is found to have a long, closed cervix and irregular uterine contractions that resolve with hydration. The fetal heart rate pattern is reassuring. UA shows 40 white blood cells (WBCs) per high-power field (HPF). What therapy is appropriate?

A. Antibiotics
B. Tocolysis
C. Amniocentesis
D. Contraction stress test (CST)

Answer: A

Antibiotic therapy for a urinary tract infection (UTI) is warranted at this time. Tocolysis at this time is controversial but may be used. The risks of amniocentesis are too high in this situation in which premature lungs may be assumed and there is no clinical evidence of amniotic infection. CST would be of little value.

Case 22B

A 29-year-old G4 P2103 presents complaining of painful uterine contractions for 2 hours and a sensation of pelvic fullness. She is in the thirtieth week of gestation age based on LMP and two ultrasound examinations. She has had three uneventful vaginal deliveries, two at term and one at 35.5 weeks.

Cervical examination shows she is 3 cm dilated and 90% effaced, her membranes are intact, and there is a cephalic presentation at zero station. On EFM she is having uterine contractions every 4 minutes, which the nurse evaluates as moder-

ate to strong in intensity; the fetal heart pattern is reassuring.

Question Case 22B

Interventions recommended at this time include all of the following EXCEPT

A. IV fluids
B. Ultrasound to evaluate for fetal anomalies
C. Tocolysis with magnesium sulfate
D. UA, C&S, and cervical cultures
E. Amniocentesis

Answer: E

Immediate intravenous hydration and tocolysis with magnesium sulfate are indicated. Urinalysis and cultures provide important information for future management that can be easily obtained. After tocolytic therapy has been started, ultrasound is appropriate. If tocolysis is successful, consideration for amniocentesis may then be in order.

Tocolysis with intravenous fluids and magnesium sulfate is successful, with cervical changes arrested for the time at 3 cm dilation and 90% effacement. For further consideration: What will you tell the patient about the risks and benefits of steroid therapy in her situation? Will you use the same or different agents if uterine contractions reoccur? Will you consider discharge if uterine contractions do not reoccur? If so, will you send the patient home on a tocolytic? Is electronic ambulatory fetal monitoring warranted in this patient?

23

PREMATURE RUPTURE OF MEMBRANES

This chapter deals primarily with APGO Objective(s):

OBJECTIVE 26 Premature Rupture of Membranes

A. Describe the factors predisposing to premature rupture of membranes.

B. Describe the signs and symptoms of premature rupture of membranes and the methods used to confirm it.

C. Describe the management of premature rupture of membranes, including expectant management vs. timely delivery, and the methods used to monitor maternal and fetal status in the case of expectant management.

Beginning early in pregnancy, amniotic fluid is produced continuously as the result of passage of fluid across the fetal membranes and across the skin, fetal urine production, and fetal pulmonary effluent. Amniotic fluid provides protection against infection, protects the fetus from trauma, and provides protection from umbilical cord compression. It also allows for fetal movement and fetal breathing, which, in turn, permits full fetal respiratory development. Decreased or absent amniotic fluid can lead to compression of the umbilical cord and decreased placental blood flow. Disruption (rupture) of these fetal membranes is associated with loss of protective effects and developmental roles of amniotic fluid.

Premature rupture of membranes (PROM) is defined as rupture of the chorioamniotic membrane before the onset of labor. PROM occurs in approximately 10% to 15% of all pregnancies. PROM is associated with about 10% of term pregnancies (37 weeks' gestational age or more) and is generally followed by the onset of labor. *The primary risk of PROM is preterm labor and delivery,* with about 75% of patients with preterm PROM (rupture of membranes before 37 weeks' gestational age) delivering within one week. Preterm PROM is associated in about 30% of preterm deliveries. PROM leading to preterm delivery is, in turn, associated with neonatal complications of prematurity such as respiratory distress syndrome, intraventricular hemorrhage, neonatal infection, necrotizing enterocolitis, neurologic and neuromuscular dysfunction, and sepsis. The second most common complication is intrauterine infection (chorioamnionitis; 30%–50% of cases), the incidence of which is increased with decreasing gestational age at PROM and positive cervical cultures for *Neisseria gonorrhoeae* and group B streptococcus. Other complications include prolapsed umbilical cord and abruptio placentae.

The consequences of preterm PROM differ substantially depending on the gestational age, increasing as gestational age decreases. Mid-trimester preterm PROM (between 16 and 26 weeks' gestational age) complicates about 1% of all pregnancies.

Nowadays, survival is increasingly likely in the 24–26 week group, although the morbidities of extreme prematurity in this group of neonates are more substantial and frequent in inverse proportion to gestational age. Oligohydramnios at this very early gestational age is associated with incomplete alveolar development and the development of pulmonary hypoplasia. Infants born with pulmonary hypoplasia cannot be adequately ventilated and soon succumb to hypoxia and barotrauma from high-pressure ventilation.

The *cause* of PROM is not clearly understood. Sexually transmitted diseases (STDs) play a role, because such *infections* are more commonly found in women with premature rupture of membranes than in those without STD. However, intact fetal membranes and normal amniotic fluid do not fully protect the fetus from infection, because it appears that subclinical intra-amniotic infection may be responsible for PROM in certain cases. Metabolites produced by bacteria may either weaken the fetal membranes or initiate uterine contractions through stimulating prostaglandin synthesis. The risk of PROM is at least doubled in *women who smoke* during pregnancy. Other risk factors for PROM include *prior PROM* (about two-fold), a short cervical length, prior preterm delivery, hydramnios, multiple gestation, and bleeding in early pregnancy.

The relation between PROM and preterm contractions also is unclear. It is theorized that preterm contractions may cause dilation of the cervix, thereby exposing the fetal membranes to infective agents, which may then cause spontaneous rupture of the membranes. There is also uncertainty about the impact of gestational age and the length of time since membrane rupture on the likelihood of intrauterine infection. This *triad of PROM, preterm labor, and infection* remains an important clinical consideration but requires further research.

Chorioamnionitis poses a major threat to the mother and may cause fetal sepsis. Patients with intra-amniotic infection can experience significant fever (generally, > 100.5° F), tachycardia (maternal and fetal),

TABLE 23.1.	Causes of False-positive and False-negative Nitrazine Tests	
False-positive	**False-negative**	
Basic urine	Remote PROM with no residual fluid	
Semen	Minimal amniotic fluid leakage	
Cervical mucus		
Blood contamination		
Some antiseptic solutions		
Vaginitis (especially trichomonas)		

PROM = premature rupture of membrane.

and uterine tenderness. Purulent cervical discharge is usually a very late finding. The maternal white blood cell (WBC) count is generally elevated, but this finding may be misleading for two reasons: (*1*) the WBC count increases somewhat in normal pregnancy, with the upper range of normal being 12,000 to 13,000/mm^3; and (*2*) the WBCs normally increase with uterine contractions and labor, at times to a level exceeding 20,000/mm^3. Patients with chorioamnionitis frequently enter spontaneous and often tumultuous labor. Once the diagnosis of chorioamnionitis is made, treatment consists of antibiotic therapy and prompt delivery by induction or augmentation of labor if needed.

DIAGNOSIS

Fluid passing through the vagina must be presumed to be amniotic fluid until proved otherwise. At times, patients describe a "gush" of fluid, whereas at other times they note a history of steady leakage of small amounts of fluid. *Intermittent urinary leakage* is common during pregnancy, especially near term, and this can be confused with PROM. Likewise, the normally increased vaginal secretions in pregnancy as well as perineal moisture (especially in hot weather) may be mistaken for amniotic fluid.

The *Nitrazine test* uses pH to distinguish amniotic fluid from urine and vaginal secretions. Amniotic fluid is quite alkaline, having a pH above 7.0; vaginal secretions in pregnancy usually have pH values of less

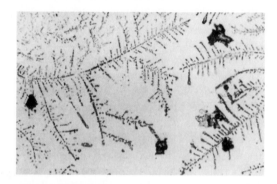

FIGURE 23.1.   Ferning.

than 6.0. To perform the Nitrazine test, a sample of fluid obtained from the vagina during a speculum examination is placed on a strip of Nitrazine paper. The paper turns dark blue in response to amniotic fluid. Cervical mucus, blood, and semen are possible causes of false-positive results (Table 23.1).

The *"fern test"* is also used to distinguish amniotic fluid from other fluids. It is named from the pattern of arborization that occurs when amniotic fluid is placed on a slide and is allowed to dry in room air. The resultant pattern, which resembles the leaves of a fern plant, is caused by the sodium chloride content of the amniotic fluid. The ferning pattern from amniotic fluid is fine with multiple branches, as shown in Figure 23.1; cervical mucus does not fern or, if it does, the pattern is thick with much less branching. This test is considered more indicative of ruptured membranes than the Nitrazine test, but as with any test, it is not 100% reliable.

Ultrasound can be helpful in evaluating the possibility of rupture of membranes. If ample amniotic fluid around the fetus is visible on ultrasound examination, the diagnosis of PROM must be questioned; however, if the amounts of amniotic fluid leakage are small, sufficient amniotic fluid will still be visible on scan. When there is less than the expected amount of fluid seen on ultrasound, the differential diagnosis of oligohydramnios must also be considered.

The differential diagnoses for PROM include urinary incontinence, increased vaginal secretions in pregnancy (physiologic), increased cervical discharge (pathologic, infection), exogenous fluids (such as semen or douche), and vesicovaginal fistula.

EVALUATION AND MANAGEMENT

Patients with PROM are *hospitalized for their initial evaluation* and further management. In the hospital environment, evaluations may proceed quickly and efficiently so that delivery may be accomplished if needed. *Factors to be considered in the management of the patient with PROM include* the gestational age at the time of rupture, the presence of uterine contractions, the likelihood of chorioamnionitis, the amount of amniotic fluid around the fetus, and the degree of fetal maturity.

The patient's history as well as the management factors listed previously must be carefully evaluated for information relevant to the diagnosis. Abdominal examination includes palpation of the uterus for tenderness and fundal height measurement for evaluation of gestational age and fetal lie.

A sterile speculum examination is performed to assess the likelihood of vaginal infection and to obtain cervical cultures for *N. gonorrhoeae*, β-hemolytic streptococcus, and possibly *Chlamydia trachomatis*. The cervix is visualized for its degree of dilation as well as for the presence of free-flowing amniotic fluid. Fluid is obtained from the vaginal vault for Nitrazine and/or fern testing. If there is fluid pooled in the vaginal vault, it may be sent for *fetal maturity test-ing* if the gestational age warrants. The test for phosphatidylglycerol (PG) is considered the most reliable indicator of fetal lung maturity, because PG is not found in vaginal secretions or blood. *Because of the risk of infection, intracervical digital examination should be avoided unless, and until, the patient is in active labor.*

Ultrasound examination can be helpful in determining gestational age, verifying the fetal presentation, and assessing the amount of amniotic fluid remaining within the uterine cavity. It has been shown that labor is less likely to occur when an adequate volume of amniotic fluid remains within the uterus.

If PROM occurs at term (37 weeks' gestational age or more), spontaneous labor will ensue in 90% of women within about 24 hours. Further, amniotic fluid inhibits bacterial growth for about 24 hours. Thus, awaiting the onset of spontaneous labor for 12–24 hours has limited risk of infection, unless there are risk factors such as previous or concurrent vaginal infection or multiple digital pelvic examinations. However, induction of labor at any time after presentation PROM is also considered appropriate with informed consent. Information that the physician shares with the patient as this decision is made includes, in addition to the risk of infection, that immediate oxytocin administration is associated with a decreased risk of chorioamnionitis and endometritis while there is a decrease in the incidence of ceasarean section in patients managed expectantly. Serial evaluation for the development of intrauterine infection and other complications of PROM is requisite with expectant management, which in most cases should not extend beyond 24 hours in term pregnancy.

The time from PROM to labor is inversely related to gestational age. At term, greater than 37 weeks, labor ensues in 90% of patients within 24 hours. Between term and about 28 weeks' gestational age, about 50% labor within 24 hours and 80% within one week, while only 50% of patients whose gestational age is 24–28 weeks labor within one week of PROM.

If the gestational age is thought to be in the transitional time of fetal maturity (i.e., from 34 to 36 weeks) or if there is clinical suspicion for the presence of uterine infection, amniotic fluid may be collected by amniocentesis from any pocket of fluid located on ultrasound. Fluid can be assessed for the presence of infection by Gram staining, culture, and glucose concentration. Tests of fetal maturity can be performed. The presence of bacteria on Gram stain is a better predictor of infection than the presence of white blood cells.

If the evaluation suggests *intrauterine infection*, antibiotic therapy and delivery are indicated. The antibiotic prescribed should have a broad spectrum of coverage, because of the polymicrobial nature of the infection. Delivery is usually accomplished by induction of labor or, if the infant is a preterm breech, possibly by ceasarean delivery. If the patient is beginning to have uterine contractions or if the cervix is dilated beyond approximately 3 cm, labor is usually allowed to proceed. As in cases of labor not related to PROM, oxytocin augmentation may be necessary. Persistent contractions after PROM may be a manifestation of infection, possibly subclinical, so that most clinicians do not attempt to inhibit labor when such contractions begin spontaneously.

If the fetus is significantly preterm and in the absence of infection, expectant management is generally chosen. Patients are assessed carefully on a daily basis for uterine tenderness as well as maternal or fetal tachycardia. WBC counts are obtained frequently, usually daily for several days. Frequent ultrasound assessment helps to determine amniotic fluid volumes, because amniotic fluid may reaccumulate around the fetus. Antibiotic therapy prolongs the latency period after preterm PROM and improves the perinatal outcome and should be used. Daily fetal movement monitoring by the mother can also be helpful to assess fetal well-being. In the absence of sufficient amniotic fluid to buffer the umbilical cord from external pressure, compression of the cord can lead to fetal heart rate decelerations. If these are frequent and severe, there should be early and expeditious delivery to avoid fetal compromise or death. Electronic fetal monitoring is used frequently during the initial evaluation period to search for any fetal heart rate decelerations, although the fetal cardiac control mechanisms are often insufficiently developed to allow meaningful evaluation for fetal heart rate variability.

To enhance fetal pulmonary maturity in patients with preterm PROM, corticosteroid therapy (such as betamethasone) is generally recommended in patients whose gestational age is 32 weeks or less. Despite the immunosuppressive property of steroids, they do not seem to predispose the mother or fetus to infection.

At times, the leakage of amniotic fluid ceases, and the fetal membranes are said to "seal over." Should this occur, patients can be monitored at home, with careful attention to temperature and uterine tenderness. Unfortunately, this circumstance is unlikely. Much more common is the onset of uterine contractions and frank labor in the first week following rupture of membranes. For this reason, it is the exceptional patient who can expect to be discharged home with documented PROM.

PROM at very early gestational ages, such as before 25 to 26 weeks of gestation, presents additional problems. Along with the risks of prematurity and infection already discussed, the very premature fetus faces the further hazards of *pulmonary hypoplasia* and the *amniotic band syndrome*. The relation of PROM with both of these entities is both interesting and important. For normal fetal lung development to occur, it is necessary that fetal breathing movements take place. During intrauterine life, the fetus normally inhales and exhales amniotic fluid. This adds substances generated in the respiratory tree to the amniotic fluid pool, including the phospholipids that form the basis for many of the fetal maturity tests. If rupture of fetal membranes occurs before 25 to 26 weeks of gestation, the lack of amniotic fluid interferes with this normal breathing process and, therefore, with pulmonary development. The result is a failure of normal growth and differentiation of the respiratory tree. If severe, the fetus is said to have *pulmonary hypopla-*

sia. Neonatal death then occurs because of an inability to maintain ventilation. The development of pulmonary hypoplasia is not necessarily an all-or-none phenomenon but rather represents a spectrum of disordered development.

The *amniotic band syndrome* is a constellation of findings associated with entanglement of fetal parts with the amniotic membranes that can collapse around the fetus once rupture of membranes occurs.

These bands may cause virtually any type of deformity or anatomic disruption, including amputation of extremities or fingers. Patients with ruptured membranes early in pregnancy are exposed to these additional risks if expectant management is chosen. On the brighter side, PROM that occurs early in pregnancy, sometimes following genetic amniocentesis, has a greater likelihood of sealing over with reaccumulation of amniotic fluid.

CASE STUDIES

Case 23A

A 25-year-old G1 at 30 weeks of gestational age by menstrual history and early pelvic and ultrasound examinations presents with a history of "water leaking from my vagina" for the last 4 hours. Her pregnancy has been unremarkable except for a positive cervical C. trachomatis culture at the time of her initial obstetric visit at 8 weeks of gestational age. The infection was treated and a repeat culture was negative.

Questions Case 23A

Which of the following should not be included in the initial evaluation of this patient?

  A. Sterile speculum examination
  B. Digital examination of the cervix
  C. External electronic fetal monitoring
  D. Cervical cultures for *N. gonorrhoeae* and *C. trachomatis*
  E. Transabdominal ultrasonography

Answer: B

The initial evaluation should be focused to determine if PROM has occurred. Thus a sterile speculum examination to look for

fluid is appropriate, but not a digital examination, which may increase the risk of infection. Fern and Nitrazine tests can be made on the fluid. Cultures from the cervix can be taken, which are especially important in this patient who has a previous history of *Chlamydia* infection. Similarly, external fetal monitoring (EFM) and ultrasonography are valuable and offer no risk.

Examination shows no fluid coming from the os or in the vaginal vault. The Nitrazine test is negative. Ultrasound shows adequate fluid. EFM shows a reassuring fetal heart rate (FHR) pattern, without evidence of uterine activity. All of the following are possible explanations of fluid coming from this patient's vagina EXCEPT

  A. Urinary incontinence
  B. Normal vaginal secretions
  C. Perineal moisture
  D. Patient anxiety
  E. Bartholin cyst drainage

Answer: E

A through *D* are sources of fluid leakage from the vagina commonly encountered in pregnancy. Bartholin cysts do not drain.

(Continued)

Case 23B

A 36-year-old infertility patient, who conceived after being administered clomiphene citrate, is now at 30 weeks of gestation based on last menstrual period (LMP) and early physical examination and ultrasonography. She presents with the history of a gush of fluid from her vagina 1 hour ago. She is now feeling "little twinges" in her uterus, a new and disturbing sensation. She is very frightened.

Speculum examination shows fluid coming from the cervical os, which is Nitrazine- and fern-positive. The patient's cervix appears to be approximately 1 cm dilated. On EFM the fetal heart rate is 170 and there are occasional uterine contractions. The patient is afebrile, and her uterus is not tender. Her WBC is found to be 16,000/mm³.

Questions Case 23B

Which of the following are likely problems in this case?

A. Premature labor
B. Intrauterine infection
C. Pulmonary hypoplasia
D. Neonatal intraventricular hemorrhage

Answer: A, B, D

Pulmonary hypoplasia is rarely seen with PROM beyond 26 weeks, because fetal lung development has advanced beyond the hypoplastic stage. All of the others are serious clinical considerations for this patient and her fetus. At 30 weeks of gestation, survival in a neonatal ICU is likely but so is significant short- and long-term morbidity.

You and your patient decide to wait 24 hours, at which time—as you hoped—there is no evidence of intrauterine infection or premature labor. Obviously, this patient has gone to great lengths to be pregnant. Now she is faced with difficult decisions and your advice is important.

Management should include all of the following EXCEPT

A. Steroids to promote fetal lung development
B. Tocolysis to stop contractions to give steroids time to work
C. Antibiotics to help prevent infection, especially group B streptococcus
D. Repeated speculum examinations to verify PROM
E. Electronic monitoring to ensure a normal FHR pattern

Answer: D

Once PROM is identified with usual procedures, testing for it need not be repeated.

SECTION C

PROCEDURES

C H A P T E R

24

OBSTETRIC PROCEDURES

CHAPTER OBJECTIVES

This chapter deals primarily with APGO Objective(s):

OBJECTIVE 34   Obstetric Procedures

The student should demonstrate a knowledge of the following procedures: ultrasound, episiotomy, cesarean delivery, forceps delivery, induction and augmentation of labor, vacuum-assisted delivery, breech delivery, antepartum fetal assessment, amniocentesis and cordocentesis, chorionic villus sampling, newborn circumcision, vaginal birth after cesarean section, spontaneous vaginal delivery, and fetal surveillance.

Some are reviewed in this chapter, and some in other topic-specific chapters.

Women's health care physicians must be familiar with the procedures common in obstetric and gynecologic practice. Whether the physician performs the procedure or not, he or she should understand the indications, contraindications, risks, benefits, and the appropriate language needed to inform the patient about her diagnoses and therapeutic options.

AMNIOCENTESIS

Amniocentesis is the withdrawal of fluid from the amniotic sac to obtain fluid and cells for a variety of tests (Figure 24.1). Biochemical studies can identify the presence of fetal physiologic markers (e.g., deficiency of hexosaminidase A or Tay-Sachs disease) or the presence of substances indicating fetal abnormalities (e.g., α-fetoprotein in neural tube defects or bilirubin in Rh incompatibility). Evaluation of the DNA of fetal cells grown in tissue culture allows genetic evaluation of the fetus.

In more advanced gestations, fluid obtained through amniocentesis is used to assess the degree of fetal lung maturity. This indication of fetal lung readiness is extremely valuable in the management of premature labor or the timing of delivery for patients with medical complications. Fluid obtained at amniocentesis may also be cultured and stained to evaluate for intrauterine infection (i.e., chorioamnionitis).

Amniocentesis is associated with a 0.5% risk of fetal loss because of bleeding, infection, preterm labor, or fetal injury. To reduce this risk, the procedure is usually performed using ultrasonographic guidance.

CHORIONIC VILLUS SAMPLING

In chorionic villus sampling (CVS), a small cannula is passed through the cervix to aspirate villus cells for genetic analysis of an early gestation (Figure 24.2). Cells may also be acquired via transabdominal aspiration. The cells that are obtained are cultured for genetic studies.

Because CVS carries approximately a 0.5% risk of fetal loss, it is usually reserved for patients with a greater than 0.5% chance of an abnormality (e.g., those over the age of 35 or with a history of genetic abnormalities). Bleeding or infections are infrequent complications.

Compared with amniocentesis, CVS can be performed earlier in pregnancy with a more rapid availability of results. This allows for an earlier decision regarding pos-

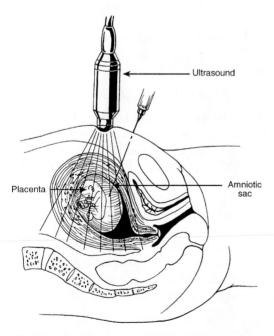

FIGURE 24.1. Amniocentesis with ultrasound guidance. Cross-section of uterus and fetus with the needle in a pocket of amniotic fluid.

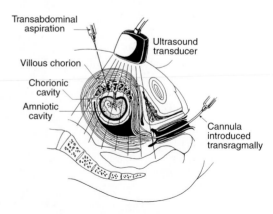

FIGURE 24.2. Chorionic villus sampling.

sible pregnancy termination in the case of significant fetal abnormality. Isolated reports of an association of CVS with limb reduction defects should be noted, but as yet an association has not been confirmed.

PERIUMBILICAL ARTERY BLOOD SAMPLING

In *periumbilical artery blood sampling* (PUBS), a fetal blood sample is obtained via a transabdominal needle aspiration of the umbilical cord under real-time ultrasonographic guidance. Various analyses may be performed on the fetal blood sample obtained, including fetal blood gas and metabolic evaluation, fetal hemogram and blood chemistries, and fetal genetics studies. The risks of this procedure are the same as those of amniocentesis plus an approximately 1% risk to the fetus from bleeding at the umbilical puncture site. This procedure is also referred to as *cordocentesis*.

FORCEPS DELIVERY AND VACUUM EXTRACTION

Vaginal delivery may be assisted with obstetric forceps or a vacuum extractor. These methods augment the expulsive forces during the second stage of labor as well as direct these forces in an optimal manner.

Obstetric forceps are designed either to provide traction to augment and/or direct the expulsive forces of the second stage of labor, or to facilitate the rotation of the fetal head (Figures 24.3 and 24.4). Each type is applied to the fetal head and is classified as low (or outlet), mid, or high, based on the level of descent of the fetal head (station) at the time the forceps are applied. In general, low, or outlet, forceps describe application when the fetal scalp is visible at the introitus; midforceps, when the head is engaged but above the pelvic outlet or in those cases in which a forceps rotation of the head is performed; and high forceps, when the presenting part is above zero station. Because of the risk of injury to fetus and mother, it is inappropriate to use high forceps.

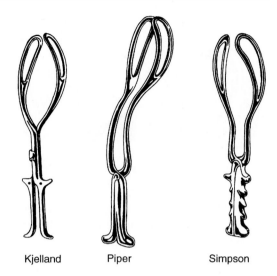

Kjelland   Piper   Simpson

FIGURE 24.3. Commonly used obstetric forceps.

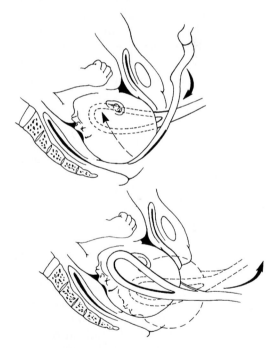

FIGURE 24.4. Correct biparietal, bimalar, cephalic forceps application.

Instead, delivery should be accomplished by cesarean section.

Although virtually any forceps may be used in a low forceps delivery (for example, *Simpson forceps*), some specific types of forceps are often chosen for midforceps deliveries. The *Kjelland (Kielland) forceps*

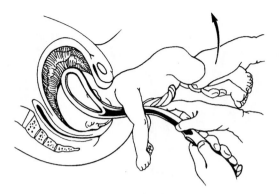

FIGURE 24.5. Use of Piper forceps on an after-coming head during breech delivery.

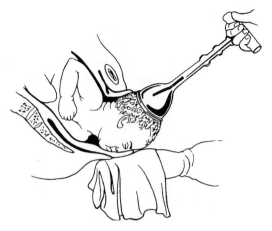

FIGURE 24.6. Vacuum extractor applied to head.

are especially suited for midforceps deliveries involving rotation of the fetal head. *Piper forceps* are specially designed to facilitate the delivery of the "after-coming head" in vaginal breech deliveries (Figure 24.5).

Forceps may cause injury to either the fetus or mother unless applied carefully and used judiciously. Transient bruising over the zygomatic arch is common and is generally of little consequence. More dangerous are lacerations of the birth canal or cervix, which may result from excessive force or improper manipulation of the forceps during delivery.

The *vacuum extractor* is a suction cup-like device that is applied to the fetal scalp (Figure 24.6). Traction is then used to aid maternal expulsive efforts and expedite delivery. Although damage to maternal structures is less likely with the use of the vacuum extractor than with forceps, hematomas or abrasions of the fetal scalp can occur. The indications and criteria for vacuum assisted vaginal delivery are the same as for the use of obstetric forceps.

CESAREAN DELIVERY

Cesarean delivery (or cesarean section) is the delivery of the fetus through an abdominal incision. This route may be chosen when rapid delivery is required and vaginal delivery is not imminent (e.g., nonreassuring fetal status—"fetal distress"), when vaginal delivery is not advisable (e.g., placenta previa, fetal anomalies, or malpresentation), or when vaginal delivery cannot be accomplished by the normal forces of labor (e.g., cephalopelvic disproportion, macrosomia, malpresentation, or uterine dysfunction). Depending on the locality, practice patterns, and level of obstetric risk, cesarean section rates range from 5–8 to 20 percent, although there is a national movement to return the overall cesarean section rate to under 10%.

Cesarean sections are not classified by the kind of abdominal incision made, but rather as *lower uterine segment* (transverse or vertical) when the incision is in the lower uterine segment or *classical* when the incision is in the upper, contractile portion of the uterus (Figure 24.7). Patients with lower uterine segment cesarean deliveries may be candidates for future vaginal delivery because these incisions are less likely to rupture in labor. *Vaginal birth after cesarean section (VBAC)* is safe and effective in reducing maternal morbidity as well as cesarean section rates if careful maternal and fetal monitoring are available as well as staff and facilities for emergency cesarean section. Patients with classical incisions and those who have had incisions of the upper uterus for other reasons (e.g., myomectomy, cornual resection) are at greater risk of rup-

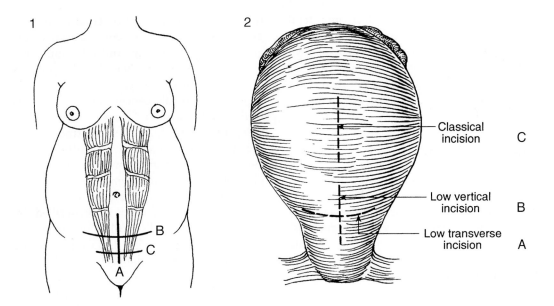

FIGURE 24.7. Incisions at cesarean section. *(1) Abdominal incisions*, including: (**A**) the midline incision through the less vascular midline space, (**B**) the Maylard incision, which involves incision of the rectus sheath and muscles, and (**C**) the Pfannenstiel incision, where the rectus sheath and muscles are retracted away rather than incised. In general, midline incisions allow somewhat more rapid access but at the expense of a less pleasing cosmetic effect and more postoperative discomfort than the transverse abdominal incisions. *(2) Uterine incisions*, by which cesarean sections are classified: (**A**) the lower segment transverse (lower segment transverse cesarean section, LSTCS), (**B**) the lower segment vertical cesarean section (LSVCS), and (**C**) the classical cesarean section where the incision is through the thick contractile upper uterine segment.

ture of the uterine scar before or during labor and are generally not allowed to labor in subsequent pregnancies.

EXTERNAL CEPHALIC VERSION

The application of gentle constant pressure to the breech fetus between 36 and 39 weeks' gestation may facilitate version to the cephalic presentation (Figure 24.8). In a woman of normal body habitus, a fetus of normal size with adequate amniotic fluid volume, and proper relaxation (which may include tocolysis), success rates of 50%–75% may be expected with half or more remaining in the cephalic presentation until labor ensues. The cesarean section rate for these patients is one half of that for those who do not undergo version, balanced against infrequent risks of cord compression

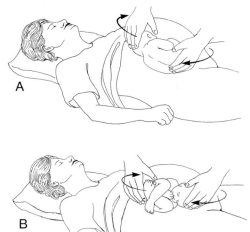

FIGURE 24.8. External cephalic version. Steady gentle pressure is applied to "squeeze" the fetus from the breech to the cephalic, more often in a "forward roll" motion as noted.

and placental abruption. Electronic fetal monitoring and/or ultrasonographic monitoring before and after the procedure is recommended, and Rh-negative women should receive Rh-immune globulin because there is a 5%–10% incidence of fetomaternal transfusion.

CIRCUMCISION

Circumcision of the newborn male (the removal of the foreskin from the penis) has been practiced for centuries as social custom and for religious and health reasons. Controversy continues over the health value of this surgical procedure. It has been argued that circumcision represents mutilation, reduces penile sensitivity, and carries a greater risk of operative complications (surgical damage, bleeding, and infection) than is warranted by its benefits. Proponents point to improved hygiene and a reduced incidence of penile cancer and phimosis, as well as social benefits. Circumcision is elective surgery and should be performed only if the newborn is stable and healthy. Local anesthesia has been shown to reduce the physiologic effect to newborn circumcision and is generally recommended today.

Female circumcision is proscribed by most of the world's health organizations and societies as having no value, serving only to mutilate and damage normal female appearance and function.

UNIT III

Gynecology

SECTION A

GENERAL GYNECOLOGY

C H A P T E R

25

CONTRACEPTION

The ability to control fertility has had a more wide-ranging impact on society than almost any other aspect of medical practice, past or present. Because the subject of contraception has personal, religious, and political overtones, it can often lead to conflict, emotionality, and confusion. Helping the patient and her partner sort through their options is both important and rewarding. Before the physician can advise a couple on their contraceptive options, he or she must understand the physiologic or pharmacologic basis of action, the effectiveness, the indications and contraindications, complications, and advantages and disadvantages of the contraceptive methods available, as well as the cultural context of the couple within which the selected method is used.

There are many methods of contraception considered reliable as well as numerous methods of dubious or no value arising from superstition or ignorance. Because no method is 100% reliable, failures are reflected in the descriptive measures of *method failure* (the failure rate inherent in the method if the patient uses it correctly 100% of the time, the *lowest expected rate*) and *patient failure* (the failure rate seen when patients actually use the method, i.e., make the mistakes in usage everyone will make from time to time, or actual noncompliance—the *typical rate*) [Table 25.1].

TABLE 25.1. Contraceptive Technique Pregnancy Rates in the First Year of Use in the United States

Method	Percentage of Women with Pregnancy	
	Lowest Expected*	Typical†
No method of contraception	85.0%	85.0%
Hormonal contraceptives		
Combination pill	0.1	3.0
Progestin-only pill	0.5	3.0
Norplant	0.2	0.2
Depo-Provera	0.3	0.3
Medroxyprogesterone and estradiol cypionate	0.3	0.3
Barrier contraceptives		
Spermicides	3.0	20.0
Condom	2.0	12.0
Cervical cap	6.0	18.0
Diaphragm and spermicide	6.0	18.0
Intrauterine contraceptive devices (IUCDs)		3.0
Progesterone IUCD	2.0	< 2.0
Copper T 380A	0.8	< 1.0
Natural family planning		
Withdrawal	4.0	18.0
Postcoital douche		40.0
Periodic abstinence		20.0
Calendar	9.0	
Ovulation method	3.0	
Symptothermal	2.0	
Postovulation	1.0	
Postcoital contraception/emergency [Yuzpe method]		25.0
Permanent—sterilization		
Male	0.1	0.15
Female	0.2	0.4

*Best performance/compliance; theoretical.
†Usual performance/compliance; usual or actual.
Modified from Speroff, Darney: *A Clinical Guide for Contraception.* 2nd ed. Baltimore, Williams & Wilkins, 1996, p. 5.

HOW CONTRACEPTIVES WORK

All available contraceptive methods act to prevent sperm and egg from uniting or prevent implantation and growth of the embryo. These goals are accomplished by (*a*) inhibiting the development and release of the egg (oral contraceptives, implantable rods, long-acting progesterone injection); (*b*) imposing a mechanical, chemical, or temporal barrier between sperm and egg (condom, diaphragm, foam, rhythm, and implantable rods); or (*c*) altering the ability of the fertilized egg to implant and grow [intrauterine devices, diethylstilbestrol, postcoital oral contraceptives, and inducing menstruation or abortion (RU 486)]. Each approach may be used successfully, individually or in combination, to prevent pregnancy, and each method has its own unique advantages and disadvantages.

FACTORS AFFECTING CHOICE OF CONTRACEPTIVE METHOD

Although efficacy is important in the choice of contraceptive methods, it is not the only factor on which the final decision is based. Factors such as safety, availability, cost, degree to which the method relies on or interferes with coitus (coital dependence), and personal acceptability to patient and partner all have a role to play in the decision. Although we tend to think of safety in terms of significant health risks, for many patients this also includes the possibilities of side effects. For a couple to use a method, it must be accessible (i.e., immediately available, especially in coitally dependent or use-oriented methods) and affordable for the patient. The effects of a method on spontaneity or modes of sexual expression may be important in some cases. The ability of a contraceptive method to provide some protection against sexually transmitted diseases may also be relevant. Furthermore, cultural, religious, or social considerations may influence a couple's choice of contraceptive method. Career or other life choices as well as plans for future fertility may influence the type and duration of the method chosen. Finally, the couple's feelings about which partner should take responsibility for contraception may be important. The clinician must be sensitive to all these factors that might influence the decision and provide factual information that fits the needs of the patient and her partner. A decision tree based on this concept is presented in Figure 25.1.

HORMONAL CONTRACEPTIVES

For many women, "*birth control*" is synonymous with the oral contraceptive pill, which in turn is synonymous with hormonal contraception. Recently, their choices have expanded to injectable hormonal preparations [injectable medroxyprogesterone; Depo-Provera; and injectable medroxyprogesterone and estradiol cypionate (MPA/E2C, or Lunelle)] and an implantable progestin mechanism (Norplant).

More than 150 million women worldwide have used oral contraceptives, and roughly one third of sexually active, fertile women in the United States use these agents. It is estimated that about one half of women in the United States 20 to 24 years old use oral contraceptives. Despite this widespread use, "the Pill" is often mistrusted or misunderstood. In some polls, up to two thirds of the respondents said that they thought the Pill was more dangerous than pregnancy, and up to one third thought that the Pill caused cancer. This lack of knowledge about such a commonly used contraceptive method makes patient education a high priority for those who care for women.

Hormone-based contraceptives provide the most effective reversible pregnancy prevention available. Theoretical failure rates for oral contraceptives are in the range of 1% or less. Long-acting hormonal methods (injections and implantable capsules) have effectiveness rates that equal or even surpass

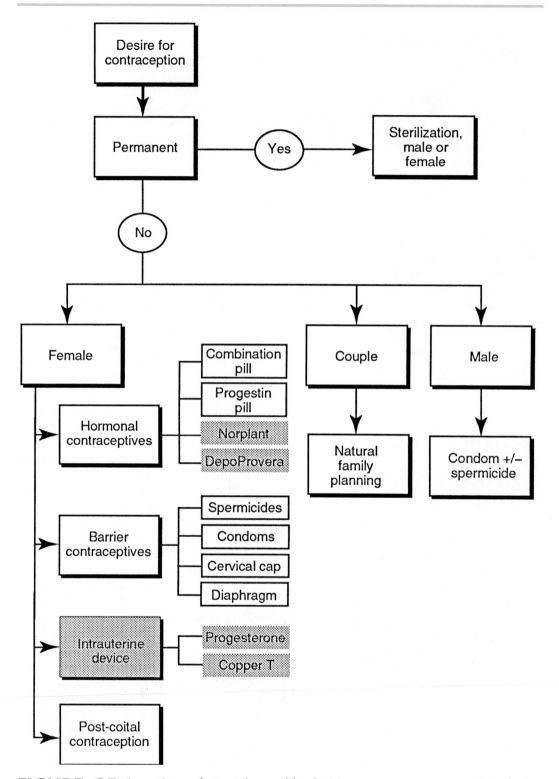

FIGURE 25.1.   One of several possible decision trees to contraceptive choice. Shaded choices are less "use oriented," that is, require minimal action on the part of the couple to be effective.

those of sterilization. Because failures are usually related to missed pills, injectable or implantable long-acting agents share the advantage of providing reliable contraception without concern for daily compliance.

Biochemistry and Methods of Action

Most of the oral contraceptive formulations are *combinations of an estrogen and a progestin*. There are also progestin-only products (Table 25.2). Combination oral contraceptive preparations contain ethinyl estradiol (estradiol with an ethinyl group at the 17 position, rendering the estradiol active orally) or *mestranol* as the estrogen component, and one of the *19-nortestosterones* as the progestin product. The progestational component provides the major contraceptive effect, acting primarily by suppression of luteinizing hormone (LH) secretion and, in turn, ovulation. The estrogenic component acts by suppression of follicle-stimulating hormone (FSH) secretion (thus preventing selection and emergence of a dominant follicle) as well as by potentiation of the action of the progestational agent, probably by increasing the number of intracellular progesterone receptors. Additional effects of the progestational component include thickening of the cervical mucus and altered fallopian tube peristalsis. Thus, the minimal estrogenic component potentiates the progestational effect and provides a modest contraceptive effect itself, but is necessary to attain the full efficacy of the combination oral contraceptive.

Based on human endometrial response and selected biochemical markers, ethinyl estradiol is thought to be about 1.7 times as potent as the same weight of mestranol. Ethinyl estradiol is absorbed by the stomach; peak serum levels are reached within 1 hour of ingestion, with mestranol peaking somewhat later. Common examples of the progestin compounds used include, in descending order of biologic progestin activity, *norgestrel, ethynodiol diacetate, norethindrone acetate, norethynodrel, and norethindrone*. Oral contraceptives using the less androgenic agents *desogestrel* and *gestodene* are also available if less androgenic activity is desired.

Most oral contraceptives contain a fixed ratio of estrogen and progestin. *"Phasic" formulations* have been introduced that vary this ratio during the course of the month. This leads to a slight decrease in the total dose of hormone used per month, but is also associated with a slightly higher rate of bleeding between periods.

Progestin-only contraceptives (progestin-only "minipill") act primarily by making the endometrium hostile to implantation and the cervical mucus thick and relatively impermeable. Ovulation continues normally in about 40% of patients. The minipill has a higher failure rate, especially in younger women compared with women older than 40 years of age. As a result, these oral contraceptives are of special usefulness in two clinical situations: lactating women and women older than 40 years. In the former group, the progestin effect coincides with the prolactin-induced suppression of ovulation; in the latter group, the inherent reduced fecundity adds to the progestin effect. There is no effect on the quality or quantity of breast milk, nor any evidence of short- or long-term adverse effects on infants, and the progestin-only pill may be started immediately after delivery in the breast-feeding mother. The progestin-only pill is also a good choice for women in whom estrogen-containing formulations are contraindicated. Because of the low dosages of progestin, the minipill must be taken at the same time each day, starting on the first day of menses. If a woman is more than 3 hours late in taking the minipill, a backup contraceptive method should be used for 48 hours.

Hormonal contraceptive agents act to prevent pregnancy through several routes. These agents *block ovulation* by interfering with the pulsatile release of FSH and LH from the pituitary. This appears to be the main effect that confers protection from pregnancy. The estrogenic components seem preferentially to inhibit FSH and are dose dependent, whereas the progestational agents preferentially inhibit the preovulatory

TABLE 25.2. Common Oral Contraceptive Preparations

Preparation	Estrogen	μg	Progestin	Days	mg
Combination oral contraceptives					
Alesse	Ethinyl estradiol	20	Levonorgestrel		1
Brevicon	Ethinyl estradiol	35	Norethindrone		0.5
Demulen	Ethinyl estradiol	50	Ethynodiol diacetate		1
Demulen 1/35	Ethinyl estradiol	35	Ethynodiol diacetate		1
Desogen	Ethinyl estradiol	30	Desogestrel		0.15
Estrostep	Ethinyl estradiol	20	Norethindrone acetate	1–5	1
		30		6–12	1
		35		13–21	1
Genora 0.5/35	Ethinyl estradiol	35	Norethindrone		0.5
Genora 1/35	Ethinyl estradiol	35	Norethindrone		1.0
Levelen	Ethinyl estradiol	30	Levonorgestrel		0.15
Loestrin 1/20	Ethinyl estradiol	20	Norethindrone acetate		1
Loestrin 1.5/30	Ethinyl estradiol	30	Norethindrone acetate		1.5
Lo/Ovral	Ethinyl estradiol	30	Norgestrel		0.3
Modicon	Ethinyl estradiol	35	Norethindrone		0.5
Nordette	Ethinyl estradiol	30	Levonorgestrel		0.15
Norlestrin 1/50	Ethinyl estradiol	50	Norethindrone acetate		1
Norlestrin 2.5/50	Ethinyl estradiol	50	Norethindrone acetate		2.5
Norinyl 1 + 35	Ethinyl estradiol	35	Norethindrone		1
Norinyl 1 + 50	Mestranol	50	Norethindrone		1
Ortho-Cept	Ethinyl estradiol	30	Desogestrel		0.15
Ortho-Cyclen	Ethinyl estradiol	35	Norgestimate		0.25
Ortho-Novum 1/35	Ethinyl estradiol	35	Norethindrone		1
Ortho-Novum 1/50	Mestranol	50	Norethindrone		1
Ortho-Novum 10/11	Ethinyl estradiol	35	Norethindrone	1–10	0.5
				11–21	1
Ortho-Novum 7/7/7	Ethinyl estradiol	35	Norethindrone	1–7	0.5
		35		8–14	0.75
		35		15–21	1.0
Ortho Tri-Cyclen	Ethinyl estradiol	35	Norgestimate	1–7	0.18
		35		8–14	0.215
		35		15–21	0.25
Ovcon	Ethinyl estradiol	35	Norethindrone		0.4
Ovral	Ethinyl estradiol	50	Norgestrel		0.5
Tri-Levlen	Ethinyl estradiol	30	Levonorgestrel	1–6	0.05
		40		7–11	0.075
		30		12–21	0.125
Tri-Norinyl	Ethinyl estradiol	35	Norethindrone	1–7	0.5
		35		8–16	1.0
		35		17–21	0.5
Triphasil	Ethinyl estradiol	30	Levonorgestrel	1–6	0.05
				7–11	0.075
				12–21	0.125
Progestin-only "minipill"					
Micronor			Norethindrone		0.35
Nor-Q D			Norethindrone		0.35
Ovrette			Norgestrel		0.075

LH surge, with a lesser effect on FSH. Hormonal agents also *alter cervical mucus*, making it thicker and more difficult for sperm to penetrate. It has been postulated that the combined estrogenic and progestational influences on the endometrium result in a thinned, unstimulated, *atrophic change in the endometrium*, inhibiting implantation. This latter effect sometimes results in scant or missed menses. For many patients the establishing of regular, highly predictable, scant, and relatively painless menses is an added benefit of oral contraceptives.

Effects of Hormonal Contraceptives

Hormonal contraception affects more than just the reproductive system. Estrogens cause alterations in glucose tolerance, affect lipid metabolism, potentiate sodium and water retention, increase renin substrate, and can reduce antithrombin III. Progestins increase sebum and facial and body hair, induce smooth muscle relaxation, and increase the risk of cholestatic jaundice. The newer progestational agents desogestrel and gestodene have less metabolic impact.

Oral contraceptives have many beneficial effects. As many as 1 in 750 women, or some 50,000 women a year in the United States, avoid hospitalization because of the beneficial effects of oral contraceptives. Oral contraceptive users have a lower incidence of endometrial and ovarian cancer, benign breast and ovarian disease, and pelvic infection. Ectopic pregnancy is prevented along with the complications of intrauterine pregnancies. Menstrual periods are predictable, shorter, and less painful, and as a result, the risk of iron deficiency anemia is reduced. There even appears to be a protective effect against rheumatoid arthritis.

Breakthrough bleeding is noted in 10% to 30% of women taking low-dose oral contraceptives during the first 3 months of use, and is an especially worrisome symptom, although it is not associated with decreased efficacy as long as the pill-taking regimen is maintained. The most common kind of breakthrough bleeding occurs in the first 3 months of use and is best managed by encouragement and reassurance because it resolves spontaneously. Breakthrough bleeding thereafter is associated with progestin-induced decidualization, with the shallow and fragile endometrium prone to asynchronous breakdown and bleeding. If the bleeding is too worrisome, a short course of exogenous estrogen, usually 1.25 mg conjugated estrogen daily for 7 days when the bleeding is present, is given while the patient continues the oral contraceptive, no matter where the patient is in her oral contraceptive cycle. Taking two or three of the low-dose oral contraceptives is not an effective therapy because the progestin component will predominate, often worsening the problem by further decidualizing already asynchronously shedding endometrium. *Amenorrhea* is another worrisome symptom, primarily because of recurrent concern about pregnancy. It is seen in approximately 1% of users of low-dose oral contraceptives in the first year of use, reaching perhaps 5% of users after several years of use. Contraceptive efficacy is maintained if the pill regimen is followed. Exogenous estrogen (1.25 mg conjugated estrogen throughout the 21 days while taking the oral contraceptive) may be used to facilitate menses if the patient wishes. A pregnancy test should precede any therapy.

Serious complications such as venous thrombosis, pulmonary embolism, cholestasis and gallbladder disease, stroke, and myocardial infarction were more likely for women using the high-dose early formulations of oral contraceptives, which are no longer used. They are seen in patients taking low-dose formulations in rare circumstances, also. Hepatic tumors have also been associated with the use of oral contraceptives. These tumors are rare and have been most closely associated with high-dose mestranol-containing drugs. Although all of these complications are from 2 to 10 times more likely in pill users, they are still rare. Factors such as age, weight, and especially smoking also represent significant risk factors.

TABLE 25.3. The Management of New Symptoms in Patients Using Oral Contraceptives

Discontinue OCP; start nonhormonal methods, immediate evaluation

Loss of vision, diplopia	(Possible retinal artery thrombosis)
Unilateral numbness, weakness	(Possible stroke)
Severe chest/neck pain	(Possible myocardial infarction)
Slurring of speech	(Possible stroke)
Severe leg pain, tenderness	(Possible thrombophlebitis)
Hemoptysis, acute shortness of breath	(Possible pulmonary embolism)
Hepatic mass, tenderness	(Possible hepatic neoplasm, adenoma)

Continue OCP; immediate evaluation

Amenorrhea	(Possible pregnancy)
Breast mass	(Possible breast cancer)
Right upper quadrant pain	(Possible cholecystitis, cholelithiasis)
Severe headache	(Possible stroke, migraine headache)
Galactorrhea	(Possible pituitary adenoma)

OCP = oral contraceptive pill.

Less serious but more common side effects also depend on the dosage and type of hormones used. Estrogens may cause a feeling of bloating and weight gain, breast tenderness, nausea, fatigue, or headache. Progestins are often blamed for symptoms such as acne or depression. Most of these minor side effects may be treated by altering the dose or composition of the agent used.

The therapeutic principle of contraception is to select the method providing effective contraception with the greatest margin of safety, and then to use it as long as the patient wishes contraception. However, after selection, new clinical situations may arise that require either further evaluation or cessation of the chosen contraceptive method and substitution of another while evaluation is undertaken (Table 25.3).

A better understanding of steroid biochemistry has led to a continuing decrease in the dosage of hormones needed to provide effective contraception, which has also decreased complications and breakthrough bleeding. Every effort should be made to take advantage of lower-dosage products, while balancing the need for reliability and freedom from menstrual disturbances.

Patient Evaluation for Oral Contraceptive Use

Before considering oral contraceptives for a patient, a careful evaluation is required. Not only is the Pill relatively or absolutely contraindicated in some patients (Table 25.4), but also factors such as previous menstrual history may have an impact on the choice of these agents.

As an example, approximately 3% of patients may experience problems with resumption of their periods after prolonged oral contraceptive use (*postpill amenorrhea*). Younger women and those with *irregular periods* before the use of oral contraceptives are more likely to experience this problem after discontinuing their use, either because of the pills or a resumption of their previous menstrual pattern. These patients deserve counseling about this potential complication, or a consideration of alternative methods.

Oral contraceptives may interact with other medications that the patient is taking. This interaction may reduce the efficacy of either the oral contraceptive or the other medications. Examples of drugs that decrease the effectiveness of oral contracep-

TABLE 25.4.   Absolute and Relative Contraindications to the Use of Combination Oral Contraceptives*

Absolute

Thrombophlebitis, thromboembolic disease
Cerebral vascular disease
Coronary occlusion
Impaired liver function
Known or suspected breast cancer
Undiagnosed abnormal vaginal bleeding
Known or suspected pregnancy
Smokers older than the age of 35 years
Congenital hyperlipidemia
Hepatic neoplasm

Relative

Severe vascular headache (migraine, cluster)
Severe hypertension (if younger than 35–40 years of age and in good medical control, can elect OCP)
Diabetes mellitus (prevention of pregnancy outweighs the risk of complicating vascular disease in diabetics younger than 35–40 years)

Gallbladder disease (may exacerbate emergence of symptoms when gallstones are present)
Obstructive jaundice in pregnancy (some patients will develop jaundice)
Epilepsy (do not exacerbate epilepsy, but antiepileptic drugs may decrease effectiveness of OCPs)
Morbid obesity (must monitor glucose and lipoprotein profiles regularly)

Conditions no longer considered contraindications

Uterine leiomyoma (low-dose formulations not associated with growth; reduced bleeding may help in management)
Sickle-cell disease or sickle C disease
Before elective surgery (theoretical association with thrombosis outweighed in most cases by avoiding pregnancy)

OCP = oral contraceptive pill.
*Risk primarily related to the estrogenic component.

tives include penicillin-based antibiotics, tetracycline, barbiturates, benzodiazepines, ibuprofen, phenytoin, and the sulfonamides. Drugs that may show retarded biotransformation when oral contraceptives are also used include anticoagulants, insulin, methyldopa, hypoglycemics, phenothiazines, reserpine, and tricyclic antidepressants. Before prescribing medications to women using oral contraceptives, the clinician should consider possible drug interactions.

Injectable and Implantable Hormonal Contraceptives

Injectable medroxyprogesterone acetate (Depo-Provera) is an injectable progestin presently available in the United States. It is given in 150-mg intramuscular injections every 3 months, with a contraceptive level of progesterone maintained for at least 14 weeks providing a useful "safety" margin. The injection should be given within the first 5 days of the current menstrual period, and, if not, a back-up method of contraception is necessary for 2 weeks. Depo-Provera is not a sustained-release preparation, relying instead on higher peaks and sustained levels of progestin, as seen in Figure 25.2. In addition to thickening of the cervical mucus and decidualization of the endometrium, Depo-Provera also acts by having a circulating level of progestin high enough to block the LH surge and hence ovulation. FSH suppression does not occur as in combination oral contraceptives, with follicular development and hence maintenance of estrogen production, so that vaginal atrophy, decrease in breast size, and other estrogen-deficiency symptoms do not occur. The efficacy of Depo-Provera is roughly equivalent to that of sterilization (see Table 25.1) and is not affected by

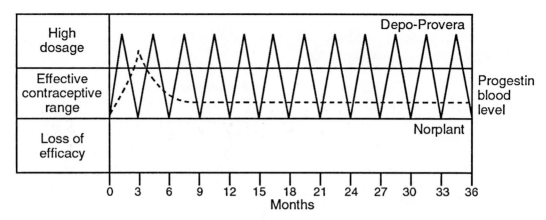

FIGURE 25.2. Rate of release of progestin for Depo-Provera.

weight or altered by patients taking medications that alter hepatic function. Depo-Provera is a popular choice for many and has special advantages for some with administration contraindicated in only a few situations, as shown in Table 25.5. The most worrisome problem with Depo-Provera is irregular vaginal spotting, which decreases with each use so that 80% of women are amenorrheic after 5 years. Because 25% of users discontinue Depo-Provera within the first year of use owing to this problem, treatment with 7 days of conjugated estrogen (1.25 mg/day) may be useful. When Depo-Provera is discontinued, about 50% resume normal menses within 6 months, although perhaps 25% do not resume menses for more than 1 year; they should be evaluated because it should not be presumed to be a drug effect. A newly released injectable formulation is a combination of medroxyprogesterone (25 mg) and estradiol cypionate (5 mg) [MPA/E2C, Lunelle], also given on a monthly basis. Its main difference may be a decreased incidence of irregular bleeding compared with medroxyprogesterone injection as a single agent.

The *Norplant system* involves the subcutaneous (Figure 25.3) implantation of six Silastic rods that permit the sustained release of levonorgestrel, leading to a sustained progestin level (see Figure 25.2) that provides contraception for 5 years. Levonorgestrel appears to exert its contraceptive effect by one or more of three mecha-nisms: suppression of the LH surge necessary for ovulation, thickening of cervical mucus, and suppression of the estradiol-induced cyclic maturation of the endometrium. The Norplant system is highly effective (see Table 25.1) and may offer advantages in women desiring longer spacing of pregnancies along with minimal user responsibility, who have contraindications to estrogen-containing contraceptive preparations or have menorrhagia-associated anemia, who are older than 35 years of age and smoke, or who have diabetes, hypercholesterolemia, hypertension, cardiovascular disease, or gallbladder disease. Norplant is contraindicated in women with active thrombophlebitis/thromboembolic disease, undiagnosed vaginal bleeding, acute liver disease, benign or malignant liver tumors, and known or suspected breast cancer. Pregnancy during Norplant use requires immediate evaluation because 30% of such pregnancies are ectopic. Circulating levels of levonorgestrel are too low to measure 48 hours after implant removal, with a prompt return to baseline fertility rates.

BARRIER CONTRACEPTIVES

Among the oldest and most widely used contraceptive methods are those that *provide a barrier between sperm and egg* and include condoms (for one or both partners), diaphragms, and cervical caps. Each of these

TABLE 25.5.   Indications and Contraindications for Depo-Provera Contraception

Indications

Desire for more than 1 year of contraception	The delay in pregnancy after the last injection averages about 9 months, with 90% of users achieving pregnancy within 18 months
Women with limited ability to remember contraceptive requirements, those with disorganized lives, and intellectually challenged women	One injection every 3 months, 2-week "safety" interval (i.e., can be delayed up to 2 weeks without loss of efficacy)
Breast-feeding	No effect on quality of breast milk or on baby; increases quantity of breast milk; can be administered immediately postpartum; should be used no later than the third postpartum week
Women for whom estrogen-containing preparations are contraindicated	See Table 25.4, Absolute Contraindications list
Women with seizure disorders	Antiseizure medications unaffected, and sedative effects of progestins may aid in seizure control
Sickle-cell anemia	Probable in vivo inhibition of sickling
Anemia secondary to menorrhagia	Decreased menstrual flow

Contraindications

Known or suspected pregnancy, or as a diagnostic test for pregnancy
Undiagnosed vaginal bleeding
Known or suspected malignancy of the breast
Active thrombophlebitis, or current or past history of thromboembolic disorders, or cerebral vascular disease
Liver dysfunction or disease
Known sensitivity to Depo-Provera (medroxyprogesterone acetate or any of its other ingredients)

---

methods *depends on proper use before or at the time of intercourse and, as such, are subject to a higher failure rate than oral contraceptives, because of inconsistent or incorrect use as well as actual damage to the barrier material itself.* Despite this, *these methods provide relatively good protection from unwanted pregnancy,* are inexpensive, and in the case of condoms, do not require medical consultation. In addition, condoms and diaphragms provide an estimated 50% reduction in the transmission of sexually transmitted diseases, including gonorrhea, herpes, and chlamydial and human papillomavirus infection. The condom is also a highly effective means of prevention of the transmission of the human immunodeficiency virus. The use of these methods, however, does not decrease the need for couples to be cautioned about high-risk behaviors.

Condoms

Condoms are sheaths usually worn over the erect penis or inside the vagina to prevent sperm from reaching the cervix and upper genital tract. Although almost one half of all condoms are sold to women, the condom is the only reliable, nonpermanent method

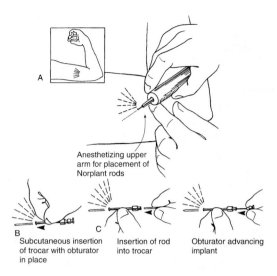

FIGURE 25.3.   Insertion of Norplant.

of contraception available to men. Condoms are widely available and inexpensive. They may be made of latex or, less commonly, animal membrane (usually sheep cecum). They are available with or without lubricants or spermicides, plain or with reservoir tips, in colors, flavors, and with ridges. There are even those that glow in the dark. Although most of these choices are of personal preference only, both lubrication and a reservoir tip reduce the likelihood of breakage.

The condom is well tolerated, with only rare reports of skin irritation or allergic reaction. Some men complain of reduced sensation with the use of condoms, but this may actually be an advantage for those with rapid or premature ejaculation. The slippage and breakage rate in normal use is estimated at 5% to 8%. Couples should be counseled to seek medical care within 72 hours of slippage or breakage so that emergency contraceptive methods may be used.

The recent introduction of the *female condom* provides another option for some couples. This is a sheath, or vaginal liner, that fits into the vagina before intercourse. Like the traditional male condom, this contraceptive relies on patient motivation to ensure proper use with each episode of intercourse. Three devices are available: a condom that looks like a G-string panty with a condom rolled within the crotch to be unrolled by the penis; the Women's

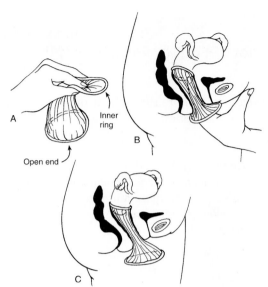

FIGURE 25.4.   The female condom. (*A*) Preparation for insertion. (*B*) Insertion. (*C*) Condom in proper position.

Choice condom, similar to a male condom, with a 2-inch flexible ring that hangs from the vaginal opening and a thickened, domed upper end that is inserted into the vagina with a tampon-like applicator; and the Reality condom, a polyurethane sheath with an open ringed end to the outside and a closed internal ring placed over the cervix, much like a diaphragm (Figure 25.4). All have slippage/breakage rates of about 3%, and like diaphragms and cervical caps, it is recommended that they be left in place 6 to 8 hours after coitus.

Diaphragms and Cervical Caps

The diaphragm is a springy ring with a dome of rubber. Proper use of a diaphragm includes applying a contraceptive jelly or cream containing spermicide to the center and rim of the device, which is then inserted into the vagina, over the cervix, and behind the pubic symphysis. In this position, the diaphragm covers the anterior vaginal wall and cervix.

There are three types of diaphragms made in sizes from 50 to 105 mm in 2.5- and 5-mm increments. Most women use 60-

to 85-mm diaphragms. The *flat or coil spring type* is suitable for women with good vaginal tone; it forms a straight line when pinched for insertion. The *arcing spring* diaphragm comes in two types: the All Flex and the hinged types. These are easier for most women to insert and are more useful for women with poor vaginal tone, cystoceles, rectoceles, a long cervix, or an anterior cervix with a retroverted uterus. The diaphragm must be inserted before intercourse (up to 1 hour before) and be left in place for 6 to 8 hours afterward. It may then be removed, washed, and stored. Should additional intercourse be desired during the 6- to 8-hour waiting time, additional spermicide should be applied without removing the diaphragm, and the waiting time restarted.

Diaphragms must be fitted to the individual patient. Fit may change with significant weight change, vaginal birth, or pelvic surgery. The diaphragm should be the largest that can be comfortably inserted, worn, and removed. If the diaphragm is too small, it may slip out during coitus because of vaginal elongation; if it is too large, it may buckle, causing discomfort, irritation, and leakage. The patient must be initially instructed in the proper positioning of the diaphragm, with the correct position subsequently verified by the patient each time it is used. If the cervix can be felt through the dome of the diaphragm, the positioning is correct. If a diaphragm is fitted in the postpartum period, its sizing should be reevaluated in 2 to 3 months because vaginal dimensions and support may change in the interval. The three types of diaphragms and correct positioning of a diaphragm are shown in Figure 25.5.

Women who use diaphragms are about twice as likely to have urinary tract infections as women using oral contraceptives. Presumably, this is related to a combination of pressure against the urethra causing a relative urinary stasis and an effect of spermicides on the normal vaginal flora, increasing the risk of *Escherichia coli* bacteriuria and infection.

Fitting a diaphragm involves two steps. The first step is a pelvic examination followed by trial-and-error fitting of various

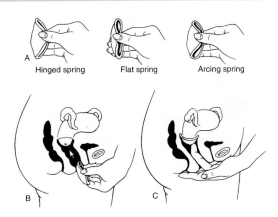

FIGURE 25.5.   Diaphragms. (*A*) The three types of diaphragms. (*B*) Insertion of the diaphragm. (*C*) Checking to ensure that the diaphragm covers the cervix.

sizes of diaphragms until one meets the criteria noted previously. The second step is to allow the patient to practice insertion, check for proper position, and remove the device, with supervision, until she is comfortable with the process and both she and the physician know that she is placing the diaphragm properly. Much of the failure associated with diaphragms may be traced to the patient not using the device because of discomfort with the method and/or improper placement.

The *cervical cap* is a smaller version of the diaphragm that is applied to the cervix itself. This method is associated with a relatively high degree of displacement and, therefore, of failure, as well as association with cervicitis and toxic shock syndrome. It also requires considerable effort to fit.

Spermicides

Although many "spermicidal" chemicals have been tried over the years, today's spermicides rely on one of two agents to immobilize or kill sperm: *nonoxynol-9 and octoxynol-3*. These compounds are inserted into the vagina before intercourse and are delivered in a variety of ways: creams, jellies, foams, films, suppositories, and tablets. They should be applied high into the vagina against the cervix, from 15 to 60 minutes before each act of intercourse, because the duration of maximal spermicidal effectiveness is usually no more than 1 hour. Douching should be avoided for at least 8 hours after use. There is no known association between spermicide use and congenital malformation.

Spermicides are inexpensive, well tolerated, and provide good protection from pregnancy. *For a well-motivated couple who wish a greater degree of protection, spermicides are often combined with condoms to achieve failure rates that approach those of hormonal methods.*

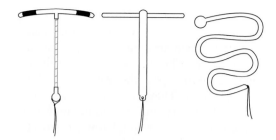

FIGURE 25.6. Intrauterine devices. The ParaGard copper-releasing IUD (approved life span 8 years) and the Progestasert progestin-releasing IUD (approved life span 1 year) are available in the United States. The flexible polyethylene Lippes loop is used throughout the world except in the United States.

INTRAUTERINE DEVICES

Intrauterine contraceptive devices (IUCDs or IUDs) are among the most commonly used and safe methods of interval contraception worldwide, and were used extensively in the United States until the 1980s. At that time a marked increase in pelvic infections in women using a specific IUD, the Dalkon Shield, led to a general rejection of all IUDs by patients and physicians. In fact, the tail of the Dalkon Shield was improperly designed, promoting infection; a design not shared by the other IUDs, which were actually safe then and remain safe and effective nowadays. In recent years new, exhaustively tested IUDs have been introduced, and these new IUDs are again, appropriately, gaining acceptance and use in the United States.

Two "medicated" IUDs are available in the United States (Figure 25.6). The *TCU-380A (ParaGard)* is a T-shaped polyethylene frame holding 380 mm² of exposed copper weighing 176 mg, to which is attached a polyethylene monofilament tied through a 3-mm ball on the stem of the IUD so that two white threads are available for detection and removal. The IUD frame is rendered radiopaque with barium sulfate. The other is the *Progestasert,* a T-shaped ethylene/vinyl acetate device whose vertical stem contains a reservoir of 39 mg of progesterone together with barium sulfate dispersed in silicone fluid. Two blue-black monofilament strings are attached at a hole

in the base of the stem. The device releases 65 μg per day of progesterone.

There are many other medicated and unmedicated IUDs used throughout the world. Perhaps the most common unmedicated variety is the Lippes loop, a barium sulfate impregnated IUD, which was also widely used in the United States until the scare of the 1980s (see Figure 25.6).

IUDs act by rendering the intrauterine environment hostile by means of what has been termed a sterile inflammatory response to the foreign IUD. This environment is spermicidal so few sperm reach the ovum in the fallopian tube, preventing fertilization, and if fertilization does occur, implantation is likewise inhibited when the cleaving ovum reaches the uterine cavity. Thus, IUDs do not act by alteration of ovulation nor are IUDs abortifacients. In the case of the copper-containing IUD, the copper and copper salts that are released enhance the inflammatory response and, in addition, exert an additional spermicidal effect in the cervical mucus. The progestin-releasing devices add progestin effects, including decidualization of the endometrium and inhibition of implantation, inhibition of sperm capacitation and survival, and thickening of the cervical mucus. An important side effect of the progestin is a decrease in menstrual blood loss (up to 50%) and severity of dysmenorrhea. Serum progesterone levels are not affected. IUD removal is followed by rapid reversal of the effects and return to a normal intrauterine environment and normal fertility.

The IUDs presently available in the United States are highly effective. The TCU-380A has a recommended life span of 8 years and demonstrates a pregnancy rate of 0.5%–0.8%. The progesterone-releasing Progestasert must be replaced yearly as the progesterone reservoir is depleted and has a pregnancy rate of 1.3%–1.6%. The overall expulsion rate for IUDs is 1%–5%, with the greatest likelihood in the first few months of use. Expulsion is often heralded by cramping, vaginal discharge, or bleeding, although it may be asymptomatic with the only evidence being the observed lengthening of the IUD string. Patients should be counseled to see their clinician if expulsion is suspected because the device is not effective in this circumstance.

Increased *vaginal bleeding and menstrual pain* are experienced by 5%–10% of women and often result in their request to discontinue IUD use. The progestin IUDs have a lesser incidence of this problem because of the progestin effect on the endometrium. The use of nonsteroidal anti-inflammatory drugs (NSAIDs) on a scheduled format during the first few cycles of IUD use is often effective in preventing or ameliorating these symptoms.

There are two categories of *pelvic infection associated with IUDs.* The first is infection within 6–8 weeks of insertion. Such "insertional" infections are presumed to arise from bacteria introduced into the uterus during IUD insertion, and are derived from the endogenous cervicovaginal flora, are polymicrobial, and have a predominance of anaerobes. Doxycycline (200 mg) or azithromycin (500 mg) administered one hour prior to insertion can provide significant protection from such infection. Women with rheumatic or valvular heart disease or with prosthetic heart valves may be acceptable candidates for IUD contraception if they are otherwise appropriate candidates. Antibiotic prophylaxis (amoxicillin 2 g orally) should be given to these women one hour before IUD insertion (or

removal). Pelvic infection occurring three or more months after IUD insertion may be presumed to be an acquired sexually transmitted disease (STD) and treated accordingly. Asymptomatic IUD users with positive cervical cultures for gonorrhea or chlamydia, or with bacterial vaginosis, should be treated promptly. The IUD may remain in place unless there is evidence of ascent of the infection to the endometrium or fallopian tubes. In the latter case, the IUD should be removed promptly and the antibiotic regimen appropriate to the patient's clinical diagnosis utilized.

IUDs do not increase the overall risk of ectopic pregnancy. However, because the IUD offers greater protection against intrauterine than extrauterine pregnancy, the relative ratio of extrauterine pregnancy is greater in an IUD user than in a woman not using contraception.

Pregnancy with an IUD in place is a vexing problem. About 40%–50% of patients will spontaneously abort in the first trimester. Because of this risk, patients should be offered IUD removal if the string is visible, and this is associated with a decreased spontaneous abortion rate of about 30%. If the IUD string is not visible, instrumental removal may be performed, but the risk of pregnancy disruption is increased. If the IUD is left in place, pregnancy may proceed uneventfully, and there is no evidence of an increased risk of congenital anomalies, with either medicated or unmedicated devices. There is, however, an approximate 2- to 4-fold increase in the incidence of preterm labor and delivery.

Patient selection and skillful insertion are crucial to successful use of the IUD as a method of contraception. The risk of STDs is the most important factor in patient selection, not age and parity. IUD use is relatively contraindicated for women with multiple sexual partners, whose partners have multiple partners, who have a history of recurrent or recent episodes of gonorrheal or chlamydial infection, or who are drug or alcohol abusers. IUD insertion is contraindicated when there is a history of current, recent, or recurrent pelvic inflammatory disease (PID). Women with heavy

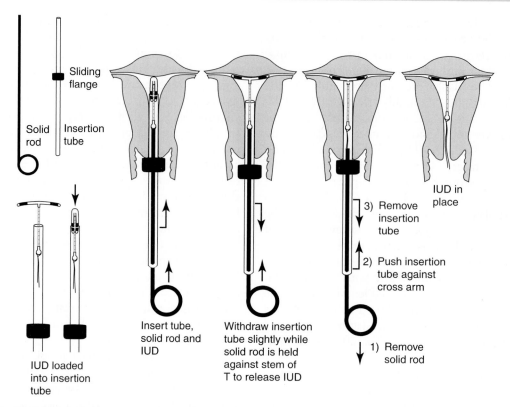

Solid rod

Insertion tube

Sliding flange

IUD loaded into insertion tube

Insert tube, solid rod and IUD

Withdraw insertion tube slightly while solid rod is held against stem of T to release IUD

3) Remove insertion tube

2) Push insertion tube against cross arm

1) Remove solid rod

IUD in place

FIGURE 25.7.   Insertion of an IUD.

menses, who are anticoagulated, or who have a bleeding disorder may benefit from a progestin IUD but should not use non-medicated or copper-bearing IUDs. Other conditions (i.e., uterine anomalies, leiomyomas, cervical stenosis) can compromise IUD success and alternate contraceptive methods may be better chosen. Immuno-suppressed patients should not use IUDs. Adolescence and nulliparity are not contraindications in properly selected young women in monogomous relationships.

IUD insertion is best accomplished when the patient is menstruating. IUDs may also be inserted in breast-feeding women who in fact demonstrate a lower incidence of postinsertional discomfort and bleeding. All IUD insertion techniques share the same basic rules: careful bimanual examination before insertion to determine the likely direction of insertion into the endometrial cavity, proper loading of the device into the inserter, careful placement to the fundal margin of the endometrial cavity, and

proper inserter removal while leaving the IUD in place. Figure 25.7 demonstrates these techniques. IUD removal is usually easy; when the patient is on her menses, pull on the IUD string. If the string is not visible, rotating two cotton-tip applicators in the endocervical canal will often retrieve the strings. If this is not possible, a fine probe may be inserted, the IUD felt, and then removed with an "IUD hook" or small forceps. Infrequently, IUDs become embedded in the uterine wall and require hystero-scopic removal.

NATURAL FAMILY PLANNING

So-called natural family planning (also called "the rhythm method") usually refers to methods that seek to *prevent pregnancy by either avoiding intercourse around the time of ovulation or using knowledge of the time of ovulation to augment other meth-*

ods, such as barriers or spermicides. These methods are safe, cost little, and are more acceptable for religious reasons or for those couples who wish a more natural method. For couples who are highly motivated and for women with a regular menstrual cycle, these methods may provide acceptable contraception.

The *estimation of the woman's "fertile" period* is based on calendar calculations, variations in basal body temperature, changes in cervical mucus, or a combination (sometimes called symptothermic method) of these methods. When the calendar is used, the fertile period would last from days 10 through 17 for a woman with an absolutely regular 28-day cycle. Additional days are added to the fertile period based on the time of shortest and longest menstrual interval. Thus, a woman with periods every 28 ± 3 days would be considered to be fertile from days 7 (10 − 3) to 20 (17 + 3). Basal body temperatures (BBTs) and changes in cervical mucus are used to detect ovulation. A rise in BBT of 0.5 to 1° F or the presence of thin, "stretchy," clear cervical mucus indicates ovulation.

Couples using these methods avoid intercourse until a suitable period after ovulation, that is, from the start of menses until 2 to 3 days after temperature rise or from the first awareness of the clear, copious mucus associated with ovulation until 4 to 5 days thereafter, indicated by the return of the milky or opaque mucus seen in the nonovulatory, or "safe," interval. These methods are especially difficult to use in the postpartum time, when menstrual regularity has not yet resumed and cervical secretions are varied in appearance. Resumption of normal pituitary function and ovulation usually occurs sometime in the 4th to 6th week postpartum but can vary with individuals, especially with breast-feeding. Ovulation has been reported as early as the 5th week postpartum, however, in a lactating patient.

These methods are less attractive to many couples because of the high level of motivation and cycle regularity required, along with the restrictions and loss of spontaneity placed on sexual relations.

POSTCOITAL/EMERGENCY CONTRACEPTION

Postcoital/emergency contraception may be needed for women who experience an act of unprotected sexual intercourse (e.g., unintended intercourse; IUCD expulsion; barrier failure such as condom breakage or diaphragm displacement; or in the case of sexual assault). Making postcoital contraception widely and easily available is one of the most important steps that can be taken to reduce the unacceptable rates of unintended pregnancy and abortion. It is estimated that the regular use of this postcoital regimen would prevent in excess of 1.5 million unintended pregnancies in the United States.

The most frequently used modern method, cited by the Food and Drug Administration (FDA) as a safe and effective method of postcoital contraception, is the relatively high-dose estrogen-progestin method of Yuzpe, oral contraceptive tablets each containing 0.05 mg ethinyl estradiol and 0.5 mg DL-norgestrel (Ovral). Two tablets are taken within 72 hours of intercourse, followed by two tablets in 12 hours. Alternatively, other regimens cited by the FDA include four tablets within 72 hours of intercourse, followed by four tablets in 12 hours of Lo/Ovral (0.03 mg ethinyl estradiol and 0.30 mg norgestrel), Nordette (0.03 mg ethinyl estradiol and 0.15 mg levonorgestrel), or Triphasil. The regimen is quite safe, and there are no recognized medical contraindications to its use. Use of an antiemetic [e.g., promethazine hydrochloride (Phenergan), one 25-mg tablet or suppository one hour before the first ECP dose and repeated as needed every 8–12 hours thereafter] before taking this regimen lessens the risk of nausea and emesis, a common side effect. The failure rate for this regimen is estimated at 25%, with up to 98% of the remaining patients menstruating within 3 weeks. Multiple unprotected coital events or an interval greater than 72 hours may be associated with an increasing failure rate.

A newly approved progestin-only oral emergency contraception method has been approved by the FDA. Called "Plan B," it consists of two tablets of levonorgestrel. It is associated with a lower incidence of nausea and emesis than the Yuzpe method while having approximately the same effectiveness. It is believed to act by preventing ovulation and fertilization and, like the Yuzpe method, will not terminate an existing pregnancy.

The total amount of hormone in these regimens is quite small compared to that when used as interval contraceptive regimens and is not associated with alterations in clotting factors and similar mechanisms. There are no evidence-based criteria studies suggesting contraindications to the use of these emergency contraceptive regimens. There is insufficient information to evaluate the teratogenic risk if treatment fails, but the use of combination oral contraceptives during the first trimester is not associated with an adverse effect in the incidence or type of common congenital anomalies, and

it is presumed that this association holds for emergency contraception as well.

IUCD insertion (ParaGard T380, Ortho Pharmaceuticals; within 7 days) is another recommended option and in limited studies has reported a failure rate of approximately 0.1%. An additional advantage of IUCD insertion is the contraceptive effect that is provided for up to 10 years.

INEFFECTIVE METHODS

Just as the clinician must provide information about effective contraception to those who request it, he or she must also counsel against routine use of less-than-effective techniques. *Folklore-based techniques* such as postcoital douching, withdrawal before ejaculation (coitus interruptus), makeshift barriers (such as food wrap), and various coital positions should all be discouraged if pregnancy is to be avoided.

CASE STUDIES

Case 25A

An 18-year-old nulligravid patient wants to know what is "the best method of birth control." She is not yet sexually active, although she and her boyfriend have been "close" on several occasions. The patient plans further education and correctly realizes that an unwanted pregnancy would spell disaster for her. She would not consider a pregnancy termination, and the fear of pregnancy has become a problem for her and her boyfriend. Her history reveals that her periods are regular with cramping, for which she takes over-the-counter medications with some relief. She is currently taking no medications and knows of no allergies.

Questions Case 25A

In listing possible options, all of the following might be appropriate EXCEPT

A. Oral contraceptives
B. Vaginal spermicides
C. Diaphragm
D. IUCD
E. Rhythm

Answer: D

All of the methods listed might be possible for the couple to use. Given the patient's history of dysmenorrhea, IUCDs are likely to be unsatisfactory.

The patient tells you that because of her fear of pregnancy, oral stimulation has become an important part of her and her boyfriend's sexual expression. Because they may not always have control over when they might have the opportunity for intercourse, they would also like to avoid methods that interfere with spontaneity. Based on this information, your best recommendation might be

A. Oral contraceptives
B. Vaginal spermicides
C. Diaphragm
D. IUCD
E. Rhythm

Answer: A

Oral contraceptive pills do not interfere with spontaneity and are effective any time the opportunity for intercourse presents itself. A diaphragm would not be a good method because it does interfere with spontaneity. The couple's preference for oral stimulation makes vaginal spermicides and diaphragms (which also use spermicides) less desirable. (These agents are not toxic, per se, but do provide an objectionable taste for most couples.) Oral contraceptives are also likely to provide relief from the patient's menstrual discomfort.

Case 25B

A 25-year-old G1 P1001 patient had six progestin-containing rods implanted after the birth of her child 3 months ago. At the time of her 6-week postpartum check she was normal, but since that time she has experienced slight random vaginal bleeding. The blood is light in amount and variable in color. She has no cramps, fever, or chills, and she is bottle feeding her infant.

Question Case 25B

The most likely cause of this condition is

A. Subinvolution of the uterus
B. Retained placental products

C. Progesterone-induced endometrial atrophy
D. Progesterone-induced endometrial hyperplasia
E. Irregular ovulation

Answer: C

Answers A and B are unlikely to be found in an asymptomatic patient 3 months after delivery. Patients using implantable progestin-containing rods usually are anovulatory and develop a thin, atrophic endometrium. Patients should be reassured that the bleeding is expected to be self-limiting.

Case 25C

A 38-year-old G3 P2012, recently divorced business executive is taking a low-dose monophasic oral contraceptive, which she has taken since the birth of her last child 6 years ago. She has had no particular problems and does not smoke. She is not currently dating but wishes to continue effective contraception. Her pelvic examination is normal with the exception of 10-week fibroids.

Question Case 25C

Acceptable methods of contraception for this patient include

A. Tubal cautery
B. Rhythm
C. Oral contraceptives
D. Condom/foam
E. IUCD

Answer: All

For a patient who is sexually active on a sporadic basis, a use-oriented method may provide excellent protection from pregnancy without the possible problems of an ongoing method. She is an educated, potentially motivated patient who could use foam/condom, a diaphragm, or even

(Continued)

rhythm quite effectively. The patient's age and finding of fibroids make oral contraceptives less desirable, although not unreasonable as long as close follow-up is maintained. The decision to undergo sterilization is an option that can be discussed, but is a decision that only the patient can make. The history suggests that this option has not been chosen, although it may also not have received consideration. An IUCD is less desirable because of possible expulsion by the uterus with fibroids and the fact that she is not necessarily going to be monogamous. This case is a good example of how contraception choices must be individualized for each patient, and the relative risks of all alternatives discussed.

Case 25D

A 25-year-old nulligravid patient requests contraception, but indicates that she does not wish to use a hormonal contraceptive method and finds barrier methods cumbersome, interfering with the spontaneity of her sexual life. She asks about IUDs. In taking her history, you learn that she has had 4 sexual partners in the last 6 years, presently with one partner for 10 months. She had chlamydia at age 20, but no illness since. She gives a history of normal pelvic examinations and negative Pap smears. She had menarche at age 13, and her periods are described as heavy and rather painful.

Question Case 25D

She asks your opinion about an IUD because she has heard that women who have not had children should not use IUDs for contraception.

Answer

You explain that IUDs are not contraindicated for nulligravidas as long as they have no history of recent infections or a history of multiple sexual partners or risky sexual practices. Because she has heavy menses that are painful, you suggest that a progestin-containing IUD may offer an additional advantage besides contraception, specifically a diminution of the pain and severity of vaginal bleeding caused by the effect of the progestin on the uterine lining, the endometrium.

26

STERILIZATION

This chapter deals primarily with APGO Objective(s):

OBJECTIVE 36   Sterilization

Describe the methods, risks and benefits, contraindications, failure rates, reversibility, financial considerations, and potential complications for each commonly used method of male and female sterilization.

Sterilization offers highly effective birth control without continuing expense, effort, or motivation. *It is the most frequent method of controlling fertility used in the United States, with close to a million procedures performed annually.* Approximately one in three married couples have chosen surgical sterilization as their method of contraception. Sterilization is the leading contraceptive method for couples when the wife is older than 30 years and for those who have been married more than 10 years.

All available surgical methods of sterilization prevent the union of sperm and egg, either by preventing the passage of sperm into the ejaculate (vasectomy) or by permanently occluding the fallopian tube (tubal ligation). Although it is possible to reverse some forms of sterilization, the difficulty of doing so, combined with the generally poor rate of success, demands that patients understand the permanent nature of the decision. The physician must be able accurately to counsel couples considering surgical sterilization and assist in determining the best method from those available. Surprisingly, twice as many women as men choose sterilization, despite the greater operative hazards involved, underscoring the need for accurate counseling of both members of the couple.

Changes in operative techniques; anesthesia methods; and attitudes of the public, insurance providers, and physicians have contributed to the rapid increase in the number of sterilization procedures performed each year. Modern methods of surgical sterilization are less invasive, less expensive, safer, and as effective—if not more effective—than those used 20 years ago. These factors have combined to decrease concern about the invasive nature of these procedures despite the reality that they are more invasive, *per se,* than vasectomy. *Counseling of patients must include discussion of the permanent nature of the procedures, the operative risks, and the chance of pregnancy (less than 1%).*

Despite careful counseling, approximately 1% of patients undergoing sterilization subsequently request reversal of the procedure because of a change in marital status, loss of a child, or desire for more children. *Successful reversal occurs in only 40% to 60% of cases.*

STERILIZATION IN MEN

About one third of all surgical sterilization procedures are performed on men. Because the vas deferens is located outside the abdominal cavity, vasectomy is safer and usually less expensive than procedures done on women. Vasectomy is also more easily reversed than most female sterilization procedures. Vasectomy is routinely performed as an outpatient procedure, under local anesthesia. The procedure takes 15 to 20 minutes and consists of mobilizing the vas through a small incision in the scrotum, excision of a short segment of vas, and sealing the ends of the vas with suture, cautery, or clips (Figure 26.1). Postoperative complications include bleeding, hematomas, and local skin infections, but these occur in less than 3% of cases. Some authors report a greater incidence of depression and change in body image after vasectomy than after female sterilization. This risk may be minimized with preoperative counseling and education. Concern has been raised about the formation of sperm antibodies in approximately 50% of patients, but no adverse long-term effects of vasectomy have been identified. Likewise, concerns about an increased risk of prostate cancer following vasectomy are not supported in literature; indeed, in countries with the highest rates of vasectomy, there is no increase in the incidence of prostate cancer.

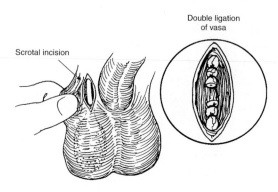

Scrotal incision

Double ligation of vasa

FIGURE 26.1. Vasectomy.

Pregnancy after vasectomy occurs in about 1% of cases. Many of these pregnancies result from intercourse too soon after the procedure, rather than from recanalization. Vasectomy is not immediately effective. Multiple ejaculations are required before the proximal collecting system is emptied of sperm. Couples should use another method of contraception until male sterility is reasonably assured (6 weeks, or after 15 ejaculations) and/or postoperative azoospermia is confirmed by semen analysis.

STERILIZATION IN WOMEN

Surgical sterilization techniques for women may be broadly divided into *postpartum* and *interval* (between pregnancies) procedures, although most techniques may be performed at either time. Factors such as parity, obesity, previous surgery or pelvic infections, and medical conditions (such as hypertension or respiratory diseases) may affect the timing and method chosen.

Laparoscopy

The development of efficient light sources, fiberoptic light guides, and smaller instruments has led to a dramatic increase in the use of laparoscopy for female sterilization. Performed as an outpatient interval procedure, laparoscopic techniques may be carried out under either local, regional, or general anesthesia. Small incisions, a relatively low rate of complications, and a degree of flexibility in the procedures possible have led to high physician and patient acceptability.

In laparoscopic procedures, a small infraumbilical incision is made in the skin and a trocar and sheath are placed into the abdominal cavity. Although most operators prefer to create a pneumoperitoneum before trocar placement, safe placement may also be accomplished without this step. The trocar is withdrawn and a laparoscope passed through the sheath into the abdominal cavity. For many procedures, two or more smaller trocars are passed (under direct vision) through the lower abdominal wall. A cannula or uterine manipulator is often used to aid in visualizing pelvic structures and moving them into position for surgery. At the close of the procedure, the pneumoperitoneum is evacuated and the skin closed with one or two buried absorbable sutures and/or skin tapes. Closure of the fascial defect is becoming more commonplace because of the possibility of hernia formation at the trocar site.

Occlusion of the fallopian tubes may be accomplished through the use of electrocautery (unipolar or bipolar) or the application of a plastic and spring clip (the Hulka clip) or Silastic band (Yoon or Falope ring) [Figure 26.2]. The choice among laparoscopic methods is often based more on operator experience, training, and personal preference than on outcome data.

Electrocautery-based methods are fast and carry the lowest failure rates, but they carry a greater risk of inadvertent electrical damage to other structures, poorer reversibility, and a greater incidence of ectopic pregnancies when failure does occur. Most operators agree that coagulation at two sites is preferable, with care being taken that the coagulation forceps is placed over the entire fallopian tube and onto the mesosalpinx so that the entire tube and its lumen are coagulated over a centimeter or so of the tube. Most operators also prefer bipolar cautery, because it has less risk of spark injury to adjacent tissue because the current is passed directly between the blades of the coagulation forceps.

The Hulka clip is the most readily reversed method because of its minimal tissue damage, but it also carries the greatest failure rate (up to 1%) for the same reason. As in coagulation, care must be taken to place the jaws of the Hulka clip over the entire breadth of the fallopian tube.

The Falope ring falls between the other two methods in both reversibility and failure rates but may have a higher incidence of postoperative pain, requiring strong analgesics. Care must be taken to draw a sufficient "knuckle" of fallopian tube into the Falope ring applicator so that the band is placed below the outer and inner borders of

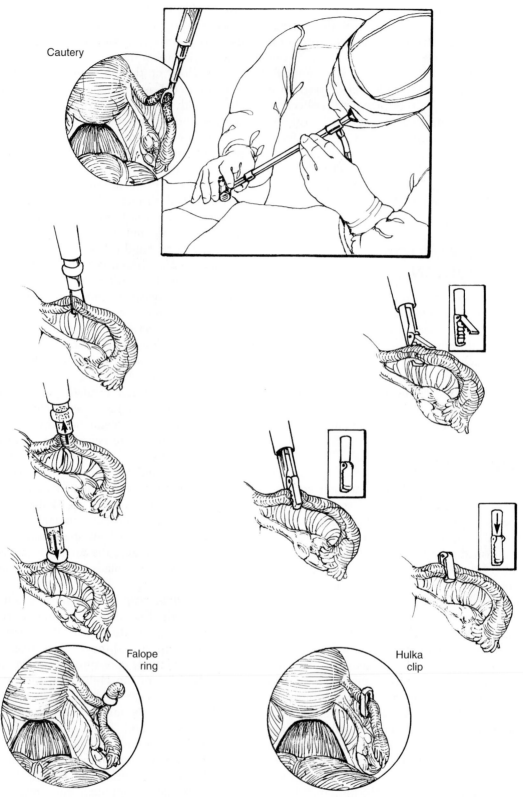

Cautery

Falope ring

Hulka clip

FIGURE 26.2. Laparoscopic sterilization.

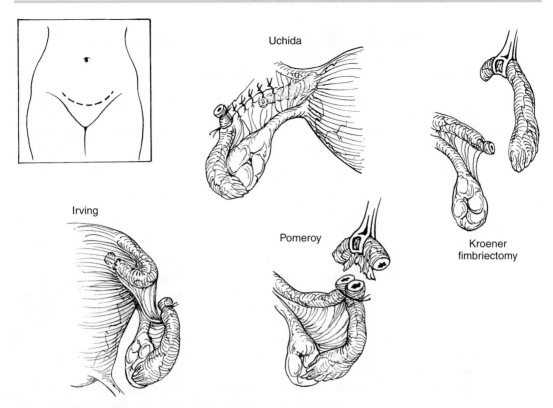

FIGURE 26.3.   Sterilization at laparotomy.

the fallopian tube, thus occluding the lumen completely.

Laparotomy

The oldest methods of female sterilization have used laparotomy. Whether it is a small infraumbilical incision made in the postpartum period or a small lower abdominal suprapubic incision (minilaparotomy) used as an interval procedure, laparotomy provides ready access to the uterine tubes. Permanent obstruction or interruption of the fallopian tubes may then be accomplished by a variety of means, such as excision of all or part of the fallopian tube or the use of clips, rings, or cautery. Laparotomy techniques do not require the special tools or training needed for laparoscopy, which makes them attractive for many more physicians or smaller hospitals.

The most common method of tubal interruption done by laparotomy is the Pomeroy tubal ligation (Figure 26.3). In this procedure, a segment of tube from the mid-portion is elevated and an absorbable ligature is placed across the base, forming a loop, or knuckle, of tube. This is then excised and sent for histologic confirmation. When healing is complete, the ends of the tube will have sealed closed, and there will be a 1- to 2-cm gap between the ends. Failure using this method is *in the range of 1 in 500 procedures.* Many modifications of this technique have been described (Table 26.1). These methods have acceptably low failure rates but are not as popular as the Pomeroy technique. Electrocoagulation or the application of clips or bands may also be accomplished through a laparotomy incision, although these are more widely used with laparoscopy.

Colpotomy

The thin wall of tissue between the vaginal canal and the posterior cul-de-sac also offers a convenient port of entry into the peritoneal cavity for sterilization procedures. All of the occlusive techniques used in

TABLE 26.1. Techniques of Tubal Ligation at Laparotomy	
Technique	**Procedure**
Madlener	Tube elevated, base crushed in clamp, crushed area ligated with nonabsorbable suture
Pomeroy	Loop of tube from middle third of tube elevated, ligated with plain gut, and excised
Irving	Tube divided, proximal stump buried in uterine wall, distal stump buried in leaves of broad ligament
Cook	Tube divided, proximal stump buried in round ligament, distal stump buried in leaves of broad ligament
Kroener	Fimbriated end of tube excised
Aldridge	Fimbriated end of tube buried in broad ligament
Uchida	Mesosalpinx injected with saline–epinephrine solution and excised to expose tube, serosa of proximal end stripped off and most of proximal segment removed, stump ligated with nonabsorbable suture and placed in broad ligament, distal end ligated, broad ligament closed with distal stump left outside the broad ligament
Partial salpingectomy	Part of tube removed
Total salpingectomy	All of tube removed
Cornual resection	Tube ligated 1 cm from cornua and excised with cornua, distal end buried in broad ligament, proximal wound covered with round ligament and broad ligament

laparoscopy, and many used with laparotomy, may be applied to the fallopian tubes by this route. Vaginal tubal procedures carry a high rate of vaginal incision site ("cuff") and ovarian infections if prophylactic antibiotics are not used. Vaginal tubal procedures require restrictions on intercourse and the use of tampons or douches for 2 weeks while healing takes place. Although less popular than in the past, this approach may have some advantage in the retroflexed and retroverted uterus.

Hysteroscopy

The possibility of transcervical obstruction of the fallopian tube avoids the inherent risks in penetration of the peritoneal cavity. Methods that have been proposed include the development of formed-in-place silicone plugs, chemical cautery (e.g., phenol), and occlusive agents such as methyl cyanoacrylate. Endometrial ablation by cautery or laser has also been suggested. Although all

of these procedures offer exciting possibilities, they remain in the developmental stage.

Hysterectomy

Vaginal hysterectomy was once a preferred means of permanent sterilization for the multigravida. Today, the morbidity of this procedure is thought to outweigh the benefits, especially with less aggressive surgical and nonsurgical means of contraception available.

Nonsurgical Methods

A great deal of interest is focused on the development of permanent contraception based on nonsurgical methods. One such approach is the creation of an antipregnancy vaccine. Based on immunization to progesterone, this experimental technique appears promising. As more is learned about the biochemistry of reproduction, other alternatives may become available.

Side Effects and Complications

No surgically based technology is free of the possibility of complications or side effects. Infection, bleeding, injury to surrounding structures, or anesthetic complications may occur with any of the techniques discussed in this chapter. The overall fatality rate attributed to sterilization is about 1.5 per 100,000 procedures, significantly lower than that for childbearing in the United States, estimated at about 10 per 100,000 births. Thus, when the risk of pregnancy from interval contraception is accounted for, sterilization is the safest of all contraceptive methods. Laparoscopic and hysteroscopic techniques carry risks that are unique to their special instrumentation, such as complications of trocar insertion or cervical damage, respectively. *Failure of surgical sterilization occurs in 1% or less of all procedures* and depends to some extent on the method chosen and operator experience.

Debate continues about the existence of a post-tubal ligation syndrome. It has been postulated that disruption of blood flow in the area of the fallopian tubes may influence ovarian function, leading to menstrual dysfunction and dysmenorrhea. Efforts to document or quantify such an effect have not been successful, and the existence of this syndrome remains conjectural.

"Pregnancy after tubal ligation is ectopic until proven otherwise" is still a wise concept for management, but the implication that each pregnancy is usually ectopic is not entirely accurate. Ectopic pregnancy does occur after tubal ligation, more commonly after cautery than mechanical tubal occlusion, probably because of microscopic fistulae in the coagulated segment connecting to the peritoneal cavity. Two or more years after tubal ligation, most pregnancies are ectopic, whereas in the first year only about 10% are ectopic; that is, the overall rate of pregnancy decreases with time after tubal ligation, whereas the ectopic pregnancy rate remains constant. Overall, it appears that approximately one third of pregnancies after tubal ligation are ectopic, and the rate of ectopic pregnancy is lower in this group than in women who have not had tubal ligation.

REVERSAL OF TUBAL LIGATION

Reversal of tubal ligation by microsurgical techniques is most successful when minimal damage is done to the smallest length of fallopian tube (e.g., Hulka clip, Falope ring), in some series approaching 50% to 75%. In most cases, however, rates of 25% to 50% are more reasonable expectations, so that many specialists in infertility recommend the use of assisted reproductive technology (e.g., in vitro fertilization) rather than attempts at tubal ligation reversal with the attendant low success rates and increased risk of tubal ectopic pregnancy. *Indeed, a patient who has undergone tubal reversal and becomes pregnant is presumed to have an ectopic pregnancy until intrauterine pregnancy is established.*

THE DECISION FOR STERILIZATION

The decision to be permanently sterilized is, obviously, important, emotionally charged, and fraught with risk if it is perceived to have been faulty because of either lack of proper explanation and information or lack of freedom in the decision. The physician has the responsibility to be certain that the following components of this decision-making process occur, and that they are appropriately documented as comprising the "consent."

1. The permanence of the procedure is explained, as well as the failure rates of the procedure and the kinds and rates of complications (e.g., ectopic pregnancy).
2. The risks and benefits and indications and contraindications of the procedure are explained.
3. The risks and benefits and indications and contraindications of alternative interval methods of contraception, including hormonal, barrier, "natural"

or timing, and other methods, as well as abstinence, are also explained.

4. The patient (and partner, if appropriate) are given opportunity to ask questions about this information, and these are fully answered.

5. Finally, given 1 through 4, the patient freely chooses a given procedure, signing the requisite consent forms.

It is important to remember that it is the patient education and decision-making process described in items 1 through 4, not the documentation described in item 5, that comprise the process of informed patient consent.

CASE STUDIES

Case 26A

A 23-year-old G3 P2002 patient is in your office for a routine prenatal visit at 34 weeks' gestation. She tells you that she and her husband of 8 years have decided that their family will be complete with the birth of this next child, and they would like to know about sterilization options. On questioning, she says that she would like something done "right away, if the baby is okay."

Questions Case 26A

Possible options for this couple include all of the following EXCEPT

A. Pomeroy tubal ligation
B. Tubal electrocautery
C. Falope ring
D. Vaginal tubal cautery
E. Vasectomy

Answer: D

Because of uterine size and the rich vascular supply induced by pregnancy, vaginal tubal sterilization techniques usually are not used within 3 months of a pregnancy. Any of the other methods, including vasectomy, would be reasonable to include in the counseling of this couple. Of the choices listed, Pomeroy tubal ligation

through a small infraumbilical incision is most commonly used for the postpartum patient. Cautery or the Falope ring is usually used during interval laparoscopy procedures.

The patient has a postpartum tubal ligation and you select the Pomeroy method. Three years later, the patient and her husband decide that they want another child and would prefer tubal ligation reversal to adoption, if possible. Hysterosalpingography confirms the clinical suspicion that the tubal ligation has occluded both fallopian tubes. Options you can offer this couple include

A. Tubal ligation reversal by microsurgical techniques
B. Assisted reproductive technology
C. Adoption counseling
D. All of the above

Answer: D

After being given information about the risks, benefits, costs, and success rates of each alternative, this couple must decide their appropriate path, which may involve a time-limited trial of one path before embarking on another. These are difficult decisions and times for the couple, who require flexibility, compassion, and understanding by their physicians and friends.

Case 26B

A 26-year-old G2 P2002 patient asks your advice in choosing a method of sterilization. She has read about the options, and she presents you with a list of things she wants from her method: It should be reliable, safe, unlikely to cause future problems, quick and inexpensive, not affect libido, and not show.

Question Case 26B

Which of the following should be included in your discussions with this patient? (Select all that apply.)

A. Reversibility
B. Operative techniques
C. Anesthetic options
D. Complications
E. Reversible alternatives (temporary methods)

Answer: All

Even though a patient has "read all about" a topic, it is imperative that a full discussion be undertaken. The likelihood of disappointment, regret, hostility, and even lawsuits can be greatly reduced by ensuring that the patient does, indeed, understand the ramifications of elective sterilization procedures and all her options. Each of the answers represents an important part of this counseling process, but by itself each is not sufficient to make an informed choice or provide an informed consent.

C H A P T E R

27

VULVITIS AND VAGINITIS

CHAPTER OBJECTIVES

This chapter deals primarily with APGO Objective(s):

OBJECTIVE 38   Vulvar and Vaginal Disease

A. Describe the physiologic variations of normal vaginal discharge and secretions.

B. Describe the evaluation and management of dermatologic disease of the vulva, vulvitis (including that due to *Candida*, atrophy, and allergy), vaginitis (including that due to bacteria, *Candida*, trichomonas, viruses, foreign bodies, and atrophy), and disorders of the Bartholin's gland.

Patients with vulvitis or vaginitis may present with acute, subacute, or indolent symptoms, ranging in intensity from minimal to incapacitating. Although generally nonspecific, the patient's history and symptoms may point to chemical, allergic, or other causes rather than infection. Irritation of the well-innervated tissues of the vulva often leads to intense pruritus. Common vaginal infections often present with characteristic patterns (Table 27.1).

Vaginal secretions are always present to some extent; the amount and character of these secretions depend on the influence of chemical, mechanical, or pathologic conditions. Understanding the physiologic processes responsible for both normal and abnormal discharge makes the diagnosis of vulvitis and vaginitis more accurate.

History taking is especially important in patients with vulvar symptoms, including hygiene and sexual practices, use of deodorants and feminine products, changes in detergents, and other contact issues such as new or unusual clothes. Thorough physical examination by inspection and palpation is also important. The physician must also be familiar with office and laboratory methods for establishing the diagnosis, especially the saline and potassium hydroxide (KOH) wet preparations for evaluations of vaginal secretions and discharges (Figure 27.1). *Inaccurate diagnosis or overtreatment of a physiologic condition is doomed to fail and may even make the patient worse.*

The vulva and vagina are covered by stratified squamous epithelium. The vulva, but not the vagina, contains hair follicles and sebaceous, sweat, and apocrine glands. The epithelium of the vagina is nonkeratinized and lacks these specialized elements. The skin of the vulva is also vulnerable to secondary irritations from vaginal secretions, and both vulva and vagina are vulnerable to contact with external irritants (such as soap residue, perfumes, fabric softeners, or infestation by pinworms).

The vulva and vagina are sites of symptoms and lesions of several sexually transmitted diseases, such as herpes genitalis, human papillomavirus, syphilis, chancroid, granuloma inguinale, lymphogranuloma venereum, and molluscum contagiosum (see Chapter 28).

TABLE 27.1.   Clinical Aspects of Physiologic Vaginal Secretions and Common Vaginal Infections

Characteristic	Physiologic Findings	Bacterial Vaginosis (BV)	Candidiasis	Trichomoniasis
Vaginal pH	3.8–4.2	> 4.5	≤ 4.5 (usually)	> 4.5
Discharge	White, clear, flocculent	Thin, homogeneous, gray, white, adherent, often increased	White, curdy, "cottage cheese-like," sometimes increased	Green–yellow frothy, adherent, increased
KOH "whiff test" (amine odor)	Absent	Present (fishy)	Absent	Possibly present (fishy)
Patient's main complaints	None	Bad odor, discharge, worse after intercourse, possible itching	Itching/burning, discharge	Frothy discharge, bad odor, dysuria, vulvar pruritus

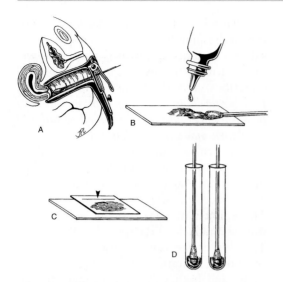

FIGURE 27.1. Saline and potassium hydroxide (KOH) preparations. A drop of physiologic saline and a drop of 10% to 20% KOH are placed on glass slides. (*A*) Vaginal discharge is collected on a cotton-tipped applicator. (*B*) The discharge is mixed in the droplets. (*C*) The preparations are then covered with a cover slide for microscopic viewing. (*D*) As an alternative, samples of discharge may be collected with two cotton-tipped applicators, which are then placed in small test tubes prepared with a few drops of NaCl and KOH solution. Material from these tubes is examined in a similar manner.

VULVITIS

Vulvar irritation and itching are the reasons for approximately 10% of all outpatient visits to gynecologists. Erythema, edema, and skin ulcers are all indications of possible *infection.* Ulcerative lesions should suggest the possibility of sexually transmitted disease such as *herpes or syphilis.* Other systemic diseases, such as *Crohn's disease,* may also present in this manner. Papillary lesions suggest *condyloma acuminatum or condyloma latum.* Screening should be done carefully for these and other sexually transmitted diseases. The vulvar skin is also subject to many common dermatoses, including intertrigo, seborrhea and seborrheic dermatitis, and psoriasis, as well as allergic reactions and infection with parasites such as *Pthirus pubis (the crab louse) and Sarcoptes scabiei (the itch mite).* Excoriation caused by the patient's scratching and fissuring of the skin of the vulva are often seen in vulvar irritation secondary to vaginal discharge. Chronic pruritus leads to itching and excoriation, and when chronic this is sometimes called neurodermatitis. In addition to treatment of the underlying cause of the pruritus, these patients may benefit from a time-limited treatment with a topical corticosteroid cream (hydrocortisone 1% twice or three times a day) to relieve inflammation and itching.

Diffuse reddening of the vulvar skin accompanied by itching and/or burning, but without obvious cause, should suggest a *secondary allergic vulvitis.* The list of possible local irritants can be quite extensive, including feminine hygiene sprays, deodorants, tampons or pads (especially those with deodorants or perfumes), tight-fitting synthetic undergarments, colored or scented toilet paper, and laundry soap or fabric softener residues. Even locally used contraceptives or sexual aids may be the source of irritation. A careful history, combined with the removal of the suspected cause, usually confirms the diagnosis and constitutes the needed therapy. In rare cases, the use of hydrocortisone cream (1% cream applied twice a day to affected areas) may be needed to decrease the local inflammatory response.

Allergic causes of vulvitis are also frequently found in the occasional pediatric patient who presents with vulvovaginal itching. However, the investigation in these cases must also include sources of irritations such as foreign bodies (especially with an accompanying vaginitis or discharge), sexual abuse, and pinworms.

Local *Candida* infection is another cause of vulvar pruritus. This etiology must be considered in diabetics and others disposed to such infection and in situations where there has been a suboptimal response to treatment for another problem. The diagnosis and treatment are described later in this chapter.

In older patients, intense itching of the vulva may occur because of *atrophic changes* brought on by reduced estrogen levels. This is typically associated with pale, thin vaginal mucosa, atrophic vaginitis, and the resultant yellowish discharge that has a pH of greater than 5.5. There will be a symmetrically reddened, smooth, and somewhat shiny look to the skin of the vulva and perineum. Biopsy will reflect the hypoplastic nature of this condition and will help to differentiate this from lichen sclerosus, which has a similar appearance. When atrophic change is the cause, estrogen replacement, either locally or systemically, is the treatment of choice (see Chapter 38). In the case of *lichen sclerosus,* local application of clobetasol proprionate 0.05% cream twice a day is generally effective. Alternatives that have been used, although with less effectiveness, include testosterone proprionate 2% in petrolatum base and progesterone cream 3%.

Vulvar itching may be caused by infestation with *P. pubis* or *S. scabiei* (Figure 27.2). This is especially true when itching of the mons is part of the patient's complaint. This itching is caused by an allergic sensitization from the parasite's bite. The crab louse is a different species from the body or head louse and is acquired by close contact or from bedding or towels. The crab louse is found exclusively in hairy areas, whereas the itch mite, although transmitted similarly, may be found anywhere in the skin surface. The diagnosis is generally made by looking for small black specks (excreta) on the skin, nits and eggs on hair shafts, or the parasites themselves. Local treatment with two applications of a γ-benzene hexachloride lotion (Kwell) is generally successful for infection from either parasite. Clothes, bedding, and those with whom close contact occurs must be disinfected/treated to break the infection cycle. More specific therapies listed in the 1998 Centers for Disease Control STD Treatment Guidelines for both pediculosis pubis and scabies include permethrin and lindane.

The vulva is subject to the same plethora of *dermatologic diseases* as other skin surfaces. *Contact dermatitis* is rela-

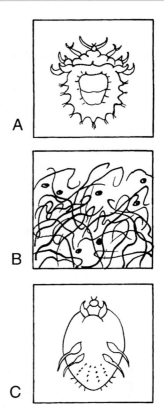

FIGURE 27.2. (A) *Pthirus pubis* (the crab louse). (B) Nits of the crab louse. (C) *Sarcoptes scabiei* (the itch mite).

tively common, with red, edematous skin surfaces and sometimes with vesicles and secondary infection. Treatment consists of removing the offending substance or material and wet compresses of Burrow's solution diluted 1 to 20, several times a day followed by drying. Hydrocortisone (0.5% to 1.0%) or fluorinated corticosteroids (Valisone, 0.1%) may be applied several times a day for symptom control. *Psoriasis* affects 1% to 3% of women and seems to have a familial pattern. This generalized pruritic skin disease of unknown cause presents with reddened skin and silvery scales, and is often refractory to simple fluorinated corticosteroids, and dermatologic consultation is required. *Seborrheic dermatitis* is another generalized skin disease of unknown cause with rare vulvar manifestations, consisting of pale to yellow–red edematous lesions covered with a fine nonadherent scale. Treatment is also with hydrocortisone cream. *Hidradenitis suppurativa* is a chronic, unrelenting skin infection causing deep, painful scars and a foul discharge. Its differential diagnosis includes Crohn's disease of the vulva. Treatment with local antibiotics and steroids is sometimes successful, but wide excision of the affected skin areas is often required.

Because of the nonspecific nature of symptoms and physical findings, patients who present with vulvitis and who do not respond to initial therapy should be offered vulvar biopsy to determine histologically the underlying etiology. Particularly in older patients, failure to obtain a tissue sample may result in missing a vulvar malignancy or significant pathology.

VAGINITIS

The most common symptom associated with infections of the vagina is discharge. *Discharge from the vagina is normal physiologically; therefore, not all discharges from the vagina indicate infection.* This distinction is important to the diagnostic process but occasionally difficult for the patient to understand or accept.

Vaginal secretions arise from several sources. The majority of the liquid portion consists of mucus from the cervix. A very small amount of moisture is contributed by endometrial fluid, exudates from accessory glands such as the Skene's and Bartholin's glands, and from vaginal transudate. Exfoliated squamous cells from the vaginal wall give the secretions a white to off-white color and provide some increase in consistency. The action of the indigenous vaginal flora also can contribute to the secretion. These components together constitute the normal vaginal secretions that provide the physiologic lubrication that prevents drying and irritation. The amount and character of this mixture vary under the influence of many factors, including hormonal and fluid status, pregnancy, immunosuppression, and inflammation. *Asymptomatic women produce, on the average, approximately 1.5 g of vaginal fluid per day. Normal vaginal secretions have no odor.*

After puberty, increased levels of glycogen in the vaginal tissues favor the growth of lactobacilli (Doderlein's bacilli) in the genital tract. These bacteria break down glycogen to lactic acid, lowering the pH from the 6 to 8 range, which is common before puberty (and after menopause), to the *normal vaginal pH range of 3.5 to 4.5* in a reproductive-aged woman. In addition to the lactobacilli, a wide range of other aerobic and anaerobic bacteria may normally be found in the vagina at concentrations of 10^8 to 10^9 colonies per milliliter of vaginal fluid. Because the vagina is a potential space, not an open tube, a ratio of 5:1 anaerobic:aerobic bacteria is normal.

Increased vaginal discharge is associated with an identifiable microbiologic cause in 80% to 90% of cases. Hormonal or chemical causes account for most of the remaining cases. Most vaginal infections are caused by three infective agents: synergistic bacteria (bacterial vaginosis, nonspecific vaginitis), fungi (candidiasis), and protozoa, such as *Trichomonas vaginalis* (trichomoniasis). Bacterial infections account for approximately 50% of infections, whereas fungi and *Trichomonas* account for roughly 25% each. Through gentle examination and simple microscopic investigation, the etiology of the patient's symptoms generally can be ascertained. *The value of microscopic examination of vaginal smears cannot be overstated. For this reason, any patient who complains of a vaginal discharge or irritation should be evaluated directly before therapy is suggested.* An increase in vaginal discharge is considered physiologic during pregnancy and at the midcycle in nonpregnant women. Although the increase in discharge amount is normal at these times, patients who complain of symptoms should be evaluated to rule out a pathologic cause.

Bacterial Vaginosis (BV)

BV is a diagnosis that has undergone a great deal of change and debate in the last few years. Once thought to be caused by the infection of *Gardnerella vaginalis* (formerly called *Haemophilus* or *Corynebacterium vaginalis*), BV is now felt to be a *symbiotic*

TABLE 27.2.	Vaginitis—Altered Ecology	
Finding	**Normal**	**Bacterial Vaginosis**
Organisms	10^8	10^{11}
Anaerobes:aerobes	5:1	1000:1
H_2O_2 production	High	Low
Lactobacillus	96%	35%
Gardnerella	5%–60%	95%
Mobiluncus	0%–5%	50%–70%
Mycoplasma hominis	15%–30%	60%–70%

infection of anaerobic bacteria (*Bacteroides*, *Peptococcus*, and *Mobiluncus* species) and *Gardnerella*, both of which contribute to the clinical findings (Table 27.2).

Women with BV generally complain of a *"musty" or "fishy" odor with an increased thin gray–white to yellow discharge.* The discharge may cause some mild vulvar irritation, but this is present in only approximately one fifth of the cases. The vaginal discharge is mildly adherent to the vaginal wall and has a pH greater than 4.5. Mixing some of these secretions with KOH (10%) liberates amines that may be detected by their fishy odor (positive "whiff test"). Microscopic examination made under saline wet mount shows a slight increase in white blood cells, clumps of bacteria, and characteristic "*clue cells,*" which are epithelial cells with numerous coccoid bacteria attached to their surface, making them appear to have indistinct borders and a "ground-glass" cytoplasm (Figure 27.3). The diagnosis of BV is defined by the presence of any 3 of the following 4 criteria: (1) homogeneous discharge, (2) pH greater then 4.5, (3) positive "whiff test," and (4) presence of clue cells.

BV may be treated with oral metronidazole (Flagyl, 500 mg twice a day for 7 days) or by intravaginal creams, using metronidazole (MetroGel) 0.75% vaginal gel twice daily for 5 days or clindamycin (Cleocin) 2% vaginal cream once a day for 7 days or a 100-mg suppository at bedtime for 3 consecutive nights. Alternative options include metronidazole 2 g in a single oral dose and clindamycin orally 300 mg twice

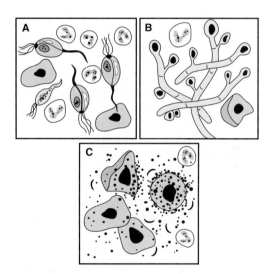

FIGURE 27.3. (*A*) Trichomonads; a flagellated protozoan is easy to identify on NaCl wet mount because of its movement. (*B*) Monilial infection; slide shows hyphae and budding yeast. (*C*) Clue cells, which are epithelial cells with clumps of bacteria on their surfaces.

daily for 7 days. Whether BV is transmitted sexually continues to be debated. Although treatment of sexual partner(s) of patients with frequent recurrences is not recommended by the Centers for Disease Control, it is common practice among physicians to treat the partners.

Trichomonas Vaginitis

Trichomonas vaginalis is a flagellate protozoan that *lives only in the vagina, Skene's ducts, and male or female urethra* and may be freely transmitted by sexual intercourse. More than 60% of partners of women with *Trichomonas* infections will also be infected. Despite the large number of cases of symptomatic vaginitis caused by the organism, up to one half of women with *Trichomonas* in the vaginal canal are asymptomatic. *Symptoms of Trichomonas infection* vary from mild to severe and may include vulvar itching or burning, copious *discharge* with rancid odor, dysuria, and dyspareunia. Although not present in all women, the discharge associated with *Trichomonas* infections is generally "frothy," thin, and yellow–green to gray in color, with a pH above 4.5. *Examination* may reveal edema or erythema of the vulva. "Characteristic" petechiae, or strawberry patches, are described as present in the upper vagina or on the cervix, but are actually found in only about 10% of affected patients.

The *diagnosis* is confirmed by *microscopic examination* of vaginal secretions suspended in normal saline. This wet smear will show large numbers of mature epithelial cells, white blood cells (WBCs), and the *Trichomonas* organism. *Trichomonas* is a fusiform protozoa just slightly larger than a WBC. The organism has three to five flagella extending from the narrow end. These flagella produce active movement that may facilitate identification of the organism (see Figure 27.3).

Treatment of Trichomonas infections is by oral *metronidazole*. Because *Trichomonas* is very sensitive to metronidazole, 1-day therapy, with 2 g orally, generally gives a 90% cure rate. Treatment with 500 mg twice a day for 7 days or 250 mg three times a day for 7 days gives comparable results. Many physicians prefer the single-day therapy because of its reduced cost and greater compliance. Vaginal metronidazole gel twice daily for 5 days is also now recommended. Treating sexual partners of women with *Trichomonas* infections is recommended and is often undertaken using the single-day therapy. Abstinence from alcohol use when taking metronidazole is necessary to avoid a possible disulfiram-like reaction. The use of metronidazole during pregnancy is not rec-

ommended because of reports of teratogenic effects. Many physicians, however, use the drug in the latter half of pregnancy for highly symptomatic patients.

Even though the pH generally associated with *Trichomonas* infections is different from that found with bacterial vaginosis, there are estimates of up to a *25% prevalence of bacterial vaginosis in those patients with Trichomonas.* Because of the overlap in metronidazole therapy for these two conditions, this debate is not significant for most patients. It may, however, be worthy of consideration in patients who receive alternative therapies or in those with frequent recurrences of vaginal infections.

Although follow-up examination of patients with *Trichomonas* for test of cure is often advocated, they are usually not cost-effective, except in the rare patient with a history of frequent recurrences. In these patients, reinfection or poor compliance must be considered as well as the possibility of infection with more than one agent or other underlying disease.

Candida (Monilial) Vaginitis

Monilial infections of the vagina are caused by ubiquitous *airborne fungi*. Approximately 90% of "yeast" infections are caused by *Candida albicans* with less than 10% caused by *Candida glabrata, Candida tropicalis,* or *Torulopsis glabrata. Candida* infections generally do not coexist with other infections and are not considered to be sexually transmitted even though 10% of male partners have concomitant penile infections. Candidiasis is more likely to occur in women who are pregnant, diabetic, obese, immunosuppressed, on oral contraceptives or corticosteroids, or have had broad-spectrum antibiotic therapy. Practices that keep the vaginal area warm and moist, such as wearing tight clothing or the habitual use of panty liners, may also increase the risk of *Candida* infections.

The most common presenting complaint for women with candidiasis is *itching,* although up to 20% of women may be asymptomatic. Burning, external dysuria, and dyspareunia are also common. The

TABLE 27.3. Topical Treatments for *Candida* Vaginitis		
Agent	**Formulation**	**Dose**
Imidazole		
Miconazole (Monistat)	2% cream	5 g bid for 14 days
	200 mg vaginal suppository	1 g qd for 3 days
Butoconazole (Femstat)	2% cream	5 g qd for 3 days
Clotrimazole		
(Gyne-Lotrimin)	1% cream	5 g qd for 7 days
	100 mg vaginal suppository	1 qd for 7 days
(Mycelex-G)	500 mg vaginal suppository	1 dose
Tioconazole (Vagistat-1)	6.5% cream	5 g in 1 dose
Polyene		
Nystatin	200,000 U vaginal tablet	1 qd for 14 days
Trazole		
Terconazole (Terazol)	0.4% cream	5 g qd for 7 days
	0.8% cream	5 g qd for 3 days
	80 mg vaginal suppository	1 qd for 3 days

vulva and vaginal tissues are often bright red in color and excoriation is not uncommon in severe cases. *A thick, adherent "cottage cheese" discharge with a pH of 4 to 5 is generally found. This discharge is odorless.*

The *diagnosis* of candidiasis is based on history and physical findings, and confirmed by the identification of hyphae and buds in wet mounts of vaginal secretions made with 10% KOH solution, which lyses most epithelial and white cells (see Figure 27.3). There is no direct correlation between the degree of symptoms and the number of organisms present. Because false-negative wet preps are not uncommon, culture confirmation may be obtained using Nickerson's or Sabouraud's media. Latex agglutination tests may be of particular use for non-*Candida albicans* strains since they do not demonstrate the pseudohyphae on wet prep.

Treatment of Candida infections is primarily with the topical application of one of the synthetic imidazoles (Table 27.3). These agents give good cure rates after 3 to 7 days of treatment. Despite greater than 90% relief of symptoms with these therapies, 20% to 30% of patients experience *recurrences* after 1 month. Treatments based on nystatin or povidone–iodine have proved to

be less effective than the imidazoles. Resistant strains of *C. tropicalis* or *T. glabrata* may respond to therapy with terconazole or gentian violet. Because noncompliance is the most frequent cause of recurrence, treatment with the oral agent fluconazole (Diflucan), 150 mg as a single dose, has become widely used. Patients with frequent recurrences should be carefully evaluated for possible risk factors such as diabetes or immune defects. For recurrence or resistance, ketoconazole 100 mg twice daily for 10 days can be effective. Prophylactic local therapy with an antifungal agent should be considered when systemic antibiotics are prescribed.

Chronic Vaginitis

A problem for both physicians and patients is "chronic" or "recurrent" vaginitis. Patients complain, often bitterly, of persistent vaginal discharge, odor, or both, without a readily identifiable cause or satisfactory response to treatment. These patients have frequently "tried everything" and visited several physicians without success. A careful history must be obtained, covering medical conditions and sexual and hygienic habits. A methodical physical examination and microscopic evaluation are also required.

In addition to the three most common causes previously listed, one must evaluate alternative explanations for the patient's complaints. Chlamydial infections may present as vulvovaginitis. Because *Chlamydia trachomatis* is the most common sexually transmitted organism in the United States, its role in recurrent/chronic cases should be evaluated (see Chapter 28). *Cytolytic vaginitis* is a common but under-recognized cause of *cyclic* vulvovaginitis. Although the exact pathophysiology is not known, it is thought to be caused by an overgrowth of the lactobacilli in the vagina, resulting in increased vaginal acidity, with subsequent cytolysis, vaginal discharge, and vulvovaginal irritation. This diagnosis should be considered when more common etiologies have been ruled out. There should be a high index of suspicion if the vaginal pH is between 3.5 and 4.5 and symptoms worsen during the luteal phase. Therapy includes using pads rather than tampons; discontinuing previous antifungal medications; and use of baking soda sitz baths (4 tablespoons in 1–2 inches of warm water) twice daily and douches (30–60 g of sodium bicarbonate in a liter of warm water) every 2–3 weeks.

Desquamative inflammatory vaginitis is characterized by purulent discharge, exfoliation of epithelial cells with vulvovaginal burning and erythema. There is a relative absence of lactobacilli and overgrowth of gram-positive cocci, usually streptococci. Vaginal pH is greater than 4.5. Initial therapy is clindamycin cream 2% applied daily for 1 week.

Victims of sexual assault (recent or quite far in the past) may present in this manner. A frank explanation of the possibility of reinfection must be carried out in individuals with true recurrent infections. The existence of additional sexual contacts for the patient or her partner should be explored in an appropriately nonjudgmental way. Alternate sources of excessive vaginal moisture, such as chronic cervical infections, must be evaluated. When the patient's complaints seem to exceed her physical and microscopic findings, the possibility of inappropriate expectations, inaccurate information, or psychological dysfunction must be entertained.

CASE STUDIES

Case 27A

A 36-year-old G3 P2012 patient calls and states that she has one of her "yeast infections" again. She has just moved to the area, but her former physician would usually "just call something in," and she would like you to do so as well. On further questioning, you find that the patient is experiencing vulvar itching, mild dysuria, a thick discharge, and a mild vaginal odor.

Question Case 27A

The most appropriate initial action would be to

A. Prescribe miconazole suppositories for 3 days
B. Prescribe metronidazole 1 g bid for 1 day
C. Ask the patient to come in for an examination
D. Refer the patient to the local STD clinic
E. Prescribe oral nystatin therapy

Answer: C

Even though this patient may have a recurrent yeast infection, the symptoms of vaginal infections overlap to such a great extent that only a thorough evaluation (history, physical, and microscopic investigation) will reliably establish the diagnosis. Without a correct diagnosis, any therapy has the potential either to fail or to make the patient worse. Especially in a patient whom you have never examined, treatment based on examination is more appropriate than calling in a prescription. The recurrent nature of her symptoms suggests an alternative etiology.

Case 27B

A 54-year-old patient comes to your office with the complaint of vaginal itching. The patient is in good health and on no medication, except for a diuretic for hypertension. Her last menstrual period was 3 years ago and she has recently begun experiencing mild hot flashes. On examination the patient's vulva is red but no edema is noted. The area of Bartholin's glands appears to be normal. The vaginal canal is also slightly reddened, and a small amount of slightly thickened discharge may be obtained from the vaginal apex.

Question Case 27B

Which of the following tests performed on the vaginal secretions would NOT be of assistance in this case?

A. Whiff test
B. 10% KOH wet prep
C. Culture on Nickerson's medium
D. Culture for bacteria
E. Saline wet prep

Answer: D

The vagina is normally populated by many species of bacteria; hence, culture of vaginal secretions for bacteria provides little useful information. Although it is likely that this patient is experiencing atrophic vulvitis and/or vaginitis, candidiasis or other infections are also possible and must be excluded.

Case 27C

A 22-year-old newlywed comes to your office with the complaint of 3 days of vaginal "wetness" that stains her underwear yellow and an excessive odor. She notes some mild vulvar irritation but no dysuria or dyspareunia. Physical examination shows diffuse redness of the vulva and vagina, with copious amount of a yellow to gray discharge on the vaginal walls. Saline wet prep shows the following: 3+ epithelium, 2+ WBCs, 1+ motile sperm, moderate small rods, and occasional motile protozoa.

Question Case 27C

The most likely diagnosis is

A. Mechanical vulvitis
B. Contact dermatitis
C. Bacterial vaginosis
D. *Trichomonas* vaginitis
E. Monilial vaginitis

Answer: D

The finding of motile protozoa is virtually pathognomonic for a *Trichomonas* infection. Although each of the other options had to be considered initially, the microscopic findings establish the diagnosis in this case.

CHAPTER

28

SEXUALLY TRANSMITTED DISEASES

OBJECTIVE 40   Salpingitis

transmitted diseases: screening programs, costs, prevention, and partner evaluation and treatment.

A. Discuss the anatomical location, causes, symptoms/physical findings, methods of diagnosis and treatment, and possible sequelae of acute and chronic salpingitis.

B. Discuss the relationship of salpingitis to tuboovarian abscess, chronic salpingitis, ectopic pregnancy, and infertility.

Sexually transmitted diseases run the gamut from vaginitis to life-threatening conditions such as acquired immune deficiency syndrome (AIDS). The increasing prevalence of sexually transmitted disease (STD) has resulted in increased awareness among physicians and patients and, in some cases, changes in attitudes about acceptable behaviors and standards. The impact of STDs for the individual and for society cannot be overlooked or overemphasized. Although some of these diseases can be acquired through nonsexual means, sexual transmission represents the major route by which most are spread.

The impact of changing sexuality has had far-reaching implications, not the least of which has been the explosive increase in the frequency and types of STDs. For example, recently there has been an increase of approximately 30% in the reported number of cases of syphilis. The physician must be alert to the possibility of STD in all patients, perform diagnostic evaluations and institute appropriate treatments promptly, and attempt to educate patients regarding the risks involved in today's sexually open society.

HISTORY AND PHYSICAL EXAMINATION

The sexual habits and modes of expression that individuals choose affect their risk of infection as well as the site and presentation by which infection is manifest. For this reason, a detailed sexual history is important for all patients and invaluable for any in whom an STD is either likely or suspected. Most of these infections require skin-to-skin contact or exchange of body fluids for transmission. Nonsexual activities that meet these criteria may also put the patient at risk.

All patients who are (or might be) sexually active should be examined with an awareness of the possibility of an STD. This is not a condemnation of the patient's lifestyle or personal choices, but rather a simple fact of life in today's society. The inguinal region should be inspected for rashes, lesions, and adenopathy. The vulva should be inspected for lesions, ulcerations, or abnormal discharge and palpated for thickening or swelling. The Bartholin's glands, Skene's ducts, and urethra cannot be overlooked because these are frequent sites of infection (e.g., gonorrhea). In patients with urinary symptoms, the urethra should be gently "milked" to express any discharge. The vagina and cervix must be inspected for lesions and abnormal discharge. When suspicion or risk is high, cultures of the urethra and cervix for gonorrhea, chlamydia, or other infections should be obtained. Last, the perineum and perianal areas must also be evaluated for signs of STDs. Cultures of the rectum for gonorrhea should be obtained in those patients who engage in anal intercourse. For completeness, the oral cavity as well as cervical and other lymph nodes must be evaluated and cultures taken if indicated by the patient's modes of sexual expression. The findings obtained by this process, combined with the patient's history, generally make the establishment of the proper diagnosis much easier. Furthermore, the sexual partner(s) of patients diagnosed with or suspected of having an STD should receive their own evaluation. It is vital to remember that *20% to 50% of patients with an STD have one or more coexisting infections.* When one venereal disease is found, others must be suspected.

SPECIFIC INFECTIONS

Herpes Genitalis

Office visits for this infection have increased tenfold in the past 10 years. It is estimated that there are approximately 500,000 new cases each year. Herpes simplex infections are highly contagious. Roughly 75% of sexual partners of infected individuals contract the disease. Approximately 85% of genital herpes lesions are caused by herpes simplex virus type 2 (HSV$_2$); this type differs slightly from the type 1 virus (HSV$_1$), which usually causes the "cold sore" lesions of the mouth but is also responsible for the balance of genital lesions. Both are DNA viruses.

CLINICAL COURSE

The development of the classic vesicular lesions is often preceded by a prodromal phase of mild paresthesia and burning beginning approximately 2 to 5 days after infection in symptomatic patients. This progresses to very painful vesicular and ulcerated lesions 3 to 7 days after exposure (Figure 28.1). Dysuria caused by vulvar lesions, or urethral and bladder involvement, may lead to urinary retention. Roughly 10% of patients with initial lesions require hospitalization for pain control or management of urinary complications. Primary infections are also characterized by malaise, low-grade

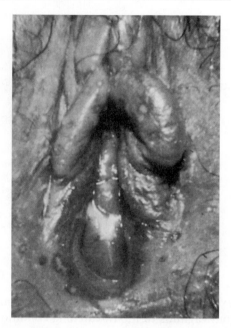

FIGURE 28.1. Herpes simplex virus infection. Note the small serpiginous, superficial lesions and edema of the vulva and urethral area.

fever, and inguinal adenopathy in 40% of patients. Aseptic meningitis with fever, headache, and meningismus can be found in some patients 5 to 7 days after the appearance of the genital lesions. This generally resolves over the period of 1 week.

PHYSICAL EXAMINATION

Findings consist of clear vesicles, which lyse and progress to shallow, painful ulcers with a red border. These may coalesce and frequently become secondarily infected and necrotic. These lesions may be found on the vulva, vagina, cervix, or perineal and perianal skin, often extending onto the buttocks. Recurrent lesions are similar in character but milder in severity and shorter in duration, generally lasting 2 to 5 days.

DIAGNOSIS

The diagnosis is based on characteristic history and physical findings. The diagnosis may be confirmed through the use of viral cultures taken by swab from the lesions. This is the most sensitive method of diagnosis and allows confirmation in as little as 48 hours. Viral shedding occurs for up to 3 weeks after lesions appear. Scrapings from the base of vesicles may be stained by immunofluorescence techniques for the presence of viral particles. This technique provides results faster than cultures and carries approximately 80% agreement with culture results. Smears may also be stained with Wright's stain to visualize the characteristic giant multinucleated cells with eosinophilic intranuclear inclusions. The lesions of herpes simplex infections should be easily distinguishable from the ulcers found in chancroid, syphilis, or granuloma inguinale by their appearance and extreme tenderness.

Treatment

Management of local lesions and symptoms is the focus. The lesions should be kept clean and dry. Sitz baths, followed by drying with a heat lamp or hair dryer, work well for this purpose. The use of a topical anesthetic, such as 2% Xylocaine jelly, may be required. If secondary infections occur, therapy with a topical antibacterial cream such as Neosporin may be of help. Oral medication can reduce the duration of viral shedding and shorten the initial symptomatic disease course. Treatments include acyclovir (Zovirax) 200 mg 5 times/day or 400 mg 3 times/day, famcyclovir (Famvir) 250 mg 3 times/day, and valacyclovir (Valtrex) 1 g 2 times/day. Topical therapy with 5% acyclovir ointment applied every 3 hours has been used, but because its effectiveness is less than that of the oral agents, its use is discouraged. These therapies do not decrease the likelihood of recurrence, and the decrease in symptom duration is often minimal.

Recurrences occur in 30% of patients. After the primary infection, the virus migrates via the nerve fibers to remain dormant in the dorsal root ganglia. Recurrences are triggered by unknown stimuli, resulting in the virus traveling down the nerve fiber to the affected area. Episodic recurrences may be treated by oral antiviral therapy, including oral acyclovir (200 mg 5 times a day, or 400 mg 3 times a day, or

800 mg twice daily, all for five days); famciclovir 125 mg twice daily for five days; or valacyclovir 500 mg twice daily for five days. For women with frequent recurrences, suppressive antiviral therapy is useful to decrease the frequency and severity of these flare-ups. Regimens include acyclovir 400 mg twice daily; or valacyclovir 250 mg twice daily, 500 mg once daily, or 1000 mg once a day; or famcyclovir 250 mg twice a day. Generally, these regimens are not thought to eliminate viral shedding nor the potential for transmission.

Severe episodes may require hospitalization for parenteral analgesia and intravenous antiviral therapy. Antiviral regimens include intravenous acyclovir (5 mg/kg infused at a constant rate over 1 hour, administered every 8 hours for 5 days in adult patients with normal renal function). Such therapy is generally recommended for immunosuppressed or otherwise compromised patients. These patients are best managed in consultation with an infectious disease specialist, and other regimens may be applied to their care, including the use of foscarnet sodium (Foscavir, 40 mg/kg intravenous every 8 hours in patients with normal renal function), or cidofovir (Vistide, 5 mg/kg intravenously every 2 weeks in patients with normal renal function).

In pregnant patients with active herpes infections and intact membranes, cesarean delivery should be considered. Vaginal delivery, when herpetic lesions are present, is associated with a 50% chance that the baby will acquire the infection, which is associated with significant morbidity and an almost 80% mortality rate.

Pelvic Inflammatory Disease

Pathogenesis

Infection of the upper female genital tract is predominantly by direct spread along the mucosal surfaces from initial infection of the cervix. The predominant organisms are *Chlamydia trachomatis* and *Neisseria gonorrhoeae*. A mucopurulent cervicitis is more common in *C. trachomatis* infection, as *N. gonorrhoeae* seems able to reside in the endocervical cells without always promoting a purulent inflammatory response. The endocervical mucus resists upward spread, especially during the progesterone-dominant part of the menstrual cycle. Oral contraceptives mimic this effect, which explains in part their action to limit pelvic inflammatory disease (PID). The cervical mucus may be penetrated by the bacteria, either directly or as riders on sperm or trichomonads or up the string of an intrauterine device. When the cervicitis traverses the cervical barrier, endometrial infection occurs, followed rapidly in most cases by spread to the fallopian tube mucosa. Occasionally, an indolent endometritis develops with further extension, more commonly with *Chlamydia* infection. Tubal ligation usually provides a barrier to spread, although in some cases small microchannels facilitate continued spread. The salpingitis that results may be localized, or it may spread causing peritonitis, adhesion formation, and abscess formation. The relative mobility of the fallopian tube probably contributes to the rapid and widespread extension of infection. In this anaerobic environment, anaerobes also thrive so that the infection in the upper portions of the genital tract is actually often polymicrobial, with a mixture of aerobic and anaerobic organisms. However, as there is poor correlation between the diverse organisms cultured and the clinical patterns of disease, the models of *C. trachomatis* and *N. gonorrhoeae* serve well as disease models.

Chlamydia Trachomatis

Infection by this obligate intracellular parasite may manifest as cervicitis (mucopurulent cervicitis), acute urethritis, salpingitis, or PID. *C. trachomatis* differs from those strains causing other chlamydial infections such as lymphogranuloma venereum (LGV). LGV has three stages: (*1*) primary lesions, consisting of papules or ulcers; (*2*) regional lymphadenopathy, the bubonic stage; and (*3*) when the buboes suppurate, they develop draining fistulas and lymphatic obstruction. More common than *N. gonorrhoeae* by as much as 10:1 in some

studies, infections by *C. trachomatis* can be the source of significant morbidity, including chronic infection, chronic pelvic pain, and infertility. Infection rates are five times higher in women with three or more sexual partners and four times higher in women using no contraception or nonbarrier methods. In industrialized countries, series report asymptomatic cervical infection in 5% to 20% of women of childbearing age, with perhaps 5% to 10% of these developing ascending infection. Between 20% and 40% of sexually active women have antibodies to *Chlamydia*.

Clinically mild cases of cervicitis or pelvic infection by *Chlamydia* may be virtually asymptomatic yet culminate in infertility or ectopic pregnancy. Infection of the fallopian tubes causes a mild form of salpingitis with insidious symptoms. Once the infection is established, it may remain active for many months, with increasing tubal damage. Perihepatitis (Fitz-Hugh-Curtis syndrome), which consists of inflammation leading to localized fibrosis with scarring of the anterior surface of the liver and adjacent peritoneum, may be caused by chlamydial infections more often than by *N. gonorrhoeae* infection, with which it was originally described (Figure 28.2). *Chlamydia* is also frequently found coexisting with or mimicking *N. gonorrhoeae* infection. Chlamydial infections are also responsible for nongonococcal urethritis and inclusion conjunctivitis.

Physical findings in infections caused by *Chlamydia* are often subtle and nonspecific. Eversion of the cervix with mucopurulent cervicitis may suggest the diagnosis. Any patient with acute PID or who is suspected of having gonorrhea should also be evaluated for *Chlamydia*.

The diagnosis of *Chlamydia* infection is suspected on clinical grounds. Cultures are generally used only to confirm the diagnosis, because it takes 48 to 72 hours to obtain culture results. Two screening tests have recently gained clinical popularity: (*1*) an enzyme-linked immunosorbent assay (ELISA) performed on cervical secretions and (*2*) a monoclonal fluorescent antibody test car-

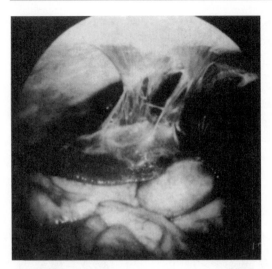

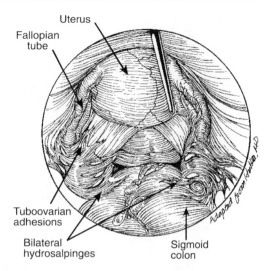

FIGURE 28.2. Fitz-Hugh-Curtis syndrome. Laparoscopic view of perihepatitis, showing scarring and string-like perihepatic adhesions associated with both gonococcal and chlamydial salpingitis.

FIGURE 28.3. Sequelae of pelvic inflammatory disease. Laparoscopic view of multiple pelvic adhesions, including tuboovarian adhesions and bilateral hydrosalpinges.

ried out on dried specimens. The immunoassay technique is easy to do and has a 95% specificity. The monoclonal technique is faster, has an 85% to 90% sensitivity and 95% specificity, but requires precision in making the slide and using the fluorescent microscope for interpretation.

Outpatient treatment of suspected or confirmed infections with *Chlamydia* is with azithromycin (Zithromax, 1 g po), doxycycline (Doxycycline or Vibramycin, 100 mg po bid for 7 days), or ofloxacin (Floxin, 300 mg bid for 7 days). Erythromycin base, 500 mg/day for 7 days or erythromycin ethylsuccinate, 800 mg qid for 7 days are also alternative treatment options. In pregnant patients, recommended treatment includes either erythromycin base 500 mg/day or amoxicillin 500 tid for 7 days. Alternative treatments in pregnancy include erythromycin base, 250 mg qid or erythromycin ethylsuccinate, 400 mg qid either for 14 days, or a one-time dose of azithromycin 1 g. Follow-up evaluation with culture or other tests as well as screening for other STDs should be performed. Partners should either be treated or referred for immediate treatment.

NEISSERIA GONORRHOEAE (GONORRHEA)

Infections with *N. gonorrhoeae,* a gram-negative intracellular diplococcus, continue to be common, and the incidence is increasing. The emergence of penicillin-resistant strains, an increased frequency of asymptomatic infections, and changing patterns of sexual behavior have all contributed to the problem. The damage caused by *N. gonorrhoeae* infections and the anaerobic organisms that grow with them in the pelvic environment can lead to recurrent infection; chronic pelvic pain; or infertility caused by adhesion formation, tubal damage, and hydrosalpinx formation (Figure 28.3). Infertility occurs in approximately 15% of patients after a single episode of salpingitis and increases to 75% after three or more episodes. The risk of ectopic pregnancy is increased 7 to 10 times in women with a history of salpingitis. It is estimated that PID results in $2.7 billion in direct medical costs and an additional $4 billion in indirect medical costs per year.

Infections with *N. gonorrhoeae* are easily acquired and can affect almost any part or organ of the body. Infection of the pharynx

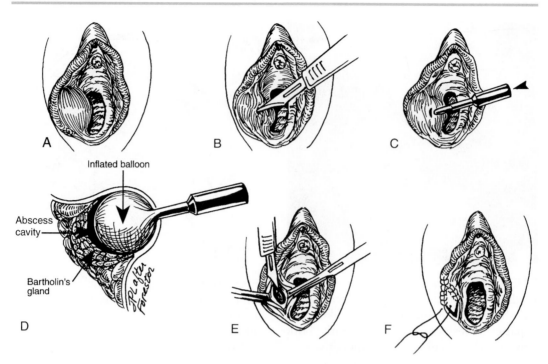

FIGURE 28.4.   Surgical treatment of Bartholin's abscess. (*A*) Unruptured right Bartholin's abscess that is "pointing" (i.e., there is a prominent area where only a thin layer of tissue covers the abscess). (*B*) A small incision is made with a scalpel on the medial aspect of the abscess. (*C*) The Word catheter, a short catheter with an inflatable balloon tip, is inserted into the incision. (*D*) The balloon is inflated while in the abscess cavity and left in place at least 1–2 weeks to allow epithelialization of the drainage tract. (*E*) An alternative technique of drainage is marsupialization, in which a larger incision is made to allow drainage. (*F*) The marsupialization technique is completed by sewing the incision open to facilitate drainage.

is found in 10% to 20% of heterosexual women with gonorrhea, and this site should not be overlooked when cultures are taken. For women, a single encounter with an infected partner leads to infection 80% to 90% of the time. Most commonly, the first signs or symptoms of infection occur 3 to 5 days after exposure but are often mild enough to be overlooked. Infection in the lower genital tract is characterized by a malodorous, purulent discharge from the urethra, Skene's duct, cervix, vagina, or anus. Anal intercourse is not always a prerequisite to anal infection. The presence of greenish or yellow discharge from the cervix ("mucopus") should alert the physician to the possibility of either *N. gonorrhoeae* or *C. trachomatis* infection. Infection of the

Bartholin's glands is frequently encountered and can lead to secondary infections, abscesses, or cyst formation. When the gland becomes full and painful, incision and drainage are appropriate (Figure 28.4).

Approximately 15% of women with *N. gonorrhoeae* infections of the cervix will develop acute pelvic infections (PID). *N. gonorrhoeae* infection of the fallopian tubes, adnexa, or pelvic peritoneum generally results in pain and tenderness, fever or chills, and an elevated white blood count (Table 28.1). Peritoneal involvement can also include perihepatitis (Fitz-Hugh-Curtis syndrome). *N. gonorrhoeae* is the causative agent in roughly 50% of patients with salpingitis. Many patients require hospitalization for adequate care (Table 28.2). In

TABLE 28.1. Clinical Criteria for Diagnosis of Acute Salpingitis

All 3 of the following necessary:
1. Abdominal tenderness with/without rebound
2. Adnexal tenderness
3. Cervical motion tenderness

PLUS

1 or more of the following:
1. Gram stain of endocervix positive for gram-negative, intracellular diplococci
2. Temperature > 38°C
3. WBC > 10,000
4. Pus on culdocentesis or laparoscopy
5. Pelvic abscess on bimanual exam or sonogram

WBC = white blood cell.

TABLE 28.2. Factors Suggesting Hospitalization for Patients with PID

Nulliparity
Peritonitis in upper abdomen
Pregnancy
Intrauterine contraceptive device use
Previous treatment failure
Significant gastrointestinal symptoms
Tuboovarian abscess
Uncertain or complicated differential diagnosis
Unreliable patient
White blood count > 20,000 or < 4000
All adolescents
Concurrent HIV infection
Immunosuppressed patients

HIV = human immunodeficiency virus; PID = pelvic inflammatory disease.

severe cases or in patients with one or more prior episodes of PID, tuboovarian abscess (TOA) formation may occur. These patients are acutely ill, with fevers of up to 39.5° C, tachycardia, severe pelvic and abdominal pain, and nausea and vomiting. Findings in PID are often nonspecific (Figure 28.5), and patients presenting with these symptoms must be differentiated from those with septic incomplete abortions, acute appendicitis, diverticular abscesses, and adnexal torsion (Table 28.3).

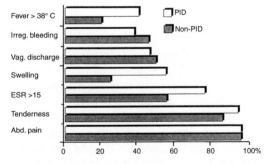

FIGURE 28.5. Frequency of symptoms in pelvic inflammatory disease (PID).

TABLE 28.3.	Correct Diagnosis in Cases of Misdiagnosis of PID
Acute appendicitis	28% of cases
Endometriosis	17% of cases
Corpus luteum bleeding	12% of cases
Ectopic pregnancy	11% of cases
Adhesions	7% of cases
"Other"	28% of cases

PID = pelvic inflammatory disease.

On examination, patients with PID may exhibit muscular guarding, and/or rebound tenderness. A purulent cervical discharge is often seen and the adnexa are usually moderately to exquisitely tender with a mass or fullness potentially palpable.

The laboratory diagnosis of *N. gonorrhoeae* infection is made by culture on Thayer-Martin agar plates kept in a CO_2-rich environment. Cultures should be obtained from the cervix, urethra, anus, and pharynx when appropriate. Cultures provide 80% to 95% diagnostic sensitivity. A solid-phase enzyme immunoassay for the detection of *N. gonorrhoeae* antigen is also available. Gram stain of any cervical discharge for the presence of this gram-negative intracellular diplococcus may support the presumptive diagnosis.

Aggressive therapy for patients with either suspected or confirmed *N. gonorrhoeae* infection should be tailored to the site of infection and the individual patient. Initial treatment should not be predicated on the results of cultures but rather on clinical suspicion. General guidelines for treatment are shown in Table 28.4. Hospitalized patients require high-dose intravenous antibiotic therapy with an antimicrobial spectrum that covers aerobic and anaerobic organisms. Surgical drainage of an abscess or even hysterectomy may be warranted in patients who fail an aggressive course of parenteral antibiotics. Rupture of a TOA, with septic shock, is a life-threatening complication and should be treated surgically. After successful medical therapy, follow-up cultures and examination of the patient should be performed 3 to 5 days after completion of therapy.

Tuberculosis

Pelvic tuberculosis (TB) may be associated with either *Mycobacterium tuberculosis* or *Mycobacterium bovis*. It almost always results from miliary hematogenous or lymphatic spread from tuberculosis elsewhere, usually the lungs. Typically, the initial involvement is tubal, with spread to ovaries and endometrium occurring in approximately 30% to 50% of cases. Tuberculosis is a relatively uncommon infection in the United States, although its incidence is increasing in some immigrant and migrant groups, in those who are immunosuppressed, and in those who abuse drugs. The diagnosis is suspected on clinical grounds and confirmed by culture, with the endometrium being the most easily accessible tissue. The TB skin test indicates exposure but not location or current infection. Medical treatment is quite effective in most cases and consists of the use of one or more of five common agents: isoniazid (INH), rifampin, streptomycin, ethambutol, and pyrazinamide. Surgical treatment is sometimes required for persistent disease, abscess formation, and pelvic pain. The operation of choice in these circumstances is total abdominal hysterectomy with bilateral salpingo-oophorectomy after stringent medical therapy.

Human Papillomavirus

Infection by the human papillomavirus (HPV) is responsible for almost as many cases of STD as *N. gonorrhoeae*. This DNA virus is found in 2.5% to 4% of women. Over the past 15 years, the number of

TABLE 28.4. Gonorrhea and PID Therapy

Disease	Preferred Treatment	Alternative Treatment
Gonorrhea	Ceftriaxone 125 mg IM (single dose) *Or* Cefixime 400 mg (single dose) *Or* Ofloxacin 400 mg (single dose) *Or* Ciprofloxacin 500 mg (single dose) *Plus* Regimen effective against *Chlamydia trachomatis* (e.g., Doxycycline 100 bid for 7 days)	Spectinomycin 2 g IM *Or* Ceftizoxime 500 mg IM *or* cefotaxime 500 mg IM *or* cefotetan 1 g IM *Or* Enoxacin 400 mg *or* lomefloxacin 400 mg *or* norfloxacin 800 mg
PID*		
Outpatient	Cefoxitin 2 g IM + probenecid *Plus* Probenecid 1 g po *Or* Ceftriaxone 250 mg IM *Plus* Doxycycline 100 mg po bid for 14 days	Ofloxacin 400 mg po bid for 14 days *Plus* Clindamycin 450 mg po qid *Or* Metronidazole 500 mg po bid for 14 days
Inpatient†	Cefoxitin 2 g IV q 6 h *Or* Cefotetan 2 g IV q 12 h *Plus* Doxycycline 100 mg IV or po q 12 h‡ *Or* Clindamycin 900 mg IV q 8 h *Plus* Gentamicin 2 mg/kg IV *or* IM loading dose followed by maintenance dose of 1.5 mg/kg q 8 h	Ofloxacin 400 mg IV q 12 h *Plus* Metronidazole 500 mg IV q 8 h *Or* Ampicillin/sulbactam 3 g IV q 12 h *Or* Ciprofloxacin 200 mg IV q 12 h *Plus* Doxycycline 100 mg IV q 12 h *Plus* Metronidazole 500 mg IV q 8–9 h *Then* Doxycycline 100 mg bid for 14 days *Or* Clindamycin 450 mg 5 × day for 10–14 days

*The indications for outpatient and inpatient treatment based on the need for parenteral administration are less clear nowadays, as parenteral medications can be given on an outpatient basis, either in outpatient care facilities or by home health agencies.
†Given for ≥ 48 hours after patient clinically improves.
‡Doxycycline to be continued for 14 days.
PID = pelvic inflammatory disease.

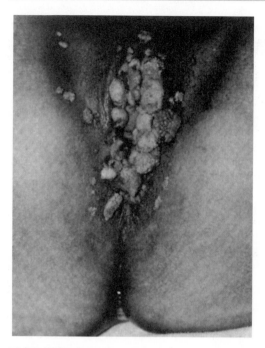

FIGURE 28.6. Condyloma acuminata.

infected individuals has increased more than fivefold. Unlike other STDs, sequelae of HPV infection may take years to develop. There have been more than 70 subtypes identified, with at least 25 identified in genital infections. Types 16, 18, 45, and 56 have a relatively higher association with cervical neoplasia.

Infection by HPV after a single contact with an infected partner results in a 65% transmission rate. Following a 6-week to 3-month incubation period, infection by HPV causes soft, fleshy growths on the vulva, vagina, cervix, urethral meatus, perineum, and anus. They may occasionally also be found on the tongue or oral cavity. These growths are termed condyloma acuminata or venereal warts (Figure 28.6). These distinctive lesions may be single or multiple and generally cause few symptoms. They are often accompanied by *Trichomonas* or other STDs. Because HPV is spread by direct skin-to-skin contact, symmetrical lesions across the midline are common (often called "kissing lesions").

Condylomas are commonly associated with HPV types 6 and 11.

The diagnosis of condyloma acuminata is made based on physical examination but may be confirmed through biopsy of the warts. Although cytologic changes typical of HPV can be found on Pap smears, Pap smears of the cervix diagnose only approximately 5% of patients with the virus. Because the condyloma lata of syphilis may be confused with venereal warts, some care must be taken in making the diagnosis in patients at high risk for both infections. Venereal warts are usually characterized by their narrower base and more "heaped-up" appearance, whereas condyloma lata lesions have a flattened top.

Management options include chemical, cautery, and immunologic treatments. Patient-applied products include Podofilox 0.5% gel or solution and Imiquimod 5% cream. The safety of use during pregnancy for either drug is yet to be established. Treatments that are administered by a health-care provider include application of trichloroacetic acid (TCA), application of podophyllin resin in tincture of benzoin, cryosurgery, surgical excision, laser surgery, or intralesional interferon injections. Lesions exceeding 2 cm respond best to cryotherapy, cautery, or laser treatment.

Lesions are more resistant to therapy during pregnancy, in diabetic patients, in patients who smoke, or in patients who are immunosuppressed. In patients with extensive vaginal or vulvar lesions, delivery via cesarean section may be required to avoid extensive vaginal lacerations and problems suturing tissues with these lesions. Cesarean delivery also decreases the possibility of transmission to the infant, which can cause subsequent development of laryngeal papillomata, although the risk is small and in and of itself not an indication for cesarean section.

Any patient with a history of condyloma should have at least yearly Pap smear evaluations of the cervix. The sexual partners of patients with HPV should also be screened for the development of genital warts.

Syphilis

Since antiquity, syphilis has been the proto-typic venereal disease. The incidence of syphilis has been increasing in the past several years. Contributing to this increase is today's increased use of nonpenicillin antibiotics to treat resistant gonorrhea; whereas in the past, penicillin treatment of gonorrhea provided treatment for coexisting syphilis.

Treponema pallidum, the causative organism of syphilis, is one of a very small group of spirochetes that are virulent for humans. Because this motile anaerobic spirochete can rapidly invade intact moist mucosa, resulting in infection and chancre formation, the most common sites of entry for women are the vulva, vagina, and cervix. Chancres may also be found in or near the anus, rectum, pharynx, tongue, lips, fingers, or other areas. Transplacental spread may occur at any time during pregnancy and can result in congenital syphilis (see Chapter 16).

Approximately 10 to 60 days after infection with *T. pallidum,* a painless ulcer appears. This is *the chancre of primary syphilis.* The chancre has a firm, punched out appearance and has rolled edges (Figure 28.7). Even though it is often accompanied by adenopathy, the chancre is commonly asymptomatic and missed. Serologic testing at this stage of syphilis generally is negative. Healing of the chancre occurs spontaneously in 3 to 9 weeks.

At 4 to 8 weeks after the primary chancre appears, manifestations of *secondary syphilis* develop. This stage is characterized by low-grade fever, headache, malaise, sore throat, anorexia, generalized lympha-denopathy, and a diffuse, symmetric, asymptomatic maculopapular rash. This rash is often seen over the palm and soles and is sometimes referred to as "money spots." Highly infective secondary eruptions, called *mucous patches,* occur in 30% of patients during this stage. In moist areas of the body, flat-topped papules may coalesce, forming condyloma lata (Figure 28.8). These may be distinguished from

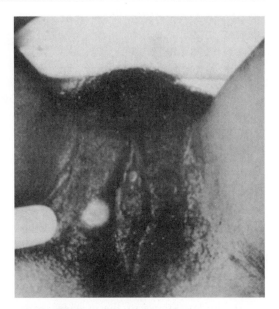

FIGURE 28.7. Chancre of the vulva. The chancre of syphilis, a rounded or ovoid raised lesion with indurated edges and a depressed center. The surface is reddish or reddish brown.

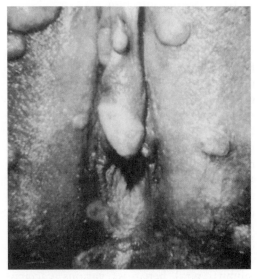

FIGURE 28.8. Condyloma lata of the vulva. The typical lesion of secondary syphilis, slightly raised, round or oval, plateau-like lesions of various sizes, often occurring in clusters. The edges are slightly indurated, and the surface is moist and covered with a grayish necrotic exudate. These lesions are highly infectious.

TABLE 28.5. Types of Serologic Tests for Syphilis

Nontreponemal	Treponemal
Venereal Disease Research Laboratory (VDRL) Rapid plasma reagin (RPR) card test Automated reagin test (ART)	Fluorescent treponemal–antibody absorption (FTA–ABS) Microhemagglutination assay for antibodies to *Treponema pallidum* (MHA–TP)

venereal warts by their broad base and flatter appearance. In untreated individuals, this stage, too, passes spontaneously in 2 to 6 weeks as the disease enters into the latent phase.

In the late stages of the disease, transmission of the infection is unlikely, except via blood transfusion or placental transfer. However, crippling damage to the central nervous system, heart, or great vessels often develops. Destructive, necrotic, granulomatous lesions called *gummas* may develop 1 to 10 years after infection.

The diagnosis of syphilis may be made by identifying motile spirochetes on dark-field microscopic examination of material from primary or secondary lesions or lymph node aspirates. For most patients, the diagnosis is established on the basis of serologic testing (Table 28.5). The Venereal Disease Research Laboratory (VDRL) and rapid plasma reagin (RPR) are nonspecific tests that are rapid, inexpensive, and useful for screening. False-positive tests may result from bacterial causes (pneumococcal pneumonia, scarlet fever, malaria, tuberculosis, mycoplasma pneumonia), viral causes (chickenpox, human immunodeficiency virus [HIV], measles, mononucleosis, mumps, viral hepatitis, various vaccinations), and noninfectious causes (chronic liver disease, pregnancy, multiple myeloma, connective tissue disease, multiple blood transfusions). These tests are used to screen for the disease and also to monitor response to treatment. The biologic false-positive

tests are associated with low titers, typically less than 1:8.

The fluorescent treponemal–antibody absorption (FTA–ABS) and microhemagglutination assay for antibodies to *T. pallidum* (MHA–TP) tests are specific treponemal antibody tests that are confirmatory or diagnostic but not used for routine screening. Even these latter tests have sources of false-positive results (e.g., Lyme disease, malaria, leprosy, mononucleosis, systemic lupus erythematosus). A woman with a positive treponemal test will usually have this positive result for life irrespective of treatment or activity of the disease. When neurosyphilis is suspected, a lumbar puncture, with a VDRL performed on the spinal fluid, is required.

The treatment of choice for syphilis is benzathine penicillin G as outlined in Table 28.6. The patient should be followed by quantitative VDRL titers and examinations at 3, 6, and 12 months.

AIDS

Acquired immune deficiency syndrome (AIDS) is the advanced manifestation of infection by HIV, an RNA retrovirus. The virus targets "helper" lymphocytes (those with CD4 marker) and monocytes. AIDS is now one of the top five causes of death in reproductive age women. It is estimated that approximately 1 in 300 people is infected with HIV. The three primary methods of contracting the virus are: (1) use of

TABLE 28.6. Treatment of Syphilis

Type	Preferred Treatment	Alternative Treatment
Primary, secondary, early latent	Benzathine penicillin G, 2.4 million units IM	Doxycycline 100 mg bid for 14 days *Or* Tetracycline 500 mg qid for 14 days *Or* Erythromycin 500 mg qid for 14 days
Late latent or syphilis of unknown duration	Benzathine penicillin G, 2.4 million units IM weekly for 3 weeks	Doxycycline 100 mg bid for 14 days *Or* Tetracycline 500 mg qid for 14 days
Neurosyphilis	Aqueous crystalline penicillin G, 3–4 million units IV q 4 h for 10–14 days	Procaine penicillin, 2.4 million units IM daily for 10–14 days *Plus* Probenecid 500 mg qid for 10–14 days

contaminated needles or blood products; (2) perinatal transmission from mother to child; and (3) intimate sexual contact.

The screening test for AIDS is an ELISA (enzyme-linked immunosorbent assay) that tests for antibodies against HIV. Although rare, false-positive tests are possible, and are more common in multiparous women and women taking oral contraceptives. Confirmation is achieved with the more specific Western blot technique. Due to the accuracy of standard HIV testing, polymerase chain reaction (PCR) and HIV viral load testing are, despite their specificity, rarely needed.

Management of HIV focuses on prevention and chemotherapy. The former emphasizes use of latex condoms and spermicides containing nonoxynol 9. The latter includes various classes of anti-HIV drugs including the nucleoside reverse transcriptase inhib-

itors (NRTI) such as zidovudine; nonnucleoside reverse transcriptase inhibitors (NNRTI); and protease inhibitors. Monotherapy is not advocated due to development of drug resistance. Instead, HAART (highly active antiretroviral therapy) combination therapy consisting of at least three agents has shown promise.

Minor Sexually Transmitted Diseases

Chancroid, granuloma inguinale, LGV, molluscum contagiosum, parasite infections (such as pediculosis pubis or scabie), enteric infections, and some types of vaginitis (e.g., trichomoniasis) are infections that are spread through sexual activities. Pertinent information about these infections, some of which are seldom seen, is summarized in Tables 28.7 and 28.8.

TABLE 28.7. Minor Sexually Transmitted Diseases

Disease	Causative Agent	Main Symptom	Diagnosis	Treatment
Chancroid	*Haemophilus ducreyi*	Painful "soft chancres," adenopathy	Clinical, smears, culture	Azythromycin, 1 g single dose Erythromycin base, 500 mg qid for 7 days *Or* Ceftriaxone, 250 mg IM *Or* Ciprofloxacin, 500 mg bid for 3 days
Granuloma inguinale	*Calymmatobacterium granulomatis*	Raised, red lesions	Clinical, smears	Doxycycline, 100 mg bid for a minimum of 3 weeks Trimethoprim/sulfamethoxazole, 1 double strength tablet bid for 3 weeks *Or* ciprofloxacin, 750 mg bid for 21 days
Lymphogranu-loma venereum (LGV)	*Chlamydia trachomatis*	Vesicle, progressing to bubo	Clinical, complement fixation test	Doxycycline, 100 mg bid for a minimum of 3 weeks Erythromycin base, 500 mg qid for 21 days
Molluscum contagiosum	*Poxviridae*	Raised papule with waxy core	Clinical, inclusion bodies	Desiccation, cryotherapy, curettage
Parasites	*Pediculus, Sarcoptes scabiei*	Itching	Inspection	Lindane 1% Permethrin cream/rinse
Enteric infections	*Neisseria gonorrhoeae, Chlamydia trachomatis, Shigella, Salmonella,* protozoa	Diarrhea	Culture	Based on agent
Vaginitis	*Trichomonas*	Odor, irritation	Microscopic examination of secretions	Metronidazole, 1 g AM and PM for 1 day or 500 mg bid for 7 days

TABLE 28.8. Genital Lesions in Sexually Transmitted Diseases*

Characteristic	Herpes	Genital Warts	Syphilis	Chancroid	LGV	Granuloma Inguinale
Organism	Herpes simplex virus	Human papillomavirus	*Treponema pallidum*	*Haemophilus ducreyi*	*Chlamydia trachomatis*	*Calymmatobacterium granulomatis*
Incubation	3–7 days	1–8 months	10–60 days	2–6 days	1–4 weeks	8–12 weeks
Primary lesion	**Vesicle**	Papule/polypoid	Papule (chancre)	Papule/pustule	Papule/pustule/vesicle	Papule
Number	**Multiple coalesce**	Variable	1	1–3	Single	Single or multiple
Pain	**Yes**	No	**Rare**	**Often**	No	**Rare**
Shape	Regular	Irregular	Regular	Irregular	Regular	Regular
Margins	Flat	Raised	Raised	**Red, undermined**	Flat	**Rolled, elevated**
Depth	Superficial	Raised	Superficial	Excavated	Superficial	Elevated
Base	Red, smooth	Normal, pink, white	Red, smooth	**Yellow, gray**	Variable	Red, **rough**
Induration	None	**Normal**	**Firm**	Rare, soft	None	**Firm**
Secretions	Serous	None	Serous	**Purulent, hemorrhagic**	Variable	Rare, hemorrhagic
Lymph nodes	Firm, tender	**Normal**	Firm, nontender	Tender, suppurative	Tender, suppurative	Pseudoadenopathy
Duration	5–10 days, **recurrent**	Months	Weeks	Weeks	Days	Weeks

*Scabies, molluscum contagiosum, *Candida*, and other dermatologic conditions (e.g., hidradenitis suppurativa) may also cause genital lesions. Items in boldface are of particular help in making a differential diagnosis. LGV = lymphogranuloma venereum.

CASE STUDIES

Case 28A

A 20-year-old college student comes to your office with the complaint of severe vulvar pain and itching, which has been present for 3 days. The patient first noted some "tingling" and irritation, followed by the development of open sores that are extremely painful. The patient also complains of extreme pain on urination. She reports a low-grade fever, but admits that she has not taken her temperature. When questioned, she concedes having broken up with her previous boyfriend and having become intimate with a new partner on one occasion approximately 1 week before the onset of symptoms. On examination, you find red, swollen labia with open ulcers that are painful to touch.

Questions Case 28A

To confirm your diagnostic suspicions, which of the following is most likely to be of help?

A. Microscopic examination of vaginal secretions mixed with 10% KOH
B. A "whiff" of vaginal secretions mixed with 10% KOH
C. Microscopic examination of material from the ulcerated lesions for giant cells
D. A cervical culture for gonorrhea
E. A serum test for syphilis (e.g., RPR)

Answer: C

The patient's history and physical findings suggest that this patient has a herpes vulvitis. If this is the case, screening for coexistent gonorrhea or syphilis is appropriate (answers D and E) but secondary to the diagnosis of the patient's complaint. Similarly, vaginal infections often occur as STDs. Although *Trichomonas* infections are common in this group, they would not be tested for with the methods given in answers A and B. Screening for a vaginal infection is appropriate if history or physical findings suggest their presence.

The most reasonable therapy for this patient would be

A. Soap and water cleansing, air drying
B. Amoxicillin, 3 g, with probenecid, 1 g
C. Podophyllin 25% in benzoin
D. Metronidazole, 500 mg twice a day
E. Local steroid cream therapy

Answer: A

For initial infections with herpes, local cleansing to decrease the risk of secondary infection is the best therapy. Amoxicillin is an option for treating gonorrhea, whereas podophyllin is useful in treating condyloma, neither of which is likely in this patient. Similarly, metronidazole is indicated for *Trichomonas*. Because of the viral nature of herpes, local steroids should be avoided. Acyclovir therapy for herpes is best started within 48 hours of the onset of lesions and is best carried out by either local cream or an oral dose of 200 mg five times per day. A three-times-a-day dosage is used for suppression of recurrences.

Case 28B

A 24-year-old married mother of three comes to the clinic with the complaint of "something growing down there." The patient first noted small growths on her labia 3 weeks previously, at the end of her menstrual period. These growths have persisted and enlarged. Several small growths have now appeared on the other side. The growths do not cause symptoms, but the patient had an aunt with breast cancer and so was concerned about what these might be. Past medical and surgical history are unremarkable. On physical examination, several small raised, shaggy lesions, ranging in size from 1 to 7 mm are noted on both labia and the perineum.

Question Case 28B

The most likely diagnosis in this patient is

A. Molluscum contagiosum
B. Genital herpes
C. Condyloma lata
D. Condyloma acuminata
E. Chancroid

Answer: D

The differential diagnosis of raised lesions must include molluscum contagiosum and condyloma lata, in addition to the more common condyloma acuminata. The lesions of molluscum contagiosum are more common over the lower abdomen and are distinguished by their central umbilication and yellowish cheesy appearance. Condyloma lata, found in syphilis, are usually flatter in appearance and have a broader base than venereal warts.

Case 28C

A 28-year-old unmarried nulligravid patient presents to you in the emergency room with a 6-hour history of diffuse lower abdominal pain. The pain was periumbilical but has now moved into the lower abdomen. She complains of a fever but has not taken her temperature. She notes mild nausea over the past hour. Past history reveals regular menstrual periods, with her last period occurring on schedule 1 week ago. She has had no previous surgeries or significant medical problems. She does note a similar episode 8 months previously for which she did not seek care. She is sexually active and has never used any contraception. On physical examination she has a pulse of 100, temperature of 38.10° C and a blood pressure of 110/65. Examination of the abdomen finds diffuse

tenderness in both lower quadrants. Pelvic examination is normal except for a yellowish discharge at the cervix, diffuse tenderness on motion of the uterus, and a tender fullness in both adnexa. You order a pregnancy test and a complete blood count (CBC) and perform cervical cultures.

Questions Case 28C

While you await the results of your laboratory tests, what is the most reasonable working diagnosis?

A. Ectopic pregnancy
B. Salpingitis (PID)
C. Appendicitis
D. Gastroenteritis
E. Threatened abortion

Answer: B

The results of the CBC return and you find a white blood cell (WBC) count of 14,000 with 82% segmented polys. The pregnancy test is negative and the culture will not be available for 48 hours. Based on this additional information, what is the most reasonable diagnosis?

A. Ectopic pregnancy
B. Salpingitis (PID)
C. Appendicitis
D. Gastroenteritis
E. Threatened abortion

Answer: B

Fever, lower abdominal pain, tachycardia, and cervical and bilateral adnexal tenderness all point to an inflammatory process in the pelvis. In a patient with infertility and a similar previous episode, recurrent salpingitis (PID) is more likely than appendicitis. This is supported by the elevated WBC count and differential. Broad-spectrum therapy should be implemented based on clinical suspicion, even if the cultures should eventually return as "negative."

CHAPTER

29

PELVIC RELAXATION, URINARY INCONTINENCE, AND URINARY TRACT INFECTION

CHAPTER OBJECTIVES

This chapter deals primarily with APGO Objective(s):

OBJECTIVE 41   Pelvic Relaxation and
Urinary Incontinence

A. Discuss the predisposing factors, anatomy including facial defects, and neuromuscular pathophysiology of pelvic relaxation and urinary incontinence, and discuss cystocele, rectocele, paravaginal defect, and vaginal and uterine prolapse.

B. Describe these diagnostic maneuvers: urine culture, post-void residual, cystoscopy, and urodynamic testing.

C. Discuss these surgical and nonsurgical treatments of pelvic relaxation and/or urinary incontinence: pessary, medical management, and reconstructive surgery.

Pelvic relaxation is a nondescript term that refers to a variety of conditions related to loss of connective tissue support adjacent to the reproductive tract organs and in the perineum. This includes loss of uterine support, paravaginal tissue support, bladder wall and urethrovesicle angle support, and support overlying the distal rectum. Patients with pelvic relaxation present in many different and often subtle ways. To identify patients who would benefit from therapy, the physician should be familiar with the types of pelvic relaxation and the approach to the patient with symptoms suggestive of this problem. The physician must also be aware of other common urinary tract conditions that affect women. Although pelvic relaxation and urinary tract disorders are frequently symptomatic, patients are often reluctant to voice their complaints. The physician must be sensitive to these complaints as well as to the physical findings that suggest a problem.

PELVIC RELAXATION AND URINARY INCONTINENCE

Although not exclusively a condition of advancing age, pelvic relaxation is more common as tissues become less resilient and the accumulated stresses of life have their effects. As a greater proportion of our patients move into their later years, more and more women will be at risk for pelvic relaxation and its attendant problems. Pelvic pressure and pain, dyspareunia, bowel and bladder dysfunction, and urinary incontinence may all result from loss of support for the pelvic organs. Almost half of all women have had the involuntary loss of small amounts of urine at some time in their life; 10% to 15% of women suffer significant, recurrent urinary loss. Loss of pelvic support can have both medical and social implications that necessitate evaluation and intervention.

Causes of Pelvic Relaxation

The pelvic organs are supported by a complex interaction of muscles (e.g., levator muscles), fasciae (e.g., urogenital diaphragm, endopelvic fascia), and ligaments (e.g., the uterosacral and cardinal ligaments). Each of these structures can lose its ability to provide support through birth trauma, chronic elevations of intra-abdominal pressure (e.g., obesity, chronic cough, or repetitive heavy lifting), intrinsic weaknesses, or atrophic changes caused by aging or estrogen loss. Underlying most of these associated factors, the most significant contribution to pelvic relaxation may be intrinsic weaknesses in collagen matrix as a result of genetic factors. Loss of adequate support for the pelvic organs may be manifest by descent or prolapse of the urethra (*urethral detachment* or *urethrocele*), bladder (*cystocele*), or rectum (*rectocele*). True herniation at the top of the vagina (*enterocele*) can also occur. These anatomic defects are illustrated in Figure 29.1. Loss of support for the uterus can lead to varying degrees of descent of the uterus (*uterine prolapse*). When the uterus descends beyond the vulva, it is termed *procidentia*. Loss of tissue support can also result in prolapse of the vaginal vault in patients who have had a hysterectomy. Although such loss of support (*pelvic relaxation*) may affect any of the pelvic organs individually, multiple organ involvement is most common.

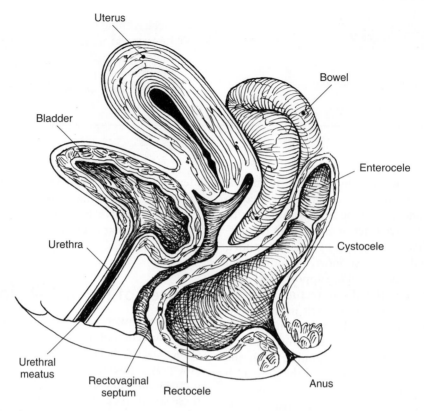

Uterus

Bowel

Bladder

Enterocele

Urethra

Cystocele

Urethral
meatus

Rectovaginal
septum

Rectocele

Anus

FIGURE 29.1.   Loss of pelvic support.

Causes of Urinary Incontinence

A common complaint of patients with a cystocele or urethrocele is urinary incontinence. This does not occur in all patients, and the degree of incontinence is often not commensurate with the degree of pelvic relaxation. There is urine flow anytime the pressure inside the bladder exceeds the pressure in the urethra. This happens physiologically during voluntary voiding when the muscles surrounding the urethra relax and the bladder contracts. It may also take place involuntarily when there is unequal transmission of intra-abdominal pressure to the bladder and urethra, as seen with the loss of pelvic support. When urethral support is lost, the urethra descends outside the influence of abdominal pressure. As a result, the bladder pressure exceeds urethral pressure briefly at times of strain or stress, resulting in *stress incontinence*. These clinical observations and assumptions regarding voiding

physiology are the basis for sophisticated urodynamic testing (see Evaluation section), which may be indicated in some patients with urinary incontinence.

If there is loss of normal innervation and control of bladder function, involuntary bladder contraction or bladder atony may result, leading to *urgency* and *overflow incontinence*, respectively. In addition, loss of urine may ensue anytime there is a breakdown of the social or emotional competence of the patient (e.g., psychosis or neurosis) or when the normal continence mechanism is physically bypassed, such as with fistulous openings.

Clinical Presentation

The symptoms caused by loss of pelvic support vary based on the structure or structures involved and the degree of prolapse. The most common symptoms are those characterized as "pressure" or "heaviness." These symptoms are diffuse, low in the abdomen or pelvis, and are often worse late in the day, after lifting, or

TABLE 29.1.   Characteristics of Urinary Incontinence

Characteristic	Stress Incontinence	Urge Incontinence	Overflow Incontinence
Associated symptoms	None (occasional pelvic pressure)	Urgency, nocturia	Fullness, pressure frequency
Amount of loss	Small, spurt	Large, complete emptying	Small, dribbling
Duration of loss	Brief, corresponds to stress	Moderate, several seconds	Often continuous
Associated event	Cough, laugh, sneeze, physical activity	None, change in position, running water	None
Position	Upright, sitting; rare supine or asleep	Any	Any
Cause	Structural (cystocele, urethrocele)	Loss of bladder inhibition	Obstruction, loss of neurologic control

when standing for long periods. Backache and dyspareunia are also common associated complaints. When support for the bladder and urethra fails, urinary (stress) incontinence, frequency, hesitancy, incomplete voiding, or recurrent infections may result. A careful history that notes the associated symptoms and events, amount and duration of urine loss, and the position in which urine losses occur is important in establishing the correct diagnosis (Table 29.1).

Loss of rectal support may lead to problems such as constipation and painful or incomplete defecation. The patient with a symptomatic rectocele may need to press down or splint the posterior vagina with her fingers to promote bowel movements. When there is complete descent, the patient may be paradoxically asymptomatic and only note the protrusion of tissue from the vagina. Vaginal, cervical, and/or uterine ulceration, bleeding, infection, or pain frequently accompanies complete descent, as a result of chronic contact with clothing and/or compromised blood supply. Symptoms of chronic constipation and difficulty passing stool are also compatible with obstructive lesions. Anoscopy or sigmoidoscopy should be considered, based on the clinical presentation or maintenance needs of the individual patient.

Evaluation

The evaluation of patients with pelvic relaxation rests primarily on the history and physical examination. Pelvic relaxation is best demonstrated by observing the vaginal area while having the patient strain. This may be done in either or both the supine and standing positions. A urethrocele or cystocele may be demonstrated by separating the labia and asking the patient to "strain down" or cough. When a urethrocele or cystocele is present, a downward movement and rotation of the anterior vaginal wall toward the introitus will be seen. To more fully evaluate the presence of a cystocele, rectocele, or enterocele, inspection should be carried out using a Sims or the lower half of a Graves speculum to retract the posterior vaginal wall. To best evaluate the extent of an enterocele, examination should be carried out with the patient in a standing position with one foot elevated on a chair. This facilitates the separate inspection of the anterior and posterior vaginal walls and allows differentiation of the structures involved. Descent of the uterus may be demonstrated either in this way or through palpation.

The degree of pelvic relaxation is often rated on a 1 to 3 scale based on the descent

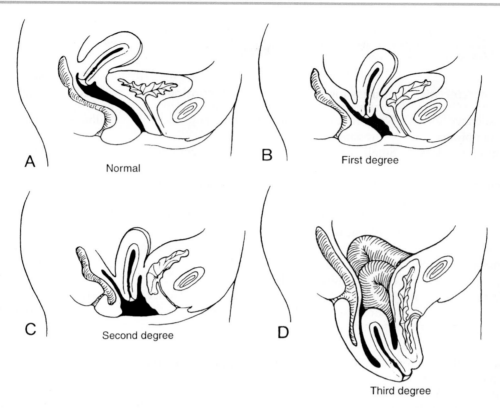

FIGURE 29.2. Degrees of pelvic relaxation.

of the structure involved (Figure 29.2). When descent is limited to the upper two thirds of the vagina, it is said to be first degree. Second-degree prolapse is present when the structure approaches the vaginal introitus. Descent of the structure to outside the vaginal opening (such as the body of the uterus in the case of procidentia) is classified as a third-degree defect. The extent of urethral detachment, commonly referred to as urethrocele, may be quantified using the Q-tip test. This is done by placing a moistened cotton swab in the urethra and measuring the angle of upward motion caused by the patient straining. Upward rotation of greater than 30° from the starting point is generally associated with urinary stress incontinence because of loss of support of the critical urethrovesical junction.

When a significant cystocele or urethrocele is found, evaluation of urinary function is advisable. Compromise of ureteral drainage may occur in cases of significant downward displacement of the trigone as is seen in some cases of second- or third-degree descent. Urinary retention and subsequent infection may also occur and should be evaluated. Because of the frequent association of more than one cause of urinary incontinence, patients with incontinence should be considered for urodynamics testing.

Urodynamics testing refers to a group of procedures that evaluate bladder structure and functions. Although these procedures vary based on the needs of the patient and the preferences of the physician, they generally include cystometrics, cystoscopy, and provocative tests such as coughing or straining. Most centers include sophisticated evaluation of bladder compliance and contractility via cystometrics as well as evaluation of the voiding process itself. Pressure profiles of the bladder and urethra as well as fluoroscopic examinations may also be included. This battery of tests is very important in the objective reproducible evaluation of proposed therapies. Clinically, these tests are useful in the evaluation of patients where "mixed" etiologies are suspected.

Differential Diagnosis

The presumptive diagnosis of pelvic relaxation is based on the evaluation of the structural integrity of pelvic support by physical examination. Often the characteristics of the patient's complaint may suggest a diagnosis. Even though the differential diagnosis of pelvic relaxation is generally simple, other processes must be considered. Urethral diverticulum or Skene's gland abscesses may mimic a cystourethrocele and, in the case of diverticula, may be a source of incontinence. These can be identified through symptoms, careful "milking" of the urethra, or cystoscopy. The complaint of urinary loss may stem from mechanical factors (such as a cystourethrocele), irritation (mechanical or inflammatory trigonitis), neurologic causes (such as diabetes or detrusor instability), the effects of medications, or mental and psychosocial conditions. In patients who have had a history of recent pelvic surgery or radiation, a vesicovaginal or ureterovaginal fistula must also be considered in the differential diagnosis. It is occasionally difficult to differentiate between a high rectocele and an enterocele. This distinction may be facilitated through rectal examination or the identification of small bowel in the hernia sac. It is common for the diagnosis of an enterocele not to be established until surgical repair is undertaken.

Most pelvic relaxation is the result of structural failure of the tissues involved, but other contributing factors should be considered in the complete care of the patient. Has there been a change in intra-abdominal pressure and why? Why does the patient have a chronic cough that has precipitated her symptoms? Is a neurologic process (such as diabetic neuropathy) complicating the patient's presenting complaint? Each of these issues should be considered prior to the selection of a diagnostic or therapeutic plan.

In the evaluation of involuntary loss of urine, the physician must also consider the possibility of fistulae. Fistulae between the vagina and the bladder (vesicovaginal), urethra (urethrovaginal), or ureter (ureterovaginal) are generally the result of surgical trauma, irradiation, or malignancy. A communication between the bladder and the uterus (vesicouterine) may also be found on rare occasions. In addition, fistulae may occur between the rectum and vagina (rectovaginal fistulae), resulting in the passage of flatus or feces from the vagina (Figure 29.3).

Nonsurgical Treatment Options

Because pelvic relaxation is a structural problem, the ultimate solutions are structural as well. These range from mechanical support (through pessaries) and exercises to strengthen the pelvic muscles, to surgical repair of the tissue defects. Estrogen replacement is also an important adjunct to other therapies in the postmenopausal woman.

In patients with urgency incontinence, effective therapy may include bladder training, biofeedback, or medical therapy. Bladder training programs are directed toward increasing the patient's bladder control and capacity by gradually increasing the amount of time between voidings. Often successful by itself, this may be augmented in difficult cases by biofeedback when available. Treatment with anticholinergic drugs [Pro-Banthine (propantheline bromide) and Ditropan (oxybutynin chloride)], β-sympathomimetic agonists [Alupent (metaproterenol sulfate)], musculotrophic drugs [Urispas (flavoxate hydrochloride) and Valium (diazepam)], antidepressants [Tofranil (imipramine hydrochloride)], or dopamine agonists [Parlodel (bromocriptine mesylate)] has had some success based on the character of the patient's problem.

The pelvic musculature may be strengthened through the use of Kegel exercises. This exercise program consists of the repetitive contraction of the pelvic floor muscles as if trying to stop the bladder from emptying. This is repeated many times throughout the day. Kegel exercises may be helpful for some patients with mild incontinence. They may also help to provide better tissues should surgical repair be attempted.

A mechanical buttress for the pelvic organs may be provided through the use of pessaries. These are devices worn in the

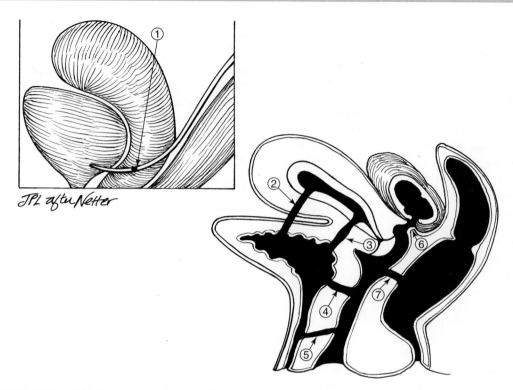

JPL after Netter

FIGURE 29.3. Female genital fistulae. (*1*) Ureterovaginal. (*2*) Vesicouterovaginal. (*3*) Vesicocervicovaginal. (*4*) Vesicovaginal. (*5*) Urethrovaginal. (*6*) Enterovaginal. (*7*) Rectovaginal.

vagina to furnish support. Pessaries come in a variety of types and sizes, all designed to replace the missing structural integrity of the pelvis or to diffuse the forces of descent over a wide area. The most common forms of pessary are the Smith-Hodge, the ring (or doughnut), the inflatable ball, and the cube (Figure 29.4). They are placed in the vagina in much the same way as a diaphragm. They occlude the vagina and hold the pelvic organs in a relatively normal position. Pessary therapy requires the cooperation and involvement of the patient but offers a good alternative to surgical repair for properly selected, well-motivated patients.

Patients who are fitted with a pessary for the control of pelvic relaxation need careful initial monitoring. Reexamination in 5 to 7 days to confirm proper placement, hygiene, and the absence of pressure-related problems (vaginal trauma or necrosis) is required. Evaluation in 24 hours may be

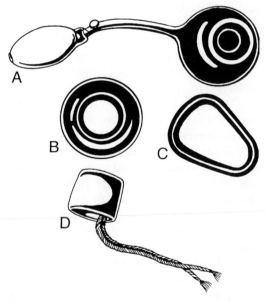

FIGURE 29.4. Pessaries. (*A*) Inflatable. (*B*) Doughnut. (*C*) Smith-Hodge. (*D*) Cube.

TABLE 29.2. Surgical Therapy for Urinary Incontinence

Type	Intent	Approach
Anterior vaginal repair (colporrhaphy, Kelly plication)	Provide support to the bladder and urethra by reinforcing the endopelvic fascia and vaginal epithelium	Vaginal
Retropubic suspension (Marshall-Marchetti-Krantz, Burch, paravaginal repair)	Repair defects in the endopelvic fascia and its attachments	Abdominal
Sling procedure (Pereyra, Stamey)	Supplement or replace the support of the bladder neck and urethra using suture or fascial slings	Combined abdominal and vaginal

advisable in patients who are debilitated or require additional assistance.

Surgical Therapy

Surgical repair of pelvic relaxation takes many forms, depending on the specific defect, ranging from hysterectomy for uterine prolapse to the creation of supportive slings for stress incontinence to occlusion of the vagina for vaginal vault prolapse in the elderly to plastic repairs to restore prolapsing structures to their original anatomic position (Table 29.2 and Figure 29.5). These procedures may be carried out from vaginal, abdominal, or laparoscopic approaches, and each has its own set of indications, advantages, disadvantages, complications, and failures. No one procedure is best, and each surgical approach must be individualized. Success is based not only on the procedure chosen but also on the skill of the surgeon, the degree of pelvic relaxation, and patient risk factors such as quality of tissues, obesity, and lifestyle (e.g., smoking).

Failure of rectovaginal support may be treated by reconstructing or reinforcing the rectovaginal space (posterior colporrhaphy). Prolapse of the vagina may be treated by suspending the vaginal vault to either the sacrospinous ligament (sacrospinous vaginal vault suspension) or to the sacrum itself (sacral colpopexy). Obliteration of the rectovaginal space (Moskowitz procedure) is also used to treat or prevent vaginal prolapse and enterocele formation. Enteroceles are treated like other hernias, with dissection and high ligation of the hernia sac.

Because of the frequent concurrence of defects in pelvic support and uterine descent, vaginal hysterectomy is often performed simultaneously with the reconstruction procedure. This corrects any symptoms referable to the descensus, provides access to the uterine support mechanisms to reinforce other repairs, and prevents the uterus from contributing to recurrence of anterior and posterior repairs should further descent occur.

For patients whose medical conditions preclude long surgical procedures and who are not sexually active, partial or complete obliteration of the vaginal canal (LeFort procedure, colpocleisis) may be done to provide support to the pelvic structures.

Therapy for fistulae is primarily surgical. Occasionally fistulae that occur following surgery spontaneously heal when adequate drainage or diversion of the urinary or fecal flow is provided. In all other cases, the only successful therapy consists of meticulous dissection of the fistulous tract and careful reapproximation of tissues. Recurrence is a common problem, especially in patients who have had radiation therapy for malignancies.

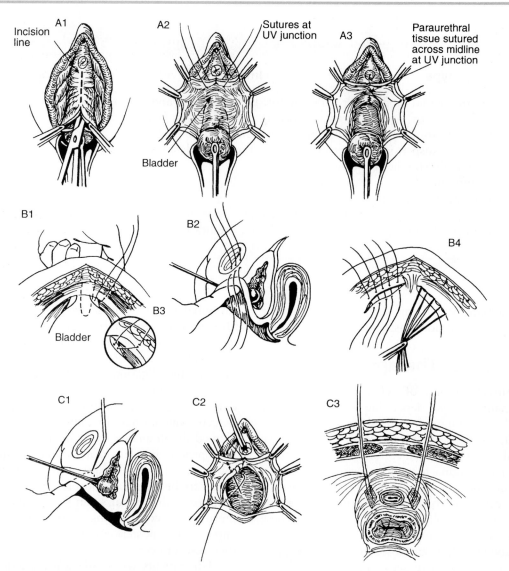

FIGURE 29.5. Surgical therapy for urinary incontinence. (*A1–A3*) Anterior vaginal wall repair, the Kelly-Kennedy procedure. (*A1*) Anterior vaginal wall is opened and undermined. (*A2*) Paraurethral tissue lateral to the urethrovesical (UV) junction is sutured. (*A3*) This creates a firm bar of tissue that supports the UV junction. (*B1–B4*) Retropubic suspension procedures, the Marshall-Marchetti-Krantz procedure. (*B1*) The suture is placed in the periurethral tissue and then into the pubic periosteum so that (*B2*) the urethra may be advanced upward into an intra-abdominal position. (*B3*) The Burch procedure, by which the tissue adjacent to the UV angle is sutured to the iliopectineal (Coopers) ligament. (*B4*) The Richardson paravaginal repair, by which the sutures are placed between the superior sulcus of the vagina and lateral pelvic side wall at the level of the iliopectineal line. (*C1–C3*) Sling procedures. (*C1*) The Pereyra procedure, by which a needle is guided transabdominally into the paraurethral tissue and back through (*C2*) to be tied suprapubically, thus supporting the UV angle. (*C3*) The Stamey procedure, by which a Dacron support material is used in the paraurethral tissue to buttress the tissue.

URINARY TRACT INFECTIONS

Women suffer urinary tract infection roughly 10 times more often than men. Approximately 15% of women experience at least one urinary tract infection in their lifetime. This necessitates the physician having a familiarity with the diagnosis and treatment of a number of urologic disorders common to women.

Most urinary tract infections in women ascend from bacterial contamination of the urethra. Except in the case of tuberculosis or immunosuppressed patients, infections are rarely acquired by hematogenous or lymphatic spread. The relatively short female urethra, exposure of the meatus to vestibular and rectal pathogens, and sexual activity that may induce trauma or introduce other organisms all increase the potential for infection. With estrogen deficiency, there is also a decrease in urethral resistance to infection, which contributes to ascending contamination. This increased susceptibility explains the almost 10% prevalence of asymptomatic bacteriuria found in postmenopausal women.

Clinical Aspects of Urinary Tract Infections

Approximately 95% of urinary tract infections are symptomatic, uncomplicated, do not ascend to the kidneys, and produce no permanent damage. Of first infections, 90% are caused by *Escherichia coli,* and these respond readily to antibiotic therapy. Anaerobic bacteria and yeasts are rare causes of infections, except in diabetic or immunosuppressed patients or those with chronic indwelling catheters.

Patients with urinary tract infections typically present with symptoms of frequency, urgency, nocturia, or dysuria. The symptoms found vary somewhat with the site of the infection. When there is irritation of the bladder or trigone, symptoms include urgency, frequency, and nocturia. Irritation of the urethra leads to frequency and dysuria. The physical examination generally is nonspecific, although some patients may report suprapubic tenderness.

Evaluation

The evaluation of the patient suspected of having a urinary tract infection should include a urinalysis and a urine culture and sensitivity. These are generally obtained through a "clean-catch midstream" urine sample, which involves cleansing the vulva and catching a portion of urine passed during the middle of uninterrupted voiding. Urine obtained from catheters or suprapubic aspiration may also be used.

Laboratory analysis of the urine may be conducted or the sample examined microscopically by the clinician. This microscopic evaluation is carried out using a drop of urine or the precipitate from a centrifuged specimen. For uncentrifuged samples, the presence of more than one white blood cell per high-power field carries a 90% accuracy in detecting infection. Centrifuged specimens may be scanned with low power for the presence of large numbers of white cells. Pyuria is defined as the presence of more than five white cells per high-power field in the centrifuged specimen. Gram stain of urine samples or sediments may also be helpful in establishing the diagnosis of infection. "Dipstick" tests for infection based on the presence of leukocyte esterase are also useful.

Cultures of urine samples that show colony counts of more than 100,000 for a single organism generally indicate infection. Colony counts as low as 10,000 for *E. coli* are associated with infection when symptoms are present. When a culture report indicates the presence of multiple organisms, contamination of the specimen should be suspected.

Recurrent urinary tract infections should prompt a reevaluation. Possible causes that must be considered include incorrect or incomplete (i.e., noncompliant) therapy, mechanical factors such as obstruction, or compromised host defenses.

Therapy

The selection of therapy for patients with urinary tract infections is simple and generally successful. Hydration, urinary acidification (with ascorbic acid, ammonium chloride, or acidic fruit juices), and urinary analgesics [Pyridium (phenazopyridine hydrochloride)] are helpful in most cases. Once confirmation by urinalysis or culture has been obtained, antibiotic therapy should be instituted. Nitrofurantoin (Macrodantin) produces good urinary antibiosis without undue alteration of other flora, although it is not effective against *Proteus* infections. Antibiotics such as ampicillin, tetracycline, and trimethoprim–sulfamethoxazole (Septra, Bactrim) provide good coverage in the urinary tract but risk more alteration of vaginal or intestinal flora. Vaginal yeast infections may result from these antibiotic treatments. When pyelonephritis is suspected, aggressive antibiotic therapy with cephalosporins such as Keflex (cephalexin) or Duricef (cefadroxil) is indicated.

Patients who have been treated for urinary tract infections should have follow-up urinalysis and culture done 10 to 14 days after the initial diagnosis. This will document cure in most patients and identify those at risk for recurrence because of incomplete or ineffective therapy.

CASE STUDIES

Case 29A

An 18-year-old nulligravid patient presents to your office with the complaint of 3 days of urinary frequency, urgency, and dysuria. She was married 2 weeks ago and the symptoms first appeared following a weekend getaway with her husband. She is using condom and foam for contraception. She reports no fever or chills, and she is aware of no vaginal discharge. Your physical examination reveals no abnormal findings. You obtain a clean-catch urine and centrifuge the specimen. You examine the sediment under the microscope and find 20 to 30 white cells, a moderate number of epithelial cells, and some bacteria in each low-power field.

Questions Case 29A

The best working diagnosis at this point is

A. Cystitis
B. Pyuria
C. Traumatic urethritis/trigonitis
D. Pyelonephritis
E. Vaginitis

Answer: C

The finding of a large number of white blood cells in the centrifuged urine specimen would normally be diagnostic of pyuria. This, combined with the patient's symptoms, supports the diagnosis of cystitis. In this case, however, the microscopic examination also showed a large number of epithelial cells, which means the specimen had had moderate contamination from vaginal secretions. Without symptoms of vaginal discharge or irritation, you cannot make the diagnosis of vaginitis, but you also cannot rely on the present urine sample to make the diagnosis of urinary tract infection. Trauma to the urethra and bladder trigone ("honeymoon cystitis") may imitate infection. The patient's recent marriage and the use of spermicides could support the possibility of mechanical or chemical irritation. Although you have not ruled out the possibility of infection, the circumstances suggest that infection may be less likely than traumatic urethritis.

To confirm your suspicions you might

A. Obtain a catheterized urine for examination
B. Request a culture and sensitivity on the specimen you have
C. Obtain a wet prep of vaginal secretions
D. Obtain a more detailed sexual history
E. Perform an intravenous pyelogram

Answer: D

Both a further exploration of the patient's sexual history and a better evaluation of the possibility of infection are indicated, but the invasive nature of urinary catheterization makes the evaluation of history a better choice. Based on the history, the need for a catheterized specimen may be better determined. You know from the presence of epithelial cells in the centrifuged specimen that the sample is contaminated and thus culture is compromised. Although a microscopic examination of vaginal secretions is easy to accomplish, there is no evidence for vaginitis in the patient's history or physical examination. Intravenous pyelography is invasive, expensive, and would not contribute to the diagnostic possibilities in this case.

Case 29B

A 64-year-old G5 P4 widowed patient comes to your office for her annual physical examination. She had a total hysterectomy 20 years ago for tumors. When you take your gynecologic history, the patient somewhat shyly admits that she is not sexually active but that she has recently met someone whom she likes. She also admits that she has begun experiencing a loss of urine when she coughs, laughs, or sneezes.

This has made her self-conscious, and she is considering giving up her seniors' aerobics class.

Your physical examination shows her to be an 87-kg woman with a blood pressure of 138/92 and a pulse of 84. Her abdomen is protuberant, but no masses or tenderness is noted. Pelvic examination reveals atrophic changes in the vulva and vagina, a second-degree cystocele, slight descensus of the vaginal vault, and no palpable adnexa.

Question Case 29B

Which of the following is probably NOT indicated at this time?

A. Weight reduction
B. Estrogen therapy
C. Kegel exercises
D. Anterior colporrhaphy
E. Low-impact exercise program

Answer: D

The history and physical examination presented are consistent with stress incontinence caused by a cystourethrocele. The patient's symptoms are mild and do not warrant surgical intervention at this time. Should the symptoms become worse, urodynamic evaluation should also be considered before scheduling a surgical repair. Estrogen therapy (systemic or vaginal) and Kegel exercises may both help to improve the patient's symptoms. Weight reduction is a worthwhile goal for general health and to decrease the possibility of progression of her pelvic relaxation. The addition of a low-impact exercise program may help the weight reduction program and support the patient's self-esteem. Reassurance is always indicated.

CHAPTER

30

ENDOMETRIOSIS

CHAPTER OBJECTIVES

This chapter deals primarily with APGO Objective(s):

OBJECTIVE 42   Endometriosis

A. Discuss the pathogenesis and associated sequelae of endometriosis.

B. Describe the signs and symptoms, pathophysiology, surgical findings, diagnosis, and medical and surgical managements of endometriosis.

The clinical impact of endometriosis relates to its association with symptoms such as infertility, dysmenorrhea, dyspareunia, and chronic pelvic pain. Endometriosis is characterized by the presence of endometrial tissue in extrauterine locations, most commonly near the ovaries, on the uterosacral ligaments, rectovaginal septum, and pelvic peritoneum. The term *endometrioma* has been used to describe an isolated collection of endometriosis involving an ovary that is large enough to be considered a tumor. The term *adenomyosis* refers to endometrial implants found deep within the uterine wall. Endometriosis and adenomyosis are benign conditions that have different clinical courses. Endometriosis is progressive, leading to ever increasing symptoms and damage. When diagnosed early, surgical and medical therapies are available to relieve the symptoms, slow the progression, or ablate the disease. Adenomyosis is confined to the uterus and presents as progressive dysmenorrhea and menorrhagia (see Chapter 31).

INCIDENCE AND PREVALENCE

The diagnosis of endometriosis may be suspected clinically and strongly supported by findings at laparoscopy or laparotomy, but histologic confirmation of endometriosis is required to make a definitive diagnosis. Therefore, the true incidence of endometriosis is difficult to establish. Because laparotomy and/or endoscopy is required to confirm the clinical diagnosis, there are patients who have asymptomatic endometriosis who are undiagnosed and patients who undergo surgery for unrelated reasons who are only then found to have incidental endometriosis.

It is estimated that 1% to 2% of women in the general population have endometriosis and that this rate increases to 30% to 50% in infertile women. Endometriosis occurs primarily in women in their 20s and 30s, although this may be a function of the frequency of evaluation of women in this age range for infertility and pelvic pain. Endometriosis is less frequently described in postmenopausal women. In adolescents, congenital anomalies that promote retrograde menstruation may be a common associated finding.

It has been thought that certain patient groups are at higher risk for developing endometriosis, such as those who delay childbearing. Middle-class white patients who are described as high achieving and perfectionist were once considered at higher risk. This stereotypical description has not been proved valid. There is evidence, however, that there is a genetic predisposition in women whose first-degree relatives have had endometriosis. A first-degree relative of a woman with endometriosis has an approximately 7% chance of being similarly affected.

PATHOGENESIS

The exact mechanism by which endometriosis develops is unknown. Three major theories are commonly cited.

1. Direct implantation of endometrial cells, typically by means of retrograde menstruation, has been postulated. This appears consistent with the occurrence of pelvic endometriosis and its predilection for the ovaries and pelvic peritoneum. This is also consistent with finding endometriosis in sites such as an abdominal incision or episiotomy scar. Direct implantation is commonly referred to as Sampson's theory because of his experimental work that showed the possibility of such a mechanism.
2. Vascular and lymphatic dissemination of endometrial cells (Halban's theory) has been postulated. Distant sites of endometriosis can be explained by this process (i.e., the presence of endometriosis in locations such as lymph nodes, the pleural cavity, and kidney).
3. Coelomic metaplasia of multipotential cells in the peritoneal cavity (Meyer's theory) states that, under certain conditions, these cells can develop into functional endometrial tissue.

This could even occur in response to the irritation caused by retrograde menstruation.

Each of these major theories has evidence to support it. It is probable that more than one theory is necessary to explain the diverse nature and locations of endometriosis. Underlying all of these possibilities is the yet undiscovered immunologic factor that would explain why some women develop endometriosis whereas others with similar characteristics do not.

PATHOLOGY

Endometriosis is found on the ovary in 60% of patients and is typically bilateral. Other common pelvic structures involved include the pouch of Douglas (particularly the uterosacral ligaments and rectovaginal septum), the round ligament, the fallopian tube, and the sigmoid colon (Table 30.1). On rare occasion, endometriosis is found in abdominal surgical scars, the umbilicus, and various organs outside of the pelvic cavity.

The gross appearance of endometriosis varies considerably. Subtle, minimal findings that have been biopsy proved to be endometriosis include 1-mm vascular hemorrhagic areas, white-opaque plaques on the peritoneal surfaces, and more classically, spots that have been described as "mulberry" or "raspberry" in appearance. These small areas may also be rust colored, dark brown, or like "powder burns" in appearance. Frequently, there is reactive fibrosis surrounding these lesions, which gives a puckered appearance. More advanced, disseminated disease causes further fibrosis and results in the typically dense adhesions found in patients whose pelvic anatomy may be obscured by the disease.

Endometriomas may reach 15 to 20 cm in size and are filled with thick, chocolate-appearing fluid, which is primarily old blood. These "chocolate cysts" are associated with endometriosis although hemorrhagic cysts of the ovary may also have this gross appearance.

The microscopic diagnosis of endometriosis is made when there are endome-

TABLE 30.1. Sites of Endometriosis	
Site	**Frequency (Percentage of Patients)**
Most common	
Ovary (frequently bilateral)	60
Pelvic peritoneum over the uterus	
Anterior and posterior cul-de-sacs	
Uterosacral ligaments	
Fallopian tubes	
Pelvic lymph nodes	30
Infrequent	
Rectosigmoid	10–15
Other gastrointestinal tract sites	5
Vagina	
Rare	
Umbilicus	
Episiotomy or surgical scars	
Kidney	
Lungs	
Arms	
Legs	
Nasal mucosa	

trial glands, stroma, and a presence of hemosiderin-laden macrophages. The glands and stroma do function histologically and physiologically like uterine mucosa, with cyclic changes in response to hormones noted. It is not, however, as well ordered as that which occurs in the endometrial cavity. In as many as one third of cases, the microscopic diagnosis is not conclusive, despite a "classic" clinical appearance.

CLINICAL FEATURES

Symptoms

Women with endometriosis demonstrate an exceptionally wide variation of symptomatology, the nature and severity of which may be surprisingly independent of both the location and extent of the disease. Women with extensive endometriosis may have few symptoms, whereas, paradoxically, those with minimal gross endometriosis may have severe pain. The classic symptoms of endometriosis include dysmenorrhea, deep thrust dyspareunia, infertility, abnormal bleeding, and pelvic pain.

The dysmenorrhea associated with endometriosis is not directly related to the amount of visible disease. Patients who present with dysmenorrhea that does not respond to oral contraceptives or nonsteroidal anti-inflammatory agents should have endometriosis considered as a possible etiology. The dyspareunia is often associated with uterosacral or vaginal involvement with endometriosis. In addition, the uterus may be retroverted and fixed in the cul-de-sac because of the extensive adhesions. The dyspareunia is typically reported on deep penetration. There is, however, no correlation between dyspareunia and the extent of endometriosis.

Infertility is more frequent in women with endometriosis than in the general population. With extensive disease, pelvic scarring and adhesions may be responsible, but the exact mechanism for the infertility is unclear in patients with minimal endometriosis. Prostaglandins and autoantibodies have been implicated, but these relations remain unproved. Infertility may, in some cases, be the only complaint. In these cases, endometriosis is discovered at the time of laparoscopic evaluation as part of the infertility workup.

Intermenstrual bleeding occurs in approximately one third of women with endometriosis. In many cases, there is premenstrual spotting, possibly the result of an associated luteal phase inadequacy.

Pelvic pain is a common finding in patients with endometriosis. In some cases, the patient's pain is not solely associated with the menstrual period (dysmenorrhea) or to coital activity (dyspareunia) but, rather, is a chronic, unremitting low pelvic discomfort. Chronic pelvic pain may be related to the adhesions and pelvic scarring found in association with endometriosis, although endometriosis may just as often be asymptomatic.

Other, less common symptoms of endometriosis include gastrointestinal symptoms such as rectal bleeding and dyschezia in patients with endometrial implants on the bowel, and urinary symptoms such as hematuria in patients with endometrial implants on the bladder or ureters. Occasionally, patients may present with an acute abdominal emergency, which may be associated with the rupture or torsion of an endometrioma.

Signs

The classic description of uterosacral nodularity on rectovaginal examination is consistent with significant gross disease involving that area, but it is not universally present. The uterus is often relatively fixed and retroflexed in the pelvis. Ovarian endometriomas may be tender, palpable, and freely mobile in the pelvis or adhered to the posterior leaf of the broad ligament, the lateral pelvic wall, or in the posterior cul-de-sac.

Physical findings in early endometriosis may be very subtle or even nonexistent. In cases of unexplained pelvic pain or infertility, the diagnosis of endometriosis should be entertained and diagnostic laparoscopy considered. It is recommended that visual and, ideally, histologic confirmation of

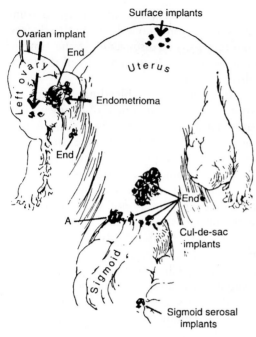

Surface implants

Ovarian implant

End

Uterus

Endometrioma

End

A

End

Cul-de-sac implants

Sigmoid

Sigmoid serosal implants

FIGURE 30.1. Clinical features of endometriosis. End = endometriosis; A = uterosacral implants.

endometriosis be obtained before institution of medical therapy for endometriosis. Typical clinical features of endometriosis are shown in Figure 30.1.

DIFFERENTIAL DIAGNOSIS

Depending on the symptoms, the differential diagnosis will change. In patients who present with chronic abdominal pain, consideration should be given to diagnoses such as chronic pelvic inflammatory disease, pelvic adhesions, gastrointestinal dysfunction, and other etiologies of chronic pelvic pain. In patients who present primarily with dysmenorrhea, both primary dysmenorrhea and etiologies for secondary dysmenorrhea should be considered. In patients who present with dyspareunia, other considerations should include chronic pelvic inflammatory disease, ovarian cysts, and symptomatic uterine retroversion. If abnormal bleeding is

the primary presentation, investigation should rule out conditions such as anovulation, hypothyroidism, and hyperprolactinemia. If premenstrual spotting is the primary symptom, luteal phase defect, polyps, or cervical lesions should be considered. If the patient presents with sudden abdominal pain, considerations other than a ruptured endometrioma include ectopic pregnancy, acute pelvic inflammatory disease, adnexal torsion, and rupture of a corpus luteum cyst or ovarian neoplasm.

DIAGNOSIS

Because of the diverse ways in which patients with endometriosis present, *history taking and physical examination can be considered only preliminary in nature. Establishing a diagnosis requires direct visualization at the time of diagnostic laparoscopy, or on occasion, at laparotomy.* The importance of diagnostic laparoscopy is underscored for adolescent patients when it is recognized that endometriosis is discovered in about one half of teenagers undergoing laparoscopy for evaluation of chronic pelvic pain or dysmenorrhea. Ideally, histologic confirmation of "endometriosis-appearing" lesions or implants should be obtained. Should rectal bleeding occur, barium enema and colonoscopy should be undertaken to exclude other primary gastrointestinal disorders and to evaluate for endometriosis involving these structures. Pelvic ultrasound cannot definitively make the diagnosis of endometriosis, nor are there any laboratory studies that are of value except to help rule out other conditions.

Once the diagnosis is made, the extent of the endometriosis should be properly documented. The most widely accepted classification system has been established by the American Fertility Society (Figure 30.2). This system standardizes the extent of the disease and aids in tracking progression or regression of endometriosis after therapy has been instituted.

THE AMERICAN FERTILITY SOCIETY
REVISED CLASSIFICATION OF ENDOMETRIOSIS

Patient's Name _____   Date _____

Stage I   (Minimal) · 1-5
Stage II (Mild)   · 6-15
Stage III (Moderate) · 16-40
Stage IV (Severe)   · >40
Total _____

Laparoscopy _____ Laparotomy _____ Photography _____
Recommended Treatment _____

Prognosis _____

	ENDOMETRIOSIS	<1cm	1-3cm	>3cm
PERITONEUM	Superficial	1	2	4
	Deep	2	4	6
OVARY	R Superficial	1	2	4
	Deep	4	16	20
	L Superficial	1	2	4
	Deep	4	16	20

	POSTERIOR CULDESAC OBLITERATION	Partial		Complete
		4		40

	ADHESIONS	<1/3 Enclosure	1/3-2/3 Enclosure	>2/3 Enclosure
OVARY	R Filmy	1	2	4
	Dense	4	8	16
	L Filmy	1	2	4
	Dense	4	8	16
TUBE	R Filmy	1	2	4
	Dense	4*	8*	16
	L Filmy	1	2	4
	Dense	4*	8*	16

*If the fimbriated end of the fallopian tube is completely enclosed, change the point assignment to 16.

Additional Endometriosis: _____ | Associated Pathology: _____

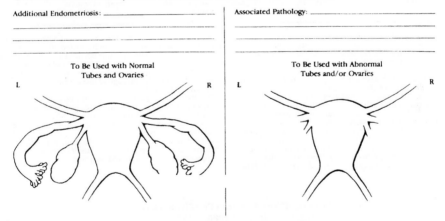

To Be Used with Normal Tubes and Ovaries

To Be Used with Abnormal Tubes and/or Ovaries

For additional supply write to: The American Fertility Society, 2131 Magnolia Avenue, Suite 201, Birmingham, Alabama 35256

FIGURE 30.2.   The American Fertility Society Revised Classification of Endometriosis.
(Continued)

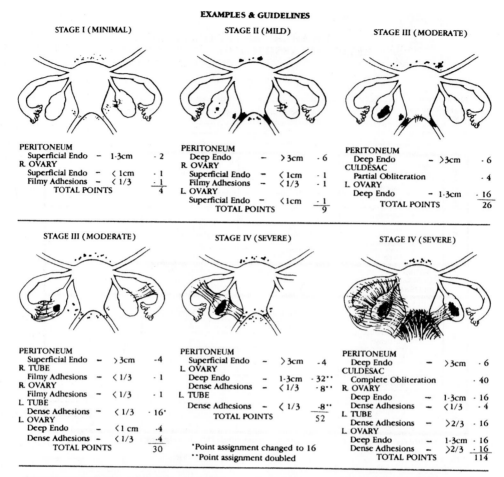

Determination of the stage or degree of endometrial involvement is based on a weighted point system. Distribution of points has been arbitrarily determined and may require further revision or refinement as knowledge of the disease increases.

To ensure complete evaluation, inspection of the pelvis in a clockwise or counterclockwise fashion is encouraged. Number, size and location of endometrial implants, plaques, endometriomas and/or adhesions are noted. For example, five separate 0.5cm superficial implants on the peritoneum (2.5 cm total) would be assigned 2 points. (The surface of the uterus should be considered peritoneum.) The severity of the endometriosis or adhesions should be assigned the highest score only for peritoneum, ovary, tube or culdesac. For example, a 4cm superficial and a 2cm deep implant of the peritoneum should be given a score of 6 (not 8). A 4cm deep endometrioma of the ovary associated with more than 3cm of superficial disease should be scored 20 (not 24).

In those patients with only one adnexa, points applied to disease of the remaining tube and ovary should be multiplied by two. **Points assigned may be circled and totaled. Aggregation of points indicates stage of disease (minimal, mild, moderate, or severe).

The presence of endometriosis of the bowel, urinary tract, fallopian tube, vagina, cervix, skin etc., should be documented under "additional endometriosis." Other pathology such as tubal occlusion, leiomyomata, uterine anomaly, etc., should be documented under "associated pathology." All pathology should be depicted as specifically as possible on the sketch of pelvic organs, and means of observation (laparoscopy or laparotomy) should be noted.

Property of The American Fertility Society
Revised 1985

FIGURE 30.2. *(Continued)*

PREVENTION

There is no known method to prevent endometriosis. Instead, the prevention of the spread of this disease should be the goal once the diagnosis has been established. A high index of suspicion can lead to early diagnosis, resulting in treatment before the endometriosis has progressed extensively. For example, conditions of the lower genital tract that may predispose to retrograde menstruation should be corrected as soon as they are found. Diagnostic procedures that require retrograde insufflation of dye or gas through the fallopian tubes (e.g., hysterosalpingography) should not be done while the patient is menstruating. Because endometriosis appears to be suppressed by the prolonged progestational effect of pregnancy, conception has traditionally been recommended as a way to prevent or minimize the effects of endometriosis. Unfortunately, there are no scientific data to support this latter recommendation. Furthermore, this recommendation potentially causes its own dilemma, because patients with endometriosis already are at greater risk for infertility.

TREATMENT

The diagnosis should be firmly established before instituting either medical or surgical therapy. The choice of therapy depends on the patient's individual circumstances, which include (a) presenting symptoms and their severity, (b) location and severity of endometriosis, and (c) desire for future childbearing. All of the medical treatments for endometriosis are temporizing measures to some extent. None can be expected to provide a permanent cure until extirpative surgery is undertaken or the hormonal stimulation is permanently removed.

Observation

There are selected cases in which patients can be treated expectantly (i.e., without either medical or surgical therapy). These include patients with very limited disease whose symptoms are minimal or nonexistent and/or those who are trying to get pregnant. In the occasional patient in her mid to late 40s with mild symptoms, consideration may be given to withholding therapy with the expectation that the decrease in menstrual hormones associated with menopause may not stimulate growth of disease.

Medical Therapy

Because the glands and stroma of endometriosis respond to both exogenous and endogenous hormones, suppression of endometriosis is based on a medication's potential ability to induce atrophy of the endometrial tissue. This is optimal for patients who are currently symptomatic, have documented endometriosis beyond minimal disease, and/or desire pregnancy sometime in the future. The patient should be aware that recurrence after the completion of medical therapy is common and that medical therapy does not have an effect on adhesions and fibrosis caused by the endometriosis.

Beneficial effects have been obtained using combined estrogen and progestin oral contraceptive agents. Commonly referred to as "pseudopregnancy," the use of oral contraceptives induces a decidual reaction in the functioning endometriotic tissue. Patients can also be maintained on oral contraceptive agents without intermittent withdrawal bleeding, thus avoiding secondary dysmenorrhea.

Progestins alone have also been administered by both the oral and parenteral routes [e.g., Provera (medroxyprogesterone acetate) 20 to 40 mg/day; Depo-Provera (depomedroxyprogesterone acetate) 100 mg IM every 2 weeks, then 200 mg monthly after 8 weeks]. Progestins suppress gonadotropin release and, in turn, ovarian steroidogenesis; they also directly affect the uterine endometrium and endometrial implants.

A state of "pseudomenopause" can also be induced with danazol, a 17 α-ethinyl testosterone derivative. Danazol suppresses both luteinizing hormone (LH) and follicle-stimulating hormone (FSH) midcycle surges so the ovary no longer produces estrogen, which stimulates endometriosis. At a dosage of up to 800 mg/day, amenorrhea occurs within 4 to 8 weeks after the onset of therapy. The desired endometrial atrophy results, but side effects are also significant. In spite of the term *pseudomenopause*, FSH and LH levels are suppressed rather than elevated as they would be in the physiologic menopausal state. Side effects of danazol are related to its hypoestrogenic and androgenic properties, including acne in 15% to 20% of patients; spotting and bleeding in

10% of patients; hot flushes in 15% of patients; oily skin, growth of facial hair, decreased libido, and atrophic vaginitis in approximately 5% of patients; and deepening of the voice, not all of which will reverse with the discontinuation of therapy. Marked alterations of lipoprotein metabolism are induced, including a 60% decrease in serum high-density lipoprotein (HDL) cholesterol level and a 40% decrease in low-density lipoprotein (LDL). Danazol provides relief from symptoms in approximately 80% of patients, with symptoms recurring in 5% to 20% of patients within one year after discontinuing the medication.

Gonadotropin-releasing hormone (GnRH) agonists such as monthly or quarterly leuprolide acetate (Lupron) injections, nafarelin acetate nasal spray, and monthly injected goserelin acetate have also been successfully used to down regulate the pituitary gland. Marked suppression of LH and FSH are noted, and the side effects are somewhat less troublesome than those of danazol as patients may have hypoestrogenic symptoms without androgenic side effects. However, the therapy is quite expensive and parenteral administration is required. Efficacy for each of these agents appears comparable with that of danazol.

Surgical Therapy

The surgical management of endometriosis can be classified as either conservative or extirpative. Conservative surgery includes excision, cauterization or ablation (by laser or electrocoagulation) of visible endometriotic lesions, and preservation of the uterus and other reproductive organs to allow for a possible future pregnancy. Conservative surgery is often undertaken at the time of the initial diagnosis. Whether the initial laparoscopy is performed for pain or infertility, attempts to remove the existent endometriosis are undertaken by the surgeon. If extensive disease is found, conservative surgery involves lysis of adhesions, removal of active endometriotic lesions, and possibly reconstruction of reproductive organs. Success rates of conservative surgery appear to correlate with the severity of the disease at the time of surgery. Medical therapy is often added either before surgery, to reduce the amount of endometriosis with which the surgeon has to contend, or after surgery, to attempt to facilitate healing and avoid recurrence of the endometriosis. Pregnancy is also possible after conservative surgical therapy, with pregnancy rates of 60%, 50%, and 40% reported after conservative surgery for mild, moderate, and severe disease, respectively.

Extirpative surgery for endometriosis is reserved only for cases in which the disease is so extensive that conservative medical or surgical therapy is not feasible or when the patient has completed her family and wishes definitive therapy. Definitive surgery includes total abdominal hysterectomy, bilateral salpingo-oophorectomy, lysis of adhesions, and removal of endometriotic implants. The ramifications of not being able to conceive in the future must be thoroughly explored with the patient. Assuming that all the ovarian tissue is removed at the time of surgery, it is unlikely that any residual endometriosis will be stimulated by further endogenous hormonal production. Occasionally, in younger patients, ovarian tissue may be left to avoid the need for long-term estrogen-replacement therapy. This should be done only with the understanding that further surgery may be necessary to remove the remaining ovary should endometriosis recur.

Estrogen replacement therapy after definitive extirpative surgery for endometriosis should not be avoided for fear of stimulating recurrent disease. Only rarely is reactivation of endometriosis noted, a far smaller risk than that associated with prolonged estrogen deficiency (i.e., osteoporosis and cardiovascular disease).

CASE STUDIES

Case 30A

A 22-year-old woman seeks treatment for infertility. She and her husband have been having intercourse without conception for 17 months. Her history includes an induced abortion at the age of 16 and two episodes of pelvic infection, which required intravenous antibiotic therapy and hospitalization. She reports significant menstrual discomfort and pain "when he pushes deep" during intercourse. On your examination you find the uterus to be retroverted and somewhat fixed. The patient reports moderate discomfort to uterine and cervical motion. There is some enlargement of the adnexa bilaterally.

Questions Case 30A

The most likely diagnosis is

  A. Acute pelvic inflammatory disease (PID)
  B. Endometriosis
  C. Primary dysmenorrhea
  D. Pelvic scarring due to pelvic infections

Answer: D

By history, this patient is most likely to have inactive scarring from the PID. The patient does not have any symptoms of an acute infection, decreasing the possibility of acute PID. The history and physical examination provide enough suspicion of pelvic pathology to make secondary rather than primary dysmenorrhea more likely. Although endometriosis might explain the retroversion of the uterus and the patient's dyspareunia, endometriosis has not been documented.

What is the best recommendation for this patient?

  A. Abdominal hysterectomy
  B. In vitro fertilization
  C. Danazol treatment
  D. Diagnostic laparoscopy
  E. Observation

Answer: D

Although the patient's most likely diagnosis based on history and physical examination is pelvic adhesions, the diagnosis of that entity as well as endometriosis can be made only by direct observation. Only with a firm diagnosis can appropriate therapeutic options be presented to the patient for consideration. At diagnostic laparoscopy, endometriosis involving the uterosacral ligaments, adnexae, and surrounding tissues is discovered. Biopsy of one implant confirms the diagnosis.

The best treatment option for this patient is

  A. Extirpative surgery
  B. Observation
  C. Medical therapy
  D. Conservative surgery
  E. None of the above

Answer: C, D

With a desire for children, medical therapy is appropriate. Conservative surgery is also an option, with the particular procedure depending on the extent and location of disease found at surgery. Counseling concerning the timing of pregnancy is also an important part of the management of this couple.

(Continued)

Case 30B

A 38-year-old woman presents for a premarital examination. She has never been pregnant, and she uses a diaphragm for contraception. Over the past 3 to 4 years she has had increasing problems with dysmenorrhea. The cramps no longer respond to over-the-counter ibuprofen. Before her wedding she would also like you to check the fit of her diaphragm because "lately it has been causing some pelvic and rectal discomfort" when she uses it. On examination she has significant cervical motion tenderness and thickening of the uterosacral ligaments. Endometriosis is suspected.

Question Case 30B

The patient should be advised that

A. An immediate pregnancy is desirable
B. Switching to an oral contraceptive might be beneficial
C. No therapy should be undertaken until exploratory surgery is performed
D. Therapy with a GnRH agonist should be started before her wedding
E. No specific therapy is needed at this time

Answer: B

Although this patient may experience problems conceiving, the decision to have a child is always up to the patient and her partner, not the physician. Although the presumptive diagnosis of endometriosis may be correct, definitive diagnosis cannot be made unless endometriosis is visualized and, preferably, biopsy proved. Nevertheless, some suggestions based on this presumption are appropriate. Because the patient is symptomatic, suppression using oral contraceptives might be beneficial, although not without risk at this patient's age and, in fact, would be contraindicated

if she were a smoker. Aggressive therapy with GnRH agonist or danazol is optimally deferred until the diagnosis is established by laparoscopy.

Case 30C

A 15-year-old nulligravida has experienced increasingly severe pelvic pain for 8 months. She is sexually active, using barrier methods of contraception, but reports that intercourse is no more or less uncomfortable now than when she became sexually active at age 13. She has been treated once for asymptomatic Chlamydia infection as was her partner. On physical examination there is mild cervical motion and uterine tenderness. There are no ovarian masses and rectovaginal examination is not rewarding.

Question Case 30C

Initial management should consist of

A. Reassurance
B. Suppressive antibiotic therapy for PID
C. Oral contraceptive therapy for presumed endometriosis
D. Diagnostic laparoscopy

Answer: D

Increasingly severe pelvic pain in a teen requires more than reassurance. In this case there is insufficient evidence to support suppressive antibiotic therapy, although significant disease may result from seemingly insignificant infection. Oral contraceptive therapy for a short interval is reasonable, but continued therapy is imprudent if there is less than marked amelioration of the symptoms. Given the incidence of endometriosis in teens with pelvic pain of this nature, diagnostic laparoscopy for definitive diagnosis should be strongly considered.

31

DYSMENORRHEA AND CHRONIC PELVIC PAIN

This chapter deals primarily with APGO Objective(s):

OBJECTIVE 43   Chronic Pelvic Pain

Define chronic pelvic pain and discuss the incidence, causes, pathophysiology, diagnostic procedures, and management of the heterogenous group of disorders which cause chronic pelvic pain.

OBJECTIVE 50   Dysmenorrhea

A. Define primary and secondary dysmenorrhea, and describe the causes of each.

B. Discuss the evaluation and management of the causes of primary and secondary dysmenorrhea.

Millions of hours each year are lost from school, work, and productive daily life, because of symptoms of dysmenorrhea and chronic pelvic pain. With single-parent families and two-income households common today, the ability to diagnose and treat dysmenorrhea and chronic pelvic pain may be critical to a woman's and a family's economic status as well as to the patient's well-being.

Painful menstruation (*dysmenorrhea*) may be caused by clinically identifiable causes (*secondary dysmenorrhea*) or by an excess of prostaglandins, leading to painful uterine muscle activity (*primary dysmenorrhea*). The term *chronic pelvic pain* is generally applied to pelvic discomfort (not solely associated with menstruation) of more than 6 months' duration.

For most patients, diagnosis can be accomplished by a careful evaluation through history and physical examination. In some instances, evaluation using other modalities, including laparoscopy, may be needed. Once the diagnosis is established, specific and usually successful therapy may be instituted.

DYSMENORRHEA

Primary and secondary dysmenorrhea represent a source of recurrent disability for approximately 10% to 15% of women in their early reproductive years. It is uncommon for primary dysmenorrhea to occur during the first three to six menstrual cycles, when rhythmic ovulation is not yet well established. *The incidence of primary dysmenorrhea is greatest in women in their late teens to early twenties and declines with age. Secondary dysmenorrhea becomes more common as a woman ages,* because it accompanies the rising prevalence of causal factors. Childbearing does not affect the occurrence of either primary or secondary dysmenorrhea.

Secondary Dysmenorrhea

The *causes of secondary dysmenorrhea* may be conveniently categorized into those processes that are outside the uterus, those

TABLE 31.1. Secondary Dysmenorrhea

Extrauterine causes
  Endometriosis
  Tumors (benign, malignant)
  Inflammation
  Adhesions
  Psychogenic (rare)
  Nongynecologic causes
Intramural causes
  Adenomyosis
  Leiomyomata
Intrauterine causes
  Leiomyomata
  Polyps
  Intrauterine contraceptive devices
  Infection
  Cervical stenosis and cervical lesions

that are within the wall of the uterus, and those that are internal or within the uterine cavity (Table 31.1). The mechanism by which these processes bring about menstrual pain is generally apparent when one considers that pain anywhere in the body occurs when there is inflammation, ischemia, stretch or distention, hemorrhage, or perforation. Pain results when these processes alter pressure in or around the pelvic structures, change or restrict blood flow, or cause irritation of the pelvic peritoneum. This may occur in combination with the normal physiology of menstruation, creating discomfort, or it may arise independently with symptoms becoming more noticeable during menstruation. *When symptoms continue between menstrual periods, these processes may be the source of chronic pelvic pain.*

Primary Dysmenorrhea

In patients with *primary dysmenorrhea*, no clinically identifiable cause of pain exists. Instead, there is *an excess of prostaglandin $F_2\alpha$ produced* in the endometrium. This potent smooth-muscle stimulant causes intense uterine contractions, resulting in

TABLE 31.2.   Pain and Associated Systemic Symptoms in Primary Dysmenorrhea

Symptom	Estimated Incidence (%)
Pain: spasmodic, colicky, labor-like; sometimes described as an aching or heaviness in lower middle abdomen; may radiate to the back and down the thighs; starts at onset of menstruation; lasts hours to days	100
Associated symptoms	
Nausea and emesis	90
Tiredness	85
Nervousness	70
Dizziness	60
Diarrhea	60
Headache	45

intrauterine pressures that can exceed 400 mm Hg and baseline intrauterine pressures in excess of 80 mm Hg. Prostaglandin $F_2\alpha$ also causes contractions in smooth muscle elsewhere in the body, resulting in the nausea, vomiting, and diarrhea reported by many women (Table 31.2). Prostaglandin production in the uterus normally increases under the influence of progesterone, reaching a peak at, or soon after, the start of menstruation. With the onset of menstruation, formed prostaglandins are released from the shedding endometrium. In addition, the necrosis of endometrial cells provides increased substrate arachidonic acid from cell walls for prostaglandin synthesis. In addition to prostaglandin $F_2\alpha$, prostaglandin E_2 is produced in the uterus. Prostaglandin E_2, a potent vasodilator and inhibitor of platelet aggregation, has been implicated as a cause of primary menorrhagia.

Clinical Evaluation

Patients with *primary dysmenorrhea* present with recurrent, month-after-month, spasmodic lower abdominal pain, which occurs on the first 1 to 3 days of menstruation. The pain is often diffusely located in the lower abdomen and suprapubic area, with radiation around or through to the back. The pain is described as "coming and going," or labor-like. The patient often illustrates her description with a fist opening and closing. This pain is frequently accompanied by moderate to severe nausea, vomiting, and/or diarrhea. Fatigue, low backache, and headache are also common. Patients often assume a fetal position in an effort to gain relief and many report having used a heating pad or hot water bottle in an effort to decrease their discomfort. Dyspareunia is generally not found in patients with primary dysmenorrhea and, if present, should suggest a secondary cause.

In patients with *secondary dysmenorrhea*, symptoms may be slightly milder and are often more general in nature. The specific complaint that an individual patient has is determined by the underlying abnormality. Frequently, a careful history suggests the possibility of an ongoing problem and helps direct further evaluations. Complaints of heavy menstrual flow, combined with pain, suggest uterine changes such as adenomyosis, myomas, or polyps.

Adenomyosis is islands of endometrial tissue within the myometrium, resulting in a usually tender, symmetrically enlarged, "boggy" uterus. Menses are especially uncomfortable. The diagnosis is supported by exclusion of other causes of secondary dysmenorrhea; but definitive diagnosis can be made only by histologic examination of a hysterectomy specimen. Pelvic heaviness or a change in abdominal contour should raise the possibility of large *leiomyomata or intra-abdominal neoplasia*. Fever, chills, and malaise should suggest the presence of an *inflammatory process*. A coexisting complaint of infertility may suggest *endometriosis or chronic pelvic inflammatory disease*.

Assessment

For patients with dysmenorrhea, the physical examination is directed toward uncovering possible causes of secondary dysmenorrhea. The presence of asymmetry or irregular enlargement of the uterus should suggest myomas or other tumors. Symmetrical enlargement of the uterus is often found in patients with adenomyosis. Painful nodules in the posterior cul-de-sac and restricted motion of the uterus should suggest endometriosis. Restricted motion of the uterus is also found in cases of pelvic scarring from adhesions or inflammation. Thickening and tenderness of the adnexal structures caused by inflammation may suggest this diagnosis as the cause of secondary dysmenorrhea. Cultures of the cervix for *Neisseria gonorrhoeae* or *Chlamydia trachomatis* should be obtained if infection is suspected.

In evaluating the patient thought to have primary dysmenorrhea, the most important differential diagnosis is that of secondary dysmenorrhea. Although the patient's history is often characteristic, a diagnosis of primary dysmenorrhea should not be made without a thorough evaluation to eliminate other possible causes. *Physical examination of patients with primary dysmenorrhea should be normal.* There should be no palpable abnormalities of the uterus or adnexa, and no abnormalities should be found on speculum or abdominal examinations. Patients examined while experiencing symptoms often appear pale and "shocky," but the abdomen is soft and nontender, with a normal uterus.

In patients with chronic pain, the clinician must always consider nongynecologic causes as a possibility. In some patients, a final diagnosis may not be established without invasive procedures, such as laparoscopy.

Therapy

In patients with dysmenorrhea in whom no other clinically identifiable cause is apparent, it is appropriate to presume a diagnosis of primary dysmenorrhea. Therapy with nonsteroidal anti-inflammatory agents is generally so successful that, if some response is not evident, the diagnosis of primary dysmenorrhea should be reevaluated. Other useful components of therapy for primary dysmenorrhea include the application of heat; exercise, psychotherapy, and reassurance; and on occasion, endocrine therapy (i.e., oral contraceptives to induce anovulation).

Patients with primary dysmenorrhea generally experience exceptional pain relief through the use of nonsteroidal anti-inflammatory drugs (NSAIDs), which are prostaglandin-synthetase inhibitors. Treatments include 500 mg of mefenamic acid (Ponstel) followed by 250 mg every 4 to 6 hours, 1200 to 1600 mg of ibuprofen (Motrin) followed by 600 to 800 mg three times a day, or 150 mg of diclofenac (Voltaren) followed by 75 mg three times a day (Table 31.3 and Table 31.4). Over-the-counter dosages of ibuprofen or other NSAIDs may be used in many patients with milder symptoms.

In the very rare patient who does not respond to medical and other therapy and whose pain is so severe as to be incapacitating, *presacral neurectomy* may be a consideration. The procedure involves surgical disruption of the "presacral nerves," the superior hypogastric plexus, which is found in the retroperitoneal tissue from the fourth lumbar vertebra to the hollow over the sacrum. It is associated with considerable morbidity if the adjacent venous structures are disrupted.

As in other areas of medicine, the best therapy is one directed toward the cause of the patient's problems. Hence, for secondary dysmenorrhea when a specific diagnosis is possible, therapy tailored to that process is the most likely to succeed. Spe-

TABLE 31.3. Nonsteroidal Anti-inflammatory Drugs for Dysmenorrhea

Drug	Initial Dose	Subsequent Dose
Diclofenac (potassium)	50–100 mg	50 mg t.i.d.
Diclofenac (sodium)	75–150 mg	75 mg t.i.d.
Diflunisal	1000 mg	500 mg q 12 h
Etodolac	400 mg	400 mg q 4–6 h
Fenoprofen calcium	200 mg	200 mg q 4–6 h
Flurbiprofen	50 mg	50 mg t.i.d.
Ibuprofen*	1200–1600 mg	600–800 mg q 4 h
Indomethacin	25 mg	25 mg t.i.d.
Ketoprofen	75 mg	75 mg t.i.d.
Ketorolac	10 mg	10 mg q 4–6 h
Meclofenamate*	100 mg	50–100 mg q 4–6 h
Mefenamic acid*	500 mg	250 mg q 4–6 h
Naproxen*	500 mg	250 mg q 4–6 h
Naproxen sodium*	550 mg	275 mg q 6–8 h
Sulindac	200 mg	200 mg b.i.d.
Suprofen	200 mg	200 mg q 4 h
Tolmetin	400 mg	40 mg t.i.d.

*FDA approved for primary dysmenorrhea.
(From Smith RP: *Gynecology in Primary Care.* Baltimore, Williams & Wilkins, 1996, p. 398.)

cific treatments for many of these processes are discussed in their respective chapters. When definitive therapy cannot be employed (e.g., in the case of a patient with adenomyosis in whom fertility is to be preserved, thereby making hysterectomy inappropriate), symptomatic therapy in the form of analgesics and/or modification of the menstrual cycle may be effective. The dysmenorrhea may be improved with the use of low-dose oral contraceptives in those patients who desire contraception and have no contraindications to their use.

CHRONIC PELVIC PAIN

The *prevalence* of chronic pelvic pain is less than that of dysmenorrhea but still represents a source of significant disability. It often demands a great deal of time and resources, from both physician and patient, to make a diagnosis and establish treatment. In these patients, the pathophysiology involved can be quite variable (Table 31.5). In many patients, the pain itself becomes the disease. Indeed, in approximately one third of patients with chronic pelvic pain who undergo laparoscopic evaluation, no identifiable cause is found. However, two thirds of these patients have potential causes identified where none was apparent before laparoscopy. A wide-ranging, often multidisciplinary approach to these patients yields the best results.

The *history* reported in chronic pelvic pain can be varied. In general, it relates to the underlying etiology. As with the evaluation of any pain, attention must be paid to the description and timing of the symptoms involved. The presence of gastrointestinal symptoms, urinary difficulties, or back problems should suggest the possibility of nongynecologic causes. The history must include a thorough medical, surgical, menstrual, and sexual history. Inquiries should be made into the patient's home and work status, social history, and family history (past and present). The patient should be questioned about sleep disturbances and other signs of depression.

TABLE 31.4. Families of Nonsteroidal Anti-inflammatory Drugs

Drug	Trade Name
Carboxylates:	
Salicylic acids	
Aspirin	Various
Diflunisal	Dolobid
Salicylate	Disalcid, Mono-Gesic, Salflex, Salsalate, Salsitabe
Indoleacetic acids	
Diclofenac potassium	Cataflam
Diclofenac sodium	Voltaren
Etodolac	Lodine
Indomethacin	Indocin
Ketorolac tromethamine	Acular, Toradol
Sulindac	Clinoril, Sulindac
Tolmetin	Tolectin, Tolmetin
Propionic acids	
Fenoprofen calcium	Nalfon, Fenoprofen
Flurbiprofen	Ansaid
Ibuprofen*	Motrin, IBU, Rufen
Ketoprofen	Orudis, Oruvail, Ketoprofen
Naproxen*	Naprosyn
Naproxen sodium*	Aflaxen, Anaprox
Fenimates	
Meclofenamate*	Mecolmen
Mefenamic acid*	Ponstel
Enolic acids:	
Pyrazolones	
Oxyphenbutazone	
Phenylbutazone	Azolid, Butazolidin
Oxicams	
Piroxicam	Feldene, Piroxicam

*FDA approved for primary dysmenorrhea.
(From Smith RP: *Gynecology in Primary Care.* Baltimore, Williams & Wilkins, 1996, p. 398.)

Assessment

As in patients with dysmenorrhea, the *physical examination* of patients with chronic pain is directed toward uncovering possible causative pathologies. The patient should be asked to indicate the location of the pain. This acts as a guide to further evaluation and provides some indication of the character of the pain by the way in which the patient points. For example, if the location of the pain is indicated with a single finger, you are probably dealing with a different process than when the patient uses a sweeping motion of the whole hand. Maneuvers that duplicate the patient's complaint should be noted, but undue discomfort should be avoided to minimize guarding, which would limit a thorough examination. Many of the same conditions that cause secondary dysmenorrhea may cause chronic pain states. As in the evaluation of patients with dysmenorrhea, cervical cultures should be obtained if infection is suspected.

For most patients, a reasonably accurate differential diagnosis can be established through the history and physical examination. *The wide range of differential diag-*

TABLE 31.5. Causes of Chronic Pelvic Pain

Gynecologic causes
  Adnexal
    Adhesive disease (adhesives from
      any cause)
    Chronic infection
    Chronic ectopic pregnancy
    Torsion of pelvic mass or organ
      (generally a cause of acute pain)
    Ovarian cyst (generally not painful
      without bleeding or growth)
  Uterine
    Fibroid tumors (uncommon cause
      of pain)
    Infection
    Retrodisplacement (rare)

Urologic causes
  Infection
  Calculi
  Tumors

Gastrointestinal causes
  Inflammatory
    Chronic appendicitis
    Gastroenteritis
    Ulcerative colitis
    Ulcer disease
    Irritable bowel syndrome
    Diverticulitis
    Mesenteric adenitis
    Biliary disease
  Mechanical
    Constipation
    Herniation

Gastrointestinal causes *(continued)*
  Mechanical *(continued)*
    Obstruction
    Torsion
    Intussusception
  Other
    Neoplasa
    Parasites

Other causes
  Aneurysm
  Musculoskeletal
    Chronic back pain
    Radiculopathy
    Spondylolisthesis
    Ankylosing spondylitis
    Strains
    Rectus hematoma
  Biochemical
    Sickle-cell crisis/disease
    Acute intermittent porphyria
    Heavy-metal poisoning
    Black widow spider bites
  Neurologic
    Tabes
    Herpes zoster (shingles)
  Psychosocial
    Somatization
    Sleep disorders
    Substance abuse
    Physical or sexual abuse
    Family or economic stress

noses possible in chronic pelvic pain lends *itself to a multidisciplinary approach,* which might include psychiatric evaluation and/or testing. Consultation with social workers, physical therapists, gastroenterologists, anesthesiologists, orthopaedists, and others should be considered. The use of imaging technologies or laparoscopy may also be required to determine a diagnosis.

The evaluation should begin with the presumption that there is an organic cause for the pain. Even in patients with obvious psychosocial stress, organic pathology can and does occur. Only when other reason-able causes have been ruled out should psychiatric diagnoses such as somatization, depression, or sleep and personality disorders be entertained.

IRRITABLE BOWEL SYNDROME

Irritable bowel syndrome (IBS) is three times more common in women than in men and symptoms of the syndrome are found in about 15% of adults. Because it is so common and more common in women, the evaluation and management of pelvic pain includes diagnosing this syndrome and treating it, or ruling it out prior to gynecologic therapy such as surgery.

The diagnosis of IBS is defined by the Rome Criteria: the presence of abdomino-pelvic pain which cannot be explained by known disease for 12 weeks (not necessarily consecutive) in the preceding 12 months, having at least two of three features. These features are pain (1) relieved with defecation, (2) associated with a change in the frequency of bowel movements (diarrhea or constipation), or (3) onset associated with a change in the form of stool (loose, watery, with mucus, or pellet-like). IBS is often usefully subcategorized for purposes of treatment depending on the predominant complaint: pain, diarrhea, constipation, or alternating constipation and diarrhea. The pathophysiology of the syndrome is not clearly identified, but factors proposed to be involved include altered bowel motility, visceral hypersensitivity, psychosocial factors (especially stress), an imbalance of neurotransmitters (especially serotonin), and infection (often indolent or subclinical.) A history of childhood sexual or physical abuse is highly correlated with the severity of symptoms experienced by those with IBS.

The diagnosis is made by history and flexible sigmoidoscopy in women less than about 50 years old, or history and colonoscopy or flexible sigmoidoscopy plus barium enema in women over about 50 years of age. When the predominant symptom is diarrhea, a biopsy of the mucosae of the descending colon should be considered to rule out microscopic colitis.

Use of a food diary to identify and eliminate foods which are associated with symptoms combined with the nurturing physician-patient relationship, to avoid "doctor shopping" and episodic care, are the mainstays of treatment. The limiting of caffeine, alcohol, fatty foods, and gas producing vegetables is often helpful. If constipation is a major symptom, the addition of 20–30 g of fiber or the use of osmotic laxatives such as lactulose (10 mg/15 ml of syrup, 15–30 ml per day) is often useful. When diarrhea is a major symptom, antidiarrheals such as Loperamide (4 mg/day initially, then 4–8 mg/day in single or divided doses) has been useful.

Therapy

Patients with chronic pelvic pain offer a therapeutic challenge. In these patients, care must be taken that the therapy offered does not potentiate the underlying problem. Analgesics may be used, but sparingly, and every effort must be made to reduce the risk of both emotional and physical dependence. When used, analgesics should be given on a fixed time schedule that is independent of symptoms. Frequent follow-up is required and should be scheduled separate of fluctuations in pain. Suppression of ovulation may be useful as either a therapeutic modality or as a diagnostic tool to assist in ruling out ovarian or cyclic processes. Surgical therapies are appropriate only when specific surgically treatable pathologies are present and thought to be the specific cause of the patient's complaints. Alternate treatment modalities such as transcutaneous electrical nerve stimulation (TENS), biofeedback, nerve blocks, laser ablation of the uterosacral ligaments, and presacral neurectomy may be used in selected patients. *In some cases, the goal in treatment may not be a cure (i.e., elimination of chronic pain), but rather successful management of the symptoms to allow maximal function and quality of life.*

FOLLOW-UP

Patients begun on therapy for pelvic pain (dysmenorrhea or chronic pain states) should be carefully monitored for success and the possibility of complications from the therapy itself. Patients on oral contraceptives for the first time should be asked to return for follow-up after 2 months and again after 6 months. Once successful therapy is established, routine periodic health maintenance visits should continue. *Patients with chronic pain should be encouraged to return for follow-up on a periodic basis, rather than only when pain is present, thus avoiding reinforcing pain behavior as a means to an end.*

Case 31A

An 18-year-old, virginal college student presents with the complaint of recurrent, severe menstrual distress, which begins a few hours after the onset of menstrual flow and lasts for the first 48 hours of menstruation. The pain is crampy, recurrent, and located in the lower abdomen, just above the symphysis. She occasionally experiences nausea with vomiting, but her pain is unchanged after she vomits. She has taken an over-the-counter pain reliever containing ibuprofen with only slight improvement. Her periods are regular, and she is taking no other medications. Pelvic examination is difficult, but normal.

Questions Case 31A

The most likely diagnosis in this patient is

A. Leiomyomata
B. Primary dysmenorrhea
C. Endometriosis
D. Irritable bowel syndrome
E. Recurrent pelvic inflammatory disease

Answer: B

In a young virginal woman, the chance of leiomyomata, pelvic infection, or endometriosis is small. The patient's history offers no hint of symptoms that might be associated with irritable bowel disease, and her physical examination does not offer evidence of other processes as a cause of secondary dysmenorrhea. This information, combined with her typical history of crampy pain, makes primary dysmenorrhea the most likely diagnosis.

The best therapy for this patient would be

A. Oral contraceptives
B. High-bulk diet

C. Tylenol (acetaminophen) with codeine, 60 mg q 4 h
D. Ampicillin, 250 mg q.i.d. for 10 days
E. Ponstel, 250 mg, two at onset of pain and one q 4–6 h p.r.n.

Answer: E

Although the patient might get some relief from the use of oral contraceptives, unless she needs contraception, this may not be the best course of therapy. Treatment with high-bulk diet or ampicillin does not appear to be supported by the patient's probable diagnosis. Even though the patient has tried NSAID therapy in the form of over-the-counter products, this is still the best option. The lack of complete response is most likely because of the low dose in over-the-counter products and not necessarily to product selection. It is probable that, in higher prescription dosages, she will obtain relief. If higher-dose NSAID therapy is unsuccessful, oral contraceptives should be considered, even though this patient is not sexually active.

Case 31B

A 23-year-old, divorced mother of three, on government assistance, seeks help for symptoms of lower abdominal pain, which began 8 months ago. This coincided with her divorce and the loss of her job at a textile mill. Her pain is located in her left lower quadrant, but spreads to the right lower quadrant and to her back. The pain is worse with menstruation, bowel movements, and intercourse. She has tried multiple medications without benefit. Past history reveals an abusive marriage and two previous laparotomies for "ovarian cysts."

(Continued)

Questions Case 31B

Based on the most likely working diagnosis, the first examination or procedure that should be performed is

A. Laparoscopy
B. Sigmoidoscopy
C. Pelvic ultrasound
D. Bimanual pelvic examination
E. Psychological profile and depression index

Answer: D

Although it is very likely that this patient has some degree of depression and multiple psychosocial stresses, a physical cause must always be considered. Sigmoidoscopy and pelvic ultrasound are not indicated based on the symptoms presented. Laparoscopy is invasive and potentially carries more risk because of the patient's previous surgeries. Although it may be needed at some point in the future, it would be premature at this point. A pelvic examination offers the most information with the least risk as an initial step in evaluation of this patient with chronic pelvic pain.

On physical examination no overt gynecologic etiology for the patient's discomfort is noted, although there is some decreased mobility of the uterus and fullness in the adnexa, which are tender to palpation. Her rectovaginal examination is negative as is her guaiac test. Her pain persists over several visits in the next 6 months, interfering with her work and life. Narcotic analgesics are only moderately successful in alleviating her discomfort, and she does not like the way she feels when using them. A routine laboratory evaluation including complete blood count (CBC), erythrocyte sedimentation rate (ESR), Pap smear, and cultures are all negative. The patient's financial and social situations have improved, but the pain is interfering with further improvement. The next most appropriate step would be

A. Laparoscopy
B. Sigmoidoscopy
C. Pelvic ultrasound
D. Bimanual pelvic examination
E. Psychological profile and depression index

Answer: A

Pelvic ultrasound adds little information, and there are no indicators that there is a significant psychological component. Without more specific bowel symptoms, sigmoidoscopy is not warranted. Diagnostic laparoscopy is appropriate, after which further therapy may be warranted, depending on the findings.

CHAPTER

32

DISORDERS OF THE BREAST

CHAPTER OBJECTIVES

This chapter deals primarily with APGO Objective(s):

OBJECTIVE 44   Disorders of the Breast

A. Describe the indications for and timing of breast self-examination, physical examination of the breast, and mammography. Describe how to teach breast self-examination.

B. Describe the diagnostic approach to a woman with a breast mass, nipple discharge, or breast pain.

C. Explain the history/physical findings associated with intraductal papilloma, fibrocystic changes of the breast, fibroadenoma, breast carcinoma, and mastitis.

Our society places special significance on the female breast, especially in matters of femininity and sexuality. In addition, there are appropriate fears of breast cancer, which are confounded by normal monthly changes that may be both uncomfortable and disconcerting. These issues make management of breast disease uniquely challenging for women and their physicians and health providers.

The adult female breast is actually a large, modified sebaceous gland, located within the superficial fascia of the chest wall (Figure 32.1). It usually weighs between 200 and 300 g and is made up primarily of fatty tissue, fibrous septa, and glandular structures. Breast tissue is organized into 12 to 20 triangular lobes with a central duct, collecting ducts, and secretory cells arranged in alveoli. Each of these lobes drains at the nipple. The breast has a rich blood supply and lymphatic system, which facilitate metastases of malignancies (Figure 32.2). Breast tissue may be located anywhere along "milk lines" that run from the axilla to the groin. Extra nipples (*polythelia*) are more common than true accessory breasts (*polymastia*).

Breast tissue is very sensitive to hormonal changes. The development of adult breast shape during puberty is a result of hormonal changes. The sensitivity to hormones is also responsible for cyclic changes that occur during the menstrual cycle and

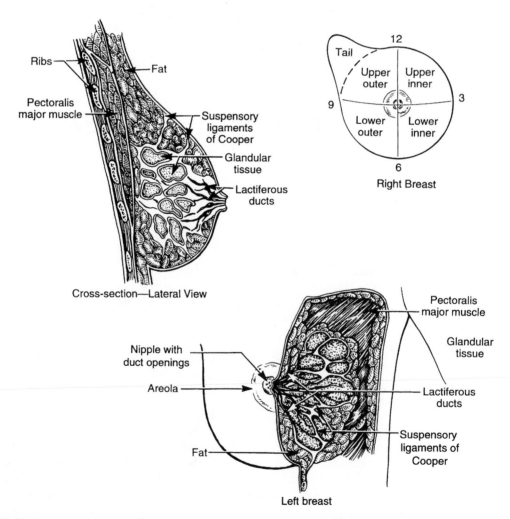

FIGURE 32.1. The structure of the mature female breast.

for the symptoms often reported by patients during therapeutic hormonal manipulations.

Each of the tissues of the breast may be the source of pathologic change. Fibrocystic changes and fibroadenomas may arise in the connective tissues of the breast. Fatty tissues may undergo necrosis in response to trauma or may harbor lipomas. The duct system of the breast may become dilated (duct ectasia or galactocele), contain papillary neoplasms, or undergo malignant change. Although more common in nursing mothers, infection of the breast (mastitis) may also occur.

Breast cancer is the most common malignancy of women, accounting for roughly one third of all women's malignancies. It is the leading cause of death from cancer for women between the ages of 35 and 54 years. With approximately 175,000 new cases and 44,500 breast cancer deaths per year in the United States, breast cancer is the most common cause of death in women in their fifth decade. *Currently a woman living in the United States has a 12.5%, or 1 in 8, lifetime risk of developing breast cancer.*

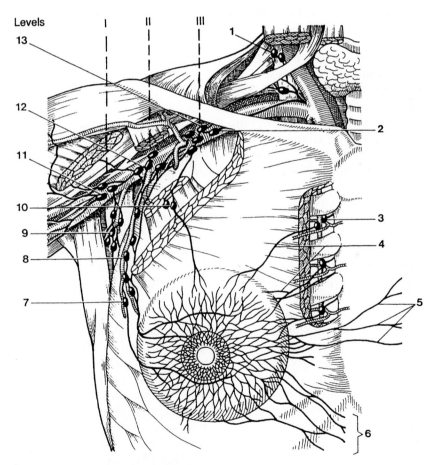

FIGURE 32.2. Lymphatic drainage of the breast. *I,* Low axillary nodes; *II,* central axillary nodes; *III,* subclavian nodes; *1,* deep cervical nodes; *2,* infraclavicular nodes; *3,* sternal nodes; *4,* pathway to the mediastinal nodes; *5,* pathway to the contralateral breast; *6,* pathway to the subdiaphragmatic nodes and liver; *7,* anterior pectoral lymph nodes; *8,* central axillary nodes; *9,* subpectoral axillary nodes; *10,* interpectoral nodes (Rotter's); *11,* brachial vein nodes; *12,* axillary vein nodes; *13,* subclavian vein nodes.

BENIGN BREAST DISEASE

Fibrocystic Change

The term *fibrocystic change* encompasses more than 35 different processes, including the misnomer "fibrocystic disease." Fibrocystic changes are the *most common of all benign breast conditions*. They may be present in one third to one half of premenopausal women and are a source of symptoms for roughly half of these women. The alterations associated with fibrocystic change may arise from an exaggerated response to hormones. Consequently, fibrocystic changes are most common during the reproductive years or occasionally during hormone replacement after menopause. Disturbed ratios of estrogen and progesterone and an increased rate of prolactin secretion have both been suggested as causes for these changes. Neither of these theories has been conclusively proven, nor is there any evidence that fibrocystic changes are caused by oral contraceptives.

Histologically, fibrocystic changes occur in three stages. Initially, there is a *proliferation of stroma,* especially in the upper outer quadrants of the breast, that leads to the induration and tenderness experienced by the patient. In the second stage, *adenosis* occurs, leading to cyst formation. During this phase, cysts range from microscopic to 1 cm in diameter. Marked proliferation of the ducts and alveolar cells occurs in this stage. In the late stages of fibrocystic change, *larger cysts* are present and *less pain* occurs (unless there is rapid change in a cyst). Proliferative changes may be marked in any of the involved tissues. When atypia are found in hyperplastic ducts or apocrine cells, there is a ten-fold increase in the risk of future carcinoma.

Fibrocystic changes most commonly present as cyclic, bilateral pain (mastalgia) and engorgement. The pain associated with fibrocystic changes is diffuse, often with radiation to the shoulders or upper arms. Occasionally, well-localized pain occurs when a cyst expands rapidly. On examination, diffuse bilateral nodularity is typical, with larger cysts taking on the character of a balloon filled with fluid. These changes are most prominent just before menstruation.

The management of fibrocystic changes may include fine-needle aspiration of cysts, which is diagnostic and often therapeutic. Open biopsy is indicated if there are mammographic findings suggesting neoplasia, or if on fine-needle aspiration (*a*) the fluid obtained is bloody, (*b*) there is a residual mass after aspiration is performed, or (*c*) the cyst recurs. Dietary restriction of caffeine and foods containing methylxanthines benefits some patients, whereas others respond to a low-salt diet, vitamin E, and/or a mild diuretic such as hydrochlorothiazide (25 to 50 mg per day for 7 to 10 days before menses). Danazol is effective in severe cases, but symptoms often resume after discontinuation of the medication. In the most severe cases, bilateral mastectomy may be required to relieve intractable, incapacitating pain.

Fibroadenoma

Fibroadenomas are the second most common form of benign breast disease, occurring in as many as 10%–20% of all women. They occur most often in young women. These firm, painless, freely movable breast masses average 1 to 3 cm in diameter and consist of a mixture of proliferating epithelial and supporting fibrous tissues. Although usually solitary, multiple fibroadenomas develop in 15% to 20% of patients. These tumors do not change during the menstrual cycle and are usually slow growing. They are often found during physical examination or during breast self-examination. The management of these usually benign lesions, like most similar lesions, is evaluation by examination and imaging techniques and then biopsy or excision, because malignancy must be ruled out by histologic evaluation. Using ultrasound and fine-needle biopsy, fibroadenomas can be distinguished from cysts. Monolayers of benign ductal cells with dense stroma on aspiration biopsy allow management by frequent clinical and mammographic evaluation, without excision. Surgical excision is indicated if the mass causes pain or grows rapidly, the fine-needle aspirate is inconclusive or suspicious for malignancy, or if the patient needs more reassurance than biopsy can provide.

Lipomas and Fat Necrosis

The fatty tissue of the breast may be the source of benign tumors that are difficult to distinguish from malignancy. Both lipomas and fat necrosis may present as ill-defined tumors of the breast. Lipomas are usually nontender, but their diffuse character may raise suspicions of malignancy. Secondary signs suggestive of cancer (e.g., skin and nipple changes) usually are absent. Biopsy or excision is often required.

Fat necrosis is uncommon and most often the result of trauma, although the causative event frequently cannot be identified. The patient usually presents with a solitary, tender, ill-defined mass. Skin retraction is present in some patients. Direct evidence of trauma is most often lacking. Even with a history of trauma, the similarity of findings between fat necrosis and cancer (on physical examination and mammography) usually requires further evaluation and biopsy or excision to establish the diagnosis.

Intraductal Papilloma

Intraductal papillomas are polypoid epithelial tumors arising in the ducts of the breast. These fibrovascular tumors are covered by benign ductal epithelium. Although these tumors may range from 2 to 5 mm in diameter, they are typically not palpable. The patient presents with a *spontaneous bloody, serous, or cloudy nipple discharge.* Although these polyps are most often benign, the similarity of symptoms to carcinoma mandates excisional biopsy for most patients.

Mammary Duct Ectasia and Galactocele

Mammary duct ectasia may arise from chronic intraductal and periductal inflammation, which causes *dilation of the ducts and inspissation of breast secretions.* Most common in the fifth decade of life, this condition presents with a thick gray to black nipple discharge, pain, and nipple tenderness. Palpation around the nipple elicits discharge and may reveal thickening that may be difficult to distinguish from cancer. Nipple retraction is common. Biopsy confirms the diagnosis, and once established, no further therapy is needed unless warranted by the patient's symptoms.

Ductal obstruction and inflammation during or soon after lactation may lead to the development of a *galactocele.* Galactoceles are cystic dilations of a duct or ducts. These ducts contain inspissated, milky secretions that may become infected and lead to acute mastitis or abscess formation. When uncomplicated by infection, needle aspiration and decompression of the ducts is curative and excision is rarely required.

BREAST CANCER

Demographics

After her gender, increasing age is a woman's greatest risk factor for developing breast cancer. A woman living in the United States has an overall risk of 1 in 8, but this risk is distributed by age with increasing risk with increasing age (Table 32.1).

Factors other than age are associated with the risk of developing breast cancer. Table 32.2 presents some of the *relative risk factors.* A relative risk compares the risk of

TABLE 32.1. Probability of Developing Breast Cancer by Age for Women

Age	Probability, 1 in
20–29	2,187
30–39	258
40–49	67
50–59	38
60–69	29
70 or more	25

TABLE 32.2. Risk Factors for Developing Breast Cancer in Women

Relative Risk	Factor
0–1.0	Menarche > 17 years old
	Menopause before age 45
	Oophorectomy before age 35
	Term pregnancy before age 35
1.1–2.0	Menarche < 12 years old
	Menopause after age 55
	First full-term pregnancy after age 35
	No full-term pregnancies (for cancer diagnosed after age 40)
	Personal history of cancer of the endometrium, ovary, or colon
	Never breast fed a child
	Recent oral contraceptive use*
	Recent hormone replacement therapy*
2.1–4.0	One first-degree relative with breast cancer (pre- or postmenopausal, unilateral disease)
	Atypical hyperplasia on breast biopsy
	Personal history of cancer of major salivary glands
	Ovaries not surgically removed at less than 35 years of age
	Nodular densities occupy more than three-fourths of breast volume on mammogram
>4	Personal history of breast cancer
	Two or more first-degree relatives with breast cancer
	Age greater than 65
	Inherited genetic mutations for breast cancer
>8	Premenopausal first-degree relative with bilateral breast cancer

*See text for discussion.

disease among people with a specific exposure to those with the same exposure. So, a relative risk above 1.0 means a higher risk. Risk factors do not allow identification of all women who will develop breast cancer, but they are useful in planning detection strategies. Mutations or alterations in the breast cancer susceptibility genes (such as BRCA1 and BRCA2) are associated with perhaps 5%–10% of breast cancers although they appear in less than 1% of the general population. Women with these mutations may benefit from earlier annual mammography (starting between ages 25 and 35). Other interventions for these women (prophylactic tamoxifen therapy or surgery) are highly individualized issues and should be considered only after careful evaluation and counseling with clinicians expert in the interpretation of these genetic data and the risks and benefits of such interventions. Oral contraceptive use and hormone replacement therapy have been suggested to have slight associations with breast cancer, although the risk seems to be resolved after cessation of use for more than 5–10 years. In addition, this small risk must be balanced against the substantial risks of unintended conception and menopausal associated conditions such as osteoporosis as women consider the appropriate use of these regimens.

Types of Breast Cancer

Although 80% of breast cancers are of the nonspecific, infiltrating, intraductal type, many different cancer types can occur

TABLE 32.3. Simplified Classification of Breast Cancer

Mammary duct cancers
Infiltrating (80%)
Papillary carcinoma
Intraductal carcinoma
Colloid carcinoma
Medullary carcinoma
Noninfiltrating (5%)
Papillary carcinoma
Intraductal carcinoma
(comedocarcinoma)
Intracystic carcinoma
Mammary lobule cancers
In situ and infiltrating (12%)

Sarcomas
Cystosarcoma phylloides
Stromal sarcoma
Liposarcoma
Angiosarcoma
Lymphoma
Rare cancers
Sweat gland carcinoma
Tubular carcinoma
Adenoid cystic carcinoma
Metaplastic lesions
Inflammatory carcinoma (2%)
Paget's disease (1%)
Metastatic cancers

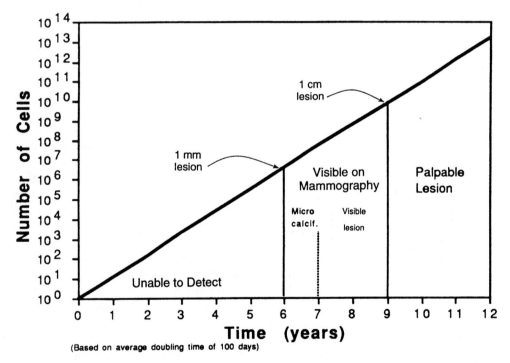

(Based on average doubling time of 100 days)

FIGURE 32.3. Mammographic and clinical detection of breast mass. With a presumed doubling time of 100 days, breast cancer may be detected by mammography significantly earlier than it can be identified clinically. *Micro calcif.* = microcalcification.

(Table 32.3). Breast cancer survival depends less on cell type than it does on the size of the tumor. Most breast tumors have a long latency from onset to clinically detectable size (Figure 32.3). For this reason, efforts to improve early detection are directed toward mammographic screening of those at high risk and increased public awareness through programs such as breast self-examination.

Symptoms

In the early stages of cancer growth, the tumor is usually painless and may feel mobile. As the tumor grows, the borders become less distinct and fixation to the supporting ligaments or underlying fascia occurs. Nipple discharge and skin changes (*peau d'orange,* or "orange peel skin") are late occurrences and are associated with a poor prognosis. Approximately 80% of breast cancers present as a mass.

History and Physical Examination

With as many as one fourth of all breast cancers found during routine examination, the role of the careful history and physical examination cannot be overemphasized. *A careful breast examination should be a part of every gynecologic examination* (see Chapter 1). All patients should be questioned on whether they practice breast self-examination. *Breast self-examination* should be done on a monthly basis. Because *90% of breast cancers are found by the patient,* this is an opportunity both to highlight an important screening test and to obtain information that may be of help clinically. A general family, medical, menstrual, and obstetric history should be obtained for all patients. Significant risk factors are also evaluated. Even though these risk factors identify only 25% of cancer patients, they are helpful in planning screening and surveillance.

When obtaining the *history* of a patient with breast problems, information about the presenting complaint such as pain, tenderness, mass, or discharge should be sought. The duration of symptoms and any changes in symptoms are also important. Any changes related to the menstrual cycle should especially be noted.

Physical examination of the breast should be performed by the physician annually and as a part of the evaluation of any breast complaint. The examination should begin with inspection of both breasts, looking for contour, symmetry, skin, or nipple changes. This should take place with the patient in both the upright and supine position, with the patient's arms above the head and also with her hands on her hips and contracting her pectoral muscles. Palpation of the breast tissue proceeds in a systematic way using the flat of the fingers, rolling the breast between the fingers and the underlying tissues. This may be carried out by quadrants or in a spiral fashion designed to ensure that the entire breast is examined. Palpation of the axilla and supraclavicular area must be included.

Evaluation

The *evaluation of any breast complaint* is based on the history and physical examination, augmented by five additional modalities: *imaging (mammography and ultrasonography), fine-needle aspiration, fine-needle biopsy (FNB), sterotatic core needle biopsy (CNB), and open biopsy.*

IMAGING

Mammography provides the best available mode of screening for early lesions and *has been credited with reducing the mortality rate from breast cancer by up to 30%. Breast cancer mortality could be reduced by as much as 50% if all women older than the age of 40 years were screened annually.* The guidelines for screening mammography have been and will probably continue to be controversial. The guidelines suggested by the American Cancer Society and American College of Obstetricians and Gynecologists in 1997 are based on an understanding that about one fifth of breast cancers are found in women in their fourth decade (Table 32.4).

Screening mammography (see Figure 33.3) involves compression of the breast tissue against an imaging plate in two projections—craniocaudad and mediolateral—and the use of a small amount of radiation to form the four images comprising the standard screening mammogram (see Figure 33.3). Compression of the breast tissue is necessary to encompass the tissue and provide clear visualization of the tissue. The axillary tail of Spence is sometimes not fully visualized, and this must be kept in mind in the interpretation of screening mammograms.

TABLE 32.4. Guidelines for Mammography Screening

Mammography every year from age 40 years
Mammography before age 40 years may be appropriate for selected high-risk patients.

Adapted from guidelines of the American Cancer Society and the American College of Obstetricians and Gynecologists, 1997.

TABLE 32.5. BI-RADS Classification of Screening Mammograms*

BI-RADS Classification	Summary Recommendation	Explanation
Category 0	Additional imaging evaluation	A finding is noted that warrants further imaging (spot compression films, magnification, special views, etc.)
Category 1	Negative	No abnormalities noted: breasts are symmetrical and no masses, architectural disturbances, or suspicious calcifications are present
Category 2	Benign finding	A negative mammogram, but the mammographer wishes to describe a finding such as a calcified fibroadenoma, multiple secretory calcifications, impants, and so forth, while still concluding that there is no mammographic evidence of malignancy
Category 3	Probably benign finding–short interval follow-up suggested	The finding has a high probability of being benign, but the mammographer would prefer to establish its mammographic stability over a short interval, usually 3 to 6 months; the interval is determined on a case basis
Category 4	Suspicious abnormality–biopsy is recommended	Lesions are noted that do not have the characteristic morphologies of breast cancer but have a definite probability of being malignant; biopsy is recommended
Category 5	Highly suggestive of malignancy–appropriate action should be taken	Lesions have morphologies characteristic of malignancy and the probability of malignancy is very high; appropriate action means referral to a gynecologic oncologist or breast surgeon

*BI-RADS: Breast Imaging Reporting and Data System, American College of Radiology, 1995.

Most reports of screening mammography include categorization according to the BI-RADS nomenclature (the Breast Imaging Reporting and Data System of the American College of Radiology; Table 32.5). This classification aids the clinician in determining the next appropriate step in management.

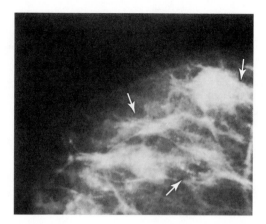

FIGURE 32.4. Multifocal duct carcinoma. Close-up shows multiple clusters of calcifications (*arrows*) and two masses. Only the larger mass was palpable.

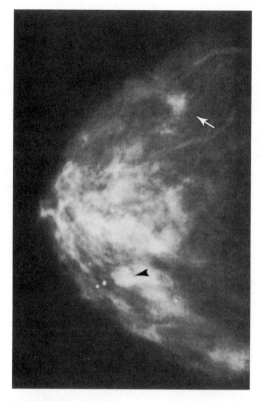

FIGURE 32.5. Cephalocaudal film-screen mammogram. Small scirrhous carcinoma (*arrow*) is contrasted with well-marginated fibroadenoma (*arrowhead*).

Mammography, with a radiation exposure of approximately 0.5 rad, provides the opportunity to identify small, nonpalpable lesions (1 to 2 mm), microcalcifications, and other changes suspect for malignancy (Figures 32.4 and 32.5). It is approximately 90% accurate in diagnosing malignancy in asymptomatic women, and therefore provides a clinically useful adjunct to clinical impressions and the definitive procedure of biopsy.

Ultrasonography has come to play an important part in the evaluation of breast lesions. It is commonly used to distinguish fluid-filled (cystic) from solid masses and help guide cyst aspiration and fine-needle biopsy. The combination of fine-needle aspiration and ultrasound guidance is especially useful in distinguishing fibroadenomas from cysts, and in the histologic evaluation of the former to exclude carcinoma.

BREAST CYST ASPIRATION

A simple and very valuable diagnostic tool is *needle aspiration* (Figure 32.6). If the patient has a breast mass that feels cystic, aspiration with a 22- to 25-gauge needle may be both diagnostic and therapeutic. In women older than 35 years of age, mammography before aspiration should be considered because of the increased incidence

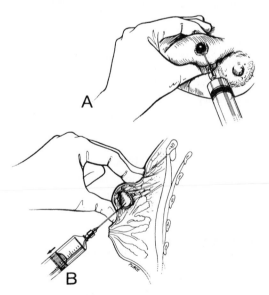

FIGURE 32.6. Needle aspiration of cystic breast mass. The needle is passed into the cyst, which is stabilized as shown. The cyst's contents are removed by gentle suction.

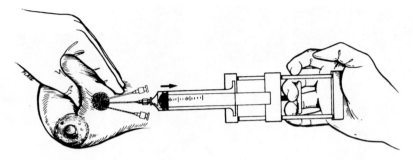

FIGURE 32.7.   Fine-needle aspiration of solid breast mass. The needle is passed into the solid mass and withdrawn at several different angles and in several different places while suction is maintained.

of malignancy. Preaspiration mammography also provides an accurate baseline appearance in the unlikely chance that bleeding into the cyst occurs as a result of the needle aspiration.

Fluid aspirated from patients with fibrocystic changes is customarily straw colored. Fluid that is dark brown or green occurs in cysts that have been present for a long time. Cytologic evaluation of the fluid obtained usually is of little value.

Fine-Needle Aspiration

Fine-needle aspiration of cells from a breast mass is gaining wide acceptance in the United States because of high sensitivity and specificity combined with avoiding the expense and morbidity of open biopsy. In this procedure, a 16- to 22-gauge needle is inserted into the mass, multiple passes are made with negative pressure applied by a syringe, and cells or tissue is obtained (Figure 32.7). The material collected is examined histologically or cytologically for signs of malignancy. This technique is 70% to 90% accurate, with a 20% false-negative rate. Therefore, if the aspiration is negative, open biopsy should still be performed. This technique depends heavily on the availability of expert cytopathology services.

Sterotatic Core Needle Biopsy

Recent advances in mammographic and computer technology have facilitated a variation in the fine-needle aspiration technique,

the *sterotatic core needle biopsy* (CNB). Information from multiple mammographic images is analyzed by a computer program that guides an automated biopsy "gun," allowing multiple cuts of core tissue from a suspicious area, often one that is not associated with physical findings.

Open Biopsy

The ultimate method of evaluation of any breast mass is open biopsy. This is often performed under local anesthesia through either radial or circumareolar incisions. For small lesions or those difficult to localize, preoperative identification and radiographically guided J-wire placement may be of value (so-called *needle-localized biopsy*). Postoperative radiography of the pathology specimen should confirm excision of the desired tissue (Figure 32.8).

Differential Diagnosis by Complaint or Finding

The most common presenting complaints are pain and the presence of a mass. Both of these complaints represent sources of great distress and perceived emergency to the patient. Therefore, they deserve prompt and considerate attention.

Diffuse, bilateral breast pain occurring before menstruation is most often caused by *fibrocystic changes. Dorsal radiculitis or inflammatory changes in the costochondral junction* (Tietze's syndrome) may also present in this way. Well-localized breast pain

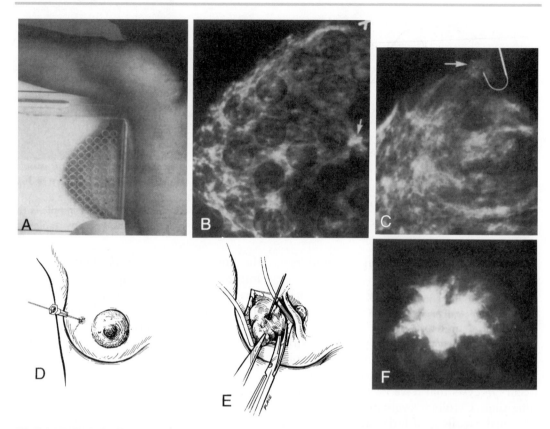

FIGURE 32.8. Prebiopsy mammographic needle localization of nonpalpable lesion. (A) A hole plate is applied to the breast surface closest to the lesion. (B) A mammogram identifies the hole over the nonpalpable stellate lesion suggestive of malignancy. (C, D) A guide wire is inserted under mammographic direction. (E) Excision of the specimen along the needle. (F) Demonstration by mammogram of the specimen that the stellate lesion has been removed for evaluation.

may result from rapid expansion of a *cyst, obstruction of a duct,* or inflammation (such as *mastitis*). Breast pain is a presenting complaint in less than 10% of patients with breast cancer.

Masses in the breast, with the attendant fear of cancer, represent one of the most emotionally charged and difficult differential diagnoses the clinician must make. Masses that are firm, round, and well demarcated are most likely to be *fibroadenomas.* Areas with a flattened, rubbery consistency are suspect for malignancy, although other conditions such as fat necrosis may cause similar changes. In either case, *further evaluation (such as tissue confirmation by open or needle biopsy) is mandatory.*

Although *bloody discharge* from the nipple is the hallmark of *intraductal papillomas,* any unilateral, spontaneous nipple discharge requires a thorough evaluation. The color or clarity of the fluid does not rule out carcinoma. Cytologic evaluation of the nipple discharge is associated with a false-negative rate of almost 20%, significantly reducing its value. Mammography and biopsy are required to establish the diagnosis.

Nipple discharge associated with burning, itching, or nipple discomfort in older patients is suggestive of *ductal ectasia.* In these patients, the discharge is thick or sticky and gray to black in color. As with other sources of nipple discharge, excisional biopsy is often required.

TABLE 32.6.	Clinical Staging of Breast Cancer	
Clinical Stage	**Description**	**Crude 5-Year Survival (%)**
Stage I	Tumor < 2 cm in diameter Nodes, if present, not felt to contain metastases Without distant metastases	85
Stage II	Tumors < 5 cm in diameter Nodes, if palpable, not fixed Without distant metastases	65
Stage III	Tumor > 5 cm or, Tumor of any size with invasion of skin or attached to chest wall Nodes in supraclavicular area Without distant metastases	40
Stage IV	With distant metastases	10

Adapted from Table 13.4. *Comprehensive Gynecology,* Herbst et al., eds. St. Louis, CV Mosby, 1992, p. 400.

GENERAL MANAGEMENT

Selection of Therapy

The treatment of patients with breast cancer is directed toward three goals: (*a*) control of local disease, (*b*) treatment of distant disease, and (*c*) improved quality of life. To this end, *most breast cancer is treated by surgical excision and adjunctive therapy. Breast cancer spreads by both vascular and lymphatic routes* with some direct infiltration. Recognition of this has led away from traditional radical surgical treatment, to therapy directed at both local and distant disease simultaneously. With local disease only, 5-year survival approaches 90%. This drops to 50% to 70% when there is regional involvement. Unfortunately, roughly 50% of patients have axillary lymph node involvement at the time of diagnosis.

Most women have an initial surgical therapy, most commonly nowadays lumpectomy (removal of the cancerous tissue plus a rim of normal tissue) or mastectomy (removal of the entire breast). Removal of the regional (axillary) lymph nodes is also often performed with these procedures to determine if disease has spread beyond the breast, allowing more informed choices for further therapy. The various radical surgical techniques, involving removal of underlying muscle and tissue, are rarely employed given the excellent outcomes obtained by less morbid and disfiguring managements. Most therapy is followed by an adjunctive therapy or a combination of such therapies, which have been shown to reduce the rates of recurrence and death over many years. Based on the stage of the disease (Table 32.6) and presence of hormone receptors, this may consist of radiation therapy (especially after lumpectomy), chemotherapy, hormonal manipulations (e.g., the anti-estrogen Tamoxifen), monoclonal antibody therapy, or a combination of all four. Like most conditions, the therapy of breast cancer must be individualized. Crude survival rates for each stage are noted in Table 32.6.

Follow-up of Therapy

Patients with diffuse tenderness and no dominant mass may be safely rechecked at a different time in the menstrual cycle. Patients who have undergone aspiration of a cyst (with clear fluid and disappearance of the palpable mass) should be rechecked in

2 weeks. Any reoccurrence of the cyst should prompt biopsy or additional evaluation. Some authors advocate a follow-up mammogram after cyst aspiration to delve for other lesions, although this is best individualized based on the needs and history of each patient.

Patients treated for breast cancer require frequent follow-up. Not only are these patients at higher risk for develop- ment of a new cancer on the opposite side, but two thirds of these patients eventually have distant metastases. Any patient who has had breast cancer must be closely followed by physical examination and mammography (where appropriate). No biologic markers yet exist to allow for either detection or monitoring of those with breast cancer.

CASE STUDIES

Case 32A

A 24-year-old G0 on triphasic oral contraceptives comes to your office with a complaint of a "lump" in her right breast. She reluctantly admits that she did not find the mass and that she would not have known that it was there had it not been for her husband. She has not had any nipple discharge and does do breast self-examination "most months." She is very worried because her mother died of breast carcinoma.

On your examination you find no change in the contour of either breast. No skin changes or nipple discharge can be found. There is a 1-cm, firm, smooth, round, mobile, nontender mass located in the upper outer quadrant of the right breast, approximately 5 cm from the areola.

Questions Case 32A

Based on the history and physical examination, you tell the patient that the most likely diagnosis is

  A. Fibrocystic change
  B. Fibroadenoma
  C. Hematoma
  D. Intraductal papilloma
  E. Fat necrosis

Answer: B

Even though this patient may have fat necrosis or a hematoma, these conditions are less likely than fibroadenomas, based on the patient's age and findings. Fibrocystic change would be expected to demonstrate a longer history and cyclic changes. Intraductal papillomas are seldom felt as a mass, but rather present with bleeding from the nipple.

The most appropriate next step would be

  A. Reexamination in 3 weeks
  B. Mammography
  C. Needle aspiration or drainage
  D. Needle biopsy
  E. Excisional biopsy

Answer: B, D, or E

Given the patient's family history and level of concern, mammography followed by histologic evaluation by needle biopsy or excision is appropriate. Some clinicians would argue that mammography is not required if excision is performed.

Case 32B

A 25-year-old G1 P1001 who delivered a son 8 weeks earlier presents with a complaint of a swollen, red, tender area on the left side of her right breast. She is breast-feeding, has no history of breast problems, and has no family history of breast cancer. On examination she is afebrile and her breasts are engorged, because she is soon scheduled to feed. There is a slightly red-dened, swollen cystic area, as described.

Questions Case 32B

The most likely diagnosis is

A. Duct ectasia
B. Galactocele
C. Fat necrosis
D. Fibrocystic change
E. Carcinoma

Answer: B

A localized, tender cystic swelling in a breast-feeding woman without evidence of infection is most consistent with a blocked excretory duct, a galactocele. Duct ectasia is the same problem in a nonlactating woman.

The best management is

A. Drainage by needle
B. Incision and drainage
C. Excision
D. Placement of word catheter
E. Radiation

Answer: A

Simple drainage is usually sufficient, with incision rarely required.

Case 32C

A worried, 26-year-old G0 nurse taking oral contraceptives presents complaining of long-standing breast pain, now so bad that it keeps her from working 3 to 6 days per month. The pain is worse with move-ment and before her menses. She tearfully relates that her mother died of breast can-

cer at the age of 42 years and her 28-year-old sister has metastatic breast cancer and is taking chemotherapy. On examination, her breasts are symmetric and dense, with multiple, tender cystic areas and sheets of dense tissue.

Questions Case 32C

The most likely diagnosis is

A. Mastitis
B. Fat necrosis
C. Carcinoma
D. Fibrocystic changes
E. None of the above

Answer: D

The prolonged time course, the complaint of cystic nodularity and pain, and the breast examination are consistent with fibrocystic changes. Unfortunately, this patient is at great risk for development of breast carcinoma, given her family history.

Your best management is

A. Mammography
B. A triphasic oral contraceptive
C. Excision of all masses for histologic evaluation
D. Bilateral mastectomies
E. None of the above

Answer: A

Mammography, however, may be of little value if there is the usual profusion of radiodense areas in the patient's breast. Needle aspiration of cysts may be helpful, as may treatment with progesterone. One of the most difficult decisions is when to sample for biopsy the patient who has mul-tiple lesions, has new ones developing all the time, and is also at high risk for cancer. Some patients in this situation choose bilateral mastectomy rather than live with the continuing risk and fear of cancer.

PROCEDURES

C H A P T E R

33

GYNECOLOGIC PROCEDURES

CHAPTER OBJECTIVES

This chapter deals primarily with APGO Objective(s):

OBJECTIVE 45   Gynecologic Procedures

The student should demonstrate a knowledge of the following procedures: colposcopy and cervical biopsy, cone biopsy, cryotherapy, culdocentesis, dilation and curettage, electrosurgical excision of cervix, endometrial biopsy, hysterectomy, hysterosalpingography, hysteroscopy, laparoscopy, laser vaporization, mammography, needle aspiration of breast mass, pelvic ultrasonography, pregnancy termination, vulvar biopsy.

Some are reviewed in this chapter, and some in other topic-specific chapters.

Women's health care physicians must be familiar with the procedures common in obstetric and gynecologic practice. Whether the physician performs the procedure or not, he or she should understand the indications, contraindications, risks, benefits, and the appropriate language needed to inform the patient about her diagnoses and therapeutic options.

IMAGING

The ability to image various parts and organs of the body has dramatically enhanced our diagnostic capabilities. These methods do not replace a careful and thoughtful history and physical evaluation, but can add more detail, which assists in both medical and surgical management. The effective use of these modalities requires that the physician be familiar with the benefits and limitations of each.

Ultrasonography

Ultrasonography is based on the use of high-frequency sound reflections to identify different body tissues and structures. The term *sonography* literally means "sound writing" and is often described as using sound waves to make a picture. Very short bursts of low-energy sound waves are sent into the body. When these waves encounter the interface between two tissues that transmit sound differently, some of the sound energy is reflected back toward the sound source (Figure 33.1). The returning sound waves are detected and the distance from the sensor is deduced using the elapsed time from transmission to reception. This information is displayed graphically as a cross-sectional view of the structure encountered by the beam.

Since ultrasonography uses low-energy sound waves, it is safe for use in pregnancy. Its reliance on subtle tissue differences limits the ability to distinguish some tissues. It is also affected by interference from substances such as bowel gas. Despite these limitations, ultrasonography is very good at distinguishing solid from cystic structures and for fetal assessments. In obstetrics, measurement of fetal anatomy to allow estimation of fetal age and weight is often performed. Detailed evaluations of fetal struc-

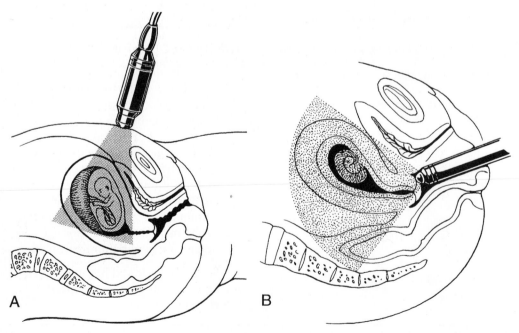

A   B

FIGURE 33.1. Transabdominal (*A*) and transvaginal (*B*) ultrasonography.

tures such as heart, brain, spinal column, and kidneys can be performed. Fetal gender may frequently be determined as well.

In gynecology, ultrasonography may be used to distinguish the character of pelvic masses (solid versus cystic) or to provide accurate measurement of tumors such as fibroids. Because of cost and limited return, ultrasonography should be used only to evaluate pelvic masses when an adequate examination is not possible (e.g., extreme obesity) or when the information gathered will alter patient management. Routine ultrasonography to confirm findings on pelvic examination is not warranted.

Improved resolution for imaging intrauterine and adnexal structures may be obtained by placing the ultrasound transducer inside the vagina, much closer to the structures to be examined than is possible with transabdominal positioning of the ultrasound transducer. The higher frequencies of sound used for transvaginal imaging allow enhanced details to be seen but limit the depth of penetration of the sound. Therefore, transvaginal ultrasound is especially useful for conditions located near the apex of the vagina (e.g., early gestations, possible ectopic pregnancies) and for ovarian follicle monitoring during assisted reproduction.

Doppler ultrasound is a form of ultrasonography that uses changes in the frequency of the reflected sound to infer motion of the reflecting surface. This can be useful in detecting cardiac motion or assessing blood flow. A growing application of Doppler ultrasound has been the evaluation of blood flow patterns in the umbilical vessels and cerebral blood vessels, because changes in these patterns may be an indication of fetal stress.

Computed Axial Tomography

Computed axial tomography (CT) scanning uses computer algorithms to construct cross-sectional images based on x-ray information (Figure 33.2). This technique involves slightly greater radiation exposure than a conventional single-exposure x-ray but provides significantly more information. With the use of contrast agents, this modality can help the physician evaluate pelvic masses, look for signs of adenopathy, or plan radiation therapy.

Magnetic Resonance Imaging

Magnetic resonance imaging (MRI) is based on the magnetic characteristics of various atoms and molecules in the body. Because of the variations in chemical composition of body tissues (especially the content of hydrogen, sodium, fluoride, or phosphorus), MRI offers exceptional images of many soft tissues. Emerging areas of clinical applicability are in the assessment of lesions in the breast and in the staging of cervical malignancy.

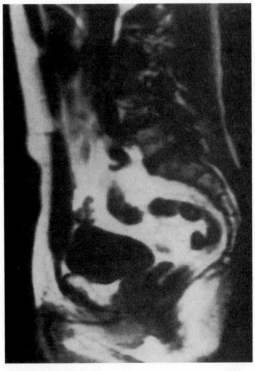

FIGURE 33.2. Computed axial tomography (CT) of the pelvis.

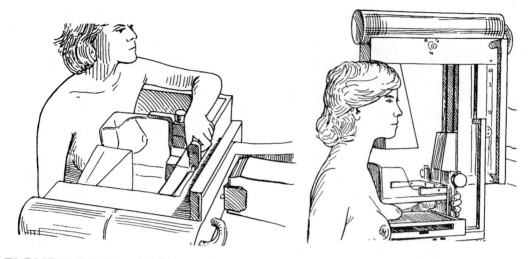

FIGURE 33.3. Technique of screening mammography.

Mammography

The need to develop an effective screening method for breast cancer has prompted the evaluation of many imaging technologies such as thermography (based on skin temperature patterns), ultrasonography, transillumination by light, and x-ray. It has been the latter (mammography) that has proved to be the most effective technique for screening and evaluation of recognized abnormalities (Figure 33.3). In mammography, breast tissue is compressed against an imaging plate, and a small amount of radiation is used to form the image. Improved films, imaging screens, and xerographic technologies have led to better images with lower radiation exposures, usually less than 0.5 rad per image set. Breast ultrasonography is a valuable adjunctive examination, especially to differentiate cystic from solid masses or lucent images on mammography.

Hysterosalpingography

For hysterosalpingography, contrast material is introduced through the cervix into the uterine cavity and x-rays are taken at specific intervals to reveal the progression of the dye through the uterus, fallopian tubes, and into the abdominopelvic cavity (Figure 33.4). This technique is useful for assessment of the size, shape, and configuration of the uterine cavity as part of the

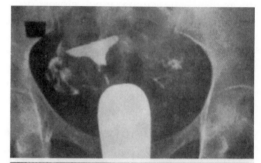
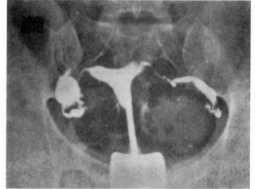
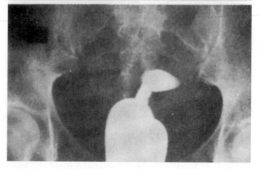

FIGURE 33.4. Hysterosalpingography.

evaluation for infertility or genital anomalies. The contrast material flows through the fallopian tubes and spills into the peritoneal cavity, which can be a good indicator of tubal patency and allow examination of tubal anatomy.

Hysterosalpingography is associated with the risk of infection of the uterus or pelvis as well as bleeding or pain. As a result, other techniques are also being used for evaluation of the uterine cavity, including hysteroscopy as well as hysterosonography (injection of saline with concurrent sonographic evaluation). Saline infusion sonohysterography is particularly useful in defining intracavitary lesions such as endometrial polyps and submucous fibroids.

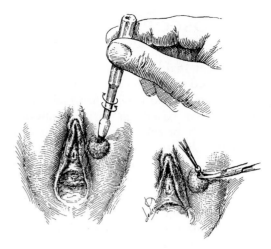

FIGURE 33.5. Biopsy of vulvar lesion with Keyes punch. Instrument is rotated in place to incise tissue.

GENITAL TRACT BIOPSY

Tissue from genital tract lesions for histologic study may be safely obtained from the vulva, vagina, cervix, and endometrial cavity. Usually performed in the office, most of these procedures require little or no anesthetics and are associated with minimal risk.

Vulvar biopsies are generally accomplished with the use of a local anesthetic. Tissue may be removed by circumscribing the biopsy specimen with a Keyes biopsy instrument (a sharp, hollow punch), elevating the tissue, and cutting across the base or by simple excision with a scalpel (Figure 33.5). This allows for full thickness histopathologic assessment and may also serve to fully excise small lesions. Local pressure or the use of styptics such as Monsel's solution (ferric subsulfate) is usually adequate for hemostasis; sutures are seldom required.

Biopsy of *vaginal* lesions is generally carried out using biopsy forceps and is most often done at the vaginal apex in cases of cellular atypica found on Pap smears in select patients who have had prior hysterectomy. The biopsy forceps is also used for cervical biopsy. Local anesthesia is usually not required for vaginal or cervical biopsies.

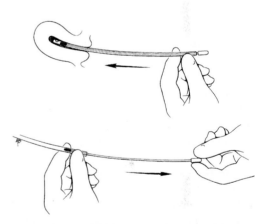

FIGURE 33.6. Endometrial biopsy using Pipelle. Hollow tube held in uterine cavity as stylet is withdrawn generating aspiration.

An *endometrial* biopsy may be obtained in several ways. A small, hollow tube may be passed through the cervix and tissue fragments aspirated using the suction pressure generated by removal of the stylet (Figure 33.6). Larger, more rigid cannula may be used to aspirate or even curette the endometrium.

COLPOSCOPY

A colposcope is a fixed stereomicroscope with an internal light source used to facilitate detailed evaluation of the surface of the cervix, vagina, and vulva when malignancy is suspected based on history, physical examination, or cytologic report. It is used to make directed biopsies of suspicious areas and is an improvement over random biopsies in the face of abnormal cytologic reports. Colposcopy may be performed in the office—almost always without the need for analgesia or anesthesia—and has minimal morbidity (see Chapter 44).

CRYOTHERAPY

Cryotherapy is the term used to describe tissue destruction by freezing. Liquid carbon dioxide or nitrogen is run through a metal probe that is placed on the tissue to be treated, allowing freezing of the tissue. Cryotherapy is most frequently used to treat dysplastic changes and benign lesions such as condyloma (Figure 33.7). The formation of ice crystals within the cells of the treated tissue leads to tissue destruction and subsequent sloughing. As a result, patients who have had cryotherapy of the cervix can be expected to have a watery discharge for several weeks as the tissue sloughs and healing occurs. Cryotherapy is inexpensive and generally effective, but it is less precise than other tissue destruction procedures such as laser ablation.

LASER VAPORIZATION

Highly energetic coherent light beams [light amplification by stimulated emission of radiation (LASER)] may be directed onto tissues, facilitating tissue destruction or incision depending on the specific wavelength of light used and the power density, or intensity, of the light beam. Great precision is possible with these systems, allowing specific tissue destruction (margins and depth of destruction) or incision selection. Infrared and CO_2 lasers are commonly used in gynecology, used alone, coupled to colposcopes, or transmitted through laparoscopes and hysteroscopes for intra-abdominal and intrauterine procedures, respectively.

DILATION AND CURETTAGE

The *dilation* of dilation and curettage (D&C) refers to opening the cervix to allow access to the endometrial cavity. This is usually done by gently using a series of graduated dilators to stretch the cervical opening. Because stretching of the cervix is painful, D&C is usually performed under a local (paracervical) or general anesthetic in an operating room. *Curettage* is a scraping of the uterine lining.

For the purpose of obtaining a representative sample of the uterine cavity (i.e., endometrial biopsy), D&C is supplanted by more easily accomplished office endometrial biopsy techniques, such as the Novak or Pipelle endometrial biopsy technique, or

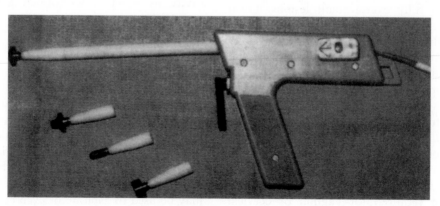

FIGURE 33.7. Cryosurgical equipment.

by biopsy under direct hysteroscopic visualization. Removal of polyps and other tumors may be accomplished by D&C, although direct removal under hysteroscopic visualization is sometimes chosen. D&C may also be useful to treat cases of incomplete spontaneous abortion.

HYSTEROSCOPY

Improved optics have led to the availability of small endoscopes that allow a direct view of the endocervix and endometrial cavity (Figure 33.8). These endoscopes may be used for diagnosis (e.g., the evaluation of bleeding or congenital malformations, the location of missing intrauterine devices) or for therapy (e.g., polypectomy, myomectomy, endometrial ablation, removal of a uterine septum). Usually done as an outpatient procedure under local or general anesthesia, hysteroscopy shares most of the same problems and complications found in D&C. Fluid may be used to distend the uterine cavity to improve visualization or the endometrium may be directly visualized (contact hysteroscopy).

PREGNANCY TERMINATION

Pregnancy termination refers to the planned interruption of a pregnancy before viability and is often referred to as induced abortion.

It is generally accomplished surgically through dilation of the cervix and evacuation of the uterine contents using local anesthetics.

Removal of the products of conception in the first and early second trimester uses either a suction or a sharp curette [*suction and curettage (S&C)*]. Suction curettes are often preferred because they are less likely to cause uterine damage such as endometrial scarring or perforation. In the second trimester, destructive grasping forceps may be used to remove the pregnancy through a dilated cervix [*dilation and evacuation (D&E)*]. Alternatively, medical induction of labor can be performed.

CERVICAL CONIZATION

Conization is a surgical procedure performed for either diagnostic or therapeutic purposes in which a cone-shaped sample of tissue, encompassing the entire cervical transformation zone and extending up the endocervical canal, is removed from the cervix (Figure 33.9). Conization is required for the definitive evaluation of patients with abnormal Pap smears for whom adequate colposcopic examinations are impossible or are inconsistent with Pap smear data.

Conization may be performed using a variety of techniques, including sharp dissection (cold knife cone), laser excision, and electrocautery [large loop excision of the

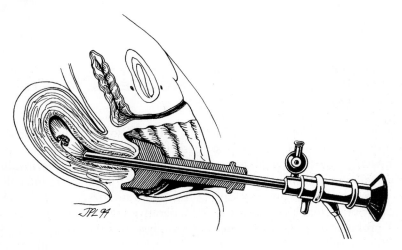

FIGURE 33.8. Hysteroscopy.

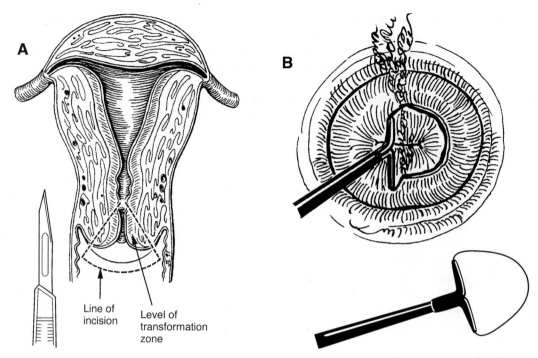

FIGURE 33.9. Conization of the cervix. (*A*) Cold knife technique. (*B*) LLETZ/LEEP (large loop excision of the transformation zone/loop electrosurgical excision procedure) technique.

transformation zone (LLETZ) or loop electrosurgical excision procedure (LEEP)]. An early complication of conization is excessive bleeding, which can occur 5 to 10 days after surgery. Cervical stenosis or incompetence is an infrequent complication.

LAPAROSCOPY

Laparoscopy (or pelviscopy) involves inspection and manipulation of tissue within the abdominal cavity using endoscopic instruments. The laparoscope is inserted into the abdominal cavity, usually through a periumbilical incision. To facilitate viewing and to decrease the chance of bowel injury, the abdominal cavity may be distended with either carbon dioxide or nitrous oxide gas. Additional incisions in the lower abdomen may be made to allow supplementary instruments to be placed into the abdominal cavity for surgical or other manipulations (Figure 33.10). A probe or other device is often inserted into the uterine cavity to facilitate uterine manipulations.

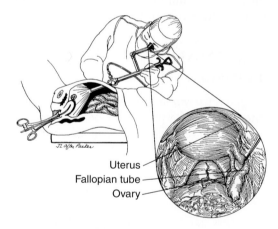

Uterus
Fallopian tube
Ovary

FIGURE 33.10. Laparoscopy.

Laparoscopy is used for diagnostic or therapeutic purposes. Laparoscopic inspection of the pelvis can be invaluable in the diagnosis of pelvic pain, infertility, congenital abnormalities, or small pelvic masses. Operative laparoscopy may be used to perform lysis of adhesions, treat endometriosis, or carry out surgical sterilizations and other gynecologic procedures.

Serious complications from injury to the bowel or great vessels can occur. Intraperitoneal bleeding or injuries such as damage to bowel during fulguration or laser also pose a risk. Anesthetic complications are possible, as are infections and bleeding at the incision site.

HYSTERECTOMY

Hysterectomy, the removal of the uterus, is still one of the most common surgical procedures performed. In the United States, approximately 500,000 hysterectomies are performed each year. Removing the uterus may be indicated for patients with benign or malignant changes in the uterine wall or cavity, abnormalities of the cervix, or menstrual disturbances that do not respond to more conservative therapy. Hysterectomy essentially eliminates the possibility of pregnancy, causes cessation of menses, and removes the risk of cervical disease. Despite these apparent advantages, hysterectomy is sufficiently expensive, time-consuming, and risky that it cannot be recommended for the sole purpose of sterilization.

In discussing hysterectomy with patients, it is important to recognize the correct use and common misuse of terms associated with the procedure. When physicians use the term *total* hysterectomy, they are referring to the removal of all of the uterus. The term does not indicate removal of the ovaries (oophorectomy) or fallopian tubes (salpingectomy). These distinctions are important and should be emphasized when taking the patient's history and providing preoperative counseling. A *subtotal*, or *supracervical*, hysterectomy is one in which the body of the uterus is removed near the level of the internal cervical os, leaving the cervix in place. A *radical* hysterectomy is a cancer surgery procedure in which the uterus is removed with very wide margins of surrounding tissues.

Removal of the uterus may be accomplished by entering the abdominal cavity from above (abdominal hysterectomy) or by extracting the uterus through the vagina (vaginal hysterectomy). Each has advantages and disadvantages that must be evaluated for each patient. With either approach, certain steps must be accomplished to allow the safe removal of the uterus. The blood supply to the uterus is interrupted by ligation of the uterine arteries and the anastomotic connections to the vaginal and ovarian blood supplies. The latter is ligated at the level of the utero-ovarian ligament (if the ovaries are to be preserved) or at the level of the infundibulopelvic ligament (if oophorectomy is planned). The supporting structures of the uterus (the round, cardinal, and uterosacral ligaments and the leaves of the broad ligament) are severed. The sequence of these steps is dictated by the route of surgery chosen (fundus to cervix for the abdominal route; cervix to fundus for the vaginal route) and the local exigencies mandated by the pathology encountered (e.g., distortion of anatomy by fibroids).

Abdominal Hysterectomy

Removal of the uterus through an abdominal incision allows the surgeon maximal exposure and latitude in performing the procedure. This approach is used when substantial pathology is anticipated (as with large fibroids or pelvic scarring), when wide margins or further exploration is required (as in cancer surgery), when additional abdominal procedures are contemplated (such as bladder suspension), or when surgery is done at the time of cesarean delivery. Abdominal hysterectomies generally involve longer operating times, because of the time spent making and repairing the abdominal wall incision. This route also is associated with a greater rate of morbidity and a longer hospital stay.

Vaginal Hysterectomy

Vaginal hysterectomy is generally associated with a faster recovery period and less patient discomfort than an abdominal hysterectomy. Offsetting this is the higher incidence of fever and infection, although the use of prophylactic antibiotics has reduced this to a minimum. Vaginal hysterectomy is often chosen when the uterus is not enlarged and other adnexal or pelvic pathology is not anticipated. This procedure is especially appropriate for patients who require repair of a cystocele, rectocele, or enterocele. Vaginal hysterectomy is typically avoided when the uterus is larger than 10 to 12 weeks' size, movement of the pelvic organs is restricted by scarring or endometriosis, or further abdominal exploration is required.

Laparoscopically Assisted Vaginal Hysterectomy

The role of laparoscopic-assisted vaginal hysterectomy (LAVH)—in which some of the initial stages of hysterectomy are done with laparoscopic instrumentation, but the uterus is ultimately removed transvaginally—remains to be fully identified. Advocates of the procedure point to the advantages of avoiding an abdominal incision by facilitating vaginal delivery of the uterus or adnexal mass in situations where such was impossible or inadvisable: pelvic adhesions, uterus size > 10–12 weeks, an adnexal mass, and poor uterine descent as may be found in women of low gravidity. Concerns that have been raised about the procedure include its technical difficulty and increased operative time and increased anesthesia exposure. More recently, laparoscopic supercervical hysterectomy (LSH) has been advocated by some in order to preserve the cervix and its attendant support of the vaginal apex. Additionally, some authors cite the advantage of cervical retention for lubrication and maintenance of sexual response.

UNIT IV

Reproductive Endocrinology and Infertility

34

REPRODUCTIVE CYCLE

There is no specific APGO objective for this chapter, although many of the chapters in this book rely on an understanding of the basic physiology discussed in this chapter.

In the female reproductive cycle, ovulation is followed by menstrual bleeding in a recurring, predictable sequence. This recurring sequence is established at puberty (around age 13) and continues until the time of menopause at around age 50. A regular, predictable reproductive cycle is usually established by age 15 and continues (except during pregnancy) until age 45. Thus a woman has approximately 30 years of optimal reproductive function. In healthy women, reproductive cycles occur at approximately 28-day intervals, and most women ovulate 13 to 14 times per year, unless ovulation is interrupted by pregnancy, lactation, hormone-based contraceptive use or other exogenous hormone or medical therapy, or illness.

The reproductive cycle depends on the cyclic interaction between hypothalamic gonadotropin-releasing hormone (GnRH), the pituitary gonadotropins follicle-stimulating hormone (FSH) and luteinizing hormone (LH), and the ovarian sex steroid hormones estradiol and progesterone. Through positive- and negative-feedback loops, these hormones stimulate ovulation, facilitate implantation of the fertilized ovum, and bring about menstruation. Feedback loops between the hypothalamus, pituitary gland, and ovaries are depicted in Figure 34.1. If any one (or more) of the above hormones becomes tonically elevated or suppressed, the reproductive cycle becomes disrupted and ovulation and menstruation cease. In the case of female reproductive dysfunction, it is essential to identify which hormones are either elevated or reduced.

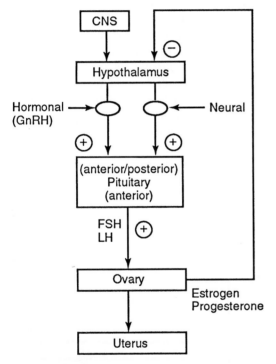

FIGURE 34.1. Traditional block diagram of feedback and control of menstruation. Traditionally, control of menstruation is based on a simple feedback loop involving the "hypothalamic-pituitary-ovarian axis." This view is giving way to evidence that the follicle itself controls the cyclic process. CNS = central nervous system; FSH = follicle-stimulating hormone; GnRH = gonadotropin-releasing hormone; LH = luteinizing hormone. (From Smith RP: *Gynecology in Primary Care.* Baltimore, Williams & Wilkins, 1996, p. 26.)

HYPOTHALAMIC GnRH SECRETION

GnRH (a decapeptide) is secreted in a pulsatile manner from the arcuate nucleus of the hypothalamus. The hypothalamus serves as the pulse generator of the reproductive clock. Surgical ablation of the arcuate nucleus in animals disrupts ovarian function, as does continuous infusion of GnRH agonists. Ovarian function can be restored by the pulsatile infusion of GnRH at 70- to 90-minute intervals. The mechanism for stimulation of GnRH secretion is unknown; however, GnRH secretion is influenced by estradiol and catecholamine neurotransmitters. The latter influence may help explain psychogenic influences on the reproductive cycle. GnRH reaches the anterior pituitary gland through the hypothalamic–pituitary portal plexus. Pituitary gonadotropin secretion is stimulated and modulated by the pulsatile secretion of GnRH.

PITUITARY GONADOTROPIN SECRETION

The pituitary gonadotropins FSH and LH are protein hormones secreted by the anterior pituitary gland. FSH and LH are also secreted in pulsatile fashion in concert with the pulsatile release of GnRH; the magnitude of secretion and the rates of secretion of FSH and/or LH are determined largely by the levels of ovarian steroid hormones and other ovarian factors. When a woman is in a state of relative estrogen deficiency, the principal gonadotropin secreted is FSH. Because the ovary responds to FSH secretion with estradiol production, there is a negative feedback to the pituitary gland to inhibit FSH secretion and facilitate LH secretion. This is discussed in more detail in association with the phases of the reproductive cycle.

OVARIAN SEX STEROID HORMONE SECRETION

Ovarian follicles respond to pituitary gonadotropin secretion by synthesizing the principal ovarian hormones *estradiol* and *progesterone*. Increasing levels of estradiol influence the pituitary gland via a negative-feedback mechanism, resulting in decreased secretion of FSH and increased secretion of LH. This results in a marked increase in LH secretion (the LH surge), which triggers ovulation. With ovulation, the ovarian follicle is converted into a corpus luteum and begins secreting progesterone.

At birth, the human ovary is filled with approximately one million *primordial follicles*. Each follicle contains an oocyte that is arrested in the prophase stage of meiosis. The oocyte is surrounded by a single layer of pregranulosa cells, which become the granulosa cells. The pregranulosa cells are surrounded by a matrix of cells that become the theca cells. Some primordial follicles partially respond to pituitary FSH during childhood, but the process of ovulation does not occur until puberty.

During a full reproductive cycle, one oocyte is brought to maturity before ovulation. In the process of bringing one oocyte to maturation, a number of oocytes are stimulated to partial maturation but subsequently undergo atresia before reaching ovulation.

During the process of follicular maturation, pregranulosa cells are stimulated by FSH to become *granulosa cells*, which begin secreting *estradiol*. Binding of FSH to receptors in the granulosa cells causes granulosa cell proliferation, increased binding of FSH, and increased production of estradiol. The follicle with the greatest number of granulosa cells, FSH receptors, and the highest estradiol production becomes the dominant follicle from which ovulation occurs.

As a primordial follicle is stimulated, the pretheca cells surrounding the granulosa cells become *theca cells*. The theca cells secrete *androgens*, which serve as the precursors for estradiol production by the granulosa cells. Current scientific theory holds that estradiol is secreted through a two-cell mechanism (Figure 34.2). Androgens are

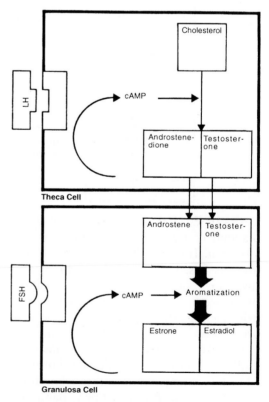

FIGURE 34.2.   Two-cell theory of estradiol production.

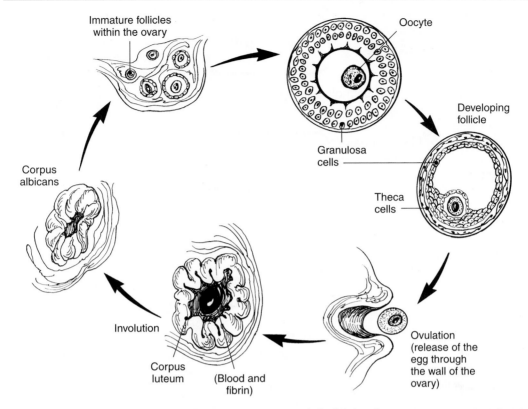

FIGURE 34.3.   Cyclic changes in ovarian follicle development. (From Smith RP: *Gynecology in Primary Care.* Baltimore, Williams & Wilkins, 1996, p. 29.)

first secreted by the theca cells. These androgens enter the granulosa cells by diffusion, where they are aromatized to estradiol.

After ovulation, the dominant follicle becomes the *corpus luteum,* which secretes *progesterone* to prepare the endometrium for implantation of a fertilized oocyte. If pregnancy does not occur, the corpus luteum undergoes involution, menstruation begins, and the cycle repeats. The changes in the follicle during the follicular phase of the cycle are presented in Figure 34.3.

REPRODUCTIVE CYCLE

For purposes of discussion, *the reproductive cycle is divided into three phases: menstruation and the follicular phase, ovulation, and the luteal phase.* These three phases refer to the status of the ovary during the reproductive cycle.

Phase I: Menstruation and the Follicular Phase

When the oocyte ovulated in the previous cycle is not fertilized, the cyclic interaction between the hypothalamus, pituitary gland, and ovaries is reset, initiating a new reproductive cycle. *The first day of menstrual bleeding is considered day 1 of the menstrual cycle.* During menstruation, the endometrium is sloughed in response to progesterone withdrawal. This is followed by the follicular phase, during which a new endometrial lining of the uterus is renewed in preparation for implantation of an embryo.

Women usually menstruate for 3 to 5 days. A woman sheds approximately 30 to 50 ml of dark, nonclotting menstrual blood during menstruation. Occasionally, tissue elements of endometrium can be identified in the menstrual effluent.

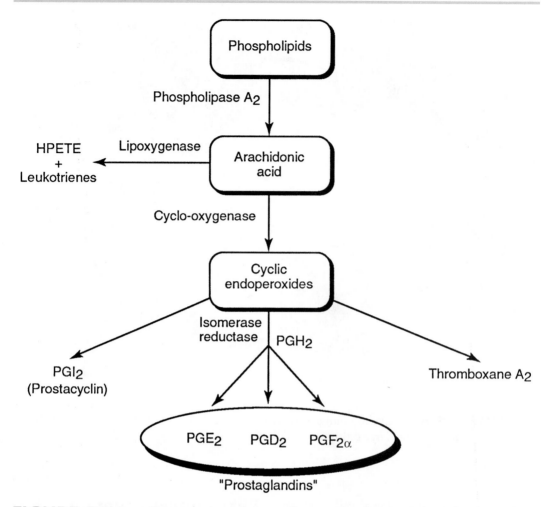

FIGURE 34.4. Biosynthetic pathways of prostaglandins (and thromboxanes) from arachidonic acid. (From Smith RP: Cyclic pelvic pain and dysmenorrhea. *Obstet Gynecol Clin North Am* 20:753–764, 1993.)

There may be uterine cramps during the first day or two of menstrual bleeding. These cramps are a result of the action of prostaglandins liberated from the endometrium during menstruation. Prostaglandins are a group of endogenous 20-carbon hydroxy-unsaturated fatty acids, whose biosynthetic pathway begins with the precursor arachidonic acid (Figure 34.4). The secretory endometrium synthesizes prostaglandins, especially prostaglandin $F_{2\alpha}$ ($PGF_{2\alpha}$), under the influence of progesterone. The endometrial content of $PGF_{2\alpha}$ is higher during the secretory than during the follicular phase and is highest during early menstruation. At this time, prostaglandins are formed and released, and produce contractions of the uterine musculature and vasculature, causing contractile and ischemic pain (Figure 34.5). These prostaglandin-associated uterine contractions also aid the normal expulsion of the menstrual effluent.

Menstruation marks the beginning of the follicular phase of the cycle. With the beginning of menstruation, plasma concentrations of estradiol, progesterone, and LH reach their lowest point. Only FSH is increased at the beginning of menstruation. The increase in FSH begins approximately 2 days before the onset of menstruation and is involved in the maturation of another group of ovarian follicles and the

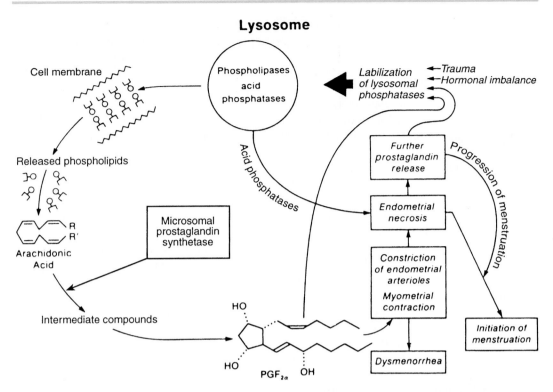

FIGURE 34.5. Menstrual-associated prostaglandin release and uterine contractions.

selection of a dominant follicle for ovulation in the next cycle. FSH binds to receptors located in the granulosa cells of the primary oocyte. As FSH is bound to the granulosa cells, it stimulates their differentiation from a stratified squamous-type cell into a cuboidal cell. Moreover, FSH stimulates mitosis of the granulosa cells, thereby increasing the number of granulosa cells surrounding the oocyte. Under the influence of FSH, the granulosa cells begin to secrete estradiol.

Estradiol begins to rise in plasma by the fourth day of the cycle. Estradiol stimulates LH receptors on the theca cells, preparing them to increase secretion of androgen precursors to estradiol and preparing the granulosa and theca cells for progesterone production after ovulation.

With rising estradiol, there is negative feedback on the pituitary gland to decrease the release of FSH and positive feedback on the pituitary gland to increase the release of LH. During the early follicular phase of the cycle, the FSH:LH ratio is > 1; as the cycle progresses, the FSH:LH ratio becomes < 1, demonstrating both positive and negative feedback effects of estradiol on the pituitary gland.

As follicles enlarge, they secrete both androgens and estrogens; however, if the estradiol:androgen ratio within the follicular fluid becomes < 1, that follicle becomes atretic and never becomes a dominant follicle. The dominant follicle is the one that has a follicular fluid estradiol:androgen ratio of > 1.

As the dominant follicle secretes more and more estradiol, there is marked positive feedback to the pituitary gland to secrete LH. By day 11 to 13 of the normal cycle, an LH surge occurs, which triggers ovulation. Ovulation occurs within 30 to 36 hours of the LH surge, causing the oocyte to be expelled from the follicle and the follicle to be converted into a corpus luteum to facilitate progesterone production during the remainder of the cycle. At the time of the LH surge just before ovulation, there is a concomitant rise in FSH. The mechanism for this FSH rise and its effect on the follicle are currently being studied.

Phase II: Ovulation

The mechanism for ovulation is poorly understood. As the dominant follicle enlarges and accumulates follicular fluid, it is said to "ripen" and become ready for release. Through animal studies, it has been demonstrated that intrafollicular prostaglandins play an essential role in release of the oocyte and that the administration of prostaglandin synthetase inhibitors causes the oocyte to be retained within the follicle during the luteal phase of the cycle. A condition of luteinized retained follicle has been recognized, in which the oocyte does not appear to be expelled from the follicle.

Many women experience a twinge of pain ("mittelschmerz") at the time of ovulation and can distinguish the time of ovulation with precision. Others do not experience pain but can appreciate the effects of changing hormone production that occur with ovulation.

The application of transvaginal ultrasound imaging has enabled physicians to follow the process of follicular growth and maturation and observe the collapse of the dominant follicle following ovulation.

Phase III: Luteal Phase

The luteal phase of the cycle is characterized by a change in secretion of sex steroid hormones from estradiol predominance to progesterone predominance. As FSH rises early in the cycle, stimulating mitosis of granulosa cells and production of estradiol, additional LH receptors are created in the granulosa cells and theca cells. With the LH surge at the time of ovulation, these LH receptors bind LH and convert the enzymatic machinery of the granulosa and theca cells to facilitate production of progesterone.

The production of progesterone begins approximately 24 hours before ovulation and rises rapidly thereafter. A maximal production of progesterone occurs 3 to 4 days

after ovulation and is maintained for approximately 11 days following ovulation. If fertilization and implantation do not occur, progesterone production diminishes rapidly, initiating events leading to the beginning of a new cycle.

Progesterone production depends on the initial FSH and LH signals from the pituitary gland. Adequate progesterone production is necessary to facilitate implantation of the fertilized oocyte into the endometrium and to sustain pregnancy into the early first trimester. If the initial rise in FSH is inadequate and if the LH surge does not achieve maximal amplitude, an "inadequate luteal phase" (i.e., luteal phase defect) can occur, resulting in inadequate progesterone production to facilitate implantation of a fertilized oocyte or to sustain pregnancy.

The corpus luteum measures approximately 2.5 cm in diameter and has a characteristic deep yellow color. It can be seen on gross inspection of the ovary if laparoscopy or laparotomy is performed during the luteal phase of the cycle. As the corpus luteum fails, it decreases in volume and loses its yellow color. After a few months, the corpus luteum becomes a white fibrous streak within the ovary called the corpus albicans.

The corpus luteum has a fixed life span of 13 to 14 days unless pregnancy occurs. If the oocyte becomes fertilized and implants within the endometrium, the early pregnancy begins secreting human chorionic gonadotropin (hCG), which sustains the corpus luteum for another 6 to 7 weeks.

Progesterone has negative feedback on pituitary secretion of both FSH and LH. During the luteal phase of the cycle, both FSH and LH are suppressed to low levels. As the corpus luteum fails and progesterone secretion diminishes, FSH begins to rise to prepare a woman for the next reproductive cycle.

The cyclic changes in FSH, LH, estradiol, and progesterone along with the changes in the follicle, endometrium, vagina, and cervix are presented in Figure 34.6. Note the cyclic interaction between the four

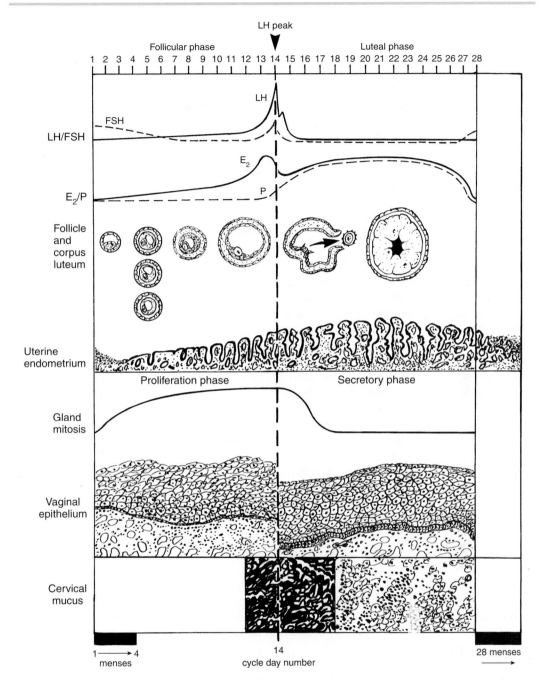

FIGURE 34.6. Composite changes in tissues and hormones during the reproductive cycle.

hormones during the course of a reproductive cycle.

Perimenopause

As a woman ages, the ovarian follicles diminish in number and become less sensitive to FSH. The process of ovulation becomes increasingly inefficient, less regular, and less predictable than in earlier years. A woman begins to notice changes in her reproductive cycle at around age 38 to 42. Initially, she notices a shortening of the cycle length. With increasing inefficiency of the reproductive cycle, the follicular phase shortens but the luteal phase is maintained at normal length. With the passing of time, some cycles become anovulatory.

As menopause approaches, the remaining follicles become almost totally resistant to FSH. The process of ovulation ceases entirely and cyclic hormone production ends with menopause.

CLINICAL MANIFESTATIONS OF HORMONAL CHANGES

The presence or absence of sex steroid hormones produces clinical manifestations that aid in establishing the phases of the reproductive cycle. The endometrium and endocervix, the breasts, the vagina, and the hypothalamic thermoregulating center all undergo cyclic changes in response to hormonal control. The changes in the endocervix and breasts can be directly observed, and the changes in the hypothalamic thermoregulatory center can be measured by recording the basal body temperature. The changes in the vagina can be identified by cytologic examination of the vaginal epithelium, and the changes in the endometrium can be evaluated by endometrial biopsy followed by histologic examination of the biopsy sample. Other changes can be ascertained through a careful history. Some of these changes include alteration of libido, abdominal bloating, fluid retention, mood changes, and uterine cramps at the onset of menstruation.

Endometrium

The endometrial lining of the uterus undergoes dramatic histologic changes during the reproductive cycle. During menstruation, the endometrium is sloughed to a basal level, consisting of compact stroma cells and short, narrow endometrial glands. Estrogen is a mitogenic hormone, which stimulates cell growth. With rising estradiol production during the follicular phase of the cycle, the endometrial stroma thickens and the endometrial glands become elongated; this is a proliferative endometrium. The endometrium reaches a maximal thickness at the time of ovulation. If ovulation does not occur and a woman remains in an estrogenic state, the endometrium continues to thicken and the endometrial glands continue to elongate until the endometrium outgrows its blood supply and sloughs. This abnormal condition is the basis for dysfunctional uterine bleeding (see Chapter 36).

When ovulation occurs, the hormonal balance changes from an estrogenic state to a progestational state. Progesterone is not a mitogen, but causes differentiation of the tissues that contain progesterone receptors. Progesterone converts the proliferative endometrium into a secretory endometrium. The endometrial stroma becomes loose and edematous, and blood vessels entering the endometrium become thickened and twisted. The endometrial glands, which were straight and tubular in the proliferative phase of the endometrium, become tortuous and contain secretory material within the lumina. Following ovulation, distinct, recognizable changes occur within the endometrium at almost daily intervals. Therefore, the quality of the corpus luteum and stage of the reproductive cycle can be evaluated by histologic examination of a small sample of endometrium.

Endocervix

The endocervix contains glands that secrete endocervical mucus in response to hormonal changes. Under the influence of estradiol, the endocervical glands secrete large quantities of thin, clear, watery, endocervical mucus. This mucus facilitates sperm capture, sperm storage, and sperm transport. Sperm can be stored in the crypts of the endocervical glands for up to 7 days and then released into the upper genital tract for fertilization of an oocyte. Endocervical mucous production is maximal at the time of ovulation. With ovulation and the shift in hormone production from estradiol to progesterone, the endocervical mucus becomes thick, opaque, and tenacious. This type of mucus is an impediment to sperm capture, storage, and transport.

Breasts

The ductal elements of the breasts, nipples, and areolae respond to estradiol secretion. After ovulation, progesterone stimulates the acinar (milk producing) glands. Because the acinar glands are located in the tails of the breasts, this gives the breasts a more rounded configuration. Moreover, progesterone makes the venous pattern on the surface of the breasts appear more prominent and accentuates the small Montgomery glands contained within the areolae. These dynamic changes can be observed during the reproductive cycle and are seen in the development states of puberty.

Vagina

Estradiol stimulates vaginal thickening and maturation of the surface epithelial cells of the vaginal mucosa. Estradiol also facilitates vaginal transudation during sexual excitement, creating a moist, lubricated vagina for sexual intercourse. During the luteal phase of the cycle, the vaginal epithelium retains its thickness but the secretory changes are markedly diminished. Women report less sexual desire and sexual enjoyment during the luteal phase. This loss of sexual desire is even more marked during the early weeks of pregnancy.

Hypothalamic Thermoregulating Center

Progesterone shifts the basal body temperature upward by 0.6° F to 1.0° F. This shift occurs abruptly with the beginning of the progesterone secretion and wanes abruptly with loss of progesterone secretion. The changes in the basal body temperature reflect the changing plasma progesterone concentration. The basal body temperature

record is a useful tool for women and their physicians who want to evaluate the reproductive cycle in a dynamic and inexpensive way (see Figure 39.3).

CLINICAL IMPLICATIONS OF THE REPRODUCTIVE CYCLE

Some women have exaggerated responses to the changing hormonal environment of the reproductive cycle and experience troublesome symptoms. The two conditions for which women seek medical attention as a result of the reproductive cycle are premenstrual syndrome (PMS) and primary dysmenorrhea.

The etiology and pathogenesis of PMS are poorly understood. There are many theories to explain this common condition, and a number of treatments have been devised for its correction. However, none of these theories has withstood scientific scrutiny. The emotional, physical, and behavioral symptoms of PMS occur during the luteal phase of the reproductive cycle, and these symptoms do not occur in anovulatory women. Thus PMS is directly associated with the reproductive cycle.

Primary dysmenorrhea is the occurrence of debilitating uterine cramps during the first 2 days of menstruation. Associated symptoms are diarrhea, nausea, vomiting, and headache. These symptoms are self-limiting and abate as menstruation ceases. The etiology of primary dysmenorrhea is linked to the endometrial production and secretion of prostaglandins just before and during menstruation. Symptoms of primary dysmenorrhea can be directly alleviated by the administration of prostaglandin synthetase inhibitors and moderately alleviated by hormonal contraceptives, which inhibit ovulation.

Case 34A

A 24-year-old woman has regular, predictable menstrual cycles that began at age 13.

Questions Case 34A

Which of the following statements about the follicular phase of her cycle are correct?

A. FSH initiates the development of a cohort of follicles, one of which becomes the dominant follicle
B. Endometrial biopsy reveals the presence of a secretory endometrium
C. Endocervical mucus is thin, clear, and watery during the late follicular phase
D. Estradiol is the predominant steroid hormone

Answer: A, C, D

The only incorrect statement is regarding the state of the endometrium, which would be proliferative. Secretory endometrium reflects a state of progesterone dominance and occurs in the luteal phase.

Which of the following statements about the luteal phase of the cycle are correct?

A. Progesterone is the predominant steroid hormone
B. Endocervical mucus is thick, sticky, and tenacious
C. Basal body temperature is elevated
D. It is during this phase of the reproductive cycle that some women develop cyclic emotional, physical, and behavioral symptoms

Answer: All

Each of the options is correct and each statement has clinical relevance in certain patients. A basic understanding of the underlying reproductive cycle physiology facilitates diagnosis as well as treatment.

Case 34B

A 45-year-old woman notices a lengthening of her cycle from the usual 29 days to 50 to 60 days. She also experiences occasional hot flushes.

Question Case 34B

Which of the following statements is correct?

A. The number of ovarian follicles is still adequate for ovulation
B. Her FSH concentration is tonically elevated
C. Her FSH has altered, and the ovarian follicles are less responsive to the altered molecule
D. Her plasma estradiol concentration is zero

Answer: A

Although the total number of follicles continues to decrease with each cycle, the woman is apparently still having ovulatory cycles. The FSH concentration is not tonically elevated until the ovary no longer responds to FSH. Until then, it continues to fluctuate. The FSH molecule itself does not change in configuration during the perimenopausal period. The estradiol concentration is not zero, because the ovary continues to produce estradiol, albeit in less efficient fashion. The occasional vasomotor symptoms suggest waning of but not lack of ovarian function.

CHAPTER

35

PUBERTY

CHAPTER OBJECTIVES

This chapter deals primarily with APGO Objective(s):

OBJECTIVE 46   Puberty

A. Describe the physiologic and psychologic events associated with normal puberty, the approximate ages they occur, and the appropriate counseling to include sexuality, sexual decision making, and social contexts.

B. Describe the types, causes, characteristics, and diagnostic and management approaches to early or delayed puberty.

Puberty is the physical, emotional, and sexual transition from childhood to adulthood. Although the transition occurs gradually, it contains a series of well-defined events and milestones. Few individuals have problems with this endocrine process. However, when puberty is delayed or advanced, an understanding of the hormonal events of puberty and the sequence of physical changes is essential for the clinician to be able to evaluate the process and progress of sexual development. Moreover, an understanding of puberty is essential for an understanding of the process of reproduction.

The endocrine events that initiate the onset of secondary sexual maturation are unknown. The hypothalamic-pituitary-gonadal axis functions during fetal life and during the first few weeks following birth, after which the axis becomes quiescent. At approximately the age of 8 in both boys and girls, the adrenal glands begin to secrete increasing quantities of dehydroepiandrosterone; approximately 2 years later, the gonads begin secreting sex steroid hormones. The process of secondary sexual maturation requires approximately 4 years from its beginning until full sexual maturation has been achieved; this process takes place in an orderly, predictable sequence. The events, age, and hormone(s) responsible for the sequence of *sexual maturation* in girls is presented in Table 35.1. The sequence of breast development (*thelarche*) and pubic hair growth (*adrenarche*) is presented in Figure 35.1.

These events are predictable and reflect the secretion and action of hypothalamic peptide hormones and pituitary protein hormones, adrenal steroid hormones, and gonadal sex steroid hormones. An alteration in the sequence of these events suggests that there is an alteration in normal hormone secretion and action.

Three known critical elements play a role in the timing of *secondary sexual maturation*. These are adequate body fat, adequate sleep, and vision (optic exposure to sunlight).

Girls must attain a *critical body weight*—irrespective of height—before breast development begins. Moreover, a body weight of *85–106 pounds* must be achieved before menses begins, and a proportion of *body fat of 16%–24%* is required to sustain ovulatory cycles. This theory of critical body weight has been challenged by a number of investigators but has held up well in clinical observations and in practice. Girls who engage in strenuous exercise programs before puberty have delayed sexual development; girls who are obese as children have early menarche. The role of body weight in male secondary sexual maturation and in sustaining male reproductive function is not defined.

Sleep has varying effects on the gonadotropin secretory pattern in prepubertal children, intrapubertal children, and sexually mature adolescents. In prepubertal children, there is no correlation between sleep cycle and gonadotropin secretion. In intrapubertal adolescents—girls who have breast development and sexual hair growth but who have not menstruated and boys who have penile and testicular enlargement

TABLE 35.1.	Sequence of Sexual Maturation in Girls	
Event	**Age (Years)**	**Hormone(s)**
Breast budding	10–11	Estradiol
Sexual hair growth	10.5–11.5	Androgens
Growth spurt	11–12	Growth hormone
Menarche	11.5–13	Estradiol
Adult breast development	12.5–15	Progesterone
Adult sexual hair	13.5–16	Androgens

Tanner stage

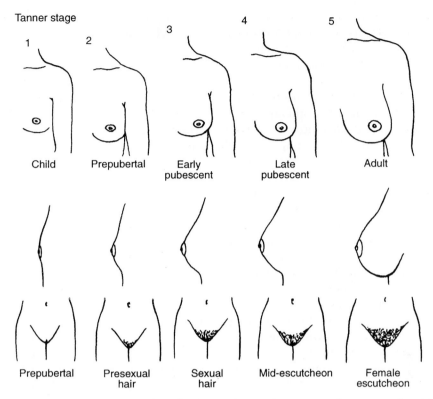

| 1 | 2 | 3 | 4 | 5 |

Child   Prepubertal   Early pubescent   Late pubescent   Adult

Prepubertal   Presexual hair   Sexual hair   Mid-escutcheon   Female escutcheon

FIGURE 35.1.   Tanner's classification of sexual maturity: breasts and pubic hair.

but who have not ejaculated—there is a sleep-entrained gonadotropin secretory cycle. That is, during sleep, there is a marked increase in the secretion of follicle-stimulating hormone (FSH) and luteinizing hormone (LH). In sexually mature adolescents, the release of gonadotropins bears no relationship to the sleep cycle. Instead, gonadotropins are released at 6- to 8-hour intervals. This pattern is maintained for the remainder of a person's reproductive life, unless reproductive dysfunction occurs.

Optic exposure to sunlight is essential for timely secondary sexual development. Blind girls have delayed menarche and blind boys have delayed spermatogenesis and ejaculation. In hibernating animals who obviously have limited optic exposure, pituitary secretion of gonadotropins is suppressed during the period of hibernation. A similar mechanism is postulated for humans with decreased exposure to sunlight for any reason.

Abrupt *mood changes* occur during the period of secondary sexual maturation in girls and boys. Periods of depression, eupho-

ria, and even violent behavior occur to some extent in many intrapubertal adolescents. Once full sexual maturation—with release of gametes—is completed, these mood changes disappear, so the physician can reassure the young person and concerned, distraught parents that the mood changes will abate with time.

ABNORMALITIES OF PUBERTAL DEVELOPMENT

The abnormalities of puberty include delayed sexual maturation, incomplete sexual maturation, primary amenorrhea, and precocious puberty. The presence of any of these disorders requires investigation of the hypothalamic-pituitary-gonadal axis and the reproductive outflow tract. The initial investigation must begin with measurement of pituitary gonadotropins (FSH and LH). These hormones distinguish a hypothalamic–pituitary etiology from a gonadal etiology.

TABLE 35.2.	Causes of Delayed Puberty or Menstruation

Premature ovarian failure
   Turner syndrome
   Long-arm X chromosomal deletion
   Alkylating chemotherapy
Inadequate gonadotropin-releasing hormone secretion
   Olfactory tract hypoplasia (Kallmann syndrome)
   Constitutional delayed puberty
   Craniopharyngioma
   Hypothalamic hamartoma
   Marijuana use
Inadequate gonadotropin secretion
   Isolated gonadotropin deficiency
   Prolactin-secreting pituitary adenoma
   Other space-occupying lesions of the sella turcica
Inadequate body fat
   Anorexia nervosa
   Exercise-induced hypothalamic dysfunction
Genital tract abnormalities
   Imperforate hymen
   Vaginal and uterine agenesis (Rokitansky-Küster-Hauser syndrome)

Delayed Sexual Maturation

The first step in sexual maturation is breast budding, which usually begins between 10 and 11 years in most girls. Some girls begin breast budding by 8 years, and this falls within the range of normal. However, if breast budding does not begin by 13 years, puberty may be delayed or may not begin spontaneously. *Failure to establish a breast bud by age 13* should cause the physician to initiate an endocrine evaluation to elucidate the cause of pubertal delay. Moreover, *if sexual hair growth precedes breast budding by more than 6 to 9 months*, the physician should likewise initiate an endocrine evaluation. The most *common causes of delayed puberty* are presented in Table 35.2.

Premature Ovarian Failure

Ovarian failure can occur anytime before the expected time of menopause. *Ovarian failure is characterized by diminished or absent estrogen production in association with elevated gonadotropins.* The most common etiology of premature ovarian failure seen in prepubertal and pubertal girls is

Turner syndrome. The features of Turner syndrome are failure to establish secondary sexual development along with somatic changes such as short stature, a webbed neck (pterygium colli), a shield chest with widely spaced nipples, and an increased carrying angle of the elbows (cubitus valgus).

The fundamental genetic defects in girls with Turner syndrome are absence of an X chromosome (Figure 35.2). No Barr bodies are seen. Genetic information that regulates the rate of ovarian follicular atresia is carried on the long arm of the X chromosome, whereas somatic information is carried on the short arm of the X chromosome. The absence of the entire X chromosome leads to loss of ovarian function and to the somatic features described above.

Partial deletions of the long arm of the X chromosome cause premature ovarian failure to occur at varying chronological ages. For example, complete loss of the long arm of the X chromosome results in premature ovarian failure before puberty, whereas a small fragmentary loss of the X chromosome may not result in ovarian failure until many years after a normal puberty.

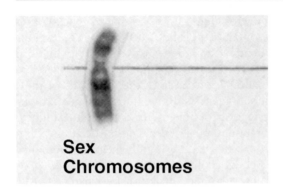

Sex Chromosomes

FIGURE 35.2. Karyotype of Turner syndrome: 45,X, one of the X chromosomes is missing. Approximately 50% of people with Turner syndrome have this 45,X karyotype; 15% have 46,X,i [Xq0]; 25% have 45,X/46,XX;46,XY;47,XXX; and 2% to 3% each have 46,X,Xp- and 46,X,r[X].

When breast development fails to occur at the expected age or when breast development begins and then fails to be completed, the clinician should consider premature ovarian failure. This diagnosis is established easily by the finding of elevated gonadotropins in association with decreased levels of ovarian sex hormones. Estrogen administration should be initiated as soon as possible. Estrogen is necessary to stimulate breast development, genital tract maturation, and the beginning of menstruation. Administration of a low dose of estrogen is used to initiate secondary sexual maturation. Estradiol-17β (Estrace), 0.5 mg/day or conjugated equine estrogens (Premarin), 0.3 mg/day is an appropriate starting dose. Once breast budding begins, the dosage may be doubled. The usual dose of estrogen to initiate menarche is estradiol-17β, 2 mg/day or conjugated equine estrogens, 1.25 mg/day. Once menarche occurs, medroxyprogesterone (Provera), 5 to 10 mg for 10 to 14 days every month will complete breast development and produce cyclic uterine bleeding. If an excessive amount of estrogen is administered initially, epiphyseal closure may begin and long bone growth will be truncated and adult height compromised. A delay in estrogen administration can lead to the development of osteoporosis beginning during the teenage years.

Hypothalamic Dysfunction

The arcuate nucleus of the hypothalamus secretes gonadotropin-releasing hormone (GnRH) in cyclic bursts, which stimulates release of gonadotropins from the anterior pituitary gland. Dysfunction of the arcuate nucleus disrupts the short hormonal loop between the hypothalamus and pituitary, resulting in absent FSH or LH secretion. Consequently, the ovaries are not stimulated to secrete estradiol and secondary sexual maturation is delayed.

An unusual cause of hypothalamic dysfunction is *Kallmann syndrome*. In this disorder, the olfactory tracts are hypoplastic and the arcuate nucleus does not secrete GnRH. Young women with Kallmann syndrome have no sense of smell and fail to have breast development and secondary sexual hair growth. The diagnosis of this condition can be made on initial physical examination by challenging olfactory function with known odors. Patients with this disorder fail to recognize common odors such as coffee or rubbing alcohol. The prognosis for successful secondary sexual maturation and reproduction is excellent in Kallmann syndrome. Secondary sexual maturation can be stimulated by the administration of exogenous hormones or by the administration of pulsatile GnRH. When pregnancy is desired, ovulation can be induced by exogenous gonadotropin administration or by administration of pulsatile GnRH. Once pregnancy is established, the lack of pituitary secretions has no adverse effects.

Less common causes of hypothalamic dysfunction are *neoplasms and inflammatory disorders of the hypothalamic–pituitary axis*. Examples are craniopharyngioma, hamartoma of the pituitary stalk, and sarcoidosis of the hypothalamus. More than 70% of cases are associated with calcifications in the suprasellar region on plain skull x-ray. If a suprasellar neoplasm is strongly suspected, a magnetic resonance image of the hypothalamic–pituitary area is indicated.

Use of marijuana by prepubertal and intrapubertal boys and girls delays the onset of puberty. Marijuana blocks the release of

GnRH from the hypothalamus; thus marijuana truncates gonadotropin secretion by the pituitary gland, which in turn delays gonadal function. With the increasing incidence of drug abuse by adolescents, this must be considered in the differential diagnosis of hypogonadotropic–hypogonadism.

Body Weight

Body weight seems to be a critical element for establishing full secondary sexual maturation, including the capacity for reproduction. Girls who are *underweight* have delayed puberty. Moreover, girls who participate in *strenuous athletics* such as gymnastics, ballet, and competitive running may experience pubertal delay. Young female athletes who have pubertal delay have the normal onset and sequence of secondary sexual maturation when they decrease their level of training. No residual harm results from this pubertal delay. Full reproductive function will be attained. However, there is risk of osteoporosis if ovarian estrogen secretion is delayed for many years.

Genital Tract Anomalies

During fetal life, müllerian ducts develop and fuse in the female fetus to form the upper reproductive tract (i.e., the fallopian tubes, uterus, and upper vagina). The lower and midportion of the vagina develop from the canalization of the genital plate. Approximately 1 in 10,000 females has a birth defect of the reproductive tract that presents as primary amenorrhea. The simplest genital tract anomaly is *imperforate hymen*. In this condition, the genital plate canalization is incomplete and the hymen is, therefore, closed. Menarche occurs at the appropriate time, but because there is obstruction to the passage of menstrual blood, it is not apparent. This condition presents with pain in the area of the uterus and a bulging vaginal introitus. Hymenotomy is the definitive therapy.

In *müllerian agenesis (Rokitansky-Küster-Hauser syndrome)*, the uterus is absent along with its cervical extremity and the vagina. All of the endocrine events of puberty occur at the proper time as ovarian development is unaffected. The young woman establishes normal breast development, sexual hair growth, and ovulation. Yet, there is no menstruation. Physical examination leads to the diagnosis of müllerian agenesis. Renal anomalies (e.g., reduplication of the ureters, horseshoe kidney, or unilateral renal agenesis) occur in 25% to 35% of cases, and skeletal anomalies such as scoliosis occur in 15% to 25% of these women. Rokitansky-Küster-Hauser syndrome is generally sporadic in expression, although families displaying autosomal recessive inheritance have been documented. If there is an affected child, the estimated risk of recurrence in future female offspring is approximately 4%; there is no way to determine whether the inheritance is familial or sporadic.

There are several therapeutic approaches to this condition. An artificial vagina may be created by repetitive pressure to the perineum or by surgical construction followed by a split-thickness skin graft. After creation of a vagina, these women are able to have sexual intercourse. With the advances in assisted reproductive technologies including in vitro fertilization (IVF) and surrogacy, it is possible for women with this condition to have a genetic child.

Precocious Puberty

If physical signs of *secondary sexual development appear before the age of 8 years*, the physician should consider the diagnosis of precocious puberty. Precocious puberty occurs in girls more frequently than in boys. Most precocious puberty is isosexual (i.e., the sequence of pubertal events is appropriate for sexual development and leads to full sexual maturation). *Idiopathic isosexual precocious puberty* has no serious pathology. It causes only an advance in sexual maturation and carries the risk of short stature because of premature closure of the epiphyseal plates.

Occasionally, isosexual precocious puberty results from *neoplasms of the hypothalamic–pituitary stalk or transient inflammatory conditions of the hypothalamus*. In these situations, although sexual development begins early, the rate of sexual development is slower than the usual rate. In the case of inflammatory conditions, sexual development may begin and end abruptly. Laboratory studies show either an appropriate rise in gonadotropins or a steady gonadotropin level in the prepubertal range.

Precocious puberty may be the result of *inappropriate secretion of androgens or estrogens.* The most common cause of inappropriate hormone secretion is *congenital adrenal hyperplasia of the 21-hydroxylase type.* In this disorder, the adrenal glands are unable to produce adequate amounts of cortisol as a result of a partial block in the conversion of progesterone to desoxycorticosterone. Because this step is mediated by the enzymatic action of 21-hydroxylase, defi-

ciency of the enzyme leads to an accumulation and release of adrenal androgens, which results in precocious adrenarche. In girls, there is premature development of pubic hair followed by axillary hair. Breast development either does not occur or is incomplete for the stage of sexual development. Measurement of adrenal androgens—such as dehydroepiandrosterone, dehydroepiandrosterone sulfate, and androstenedione—leads to the diagnosis. Medical therapy consists of steroid replacement, a standard regimen being hydrocortisone (25 mg/m^2/day) in divided doses, with 9-α-fluorocortisone at a dosage of 15 to 75 mg twice a day for those afflicted with salt wasting. Therapy should be instituted as early as possible to achieve maximum benefit (Figure 35.3). Surgical

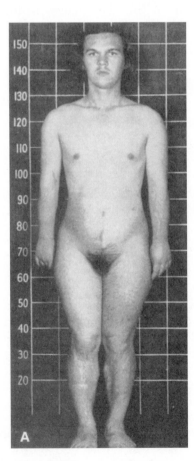
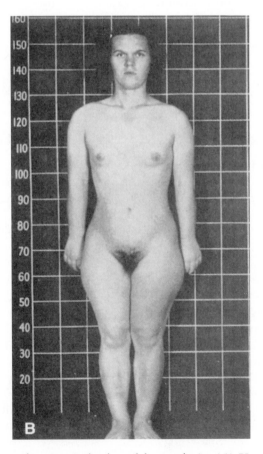

FIGURE 35.3. Medical treatment of congenital adrenal hyperplasia. (*A*) Untreated 16-year-old with characteristic short stature, short arms and legs, absence of breast development, and growth of hair on body and face. (*B*) Same patient after 3 months of cortisone therapy. Note alteration of body habitus to a more feminine configuration and reduction of hirsutism.

therapy is often also required, depending on the degree and nature of the effect, including removal of redundant erectile tissue, provision of an exteriorized vagina to allow for menstruation and sexual intercourse, and preservation of the sexually sensitive glans clitoris.

In boys with this condition, there is premature enlargement of the phallus and the appearance of axillary and pubic hair. However, the testicles remain small because the source of androgens is of adrenal rather than of testicular origin. Again, adrenal hormones are elevated. Once the diagnosis is established, treatment should commence immediately to avoid or minimize short stature.

Rarely, there is *inappropriate secretion of estrogens* in girls. This can result from ovarian neoplasms or from inappropriate secretion of chorionic gonadotropin by hepatic or gonadal neoplasms. In these con-

ditions, there is rapid breast development without sexual hair growth. Menarche may be established within a few months of thelarche. This deviation from the expected pattern of secondary sexual maturation suggests an abnormality.

Isosexual precocious puberty can be treated by the tonic administration of an exogenous GnRH agonist. These agents block the periodic secretion of GnRH and suppress pituitary gonadotropin secretion. If precocious puberty is within a few months of the expected time of normal puberty, it is probably wise to allow puberty to progress. However, if puberty is advanced by several years, the process should be arrested. If the events of puberty do not progress in the expected way, an evaluation for hormonal abnormalities and/or hypothalamic–pituitary tumors is advised. If an abnormality is found, it should be treated specifically.

CASE STUDIES

Case 35A

A 15-year-old girl is brought by her mother for evaluation because she has never menstruated.

Questions Case 35A

Which of the following is the normal sequence in secondary sexual maturation?

A. Hair growth, growth spurt, thelarche, menarche
B. Growth spurt, hair growth, thelarche, menarche
C. Thelarche, hair growth, growth spurt, menarche
D. Thelarche, growth spurt, menarche, hair growth

Answer: C

Secondary sexual maturation should occur in an orderly sequence. Table 35.1 summarizes these events.

Which of the following laboratory studies would be indicated on initial evaluation on this patient?

A. Chromosomal karyotype
B. Computed tomography (CT) scan of the pituitary gland
C. FSH and LH
D. Progesterone

Answer: C

Although all the tests listed may be used as part of the evaluation in different situations, for the initial evaluation of the patient described, gonadotropin measurement is the most cost-effective.

Initial laboratory studies suggest premature ovarian failure. Which of the following would be the most useful diagnostic test for establishing this diagnosis?

A. Chromosomal karyotype
B. CT scan of the pituitary gland
C. Dehydroepiandrosterone, dehydroepiandrosterone sulfate
D. Progesterone

Answer: A

Premature ovarian failure is diagnosed by finding elevated (i.e., menopausal) gonadotropin levels. The most common etiology of this in prepubertal girls is Turner syndrome in which one X chromosome is absent. Chromosomal karyotype is, therefore, the most appropriate test.

Case 35B

A 16-year-old girl presents with primary amenorrhea. She has normal secondary sexual development including breast development, pubic and axillary hair growth, and adult height.

Questions Case 35B

The differential diagnosis would include all of the following EXCEPT

A. Müllerian agenesis
B. Pregnancy
C. Premature ovarian failure
D. Kallmann syndrome

Answer: D

Patients with Kallmann syndrome do not have spontaneous breast development or sexual hair growth and, therefore, would not fit this clinical presentation.

A physical examination reveals absence of the vagina. Based on this additional information, which management would you institute?

A. Creation of an artificial vagina
B. Administration of exogenous estrogen
C. Administration of pulsatile GnRH
D. Counseling to decrease strenuous physical activity

Answer: A

The patient described has müllerian agenesis (Rokitansky-Küster-Hauser syndrome). Because there is no uterus, the patient never has menstrual periods. Once the vagina is developed, either by surgical construction or by a series of perineal pressure exercises, normal sexual activity can be anticipated.

36

AMENORRHEA AND DYSFUNCTIONAL UTERINE BLEEDING

This chapter deals primarily with APGO Objective(s):

OBJECTIVE 47   Amenorrhea

A. Define primary amenorrhea, secondary amenorrhea, and oligomenorrhea.

B. Describe the physical, endocrinologic, and psychological causes of amenorrhea and the approach to the diagnosis and management of each.

OBJECTIVE 49   Normal and Abnormal Uterine Bleeding

A. Discuss the physiology and endocrinology of the normal menstrual cycle.

(Continued)

B. Define abnormal uterine bleeding and dysfunctional uterine bleeding, and describe the causes, pathophysiology, diagnosis and management options for each.

Menstruation (cyclic uterine bleeding) is usually established by age 13 and continues until approximately age 45 to 50. Once established at puberty, in most women menstrual cycles remain regular and predictable until menopause approaches, at which time some menstrual irregularity may be experienced.

Amenorrhea and dysfunctional uterine bleeding are the most common gynecologic disorders of reproductive-age women. *Absence of menstruation is amenorrhea; irregular menstruation without anatomic lesions of the uterus is dysfunctional uterine bleeding.* Amenorrhea and dysfunctional uterine bleeding are discussed as separate topics in this chapter. However, the pathophysiology underlying amenorrhea and dysfunctional uterine bleeding are often the same.

AMENORRHEA

If a young woman has never menstruated, she is classified as having *primary amenorrhea*. If a menstrual aged woman has previously menstruated but has failed to menstruate within 6 months, she is classified as having *secondary amenorrhea*. The designation of primary or secondary amenorrhea has no bearing on the severity of the underlying disorder or on the prognosis for restoring cyclic ovulation. Terms often confused with these include *oligomenorrhea*, defined as a reduction of the frequency of menses, with the interval being more than 40 days but less than 6 months, and *hypomenorrhea*, defined as a reduction in the number of days or the amount of menstrual flow. Amenorrhea not caused by pregnancy probably occurs in 5% or less of all women during their menstrual lives.

The physiology of ovulatory menstrual cycles is presented in Chapter 34. When there is disruption of hypothalamic-pituitary-ovarian endocrine function or alteration of the genital outflow tract (obstruction of the uterus, cervix, or vagina or scarring of the endometrium), menstruation ceases. Causes of amenorrhea are divided into those arising from (1) pregnancy, (2) hypothalamic–pituitary dysfunction, (3) ovarian dysfunction, and (4) alteration of the genital outflow tract.

Pregnancy

Because the most common cause of amenorrhea is pregnancy, it is essential to exclude pregnancy in the evaluation of amenorrhea. Often, a history of breast fullness, weight gain, nausea, and a "feeling of being pregnant" suggest the diagnosis of pregnancy. The diagnosis can be confirmed by a pregnancy test. It is important to rule out pregnancy to allay the patient's anxiety and to avoid unnecessary testing. Also, some of the treatments for other causes of amenorrhea can be harmful to an ongoing pregnancy.

Hypothalamic–Pituitary Dysfunction

Release of hypothalamic gonadotropin-releasing hormone (GnRH) occurs in a pulsatile fashion. When this pulsatile secretion of GnRH is disrupted or altered, the anterior pituitary gland is not stimulated to secrete follicle-stimulating hormone (FSH) and luteinizing hormone (LH). The result is an absence of regular ovulation and menstruation.

GnRH release is modulated by catecholamine secretion from the central nervous system and by feedback of sex steroids

TABLE 36.1. Causes of Hypothalamic–Pituitary Amenorrhea

Functional causes
  Weight loss
  Excessive exercise
  Obesity
Drug-induced causes
  Marijuana
  Tranquilizers
Neoplastic causes
  Prolactin-secreting pituitary adenomas
  Craniopharyngioma
  Hypothalamic hamartoma

Psychogenic causes
  Chronic anxiety
  Pseudocyesis
  Anorexia nervosa
Other causes
  Head injury
  Chronic medical illness

from the ovaries. Alterations in catecholamine secretion and metabolism and in sex steroid hormone feedback disrupt ovulation and menstruation. In addition, alteration of blood flow from the hypothalamus to the pituitary gland through the hypothalamic–pituitary portal plexus can disrupt the signaling process that leads to ovulation. This alteration can be caused by tumors that alter blood flow.

The most common causes of hypothalamic–pituitary dysfunction are presented in Table 36.1. Most hypothalamic–pituitary amenorrhea is of functional origin and can be corrected by modifying causal behavior or by stimulating gonadotropin secretion.

In each of the disorders resulting in hypothalamic–pituitary amenorrhea, there is interference with the hypothalamic release of GnRH or interference with the pituitary secretion of FSH and LH. The physician cannot differentiate hypothalamic–pituitary causes of amenorrhea from ovarian or genital outflow causes by medical history or even physical examination alone. For example, women with hypothalamic–pituitary dysfunction usually do not complain of hot flushes and sleep problems as do women who have ovarian failure. However, there are some clues in the medical history and physical examination that would suggest a hypothalamic–pituitary etiology for amenorrhea. A history of any condition listed in Table 36.1 should cause the physi-

TABLE 36.2. Signs and Symptoms of Ovarian-associated Estrogen Deficiency

Symptoms	Signs
Hot flushes	Vaginal dryness
Mood changes	Thin vaginal
Sleep disturbances	epithelium
Vaginal dryness	Thinning of skin
Dyspareunia	Hot flushes

cian to consider hypothalamic–pituitary dysfunction.

The way to definitively identify hypothalamic–pituitary dysfunction is to measure FSH, LH, and prolactin in blood. In these conditions, FSH and LH are in the low range. Prolactin is normal in most conditions but is elevated in prolactin-secreting pituitary adenomas.

Ovarian Failure

In ovarian failure, the ovarian follicles are either exhausted or are resistant to stimulation by pituitary FSH and LH. As the ovaries fail, *blood concentrations of FSH and LH increase.* This is the basis for the chemical diagnosis of ovarian failure. Women with ovarian failure experience the symptoms and signs of estrogen deficiency that are listed in Table 36.2.

TABLE 36.3.	Causes of Ovarian Failure

Chromosomal causes
  Turner's syndrome (45,X gonadal dysgenesis)
  X chromosome long-arm deletion (46,XX q5)
Unknown causes
  Gonadotropin-resistant ovary syndrome (Savage's syndrome)
  Premature natural menopause

Immunologic cause
  Autoimmune ovarian failure (Blizzard's syndrome)
Iatrogenic causes
  Ovarian failure because of effects of alkylating chemotherapy
  Menopause ("normal, or physiologic")

Women with estrogen deficiency caused by ovarian failure usually experience hot flushes, whereas those with estrogen deficiency caused by hypothalamic–pituitary dysfunction usually do not experience hot flushes. This is an important differential point in the medical history. A summary of causes is presented in Table 36.3. A detailed description of these causes is presented in Chapter 38.

Obstruction of the Genital Outflow Tract

Obstruction of the genital outflow tract prevents menstrual bleeding even if ovulation occurs. Most cases of outflow obstruction result from congenital *abnormalities in the development and canalization of the müllerian ducts.* Imperforate hymen and absence of a uterus and/or vagina are the most common anomalies that result in primary amenorrhea. Even with attempted surgical correction, menstruation and fertility are often not restored.

Scarring of the uterine cavity (Asherman's syndrome) is the most frequent anatomic cause of secondary amenorrhea. Women who undergo dilation and curettage (D&C) for retained products of pregnancy are at particular risk for developing scarring of the endometrium. Moreover, scarring may occur as the result of infection of the uterine cavity. Cases of mild scarring can be corrected by surgical lysis of the adhesions performed by D&C or hysteroscopy. However, severe cases are often refractory to

therapy. Estrogen therapy should be added to the surgical treatment to stimulate endometrial regeneration of the denuded areas.

Treatment of Amenorrhea

It is essential to first establish a cause for the amenorrhea. The progesterone "challenge test" is commonly used to determine whether or not the patient has adequate estrogen. An injection of 100 mg of progesterone in oil or a course of oral medroxyprogesterone acetate is expected to induce progesterone withdrawal bleeding within a few days. If this does occur, the patient is likely to be chronically anovulatory or oligo-ovulatory. If withdrawal bleeding does not occur, the patient is felt to be hypoestrogenic or have an anatomic condition such as Asherman's syndrome or outflow tract obstruction.

In hypothalamic amenorrhea, ovulation can usually be restored by changing behavior in women who have functional amenorrhea. Women with central nervous system tumors should be considered on an individual basis for surgical therapy. Often, central nervous system tumors are benign and need not be removed. The *hyperprolactinemia associated with some pituitary adenomas* results in amenorrhea and galactorrhea. Approximately 80% of all pituitary tumors secrete prolactin, causing galactorrhea, and these are treated with either cabergoline (Dostinex) or the dopamine agonist *bromocriptine (Parlodel).* In approximately 5% of patients with hyperprolactinemia and galactorrhea, the underlying etiology is hypothyroidism. A low serum thyroxine (T_4) level results in a lack of negative feedback to the hypothalamic–pituitary axis. In addition, there is a lack of positive feedback on dopamine. The reduced dopamine secretion results in elevated levels of TSH (thyroid-stimulating hormone) and prolactin. Treatment for hypothyroidism is thyroid replacement therapy.

Ovulation can also be induced by the administration of gonadotropins (see Chapter 39). Women with genital tract obstruction require surgery to create a vagina or to restore genital tract integrity. Menstruation will never be established if the uterus is absent. Women with premature ovarian failure require exogenous estrogen replacement. Hormone replacement regimens are discussed in Chapter 38.

DYSFUNCTIONAL UTERINE BLEEDING

Failure to ovulate results in either amenorrhea or irregular uterine bleeding. *Irregular bleeding, unrelated to anatomic lesions of the uterus, is referred to as dysfunctional uterine bleeding.* Dysfunctional uterine bleeding is most likely to occur in association with anovulation as found in polycystic ovarian disease, exogenous obesity, and adrenal hyperplasia.

Patients with amenorrhea do not ovulate at all, and those with dysfunctional bleeding do so only periodically. However, although women with amenorrhea do not menstruate, women with dysfunctional uterine bleeding have irregular, often heavy, uterine bleeding. This difference relates to estrogen levels. *Women with amenorrhea and no genital tract obstruction are in a state of estrogen deficiency.* There is inadequate estrogen to stimulate growth and development of the endometrium. Therefore, there is inadequate endometrium for uterine bleeding to occur. In contrast, *women with dysfunctional uterine bleeding are in a state of chronic estrus.* They have constant, noncyclic blood estrogen concentrations that stimulate growth and development of the endometrium. Without the predictable effect of ovulation, there is an absence of progesterone-induced changes. Eventually, the endometrium outgrows its blood supply and sloughs from the uterus, at irregular times and in unpredictable amounts.

When there is chronic stimulation of the endometrium from low plasma concentrations of estrogens, the episodes of dysfunctional uterine bleeding are infrequent and light. Alternatively, when there is chronic stimulation of the endometrium from increased plasma concentrations of estrogens, the episodes of dysfunctional uterine bleeding can be frequent and heavy. In this situation, the dysfunctional uterine bleeding can result in hemorrhage so heavy that it requires hospitalization for medical treatment or even minor surgical therapy (dilation of the cervix and curettage of the uterine cavity) if medical therapy is not successful.

Women who develop secondary amenorrhea may first experience a phase of dysfunctional uterine bleeding. This can occur because of weight loss, prolactin-secreting pituitary adenomas, premature ovarian failure, and other causes of amenorrhea. Because amenorrhea and dysfunctional uterine bleeding both result from anovulation, it is not surprising that they can occur at different times in the same patient.

Dysfunctional uterine bleeding can occasionally occur in association with ovulation. Although this may seem a contradiction, subtle alterations in the mechanisms of ovulation can produce abnormal cycles even when ovulation occurs (e.g., the luteal phase defect). In the *luteal phase defect,* ovulation does occur; however, the corpus luteum of the ovary is not fully developed to secrete adequate quantities of progesterone to support the endometrium for the usual 13 to 14 days and is not adequate to support a pregnancy if conception does occur. The menstrual cycle is shortened, and menstruation occurs earlier than expected. Although this is not classical dysfunctional uterine bleeding, it is considered to be in the same category.

Another example is midcycle spotting in which patients report bleeding at the time

TABLE 36.4. Anatomic Causes of Irregular Bleeding	
Uterine lesions	Vaginal lesions
Myomas	Carcinoma, sarcoma, or adenosis
Polyps	Laceration or trauma
Endometrial carcinoma	Infections
Cervical lesions	Foreign bodies (diaphragm, tampons)
Neoplasia	Pessaries
Polyps	Bleeding from other sites
Cervical eversion	Urethral caruncle
Cervicitis	Infected urethral diverticulum
Cervical condyloma	Gastrointestinal bleeding
	Labial lesion (neoplasm, trauma, infection)

of ovulation. In the absence of demonstrable pathology, this self-limited bleeding can be attributed to the sudden drop in estrogen level at this time of the cycle.

Diagnosis of Dysfunctional Uterine Bleeding

Dysfunctional uterine bleeding should be suspected when menstrual cycles are not regular and predictable and when cycles are not associated with the premenstrual molimina accompanying ovulatory cycles. These include breast fullness, abdominal bloating, mood changes, edema, weight gain, and menstrual cramps.

Before a diagnosis of dysfunctional uterine bleeding is made, anatomic causes of abnormal uterine bleeding must be excluded. These include uterine leiomyomata, inflammation/infection of the genital tract, carcinoma of the cervix or endometrium, cervical erosions, cervical polyps, and lesions of the vagina (Table 36.4). Women with these organic causes for bleeding typically have regular, ovulatory cycles with superimposed irregular bleeding.

If the diagnosis is uncertain from history and physical examination alone, a woman may keep a basal body temperature chart for 6 to 8 weeks to look for the shift in the basal temperature that occurs with ovulation. A luteal phase progestin may also be measured. In the cases of anovulation and irregular bleeding, an endometrial biopsy may reveal endometrial hyperplasia. Because dys-

functional uterine bleeding results from chronic, unopposed estrogenic stimulation of the endometrium, the endometrium appears proliferative or, with prolonged estrogenic stimulation, hyperplastic.

Treatment of Dysfunctional Uterine Bleeding

The risks to a woman with dysfunctional uterine bleeding are incapacitating blood loss, endometrial hyperplasia, and/or carcinoma. Uterine bleeding can be severe enough to require hospitalization. Both hemorrhage and endometrial hyperplasia can be prevented by appropriate management.

The primary goal of treatment of dysfunctional uterine bleeding is to convert the proliferative endometrium into secretory endometrium, which results in predictable uterine withdrawal bleeding. This goal can be achieved by administration of a progestational agent for a minimum of 10 days, the most commonly used being medroxyprogesterone acetate (Provera; Table 36.5). When the progestational agent is discontinued, uterine withdrawal bleeding ensues, thereby mimicking physiologic withdrawal of progesterone.

As an alternative, administration of oral contraceptives suppresses the endometrium and establishes regular, predictable withdrawal cycles. No particular oral contraceptive preparation is better than any of the others for this purpose. Women who take oral contraceptives as treatment of

TABLE 36.5. Progestational Therapy for Anovulatory Uterine Bleeding

Drug	Dose
Norethindrone (Aygestin)	5–10 mg qid for the first 7–10 days of each month
Norethindrone acetate (Norlutate)	5–10 mg qid for the first 7–10 days of each month
Medroxyprogesterone acetate (Provera; other names for Provera include Cycrin and Amen)	10–20 mg qid for the first 7–10 days of each month
Megestrol acetate (Megace)	40 mg qid for 3 months
Progesterone in oil (Lipolutin)	50–100 mg IM monthly
Progesterone, micronized (Prometrium)	400 mg qid for the first 7–10 days of each month
17α-Hydroxyprogesterone (Delalutin)	125 mg IM monthly

dysfunctional uterine bleeding often resume dysfunctional uterine bleeding after therapy is discontinued.

If a patient is being treated for a particularly heavy bleeding episode, once organic pathology has been ruled out, treatment should focus on two issues: (1) control of the acute episode and (2) prevention of future recurrences. Both high-dose estrogen and progestin therapy as well as combination treatment (oral contraceptive pills, 4 per day) have been advocated for management of heavy dysfunctional bleeding in the acute phase. Long-term preventive management may include either intermittent progestin treatment or oral contraceptives.

If there is an associated anemia, it should be appropriately evaluated and treated.

CASE STUDIES

Case 36A

A 27-year-old woman complains of 6 months of amenorrhea.

Questions Case 36A

All of the following could affect her menstrual cycles except

A. Change in body weight
B. Marijuana use
C. Müllerian agenesis
D. Pregnancy

Answer: C

Patients with müllerian agenesis present with primary amenorrhea, not secondary amenorrhea as this patient does. In all patients of reproductive age, pregnancy should be ruled out as the first stage of evaluation.

If evaluation reveals elevated gonadotropins, which of the following statements are correct?

A. The patient may have a loss of chromosomal material on the long arm of the X chromosome
B. Her ovaries may be depleted of ovarian follicles
C. She may have numerous ovarian follicles that are resistant to FSH and LH
D. She may have hypothalamic dysfunction

Answer: A, B, C

A, B, and C are all clinical circumstances that can result in elevated gonodatropins. Each can be described as ovarian failure. The elevated gonadotropins are a result of the ovary not producing adequate amounts of hormones to feed back to the pituitary. Hypothalamus dysfunction would result in lower or normal gonadotropins.

If evaluation reveals low gonadotropins, which of the following statements are correct?

A. The patient has decreased hypothalamic release of gonadotropin-releasing hormone
B. Her ovaries are depleted of ovarian follicles
C. Ovulation can be induced by administration of exogenous FSH and LH
D. The examiner should inquire about changes in body weight, stress, and marijuana use

Answer: C, D

A low level of gonadotropins does not usually suggest decreased GnRH release, because any aberration in the normally delicate pulsatile release can result in loss of physiologic mechanisms. The importance of low gonadotropin levels is that it is not ovarian failure that has caused amenorrhea.

Case 36B

A 33-year-old woman gives a history of irregular menstrual cycles. She has basal body temperature records of 12 months' duration that reveal ovulation occurring three times during that period.

Questions Case 36B

Which of the following statements are correct?

A. The patient has interruption of the cyclic interaction between gonadotropins and sex steroid hormones

B. The endometrium varies between a proliferative endometrium and a secretory endometrium every month
C. The patient is at high risk for endometrial hyperplasia
D. She does not need to use contraception to prevent pregnancy

Answer: A

This is a good example of intermittent ovulation resulting in dysfunctional bleeding. The patient's risk of endometrial hyperplasia is very low because the intermittent progestational effect of ovulatory cycles is protective. The endometrium becomes secretory only when ovulation has occurred, which in this patient was three times in 1 year. Contraception is still needed, because there is no way to predict when she will ovulate.

Further evaluation reveals tonic elevation of LH. Based on this additional data, which of the following statements are correct?

A. LH can be suppressed by administration of oral contraceptives
B. Ovulation can probably be induced by administration of clomiphene citrate
C. The patient may have elevated androgens
D. Obesity frequently coexists with dysfunctional uterine bleeding

Answer: All

This clinical picture is commonly seen in patients with oligo-ovulation and oligomenorrhea. If the patient wants to conceive, medical induction of ovulation can usually be accomplished. Otherwise, oral contraceptives are commonly used to regulate menstrual periods. Hyperandrogenism may be a contributory factor to the irregular ovulation (see Chapter 37). Obesity can also contribute, because peripheral fat stores convert androstenedione to estrone, thereby chemically increasing estrogen production and adversely affecting cyclic estrogen feedback.

37

HIRSUTISM AND VIRILIZATION

CHAPTER OBJECTIVES

This chapter deals primarily with APGO Objective(s):

OBJECTIVE 48   Hirsutism and Virilization

A. Describe the normal variations of secondary sexual characteristics.

B. Define hirsutism and virilization, and describe the causes (ovarian, adrenal, pituitary, and pharmacological) of each as well as their diagnosis and managements.

A woman who complains of being too hairy or too masculine presents a diagnostic and therapeutic challenge for the physician. Hirsutism and virilization may be clinical clues to an underlying *androgen excess disorder.* The physician should consider the sites of androgen production and the mechanisms of androgen action when evaluating and treating hirsutism and virilization. Idiopathic (constitutional or familial) hirsutism is the most common nonpathologic etiology, representing about one half of all cases. This is a diagnosis of exclusion. *The most common pathologic cause of hirsutism is polycystic ovarian syndrome; the second most common, adrenal hyperplasia.* These conditions must be established by laboratory diagnosis. *Treatment of androgen excess should be directed at suppressing the source of androgen excess or blocking androgen action at the receptor site.*

Androgens play three key roles as precursors for estrogen biosynthesis and also as stimuli to sexual hair growth. However, exposure to excess androgens, through either excess production or increased action, results in increased body hair and acne.

Hirsutism is defined as excess body hair. It is manifested initially by the appearance of midline *terminal hair.* Terminal hair is darker, coarser, somewhat kinkier than vellus hair, which is soft, downy, and fine. Care must be taken to evaluate the possibility that excess terminal hair is familial, not medical in origin. When a woman is exposed to excess androgens, terminal hair first appears on the lower abdomen and around the nipples, next around the chin and upper lip, and finally between the breasts and on the lower back. Usually a woman with hirsutism also has *acne.* In Western cultures, terminal hair on the abdomen, breasts, and face is considered unsightly and presents a cosmetic problem for women. At the first sign of hirsutism, women often consult their physician to seek a cause for the excess hair growth and seek treatment to eliminate it.

Virilization is defined as masculinization of a woman. It is associated with marked increase in circulating *testosterone.* As a woman becomes virilized, she first notices enlargement of the clitoris followed by tem-

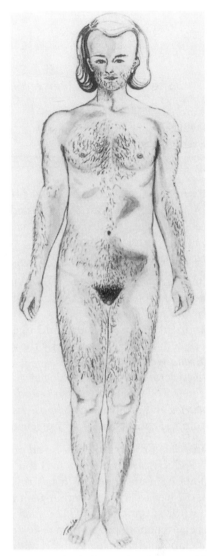

FIGURE 37.1.   A woman with **virilization.** Note the clitoral enlargement, temporal balding, masculine body habitus, and hirsutism.

poral balding, deepening of the voice, involution of the breasts, and a remodeling of the limb-shoulder girdle as well as hirsutism. Over time, she takes on a more masculine appearance, as shown in Figure 37.1.

ANDROGEN PRODUCTION AND ANDROGEN ACTION

In women, *androgens are produced in the adrenal glands, the ovaries, and adipose*

TABLE 37.1. Sites of Androgen Production			
Site	DHEA-S (Percent)	Androstenedione (Percent)	Testosterone (Percent)
Adrenal glands	90	50	25
Ovaries	10	50	25
Extraglandular	0	0	50

tissue where there is extraglandular production of testosterone from androstenedione. The following three androgens may be measured in evaluating a woman with hirsutism and virilization.

1. *Dehydroepiandrosterone* (DHEA): a weak androgen secreted principally by the *adrenal glands.*
2. *Androstenedione:* a weak androgen secreted in equal amounts by the *adrenal glands and ovaries.*
3. *Testosterone:* a potent androgen secreted by the *adrenal glands and ovaries* and produced in *adipose tissue* from the conversion of androstenedione.

The sites of androgen production and proportions produced are presented in Table 37.1. In addition, testosterone is also converted within the hair follicle and within genital skin to *dihydrotestosterone* (DHT), which is an androgen even more potent than testosterone. This metabolic conversion is the result of the local action of 5α-reductase on testosterone at these sites. This is the basis for constitutional hirsutism, which is discussed later.

Adrenal androgen production is regulated by pituitary secretion of adrenocorticotropic hormone (ACTH). ACTH stimulates the adrenal cortical production of cortisol. In the metabolic sequence of cortisol production, DHEA is one precursor hormone. In enzymatic deficiencies of adrenal steroidogenesis (21-hydroxylase deficiency and 11β-hydroxylase deficiency), DHEA accumulates and is further metabolized to androstenedione and testosterone. The flow of adrenal hormone production is shown in Figure 37.2.

Ovarian androgen production is largely under the control of luteinizing hormone (LH) secretion from the pituitary gland. LH stimulates theca-lutein cells surrounding the ovarian follicles to secrete androstenedione and, to a lesser extent, testosterone. These androgens are precursors for estrogen production by granulosa cells of the ovarian follicles. In conditions of sustained or increased LH secretion, androstenedione and testosterone increase. The metabolic relationship between androgens and estrogens is shown in Figure 37.3.

Extraglandular testosterone production occurs in adipocytes (fat cells) and depends on the magnitude of adrenal and ovarian androstenedione production. When androstenedione production increases, there is a dependent increase in extraglandular testosterone production. When a woman becomes obese, the conversion of androstenedione to testosterone in adipocytes increases.

Testosterone is the primary androgen that causes increased hair growth, acne, and the physical changes associated with virilization. After testosterone is secreted from its site of production, it is bound to a carrier protein—*sex hormone–binding globulin* (SHBG)—and circulates in plasma as a bound steroid hormone. Only a small fraction (1% to 3%) of testosterone is unbound (free). Bound testosterone is unable to attach to testosterone receptors and is, therefore, metabolically inactive. It is the small fraction of free hormone that exerts the effects. SHBG is produced by the liver. Estrogens stimulate hepatic production of SHBG. Greater estrogen production is associated with less free testosterone, whereas decreased estrogen production is associated with increased free testosterone. Therefore, measurement of total testosterone alone may not reflect the amount of biologically active testosterone.

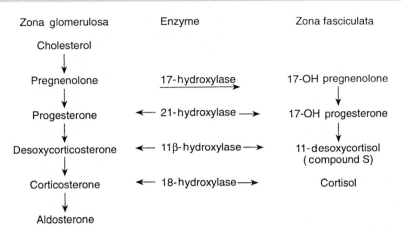

Zona glomerulosa	Enzyme	Zona fasciculata

Cholesterol

↓

Pregnenolone   17-hydroxylase →   17-OH pregnenolone

↓   ↓

Progesterone   ← 21-hydroxylase →   17-OH progesterone

↓   ↓

Desoxycorticosterone   ← 11β-hydroxylase →   11-desoxycortisol
(compound S)

↓   ↓

Corticosterone   ← 18-hydroxylase →   Cortisol

↓

Aldosterone

FIGURE 37.2. A schematic flow chart of adrenal steroidogenesis.

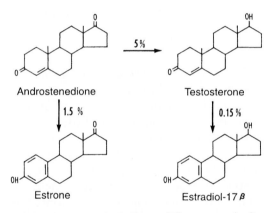

Androstenedione   —5%→   Testosterone

↓1.5 %   ↓0.15 %

Estrone   Estradiol-17β

FIGURE 37.3. The metabolic interrelationships between androgens and estrogens. The percentages indicate the extent of metabolism in adipocytes.

Testosterone receptors are scattered throughout the body. For the purpose of this discussion, testosterone receptors are considered only in hair follicles, sebaceous glands, and genital skin. Free testosterone enters the cytosol of testosterone-dependent cells. There it is bound to a testosterone receptor and carried into the nucleus of the cell to initiate its metabolic action. *When testosterone is excessive,* there is increased hair growth, acne, and rugation of the genital skin. Some individuals have increased 5α-reductase within hair follicles, resulting in excessive local production of DHT.

CONDITIONS CAUSED BY OVARIAN ANDROGEN EXCESS

Polycystic Ovarian Syndrome

Polycystic ovarian syndrome (PCOS) is the *most common cause of androgen excess and hirsutism.* The etiology of this disorder is unknown. Some cases appear to result from a genetic predisposition, whereas others seem to result from obesity or other causes of LH excess. One proposed mechanism for PCOS is shown in Figure 37.4.

PCOS is related to obesity by the following mechanism. LH stimulates the theca-lutein cells to increase androstenedione production. Androstenedione undergoes aromatization to estrone within adipocytes. Although estrone is a weak estrogen, it has a positive-feedback action or stimulating effect on the pituitary secretion of LH. LH secretion is, therefore, stimulated by increased estrogen. With increasing obesity, there is increased conversion of androstenedione to estrone. In many women with PCOS, obesity seems to be the common factor, and the acquisition of body fat coincides with the onset of PCOS. With the increased rise in androstenedione, there is coincident increased testosterone production, which causes acne and hirsutism.

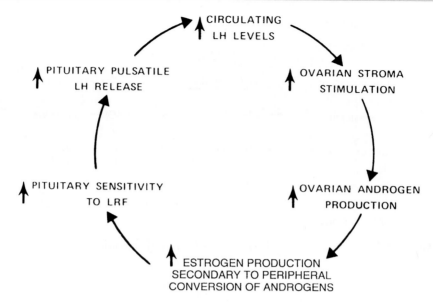

FIGURE 37.4. A mechanism for polycystic ovarian syndrome proposed by Yen. LH = luteinizing hormone; LRF = luteinizing-releasing factor.

Hormonal studies in women with PCOS show the following: (1) increased LH:FSH (follicle-stimulating hormone) ratio, (2) estrone in greater concentration than estradiol, (3) androstenedione at the upper limits of normal or increased, and (4) testosterone at the upper limits of normal or slightly increased. One possible scheme for the evaluation of these women is shown in Figure 37.5.

The symptoms of PCOS include *oligomenorrhea or amenorrhea, anovulation, acne, hirsutism, and infertility.* The disorder is characterized by chronic anovulation or extended periods of infrequent ovulation.

Approximately 30% of patients with PCOS have impaired glucose tolerance and 8% have overt type 2 diabetes mellitus. Screening for diabetes with a fasting glucose level or glucose tolerance test in these patients is a cost-effective test. Acanthosis nigricans has also been found in a significant percentage of these patients. The HAIR-AN syndrome (hyperandrogenism, insulin resistance, acanthosis nigricans) constitutes a defined sub-group of patients with PCOS. Administration of the antihyperglycemic agent metformin also reduces androgen and insulin levels.

PCOS is a functional disorder whose treatment should be targeted to interrupt the disorder's positive-feedback cycle. The most common therapy for PCOS is the *administration of oral contraceptives,* which suppresses pituitary LH production. By suppressing LH, there is decreased production of androstenedione and testosterone. The ovarian contribution to the total androgen pool is thereby decreased. Acne clears, new hair growth is prevented, and there is decreased androgenic stimulation of existing hair follicles. By preventing estrogen excess, oral contraceptives also prevent endometrial hyperplasia. In addition, the women have cyclic predictable withdrawal bleeding episodes.

If a woman with PCOS wishes to conceive, oral contraceptive therapy is not a suitable choice. If the patient is obese, a *weight reduction* diet designed to restore the patient to a normal weight should be instituted. With body weight reduction alone, many women resume regular ovulatory cycles and conceive spontaneously. In some women who desire pregnancy, ovulation induction with clomiphene citrate is needed. Ovulation induction is facilitated by weight reduction in obese women.

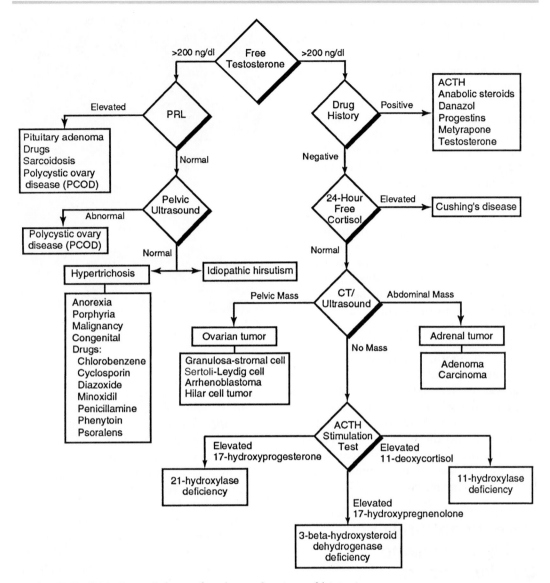

FIGURE 37.5. Scheme for the evaluation of hirsutism.

Hyperthecosis

Hyperthecosis is a *more severe form of polycystic ovarian syndrome.* In cases of hyperthecosis, *androstenedione* production may be so great that testosterone reaches concentrations such that early signs of *virilization* appear. Women with this condition may exhibit some temporal balding, clitoral enlargement, deepening of the voice, and remodeling at the limb-shoulder girdle. Hyperthecosis is refractory to oral contraceptive suppression. It is also more difficult to successfully induce ovulation in women with this condition.

Sertoli-Leydig Cell Tumors

Sertoli-Leydig cell tumors (also called androblastoma and arrhenoblastoma) are ovarian neoplasms that secrete testosterone. These tumors constitute less than 0.4% of ovarian tumors and usually occur in women between the ages of 20 and 40. The tumor is most often unilateral and may reach a size of 7 to 10 cm in diameter.

Women with a Sertoli-Leydig cell tumor have a rapid onset of *acne, hirsutism* (three fourths of patients), *amenorrhea* (one third of patients), and *virilization.* A characteristic clinical course of two overlapping stages is described: first, the stage of *defeminization,* characterized by amenorrhea, breast atrophy, and loss of the subcutaneous fatty deposits responsible for the rounding of the feminine figure; second, the stage of *masculinization,* characterized by clitoral hypertrophy, hirsutism, and deepening of the voice. These changes may occur over 6 months or less.

Laboratory studies of this disorder show suppression of FSH and LH, a low plasma androstenedione, and a marked elevation of testosterone. An ovarian mass is usually palpable on pelvic examination and confirmed by sonography. Once the diagnosis is suspected, there should be no delay in *surgical removal* of the involved ovary. The contralateral ovary should be inspected, and if it is found to be enlarged should be bisected for gross inspection.

Following surgical removal of a Sertoli-Leydig cell tumor, ovulatory cycles return spontaneously and further progression of hirsutism is arrested. If the clitoris has become enlarged, it does not revert to its pretreatment size. However, temporal hair is restored, and the body habitus becomes feminine once again. The 10-year survival rates for this low-grade malignant ovarian tumor approximate 90% to 95%.

Uncommon Virilizing and Masculinizing Ovarian Tumors

Gynandroblastoma is a very rare ovarian tumor, having both granulosa cell and arrhenoblastoma components. The predominant clinical feature is masculinization, although estrogen production may simultaneously produce endometrial hyperplasia and irregular uterine bleeding. Treatment is surgical as in Sertoli-Leydig cell tumors.

Lipid (lipoid) cell tumors are usually small ovarian tumors, containing sheets of round, clear pale-staining cells with a differential histologic diagnosis of hilus cell tumors, stromal luteoma or pregnancy, and Sertoli-Leydig cell tumors. The clinical presentation is *masculinization or defeminization* associated with elevated 17-ketosteroids

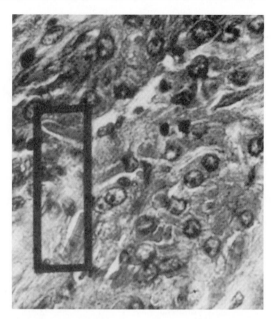

FIGURE 37.6. Reinke crystalloid of the hilus cell tumor.

in many cases. Treatment is surgical as in Sertoli-Leydig cell tumors.

Hilus cell tumors arise from an overgrowth of mature hilar cells or from ovarian mesenchyme. They are characterized clinically by masculinization which supports the idea that hilar cells are the homologs of the interstitial or Leydig cells of the testis. Histologically, the tumors contain pathognomonic Reinke albuminoid crystals in most cases (Figure 37.6), and grossly, they are always small, unilateral, and benign. Treatment is surgical removal.

ADRENAL ANDROGEN EXCESS DISORDERS

Congenital Adrenal Hyperplasia

In the sequence of adrenal steroidogenesis, DHEA is a key hormone. DHEA is a precursor for androstenedione and testosterone. The most common cause of increased adrenal androgen production is adrenal hyperplasia as a result of *21-hydroxylase deficiency.* 21-hydroxylase catalyzes the conversion of progesterone and 17α-hydroxyprogesterone to desoxycorticosterone and compound S.

When 21-hydroxylase is deficient, there is an accumulation of progesterone and 17α-hydroxyprogesterone, which are metabolized subsequently to DHEA. This disorder affects approximately 2% of the population and is caused by an alteration in the gene for 21-hydroxylase, which is carried on chromosome 6. The genetic defect is autosomal recessive and has variable penetrance.

In the most severe form of 21-hydroxylase deficiency, the newly born female infant is virilized (ambiguous genitalia) and suffers from life-threatening salt wasting. However, milder forms are more common and can appear at puberty or even later in adult life. A mild deficiency of 21-hydroxylase is frequently associated with terminal body hair, acne, subtle alterations in menstrual cycles, and infertility. *When 21-hydroxylase deficiency is manifested at puberty,* adrenarche may precede thelarche. The history of pubic hair growth occurring before the onset of breast development may be a clinical clue to this disorder. The *diagnosis of 21-hydroxylase deficiency* is made by measuring *increased dehydroepiandrosterone sulfate (DHEA-S) and androstenedione* in plasma.

A less common cause of adrenal hyperplasia is *11β-hydroxylase deficiency.* 11β-hydroxylase catalyzes the conversion of desoxycorticosterone to cortisol. A deficiency in this enzyme also results in increased androgen production. The clinical features of 11β-hydroxylase deficiency are mild hypertension and mild hirsutism. The *diagnosis* of 11β-hydroxylase deficiency is made by demonstrating increased plasma desoxycorticosterone.

Treatment of Adrenal Hyperplasia

In adrenal hyperplasia, the adrenal glands require increased ACTH secretion to stimulate adequate cortisol production. To maintain normal cortisol production, the adrenal glands oversecrete androgens.

This condition can be managed easily by *supplementing glucocorticoids.* Usually, prednisone, 2.5 mg daily, suppresses adrenal androgen production to within the normal range. When this therapy is instituted, facial acne usually clears promptly, ovulation is restored, and there is no new terminal hair growth.

Medical therapy for adrenal and ovarian disorders cannot resolve hirsutism; it can only suppress new hair growth. Hair that is present must be controlled by shaving, by use of depilatory agents, or by electrolysis.

Cushing Syndrome

In addition to congenital adrenal hyperplasia, Cushing syndrome is a major adrenal disease resulting in adrenal excess. As a result of an adrenal neoplasm or ACTH-producing tumor, the patient demonstrates signs of corticosteroid excess (i.e., truncal obesity, moon-like facies, glucose intolerance, skin thinning with striae, osteoporosis, and proximal muscle weakness in addition to evidence of hyperandrogenism and menstrual irregularities).

Adrenal Neoplasms

An adrenal adenoma is a rare cause of hirsutism. In androgen-secreting adrenal adenomas, there is a rapid increase in hair growth associated with severe acne, amenorrhea, and sometimes virilization. In androgen-secreting adenomas, DHEA-S is usually elevated above 6 mg/ml. The diagnosis is established by computed axial tomography or magnetic resonance imaging of the adrenal glands, which shows the adrenal adenoma. Adrenal adenomas must be removed surgically.

CONSTITUTIONAL HIRSUTISM

Occasionally after a diagnostic evaluation for hirsutism, there is no explanation for the cause of the disorder. By exclusion, this condition is often called *constitutional hirsutism.* Data support the hypothesis that women with constitutional hirsutism have *greater activity of 5α-reductase* than do unaffected women. Treatment of constitutional hirsutism depends on the source of excess androgens. If serum testosterone levels are elevated, thereby suggesting an ovarian source, oral contraceptives are most appropriate. If DHEA-S levels are increased, implicating the adrenal gland as the source of excess androgens, dexamethasone therapy is warranted. If neither is elevated, spironolactone 100 mg/dl is indicated. This latter agent is an androgen receptor blocker, decreases testosterone production by the ovary, and also reduces 5α-reductase activity.

IATROGENIC ANDROGEN EXCESS

Danazol

Danazol is an *attenuated androgen used for the suppression of pelvic endometriosis*. It has androgenic properties, and some women develop hirsutism, acne, and deepening of the voice while taking the drug. If these symptoms develop, the value of the danazol should be weighed against the side effects before continuing therapy. Pregnancy should be ruled out before initiating a course of danazol therapy, because it can produce virilization of the female fetus.

Oral Contraceptives

The progestins in oral contraceptives are impeded androgens. Rarely, a woman taking oral contraceptives develops acne and even hirsutism. If this occurs, another product with a less androgenic progestin should be selected or the Pill should be discontinued. Moreover, evaluation for the coincidental development of late-onset adrenal hyperplasia should be done.

CASE STUDIES

Case 37A

A 19-year-old unmarried woman presents with a complaint of being "too hairy." Her history includes severe irregular menstrual cycles, worsening acne, and hair growth on the face, breasts, and lower abdomen. She is on no medication, is sexually active, uses condoms for contraception, and otherwise feels well. She is depressed about the new hair growth.

Questions Case 37A

The most likely cause for this group of symptoms is

A. Congenital adrenal hyperplasia
B. Sertoli-Leydig cell tumor of the ovary
C. Polycystic ovarian syndrome
D. Constitutional hirsutism

Answer: C

PCOS is the most common cause of this patient's complaints. Although she was focused on the increased hair growth, further history revealed androgen excess in general, with symptoms comparable with those of PCOS.

Which of the following laboratory studies should be performed?

A. DHEA-S
B. Progesterone
C. Androstenedione
D. Testosterone

Answer: A, C, D

LH stimulates androstenedione production, which is aromatized in the fat cells to estrone, which stimulates pituitary LH production: a positive-feedback loop. Very high testosterone levels may suggest the need for a Gyn ultrasound examination of the ovaries, because such levels are associated with Sertoli-Leydig cell tumors. DHEA is the "key hormone" in adrenal hyperplasia. Progesterone levels are not helpful in the workup of hirsutism.

A diagnosis of polycystic ovarian syndrome is made. An initial treatment plan should include

A. Clomiphene citrate
B. Oral contraceptives
C. Prednisone
D. Spironolactone

Answer: B

Because this patient does not wish to get pregnant, oral contraceptive therapy is the best choice of therapy, because it provides effective contraception and also suppresses LH production.

Case 37B

A 27-year-old woman G0 complains of the gradual appearance of terminal hair on the face and lower abdomen. She has noted subtle changes in her menstrual cycle length. She has tried to conceive for 1 year but has been unsuccessful. Her blood pressure is normal.

QUESTIONS CASE 37B

Of the following, which is the most likely cause for these symptoms?

A. Hyperthecosis
B. Constitutional hirsutism
C. Late-onset adrenal hyperplasia (21-hydroxylase type)

D. Late-onset adrenal hyperplasia (11α-hydroxylase type)

Answer: C

Late-onset adrenal hyperplasia should be suspected in women with hirsutism, acne, and menstrual irregularities. Infertility is also common.

Initial laboratory studies show an elevated DHEA-S. Which of the following is the most appropriate next diagnostic study?

A. Gonadotropin-releasing hormone (GnRH) stimulation test
B. ACTH stimulation test
C. FSH and LH measurement
D. Thyroid stimulation test

Answer: B

DHEA-S and androstenedione are elevated in 21-hydroxylase deficiency, the most common disorder causing adrenal hyperplasia. ACTH stimulation confirms this diagnosis.

A diagnosis of late-onset adrenal hyperplasia (21-hydroxylase type) is made. Which of the following therapies should be initiated?

A. Clomiphene citrate
B. Oral contraceptive suppression
C. Prednisone
D. Thyroid-replacement therapy

Answer: C

Glucocorticoid supplementation suppresses adrenal androgen production. Facial acne usually clears, and ovulation resumes.

38

MENOPAUSE

CHAPTER OBJECTIVES

This chapter deals primarily with APGO Objective(s):

OBJECTIVE 51   Climacteric

A. Describe the physiologic changes in the hypothalamic-pituitary-ovarian axis related to the climacteric and menopause and the associated physical, emotional, and sexual symptoms/physical findings. Describe the long-term changes associated with hypoestrogenism.

B. Describe the indications, contraindications, risks and benefits of the treatments of menopause, including hormone replacement, nutrition including calcium intake, exercise, and non-hormonal therapeutic options.

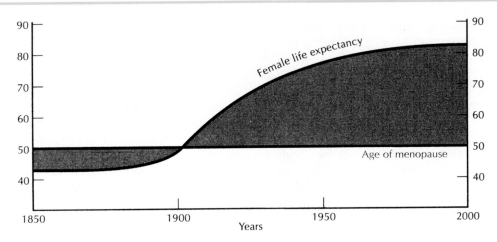

FIGURE 38.1.   Age of menopause and female life expectancy.

The cessation of menses is *menopause*. The *climacteric* and perimenopausal are the periods of waning ovarian function (i.e., the transition from the reproductive to the nonreproductive years). An increasing number of Americans are included in these groups, because the female life expectancy has lengthened and the number of women in this age group is expanding (Figure 38.1). If a woman reaches the menopausal age of approximately 50 years, she can expect to live another 30 to 35 years and thus spend approximately one third of her life after menopause. If for no other reasons than these, understanding the health issues of these women, including the evaluation and treatment of menopause, is important.

MENSTRUATION AND MENOPAUSE

Unlike the male who is able to renew gametes on a daily basis, the female has a fixed number of gametes for her reproductive life. At the time of birth, the female infant has approximately 1 to 2 million oocytes; by puberty, she has approximately 400,000 oocytes remaining. By age 30 to 35, the number of oocytes has decreased to approximately 100,000. For the remaining reproductive years, the process of oocyte maturation and ovulation becomes increasingly inefficient.

A woman ovulates approximately 400 oocytes during her reproductive years. The

TABLE 38.1.   Relative Changes in FSH as a Function of Life Stages

Life Stages	FSH (mIU/ml)
Childhood	< 4
Prime reproductive years	6–10
Perimenopause	14–24
Menopause	> 30

process of *oocyte selection* is poorly understood. During the reproductive cycle, a cohort of oocytes is stimulated to begin maturation, but only 1 or 2 dominant follicles complete the process and are eventually ovulated.

Follicular maturation is induced and stimulated by the pituitary release of follicle-stimulating hormone (FSH) and luteinizing hormone (LH). FSH binds to its receptors in the follicular membrane of the oocyte and stimulates follicular maturation, providing estradiol (E_2), which is the major estrogen of the reproductive years. LH stimulates the theca luteal cells surrounding the oocyte to produce androgens as well as estrogens and serves as the triggering mechanism to induce ovulation. With advancing reproductive age, the remaining oocytes become increasingly resistant to FSH. Thus plasma concentrations of FSH begin to increase several years in advance of actual menopause, when the FSH is generally found to be > 30 mIU/ml (Table 38.1).

Menopause marks the end of a woman's reproductive life. *The average age for menopause in the United States is between 50 and 52 years of age (median 51.5),* with 95% of women experiencing this event between the ages of 44 and 55 (Figure 38.2). The age of menopause is not influenced by the age of menarche, number of ovulations or pregnancies, lactation, or the use of oral contraceptives. Race, socio-economic status, education, and height also have no effect on the age of menopause. Undernourished women and smokers do tend to have an earlier menopause, although the effect is slight. Approximately 1% of women undergo menopause before the age of 40. When this happens, it is generally referred to as "premature ovarian failure" rather than "menopause" because of the social implications inherent in the latter.

Menopause is a physiologic process. However, the consequences of ovarian failure can diminish a woman's quality of life and can predispose her to osteoporosis and an increased risk of cardiovascular disease.

The postmenopausal ovary is not quiescent. Under the stimulation of LH, theca cell islands in the ovarian stroma produce hormones, primarily the androgens testosterone and androstenedione. Testosterone appears to be the major product of the postmenopausal ovary. Testosterone concentrations decline after menopause but remain two times higher in menopausal women with intact ovaries than in those whose ovaries have been removed or are premenopausal. Estrone is the predominant endogenous estrogen in postmenopausal women and is termed extragonadal estrogen because the concentration is directly related to body weight, because androstenedione is converted to estrone in fatty tissue (Table 38.2).

SYMPTOMS AND SIGNS OF OVARIAN FAILURE

Menstrual Cycle Alterations

Soon after an adolescent woman has her first menstrual cycle, regular, predictable menstrual cycles are established that continue until approximately 40 years of age.

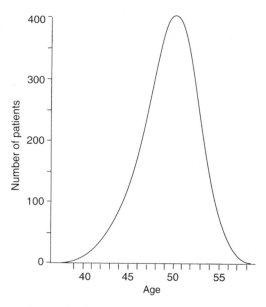

FIGURE 38.2.   Age of menopause.

Hormone	Premenopausal (Normal Ranges in Parentheses)	Postmenopausal	Postoophorectomy
Testosterone (ng/dl)	325 (200–600)	230	110
Androstenedione (ng/dl)	1500 (500–3000)	800–900	800–900
Estrone (pg/ml)	30–200	25–30	30
Estradiol (pg/ml)	35–500	10–15	15–20

TABLE 38.2. Steroid Hormone Serum Concentrations in Premenopausal Women, Postmenopausal Women, and Women After Oophorectomy

Around 40 years, the number of ovarian follicles becomes substantially depleted and subtle changes occur in the frequency and length of menstrual cycles. A woman may note shortening or lengthening of her cycles. The luteal phase of the cycle remains constant at 13 to 14 days, whereas the variation of cycle length is related to a change in the follicular phase. Women in their 20s and 30s ovulate 13 to 14 times per year. Several years in advance of menopause, the frequency of ovulation decreases to 11 to 12 times per year and, with advancing reproductive age, may decrease to 3 to 4 times per year.

With the change in reproductive cycle length and frequency, there are concomitant changes in the plasma concentration of FSH and LH. More *FSH* is required to stimulate follicular maturation. Beginning in the late 30s and early 40s, the concentration of FSH begins to increase. This is the first chemical evidence of ovarian failure. The 5- to 10-year period before menopause is termed *perimenopause*. During the perimenopausal years, women begin to experience symptoms and signs of estrogen deficiency as reproductive function becomes increasingly inefficient (Table 38.3). Relative changes in FSH as a function of stage of life are presented in Table 38.1.

Hot Flushes and Vasomotor Instability

Coincident with the change in reproductive cycle length and frequency, *the hot flush is the first physical manifestation of ovarian failure.* Occasional hot flushes begin several years before actual menopause. *The hot flush is the most common symptom of impending ovarian failure.* More than 95% of perimenopausal and menopausal women experience hot flushes.

Hot flushes have rapid onset and resolution. When a hot flush occurs, a woman experiences a sudden sensation of warmth. The skin of the face and the anterior chest wall become flushed for approximately 90 seconds. With resolution of the hot flush, a woman feels cold and breaks out

TABLE 38.3. Signs and Symptoms Associated with Menopause in Women Not on Estrogen-Replacement Therapy

Vulva and vagina
   Dyspareunia (atrophic vaginitis)
   Blood: stained discharge (atrophic vaginitis)
   Pruritus vulvae
Bladder and urethra
   Frequency, urgency
   Stress incontinence
Uterus and pelvic floor
   Uterovaginal prolapse
Skin and mucous membranes
   Dryness or pruritus
   Easily traumatized
   Loss of resilience and pliability
   Dry hair or loss of hair
   Minor hirsutism of face
   Dry mouth
   Voice changes: reduction in upper register
Cardiovascular system
   Angina and coronary heart disease

Skeleton
   Fracture of hip or wrist
   Backache
Breasts
   Reduced size
   Softer consistency
   Reduced support
Emotional symptoms
   Fatigue or diminished drive
   Irritability
   Apprehension
   Altered libido
   Insomnia
   Feelings of inadequacy or
      nonfulfillment
   Headache, tension
Metabolic
   Vasomotor symptoms: hot flushes
   Diaphoresis

into a "cold sweat." The entire phenomenon lasts less than 3 minutes. The hot flush is the result of declining estradiol-17β secretion by the ovarian follicles. As a woman approaches menopause, the frequency and intensity of hot flushes increase. Hot flushes may be disabling, producing *diaphoresis*, especially at night. When perimenopausal and postmenopausal women receive estrogen replacement, hot flushes usually resolve in 3 to 6 weeks. If a menopausal woman does not receive estrogen-replacement therapy, hot flushes usually resolve spontaneously within 2 to 3 years.

Sleep Disturbances

Ovarian failure with consequent declining estradiol induces a change in a woman's sleep cycle so that restful sleep becomes difficult and for some, impossible. The latent phase of sleep (i.e., the time required to fall asleep) is lengthened; the actual period of sleep is shortened. Therefore, perimenopausal and postmenopausal women complain of having difficulty falling asleep and of waking up soon after going to sleep. This is one of the most disabling and least appreciated adverse effects of menopause. Women with marked sleep aberration are often tense and irritable and have difficulty with concentration and interpersonal relationships. The sleep cycle is restored to the premenopausal state by the administration of replacement estrogens.

Vaginal Dryness and Genital Tract Atrophy

The vaginal mucosa, cervix, endocervix, endometrium, myometrium, and uroepithelium are estrogen-dependent tissues. With decreasing estrogen production, these tissues become atrophic, resulting in various symptoms. The vaginal epithelium becomes thin and cervical secretions diminish. Women experience vaginal dryness while attempting or having sexual intercourse, leading to diminished sexual enjoyment and dyspareunia. *Atrophic vaginitis* also may present with itching and burning. The

thinned epithelium is also more susceptible to becoming infected by local flora.

The endometrium also becomes atrophic, sometimes resulting in postmenopausal spotting. The paravaginal tissues that support the bladder and rectum become atrophic, resulting in loss of support for the bladder (cystocele) and rectum (rectocele). In addition, uterine prolapse is more common in the hypoestrogenic patient. Because of atrophy of the lining of the urinary tract, there may be symptoms of dysuria and urinary frequency. *Senile urethritis* often improves dramatically with estrogen-replacement therapy, leading to loss of the symptoms of urgency, frequency, and dysuria. Loss of support to the urethrovesical junction may result in stress urinary incontinence.

Therapy with replacement estrogens restores the integrity of the vaginal epithelium, relieving symptoms of vaginal dryness and dyspareunia. Sexual pleasure is often restored. Estrogen-replacement therapy partially restores the integrity and support of the tissues surrounding the vagina. If a menopausal woman has symptomatic pelvic relaxation, estrogen-replacement therapy should be administered for several months before surgical correction is considered. In some cases, estrogen replacement plus pelvic muscle (Kegel) exercises reverse the changes sufficiently to reestablish continence without surgery.

Mood Changes

Perimenopausal and postmenopausal women often complain of volatility of affect. Some women experience depression, apathy, and "crying spells." These may be caused directly by estrogen deficiency, by estrogen-deficiency associated sleep disturbance, or by both. Not only are these emotional symptoms disturbing to a woman but also her inability to control these feelings is equally of concern. The physician should provide counseling and emotional support as well as medical therapy. The role of estrogens in central nervous system function is unknown. However, it is well established that sex steroid hormone receptors are present in the central nervous system. Estrogen replacement in perimenopausal and post-menopausal women often diminishes these mood swings.

Skin, Hair, and Nail Changes

Estrogen influences *skin* thickness. With declining estrogen production, skin tends to become thin, less elastic, and eventually more susceptible to abrasion and trauma. Estrogen replacement helps restore the thickness and elasticity of skin. Estrogen therapy also helps to slow the formation of wrinkles.

Some women notice *changes in their hair and nails* with the hormonal changes of menopause. Estrogen stimulates the production of sex hormone–binding globulin, which binds androgens and estrogens. With declining estrogen production, there is less available sex hormone–binding globulin, which results in more free testosterone. This may result in *increased facial hair*. More-over, changes in estrogen production affect the rate of hair shedding. Hair from the scalp is normally lost and replaced in an asynchronous way. With changes in estrogen production, hair is shed and replaced in a synchronous way, resulting in the appearance of increased scalp hair loss. This is a self-limiting condition and requires no therapy, but patients do require reassurance. *Nails become thin and brittle* with estrogen deprivation, but are restored to normal with estrogen replacement.

Osteoporosis

Bone demineralization is a natural consequence of aging. Diminishing bone density occurs in both men and women. However, the onset of bone demineralization occurs 15 to 20 years earlier in women than in men by virtue of acceleration after ovarian function ceases. Bone demineralization not only occurs with natural menopause but also has been reported in association with decreased estrogen production in certain groups of young women. Other factors contribute to the risk of osteoporosis (Table 38.4).

TABLE 38.4. Risk Factors for Osteoporosis
Reduced weight for height
Family history of osteoporosis
Early menopause or oophorectomy
Low calcium intake
Cigarette smoking
Nulliparity
High alcohol intake
High caffeine intake

Estrogen receptors have been demonstrated in osteoblasts. This finding suggests a permissive and perhaps even essential role for estrogen in bone formation. Bone density diminishes at the rate of approximately 1% to 2% per year in postmenopausal women compared with approximately 0.5% per year in perimenopausal women. Of all the therapies used for the prevention and treatment of osteoporosis, estrogen replacement seems to be most effective, especially when combined with appropriate calcium supplementation and judicious exercise. Indeed, weight bearing activity, such as walking, for as little as 30 minutes a day increases the mineral content of older women.

If a woman does not receive estrogen in the first 5 years following menopause, she will have a progressive, linear decrease in bone mineral mass. However, if estrogen replacement is initiated before or at the time of menopause, bone density is maintained at the premenopausal levels. Starting estrogen replacement in a woman 5 or more years after menopause may still have an effect on bone density and is generally recommended.

Calcium supplementation is not a substitute for estrogen replacement. In several studies comparing estrogen with calcium, patients who received calcium alone had continued loss of bone mineral mass, whereas those who received estrogens had a stabilization of bone mineral mass. It is appropriate, however, to recommend

1000 to 1500 mg of daily calcium intake for menopausal women.

The recent approval of several bisphosphonates such as alendronate (Fosamax) for the treatment of postmenopausal osteoporosis has introduced an additional option for those patients who are not candidates for estrogen therapy. These agents reduce bone resorption through the inhibition of osteoclastic activity and provide good bone response but they do not provide the other benefits of estrogen therapy (i.e., they have no effect on cardiovascular disease, hot flushes, or atrophic changes). As a result, estrogen-replacement therapy remains the most desirable treatment for the prevention of osteoporosis when there is no contraindication to estrogen-replacement therapy.

Cardiovascular Lipid Changes

With approaching ovarian failure, changes occur in the cardiovascular lipid profile. Total cholesterol increases, high-density lipoprotein (HDL) cholesterol decreases, and low-density lipoprotein (LDL) cholesterol increases.

The administration of exogenous estrogens to perimenopausal and postmenopausal women promotes normalization of the cardiovascular lipid profile. It is still unclear whether women who take hormone replacement therapy are afforded protection against myocardial events and stroke. Retrospective case control studies suggest a cardioprotective effect. However, recent data suggest that no such protection exists in placebo control clinical trials. At this time, hormone replacement should not be offered to patients with the primary goal of protection against heart disease.

PREMATURE OVARIAN FAILURE

The diagnosis of premature ovarian failure applies to the approximately 1% of women who experience *menopause before the age of 40 years*. The diagnosis should be suspected in a young woman with hot flushes and other symptoms of hypoestrogenism and secondary amenorrhea. The diagnosis is confirmed by the laboratory findings of menopausal FSH levels. Interestingly, hot flushes are not as common as might be expected in this group of patients. The diagnosis has profound emotional implications for most patients, especially if their desires for childbearing have not been fulfilled, as well as metabolic and constitutional implications. For some, premature ovarian failure may be the cause of infertility, and for others, the cause for the menopausal symptoms. There are many causes of premature loss of oocytes and premature menopause (Table 38.5), some of the more common of which are discussed below.

Genetic Factors

There are several factors that influence a woman's reproductive life span. Genetic information that determines the length of a woman's reproductive life is carried on the distal long arm of the X chromosome. Partial deletion of the long arm of one X chromosome results in premature ovarian failure. Total loss of the long arm of the X chromosome, as seen in Turner's syndrome, results in ovarian failure at birth or in early childhood. When suspected, these diagnoses can be established by careful mapping of the X chromosome.

Gonadotropin-resistant Ovary Syndrome (Savage's Syndrome)

Some women with premature ovarian failure have an adequate number of ovarian follicles, yet these follicles are resistant to FSH and LH. A number of pregnancies have been reported in women with the gonadotropin-resistant ovary syndrome during the administration of exogenous estrogen. This fact suggests a role for estrogens in stimulating FSH receptors in the ovarian follicles.

TABLE 38.5.	Causes of Premature Loss of Oocytes	

Decreased number of germ cells
   Failure of germ cell migration
   Inherited reduction in germ cell number
Accelerated atresia
   Inherited tendencies
   Chromosomal abnormalities
     Gonadal dysgenesis
     With stigmata of Turner's syndrome
     Pure (46,XX or 46,XY)
     Mixed disorder
     Trisomy X with or without
       chromosomal mosaicism
   Defects in gonadotropin secretion
     Secretion of biologically inactive forms
     Subunit a or b defects

Congenital thymic aplasia
Gonadotropin receptor and/or
   postreceptor defects (resistant ovary
   or Savage's syndrome)
Postnatal destruction of germ cells
   Physical causes
     Chemotherapeutic agents
     Viral agents
     Surgical extirpation
   Autoimmune disorders
     With associated endocrine disorders
     Isolated

Autoimmune Disorders

Some women develop autoantibodies against thyroid, adrenal, and ovarian endocrine tissues. These autoantibodies may cause ovarian failure. Some women respond to estrogen-replacement therapy with subsequent resumption of ovulation.

Smoking

Women who smoke tobacco can undergo ovarian failure some 3 to 5 years earlier than the expected time of menopause. It is established that women who smoke metabolize estradiol primarily to 2-hydroxyestradiol. The 2-hydroxylated estrogens are termed *catecholestrogens* because of their structural similarity to catecholamines. The catecholestrogens act as antiestrogens and block estrogen action. The mechanism for premature ovarian failure in women smokers is unknown. However, the effects of smoking should be considered in smokers who are experiencing symptoms of estrogen deficiency.

Alkylating Cancer Chemotherapy

Alkylating cancer chemotherapeutic agents affect the membrane of ovarian follicles and hasten follicular atresia. One of the consequences of cancer chemotherapy in reproductive-age women is loss of ovarian function. Young women being treated for malignant neoplasms should be counseled of this possibility, and advised that they may be candidates for follicular retrieval and cryopreservation as a means for attempting future pregnancy.

Hysterectomy

Surgical removal of the uterus (hysterectomy) in reproductive-age women is associated with ovarian failure some 3 to 5 years earlier than the expected age. The mechanism for this occurrence is unknown. It is likely to be associated with alteration of ovarian blood flow resulting from the surgery.

Low Body Weight

Because adipocytes play a role in estrogen production and estrogen storage, slender women experience menopausal symptoms earlier than do women of normal body habitus and obese women. Moreover, slender women tend to be more difficult to normalize with exogenous estrogen replacement during the menopausal years. Women who are less than their ideal body weight at

TABLE 38.6. Common Estrogen Preparations and Dose Equivalence of Estrogenic Components

Estrogen	Preparation	Dose Equivalency
Conjugated estrogen		
Premarin	Oral: 0.3, 0.625, 0.9, 1.25, and 2.5 mg Vaginal: 0.625 mg/g of cream	0.625 mg
Esterified estrogen		
Estratab	Oral: 0.3, 0.625, 1.25, and 2.5 mg	0.625 mg
Estratest h. s.	Oral: 0.625 and 1.25 mg methyltestosterone	
Estratest	1.25 and 2.5 mg methyltestosterone	
Estradiol-17β		
Climara, Vivelle (transdermal patch)	0.05, 0.10 mg	0.05 mg
Micronized estradiol		
Estrace	Oral: 0.5, 1.0, and 2.0 mg Vaginal: 0.1 mg/g	1.0 mg
Estropipate (piperazine estrone sulfate)		
Ogen, Ortho-est	Oral: 0.3, 0.625, 1.25, 2.5, and 5.0 mg	0.75 mg
Ogen	Vaginal: 1.5 mg/g	

the time of menopause should be counseled regarding the clinical implications of their weight.

MANAGEMENT OF MENOPAUSE

All of the signs and symptoms, and adverse effects, of menopause result from declining estradiol-17β production by the ovarian follicles. *Exogenous estrogen administration* to the perimenopausal and postmenopausal woman obviates most of these changes. Estradiol-17β and its metabolic byproducts, estrone and estriol, are used for replacement.

The *objective of estrogen-replacement therapy* should be to diminish the signs and symptoms of ovarian failure and restore estrogen levels. There are several different estrogen preparations available through various routes of administration (Table 38.6). Conjugated estrogens (Premarin, Ogen) have been used as oral medication for decades as primary hormone preparations for estrogen replacement. Conjugated estrogens are unconjugated in the gastrointestinal tract and delivered to the target tissues as estrone. Conjugated estrogens are effective in diminishing the symptoms of estrogen deficiency, in maintaining bone mass, and restoring plasma lipids to more normal levels.

Estradiol-17β can be administered orally; however, it then is oxidized in the enterohepatic circulation to estrone. Estradiol-17β remains unaltered if it is administered transdermally, transbucally, transvaginally, intravenously, or intramuscularly. Unfortunately, intramuscular estradiol administration results in unpredictable fluctuations in plasma concentration. When estradiol is administered across the vaginal epithelium, absorption is poorly controlled and pharmacologic plasma concentrations of estradiol can result. The *transdermal administration* of estradiol results in steady, sustained estrogen blood levels and is the preferred alternative method (instead of oral dosing) of estrogen administration (Estraderm Climera).

TABLE 38.7. Common Progestin Preparations and Dose Equivalence of Progestin Components

Progestin	Preparation	Dose Equivalency
Medroxyprogesterone		
Provera, Cycrin, Amen	Tablets in 2.5, 5.0, and 10.0 mg	10.0 mg
Depo-Provera	Injectable, 100 and 400 mg/ml	
Norethindrone acetate		
Aygestin	Tablet, 5 mg	5.0 mg
Norlutate	Tablet, 5 mg	
Micronized progesterone	Capsules, 100 and 200 mg	
Prometrium		
Norgestimate		

The administration of continuous *unopposed estrogens* can result in endometrial hyperplasia and an increased risk of endometrial adenocarcinoma. Therefore, it is essential to administer a progestin, most commonly medroxyprogesterone acetate (Provera), in conjunction with estrogens in women who have not undergone hysterectomy. To achieve this protective effect, the progestin chosen must be administered a minimum of 10 days each month (Table 38.7). If estrogen is administered alone because of unacceptable side effects of progestins, then it is imperative to counsel the patient as to the need for yearly endometrial biopsy.

There are two principal *regimens for estrogen-replacement therapy.* Continuous estrogen replacement with cyclic progestin administration results in excellent resolution of symptoms and cyclic withdrawal bleeding from the endometrium. One of the difficulties of this method of therapy is that many postmenopausal women do not want to continue having menstrual cycles. As a result, many physicians and patients choose to avoid the problem of cyclic withdrawal bleeding by the daily administration of both an estrogen and a low-dose progestin.

There is a wide *variety of estrogen preparations available.* The following are comparable dosages: conjugated equine estrogens, 0.625 mg; estrone sulfate, 0.625 mg; estradiol-17β, 1 mg; and transdermal estradiol-17β, 50 mg. Most perimenopausal and menopausal women respond to one of these preparations, all of which are adequate to prevent osteoporosis and to provide protection from cardiovascular disease. Most women experience relief from hot flushes, vaginal dryness, sleep disturbances, and mood changes. The administration of 5 to 10 mg of *medroxyprogesterone acetate* (Provera) given for 10 to 12 days each month converts the proliferative endometrium into a secretory endometrium, brings about endometrial sloughing, and prevents endometrial hyperplasia or cellular atypia. If continuous progestin therapy is used to produce endometrial atrophy, 2.5 mg of medroxyprogesterone acetate per day is used.

Three new preparations combining estrogen and progesterone are available in a single tablet. Prempro consists of tablets containing 0.625 mg of conjugated estrogen and 2.5 mg medroxyprogesterone acetate, which are taken daily. Premphase consists of two packets of 14 tablets, the first taken the first fourteen days of the month containing 0.625 mg conjugated estrogen and the second taken the last fourteen days of the month containing 0.625 mg conjugated estrogen and 5 mg of medroxyprogesterone acetate. A more recent method is pulsed therapy (Prefest), which employs intermittent short bursts (3 days) of progestin (norgestimate) in combination with daily low-dose estrogen (estradiol, 1 mg). Pulsed therapy is thought to reduce the incidence of bothersome bleeding by not contributing to as much endometrial atrophy as continuous combined therapy.

An annual pelvic examination with Pap smear and mammogram (after age 50) is advisable for all women whether they are taking hormone-replacement therapy or not.

CAUTIONS IN ESTROGEN REPLACEMENT

Patients with unexplained abnormal vaginal bleeding should not receive estrogen-replacement therapy until the cause of the bleeding is ascertained and treated appropriately. In addition, patients with active liver disease or chronically impaired liver function should generally not receive estrogen replacement.

Carcinoma of the Breast

Carcinoma of the breast has been a contraindication to estrogen replacement. In light of the benefits of estrogen-replacement therapy in regard to osteoporosis and cardiovascular disease, selected patients may not be considered inappropriate for estrogen-replacement therapy. It may be reasonable to administer estrogen replacement to women who have documented breast tumors and negative axillary lymph nodes. Any such patients should be several years removed from their original diagnosis and treatment to minimize risks. Because this is still controversial, *caution must be exercised when making the decision to administer estrogen to women with a history of breast cancer.*

Thromboembolic Disease

Oral estrogens stimulate the production of clotting factors, but estradiol administered by the transdermal route has no effect on clotting. Therefore, women with a history of thromboembolic disease can safely receive transdermal estradiol therapy.

Endometrial Carcinoma

There is little evidence to suggest that estrogens should be withheld from women with a history of carcinoma of the endometrium if the tumor was limited to the endometrium and myometrium. Women with metastatic endometrial carcinoma should not receive exogenous estrogens.

CASE STUDIES

Case 38A

A 46-year-old woman complains of increasing irritability, hot flushes, and an increasingly irregular menstrual cycle over the last 12 months. Her mother died of breast cancer. She had three uncomplicated pregnancies and has been well, with no other problems other than varicose veins.

Questions Case 38A

Which of the following signs and symptoms would be expected?

A. Sleep disturbance
B. Dry skin
C. Loss of hair
D. Vaginal irritation after coitus
E. Oily skin

Answer: A, B, C, D

The loss of estrogen can result in many physiologic changes. Of those listed, only oily skin is not caused by estrogen deprivation.

Which of the following findings would be expected?

A. Increased FSH
B. Decreased FSH
C. Increased LH
D. Decreased LH
E. Increased bone density
F. Decreased bone density
G. Increased total cholesterol
H. Decreased total cholesterol

Answer: A, C, G

If this patient is experiencing early menopause, FSH and LH are elevated and total cholesterol may be increased. Untreated, bone density declines over several years, but the findings now would most likely be normal.

Which are appropriate therapeutic steps?

A. Oral progestin
B. Oral estrogen
C. Oral calcium
D. Oral tranquilizers
E. Parenteral progesterone
F. Parenteral estrogen
G. Parenteral calcium
H. Parenteral tranquilizers

Answer: A, B, C

Oral estrogen replacement is appropriate for treatment of menopausal symptoms. Progestin therapy is indicated in addition to estrogen whenever the patient still has a uterus. Calcium supplementation is also a good idea as additional therapy to prevent osteoporosis. Parenteral preparations of any of these drugs are rarely needed. Tranquilizers are not routinely indicated, because estrogen-replacement therapy usually successfully treats the mood changes. Because of the first-degree relative with breast carcinoma, yearly breast examination by a physician and yearly screening mammography are indicated.

Case 38B

A 27-year-old woman presents with a history of amenorrhea and hot flushes for the last 6 months. Laboratory studies reveal elevated FSH and LH.

Questions Case 38B

The differential diagnosis would include all of the following EXCEPT

A. Gonadotropin-resistant ovary syndrome
B. 46,XX q-ovarian dysgenesis
C. Idiopathic ovarian failure
D. Pituitary prolactinoma

Answer: D

A pituitary prolactinoma would present with amenorrhea, but the gonadotropins would not be elevated as seen in this case. An elevated prolactin level would be expected if a prolactinoma were present.

Which of the following is not a potential therapy for this patient?

A. Estrogen and progestin replacement
B. Securing a donor oocyte
C. Biopsy of the ovaries
D. Maintaining ideal body weight

Answer: D

The vasomotor symptoms of premature ovarian failure should respond to estrogen replacement. Progestin is a part of the therapeutic regimen to prevent endometrial hyperplasia. The use of donor oocytes could be used if assisted reproductive technology were to be tried in the future. Biopsy of the ovary may be considered if ovarian dysgenesis is a possibility. Body weight is often associated with anovulation and amenorrhea but is not a factor in premature ovarian failure.

CHAPTER

39

INFERTILITY

CHAPTER OBJECTIVES

This chapter deals primarily with APGO Objective(s):

OBJECTIVE 52   Infertility

Define primary and secondary male and female infertility, describing for each the causes and approach to diagnosis and management.

Infertility affects 15% of reproductive age couples in the United States. Infertility is defined as a couple's failure to conceive following 1 year of unprotected sexual intercourse. This definition is emphasized in the cumulative monthly conception rates for fertile couples engaging in unprotected coitus (Figure 39.1).

Reproductive age is synonymous with a woman's reproductive years (*generally defined as ages 15 to 44 years,* although menarche and pregnancy before age 15 are not uncommon and pregnancy after 44 is no longer rare). Because this 15- to 44-year-old cohort is generally among the healthiest among women, it is surprising that 15% of this group experiences reproductive dysfunction. One must look not only for disease, such as endometriosis, which causes infertility, but also causes resulting from environmental and life-style issues. Infertility may be related to life-style changes such as maintaining a low body weight associated with dieting and/or exercise, smoking, the use of drugs such as marijuana, deferred childbearing, and increased sexual contacts associated with increased incidence of pelvic inflammatory disease. Deferred childbearing is a factor of increasing importance in a society where both husband and wife may have careers outside the home, because female fertility decreases with increasing age. Indeed, fertility is approximately halved between about the 37th and 45th year of a woman's life, primarily because of age-associated alterations in ovulation.

Formerly, there was little hope for the infertile couple; today, 85% of couples can expect to have a child with appropriate diagnosis and treatment of "infertility."

The inability to conceive a child or carry a pregnancy places a great emotional burden on infertile couples. The quest to have a child becomes the driving force in the infertile couple's life. Friends, family, and often occupation can be subordinated to this medical problem. Unlike dysfunction of other organ systems, dysfunction of the reproductive system does not directly produce physical or mental abnormalities. Yet, the mental anguish of infertility is nearly as incapacitating as the pain or life restrictions of other diseases. *The emotional needs of infertile couples must be recognized and fully addressed.*

CAUSES OF INFERTILITY

Infertility can be reduced to three generic causes that account for 90% of reproductive dysfunction. These causes are *(1) anovulation (30%), (2) anatomic defects of the female genital tract (30%), and (3) abnormal spermatogenesis (40%).* Each of these categories can be investigated by a simple diagnostic procedure that gives a high probability of establishing a cause. In the initial investigation of the infertile couple, it is important for the physician to establish, as rapidly as possible, the major cause(s) of the infertility, using initially the least invasive tests possible. For this reason, the sequence generally chosen is based on the most commonly observed causes of infertility: male factors and ovulation disorders (Figure 39.2).

Basal body temperature measurement is an excellent screening test for ovulation, and is also often useful in the timing of coitus. The characteristic biphasic temperature shift occurs in more than 90% of ovulating women: The temperature drops at the time of menses, then rises two days after the peak of the luteinizing hormone (LH) surge, coinciding with a rise in peripheral levels of

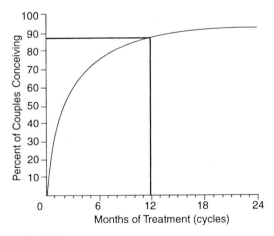

FIGURE   39.1.   Conception rates for fertile couples.

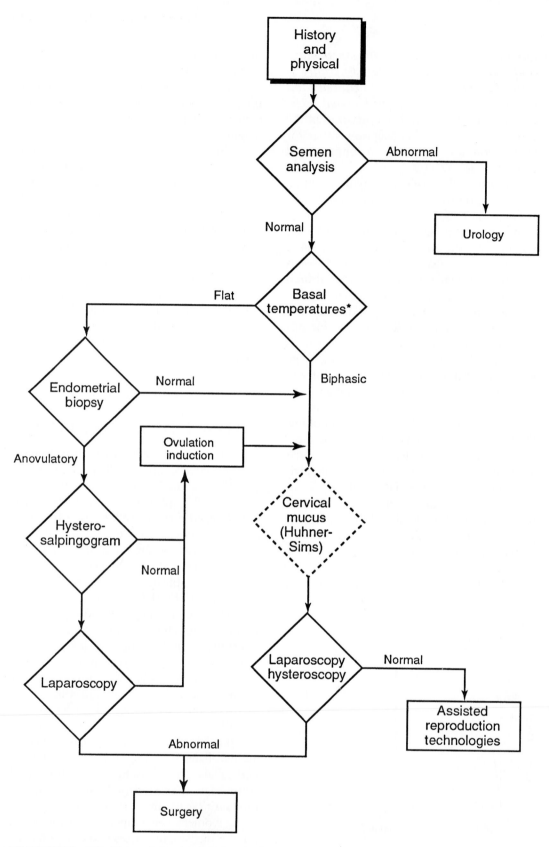

FIGURE 39.2. Scheme for the evaluation of the infertile couple. (Modified from Smith RP: *Gynecology in Primary Care.* Baltimore, Williams & Wilkins, 1996, p. 344.)
*A luteal phase progestin may also be used.

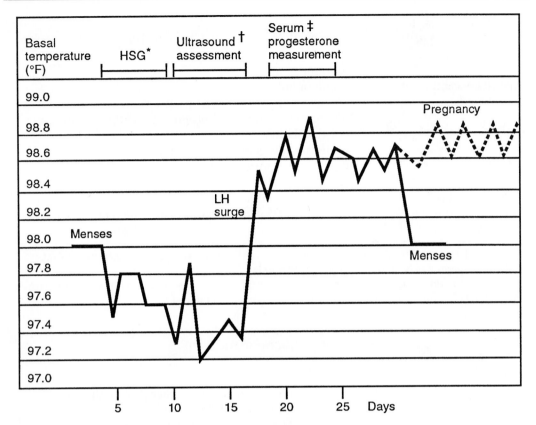

FIGURE 39.3. Ovulation associated biphasic basal body temperature pattern.
*Preferred time for hysterosalpingogram (HSG) testing.
†Preferred timing for sonographic assessment for ovulation.
‡Optimal interval for serum progesterone measurement for ovulation.

progesterone to greater than 4 ng/ml. Ovum release probably occurs one day before the first temperature elevation, and the temperature remaining elevated for 13–14 days, then dropping with menses beginning 14–36 hours thereafter. A temperature elevation of more than 16 days is quite suggestive of pregnancy (Figure 39.3). Serum progesterone levels drawn in mid-luteal phase are sometimes useful. A value above 15 ng/ml is 80% accurate in distinguishing a normal from abnormal cycle, whereas values less than 10 ng/ml are rarely associated with normal cycles.

Analysis of a semen specimen obtained by masturbation provides immediate information about the quantity and quality of seminal fluid, the density of the sperm, the morphology of sperm, and the motility of sperm. The man is instructed to abstain from coitus for 2 to 3 days before the test,

because coitus during this time interval lowers the sperm count in some cases. It is important to collect all the ejaculate, because the first part contains the greatest density of sperm. The analysis should be performed no more than 2 hours after the specimen is collected, preferably sooner; thus collection of the specimen at the site of analysis is preferable. A normal semen specimen should contain motile, morphologically normal sperm. Table 39.1 presents common values for a normal semen analysis. A normal semen analysis excludes a male cause for infertility in more than 90% of couples. The causes of abnormal semen analyses are presented in Table 39.2.

The *hysterosalpingogram,* an x-ray study of the internal female genital tract, provides important information about the tract's architecture and integrity. A radiopaque dye is injected through the cervix

TABLE 39.1. Commonly Accepted Values for a Normal Semen Analysis

Volume	2.0 ml or more
Sperm concentration	20 million/ml or more
Motility	50% or more with forward progression
	25% or more with rapid progression within 60 minutes of ejaculation
Viscosity	Liquification within 30–60 minutes
Morphology	30% or more normal forms
pH	7.2–7.8
White blood cells	Fewer than 1 million/ml
Immunobead test*	Fewer than 20% spermatozoa with adherent particles
SpermMar Test†	Fewer than 10% spermatozoa with adherent particles

*Sperm incubated with beads labeled with anti-IgG, anti-IgA, or anti-IgM; beads with anti-IgG adhere to sperm heads, with anti-IgA to sperm tails.

†Mixed agglutination test; uses antiserum to IgG to bridge antibody-coated sperm and latex particles that have been conjugated with human IgG, end point clumping.

TABLE 39.2. Causes of Abnormal Semen Analysis

Abnormal sperm count	
No sperm (azoospermia)	Klinefelter's syndrome or other genetic disorders
	Sertoli cell only syndrome
	Seminiferous tubule or Leydig cell failure
	Hypogonadotropic-hypogonadism
	Ductal obstruction (e.g., vasectomy)
	Varicocele
Few sperm (oligospermia)	Genetic disorder
	Endocrinopathies, including androgen receptor defects
	Varicocele and other anatomic disorders
	Maturation arrest
	Hypospermatogenesis
	Exogenous factors (e.g., heat)
Abnormal sperm morphology	Varicocele
	Stress
	Infection (mumps)
Abnormal motility	Immunologic factors, male–female incompatibility
	Infection
	Defect in sperm structure or metabolism
	Poor liquefaction of semen
	Varicocele
Abnormal volume	
No ejaculate	Ductal obstruction
	Retrograde ejaculation
	Ejaculatory failure
	Hypogonadism
Low volume	Obstruction of ejaculatory ducts
	Absence of seminal vesicles and vas deferens
	Partial retrograde ejaculation
	Infection

TABLE 39.3. Tests in the Infertility Work-Up

Possible Cause	Test	Comments
Anovulation	Basal body temperature	Patient must do each morning
	Endometrial biopsy	Office procedure in late luteal phase
	Serum progesterone	Blood test (done in luteal phase)
	Urinary ovulation-detection kit	Home use at midcycle
Anatomic disorder	Hysterosalpingogram	X-ray in proliferative phase
	Diagnostic laparoscopy	View external surfaces of pelvic organs
	Hysteroscopy	Visualize endometrial cavity
Abnormal spermatogenesis	Semen analysis	Normal value > 20 million/ml, 2 ml volume, 60% motility
	Postcoital test	Midcycle timing
Immunologic disorder	Antisperm antibodies	Male and female tested

into the uterine cavity and fallopian tubes and then into the peritoneal cavity, assuming that the tubes are patent. The internal architecture of all of these structures is then outlined on x-ray. The hysterosalpingogram has a diagnostic accuracy of approximately 70% for detecting anatomic abnormalities of the genital tract. A diagnostic laparoscopy is another method of evaluating the genital tract but is complementary to the hysterosalpingogram (Table 39.3). The pelvic cavity, including visualization of the "external surfaces" of the uterus, ovaries, fallopian tubes, and support structures, is evaluated by this method.

Anovulation

A healthy woman between age 18 and 36 is presumed to ovulate 13 to 14 times per year. The typical menstrual cycle is 28 days long, with ovulation occurring on the fourteenth day. The *luteal phase* of the menstrual cycle is dominated by the secretion of progesterone by the corpus luteum. Progesterone acts on the endocervix to convert the thin, clear endocervical mucus into a sticky mucoid material. Progesterone shifts the thermoregulatory center and increases the set point of the basal body temperature.

Following ovulation, the basal body temperature increases by approximately 0.6° F and remains elevated until menstruation begins. With involution of the corpus luteum, progesterone production abruptly decreases and the basal body temperature shifts downward; menstruation ensues soon after.

A history of regular menstrual periods strongly suggests regular ovulation. Characteristically, following ovulation and preceding menstruation, an ovulating woman experiences some fullness and heaviness of the breasts, decreased vaginal secretions, abdominal bloating, mild peripheral edema with slight increase in body weight, and occasional episodes of depression. In a minority of patients, the physical and emotional changes may be debilitating, the so-called *premenstrual syndrome.* These changes do not occur in anovulatory women. Therefore, *a history of these cyclic changes may be interpreted as presumptive evidence of ovulation.*

Diagnostic studies to confirm ovulation, in addition to recording the basal body temperature, include the endometrial biopsy, measurement of serum progesterone, and the urinary ovulation-detection kit. The *endometrium* undergoes specific histologic changes on an almost daily basis following ovulation. These changes can be detected from an endometrial biopsy. This is a useful procedure for evaluating certain causes of infertility, but it is expensive and provides only static information. *Progesterone* increases in plasma following ovulation and can be measured to confirm that ovulation has occurred. However, a single measurement provides little information that cannot be obtained by a well-kept basal body temperature chart. Ovulation-detection kits are available that measure changes in urinary LH. As the LH surge begins, more LH is excreted in the urine, which can be measured by qualitative detection kits. This is useful in helping to predict ovulation, but it does not confirm ovulation. Ovulation-detection kits should not be used routinely, but can be useful when ovulation prediction is needed, such as in the timing of artificial insemination.

Symptoms such as irregular, unpredictable menstrual cycles and episodes of *amenorrhea* as well as signs of hirsutism, acne, galactorrhea, and increased or decreased vaginal secretions *suggest anovulation*. A woman with irregular menstrual cycles can be presumed to be anovulatory. In this case, maintaining a basal body temperature record is not necessary.

Given a history of irregular menstrual cycles, the physician should look for signs of abnormal androgen, prolactin, and gonadotropin secretion. A woman who is anovulatory should have some or all of the following tests drawn, depending on individualized evaluation of the case: follicle-stimulating hormone (FSH), LH, prolactin, androstenedione, total testosterone, and dehydroepiandrosterone sulfate (DHEAS). If thyroid dysfunction is suspected, thyroxin (T_4) and thyroid-stimulating hormone (TSH) should be measured as well. The results of these hormonal studies help the physician understand the etiology of the chronic anovulation. Once the etiology of anovulation is established, a treatment regimen designed to induce ovulation can be developed for the patient. Any agent that sets in cyclic motion the secretion of gonadotropins or estradiol stimulates ovulation.

Anatomic Disorders of the Female Genital Tract

SPERM TRANSPORT, FERTILIZATION, AND IMPLANTATION

The internal anatomic genital tract serves as more than a simple conduit for sperm and eggs. Indeed, these are dynamic structures that are essential for normal transportation, fertilization, and implantation. The female genital tract *facilitates* the migration of sperm from the posterior vaginal fornix toward the unfertilized egg. *Cervical mucus* secreted by the endocervix traps the coagulated ejaculate, where the sperm are stored and capacitated for immediate or later migration into the endometrial cavity and fallopian tubes.

At the time of ovulation, the oocyte is either picked up directly or retrieved from the pelvic cul-de-sac by the fimbriated end of the fallopian tube. The oocyte is then transported to the proximal portion of the fallopian tube, where fertilization occurs. The fertilized oocyte cleaves and forms a zygote and then an embryo. At 3 to 5 days following fertilization, the embryo enters the *endometrial cavity,* where it implants into the secretory endometrium for subsequent growth and development.

ACQUIRED AND CONGENITAL DISORDERS

The most *common disorders* of the female genital tract are acquired during the early reproductive years. The most common cause of fallopian tube disease is *acute salpingitis*. Organisms that infect the fallopian tubes include *Neisseria gonorrhoeae* and *Chlamydia trachomatis*. These organisms alter the functional integrity of the fallopian tubes and can lead rapidly to fallopian tube obstruction. An example of an acquired uterine disorder would be intrauterine scarring (Asherman's syndrome, intrauterine synechiae) often associated with the denuding of the endometrial lining at the time of curettage. This scarring leads to irregular bleeding and impaired implantation.

Endometriosis, scarring and adhesions from pelvic inflammation or surgery, tumors of the uterus (e.g., leiomyoma) and ovary,

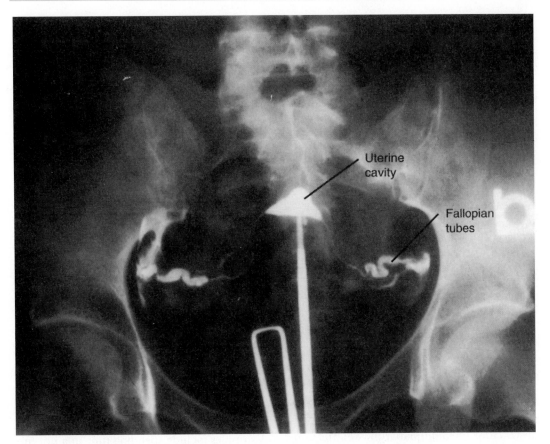

Uterine
cavity

Fallopian
tubes

FIGURE 39.4.   A hysterosalpingogram showing normal genital tract anatomy and architecture.

and (rarely) sequelae of trauma may also distort the reproductive tract anatomy. Less common congenital anatomic abnormalities of the female genital tract can range from a simple septum of the upper uterine cavity to a complete reduplication of the genital tract with a double vagina, double cervix, and double uterus.

HYSTEROSALPINGOGRAPHY

The hysterosalpingogram is an essential diagnostic tool for evaluation of the internal genital structures. The hysterosalpingogram should be performed between the seventh and eleventh day of the menstrual cycle. If it were performed during menses, the risk of iatrogenic retrograde menstruation would be increased. If performed later, it could interfere with the possible ovum transport, fertilization, or implantation.

There are several important characteristics of the normal hysterosalpingogram (Figure 39.4). The endometrial cavity should be smooth and symmetrical. Indentations and irregularities of the endometrial cavity suggest uterine leiomyomata or chronic scarring of the endometrium from previous surgery. The proximal two thirds of the fallopian tubes should be slender, approximating the diameter of a pencil lead. The distal one third of the fallopian tubes is the ampulla and should appear dilated compared with the proximal two thirds. The fimbrial folds should appear as linear radiolucencies along the longitudinal axis of the tube. Examples of hysterosalpingograms, demonstrating two common abnormalities, are shown in Figure 39.5.

During the radiographic study, dye should *spill* promptly from the fallopian tubes into the peritoneal cavity. In a pelvis

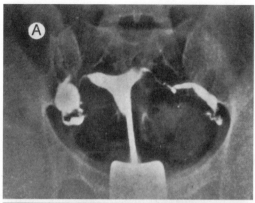

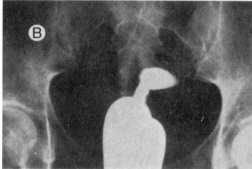

FIGURE 39.5.   Abnormal hysterosalpingograms. (*A*) Bilateral hydrosalpinx obstructing the fallopian tubes at the fimbriated ends. Arcuate uterus. (*B*) Bilateral tubal occlusion at the cornu; uterus over distended with radiopaque medium.

free of adhesions, dye intersperses between loops of bowel, producing characteristic crescents throughout the pelvis. Moreover, dye should spill freely into the cul-de-sac and dispense throughout the pelvis. Failure to observe these late changes in the hysterosalpingogram suggests the possibility of peritubal adhesions or endometriosis, which restrict normal fallopian tube mobility.

A hysterosalpingogram that shows an abnormality of the fallopian tubes should be followed with a *diagnostic laparoscopy. The hysterosalpingogram provides information about the inner surfaces of the genital tract organs, whereas diagnostic laparoscopy provides information about the external surfaces of these organs.* Hysteroscopy can provide direct visualization of the endometrial cavity as well as access to possible correction of lesions found.

Abnormalities of Spermatogenesis

Problems of spermatogenesis account for more than *40% of cases of infertility.* Unlike oocytes, which are ovulated periodically, sperm are being constantly produced by the germinal epithelium of the testicles. As sperm develop within the germinal epithelium, they are released into the epididymis where maturation occurs before ejaculation.

The *sperm generation time* is approximately 73 days. Thus an abnormal sperm count is a reflection of events that occurred 73 days before the collection of a semen specimen. Alternatively, a minimum of 73 days is required to observe the change in sperm production following therapy for oligospermia.

Sperm production is thermoregulated. Intratesticular temperature is regulated by contraction and relaxation of the scrotum. Sperm production occurs at a temperature of approximately 1° F less than body temperature. External thermal shock to the testicles can result in reduced sperm production. Examples include spending time in a hot tub, sitting on the testicles for long periods of time with poor heat dispersion, and wearing tight clothing that pulls the testicles against the body for extended periods of time. In many cases, one of these causes can be discovered from a carefully obtained history. As the follicle of the ovary responds to FSH and LH, the Leydig cells and germinal epithelium of the testicles also respond to gonadotropic stimulation. In some men, the germinal epithelium becomes fibrotic and sperm production is diminished. In others, testosterone production by Leydig cells is decreased. Men with oligospermia should have gonadotropin hormones measured to exclude testicular failure. Suspected testicular failure should be confirmed by testicular biopsy.

Some men with marginal testicular failure or poor gonadotropic production respond to the administration of clomiphene citrate. This is appropriate therapy for a limited time. The man who has *poor sperm production* as a result of hormonal abnormalities does not respond well to induction of spermatogenesis.

Besides sperm analysis, another method to evaluate sperm density and sperm motility has historically been the *postcoital test (Huhner-Sims test)*. The test should be timed to take place during the late follicular phase of the menstrual cycle just before ovulation. At this time of the cycle, cervical mucus is abundant and facilitates sperm survival and transport. The couple should have intercourse approximately 8 hours before the test is scheduled. The female partner undergoes a speculum examination to expose the cervix. With a tuberculin syringe, a small sample of endocervical mucus is aspirated from the endocervical canal. This is placed on a glass side and examined under a microscope. Normally, 8 to 10 motile sperm per high-powered field are seen in the cervical mucus. This simple test provides important information about coitus, ejaculation, sperm pickup, sperm motility, and sperm storage within the endocervical canal. Because scientific support for the usefulness of the postcoital test is lacking, it is no longer as widely used as it once was.

Both men and women can produce *antisperm antibodies*. If the woman produces antisperm antibodies, sperm are immobilized in the cervical mucus. If the man produces antisperm antibodies (3% to 20% of "infertile" men), sperm agglutinate and are unable to penetrate the cervical mucus. The diagnosis of antisperm antibodies is made by performing immunologic studies on both partners and as part of the semen analysis. If antisperm antibodies exist in the woman, timed intrauterine insemination using washed sperm may produce a pregnancy. There is no known effective treatment for men with antisperm antibodies, although attempts at therapy include washing and concentration of sperm with either intracervical or intrauterine insemination and high-dose steroid therapy.

For some couples, there may be no biologic explanation for their infertility. Physicians must consider low body weight, individuals or couples who use marijuana, or something else in their life-style that may compromise reproduction. These "normal" infertile couples may comprise up to 10% of those seeking treatment of infertility.

TREATMENT OF THE INFERTILE COUPLE

Anovulation

If *anovulation* is the cause of infertility, therapy should be directed to *restore ovulation by the administration of ovulation-inducing agents*. The most frequently used therapy is *clomiphene citrate*. Clomiphene citrate is an antiestrogen, which combines with and blocks estrogen receptors at the hypothalamic and pituitary level, thus inducing, by negative-feedback inhibition of estrogens, an increase in FSH release from the pituitary. FSH in turn is one of the major signals stimulating the development of follicles. Before therapy, the patient should be taking basal body temperature measurements, which are used to monitor therapy. Progesterone (50 to 100 mg) is given intramuscularly, and clomiphene is begun on the fifth day of menses. Depending on the hormonal milieu of the patient, 50 to 100 mg are given from day 5 to day 9. If the patient ovulates, it occurs approximately 14 days after the first day of clomiphene administration. In the absence of ovulation, the schedule of medication may be altered by increasing the daily dosage of clomiphene, increasing the duration of administration, or administering human chorionic gonadotropin (hCG) timed to substitute for the absent LH surge. This is commonly given as 5000 IU of hCG at the time of optimum cervical mucus. The maximum dosage of clomiphene is usually 150 mg/day.

If a woman fails to respond to clomiphene citrate, *FSH* can be administered directly to stimulate follicular growth. A purified preparation of gonadotropins from the urine of postmenopausal women [Pergonal (menotropins)] is usually used. Pergonal contains approximately 75 or 150 IU of both FSH and LH per dose and must be given parenterally, because it is inactivated if given orally. If exogenous FSH is administered, monitoring requires frequent measurement of estradiol-17β and frequent ultrasound imaging of the ovarian follicles. The therapy is expensive and includes significant risk of three complications: hyperstimulation of the ovaries, multiple gestation, and fetal wastage.

Anatomic Abnormalities

In the event an anatomic abnormality of the genital tract is discovered, a *surgical treatment* is usually recommended. Lysis of pelvic adhesions results in freeing of entrapped internal genital structures. In case of fallopian tube obstruction, the obstruction can be corrected surgically. However, for these operations to be successful, the endosalpinx must be healthy. If the endosalpinx has been altered such that ovum pickup and transport cannot occur, one of the assisted reproductive technologies—primarily in vitro fertilization—must be considered as an option. Correction of abnormalities of the endometrial cavity can also be accomplished, often at the time of hysteroscopic diagnosis.

Inadequate Spermatogenesis

Problems of spermatogenesis should be addressed by trying to eliminate alterations of thermoregulation. Attempts at induction of spermatogenesis can be made by the administration of clomiphene citrate. However, the response to this therapy is usually less than 20%.

If spermatogenesis cannot be improved, couples may choose to use *artificial insemination using donor sperm* (AID); several techniques are in common use (Figure 39.6). Couples may also choose one of the assisted reproductive technologies such as gamete intrafallopian tube transfer (GIFT) or in vitro fertilization (IVF) to facilitate fertilization using the infertile partner's sperm.

Assisted Reproductive Technologies

An explosion of assisted reproductive technologies has occurred in the last decade (Table 39.4). These include IVF, GIFT, and

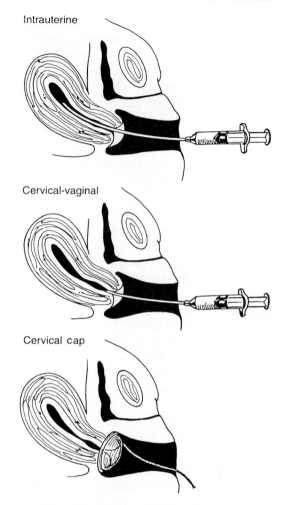

Intrauterine

Cervical-vaginal

Cervical cap

FIGURE 39.6.   Techniques of artificial insemination.

zygote intrafallopian tube transfer (ZIFT). These technologies provide infertility specialists with tools to bypass the normal mechanisms of gamete transportation and fertilization. However, IVF, GIFT, and ZIFT are expensive and place infertile couples on an emotional roller coaster. The expected successful outcome from IVF in properly selected couples is approximately 18% to 22% per cycle. The expected successful outcome for properly selected couples for GIFT and ZIFT is approximately 22% to 28% per cycle. Strict indications for the use of these procedures must be maintained to prevent misuse and exploitation of couples. The probability of pregnancy in a healthy couple is approximately 18% to 20% per cycle. Assisted reproductive technologies do

TABLE 39.4.	Commonly Encountered Abbreviations Associated with Assisted Reproduction

Abbreviation	Technique
AID	Artificial insemination, donor [using donor sperm, occasionally referred to as therapeutic donor insemination (TDI)]
AIH	Artificial insemination, homologous (using the partner's sperm)
BBT	Basal body temperature
GIFT	Gamete intrafallopian transfer (gametes are placed in the fallopian tube for fertilization)
HSG	Hysterosalpingogram, or uterine cavity x-ray
ICSI	Intracytoplasmic sperm injection
IUI	Intrauterine insemination, placement of either donor's or husband's sperm directly into the uterine cavity
IVF/ET	In vitro fertilization with embryo transfer
PCT	Postcoital test or Huhner-Sims test
SPA	Sperm penetration assay (also known as a hamster egg test, or zona-free egg penetration test)
ZIFT	Zygote intrafallopian transfer (fertilization takes place in vitro and the zygote is transferred to the fallopian tube to be transported into the uterine cavity)

From Smith RP: *Gynecology in Primary Care*. Baltimore: Williams & Wilkins, 1996, p. 352.

not enhance the possibility of pregnancy in couples who do not have appropriate indications for their use and they should be used only in carefully selected cases.

With the array of imaging techniques, pharmacologic agents, and surgical procedures available to the physician, there are many treatment options for infertile couples. Thus the physician can be optimistic in counseling infertile couples about the prognosis for having a child. At the same time, although offering encouragement, the physician must be aware of the psychological impact that infertility has on both partners and their family. Appropriate therapy must include psychological support.

CASE STUDIES

Case 39A

A couple in their late 20s presents for evaluation of infertility. The woman is nulligravid and has regular menses. The husband has never fathered a child. They have had unprotected sexual intercourse for 18 months. Neither has a history of sexually transmitted disease or major illness. The husband reports no difficulty with erection or ejaculation.

Questions Case 39A

Which of the following is the most likely cause of their infertility?

A. An ovulation disorder
B. An abnormality of spermatogenesis
C. An anatomic disorder of the woman's reproductive tract
D. Immunologic disorder

(Continued)

Answer: B

Problems with spermatogenesis are found in approximately 40% of couples with infertility, whereas abnormalities of ovulation and anatomic disorders of the female reproductive tract each account for approximately 30% of infertility cases. An ovulation disorder is unlikely, given her regular menstrual history. There is no reason to expect an anatomic abnormality, but this needs to be evaluated along with the possibility of infertility of immunologic etiology.

Which of the following diagnostic studies would not be indicated as part of this couple's initial evaluation?

A. Basal body temperature record
B. Semen analysis
C. Hysterosalpingogram
D. Diagnostic laparoscopy

Answer: D

Basal body temperature records are an excellent method of confirmation of ovulation, and semen analysis, of confirmation of spermatogenesis. Hysterosalpingography should be a part of initial infertility evaluations to rule out possible endometrial or tubal pathology. Diagnostic laparoscopy is used to evaluate the external surfaces of the female reproductive tract but requires a hospital surgical procedure. It should, therefore, be reserved until other initial tests are completed. Hysteroscopy may also be used for detailed evaluation of the intrauterine cavity and is commonly performed in conjunction with laparoscopy.

The female partner is found to have anovulation, despite her history of regular menses. The next step in the evaluation is to

A. Induce ovulation with clomiphene citrate
B. Perform artificial insemination

C. Induce ovulation with exogenous gonadotropins
D. Perform diagnostic laparoscopy to rule out other causes of infertility

Answer: A

Initial treatment with clomiphene citrate often is sufficient to induce ovulation. Occasionally, other agents such as Pergonal and hCG may be necessary. If ovulation does not occur, evaluation as to the etiology is indicated. Artificial insemination is not yet indicated, because it does not address the identified dysfunction. Laparoscopy would also be premature at this point.

Case 39B

A 37-year-old woman with a history of gonococcal salpingitis presents with her husband and expresses a complaint of infertility.

Questions Case 39B

Which of the following studies is indicated on initial evaluation?

A. Basal body temperature record
B. Semen analysis
C. Hysterosalpingogram
D. Endometrial biopsy

Answer: A, B, C

Without evidence of anovulation, the endometrial biopsy is not indicated, whereas evaluation of the man (semen analysis) is routine and the hysterosalpingogram is performed to rule out fallopian tube obstruction.

The hysterosalpingogram reveals bilateral tubal obstruction. A consultant advises against corrective surgery because of the very poor prognosis for successful outcome from reconstructive pelvic surgery.

Which of the following should be recommended?

A. Gamete intrafallopian tube transfer
B. Homologous intrauterine insemination
C. In vitro fertilization
D. Adoption

Answer: C

Because of the tubal obstruction, transfer of a gamete to the fallopian tube would not be appropriate. Similarly, intrauterine insemination would not overcome the anatomic block. IVF, if economically feasible for the couple, could provide a solution to the problem by bypassing the blocked fallopian tube. By obtaining the woman's eggs and fertilizing them with the man's sperm, then placing them into the prepared uterus, the couple has the opportunity of having a child that is genetically theirs. Adoption is always an option in cases when the couple is unable to conceive.

CHAPTER

40

PREMENSTRUAL SYNDROME

Premenstrual syndrome (PMS) is a group of physical, mood, and behavioral changes that occur in a regular, cyclic relationship to the luteal phase of the menstrual cycle. These symptoms occur in most cycles, resolving near the end of menses with a symptom-free interval of at least 1 week. This cyclic symptom complex may be minimally to totally disruptive of the patient's normal daily activities. First described in 1931, premenstrual syndrome is still a poorly understood condition, because there is no consensus on critical issues such as its pathophysiology, its diagnostic criteria, and optimal therapies. In fact, it has been suggested that PMS is actually more than a single clinical entity. For example, the *Diagnostic and Statistical Manual of Mental Disorders, fourth edition* (DSM-IV) lists the *premenstrual dysphoric disorder (PMDD)* as a type of depression in which symptoms such as depressed mood, marked anxiety, affective lability, and decreased interest in activities (anhedonia) regularly occur during the last week before the onset of menses. Despite these areas of confusion, it is clear that patients do present with symptoms that wax and wane in relationship to their menstrual cycles. Physicians must, therefore, be aware of potential causes for these changes, including the possibility of PMS.

INCIDENCE

Because of the wide variability in the signs and symptoms that are considered in making a diagnosis of PMS, the reported incidence of the syndrome ranges from 10% to 90%. Severe, debilitating PMS is reported in less than 10% of patients, although 70% of all women have some physical or emotional premenstrual symptoms. PMS appears to be most prevalent in women in their 30s and 40s, with a greater incidence in women with a past history of postpartum depression or other affective disorders. Accurate diagnosis is further confused by the similarity between some PMS symptoms and some psychiatric conditions.

SYMPTOMS

There have been well over 150 symptoms attributed to PMS. Each patient presents with her own constellation of symptoms, thus making *specific symptomatology less important than the cyclic occurrence of the symptoms.* Attempts have been made to classify PMS symptoms into subgroups, but none of these classification systems has been accepted universally. *Somatic symptoms* that are most common include breast swelling and pain (mastodynia), bloating, headache, constipation and/or diarrhea, and fatigue. The most common *emotional symptoms* include irritability, depression, anxiety, hostility, and changes in libido. Common *behavioral symptoms* include food cravings, poor concentration, sensitivity to noise, and loss of motor skills. *Situational depression* is associated with PMS in some cases and aggravates PMS in others. Table 40.1 presents a rational approach to the diagnostic criteria for premenstrual dysphoria disorder. Consequently, the recognition of coexisting situational depression must be made by careful questioning of marital and relationship problems, occupational difficulties or change, recent childbirth or child-rearing difficulties, and family or personal problems.

ETIOLOGY

Many theories have been proposed to explain PMS, but none provides a single, unified explanation that accounts for all the variations that are seen.

Psychiatric Basis

The high incidence of anxiety, depression, and other symptoms that simulate psychiatric disorders led to the theory that PMS is merely cyclic manifestations of underlying psychopathology.

Endocrinologic Basis

It was originally thought that PMS was related to abnormal luteal-phase steroid levels, predominantly higher estradiol levels relative to progesterone levels. Significant

TABLE 40.1. Diagnostic Criteria for Premenstrual Dysphoric Disorder

All of the following:
    Symptoms NOT an exacerbation of another underlying psychiatric disorder
    Symptoms clustered in luteal phase; absent within first few days of the follicular phase
    Symptoms cause significant disability
Plus, five or more of the following:
    At least one:
        Marked affective lability
        Marked anxiety, tension, feelings of being "keyed up" or "on edge"
        Markedly depressed mood, feelings of hopelessness, or self-deprecating thoughts
        Persistent and marked anger or irritability
    One or more of the following:
        Avoidance of social activities
        Decreased interest in usual activities
        Decreased productivity and efficiency
        Increased sensitivity to rejection
        Interpersonal conflicts
        Lethargy, easy fatigability, lack of energy
        Marked change in appetite, cravings
        Physical symptoms (reproducible pattern of complaints)
        Sleep disturbances (hypersomnia, insomnia)
        Subjective sense of being "out of control"
        Subjective sense of being overwhelmed
        Subjective sense of difficulty in concentration

Modified from Reid RL, Yen SSC. Premenstrual syndrome. *Am J Obstet Gynecol* 139:85, 1981.

alterations in estradiol and/or progesterone levels have not been found. This theory remains viable, however, because of the cyclic nature of symptoms. It is known that progesterone does have a sedative effect on the central nervous system and that both estrogen and progesterone receptors exist in the brain.

Diet Basis

Some patients with PMS seem to have a high intake of salt and refined carbohydrates, resulting in premenstrual hypoglycemic episodes, sometimes associated with outbursts of crying and violent behavior. Diet and evaluation for glucose intolerance are advocated in this subset of patients.

Endorphin Basis

There is a relative decrease in the luteal-phase endorphin levels in some patients who suffer from PMS. Because these endogenous opiates are associated with a sense of well-being, a decline in their production is seen as a cause for some of the findings in these patients. In addition, PMS symptoms are mimicked by some symptoms of opiate withdrawal. A strong argument in favor of the endorphin basis of PMS comes from patients who describe alleviation of symptomatology when moderate exercise is undertaken, presumably because of an exercise-associated increase in endorphin production.

Serotonin Basis

Premenstrual serotonin levels in PMS patients have been reported to be lower than in control patients. Because lower serotonin levels have been associated with clinical depression, affective changes in PMS may be explained on this basis. In addition, anxiety has been described as a possible state of serotonin excess. Therefore, dysfunction in serotonin neurotransmission is an attractive explanation for many PMS symptoms.

Prostaglandin Basis

Because prostaglandins are produced in the breast, brain, gastrointestinal tract, kidney, and reproductive tract and because these are areas that often present with physical symptoms in patients with PMS, a prostaglandin-associated basis for PMS remains attractive. Nonsteroidal anti-inflammatory agents have provided relief for some symptoms in some studies.

Fluid Retention Basis

Many women both with and without PMS report some premenstrual weight gain and edema. Although studies do not demonstrate an increased body weight in these patients, alterations of the renin-angiotensin-aldosterone axis as well as antidiuretic hormone have been suggested as a basis for PMS.

Vitamin Basis

Particular focus has also been placed on deficiency of vitamins A, B, and E as possible causes of PMS. Of note, vitamin B_6 (pyridoxine) is a cofactor in the production of serotonin as well as prostaglandin.

Other Bases

Other suggested bases for PMS include thyroid disorders, prolactin disorders, endometrial infection, and hypoglycemia.

DIFFERENTIAL DIAGNOSIS

Virtually any condition that results in mood or physical changes in any cyclic fashion may be included in the differential diagnosis of PMS. As a result, the physician must remain open-minded at the outset in order not to prematurely exclude the primary problem (Table 40.2).

DIAGNOSIS

Because the etiology of PMS is unknown, there are no definitive historical, physical examination, or laboratory markers to aid in diagnosis. At present, the diagnosis of PMS is based on documentation of the relationship of the patient's symptoms to the luteal phase. This is best done by prospective documentation of symptoms using a *menstrual diary.* Because the patient's memory of daily symptoms cannot be depended on for accuracy given the wide variety of and sometimes subtle nature of the symptoms, she is asked to monitor and record key symptoms and their severity on a daily basis. *To confirm the diagnosis of PMS, the patient must demonstrate a symptom-free follicular phase in contrast to the problems seen in the luteal phase.*

A thorough physical examination for specific organic pathology is requisite, although it is also important to understand that no specific physical findings are diagnostic of PMS.

TREATMENT

Because of the diverse symptoms of patients with PMS, a multidisciplinary team of providers, including a gynecologist, psychiatrist, psychologist, endocrinologist, nutritionist, and social worker, is often advocated. In addition, because the underlying pathophysiology is yet to be determined, a wide range of treatment protocols has been recommended (Figure 40.1). A major portion of any management scheme should include *education of the patient as well as her family* to clarify what is known about PMS as well as what to expect from possible therapies. Education can, in and of itself, be therapeutic for patients who are otherwise lacking insight into the possible causes of their symptoms.

As part of the educational process, prospective charting of symptoms not only documents the cyclic or noncyclic nature of the patient's symptoms but also allows the patient to become a part of the diagnostic effort, thus helping her to take an active

TABLE 40.2.	Differential Diagnosis of Premenstrual Syndrome

Allergy	Gastrointestinal conditions
Breast disorders (fibrocystic change)	Inflammatory bowel disease (Crohn's
Chronic fatigue states	disease, ulcerative colitis)
Anemia	Irritable bowel syndrome
Chronic cytomegalovirus infection	Gynecologic disorders
Lyme disease	Dysmenorrhea
Connective tissue disease (lupus	Endometriosis
erythematosus)	Pelvic inflammatory disease
Drug and substance abuse	Perimenopause
Endocrinologic disorders	Uterine leiomyomata
Adrenal disorders (Cushing's	Idiopathic edema
syndrome, hypoadrenalism)	Neurologic disorders
Adrenocorticotropic hormone-	Migraine
mediated disorders	Seizure disorders
Hyperandrogenism	Psychiatric and psychological disorders
Hyperprolactinemia	Anxiety neurosis
Panhypopituitarism	Bulimia
Pheochromocytoma	Personality disorders
Thyroid disorders (hypothyroidism,	Psychosis
hyperthyroidism)	Somatoform disorders
Family, marital, and social stress	Unipolar and bipolar affective
(physical or sexual abuse)	disorders

From Smith RP: *Gynecology in Primary Care*. Baltimore, Williams & Wilkins, 1996, p. 434.

part in the diagnosis and management of her condition. In some cases, giving the symptoms a diagnostic label helps relieve the patient's concern that she may be "going crazy." Often a patient's symptoms become less unbearable because she begins to understand her condition.

In addition to patient education, the following interventions have been shown to be helpful in selected groups of patients. Patients should be advised that no one therapy works for all patients and that a logical sequence of therapeutic manipulations may have to be done to achieve resolution of symptoms.

Diet recommendations emphasize fresh rather than processed foods. The patient is encouraged to eat more fresh fruits and vegetables and minimize refined sugars and fats. Some patients benefit by eating frequent small meals during the day rather than having three large meals, thereby minimizing hypoglycemia symptoms. Minimiz-

ing salt intake may help with bloating, and eliminating caffeine from the diet can reduce nervousness and anxiety.

Exercise has been found to be helpful in some patients, possibly by increasing endogenous production of endorphins.

Medications to induce anovulation have been reported to be of benefit in PMS. Because premenstrual symptoms are typically associated with ovulatory cycles, inducing an anovulatory state should be beneficial. This can be accomplished by using oral contraceptives, danazol, or gonadotropin-releasing hormone (GnRH) agonist. Oral contraceptives are a logical first choice for patients who also require contraception. Some patients, however, find a worsening of their symptoms when taking oral contraceptives. The use of *danazol and GnRH* agonists has been demonstrated to be beneficial in short-term studies, but long-term effects of such drugs for PMS have not been fully evaluated. The use of either

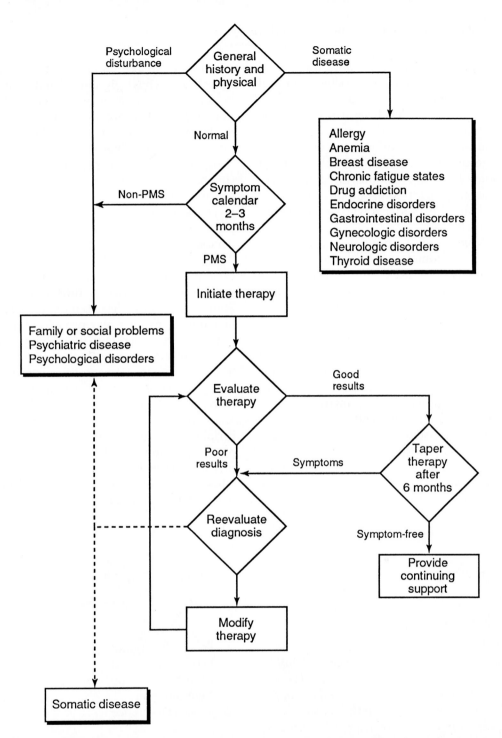

FIGURE 40.1. Algorithm for the management of premenstrual syndrome (PMS). The diagnosis of PMS is predicated on the elimination of other mimicking physical and psychological conditions, and the use of a two- to three-month, prospective calendar of symptoms. Once the diagnosis of PMS is established, pharmacologic and supportive (nonpharmacologic) therapy is begun. If successful, the pharmacologic therapy is withdrawn after six months and careful, supportive follow-up continued. Failure of any therapy suggests the need for a critical reevaluation of the diagnosis. If this reassessment continues to support the diagnosis of PMS, the therapy is modified and the process of monitoring begins anew. (From Smith RP: *Gynecology in Primary Care.* Baltimore, Williams & Wilkins, 1996, p. 433.)

constitutes a "medical oophorectomy" and may be used as a trial before surgical oophorectomy is considered.

Progesterone has been described to be effective delivered either as a vaginal or rectal suppository or as oral micronized progesterone. Although well-designed studies have not demonstrated its effectiveness, progesterone suppositories are widely used by patients who describe beneficial results.

Nonsteroidal anti-inflammatory agents have been found to be useful for more symptoms than just dysmenorrhea. This is possibly related to prostaglandin production in various sites in the body.

Diuretics—such as *spironolactone* (25 mg orally two or three times daily), an aldosterone antagonist; *hydrochlorothiazide* (25–50 mg orally four times daily) with potassium supplementation; or *Dyazide* (hydrochlorothiazide 25 mg/triamterene 50 mg four times daily without the requirement for potassium supplementation)—have been found to help control weight gain as well as some psychological symptoms. Bloating is also minimized in patients taking diuretics.

Anxiolytic and antidepressant medications have been widely studied and found to be useful in some patients, especially those not responsive to other regimens. These medications have often been used in consultation with a psychiatrist, especially when there is significant depression. *Buspirone* (BuSpar) is a nonsedating, nonaddictive anxiolytic found effective in some cases. It is given as an initial dosage of 5 mg orally three times daily with meals but does not demonstrate its effect for approximately 2 weeks. *Alprazolam* (Xanax) is also an efficacious anxiolytic given in an initial dosage of 0.25 mg orally two or three times daily. Fluoxetine (Prozac) has been found effective in reducing psychic and behavioral symptoms in a well-tolerated 20-mg daily dose.

Vitamin therapy, including administration of pyridoxine (vitamin B_6), a cofactor in the synthesis of serotonin, has been shown to be helpful in some patients. There are reported side effects, including reversible peripheral neuropathy when large doses of pyridoxine are taken. Evening primrose oil, rich in vitamin E, has also been helpful in relieving both breast tenderness and depressive symptoms associated with PMS.

CASE STUDIES

Case 40A

A 29-year-old G2 P2 complains of periodic anxiety, depression, and irritability for 2 years. Her gynecologic history includes regular menses with mild cramps. Her breasts are also mildly tender before each period. She is presently using a diaphragm for contraception. Physical examination is normal.

Question Case 40A

What initial evaluation(s) should be recommended?

A. Pelvic ultrasound
B. Psychiatric consult
C. Monthly symptom calendar
D. Mammogram
E. Glucose tolerance test

Answer: C

Because of the periodic nature of these emotional symptoms, they may or may not be temporally related to the menstrual cycle. A prospective documentation of symptoms aids in determining whether this is PMS or not. Pelvic ultrasound is unnecessary given the normal examination. A psychiatric consult may be needed if the patient's symptoms are severe, refractory to care, or causing significant emotional or interpersonal distress. A mammogram in this age group has little to offer in a patient with cyclic mastalgia. A glucose tolerance test is sometimes used to identify a patient with hypoglycemic episodes who might present with PMS-like symptoms, but would not be appropriate here.

Case 40B

A 40-year-old G4 P4 has struggled with documented PMS for several years. Despite treatments including vaginal progesterone, tranquilizers, vitamin B, and diuretics, she continues to have 10 days of premenstrual bloating, headaches, and mood swings. She requests a hysterectomy as definitive treatment.

Question Case 40B

Which of the following medical therapies is most appropriate instead of hysterectomy?

A. Fluoxetine
B. Oral progesterone
C. Bromocriptine
D. GnRH agonist
E. Ibuprofen

Answer: D

GnRH agonist is the most appropriate of the drugs listed. The patient believes that removing the uterus will be a cure to her problems. Unfortunately, it is the ovaries, not the uterus, which may be linked with the symptoms. The uterus and monthly menses serve only as a reference point to which her symptoms are related. The GnRH can provide a temporary oophorectomy as a trial before any consideration for surgical oophorectomy. If the patient improves with GnRH agonist, then symptoms return when the medication is discontinued, bilateral oophorectomy might be a consideration. All the other therapies have been utilized for patients with PMS, but will not affect the physiologic changes she is seeking. Each may have a role, however, in treatment of specific symptoms of PMS.

UNIT V

Neoplasia

41

CELL BIOLOGY AND PRINCIPLES OF CANCER THERAPY

CHAPTER OBJECTIVES

There is no specific APGO objective for this chapter, although many chapters, especially in Unit V, Neoplasia, rely on an understanding of the information in this chapter.

Treatment of cancers involving the breast and genital organs can involve surgery, chemotherapy, radiation therapy, and hormone therapy, used alone or in combination. The specific treatment plan depends on the type of cancer, the stage of the cancer, and the characteristics of the individual patient. Individualizing treatment is an important characteristic of cancer therapy.

CELL CYCLE AND CANCER THERAPY

Knowledge of the cell cycle is important in understanding cancer therapies. Many treatments are based on the fact that cancer cells are constantly dividing, making them more vulnerable to agents that interfere with the cell division process.

The cell cycle consists of four phases (Figure 41.1). During the G_1 phase, there is synthesis of RNA and protein that prepares the cell for DNA synthesis, which occurs in the S phase. The G_2 phase is a period of additional RNA, protein, and specialized DNA synthesis. This leads to mitosis (M phase), during which cell division occurs. After mitosis, cells can again enter the G_1 phase or can "drop out" of the cell cycle and enter a resting phase (G_0). Cells in G_0 do not engage in the synthetic activities characteristic of the cell cycle and, therefore, are not vulnerable to therapies aimed at actively growing and dividing cells. The *growth fraction* is the number of cells in a tumor that are actively involved in cell division (i.e., not in the G_0 phase). The growth fraction of tumors decreases as they enlarge, because vascular supply and oxygen levels are decreased. *Surgical removal of tumor tissue* (cytoreductive debulking surgery) can result in G_0 cells reentering the cell cycle, thus making them more vulnerable to chemotherapy and radiation therapy.

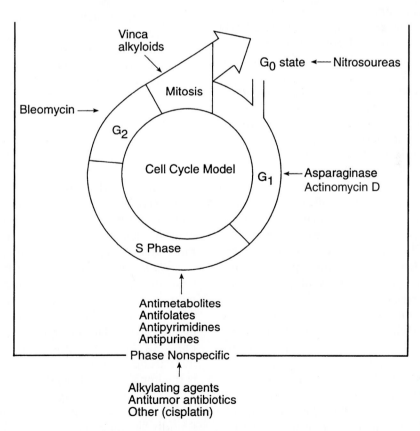

FIGURE 41.1. Actions of antineoplastic agents within the cell cycle.

The generation time is the length of the cell cycle, from M phase to M phase. For a given cell type, the lengths of the S and M phases are relatively constant, whereas G_2 and, especially, G_1 vary. The variable length of G_1 can be explained by cells entering G_0 for a period and then reentering the cycle.

Chemotherapeutic agents and radiation kill cancer cells by first-order kinetics. This means that each dose kills a constant fraction of tumor cells, instead of a constant number. The implication of this is that a number of intermittent doses are more likely to be curative than a single large dose.

CHEMOTHERAPY

Chemotherapeutic agents can be (a) cell-cycle (phase) nonspecific, which means that they can kill in all phases of the cell cycle and are useful in tumors with a low growth index, or *(b) cell-cycle (phase) specific,* which means that they kill in a specific phase of the cell cycle and are most useful in tumors that have a large proportion of cells actively dividing. Figure 41.1 contains examples of common drugs and their sites of action within the cycle.

There are several *classes of antineoplastic drugs* (Table 41.1). *Alkylating agents* primarily interact with DNA molecules to interfere with base pairing, produce interstrand and intrastrand cross-links, and cause single- and double-strand breaks. This interferes with DNA, RNA, and protein synthesis. Dividing cells are most sensitive to the effects of these drugs. The late G_1 and S phases are the times of maximum sensitivity. The major side effects of the alkylating agents are myelosuppression and immunosuppression. They also may result in amenorrhea.

The *antitumor antibiotics* intercalate between DNA base pairs to inhibit DNA-directed RNA synthesis and also are involved in the formation of free radicals, causing strand breakage. They are phase nonspecific (i.e., they are effective in all phases of the cell cycle). Their general side effects are similar to those of the alkylating agents. Other side effects are drug specific.

TABLE 41.1. Examples of Antineoplastic Drugs

Alkylating agents
  Carboplatin
  Cyclophosphamide
  Chlorambucil (Leukeran)
  Busulfan (Myleran)
  Melphalan (Alkeran, L-PAM)
  Ifosfamide (Ifex)
Antitumor antibiotics
  Doxorubicin (Adriamycin)
  Bleomycin (Blenoxane)
  Actinomycin D (Dactinomycin, Cosmegen)
  Mitomycin C (Mutamycin)
  Mitoxantrone
Antimetabolites
  Methotrexate (MTX, Amethopterin)
  6-Mercaptopurine (6-MP, Purinethol)
  5-Fluorouracil (Fluorouracil, 5-FU)
  Hydroxyurea (Hydrea)
Plant alkaloids
  Cis-diaminedichloroplatinum (cisplatin)
  Vinblastine (Velban)
  Vincristine (Oncovin)
  Paclitaxel (Taxol)

The *antimetabolites* are structural analogs of normal molecules necessary for cell function. They competitively interfere with the normal synthesis of nucleic acids and, therefore, are most active during the S phase of cell division. They may cause bone marrow suppression or gastrointestinal-mucositis when given in a bolus.

Plant (vinca) alkaloids primarily prevent the assembly of microtubules, thus interfering with the M phase of cell division. They may cause bone marrow suppression or an anaphylactoid reaction. Cisplatin binds to DNA to cause interstrand and intrastrand cross-links. A major side effect is the impairment of renal tubular function.

Antineoplastic drugs are toxic because they act on normal as well as cancer cells. Rapidly dividing cell types are most sensitive. For example, the cells of the erythroid, myeloid, and megakaryocytic series are damaged by common neoplastic drugs. Granulocytopenia and thrombocytopenia are predictable side effects. Patients with low granulocyte counts are at high risk for fatal sepsis, and those with sustained thrombocytopenia are at risk for spontaneous gastrointestinal or acute intracranial hemorrhage. Prophylactic antibiotics are usually administered to febrile patients to prevent serious infection, and platelet transfusions are used to decrease the risk of hemorrhage. Table 41.2 describes the major side effects of antineoplastic agents.

There are limitations in the use of single agents. These include the development of drug resistance and toxicity. As a consequence, combination chemotherapy has come into use.

There are several strategies that can be used to select drugs for combination chemotherapy. In *sequential blockade,* the drugs block sequential enzymes in a single biochemical pathway. In *concurrent blockade,* the drugs attack parallel biochemical pathways leading to the same end product. *Complementary inhibition* interferes with different steps in the synthesis of DNA, RNA, or protein.

The *interactions between drugs used in combination* are defined as *synergistic* (result in improved antitumor activity or decreased toxicity than with each agent alone), *additive* (result in enhanced antitumor activity equal to the sum of each individual agent), or *antagonistic* (result in less antitumor activity than each individual agent). Drugs used in combinations should (*a*) be effective when used singly, (*b*) have different mechanisms of action, and (*c*) be additive or, preferably, synergistic in action.

Chemotherapy is administered in a variety of regimens. *Adjuvant chemotherapy* is usually a short course of combination chemotherapy that is given in a high dose to patients with no evidence of residual cancer after radiotherapy or surgery. The purpose is to eliminate any residual cancer cells. *Induction chemotherapy* is usually a combination chemotherapy given in a high dose to cause a remission. *Maintenance chemotherapy* is a long-term and low-dose regimen

TABLE 41.2. Major Side Effects of Antineoplastic Drugs

Hematologic
   Granulocytopenia
   Thrombocytopenia
Gastrointestinal
   Mucositis
   Necrotizing enterocolitis
Immunosuppression
Dermatologic
   Alopecia
   Local necrosis
   Allergic/hypersensitivity reactions
Hepatic
Pulmonary
   Interstitial pneumonitis
Cardiac
   Cardiomyopathy
Urinary
   Chronic azotemia
   Acute renal failure
Neurologic
   Peripheral neuropathies
   Ototoxicity
   Paresthesias
Reproductive
   Amenorrhea
Metabolic abnormalities
   Tumor lysis syndrome

that is given to a patient in remission to maintain the remission by inhibiting the growth of remaining cancer cells.

RADIATION THERAPY

Ionizing radiation causes the production of free hydrogen ions and hydroxyl (OH^-) radicals. In the presence of sufficient oxygen, H_2O_2 is formed, which affects DNA and, eventually, the cell's ability to divide. As with chemotherapy, killing is by first-order kinetics. Because dividing cells are more sensitive to radiation damage and because not all cells in a given tumor are dividing at any one time, *fractionated doses of radiation are more likely to be effective than a single dose.* Providing multiple lower doses of radiation also reduces the deleterious effects on normal tissues.

The basis of fractionated dosage comes from the *"four Rs" of radiobiology.*

1. *Repair of sublethal injury.* When a dose is divided, the number of normal cells that survive is greater than if the dose were given at one time (higher total amounts of radiation can be tolerated in fractionated as opposed to single doses).
2. *Repopulation.* Reactivation of stem cells occurs when radiation is stopped; thus regenerative capacity depends on the number of available stem cells.
3. *Reoxygenation.* Cells are more vulnerable to radiation damage in the presence of oxygen; as tumor cells are killed, surviving tumor cells are brought into contact with capillaries, making them radiosensitive.
4. *Redistribution in the cell cycle.* Because tumor cells are in various phases of the cell cycle, fractionated doses make it more likely that a given cell is irradiated when it is most vulnerable.

The *rad* has been used as a measure of the amount of energy absorbed per unit mass of tissue. A standard measure of absorbed dose is the *Gray,* which is defined as 1 joule per kilogram; *1 Gray is equal to 100 rad.* Radiation is delivered in two general ways: external irradiation (teletherapy) and local irradiation (brachytherapy). *Teletherapy* depends on the use of high-energy (> 1 million eV) beams, because this spares the skin and delivers less toxic radiation to the bone. Tolerance for external radiation depends on the vulnerability of surrounding normal tissues. Teletherapy usually is used to shrink tumors before localized radiation.

Brachytherapy depends on the inverse square law: the dose of radiation at a given point is inversely proportional to the square of the distance from the radiation source. To put the radioactive material at the closest possible distance, brachytherapy uses encapsulated sources of ionizing radiation implanted directly into tissues (intersti-tial) or placed in natural body cavities (intracavity). *Intracavity devices* can be placed within the uterus or vagina and then afterloaded with radioactive sources (phosphorus-32, cesium-137). This method protects health personnel from radiation exposure. *Interstitial implants* use isotopes (iridium-192, iodine-125) formulated as wires or seeds. These implants are usually temporary.

Complications associated with radiation therapy can be acute or late (chronic). *Acute reactions* affect rapidly dividing tissues, such as epithelia (skin, gastrointestinal mucosa, bone marrow, and reproductive cells). Manifestations are cessation of mitotic activity, cellular swelling, tissue edema, and tissue necrosis. Early problems associated with irradiation of gynecologic cancers include enteritis, acute cystitis, vulvitis, proctosigmoiditis, and occasionally, bone marrow depression. *Chronic complications* occur months to years after completion of radiation therapy. These include obliteration of small blood vessels or thickening of the vessel wall, fibrosis, and reductions in epithelial and parenchymal cell populations. This results in chronic proctitis, hemorrhagic cystitis, formation of uterovaginal or vesicovaginal fistula, and rectal or sigmoid stenosis as well as gastrointestinal fistulae.

HORMONAL THERAPY

The therapeutic importance of the presence of cellular *estrogen receptors (ER)* has been well established in breast cancers. There is a good relationship between the presence of ER and the response of patients to endocrine therapy. Normally, estrogen enters cells and binds to ER in the cytoplasm. The complex is translocated to the nucleus, where it binds to acceptor sites on chromosomes, resulting in activation of RNA and protein synthesis. The drug tamoxifen acts as a competitive inhibitor of estrogen binding. The tamoxifen–ER complex also binds to chromosomes but does not activate cell metabolism. This decreases cellular activity and cell division, thus reducing tumor growth. Tamoxifen is used in the adjunct treatment of breast cancer.

There also are *progestin receptors (PR),* which are located in the nucleus of progestin-sensitive cells. The PR complex binds to acceptor sites on DNA. This, in turn, reduces the synthesis of both ER and PR. Like the presence of estrogen receptors, the presence of receptors for progesterone is useful in identifying patients who will benefit from hormonal therapy. In addition, androgen receptors have been identified in epithelial ovarian cancer.

Luteinizing hormone-releasing hormone (LH-RH) antagonists are being evaluated in the treatment of breast and ovarian cancers. Cytotoxic analogs of LH-RH could be used to competitively inhibit LH-RH binding to receptors on tumors.

GENE THERAPY

In the next decade, it is anticipated that there will be significant progress in so-called "gene therapy," therapies designed to modulate gene function and thus many biological processes, including the abnormal cellular proliferation we term cancer. The potential benefits of this therapeutic concept are manifold, whether considered as primary or adjunctive therapy.

CASE STUDIES

Case 41A

A patient with a large ovarian tumor undergoes total abdominal hysterectomy with bilateral salpingo-oophorectomy for widespread disease. Most of the tumor mass is removed.

Question Case 41A

Which of the following is a likely result of this operation?

A. The proportion of tumor cells in G_0 will increase

B. The growth fraction of the remaining tumor will decrease

C. The proportion of tumor cells that are sensitive to antineoplastic agents will increase

D. A single dose of chemotherapy will be able to kill the remaining tumor cells

Answer: C

Removal of part of a tumor mass increases the growth fraction (the number of cells that are actively dividing). Therefore, the proportion of cells in G_0 (the nondividing phase) will decrease and the proportion of cells sensitive to antineoplastic agents will increase (because dividing cells are more sensitive). A single dose of chemotherapy will probably not be sufficient to kill the remaining tumor cells, because cells still will be killed by first-order kinetics.

42

GESTATIONAL TROPHOBLASTIC DISEASE

CHAPTER OBJECTIVES

This chapter deals primarily with APGO Objective(s):

OBJECTIVE 54   Gestational
Trophoblastic Neoplasia

A. List the symptoms/physical findings
found in gestational trophoblastic
disease.

B Describe the diagnostic methods used
to confirm this condition and the
management and follow-up options
which are available.

Gestational trophoblastic neoplasia (GTN), which represents a *rare variation of pregnancy,* is limited in most instances to a benign disease called *molar pregnancy.* This disorder includes neoplasms that are derived almost entirely from abnormal placental (trophoblastic) proliferation. Molar pregnancy may in turn be divided into *complete mole* (no fetus) and *incomplete mole* (fetus plus molar degeneration). *Persistent or malignant disease* will develop in approximately 20% of patients with molar pregnancy. Fortunately, persistent or malignant GTN is very responsive to effective chemotherapy.

Key clinical features of GTN include its consistent clinical presentation, reliable means of diagnosis with pathognomonic ultrasound findings, presence of specific tumor marker [quantitative serum human chorionic gonadotropin (hCG)], availability of effective surgical treatment, sensitivity to chemotherapy when GTN is persistent or malignant, and reliable long-term follow-up through assessment of quantitative hCG levels.

The disease has a number of *characteristic features,* including *(a)* the potential for malignant transformation, *(b)* clinical presentation as a pregnancy, *(c)* profound hormonal changes found in association with the abnormal proliferation of trophoblastic tissue, *(d)* genetic makeup, and *(e)* high sensitivity to chemotherapeutic agents.

The *etiology* of this disorder is unknown. It has been observed that the incidence varies among different national and ethnic groups, with the highest occurring among Asian women living in Asia (up to 1 in 200 pregnancies) and the lowest incidence occurring in white women of Western European and U.S. origins (approximately 1 in 2000 pregnancies). The recurrence rate is approximately 2%. It is more common in very young women and in women at the end of their reproductive years. It is also associated with dietary deficiencies, such as folic acid deficiency. The classification of gestational trophoblastic disease is described in Table 42.1. Because persistent GTN may follow simple molar pregnancy, an appreciation of the latter's clinical presentation,

TABLE 42.1. Classification of Gestational Trophoblastic Disease
Molar pregnancy
Complete mole
Partial mole
Persistent gestational trophoblastic neoplasia
Histologically benign
Persistent histologically benign
Persistent histologically malignant
Placental site tumors

histology, clinical risk factors, and long-term follow-up is necessary to thoroughly treat the patient with this unusual tumor.

HYDATIDIFORM MOLE (MOLAR PREGNANCY)

A *complete hydatidiform mole* includes abnormal proliferation of the syncytiotrophoblast and replacement of normal placental trophoblastic tissue by *hydropic placental villi.* Complete moles do not include the formation of a fetus, and fetal membranes are characteristically absent. *Partial moles* are characterized by focal trophoblastic proliferation and degeneration of the placenta and are associated with a chromosomally abnormal fetus. In this form of molar pregnancy, trophoblastic proliferation is largely from the cytotrophoblast (Figure 42.1).

The *genetic constitutions* of these two types of molar pregnancy are different (Table 42.2). Complete moles are entirely of paternal origin as a result of the fertilization of a blighted ovum by a haploid sperm, which then reduplicates. Accordingly, the karyotype of a complete mole is 46,XX. The fetus of a partial mole is usually a triploidy, the most common being 69,XXY. The triploidy comprises one haploid set of maternal chromosomes and two haploid sets of paternal chromosomes, which arise from dispermic fertilization. Of the two varieties, the complete mole is more common (approximately 90% of molar pregnancies). Although the potential for malignant transformation is greater in complete moles, partial moles may also undergo this change, and therefore both varieties should be followed in a similar fashion to minimize the chance for malignant sequelae.

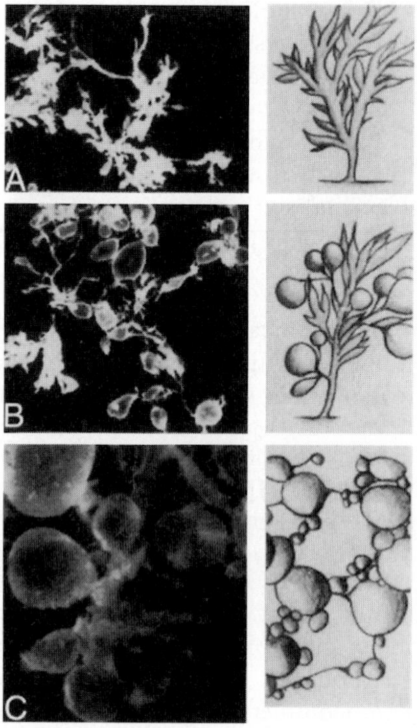

Clinical Presentation

Clinically, patients with molar pregnancy of either variety may present with findings consistent with pregnancy but also with uterine size/dates discrepancy, exaggerated subjective symptoms of pregnancy, and bleeding suggestive of spontaneous abortion. Of these symptoms, *bleeding* is the most characteristic and occurs in most patients early in the second trimester of pregnancy. The bleeding is usually painless. The patient also may experience the passage of tissue, as fragments of the edematous trophoblast are passed through the dilated cervical os. Most patients have already been *diagnosed as pregnant*, having had a positive pregnancy test. There is a *uterine dates/size discrepancy* in two thirds of patients. The uterus may be either too large or too small for gestational age, usually larger than expected. This discrepancy, coupled with late first or early second trimester bleeding, usually leads the clinician to perform ultrasound imaging of the uterus, which confirms the diagnosis of molar pregnancy by its characteristic "snowstorm" appearance (Figure 42.2).

Molar pregnancies may present with *other signs and symptoms*, including visual disturbances, severe nausea and vomiting, marked pregnancy-induced hypertension (preeclampsia), proteinuria, and rarely, clinical hyperthyroidism. Some patients experi-

FIGURE 42.1. Villi gross morphology. (A) Normal chorionic villi. (B) Partial mole with normal villi admixed with swollen ones (case of triploidy, 69,XXY). (C) Complete mole with swollen, vesicular villi.

TABLE 42.2. Complete and Incomplete Hydatidiform Moles

Characteristic	Complete	Incomplete
Synonyms	True; classic	Partial
Uterus large for dates	About 50%	Not usually
Villi	All edematous	Some normal
Capillaries	Few, no fetal RBCs	Some; fetal RBCs
Embryo	None	Abnormal fetus
hCG titer	High	Moderately elevated to high
Karyotype	Mostly 46,XX	Triploid (69,XXY)
Malignant potential	15%–30%	Slight (<5%)

hCG = human chorionic gonadotropin; RBCs = red blood cells.

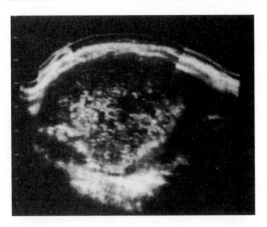

FIGURE 42.2. "Snowstorm" appearance of complete mole on ultrasound examination.

ence tachycardia and shortness of breath, arising from intense hemodynamic changes associated with acute hypertensive changes. In these patients, hyperreflexia may also be found. Physical examination reveals not only the dates/size discrepancy of the uterine fundus and absent fetal heart tones, but changes associated with developing preeclampsia. Occasionally, bimanual pelvic examination may reveal large *adnexal masses* (theca lutein cysts), which represent marked enlargement of the ovaries as a result of high levels of hCG stimulation.

Histologically identical to complete mole, *invasive mole (chorioadenoma destruens)* is a complete mole invading the myometrium without any intervening endometrial stroma on histologic sample. It is often diagnosed months after evacuation of a complete mole following evaluation for hCG levels that do not fall appropriately, although it may be diagnosed on curettage at the time of initial molar evacuation. Untreated, its natural course includes local invasion and, on occasion, vascular invasion and metastasis. It is reported to follow 5%–15% of complete hydatidiform moles.

The clinical presentation of partial molar pregnancy is similar to that for complete mole, although typically the patient presents at a more advanced gestational age (after the 20th week of pregnancy). Vaginal bleeding is less common than with complete moles. Uterine growth that is less than that

expected for the gestational age, especially if coupled with rapidly developing hypertension, may be the first clinical indication. Because of the growth/dates discrepancy, ultrasonography is obtained, which reveals molar degeneration of the placenta and frequently a grossly abnormal fetus.

Laboratory Assessment

The laboratory assessment of molar pregnancy is critical for both treatment and follow-up. After the molar pregnancy has been confirmed by imaging studies, laboratory documentation is necessary to ascertain the *level of hCG*. These levels are extremely high in molar pregnancy and not only *help classify risk category but also serve as a sensitive tumor marker in the follow-up* of these patients. Other valuable studies include a baseline chest radiograph to check for metastatic disease, assessment of hemoglobin and hematocrit, and selected other tests depending on clinical evidence of other conditions such as preeclampsia and/or hyperthyroidism. Before treatment, blood should be obtained for blood type and Rh and screened for antibodies in case blood replacement is necessary. This is particularly important for patients who undergo uterine evacuation because there is the potential for extensive blood loss during the procedure. Similar laboratory studies should be obtained whether the patient has partial or complete mole.

Treatment

In most cases of *molar pregnancy,* the definitive treatment is prompt *removal of the intrauterine contents.* Uterine evacuation is done most expeditiously by dilation of the cervix followed by *suction curettage.* After suction curettage with an atraumatic plastic cannula, *gentle sharp curettage* may be performed to provide small amounts of myometrial tissue for separate pathologic assessment. This is used to ascertain whether there has been myometrial invasion. The evacuation of larger moles is sometimes associated with uterine atony and excessive blood loss, so that appropriate preparations

TABLE 42.3. Conditions That Define High-Risk Gestational Trophoblastic Disease

Uterus > 16-week size
Theca lutein cysts
Marked trophoblastic proliferation
    and/or anaplasia
Hyperthyroidism

TABLE 42.4. Posttreatment Follow-up for Molar Pregnancy

General physical and pelvic examination
    and baseline chest radiograph at
    2 weeks
Serum quantitative hCG level every
    2 weeks until normal (0–5 mIU)
Serum quantitative hCG monthly for
    1 year after obtaining first normal level
Assurance of contraception for 1 year
    (oral contraceptives preferred unless
    contraindicated)
Early ultrasound examination and
    quantitative hCG level for future
    pregnancy

hCG = human chorionic gonadotropin.

should be made for oxytocin administration and blood transfusion if they are needed.

In cases of *partial mole,* a similar procedure may be carried out, with the additional need for larger grasping instruments to remove the abnormal fetus. With cases involving enlargement of the uterus beyond 24 weeks' gestational size, an alternative to suction evacuation is induction of labor with prostaglandin vaginal suppositories. In general, *the larger the uterus, the greater the risk of pulmonary complications* associated with trophoblastic emboli, fluid overload, and anemia. This is particularly true in patients with extreme degrees of associated pregnancy-induced hypertension (preeclampsia), because patients may experience concomitant hemoconcentration and alteration in vascular hemodynamics. In these patients, uterine evacuation by prostaglandin stimulation may be safer.

Occasional patients in the older reproductive age group may be best served by hysterectomy, which ensures removal of the entire primary neoplasm. This is especially true in patients with "high-risk" disease, as described in Table 42.3. This treatment should be reserved for patients who have no interest in further childbearing and/or have other indications for hysterectomy.

The *bilaterally enlarged multicystic ovaries (theca lutein cysts),* arising from massive follicular stimulation by large amounts of systemic hCG, do not represent malignant changes. This enlargement invariably regresses within a few months after the molar pregnancy has been evacuated, and therefore does not require surgical removal. Understanding the physiology of

these cysts is especially important in the patient undergoing abdominal hysterectomy as the primary treatment.

Postevacuation Management

Because of the predisposition for recurrent nonmalignant or malignant disease, patients should be followed closely for at least 1 year. The *removed molar tissue* should be examined carefully to identify hyperplastic and/or anaplastic proliferation. The small tissue sample provided by the sharp curettage specimen is pivotal in determining myometrial invasion. RhoGAM should be given in cases of incomplete mole.

Follow-up consists primarily of *periodic physical examination,* including pelvic examination and the *assessment of quantitative hCG levels,* according to the schedule outlined in Table 42.4. Quantitative serum β-hCG values fall after evacuation in a characteristic manner (Figure 42.3), with plateauing being an indication of persistent disease and the need for further treatment. Following this guideline assures the physician that recurrent disease is not developing; that an intercurrent pregnancy (within 1 year) is not causing an increase in hCG levels; and that for future pregnancy

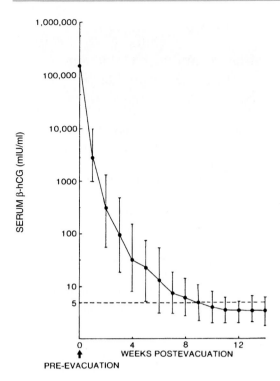

FIGURE 42.3. Normal regression curve and smoothed 95% confidence limits of serum β-hCG after evaluation of a hydatidiform mole. Time 0 is time of evacuation.

another molar pregnancy is ruled out early, because the *recurrence rate* for these patients is approximately five times the initial rate (1 in 400 in the United States). Effective contraception is recommended in the first year of follow-up.

There is little or no increased risk of congenital anomalies in subsequent pregnancies, but the risk of major obstetric complications is higher in this group, approaching 5%–9%. The incidence of placental accreta in particular appears to be increased.

METASTATIC/MALIGNANT GESTATIONAL TROPHOBLASTIC NEOPLASIA

Recurrent benign GTN occurs in less than 10% of patients with antecedent molar pregnancy. Malignant transformation of

hydatidiform mole, *choriocarcinoma,* is an aggressive pathology characterized by rapid myometrial and uterine vessel invasion and systemic metastasis resulting from hematogenous embolization. Lung, vagina, central nervous system, kidney, and liver are common metastatic locations for this tumor. There are no chorionic villi; rather, the tumor has a red, granular appearance on cut section and consists of intermingled syncytioblastic and cytotrophoblastic elements with many abnormal cellular forms. Choriocarcinoma may also follow a normal antecedent term pregnancy, an abortion, or an ectopic pregnancy. In the United States, *choriocarcinoma is associated with approximately one in 150,000 pregnancies, one in 15,000 abortions, one in 5000 ectopic pregnancies, and one in 40 moles.* Early identification and treatment of recurrence are critically important in both cases. Failure of quantitative hCG levels to regress after initial therapy suggests that further treatment is needed. Common sites of persistent or metastatic disease include the uterus, adjacent pelvic structures, the lungs, and the brain. Treatment of persistent gestational trophoblastic disease may involve the use of a number of potentially effective chemotherapeutic agents. What should be remembered is that GTN, even in its malignant form, is highly sensitive to chemotherapy and is considered a "prototype" for tumors that are sensitive to these agents. The indications for chemotherapy for persistent or malignant trophoblastic disease are presented in Table 42.5.

In general, nonmetastatic persistent GTN is completely treated by single-agent chemotherapy. The prognosis for malignant GTN is more complex, divided into good and poor prognostic categories (Table 42.6). The World Health Organization (WHO) has developed a prognostic scoring system for GTN that takes into account a number of epidemiologic and laboratory findings (Table 42.7). Chemotherapeutic agents used include both single-agent treatment with methotrexate and actinomycin as well as combination chemotherapy ("triple therapy"), which includes methotrexate, actinomycin, and chlorambucil (MAC; Table 42.8).

Other chemotherapeutic agents are being tested and may be effective as well. Where chemotherapy is indicated, the treatment protocol depends on whether patients fall into the "good" or "poor" prognosis metastatic group. Adjunctive radiation therapy is usually recommended for patients with brain or liver metastases, although the data in support of this therapy are scant.

TABLE 42.5. Indications for Chemotherapy for Trophoblastic Disease

Histologic diagnosis of choriocarcinoma
Evidence of metastatic disease
Indications based on quantitative serum β-human chorionic gonadotropin levels
  Plateaued or rising titer after evacuation
  Titer that has not returned to normal after 12 weeks postevacuation
Re-elevated level after a normal level has been obtained, exclusive of a new pregnancy

TABLE 42.6. Clinical Classification of Malignant Gestational Trophoblastic Neoplasia (GTN)

Nonmetastatic GTN (not defined in terms of good versus poor prognosis)
Metastatic GTN
  Good prognosis: absence of high-risk factors
    Pretreatment hCG level < 40,000 mIU/ml serum β-hCG
    < 4 months' duration of disease
    No evidence of brain or liver metastasis
    No significant prior chemotherapy
    No antecedent term pregnancy
  Poor prognosis: any single high-risk factor
    Pretreatment hCG level > 40,000 mIU/ml serum β-hCG
    > 4 months' duration of disease
    Brain and/or liver metastases
    Failed prior chemotherapy
    Antecedent term pregnancy

hCG = human chorionic gonadotropin.

TABLE 42.7. WHO Prognostic Scoring System for Gestational Trophoblastic Disease*

Prognostic Factor	0	1	2	3
Age	< 39	> 39		
Antecedent pregnancy	HM[†]	Abortion; ectopic	Term	
Interval (months)[‡]	< 4	4–6	7–12	> 12
hCG level (IU/liter)	< 10^3	10^3–10^4	10^4–10^5	> 10^5
ABO blood groups (female × male)		O × A	B	
		A × O	AB	
Largest tumor (cm)	< 3	3–5	> 5	
Site of metastasis		Spleen, kidney	GI[†] tract, liver	Brain
Number of metastases		1–3	4–8	> 8

*Low risk, 4; intermediate risk, ≤ 5–7; high risk, ≥ 8.
[†]GI = gastrointestinal; hCG = human chorionic gonadotropin; HM = hydatidiform mole.
[‡]Time between antecedent pregnancy and start of chemotherapy.

TABLE 42.8.	Chemotherapy for Gestational Trophoblastic Disease

Single agent
    Methotrexate (15–25 mg IM or IV daily for 5 days)
    Actinomycin D (0.015 mg/kg or 0.5 mg IV daily for 5 days)
    Treatment courses are repeated as often as toxicity will allow
Triple therapy
    Methotrexate (15–25 mg IV daily for 5 days)
    Actinomycin D (0.5 mg IV daily for 5 days)
    Chlorambucil (10 mg orally daily for 5 days)
    or
    Cytoxan (150–250 mg IV daily for 5 days)
Leucovorin "rescue"
    Methotrexate (1.0 mg/kg IM) followed in 12–24 hr by citrovorum factor
      (0.01 mg/kg IM); the methotrexate is given every other day for four doses
      or until toxicity develops

PLACENTAL SITE TUMORS

Placental site tumor is a rare form of trophoblastic disease. The tumor is comprised of monomorphic populations of intermediate cytotrophoblastic cells that are locally invasive at the site of placental implantation. It is different in that it secretes placental lactogen but only small amounts of hCG, is rarely metastatic, and unfortunately is much more resistant to standard chemotherappy. Hysterectomy is the appropriate initial therapy in most cases, although curettage has apparently been effective in some situations.

CASE STUDIES

Case 42A

A 38-year-old woman presents for prenatal care. Her last normal menstrual period was approximately 10 weeks ago. For the past 5 or 6 days, she has experienced light vaginal spotting, and she has been bothered by rather intense "morning sickness" for the past 4 weeks. She has been able to tolerate fluids and a few small meals, but in general does not have a normal appetite.

Physical examination reveals a blood pressure of 150/100, urine shows 3+ protein, the uterine fundus is approximately 16 weeks' size, and there is an absence of fetal heart tones. Pelvic examination shows the cervix to be fingertip dilated with a small amount of blood at the os. Bimanual examination confirms an enlarged uterus consistent with approximately 16-week size, and there is a suggestion of bilateral adnexal masses.

Question Case 42A

Which of the following should be done immediately?

A. Obtain quantitative serum hCG
B. Obtain pelvic ultrasound

(Continued)

C. Begin 24-hour urine collection for total protein
D. Obtain fetal heart rate reading with fetal monitor
E. Initiate hypertension work-up

Answer: A, B

This problem typifies a number of features of molar pregnancy, including uterine dates/size discrepancy, acute pregnancy-induced hypertension (preeclampsia), absence of fetal development, and bilateral theca lutein cysts. The diagnosis can be most readily made by obtaining an ultrasound. This should be done first to confirm the diagnosis, after which management includes treatment of the preeclampsia to prevent seizures and plans for expeditious uterine evacuation. A quantitative serum β-hCG is drawn as a baseline value against which postevacuation β-hCG evaluations may be compared.

Case 42B

A 22-year-old woman returns for her fourth postoperative follow-up examination since undergoing a suction curettage for an incomplete mole (trophoblastic degeneration of the triploid fetus) 5 weeks ago. The initial quantitative hCG titer drawn at the time of her diagnosis was 40,000 mIU. The serum titer drawn 2 weeks ago was 1500 mIU. The serum titer obtained yesterday shows a quantitative hCG level of 4500 mIU.

Question Case 42B

The most appropriate therapy at this point should be

A. A simple hysterectomy
B. Hysterectomy and bilateral salpingo-oophorectomy
C. Radiation therapy
D. Dilation and curettage
E. Chemotherapy

Answer: D, then E

This case is typical of a patient with persistent trophoblastic disease, as illustrated by rapidly falling serum β-hCG titers followed by resurgence a few weeks later. Given her young age and low-risk category, single-agent chemotherapy is most appropriate to treat this problem. Before beginning chemotherapy, she should have another dilation and curettage to obtain enough tissue to characterize the type of persistent trophoblast. It should be remembered, however, that dilation and curettage may not always reveal the presence of persistent trophoblast, because it can be present outside the uterine cavity and/or in metastatic sites.

C H A P T E R

43

VULVAR AND VAGINAL DISEASE AND NEOPLASIA

CHAPTER OBJECTIVES

This chapter deals primarily with APGO Objective(s):

OBJECTIVE 55   Vulvar Neoplasia

A. Define the risk factors for vulvar neoplasia and disease.

B. Describe the diagnostic approaches (including vulvar punch biopsy) and management for the various vulvar diseases and neoplasms.

VULVAR DISEASE

Appreciation of vulvar symptoms and examination for vulvar disease and neoplasia constitute a significant part of primary health care for women. Noninflammatory vulvar pathology is found in women of all ages, but is particularly significant in perimenopausal and postmenopausal women because of concern regarding the possibility of vulvar neoplasia. *The major symptoms of vulvar disease are pruritus, burning, and nonspecific irritation; and/or appreciation of a mass.* Diagnostic aids for the assessment of noninflammatory conditions are likewise relatively limited in number and include, in addition to careful history, inspection and biopsy. *Because vulvar lesions are often difficult to diagnose, liberal use of vulvar biopsy is central to good care.*

In this chapter there are discussions of a range of vulvar pathologic conditions, including nonneoplastic dermatoses, white lesions (atrophic and hyperkeratotic lesions), benign vulvar mass lesions, vulvar intraepithelial neoplasia, and vulvar cancer. Inflammatory conditions of the vulva are discussed in Chapter 27. Table 43.1 outlines common vulvar diseases.

TABLE 43.1. Common Vulvar Diseases

Common vulvar dermatoses
  Lichen simplex chronicus (LSC)
  Lichen planus
  Psoriasis
  Seborrheic dermatitis
  Vestibulitis
White lesions
  Hyperplastic vulvar dystrophy
  Lichen sclerosis (atrophic vulvar
    dystrophy)
Vulvar intraepithelial neoplasia (VIN)
  Without atypia
  With atypia, including carcinoma
    in situ
Vulvar carcinoma
  Paget disease
  Squamous cell carcinoma

Common Vulvar Dermatoses

LICHEN SIMPLEX CHRONICUS

In contrast to many dermatologic conditions that may be described as "rashes that itch," lichen simplex chronicus (LSC) can be described as *"an itch that rashes."* Although oversimplified, this dermatologic maxim adequately describes the condition. It is thought that the majority of patients develop this disorder secondary to *an irritant dermatitis, which progresses to LSC as a result of the effects of chronic mechanical irritation* from scratching and rubbing an already irritated area. The mechanical irritation contributes to epidermal hyperplasia, which, in turn, leads to heightened sensitivity that triggers more mechanical irritation.

Accordingly, the history of these patients is one of *progressive vulvar pruritus and/or burning*, which is temporarily relieved by scratching or rubbing with a washcloth or some similar material. *Etiologic factors* for the original pruritic symptoms often are unknown but may include sources of skin irritation such as laundry detergents, fabric softeners, scented hygienic preparations, and the use of colored or scented tissue. These potential sources of symptoms must be investigated. Any domestic or hygienic irritants must be removed, in combination with treatment, to break the cycle described above.

On *clinical inspection*, the skin of the labia majora, labia minora, and perineal body often shows diffusely reddened areas with occasional hyperplastic or hyperpigmented plaques of red to reddish brown. One may also find occasional areas of linear hyperplasia, which show the effect of grossly hyperkeratotic ridges of epidermis. Biopsy of patients who have these characteristic findings is usually not warranted.

Empiric *treatment* to include antipruritic medications such as Benadryl (diphenhydramine hydrochloride) or Atarax (hydroxyzine hydrochloride) that inhibit nighttime, unconscious scratching, combined with a mild to moderate topical steroid cream applied to the vulva, usually provides relief. A *steroid cream* such as hydrocortisone (1% or 2%) or, for patients with significant areas of obvious hyperkeratosis, triamcinolone acetonide (0.1%; Kenalog) or betamethasone valerate (0.1%; Valisone) may be used. *If significant relief is not obtained within 3 months, diagnostic vulvar biopsy is warranted.*

The prognosis for this disorder is excellent when there is removal of the offending irritating agents and appropriate use of a topical steroid preparation. In most patients, these measures cure the problem and eliminate future recurrences.

LICHEN PLANUS

Although lichen planus is usually a desquamative lesion of the vagina, occasional patients develop lesions on the vulva near the inner aspects of the labia minora and vulvar vestibule. Patients may have areas of whitish, lacy bands of keratosis near the reddish ulcerated-like lesions characteristic of the disease. Typically, complaints include *chronic vulvar burning and/or pruritus* and *insertional* (i.e., entrance) *dyspareunia* and a *profuse vaginal discharge.* Because of the patchiness of this lesion and the concern raised by atypical appearance of the lesions, *biopsy may be warranted* to confirm the diagnosis in some patients. In lichen planus, biopsy shows an absence of atypia. Examination of the vaginal discharge in these patients frequently reveals large numbers of acute inflammatory cells in the absence of significant numbers of bacteria. Accordingly, most often the diagnosis can be made by the typical history of vaginal/vulvar burning and/or insertional dyspareunia coupled with a physical examination that shows the bright red patchy distribution and a wet prep that shows large numbers of white cells.

Treatment for lichen planus is topical *steroid preparations* similar to those used for LSC. This may include the use of intravaginal 1% hydrocortisone douches. Length of treatment for these patients is often shorter than that required to treat LSC, although lichen planus is more likely to reoccur.

PSORIASIS

Psoriasis may involve the vulvar skin as part of a generalized dermatologic process. With approximately 2% of the general population suffering from psoriasis, the physician should be alert to its prevalence and likelihood of vulvar manifestation. Moreover, because it may appear at menarche, pregnancy, and menopause, the physician may be consulted by the patient for what she perceives to be a gynecologic disorder.

The *lesions* are typically slightly raised round or ovoid patches with a silver scale appearance atop an erythematous base. These lesions most often measure approximately 1×1 to 1×2 cm. Most patients are concerned by the appearance of this lesion, as pruritus is usually not marked. *The diagnosis is generally known because of psoriasis found elsewhere on the body, obviating the need for vulvar biopsy to confirm the diagnosis.* The occurrence of isolated vulvar lesions is rare.

Treatment often occurs in conjunction with consultation by a dermatologist. Like lesions elsewhere, vulvar lesions usually respond to topical cold tar preparations, followed by exposure to ultraviolet light as well as corticosteroid medications, either topically or by intralesional injection. Coal tar preparations are extremely irritating to the vagina and labial mucous membranes and should be avoided in these areas. Because vulvar application of some of the photoactivated preparations can be somewhat awkward, topical steroids are most effective, using compounds such as betamethasone valerate 0.1% (Valisone).

SEBORRHEIC DERMATITIS

Isolated vulvar seborrheic dermatitis is rare. The diagnosis is usually made in patients complaining of vulvar pruritus who are known to have seborrheic dermatitis in the scalp or other hair-bearing areas of the body. The lesion may mimic other entities such as psoriasis, tinea cruris (jock itch), or LSC. *The lesions are pale red to a yellowish pink and may be covered by an oily appearing, scaly crust.* Because this area of the body remains continually moist, occasional exudative lesions include raw "weeping" patches, caused by skin maceration, which are exacerbated by the patient's scratching. As with psoriasis, *vulvar biopsy is usually not needed* when the diagnosis is made in conjunction with known seborrheic dermatitis in other hair-bearing areas.

For patients with acute exudative variations of seborrheic dermatitis, initial perineal hygiene includes the use of *Burrow's solution soaks* (5% solution of aluminum acetate). After remediation of the exudative phase, standard treatment includes *topical corticosteroid lotions or creams* containing a mixture of an agent that penetrates well such as betamethasone valerate in conjunction with Eurax (crotamiton) to control the intense pruritus. As with LSC, the use of antipruritic agents such as Atarax or Benadryl as a bedtime dose in the first 10 days to 2 weeks of treatment frequently helps break the sleep/scratch cycle and allows the lesions to heal.

VESTIBULITIS

Vulvar vestibulitis is a condition without known etiology. It involves the acute and chronic inflammation of the vestibular glands, which lie just inside the vaginal introitus near the hymeneal ring. The involved glands may be circumferential to include areas near the urethra, but this condition most commonly involves posterolateral vestibular glands in the 4 and 8 o'clock positions (Figure 43.1). The diagnosis should be suspected in all patients who present with *new onset insertional dyspareunia*. Patients with this condition frequently complain of progressive insertional dyspareunia to the point where they are unable to have intercourse. The history may go on a few weeks but most typically involves progressive worsening over the course of 3 or 4 months. Patients also complain of pain upon tampon insertion and at times during washing or bathing the perineal area.

Physical examination is the key to diagnosis. Because the vestibular glands lie between the folds of the hymenal ring and the medial aspect of the vulvar vestibule, diagnosis is frequently missed when inspection of the perineum does not include these areas. Once the speculum has been placed in the vagina, the vestibular gland area becomes impossible to identify. After carefully inspecting the proper anatomic area,

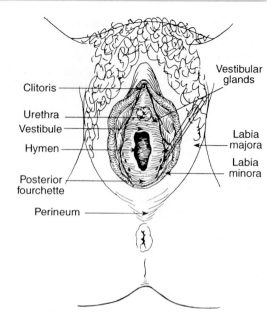

FIGURE 43.1. Vestibular glands.

light touch with a moistened cotton applicator recreates the pain exactly for those patients who have vulvar vestibulitis. In addition, the regions affected are most often evident as small, reddened, patchy areas.

Because the cause of vestibulitis is unknown, treatments are varied and range from temporary sexual abstinence and application of cortisone ointments and topical Xylocaine jelly to more radical treatments such as surgical excision of the vestibular glands. No single treatment has proved highly efficacious, and treatment must be individualized based on the severity of patient symptoms and the sexual disability that is present.

Recent limited data suggest that some patients may benefit from low-dose tricyclic medication (amitriptyline and imipramine) to help break the cycle of pain, while other limited reports suggest the use of calcium citrate to change the urine composition by removing oxalic acid crystals. Those advocating changing the urine chemistry cite evidence to suggest that oxalic acid crystals are particularly irritating when precipitated in the urine of patients with high urinary oxalic acid composition. The efficacy of calcium citrate use needs to be studied in prospective randomized trials but preliminary data look promising.

Benign Vulvar Lesions

Sebaceous or inclusion cysts are caused by inflammatory blockage of the sebaceous gland ducts and are small, smooth nodular masses, usually arising from the inner surfaces of the labia minora and majora, that contain cheesy, sebaceous material. They may be easily excised if their size or position is troublesome.

The round ligament inserts into the labium majus, carrying an investment of peritoneum. On occasion, peritoneal fluid may accumulate therein, causing a *cyst of the canal of Nuck or hydrocele.* If such cysts reach symptomatic size, excision is usually required.

Fibromas (fibromyomas) arise from the connective tissue and smooth muscle elements of vulva and vagina and are usually small and asymptomatic. Sarcomatous change is extremely uncommon, although edema and degenerative changes may make such lesions suspicious for malignancy. If they are large, however, they may become pedunculated. Of historical interest is the almost unbelievable 268-lb pedunculated vulvar fibroma reported by Buckner in 1851. Treatment is, of course, surgical excision when the lesions are symptomatic or when there is concern about malignancy. *Lipomas* appear much like fibromas, are quite rare, and are also treated by excision.

Hidradenoma is a rare lesion arising from the sweat glands of the vulva. It is almost always benign, is usually found on the inner surface of the labia majora, and is treated with excision.

Nevi are benign, usually asymptomatic, pigmented lesions whose importance is that they must be distinguished from malignant melanoma, 3% to 4% of which occur on the external genitalia in females. Biopsy of pigmented vulvar lesions may be warranted depending on clinical suspicion.

VULVAR NEOPLASIA

The classification of vulvar disease used descriptive terminology based on gross morphologic appearance: leukoplakia, kraurosis vulvae, and vulvar dystrophy. Standard-

TABLE 43.2. ISSVD Classification of Vulvar Disease

	Description
I	Squamous cell hyperplasia
II	Lichen sclerosis
III	Other dermatoses

ISSVD = International Society for the Study of Vulvar Disease.

ization of nomenclature and classification by symptoms, gross appearance, and histology were lacking. To improve standardization and thus treatment of these disorders, the International Society for the Study of Vulvar Disease (ISSVD) established a modified classification in 1987 based on both gross and microscopic morphology (Table 43.2).

Vulvar dermatoses have been described previously. The following discussion includes a description of squamous cell hyperplasia (formerly hyperplastic dystrophy) and lichen sclerosis.

Squamous Cell Hyperplasia (Hyperplastic Dystrophy)

In considering the various types of vulvar neoplasia, the clinician should be aware that gross appearance may not be consistent with underlying cellular architecture and that often atrophic lesions, such as lichen sclerosis, may appear grossly to be hyperplastic. Furthermore, *within the group of true hyperplastic lesions, there is a need to confirm whether the hyperplasia is accompanied by atypia.* As a result, classification of intraepithelial vulvar disease becomes a matter of close cooperation between the clinician, who must first appreciate the need for thorough investigation, and the pathologist, who is called on to confirm the presence of lesions that may have premalignant or malignant potential. Because these distinctions cannot always be made on physical examination alone and because many of these lesions present with similar symptoms, *liberal use of vulvar biopsy is encouraged to provide definitive diagnosis and ensure rational treatment.*

Many hyperplastic lesions without atypia evolve from chronic irritation and secondary thickening of the vulvar skin and are classified under the LSC group (which were discussed earlier in this chapter). As with many of the other lesions, vulvar pruritus is the main presenting symptom. On gross inspection of the vulva, areas may be isolated and include obviously hyperkeratotic skin with secondary excoriation. These changes may diffusely involve the vulva or may occur as isolated ridges or patches. In the presence of gross abnormalities of the vulvar skin, directed biopsies of the lesions are warranted.

The microscopic appearance confirms the diagnosis. *Squamous cell hyperplasia without atypia* characteristically shows hyperkeratosis as well as acanthosis with an absence of mitotic figures. These lesions are usually treated as described in the previous discussion of LSC, using various types of *topical, highly penetrating corticosteroid creams.* The patient can be reassured that these lesions usually respond to treatment with complete resolution and do not predispose to further premalignant or malignant vulvar disease.

Lichen Sclerosis

Lichen sclerosis, previously called lichen sclerosis et atrophicus, has confused clinicians and pathologists because of inconsistent terminology and because it is associated with other types of vulvar pathology, including those of the hyperplastic variety. As with the other disorders, *chronic vulvar pruritus* occurs in most patients. Typically, *the vulva is diffusely involved with very thin, whitish epithelial areas* termed "onion skin" epithelium. Most patients have involvement on both sides of the vulva, with the most common sites being the labia majora, labia minora, the clitoral and periclitoral epithelium, and the perineal body. The lesion may extend to include a perianal "halo" of atrophic, whitish epithelium. In severe cases, there is loss of many normal anatomic landmarks, including obliteration

of labial and periclitoral architecture as well as severe stenosis of the vaginal introitus. Some patients have areas of cracked skin, which are prone to bleeding with minimal trauma. Patients with these severe anatomic changes complain of difficulty in having normal coital function.

Microscopic confirmation of lichen sclerosis is often necessary and very useful because it allows specific therapy. The histologic features are pathognomonic and include areas of hyperkeratosis, despite epithelial thinning; a zone of homogeneous, pink-staining collagenous-like material directly under the epithelial layer; and a band of chronic inflammatory cells, consisting mostly of lymphocytes.

It is important to remember that there may be associated areas of hyperplasia mixed throughout or adjacent to these typically atrophic-appearing areas. In patients with this so-called *mixed dystrophy,* there is a need to treat both components to effect resolution of symptoms. Patients with histologic confirmation of a large hyperplastic component should initially be treated with well-penetrating corticosteroid creams. With improvement of these areas (usually 2 to 3 weeks), therapy can then be directed to the lichen sclerosis component.

The treatment of choice for lichen sclerosis includes the use of topical steroid preparations in an effort to ameliorate symptoms. Patients need to be reassured that this disorder is not premalignant, but that the lesion is unlikely to resolve totally. Intermittent treatment may be needed indefinitely. This is in marked contrast to the hyperplastic lesions without atypia, which usually totally resolve within 6 months.

Neither lichen sclerosis nor hyperplastic dystrophy without atypia significantly increases the patient's risk of developing cancer. It has been estimated that this risk is in the 2% to 3% range when there is no preexisting atypical hyperplasia. However, because patients who have had these disorders are more likely to eventually develop atypical hyperplasia, they need to be followed carefully and rebiopsied liberally if there is a return of vulvar symptoms or new lesions.

Vulvar Intraepithelial Neoplasia

Vulvar intraepithelial neoplasia (VIN) may be classified as VIN-I, mild dysplasia; VIN-II, moderate dysplasia; or VIN-III, severe dysplasia, carcinoma in situ. Also included in the category of intraepithelial neoplasia lesions are vulvar condylomata. Other lesions represented include Paget disease and level I melanomas. Condylomata are discussed in the section on inflammatory vulvar lesions, and Paget disease and level I melanomas are mentioned briefly later in this section.

VIN-I and VIN-II

Early vulvar intraepithelial neoplasia (VIN-I and VIN-II) represents *true neoplastic lesions* that, as with their counterparts in the cervix, are thought to have a *high predilection for progression* to severe intraepithelial lesions and eventually carcinoma.

Presenting complaints include *vulvar pruritus, chronic irritation, and a development of raised mass lesions.* Normally, the lesions are localized, fairly well isolated, and raised above the normal epithelial surface to include a slightly rough texture. These lesions are usually found along the posterior vulva and in the perineal body, although they may occur anywhere on the vulva. They typically have a whitish cast or hue. As with other vulvar lesions, diagnosis by biopsy is mandatory.

Microscopically, these lesions mimic intraepithelial neoplasia elsewhere, including mitotic figures and nuclear pleomorphism, with loss of normal differentiation in the lower one third to one half of the epithelial layer. As with the cervix, the degree of dysplasia increases to a point where full-thickness change indicates severe intraepithelial neoplasia and/or carcinoma in situ. Changes consistent with human papillomavirus (HPV) infection are occasionally seen with these lesions and suggest an association between certain types of HPV and the occurrence of VIN. Lesions that are typically condyloma in origin do not have features of attenuated maturation and have an absence of pleomorphism and atypical mitotic figures.

VIN-III (Carcinoma in Situ)

Full-thickness loss of maturation indicates lesions that are at least severely dysplastic, including areas that may represent true carcinoma in situ. Common presenting complaints include *intractable pruritus and nonspecific vulvar irritation with gross lesions that are similar to earlier grades of VIN* occurring in patchy, fairly well-isolated areas. Occasional patients may have extensive vulvar involvement. The color changes in these lesions range from white, hyperplastic areas to reddened or dusky patch-like involvement, depending on whether there is associated hyperkeratosis.

As with the other vulvar disorders, *diagnosis of VIN is made by biopsy.* In patients without obvious raised or isolated lesions, careful inspection of the vulva is warranted using a magnifying device such as a hand lens or visor. Washing the vulvar skin with a dilute solution of 3% acetic acid often accentuates the white lesions and may also help in revealing abnormal vascular patterns. When present, these areas should be selectively biopsied in multiple sites to thoroughly investigate the grade of VIN and reliably exclude the presence of invasive carcinoma.

The goal in treating VIN is to quickly and completely remove all involved areas of skin. A variety of treatments are available, depending on the extent of the lesion and the severity of the dysplasia. Most *isolated and limited VIN-I or VIN-II lesions* may be removed by local excision in the office or by *cryocautery, electrodesiccation, or laser cautery* with local anesthetic. Extended lesions showing VIN-I or VIN-II are usually treated with laser ablation in an ambulatory surgery area using a general anesthetic.

VIN-III, including carcinoma in situ, is best treated by wide local excision with or without combination laser ablation, depending on the area of involvement. Surgical excisional treatment of this disorder also has an advantage of pathologic examination of the tissue, which is not available

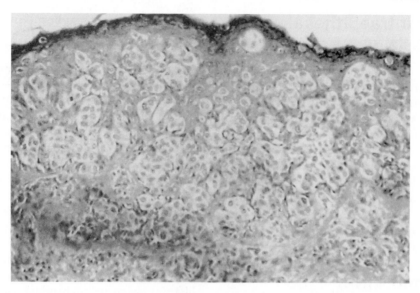

FIGURE 43.2. Paget disease. Large, pale cells of apocrine origin involving the surface epithelium. From Scott JR, Di Saia PJ, Hammond CB, et al. *Danforth's Obstetrics and Gynecology,* 8th ed. Philadelphia, Lippincott Williams & Wilkins, 1999, p. 794.

with laser treatment. This usually requires a general or regional anesthetic and may require hospitalization, depending on the extent of the vulvar surgery. Occasionally, for diffuse or recurrent disease, simple vulvectomy is warranted.

Paget Disease

Paget disease is characterized by extensive intraepithelial disease whose gross appearance is described as a fiery red background mottled with whitish hyperkeratotic areas. The histology of these lesions is similar to that of the breast lesion, with large pale cells of apocrine origin below the surface epithelium (Figure 43.2). Although not common, Paget disease of the vulva may be associated with carcinoma of the skin. Similarly, patients with Paget disease of the vulva have a higher incidence of underlying internal carcinoma, particularly of the colon and breast.

The treatment for vulvar Paget disease is wide local excision or simple vulvectomy, depending on the amount of involvement. Recurrences are more common with this disorder than with VIN, necessitating wider margins when local excision or vulvectomy is performed.

Melanoma

Vulvar melanoma usually presents with *a raised, irritated, pruritic, pigmented lesion.* Melanoma accounts for only 5% of all vulvar malignancies, and when suspected, *wide local excision* is necessary for diagnosis and staging. Survival approaches 100% when the lesions are confined to the intrapapillary ridges, decreasing rapidly as involvement includes the papillary dermis, reticular dermis, and finally subcutaneous tissues. In the latter instance, survival is generally less than 20%, as there is a substantial incidence of nodal involvement. Because early diagnosis and treatment by wide excision are so crucial, it is important to recognize that *irritated, pigmented, vulvar lesions mandate excisional biopsy for definitive treatment.*

VULVAR CANCER

Vulvar carcinoma accounts for approximately 4% of all gynecologic malignancies, with 90% of these carcinomas being of the *squamous cell* variety. The typical clinical profile includes women in their *postmenopausal years,* most commonly between the ages of 65 and 70. About 10% of these malignancies are, however, discovered in the third and fourth decades of life. *Vulvar pruritus* is the most common presenting complaint. In addition, patients may notice a red or white ulcerative or exophytic lesion arising most commonly on the posterior two thirds of either labium majus. An exophytic ulcerative lesion need not be present, further underscoring the need for thorough biopsy in patients of the age group who complain of vulvar symptoms. *There is often a delay in treatment of these patients because of reluctance of patients in this age group to present to their physicians and further reluctance on the physicians' part to investigate the symptoms and findings thoroughly via vulvar biopsy.*

Although a *specific etiology* for vulvar cancer is not known, it has been shown that there may be progression from prior intraepithelial lesions, including those that are associated with certain types of HPV.

Natural History

Squamous cell carcinoma of the vulva generally *remains localized for long periods of time and then spreads in a predictable fashion to the regional lymph nodes,* including those of the inguinal and femoral chain. Lesions of greater than 2 cm in diameter and 0.5 cm in depth have an increased chance of nodal metastases. The overall incidence of lymph node metastasis is approximately 30%. Lesions arising in the anterior one third of the vulva may spread to the deep pelvic nodes, bypassing regional inguinal and femoral lymphatics.

Evaluation

After suspicious lesions are biopsied and the diagnosis of invasive squamous cell carcinoma of the vulva confirmed, other studies that may be obtained include *chest x-ray and intravenous pyelogram.* For patients with lesions near the urethra and/or patients with lesions involving the anus or perineal area, preoperative *cystoscopy and proctoscopy,* respectively, are indicated.

The *staging classification* was altered by the Federation of Gynecology and Obstet-

rics (FIGO) in 1988 (Table 43.3). This staging convention uses the analysis of the removed vulvar tumor and microscopic assessment of the regional lymph nodes as its basis. The change from clinical staging to this surgical staging convention was necessitated by the observation that clinical assessment of this disease contained many errors, in particular, the assessment of inguinal and femoral adenopathy.

Treatment

Although the mainstay for the treatment of invasive vulvar cancer is surgical, a number of advances have been made to help individualize patients into treatment categories in an effort to reduce the amount of radical surgery while not compromising survival. Accordingly, not all patients undergo radical vulvectomy with bilateral nodal dissections. Individualized approaches include the following.

- Conservative vulvar operations for patients with unifocal lesions
- Elimination of routine pelvic lymphadenectomy
- Avoidance of groin dissection in patients with unilateral lesions less than 1 mm in depth
- Elimination of contralateral groin dissection in patients with unilateral T1 lesions who have negative ipsilateral nodes
- Separate groin incisions for those patients with indicated bilateral groin dissection
- Use of postoperative radiation therapy to decrease incidence of groin recurrence in patients with 2 or more positive groin nodes

Adjunctive treatment with chemotherapy in cases of recurrent vulvar cancer has only limited value.

Prognosis

The corrected 5-year survival rate for all vulvar carcinoma is approximately 70%, with cure rates approaching 90% if the patient has negative inguinal and femoral

TABLE 43.3. Staging for Carcinoma of the Vulva

FIGO surgical staging:

Stage 0

Tis — Carcinoma in situ; intraepithelial carcinoma

Stage I

T1 N0 M0 — Tumor confined to the vulva and/or perineum; < 2 cm in greatest dimension; nodes are not palpable

Stage II

T2 N0 M0 — Tumor confined to the vulva and/or perineum; > 2 cm in greatest dimension; nodes are not palpable

Stage III

T3 N0 M0 — Tumor of any size with:

T3 N1 M0 — 1. Adjacent spread to the lower urethra and/or the vagina, or the anus, and/or

T1 N1 M0 — 2. Unilateral regional lymph node metastasis
T2 N1 M0

Stage IVA

T1 N2 M0 — Tumor invades any of the following: upper urethra, bladder mucosa, rectal mucosa, pelvic and/or bilateral regional node metastasis

T2 N2 M0
T3 N2 M0
T4 any N M0

Stage IVB

Any T — Any distant metastasis including pelvic lymph nodes
Any N, M1

TNM clinical staging
(rules for staging are similar to those for carcinoma of the cervix):

T — Primary tumor

Tis — Preinvasive carcinoma (carcinoma in situ)

T1 — Tumor confined to the vulva and/or perineum; < 2 cm in greatest dimension

T2 — Tumor confined to the vulva and/or perineum; > 2 cm in greatest dimension

T3 — Tumor of any size with adjacent spread to the urethra and/or vagina and/or to the anus

T4 — Tumor of any size infiltrating the bladder mucosa and/or the rectal mucosa, including the upper part of the urethral mucosa and/or fixed to the bone

N — Regional lymph nodes

N0 — No lymph node metastasis

N1 — Unilateral regional lymph node metastasis

N2 — Bilateral regional lymph node metastasis

M — Distant metastasis

M0 — No clinical metastasis

M1 — Distant metastasis (including pelvic lymph node metastasis)

FIGO = Federation of Gynecology and Obstetrics; TNM = tumor, node, metastasis.

lymph nodes at the time of her first surgery. If metastatic disease is found in the regional nodes, survival falls off dramatically to as low as 20% if the deep pelvic nodes are involved.

Carcinoma of Bartholin's Gland

Carcinoma of Bartholin's gland is uncommon, arising from either the squamous epithelium of the ducts or the glandular epithelium of the greater vestibular glands. This cancer is usually diagnosed in the fifth decade or afterward upon presentation as an asymptomatic vulvar mass. Therefore, a new, asymptomatic mass in the area of the Bartholin gland in a postmenopausal woman is suspect and should be investigated aggressively. Treatment is radical vulvectomy and bilateral lymphadenectomy and radiation therapy if the pelvic nodes are positive. Recurrence is a disappointingly common event and a 5-year overall survival rate of 50% to 60% is noted.

VAGINAL DISEASE

Benign Vaginal Masses

Gartner duct cysts arise from vestigial remnants of the wolffian or mesonephric system that course along the outer anterior aspect of the vaginal canal. These cystic structures are usually small and asymptomatic, but on occasion they may be larger and symptomatic so that excision is required.

Inclusion cysts are usually seen on the posterior lower vaginal surface, resulting from imperfect approximation of childbirth lacerations or episiotomy. They are lined with stratified squamous epithelium, their content is usually cheesy, and they may be excised if symptomatic.

VAGINAL NEOPLASIA

Carcinoma in situ of the vagina and invasive vaginal cancer are among the rarest of gynecologic neoplasms. They are often mul-

tifocal, associated with other lower genital tract intraepithelial or invasive neoplasms.

Carcinoma in Situ of the Vagina

Carcinoma in situ (CIS) appears to occur more commonly in the third decade of life onward, although its exact incidence is unknown. One half to two thirds of patients with vaginal CIS have an antecedent or coexistent neoplasm of the lower genital tract. Approximately 1% to 2% of patients who undergo hysterectomy for cervical CIS and many patients who undergo radiation therapy for other gynecologic malignancy ultimately develop CIS of the upper vagina. This is one of the arguments for yearly Pap smears after hysterectomy. The importance of vaginal CIS is its potential for progression to invasive vaginal carcinoma, as the lesions themselves are usually asymptomatic and have no intrinsic morbidity.

CIS of the vagina must be differentiated from other causes of red ulcerated or white hyperplastic lesions of the vagina such as herpes, traumatic lesions, hyperkeratosis associated with chronic irritation (e.g., from a poorly fitting diaphragm), or adenosis. Inspection and palpation of the vagina are the mainstays of diagnosis, but unfortunately, this is often done in a cursory fashion during the routine pelvic examination. *Pap smears of the vaginal mucosa are sometimes rewarding*, although *colposcopy with directed biopsy is the definitive diagnostic maneuver*, just as it is in cervical intraepithelial neoplasia.

The goals of treatment of CIS of the vagina are ablation of the intraepithelial lesion while preserving vaginal depth, caliber, and sexual function. Laser ablation, local excision, and chemical treatment with 5-fluorouracil cream (Efudex 5%) are all used for limited lesions; total or partial vaginectomy with application of a split thickness skin graft is usually reserved for failure of the previously described treatments. Cure rates of 80% to 95% may be expected.

TABLE 43.4. Clinical Staging of Vaginal Carcinoma	
Stage	**Description**
0	Carcinoma in situ
I	Carcinoma limited to the vaginal mucosa
II	Carcinoma involving the subvaginal tissue but not extending onto the pelvic wall
III	Carcinoma extending onto the pelvic wall
IV	Carcinoma extending into the mucosa of the bladder or rectum or distant metastases

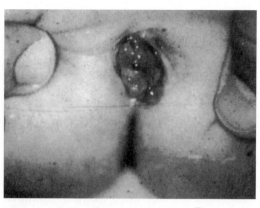

FIGURE 43.3. Sarcoma botryoides in a 6-month-old child. The grape-like polypoid tumors protruding through the vaginal introitus are asymptomatic, except for a slight bloody discharge.

Invasive Vaginal Cancer

Invasive vaginal cancer accounts for approximately 1% to 2% of gynecologic malignancies. *Squamous cell carcinoma* makes up approximately 95% of these malignancies, occurring primarily in women over 55 years old. The remainder of vaginal carcinomas consists of *adenocarcinoma of the vagina [clear cell adenocarcinoma, usually related to diethylstilbestrol (DES) exposure before 18 weeks' gestation while in utero] and vaginal melanoma.*

The staging of vaginal carcinoma is nonsurgical (Table 43.4). Radiation therapy is the mainstay of treatment for squamous cell carcinoma of the vagina. Radical hysterectomy combined with upper vaginectomy and pelvic lymphadenectomy are used for selected patients. Upper vaginal lesions and pelvic exenteration and radical vulvectomy are used for selected patients with lower vaginal lesions involving the vulva. Most young women with clear cell carcinoma have lesions located in the upper one half of the vagina and wish to maintain ovarian and vaginal function. Radical hysterectomy with upper vaginectomy combined with pelvic lymphadenectomy is often the primary treatment for these patients, with radiation therapy following. The overall 5-year survival rate for squamous cell carcinoma of the vagina is 50% and for clear cell adenocarcinoma of the vagina, 80%, with stage I and II patients having the best prognosis. Melanoma is treated with radical surgery; radiation and chemotherapy have little efficacy.

Sarcoma botryoides (or embryonal rhabdomyosarcoma) presents as a mass of grape-like polyps arising from the undifferentiated mesenchyme of the lamina propria of the anterior vaginal wall and protrudes from the introitus of very young girls and infants (Figure 43.3). There is often an associated bloody discharge in these frightening tumors. The tumor spreads locally, although it may have distant hematogenous metastases. This tumor was treated in the past with pelvic exenteration, but because this procedure was so unpalatable in this age group, wide excision combined with chemotherapy is often used in an attempt to salvage as much bowel and bladder function as possible.

CASE STUDIES

Case 43A

A 72-year-old woman comes in with a complaint of vulvar itching for the past 8 months. This has become progressively worse over the last 2 months to the point where it awakens her two or three times at night as she finds herself scratching unconsciously. Her past gynecologic history is unremarkable. She underwent normal menopause in her early 50s and is on no chronic medication. Her general health is excellent.

Examination reveals external genitalia that are somewhat atrophic as appropriate for her age. Circumferentially around the inner aspect of the labia majora, the lateral aspect of the labia minora, and the skin over the clitoral hood there is a diffuse whitish epithelial change. This coalesces in the perineal body and extends to within a centimeter of the anal verge. Scattered throughout this area are patches of what appear to be reddish ulcerations approximately 1 × 1 cm each in the perineal body and left labium majus. The remainder of the gynecologic examination is normal.

Question Case 43A

What is the next step in the management of this patient?

A. Administer topical testosterone propionate
B. Administer topical corticosteroid cream
C. Administer topical antifungal preparations
D. Administer Benadryl at bedtime
E. Perform directed vulvar biopsy(ies)

Answer: E

This case illustrates a postmenopausal patient with inflammation of the vulva secondary to one of the so-called vulvar dystrophies. Because the histologic variation is unclear and because neoplasia cannot be ruled out by gross examination, it is mandatory to perform a vulvar biopsy in this patient. With areas of heterogeneity (hyperkeratosis and/or ulceration or excoriation), two or three biopsies may be warranted to make the diagnosis. Application of the appropriate medication and/or surgical treatment can then be offered after histologic verification of the problem.

Case 43B

A 67-year-old patient presents to the office having noticed a "sore" on her vulva. She has been aware of this for approximately 8 months but has not come in hoping it would go away. Currently, it is bleeding slightly and is irritated by her underclothing. Vulvar examination reveals a 1 × 1 cm slightly raised but "cratered lesion" in the posterior left labium majus. There are no other apparent abnormalities. Examination of her groin reveals two "marble size" lymph nodes in her left inguinal ligament area.

Question Case 43B

The most likely diagnosis is

A. Epidermoid carcinoma of the vulva
B. Chancroid
C. Amelanotic melanoma
D. Granuloma inguinale
E. Lymphogranuloma venereum

(Continued)

Answer: A

Given the patient's age and physical findings, she most probably has squamous cell carcinoma of the vulva. This is suggested by an exophytic but cratered lesion in the posterior two thirds of the vulva with a highly suspicious groin examination. It is mandatory in this patient to obtain one or two vulvar biopsies at the margin of the puckered epithelium to confirm the diagnosis.

CHAPTER

44

CERVICAL NEOPLASIA AND CARCINOMA

CHAPTER OBJECTIVES

This chapter deals primarily with APGO Objective(s):

OBJECTIVE 56   Cervical Disease and
 Neoplasia

A. Describe the risk factors, symptoms, and physical findings characteristic of cervicitis and cervical neoplasia.

B. Describe the rationale and means of Pap smear screening, and the management of an abnormal Pap smear, including the Bethesda system of Pap smear classification and colposcopy.

C. Explain the common course, diagnosis, and management of cervical neoplastic disease, including histologic categories of cervical neoplasia and the FIGO staging of cervical carcinoma.

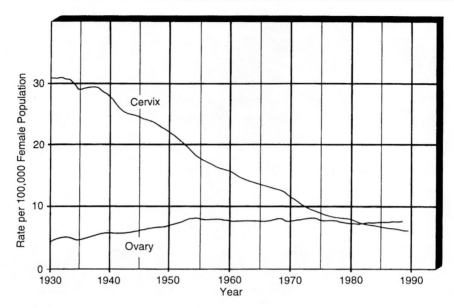

FIGURE 44.1. Age-adjusted death rate for cervical cancer in the United States, 1930–1996.

Cervical carcinoma serves as the model of a "controllable" cancer, controllable in the sense that (*a*) there is an identifiable precursor lesion (cervical intraepithelial neoplasia, CIN) with a natural history of usually slow progression to frank cervical cancer, (*b*) there is a cheap and noninvasive screening test (Pap smear) which may be augmented with adjunctive tests such as HPV DNA typing, and a follow-up diagnostic procedure (colposcopy) for diagnosis, and (*c*) there are simple and effective treatments of the precursor lesion (cryotherapy, laser ablation, loop electrosurgical excision procedure [LEEP], and cold knife cone biopsy) with high cure rates.

Because it is usually possible to identify and treat the asymptomatic precursor lesion so that there is no progression to actual cancer of the cervix, cervical cancer is now the second rather than the first most common malignancy in women. Clearly, the most important factor for the substantial improvement in the morbidity and mortality of cervical cancer is the annual Pap smear, allowing identification of women who will benefit from colposcopy and histologic evaluation of their cervix, leading to specific, appropriate, early therapy. This pattern of care is one of the great success stories of modern medicine. Furthermore, with improved treatment of cervical cancer when disease progression has gone beyond the precursor lesion, cure rates of up to 90% are seen in early stage disease (stages IA and IB) and increased life expectancy is seen in advanced stage disease. The gratifying effect of these interventions is graphically seen in the fall in the mortality rate for cervical cancer compared with that of ovarian carcinoma, for which no treatable precursor lesion can be easily identified (Figure 44.1). It is hoped that similar progress will be made in further identification of the causes of CIN/cervical cancer and development of a preventive treatment.

Within the clinical context, certain *epidemiologic factors* relating to cervical neoplasia are significant (Table 44.1). Of the factors listed, special emphasis should be placed on those factors relating to early sexual intercourse with multiple partners; the role of cigarette smoking; male factors, including the "high-risk" consort; immunologically deprived patients, such as those who are receiving immunosuppressive therapy and those infected with the HIV virus; of particular note, human papillomavirus

TABLE 44.1. Potential Factors in Cervical Neoplasia
Epidemiologic characteristics
Early intercourse
Multiple sex partners
Early childbearing
Male factors: "high-risk" consort
Socioeconomic status, race
Venereal infection
Other factors
Immune status
Oral contraceptives
Cigarette smoking
Intrauterine DES exposure
Viral relations
Papillomavirus

DES = diethylstilbestrol.

(HPV); and clinical care designed to eliminate or decrease the incidence or effect of these factors.

CERVICAL INTRAEPITHELIAL NEOPLASIA

Pathology: The Squamocolumnar Junction

Understanding the pathophysiology of CIN and its association with the *squamocolumnar junction* (SCJ) and *transformation zone* (TZ) of the cervix provides the rationale for cervical Pap smear screening, diagnostic colposcopy, and the treatment of CIN. As the uterus and cervix grow during puberty and adolescence, the original SCJ "rolls out," or everts, from its position just inside the cervical os to a position on the enlarged cervical surface. In this process, original columnar endocervical tissue is also rolled to the cervical surface. This fleshy, reddened tissue area is often misnamed erosion (as it looks like a pathologic, or eroded, tissue), although it is actually normal endocervical tissue in a new location. This area is exposed to vaginal secretions and irritants

and to a changing hormonal milieu, and the process of squamous metaplasia begins as a new SCJ is formed farther inward from the old one.

The area between the old and new SCJs, where squamous metaplasia occurs, is called the transformation zone. In the menopausal years, the uterus and cervix again decrease in size, and the new SCJ comes to lie upward into the endocervical canal, often out of direct visual contact (Figure 44.2). Approximately 95% of squamous intraepithelial neoplasia occurs within the transformation zone.

The most important risk factor for the development of cervical neoplasia and cancer is the presence of the human papillomaviris (HPV). Of the some 80 types, about 30 may infect the anogenital tract and about 15 are associated with cervical neoplasia and cancer. HPV types 16, 18, 31, 33, and 45 are the most important in this regard, with types 6 and 11 associated with genital warts (condylomata accuminata). When the double-stranded DNA HPV virus infects the reproducing cells of the basal cell layer and are not integrated into the host genome, entire encapsulated virions are produced which are expressed morphologically as "koilocytes." When, however, the HPV is integrated into the DNA, the expression of the cell's regulatory genes may be altered, leading to the transformation of the cells to high grade intraepithelial lesions or carcinoma. Because HPV infection is very much more common than cervical intraepithelial neoplasia or carcinoma, it is likely that several as yet not fully identified host or environmental factors act as cofactors. A higher incidence of HPV infection and progression of intraepithelial neoplasia is seen in immunosuppressed patients, including those infected with HIV as well as those who are organ transplant recipients, who have chronic renal failure or a history of Hodgkin's lymphoma or immunosuppressive therapy for other reasons. Another factor is cigarette smoking which is associated with a 50% higher risk for developing cervical carcinoma.

HPV DNA testing is now being used with increasing frequency, with more accurate

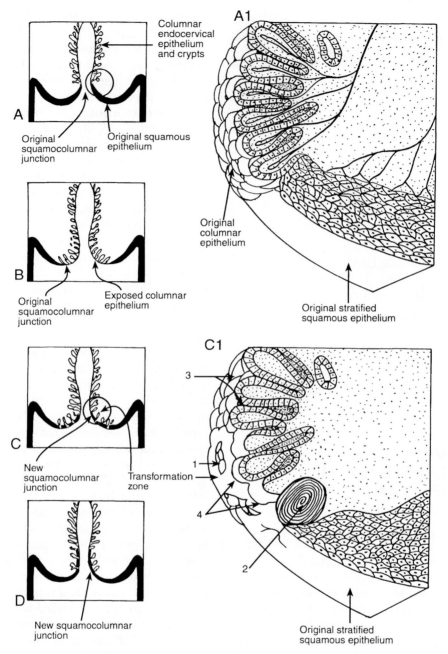

FIGURE 44.2. Squamocolumnar junction (SCJ) and transformation zone. (*A*) Before puberty and adolescence, the original SCJ is at or just above the external os, with the original squamous epithelium being outside and the original columnar endocervical epithelium, inside. (*A1*) Three-dimensional representation of the original SCJ. (*B*) As the cervix matures and grows, the original SCJ rolls outward, followed by endocervical columnar epithelium, which is now exposed to the vagina and its contents. (*C*) As the endocervical tissue is exposed and comes under the influence of mature hormone levels, the process of squamous metaplasia occurs, with a new SCJ forming inward from the old one. The area in between is the transformation zone, the site of this squamous metaplasia. (*C1*) Three-dimensional representation of mature SCJ, showing islets of columnar epithelium (*1*), nabothian cyst (*2*), gland openings (*3*), and metaplastic epithelium (*4*). (*D*) In menopause, the process reverses, and the new SCJ rolls inward to lie at or above the cervical os, often out of direct visual observation.

and encompassing tests being introduced regularly. Controversy remains as to how the information is best used, however, as the experience with such testing and its correlation to histology and management outcomes are just starting to develop. HPV DNA testing is generally done as a separate although coincident test with the Pap smear, either as an entirely separate test if a slide Pap smear system is used, or if appropriate, from the supernatant fluid of a liquid based Pap smear system. The test may be used as an adjunctive test in the ASC-US group. Patients who have ASC-US Paps and are HPV DNA negative for high risk types of HPV may be followed, whereas those positive for high risk types of HPV are referred for colposcopy. Patients with LGSIL and HGSIL Paps do not benefit from HPV DNA adjunctive testing as it does not discriminate sufficiently to suggest different managements.

Screening: The Pap Smear

In the early 1940s and before, cervical cancer was usually diagnosed at an advanced stage with substantial morbidity and mortality compared to that which might be obtained from earlier diagnosis. The diagnosis was made by biopsy of a symptomatic patient (histological sample; symptoms such as bleeding, pain, cervical mass). The Greek physician George Papanicolaou reasoned that diagnosis in the relatively long asymptomatic interval before the lesions reached advanced stage would improve the dismal outcomes common at that time. With great insight, Papanicolaou proposed that the examination of cells scraped from the cervix might facilitate accurate and earlier diagnosis. This use of exfolative cytology as a screening test became the Pap Smear. This "new technology" at the time, is now the basis of the modern screening for cervical carcinoma and its asymptomatic precursor lesions. The Pap smear represents one of the most dramatic success stories in all of medicine!

As described in Chapter 1, cells are scraped from the exocervix and endocervix with wooden spatulae and various brushes.

These cells are then either spread on a glass slide and fixed with a spray cytologic fixative agent, or swirled into a liquid medium from which the cells are separated and evaluated. Liquid based cytology also allows testing of the fluid for HPV DNA up to three weeks after the study, whereas separate HPV specimens must be obtained at the time of the Pap smear if a Pap slide is used. The cytologic specimens are read by cytopathologists and reported. Recently, automated Pap smear assessment devices have been introduced. At present their use is not for primary Pap smear evaluation, but rather rescreening of large numbers of previously screened slides as a quality control measure.

Annual Pap smear screening will reduce the incidence of invasive cervical carcinoma by more than 95%. As a result, for a long time the recommendation for Pap smear screening was to obtain the first Pap smear at the time a woman becomes sexually active or by the age of 18 years, and yearly thereafter. The rationales for this recommendation include the ease and low cost of the study, the unquestioned improvements in morbidity and mortality from cervical cancer and its precursor lesions, and the health promotion and other primary health care opportunities inherent in a yearly examination. Desipite these benefits, various organizations have advocated triannual Pap smears for sexually active women with intact cervices after three consecutive annual satisfactory Pap smears negative for epithelial cell abnormality. The rationale for this schedule is that cervical intraepithelial neoplasia is generally slow growing so that a lesion missed one year (false negative rate for Pap smears of about 10% to 20%) will be identified the following year, still within time for appropriate low-risk management. The American College of Obstetricians and Gynecologists supports the concept of triannual screening, but with more frequent Pap smears in women with recognized risk factors. (See Table 44.1.) The debate between annual, triannual, or other schedules for Pap smear screening is ongoing.

Pap smears were originally classified into Papanicolaou classes, from Class I, normal, through V, cancer. Subsequently other classifications were used, including the cervical intraepithelial lesion (CIN) and the squamous intraepithelial lesions (SIL) systems. In 1988 experts convened in Bethesda, Maryland, formulating the Bethesda Classification designed to better describe the quality of the Pap smear as well as its abnormalities. In 1991 a second meeting led to the Bethesda II system which was widely used through 2001. In the latter half of 2001, a third series of meetings, were held to upgrade the classification system and re-evaluate management. These resulted in Bethesda 2001, the present recommended classification, and revised management suggestions. (See Tables 44.2, 44.3, and 44.4.) The basis of all the classifications including Bethesea 2001 is the likelihood of progression of precursor lesions to more advanced lesions, and eventually to cervical carcinoma, and hence the window of opportunity for diagnosis and treatment in the asymptomatic precursor stage when outcomes are very good.

BETHESDA 2001

The Bethesda 2001 Classification begins by indicating *Specimen Type*, whether the specimen was fixed by conventional means on a slide or whether liquid based techniques were used. Next, there is an optional *General Categorization* with three options: negative for intraepithelial lesion or malignancy, epithelial cell abnormality, or other. This summary information may be provided, or simply included in the Interpretation/Result section. Next is a statement of *Specimen Adequacy* where the study is classified as Satisfactory and Unsatisfactory, with specific information to explain why a given evaluation of adequacy was made. The importance of repeating an unsatisfactory study is underscored upon realizing that patients with unsatisfactory Pap studies are significantly more likely to have SIL or cancer on follow-up compared to those with satisfactory studies negative for intraepithelial lesion or malignancy.

The *Interpretation/Results* section of Bethesda 2001 is the most substantial section of the report in that it directly speaks to the issue of cervical carcinoma and its precursor lesions. It contains three sections: First, *Negative for Intraepithelial Lesion or Malignancy,* if indeed that is the finding; if not, the epithelial cell abnormality which is discovered is discussed in a section which follows. This section also contains discussions of findings associated with infectious diseases (the Organisms subsection) and other findings (the Other non-neoplastic findings subsection). The second is *Other,* which includes the finding of endometrial cells in a woman over 40 years of age. It is controversial whether further evaluation is advisable because of a possible association with endometrial carcinoma, tubal carcinoma, and ovarian carcinoma. The third is the crucial section dealing with *Epithelial Cell Abnormalities.* 90 to 95% of epithelial cell abnormalities are squamous cell, and are reported in the Squamous Cell section in four categories. *Atypical squamous cells (ASC)* should comprise about 5% or less of smears and are defined as cytological changes suggestive of a squamous intraepithelial lesion that are quantitatively or qualitatively insufficient for a definitive interpretation. Because this is an "I don't know" classification, it contains situations where the suspicion of squamous intraepithelial lesion is low or predominately of a low-grade squamous intrapeithelial lesion (LSIL) and a smaller number of cases where there are cytological features suggestive of HSIL, but definite evidence is lacking. The former sub-group of ASC is called atypical squamous cells of undetermined significance (ASC-US) and the latter, atypical squamous cells, cannot exclude high grade squamous intraepithelial lesion (ASC-H). The importance of this division is in how much evaluation and management is warrented. *In general, ASC-H warrents colposcopic evaluation whereas ASC-US has several appropriate managements.*

The Interpretation/Results section of Bethesda 2001 continues with three sections

TABLE 44.2. The PAP Smear Report: Bethesda 2001

SPECIMEN TYPE Indicate conventional smear (Pap smear) vs. liquid-based study vs. other

GENERAL CATEGORIZATION (optional; information also in Interpretation/Results)
Negative for intraepithelial Lesion or Malignancy
Epithelial Cell Abnormality
Other

SPECIMEN ADEQUACY

Satisfactory for evaluation	Includes whether endocervical/transformation zone components are present or absent. Includes other quality indicators (for example, Inflammation, partially obscuring blood, etc.)
Unsatisfactory for evaluation	Indicates reason smear classified unsatisfactory (either without processing or after processing)

INTERPRETATION/RESULT

Negative for intraepithelial lesion or malignancy	No cellular evidence of neoplasia

Organisms
Trichomonas vaginalis
Fungal organisms norphologically consistent with *Candida sp.*
Sift in floral suggestive of bacterial vaginosis
Bacteria morphologically consistent with *Actinomyces sp.*
Cellular changes associated with herpes siplex virus
Other non-neoplastic findings
Reactive cellular changes associated with inflammation, Radiation, or intrauterine contraceptive device
Glandular cells status post hysterectomy
Atrophy
Other
Endometrial cells in a woman ≥ 40 years of age, specify if negative for Squamous intraepithelial lesion
Epithelial cell abnormalities
SQUAMOUS CELL
Atypical squamous cells
—of undetermined significance (ASC-US) (encompassing cells "suggestive" of SIL)
—cannot exclude HSIL (ASC-H)
Low-grade squamous intraepithelial lesion (LSIL)
Encompassing: HPV/mild dysplasia/CIN-I
High-grade squamous intraepithelial lesion (HSIL)
Encompassing: moderate and severe dysplasia, CIS/CIN-2, and CIN-3
—with features suspicious for invasion
Squamous cell carcinoma
GLANDULAR CELL
Atypical
—endocervical cells (NOS or specify in comments)
—endometrial cells (NOS or specify in comments)
—glandular cells (NOS or specify in comments)

(Continued)

TABLE 44.2.   (Continued)

Atypical
—endocervical cells, favor neoplastic
—glandular cells, favor neoplastic
Endocervical adenocarcinoma in-situ
Adenocarcinoma
—endocervical
—endometrial
—extrauterine
—not otherwise specificed (NOS)
Other malignant neoplasms (specify)

Automated Review	If case examined by automatic device, specificy device and result
Ancillary Testing	Brief description of test methods and results so as to be easily understood by clinician
Educational Notes and Suggestions	Suggestions for patient education should be consistent with other standard guidelines.

TABLE 44.3.   Comparison of Pap Smear Descriptive Conventions

Descriptive Convention			Class III		Class IV severe dysplasia CIS	Class V suggestive of cancer or CIS
Class system	Class I (normal)	Class II inflammation	Mild dysplasia or Moderate dysplasia			
CIN system	Normal	Inflammatory	CIN I or CIN II		CIN III	Suggestive of cancer
Bethesda II system	Within normal limits	a. Without atypia b. With atypia or cellular changes associated with HPV	LSIL	HSIL	HSIL	Squamous cell cancer
Bethesda 2001	Negative for intraepithelial lesion or malignancy	ASC-US ASC-H	LSIL	HSIL		Squamous cell Carcinoma
Histology	Basal cells	WBCs	Basement membrane			Invasive cervical cancer

CIN = cervical intraepithelial neoplasia; CIS = carcinoma in-situ; HPV = human papillomavirus; WBCs = white blood cells. ASC-US = atypical squamous cells of undetermined significance; ASC-H = atypical squamous cells, cannot exclude HSIL; LSIL = low grade squamous intraepithelial lesion; HSIL = high grade squamous intraepithelial lesion.

TABLE 44.4. Evaluation of Epithelial Cell Abnormalities—Bethesda 2001 Classification

(In all cases, if evaluation leads to histologic diagnosis, management is as appropriate to the histologic lesion which is identified.)

Classification	Evaluation
SQUAMOUS CELL	
ASC-US	HPV DNA testing
	If positive for high risk HPV DNA, colposcopy
	If negative, may repeat Pap in 12 months
	Colposcopy
	Repeat Pap is acceptable but not preferred
	Repeat Pap every 3–4 months until three consecutive "negative for squamous intrapeithelial lesions/malignancy" Pap smears
	Special Circumstances
	Menopausal woman: intravaginal estrogen cream nightly for 3–6 weeks, then repeat Pap; if negative, repeat in 3–4 months and if again negative, may return to routine Pap sequence; if positive, colposcopy
	Infection/severe inflammation: acceptable to treat infection and repeat Pap in 4–6 weeks; if negative, repeat in 3–4 months and if again negative, may return to routine Pap sequence; if positive, colposcopy
	Immunosuppressed woman: colposcopy
ASC-H	Colposcopy
LSIL	Colposcopy
	With follow-up Pap smears
	With treatment and then follow-up Pap smears
	Colopscopy is recommended if:
	Prior high grade lesion/dysplasia/CIN 2 or 3/CIS (treated or untreated)
	Prior ASC-US, LSIL/HSIL Pap without history of Therapy
	Inability to follow-up patient
	Immunusuppressed patient
	Postmenopausal patient without atrophy
	Strong family history of cervical or lower genital carcinoma
	Heavy smoking history
	Repeat Pap smear (if colopscopy not general scheme and none of the indications for colposcopy present)
	Repeat Pap smears every 4–6 months with return to routine screening after 3 consecutive repeat smears without evidence of intraepithelial neoplasia or cacinoma and referral for colposcopy if any repeat smear shows evidence of these abnormalities.
HSIL	Colposcopy with ECC and directed biopsy of most abnormal lesion(s) as determined colposcopically;
HSIL with features suspicious for invasion	Colposcopy with ECC and directed biopsy of most abnormal lesion(s) as determined colposcopically
Squamous Cell	Colposcopy with ECC and directed biopsy of most abnormal lesion(s) as determined colposcopically

(Continued)

TABLE 44.4. (Continued)

GLANDULAR CELL

Atypical
—endocervical cells
  (NOS or specify in comments)
—endometrial cells
  (NOS or specify in comments)
—glandular cells
  (NOS or specify in comments)
	Colposcopy, endocervical sampling

Atypical —endocervical cells, favor neoplastic —glandular cells, favor neoplastic	Colposcopy, endocervical sampling, and diagnostic excisional cervical procedure (conization, preferably cold knife conization); exception: if initial histology shows invasive carcinoma, conization should be deferred with individualized management by a gynecologic oncologist.
Endocervical adenocarcinoma in-situ	as above
Adenocarcinoma —endocervical —endometrial —extrauterine —not otherwise specified (NOS)	as above

Special circumstances
AGC (any kind)
Women over 35 years of age
  with unexplained vaginal
  bleeding
Postmenopausal women not on
  estrogen replacement therapy
	Endometrial sampling (pipelle endometrial sampling, D&C)

Repeat AGC, AGC "favor Neoplasia," and atypical endocervical cells "suggestive of AIS" where colposcopy, cervical biopsy, endocervical sampling, and cervical excisional procedure fail to elicit the source of the cellular abnormality.	Pelvic ultrasund, abdominopelvic CT scan to evaluate for non-gynecologic sources of abnormal cells. Women over 35 years of age should also have hysteroscopic evaluation to reduce the risk of missed endometrial lesions. Before proceeding with this extensive evaluation, a review of all slides is recommended.
Other	Colposcopy and endocervical evaluation followed by appropriate procedures to evaluate the suggested site of origin (e.g., ovary, fallopian tube, etc.)

which deal with more clearly identified cell abnormalities. The first is Low-Grade Squamous Intraepithelial Lesion (LSIL) which generally encompasses cells from lesions which will prove on histological evaluation to be HPV associated lesions, mild dysplasia, or cervical intrapeithelial neoplasia–1.

The second is High-Grade Squamous Intrapeithelial Lesion (HSIL) which generally encompasses cells from lesions which prove on histological evaluation to be moderate to severe dysplasia, cervical intraepithelial neoplasia–2 or –3, or carcinoma in-situ. A sub-classification is also provided,

HSIL with features suspicious for invasion. The final group is Squamous Cell Carcinoma, with cells consistent with exfoliation from frank cervical carcinoma.

The Interpretation/Results section of Bethesda 2001 concludes with a section addressing the 5%–10% of epithelial cell abnormalities which are Glandular Cell. The importance of Pap smears with these abnormalities is disproportionate to their number because about 40% are found upon evaluation to be associated with squamous intraepithelial lesions, 6% with adenocarcinoma in-situ, and another 6% with frank carcinoma. This classification harbors special importance for women over 35 years of age, as the majority of cancers in this age group are endometrial in origin. There are four sub-sections. The first consists of atypical endocervical cells (either not otherwise specified or favor neoplastic), atypical endometrial cells, or atypical glandular cells (either not otherwise specified or favor neoplastic, or probably AIS [adenocarcimoma in-situ]). The second is Endocervical adenocarcinoma in-situ (AIS). The third is Adenocarcinoma, either endocervical, endometrial, extrauterine (tubal, ovarian, other), or not otherwise specified (NOS). The fourth is Other which encompases cells which may be of tubal or ovarian origin. At present, HPV DNA typing has not been found to be of similar value as in ASC, although this may change with the acquisition of further information.

EVALUATION OF THE "ABNORMAL" PAP SMEAR—EPITHELIAL CELL ABNORMALITIES
Evaluation of Abnormal Pap Studies (See Table 44.4.)

The evaluation of atypical squamous cells is challenging because of the imprecision with which they are classified and the often conflicting information about their appropriate evaluation and treatment. ASC-US Paps, have a 3% to 10% chance of harboring a higher grade lesion, and are associaed with a sub-

stantial lack of reproducibility of the classification itself and the variable natural history of the lesions which may underlie this Pap result. As a result, two evaluation schemes are recommended and one is considered acceptable. There are special circumstances involving ASC-US as well. Menopausal women with these Pap results may have an atrophic component, even if on systemic estrogen replacement therapy, so that intravaginal estrogen therapy and a repeat Pap smear may be an appropriate management. Likewise, inflammation associated with intravaginal infection may be appropriately managed by treatment and repeat Pap smear. Because of the high risk of a higher grade lesion and/or more rapid progression, these Pap results in an immunosuppressed woman warrant colposcopy. ASC-H is evaluated by colposcopy because of the higher likelihood of underlying CIN 2-3 lesions (variously reported at an incidence of 25% to 75% of cases) or worse, compared to ASC-US.

About 1½ % of Pap smears are reproducibly classified as LSIL. About ¾ of these will be found to have a squamous intraepithelial lesion (1 in 5 CIN 2-3, and 1 in 500 squamous cell carcinoma) and the other ¼ will have no identifiable lesion. Further, about 50% of patients with CIN 1 will regress to negative, 30% will persist as CIN 1, and only 10% will progress to higher-grade CIN. Also, even if the CIN 1 does progress to a higher-grade CIN, the treatment and cure rates for low-grade and higher-grade CIN are very similar. The overall rate of progression to actual cancer is approximated at about ¼ of one percent, and over a longer time span than that for follow-up Pap smears. As a result, two evaluation schemes are recommended: colposcopy, allowing histologic diagnosis but arguably more costly; repeat Pap smear, less costly but with delay which will not be significant in terms of morbidity in most, but not all, cases. Because 80% to 90% of women with LSIL Paps are positive for oncogenic HPV at HPV DNA testing, the testing is not cost effective for the general population of LSIL patients.

The evaluation of squamous cell epithelial cell abnormalities reported as HSIL and

Carcinoma is relatively straightforward, involving colposcopy and directed biopsy or conization, endocervical sampling, and in some cases, endometrial sampling. This is because the likelihood of the presence of a more severe lesion or the progression of extant lesions is high. The goal of evaluation is to determine whether there is invasive cancer or a high grade preinvasive lesion. If there is evidence of invasion, conization is generally indicated if the depth of invasion is < 3mm or if the depth of the invasion cannot be determined, whereas treatment for invasive cancer is persued if the depth of invasion is determined to be > 3 mm.

While glandular cell abnormalities comprise less than 0.5% of epithelial cell abnormalities, their appropriate evaluation is especially important because of their association with squamous and glandular precursor lesions and carcinoma. All women with AGC of any variety should have colposcopy and endocervical sampling regardless of qualification (that is, NOS probably favor neoplasia). Repeat Pap smear is not acceptable. In all cases where the qualifiations "favor neoplasia," "probably AIS," or AIS are noted, a diagnostic cervical excisional procedure should always follow colposcopy and endocervical sampling. The choice of which type of conization is controvercial, but the preponderance of evidence supports cold conization over loop electrosurgical excision because of thermal distortion of possible glandular cell abnormalities. The exception to the cervical excisional procedure recommendation is for women with the diagnosis of invasive carcinoma on biopsy or endocervical sampling. These patients require individualized management by a gynecologic oncologist. There are also additional special situations. Women with AGC on their Pap smear and who are (1) over the age of 35 years and have unexplained vaginal bleeding or (2) are postmenopausal, and not on estrogen replacement therapy should have endometrial evaluation, either by endometrial pipelle endometrial sampling, or by D&C. Table 44.5 presents an outline of recommended evaluations for abnormal Pap smears using the Bethesda 2001 classification.

Colposcopy and Cervical Conization

Colposcopy is the most common management approach when histological evaluation is required. A colposcope is a binocular stereomicroscope with variable magnification (usually × 1 to 14) and a variable intensity light source with green filters, which aid in the identification of abnormal appearing blood vessels which may be associated with intraepithelial neoplasia. With colposcopy, areas with changes consistent with dysplasia are identified, allowing directed biopsy (that is, biopsy of the area where dysplasia is most likely). Colposcopic criteria such as white epithelium, abnormal vascular patterns, and punctate lesions help identify such areas. To facilitate the examination, the cervix is washed with a 3% to 4% acetic acid solution, which acts as an epithelial desiccant, enhancing visualization of dysplastic lesions, which usually appear with relatively discrete borders at or near the SCJ. *Visualization of the entire SCJ is required for a colposcopy to be considered a satisfactory colposcopic examination.* If the SCJ is not visualized in its entirety or if the margins of abnormal areas are not seen in their entirety, the colposcopic assessment is termed unsatisfactory and other evaluation is needed, in some cases cervical conization. This is the *first reason for cervical conization: unsatisfactory colposcopy.* When the Pap is LSIL and the colposcopy is unsatisfactory, there are two possibilities. A lesion is identified in the transformation zone or no lesion is identified. In the former case, directed biopsy and ECC allow treatment if the diagnosis is CIN 1, as the management of CIN 1 is different from that of CIN 2 and above; if the diagnosis is CIN 2 or worse, conization is considered. In the latter case, ECC is performed and if a CIN 1 lesion or worse is discovered, conization is recommended.

The number of colposcopically directed biopsies obtained will vary, depending on

TABLE 44.5. Clinical Stages of Carcinoma of the Cervix Uteri*

Stage	Characteristics
I	Carcinoma is strictly confined to cervix (extension to corpus should be disregarded)
IA	Preclinical carcinoma
IA1	Minimal microscopically evident stromal invasion
IA2	Microscopic lesions no more than 5 mm depth measured from base of epithelium surface or glandular from which it originates; horizontal spread not to exceed 7 mm
IB	All other cases of stage I: Occult cancer should be marked "occ"
II	Carcinoma extends beyond cervix but has not extended to pelvic wall; involves vagina but not as far as lower third
IIA	No obvious parametrial involvement
IIB	Obvious parametrial involvement
III	Carcinoma has extended to pelvic wall; on rectal examination there is no cancer-free space between tumor and pelvic wall; tumor involves lower third of vagina; all cases with hydronephrosis or nonfunctioning kidney should be included, unless they are known to have another cause
IIIA	No extension to pelvic wall, but involvement of lower third of vagina
IIIB	Extension to pelvic wall, hydronephrosis, or nonfunctioning kidney caused by tumor
IV	Carcinoma has extended beyond true pelvis or has clinically involved mucosa of bladder or rectum
IVA	Spread of growth to adjacent pelvic organs
IVB	Spread to distant organs

*International Federation of Gynecology and Obstetrics (FIGO) Staging Classification, revised 1985.

the number and severity of abnormal areas found. After sampling the identified lesions, an *endocervical curettage* (ECC), using a small curette, is performed, often followed by the use of a endocervical brush to retrieve additional cells dislodged but not trapped in the curette specimen. This simple sampling procedure may be performed without cervical dilation in most instances. This endocervical sample is obtained so that potential disease farther inside the cervical canal, which is not visualized by the colposcope, may be detected. The cervical biopsies and ECC are then submitted separately for pathologic assessment. ECC is positive for dysplasia in 5% to 10% of women with abnormal Pap smear. Because of the absence of tissue orientation from endocervical curettings, the degree of dysplasia determined from them is difficult to assess. This

is the *second reason for cervical conization: positive ECC.*

In approximately 10% of colposcopies with directed biopsies and ECC, there will be a substantial discrepancy between the screening Pap smear and the histologic data from biopsy and ECC (e.g., if the Pap smear is read as HSIL and the directed biopsies are read as normal with evidence of intraepithelial lesion). When such a discrepancy occurs, further tissue diagnosis by repeat colposcopy or by cervical conization will probably be necessary so that the most severe abnormality can be explained histologically. With conization, cone-shaped biopsy of the entire SCJ and identified lesions as well as a portion of the endocervical canal, the pathologist can determine the most severe lesions by histologic, hence diagnostic, criteria. Often, the cone biopsy may prove to be therapeutic as well as diagnostic, because the entire lesion is removed. This is the *third indication for cervical conization: a substantial discrepancy between Pap smear and biopsy results.*

Cervical conization, or cone biopsy of the cervix, is a minor surgical procedure performed under general or regional anesthesia. Usually performed with scalpel and scissors *(cold knife conization, CKC),* conization is now also performed with a laser or with a heated wire loop, the *LLETZ (large loop excision of the transformation zone)* or *LEEP (loop electrosurgical excision procedure).* As seen in Figure 44.3, a cone-shaped specimen is removed from the cervix, which encompasses the SCJ, all identified lesions on the ectocervix, and a portion of the endocervical canal, the extent of which depends on whether the ECC was positive or negative. Because LEEP uses an electrically heated wire, concern is often raised about thermal damage at the margins of the specimen obscuring the histology. This is usually not considered a substantial problem in the evaluation of squamous epithelial abnormalities, but it may be a more substantial issue in the evaluation of glandular epithelial lesions where abnormal cells in the bottom of glandular crypts may be altered so that evaluation is difficult if not impossible. In the latter case, cold knife conization may be more appropriate.

If the margins of the biopsy are positive or cannot be established, the patient should have either repeat conization or very close follow-up with either Pap smears at increased frequency or repeat colposcopy. If the margins are positive for either a high-grade epithelial lesion or carcinoma in-situ, treatment may include hysterectomy or close follow-up regimens depending on the patient's desires for future fertility and her views about the value of maintaining her cervix and uterus. The risks of the procedure include infection, blood loss, and the risks of anesthesia. For women who may want children in the future, there are the additional risks of cervical incompetence, if the internal cervical os is compromised, and reduced cervical capacity to facilitate sperm transport, because of loss of mucous-

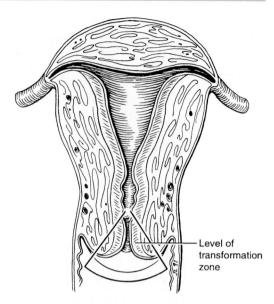

FIGURE 44.3. Cervical conization.

secreting glands. Conversely, in some women the issue is not cervical incompetence, but rather cervical stenosis which may not allow easy entrance of sperm or exit of menstrual blood, and maybe be associated with protraction disorders of labor.

Treatment

The underlying concept in the treatment of CIN is that excision or ablation of the superficial precursor lesion avoids progression to carcinoma. Because these lesions are superficial and usually confined to the visible and easily accessible SCJ, simple office techniques that require minimal or no anesthesia and that have little risk usually suffice. In general, the therapy for CIN 1 is either observation with follow-up cytology or local abalation. Therapies which are not recommended for histologically proven CIN 1 include topical acid treatment (trichloroacetic acid, TCA), topical podophyllin or podophyllin related products, single biopsy of the lesion only, or hysterectomy. The specific patterns of each CIN 1 management are presently in the form of related but diverse recommendations which reflect the still incomplete data base about each grade of lesion and its response to therapy. For preinvasive high-grade lesions

(HSIL, CIN 2 and 3, CIS), abalation or excision is generally recommended because a substantial portion of these are likely to progress to invasive carcinoma of the cervix. Ablative procedures may only be used with an adequate colposcopy and appropriate correlation between Pap smear and colposcopically directed biopsy.

Cryocautery is a popular outpatient method used to treat low-grade CIN. The procedure involves covering the SCJ and all identified lesions with a stainless-steel probe, which is then supercooled with liquid nitrogen or compressed gas (carbon dioxide or nitrous oxide). The size and shape of the probe depends on the size and shape of the cervix and the lesion to be treated. The most common technique involves a 3-minute freeze followed by a 5-minute thaw, with a repeat 3-minute freeze (Figure 44.4). The thaw period between the two freezing episodes allows the damaged tissue from the first freeze to become edematous and swell with intracellular fluid. With the second freeze, the edematous cellular architecture is refrozen and extends the damaged area slightly deeper into the tissue. Healing after cryotherapy may take up to 4 or 5 weeks, because the damaged tissue slowly sloughs and is replaced by new cervical epithelium. This process is associated with profuse watery discharge often mixed with necrotic cellular debris. It can be assumed that the entire healing process has been completed within 2 months, and usually the next follow-up Pap smear is done 12 weeks following the freezing to ascertain the effectiveness of the procedure. The cure rates for low-grade CIN using this technique approach 90%.

Colposcopically directed *laser therapy* may be employed to ablate lesions involving CIN. Because of the precision imparted by the colposcopic direction of the fine laser beam as well as the precise control of depth of ablation available, many physicians prefer laser ablation to "less precise" techniques. Each lesion may be addressed separately and ablated. In addition, ablation of the entire SCJ is often performed (see Figure 44.4). Although the technology is more sophisticated than cryocautery, long-term

cure rates with this technique are similar to that for cryocautery. An advantage of laser therapy is that it can be used for high-grade intraepithelial lesions, because the depth of ablation can be adjusted to accommodate the extent of the lesion.

Conization, either "cold knife" or by electro-loop excision, may be used as a therapeautic modality as well as for diagnosis, and indeed, often may serve both goals simultaneously. Hysterectomy may be indicated as an excisional modality in the case of high grade non-invasive lesions when further fetility is not desired and the patient is fully aware of the risks and benefits of this procedure as compared to less morbid excisional or abalative alernatives.

Follow-Up to Treatment

After treatment for non-invasive epithelial cell abnormalities, either by abalation or excision, a period of follow-up Pap smears every 4 to 6 months for about 2 years is generally recommended, with variations depending on the specifics of the case including histology, risk factors, compliance, and so forth. Most patients may return to a yearly evaluation thereafter, again depending on the same issues. If a repeat Pap smear is abnormal, it is evaluated anew in the same manner of a new abnormal Pap smear. The importance of follow-up should be stressed to the patient because of the greater risk of recurrent abnormalities.

CERVICAL CARCINOMA

Until approximately 20 years ago, cervical cancer was the most common gynecologic malignancy, with a ratio of 2:1 over endometrial carcinoma. Now the cervical carcinoma:endometrial carcinoma ratio has almost reversed; endometrial carcinoma rates are twice that for invasive cervical carcinoma. Approximately 15,000 new cases of invasive cervical carcinoma are diagnosed annually.

The average age at diagnosis for invasive cervical cancer is approximately 50 years,

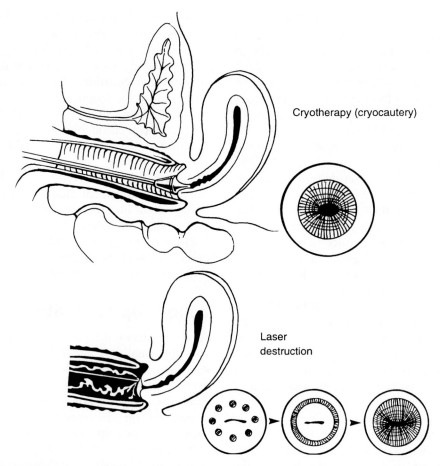

Cryotherapy (cryocautery)

Laser
destruction

FIGURE 44.4.   Ablation of cervical intraepithelial neoplasia: cryotherapy and laser ablation.

although the disease may occur in the very young as well as the very old patient. In studies following patients with advanced CIN, this precursor lesion precedes invasive carcinoma by approximately 10 years. In some patients, however, this time of progression may be considerably less.

The *etiology* of cervical cancer is unknown. There is ample evidence that advanced *CIN* arising in the squamous epithelium of the cervical transformation zone often progresses to invasive squamous cell cervical carcinoma. Similarly, *HPV* has been implicated as an etiologic cofactor in the development of cervical carcinoma. Studies involving genetic probes have identified papillomavirus DNA fragments within areas of invasive cervical carcinoma. Other etiologic associations are also similar to those for CIN, including *factors related to the male ejaculate, the immature trans-*

formation zone, the number of different sexual partners, and cigarette smoking. Immunocompromised patients (e.g., transplant patients or patients with human immunodeficiency virus [HIV] infection) are a special group who seem more susceptible to this disease.

Approximately 85% of cervical cancer is of the squamous cell variety. Approximately 15% of cervical cancers are adenocarcinomas, arising from the endocervical glands.

Three rare types of cervical cancer are also encountered: *clear cell carcinoma* associated with diethylstilbestrol (DES) exposure in utero, *sarcoma,* and *lymphoma.* In general, the evaluation and treatment of squamous cell and adenocarcinoma of the cervix are similar. The discussions that follow reflect this similarity and apply to these two most common cervical carcinomas.

Survival rates for cervical carcinoma reflect the extent of disease at the time of diagnosis. Stage I has more than 91% 5-year survival, whereas 5-year survival for stages IIA, IIIA, and IV are 83%, 45%, and 14%, respectively.

Clinical Evaluation

There is *no classic historical presentation* for cervical cancer. Two symptoms are often associated with cervical carcinoma, although both have other more common causes: *postcoital bleeding and abnormal uterine bleeding*. Other symptoms are determined by the organs or organ systems involved as the cancer spreads, and hence by the pattern of spread: direct invasion to contiguous structures and by lymphatics to distant sites of metastasis.

Visible lesions on the cervix should be biopsied. Lesions that should be considered for immediate biopsy include all new exophytic, friable, or bleeding lesions. These are readily differentiated from more common, normal variations of cervical anatomy such as nabothian cysts or condylomata. Pap smears are sometimes negative in this situation because exfoliative cells from frank cancer may be so distorted as to be uninterpretable. *When a visible lesion is present, colposcopic assessment need not be done unless the results of the direct biopsy do not confirm cancer.*

Staging is based on the International Federation of Gynecology and Obstetrics (FIGO) Staging Classification of 1985 (Table 44.5). This is a convention based both on the histologic assessment of the tumor sample and on physical and laboratory examination to ascertain the extent of disease. It is useful because of the very predictable manner in which *cervical carcinoma spreads by direct invasion and by lymphatic metastasis.*

Cervical carcinoma spreads through the cervical and paracervical lymphatics, through the parametria, and into the regional lymph nodes. Cervical carcinoma also spreads by direct extension proximally into the endocervical canal or distally into the vagina. In patients with primary lymphatic spread, the ascent of disease from the regional lymph glands proceeds to the deep pelvic nodes, including the external and internal iliac node chain, the common iliac node chain, and periaortic node chain (Figure 44.5). Accordingly, advanced stages include a description of tumor beyond the cervix, into the vagina or parametria (stage II); directly to the lateral pelvic wall or the lower third of the vagina (stage III); or widespread disease, including but not limited to the bladder or rectum (stage IV).

Other studies that may be used in staging include intravenous pyelography and cystoscopy, proctosigmoidoscopy or barium enema, blood chemistries with emphasis on liver and renal function, and computed tomography studies on a selective basis. Computed tomography has been of special value in evaluating the extent of lymphatic involvement.

Management

Once there has been histologic confirmation of invasive cervical carcinoma, it is imperative to refer the patient to a gynecologic oncologist for appropriate surgical and/or radiation therapy.

The mainstays of treatment for invasive cervical carcinoma include *radical surgical therapy and/or pelvic irradiation.* In general, surgical therapy is indicated for most patients with stage I disease and selected patients with stage II disease, because of the limited yet predictable extent of spread in these early stages. *Radical surgical therapy* includes radical hysterectomy aimed at removing all of the central disease (i.e., disease not only in the cervix itself but in all the adjacent paracervical, parametrial, and vaginal tissue). In addition, surgical eradication of the local and regional lymph nodes is an important part of radical surgical therapy (pelvic lymphadenectomy). The presence or absence of tumor in the lymph nodes sampled defines, in part, the extent of disease and the need for further therapy, either radiation therapy or perhaps chemotherapy. It should be emphasized that simple hysterectomy with removal of the cervix is inadequate treatment for invasive cervical carcinoma. In young women who are treated surgically, ovarian preservation is

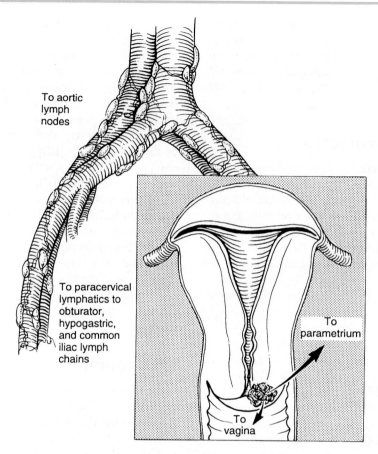

To aortic
lymph
nodes

To paracervical
lymphatics to
obturator,
hypogastric,
and common
iliac lymph
chains

To
parametrium

To
vagina

FIGURE 44.5. Spread patterns of cervical carcinoma.

usually advisable to provide the patient with the long-term benefits from endogenous estrogen secretion. Ovarian retention presents no additional risk to the patient, because cervical carcinoma neither spreads through the adnexal structures nor is estrogen dependent.

Radiation therapy is reserved for patients with stage IB or IIA disease who are poor surgical candidates and for all patients with more advanced disease. The basis for radiation therapy in more advanced disease is the likelihood for more extensive regional nodal involvement. Even with stage III disease extending to the lateral pelvic wall, approximately one third of patients are cured with primary radiation therapy. Both high-dose external beam therapy and intracavitary irradiation are used for most patients. Intrauterine and intravaginal applicators containing radioactive materials are placed to direct treatment of the uterus, cervix, and vagina as needed, and external

beam radiation is applied primarily along the paths of lymphatic extension of cervical carcinoma (Figure 44.6).

Fortunately, the adjacent nongynecologic structures, such as the bladder and distal colon, tolerate these treatments fairly well, without significant untoward effects. Radiation therapy doses are calculated by individual patient needs to maximize radiation to the tumor sites and potential spread areas, while minimizing the amount of radiation to adjacent uninvolved tissues. *Complications of radiation therapy* include radiation cystitis and proctitis, which are usually relatively easy to manage. Other more unusual complications include intestinal or vaginal fistulae, small bowel obstruction, or difficult to manage hemorrhagic proctitis or cystitis. It should be remembered that the tissue damage and fibrosis incurred by radiation therapy progresses over many years, and that these effects may complicate long-term management.

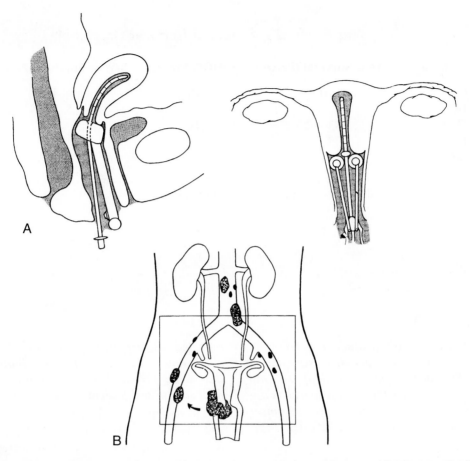

FIGURE 44.6.   Radiation therapy for cervical carcinoma. (*A*) Intravaginal and intrauterine applicators are inserted to irradiate the cervix, vagina, and uterus. (*B*) External beam radiation is used along the paths of lymphatic spread of the tumor.

Most authorities believe that radical surgical excision and pelvic lymphadenectomy offer distinct advantages over radiation therapy for earlier stage disease. These include the potential for preservation of ovarian function in young women, preservation of sexual function, and avoidance of long-term radiation effects. On the other hand, certain operative complications such as hemorrhage, damage to local nerves supplying the bladder, and urinary vaginal fistula may develop from radical pelvic surgery. It is important for the risks and benefits of each form of therapy to be explained to the patient, and treatment should be performed based on individual patient selection.

Follow-up of patients with cervical carcinoma is best done by gynecologic oncologists who use established protocols. Most oncology centers follow patients in a specialized clinic for at least 5 years. When there is recurrence, 90% reoccurs within this time period. The 5-year survival rates for various stages of cervical carcinoma are shown in Table 44.6.

Treatment for recurrent disease is associated with poor cure rates. Most chemotherapeutic protocols have only limited usefulness and are reserved for palliative efforts. Likewise, specific "spot" radiation to areas of recurrence also provides only limited benefit. Occasional patients with central recurrence (i.e., recurrence of disease in the upper vagina or the residual cervix and uterus in radiation patients) may benefit from ultraradical surgery with partial or total pelvic exenteration. These candidates are few, but when properly selected, may benefit from this aggressive therapy.

TABLE 44.6.	Five-Year Survival for Treated Cervical Carcinoma		
FIGO Stage	**5-Year Survival (Percent)**	**FIGO Stage**	**5-Year Survival (Percent)**
0	100	IIIA	45
IA	99	IIIB	36
IB	85–90	IVA	15
IIA	73–80	IVB	2
IIB	68		

FIGO = International Federation of Gynecology and Obstetrics.

CASE STUDIES

Case 44A

A 24-year-old college student, G1 P0010, presents for her annual pelvic examination and Pap smear and renewal of her oral contraceptive. History and physical examination are unremarkable. Her Pap smear is subsequently reported as HGSIL.

Questions Case 44A

The most appropriate next step in this patient's management is

A. Repeat Pap smear in 1 year
B. Repeat Pap smear now
C. Colposcopy with ECC and directed biopsy
D. Excisional biopsy
E. Cervical conization

Answer: C

HGSIL on screening examination requires histologic diagnosis so that appropriate treatment can be selected. Repeat Pap smear is another screening test and is thus inappropriate. Conization for diagnostic purposes is needed only if colposcopy and biopsy prove inadequate.

The colposcopy was satisfactory with areas of whitened epithelium. Subsequently, the ECC done at colposcopy was reported as negative for epithelial cell abnormalities as were the two biopsies that were taken. The most appropriate next step in this patient's management is

A. Repeat Pap smear in 1 year
B. Repeat Pap smear now
C. Colposcopy with ECC and directed biopsy
D. Excisional biopsy
E. Cervical conization

Answer: E

There is a substantial discrepancy between the screening Pap smear (HGSIL) and the diagnostic biopsy results ("normal"), that is, the source of the original abnormal Pap smear has yet to be found. This must be resolved before appropriate therapy can be suggested. Conization is appropriate and may, in addition, be curative.

A conization is performed and subsequently reported as three foci of moderate to severe dysplasia without extension beyond the surgical limits. The most appropriate next step in this patient's management is

A. Repeat Pap smear in 3 months
B. Repeat Pap smear now

C. Repeat colposcopy with ECC and directed biopsy
D. Excisional biopsy at four quadrants
E. Repeat cervical conization

Answer: A

The antecedent colposcopy was satisfactory, the conization has uninvolved surgical margins and is reported as CIN 2–3, so that the conization has also been therapeutic. Follow-up with Pap smears every 3 months for at least 1 year is indicated, with further evaluation if new cytologic abnormalities are discovered.

Case 44B

A 46-year-old mother of four presents with a complaint of postcoital spotting. Her last Pap smear was 2 years ago and was normal. On physical examination, a 1 × 0.5 cm friable mass is found on the anterior lip of her cervix. The remainder of her physical examination is normal.

Questions Case 44B

The most appropriate next step in this patient's management is
  A. No further management indicated
  B. Pap smear
  C. Colposcopy with ECC and directed biopsy
  D. Biopsy
  E. Cervical conization

Answer: B, D

Both a Pap smear and immediate biopsy are indicated. If cervical carcinoma is discovered, staging and appropriate therapy may be begun immediately. The Pap smear may be unreliable in frank carcinoma and should not be relied on solely in the presence of a grossly visible lesion.

*The Pap smear is reported as squamous cell carcinoma. The biopsy is reported as squamous cell carcinoma extending to the mar-*gins of the specimen. The most appropriate next step in this patient's management is
  A. Radical hysterectomy
  B. Radiation therapy
  C. Colposcopy with ECC and directed biopsy
  D. Repeat excisional biopsy to go past previous biopsy margins
  E. Cervical conization

Answer: A or B

Invasive cervical carcinoma has been diagnosed and now requires treatment. Radical hysterectomy or radiation therapy may be indicated, depending on the patient's staging evaluation.

Case 44C

A 24-year-old G0 presents for annual physical examination and renewal of oral contraceptives, which she has used without difficulty since age 15. She has no history of sexually transmitted diseases and reports sexual relations with three partners during her life.

The patient's physical examination is normal and routine screening tests are performed with renewal of her oral contraceptive. The Pap smear is reported as satisfactory, LGSIL.

Question Case 44C

The most appropriate next step in this patient's management is
  A. No further management indicated
  B. Colposcopy with ECC and directed biopsy
  C. Excisional biopsy
  D. Cervical conization

Answer: B

Colposcopy with biopsy is a recommended evaluation of LGSIL. Most often, depending on the pathologic assessment of the biopsy, treatment can be limited to local destruction by cryocautery.

45

UTERINE LEIOMYOMA
AND NEOPLASIA

Uterine enlargement as a result of leiomyoma (fibroids, myomas) is common in clinical practice. It is estimated that up to 30% of American women have these benign tumors, although the majority do not present with significant symptoms and do not require therapy. Despite this, leiomyomata are the most common indication for hysterectomy, accounting for approximately 30% of all such cases. Additionally, leiomyomata account for a large number of more conservative operations including myomectomy, uterine curettage, and operative hysteroscopy.

Histologically, these benign tumors represent localized proliferation of smooth muscle cells surrounded by a pseudocapsule of compressed muscle fibers. When these tumors are symptomatic, the most frequent clinical manifestations include:

1. Pain, including secondary dysmenorrhea
2. Bleeding, most commonly menorrhagia (increased amount and duration of flow)
3. Pressure symptoms, related to the size and number of tumors filling the pelvic cavity; pressure against bladder, bowel, and pelvic floor

Leiomyoma also represents an important clinical entity because, as pelvic masses, there may be a necessity to investigate them as if they were a malignancy. They are considered hormonally responsive tumors because the growth potential of these tumors is related to estrogen production, often with rapid growth occurring in pregnancy or high estrogen states. Data suggest that estrogen may work by stimulation of the production of progesterone receptors in the myometrium, and, in turn, progesterone binding to these sites stimulates the production of several growth factors causing the growth of myomas. Menopause generally brings about cessation of tumor growth and even some atrophy.

Although exact mechanisms are unknown, some investigators have implicated chromosomal translocations and deletions as potential pathogenic factors of leiomyomata. Peptide growth factors and induc-

tion of DNA synthesis by epidermal growth factors have also been implicated. Sensitive DNA studies suggest that each myoma arises from a single smooth muscle cell and that, in many cases, the smooth muscle cell is vascular in origin.

In 0.1% of cases, malignancy such as leiomyosarcoma may develop. These are not thought to represent "degeneration" of a fibroid but, rather, a new neoplasm. Uterine malignancy is more typical in older patients, especially postmenopausal patients who present with rapidly enlarging uterine masses and postmenopausal bleeding, unusual vaginal discharge, and pelvic pain. An enlarging uterine mass in a postmenopausal patient should be evaluated with considerably more concern for malignancy than one in a younger woman. Other cell types may be involved in this form of malignancy. These heterologous mixed tumors contain other sarcomatous tissue elements not necessarily found only in the uterus.

There are three quite rare variants of apparently benign uterine myomas. All are generally thought to be benign and somewhat estrogen dependent. Intravenous leiomyomatosis is described as invasion of the pelvic veins and even vena cava with histologically mature and benign smooth muscle tumor. Benign metastasizing leiomyoma has been reported in cardiac, lymphatic, and pulmonary nodules, presumed to be the result of either intravenous or lymphatic embolization. Leiomyomatosis peritonealis disseminata involves implants on peritoneal surfaces identical to uterine myomas.

LEIOMYOMAS

Symptoms

The symptoms associated with uterine fibroids frequently lead women to seek medical advice. Although smooth muscle tumors may occur anywhere in the body in women, they most commonly occur within the uterus or as an appendage to the uterus (Figure 45.1). Gross and histologic changes may occur in uterine fibroids, and historically, these changes have been termed forms

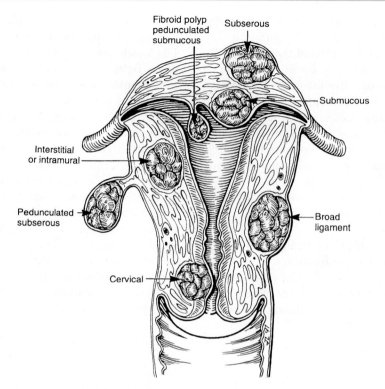

FIGURE 45.1. Common types of uterine fibroids.

of "degeneration." The most common types of change include *red degeneration,* hemorrhagic changes associated with rapid growth; *hyaline degeneration,* hyalinization of the smooth muscle elements, occurring commonly after menopause; and *calcification* and calcific replacement of inactive smooth muscle elements, also occurring after menopause.

Bleeding is the most common presenting symptom in uterine fibroids. Although the kind of abnormal bleeding may vary, the most common presentation includes the development of progressively heavier menstrual flow that lasts longer than the normal duration (*menorrhagia,* defined as menstrual blood loss of more than 80 ml). This bleeding may result from significant distortion of the endometrial cavity by the underlying tumor. This contributes to three generally accepted but unproved *mechanisms for increased bleeding:*

1. Alteration of normal myometrial contractile function in the small artery and arteriolar blood supply underlying the endometrium

2. Inability of the overlying endometrium to respond to the normal estrogen/progesterone menstrual phases, which contribute to efficient sloughing of the endometrium

3. Pressure necrosis of the overlying endometrial bed, which exposes vascular surfaces that bleed in excess of that normally found with endometrial sloughing

Characteristically, the best example of a type of leiomyoma contributing to this bleeding pattern is the so-called submucous leiomyoma. In this variant, the majority of the distortion created by the smooth muscle tumor projects toward the endometrial cavity rather than toward the serosal surface of the uterus. Enlarging intramural fibroids likewise may contribute to excessive bleeding if they become large enough to significantly distort the endometrial cavity.

Blood loss from this type of menstrual bleeding may be heavy enough to contribute to chronic iron-deficiency anemia and, rarely, to profound acute blood loss. The occurrence of isolated submucous (suben-

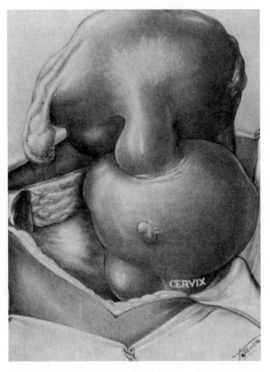

FIGURE 45.2. Large uterine fibroids at time of abdominal hysterectomy.

dometrial) leiomyomata is unusual. Commonly, these are found in association with other types of leiomyomata (see Figure 45.1).

Another common presenting complaint from uterine leiomyomata is that of a *progressive increase in "pelvic pressure."* This may be a sense of progressive pelvic fullness, "something pressing down," and/or the sensation of a pelvic mass. Most commonly, this is caused by slowly enlarging intramural or subserous myomas, which on occasion may attain a massive size (Figure 45.2). This type of leiomyoma is the most easily palpated on bimanual or abdominal examination and contributes to a characteristic "lumpy-bumpy," or cobblestone, sensation when multiple myomas are present. Occasionally, these large myomas present to the physician as a large asymptomatic pelvic or even abdominopelvic mass. Such very large leiomyomas may cause an uncommon but significant clinical problem: pressure on the ureters as they traverse the pelvic brim leading to *hydroureter and, on occasion, hydronephrosis.*

Another spectrum of presentation includes patients who develop progressively worsening *pelvic pain.* For many patients, this pain is manifest by the onset of secondary dysmenorrhea. Other pain symptoms, although rare, may be the result of rapid enlargement of a leiomyoma. This can result in areas of tissue necrosis or areas of subnecrotic vascular ischemia, which contribute to alteration in myometrial response to prostaglandins similar to the mechanism described for primary dysmenorrhea. Occasionally, torsion of a pedunculated myoma can occur, resulting in acute pain. Dull, intermittent low midline cramping pain is the clinical presentation when a submucous (subendometrial) myoma becomes pedunculated and progressively prolapses through the internal os of the cervix.

Diagnosis

The *diagnosis* of these tumors is usually made by clinical examination, including abdominal and bimanual palpation, or incidental imaging studies. In addition, irregularities of the uterine cavity can be detected at the time of endometrial curettage. Often the diagnosis is made incidentally by pathologic assessment of a uterine specimen removed for other indications.

When appreciated clinically by *abdominopelvic examination,* uterine leiomyomata have characteristic qualities. These include the presence of a large midline mobile pelvic mass with an irregular contour; the mass usually has a characteristic "hard feel" or solid quality. The degree of enlargement is usually stated in terms (weeks' size) that are used to estimate equivalent gestational size. This is often appreciated as separate from adnexal disease, although on *occasion a subserosal pedunculated myoma may be difficult to distinguish from a solid adnexal mass.*

Of the available *imaging studies, pelvic ultrasound* is the most commonly used for confirmation of uterine myomas. The ultrasonographer can demonstrate areas of acoustic shadow hypoechogenicity amid otherwise normal myometrial patterns and can see a distorted endometrial stripe. Although solid leiomyomata share these characteristics, occasionally cystic components may also be seen as hypoechogenic areas and are consistent in appearance with myomas undergoing degeneration. Adnexal structures, including the ovaries, are usually identifiable separate from these masses. This is reassuring information (i.e., the pathology is uterine in nature and not adnexal, which has an associated higher risk of malignancy). Other studies that may be used include *computerized axial tomography and magnetic resonance imaging*, neither of which is cost-effective in diagnosing uterine myomas. They are expensive, time-consuming tests that usually give no more information than can be obtained with clinical examination alone or clinical examination plus ultrasonography.

Endometrial cavity tissue sampling, through either office biopsy or dilation and curettage, usually does not provide additional information toward making the diagnosis of leiomyomata uteri. Office sampling is unreliable to confirm this diagnosis, because most of the sampling devices are not large enough to obtain the leiomyomatous elements and only scratch the surface of the endometrial cavity. However, an indirect appreciation for uterine enlargement may be gained by uterine sounding, which is part of this procedure. If there is irregular uterine bleeding and the patient's clinical presentation or age makes endometrial carcinoma a significant probability, endometrial sampling is useful to evaluate for this possibility independent of the presence of myomas.

Hysteroscopy may be used to evaluate the enlarged uterus by directly visualizing the endometrial cavity. The increased size of the cavity can be documented and submucous fibroids can be visualized and removed. Although the efficacy of hysteroscopic removal (resection) of submucous myomas has been documented, long-term follow-up suggests that up to 20% of patients require additional treatment when reexamined 10 years later.

Laparoscopic resection of subserosal or intramural myoma has gained in popularity although the long-term benefit of this procedure has not been well established. More often, laparoscopy may be used in cases in which physical examination and ultrasound imaging techniques are not clear as to whether the patient has a leiomyomata or other potentially more serious disease such as adnexal neoplasia.

Treatment of Uterine Fibroids

The majority of patients with uterine myomas do not require surgical (or medical) treatment. For example, if patients present with menstrual aberrations, the endometrial cavity may be sampled to rule out endometrial hyperplasia or cancer. This is of particular importance for patients in the late reproductive or perimenopausal years. If the patient's bleeding is not heavy enough to cause significant alteration in hygiene or lifestyle and is not contributing to iron-deficiency anemia, reassurance and observation may be all that are necessary. Assessment of further uterine growth may be done by repeat pelvic examinations and assisted by serial pelvic ultrasound measurements. Rarely, uterine fibroids impinge on the ureter, causing hydroureter and hydronephrosis. This is more likely the case when the fibroid grows laterally from the uterus between the leaves of the broad ligament.

An attempt may be made to minimize uterine bleeding by using intermittent progestin supplementation and/or prostaglandin synthetase inhibitors, which decrease the amount of secondary dysmenorrhea and in some cases the amount of menstrual flow. If there is significant endometrial cavity distortion by intramural or submucous myomas, hormonal supplementation is of minimal benefit, because the excessive bleeding is usually related to profound anatomic and vascular distortion. This conservative approach can potentially be utilized until the time of menopause.

Of the surgical options available, *myomectomy* is occasionally warranted in younger patients whose fertility is compromised by the presence of myomas, creating significant intracavitary distortion. However, there are potential complications of

TABLE 45.1. Criteria for Myomectomy*

Indication
  Leiomyomata in infertility patients, as a probable factor in failure to conceive or in recurrent pregnancy loss

Confirmation of indication
  In the presence of failure to conceive or recurrent pregnancy loss:
  1. Presence of leiomyomata of sufficient size or specific location to be a probable factor
  2. No more likely explanation exists for the failure to conceive or recurrent pregnancy loss

Actions before procedure
  1. Evaluate other causes of male and female infertility or recurrent pregnancy loss
  2. Evaluate the endometrial cavity and fallopian tubes (e.g., hysterosalpingogram)
  3. Document discussion that complexity of disease process may require hysterectomy

*Modified from the American College of Obstetricians and Gynecologists. Quality assessment and improvement in obstetrics and gynecology. Washington, DC, 1994.

myomectomy, including excessive intraoperative blood loss and risk of postoperative hemorrhage, which are slightly greater than the complications associated with hysterectomy. Recently, criteria for myomectomy have been published to help guide the clinician's decision making (Table 45.1).

Although *hysterectomy* is commonly performed for uterine myomas, it should be considered as definitive treatment only in symptomatic women who have completed childbearing. *Indications* should be specific and well documented (Table 45.2).

Because uterine leiomyomata are "estrogen-dependent" benign neoplasms, newer treatments that include *pharmacologic inhibition of estrogen secretion have been used as temporizing measures.* This is particularly applicable in the perimenopausal years when women are more likely anovulatory with relatively more endogenous estrogen. Pharmacologic removal of the ovarian estrogen source can be achieved by suppression of the hypothalamic-pituitary-ovarian axis through the use of gonadotropin-releasing hormone agonists (GnRH analogs). This treatment is commonly used for 3 to 6 months before planned hysterectomy, but it can also be used as a temporizing medical therapy until natural menopause occurs. GnRH agonists not only can result in a

reduction in uterine size, often by as much as 40% to 60%, but also can lead to a technically easier surgery with markedly diminished blood loss should surgery be undertaken.

In patients with an adequate endogenous estrogen source, this treatment does not permanently reduce the size of uterine myomas, as withdrawal of the medication predictably results in regrowth of the myomas. Although less successful, other pharmacologic agents such as danazol have also been used as medical treatment for myomas by reducing endogenous production of ovarian estrogen.

Recently several new therapeutic modalities have been in use, although their efficacy is yet to be demonstrated. Included in these are myolysis and arterial embolization. Further investigation is required before they may be considered a "mainstream" therapeutic modality, although both are being used with increasing frequency.

The ultimate decision to perform a hysterectomy or not should include an assessment of the patient's future reproductive plans as well as careful assessment of clinical factors, including the amount and timing of bleeding, the degree of enlargement of the tumors, and the associated disability rendered to the individual

TABLE 45.2.	Criteria for Hysterectomy for Leiomyomata*

Indication
  Leiomyomata
Confirmation of indication
  Presence of 1, 2, or 3:
    1. Asymptomatic leiomyomata of such size that they are palpable abdominally and are a concern to the patient
    2. Excessive uterine bleeding evidenced by either of the following:
        a. Profuse bleeding with flooding or clots or repetitive periods lasting > 8 days
        b. Anemia caused by acute or chronic blood loss
    3. Pelvic discomfort caused by myomata (a, b, or c):
        a. Acute and severe
        b. Chronic lower abdominal or low back pressure
        c. Bladder pressure with urinary frequency not caused by urinary tract infection
Actions before procedure
    1. Confirm the absence of cervical malignancy
    2. Eliminate anovulation and other causes of abnormal bleeding
    3. When abnormal bleeding is present, confirm the absence of endometrial malignancy
    4. Assess surgical risk from anemia and need for treatment
    5. Consider patient's medical and psychological risks concerning hysterectomy
Contraindications
    1. Desire to maintain fertility, in which case myomectomy should be considered
    2. Asymptomatic leiomyomata of size < 12 weeks' gestation determined by physical examination or ultrasound examination

*Modified from the American College of Obstetricians and Gynecologists. Quality assessment and improvement in obstetrics and gynecology. Washington, DC, 1994.

patient. The presence of uterine myomas alone does not necessarily warrant hysterectomy.

Although leiomyomas are equivocally associated with infertility, patients with leiomyoma do become pregnant. *Pregnancy with leiomyoma* is usually unremarkable, with a normal antepartum course, labor, and delivery. Myomas may grow or become symptomatic, sometimes associated with *red or carneous degeneration*. Bed rest and strong analgesics are usually sufficient as treatment, although on occasion myomectomy may be needed. The risk of abortion or preterm labor following myomectomy is relatively high, so that prophylactic β-adrenergic tocolytics are sometimes used. *Vaginal birth after myomectomy* is controversial and must be decided on a case-by-case basis. Rarely, myomas are located below the fetus, in the lower uterine seg-ment or cervix, causing a soft tissue dystocia, leading to a need for cesarean birth.

LEIOMYOSARCOMA

Uterine sarcomas represent an *unusual gynecologic malignancy* accounting for approximately 3% of cancers involving the body of the uterus. Progressive uterine enlargement occurring in the postmenopausal years should not be assumed to be the result of simple uterine leiomyomata, because appreciable endogenous ovarian estrogen secretion is absent, thereby minimizing this as a potential cause for progressive uterine enlargement. In addition, postmenopausal women on low-dose hormone-replacement therapy are not at risk for stimulation of uterine enlargement. In this situation, uterine sarcoma (leiomyosarcoma) should be considered. Other symptoms of uterine sarcoma include postmenopausal bleeding, unusual pelvic pain coupled with uterine enlargement, and an increase in unusual vaginal discharge. Surgical removal is the method of most reliable diagnosis. Accordingly, hysterectomy is usually indicated in patients with documented, and especially progressive, uterine enlargement.

The *virulence of uterine sarcoma* is directly related to the number of mitotic figures and cellular proliferation as defined histologically. In addition, these tumors are more likely to spread hematogenously than endometrial adenocarcinoma. When uterine sarcoma is suspected, patients should undergo typical tumor survey to include assessment for distant metastatic disease. At the time of hysterectomy, it is necessary to thoroughly explore the abdomen and sample commonly affected node chains, including the iliac and periaortic areas. The staging for uterine sarcoma is surgical and identical to that for endometrial adenocarcinoma.

The overall rate of survival for patients with uterine sarcoma is considerably worse than that for those with endometrial adenocarcinoma. Only 50% of patients survive 5 years. Adjunctive radiation therapy and chemotherapy provide little additional benefit as primary adjuvant therapy or as therapy for recurrent disease. Unlike the adenocarcinoma endometrial counterparts, these tumors are not responsive to hormonal treatment with high-dose progestins.

CASE STUDIES

Case 45A

A 47-year-old G3 P3 woman presents with an 8-month history of progressively longer and heavier menstruation. Her last two cycles have included clotted blood flow for the first 5 days of each menstrual period with another 5 days of relatively normal menstrual flow. Before 8 months ago, her menstruation included 6 days of "average flow." She has no other problems except that in the last few months she has felt tired.

Physical examination reveals a woman of normal height and weight with a resting pulse of 76. Her blood pressure is normal. General physical examination is unremarkable with the exception of a suprapubic "fullness." On pelvic examination, there is old menstrual blood in the vault. The cervix is smooth and on bimanual examination the uterus is consistent with approximately 14-week gestational size with multiple surface irregularities.

Finger stick hematocrit done by the office nurse is 27%.

Questions Case 45A

The most likely diagnosis is

A. Endometrial hyperplasia
B. Uterine fibroids
C. Endometrial carcinoma
D. Gestational trophoblastic disease
E. Leiomyosarcoma of the uterus

Answer: B

This patient typifies the history and physical findings of a perimenopausal woman with probable fibroid tumors of the uterus. Significant aspects of her history include progressive menorrhagia with associated anemia as detected in your office. Physical examination is consistent with uterine fibroids as the most likely diagnosis.

(Continued)

What studies are appropriate to adequately evaluate this patient?

A. Pelvic ultrasound
B. Pap smear
C. Endometrial biopsy
D. Complete blood count (CBC) and reticulocyte count
E. Iron/total iron-binding capacity (Fe/TIBC) and folate/B_{12}
F. Computed tomography (CT) scan of pelvis

Answer: A, B, C, D

Ultrasound is primarily indicated to evaluate the adnexae for ovarian pathology and to evaluate the ureters for hydroureter secondary to obstruction by the pelvic mass. A Pap smear and endometrial biopsy are requisite to evaluate for malignancy. A blood count and reticulocyte count will be consistent with an iron-deficiency anemia or will point to additional diagnoses. Fe/TIBC and folate/B_{12} are acceptable tests but add little to the management in most instances. A CT scan is not needed in these circumstances.

The Pap smear is satisfactory, the endometrial biopsy shows disordered normal endometrium, the pelvic ultrasound is consistent with a large fibroid uterus with no adnexal abnormalities. The possibility of hormonal suppression should be discussed. Finally, a risk/benefit discussion regarding the possibility of hysterectomy should be undertaken, particularly in light of her age and severity of symptoms.

Case 45B

A 64-year-old woman is referred to you by another physician requesting a second opinion. This patient had an uneventful menopause at the age of 54 and has not been on hormone-replacement therapy. In the last 3 months she has had intermittent vaginal bleeding, and on physical examination the referring physician detected a uterus that he thought was consistent with approximately 12-week gestational size and somewhat irregular. A previous examination done by him 1.5 years ago was entirely normal. Endometrial sampling done by him last week revealed atrophic endometrium. The uterine cavity sounded to 11 cm at that time. Your physical examination confirms his findings.

Question Case 45B

Definitive treatment for this patient should include

A. Long-term progestin hormonal suppression
B. Gonadotropin-releasing hormone agonists
C. Dilation and curettage
D. Total abdominal hysterectomy and bilateral salpingo-oophorectomy
E. Vaginal hysterectomy

Answer: D

This patient illustrates features highly suggestive of uterine sarcoma. She is postmenopausal and has little potential for endogenous stimulation of preexisting fibroids. Knowledge of a normal examination 1.5 years earlier with current findings of a markedly enlarged uterus in this age group should alert the clinician to the possibility of uterine leiomyosarcoma. Although imaging studies might be useful and endometrial sampling is mandatory, definitive treatment for this patient is an abdominal hysterectomy with bilateral salpingo-oophorectomy.

CHAPTER

46

ENDOMETRIAL HYPERPLASIA AND CANCER

CHAPTER OBJECTIVES

This chapter deals primarily with APGO Objective(s):

OBJECTIVE 58   Endometrial Carcinoma

A. Describe the approach to the patient with postmenopausal bleeding.

B. Describe the risk factors and symptoms/physical findings characteristic of endometrial carcinoma, the FIGO staging of endometrial carcinoma, the methods used in diagnosis and staging of the disease, and the typical disease course.

Endometrial carcinoma is the most common genital tract malignancy and the fourth most common cancer after breast, bowel, and lung carcinoma. Approximately 34,000 new cases of endometrial carcinoma are diagnosed annually in the United States, resulting in over 6000 deaths. *About 2%–3% of women develop endometrial carcinoma, usually in their postmenopausal years.* Fortunately, patients with this disease usually present early in the disease course with some form of abnormal uterine bleeding, particularly postmenopausal bleeding. Accordingly, *the identification of women at increased risk (women with abnormal uterine bleeding, women with endogenous or exogenous estrogen excess, and postmenopausal women) and their evaluation is very important. The detection of endometrial carcinoma or its precursor lesions is facilitated by several diagnostic maneuvers, especially endometrial sampling, which is highly accurate and should be used liberally when indicated.* With early diagnosis and medical or surgical treatment, survival rates can be excellent.

ENDOMETRIAL HYPERPLASIA/ CARCINOMA

Pathogenesis and Risk Factors

There are two kinds of endometrial hyperplasia/carcinoma. The first is *"estrogen-dependent"* endometrial carcinoma, common to younger perimenopausal women with a history of unopposed endogenous or exogenous estrogen stimulation. In these women endometrial hyperplasia develops, progressing in some women through atypical forms to endometrial carcinoma, which is usually well differentiated and hence has a more favorable prognosis. The second type, *"estrogen-independent"* endometrial carcinoma, occurs spontaneously, characteristically in thin, older postmenopausal women without unopposed estrogen excess, arising in an atrophic endometrium rather than a hyperplastic one. These cancers tend to be less well differentiated with a poorer prognosis.

Many of the risk factors for endometrial carcinoma and hyperplasia are identified, are related to prolonged hyperestrogenism, and identify women who require special evaluative attention (Table 46.1). When an endometrial biopsy shows atypical endometrial hyperplasia, the relative risk is very large, from 8 to 30 times.

Estrogen-Dependent Endometrial Hyperplasia/ Carcinoma

The *underlying pathophysiologic process* in the development of endometrial hyperplasia and endometrial cancer is overgrowth of the endometrium in response to an estrogen-dominant hormonal milieu. Sources of estrogen may be glandular (ovarian) or extraglandular (peripheral conversion or exogenous source; Table 46.2).

This relationship between estrogen and endometrial growth (proliferation) is clear. Endometrial proliferation represents a normal part of the menstrual cycle and occurs during the follicular or estrogen-dominant phase of the cycle. With continued estrogen stimulation through either endogenous mechanisms or by exogenous administration, simple endometrial proliferation will become endometrial hyperplasia (Figure 46.1). *Endometrial hyperplasia is the "abnormal proliferation of both glandular and stromal elements showing altered histologic architecture."* True endometrial proliferation is a simple overabundance of normal endometrium, whereas endometrial hyperplasia involves histologic features with cellular architectural abnormalities. When proliferation becomes hyperplasia is not clear, although studies showing sequential change suggest it requires 6 months or longer of "unopposed estrogen" stimulation.

Histologic *variations of endometrial hyperplasia include cystic glandular hyperplasia, adenomatous hyperplasia, and atypical adenomatous hyperplasia.* Unlike with cervical carcinoma precursors, there is no uniform agreement that each of these

TABLE 46.1. Risk Factors for Endometrial Hyperplasia and Carcinoma

Factor	Discussion	Relative Risk
Menopause	2.4 times more likely for women undergoing menopause after age 52 than between 49 and 52	2–3
Unopposed estrogen therapy	Estrogen replacement without progestins; risk increased with dosage and duration of use	4–8
Nulliparity		2–3
Obesity	3 times more likely at 20–50 pounds overweight, up to 10 times if more than 50 pounds overweight; associated with aromatization of adrenally produced androstenedione to estrone in fat cells	3–10
Tamoxifen therapy		2–3
Diabetes mellitus		3

TABLE 46.2. Estrogen Sources

Endogenous
  Glandular
    Estradiol (ovary)
    Estrone (ovary)
  Peripheral
    Estrone (fat, conversion of
    androstenedione)
  Tumor
    Granulosa cell of ovary (an
    uncommon tumor and source)
Exogenous
  Medications
    Conjugated estrogen (mostly
    estrone)
    Lyophilized estradiol
    Cutaneous patches
    Vaginal creams

lesions will progress to endometrial cancer if left untreated. In addition, these histologic variants can occur in only small foci of an otherwise normal endometrium, revealing that these changes may not necessarily involve the entire endometrial cavity at the same time. Therefore, the microscopic picture as judged by a pathologist may not represent the complete anatomic picture.

There are two different terminologies used to describe endometrial hyperplasia. The parameters used by both include amount of endometrium, density of glands, structural abnormalities of glands, and cytologic features of glandular epithelium. *Traditional terminology uses descriptive terms: cystic hyperplasia, adenomatous hyperplasia, and atypical adenomatous hyperplasia,* with degrees of architectural or cytologic atypia. The most recent terminology adopted by the International Society of Gynecologic Pathologists (ISGYP) presents the endometrial hyperplasias in a slightly different way to describe better their premalignant potential: *simple hyperplasia, complex hyperplasia without cytologic atypia, and atypical hyperplasia,* which includes adenomatous hyperplasia with cytologic atypia. The classifications are compared in Table 46.3.

CYSTIC ENDOMETRIAL HYPERPLASIA (SIMPLE HYPERPLASIA)

Cystic endometrial hyperplasia is the *least significant form* of endometrial hyperplasia. It is not commonly associated with progression to or the occurrence of endometrial carcinoma, although it is considered a modest risk factor as a precursor lesion. *In this variety of hyperplasia, both glandular*

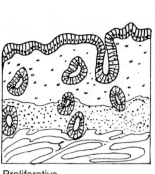

Proliferative
endometrium

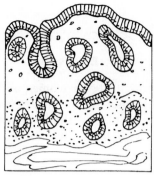

Simple
hyperplasia

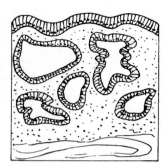

Cystic
hyperplasia (simple hyperplasia)

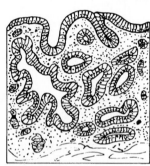

Adenomatous
hyperplasia (complex
hyperplasia)

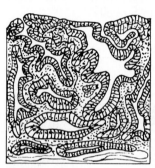

Atypical
adenomatous hyperplasia
(atypical hyperplasia with
cellular atypia)

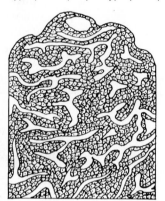

Cancer of the
endometrium

FIGURE 46.1.   Endometrial histology: hyperplasia to carcinoma (ISGYP terminology).

TABLE 46.3.   Classifications of Endometrial Hyperplasia

Traditional Histologic	ISGYP
Cystic hyperplasia	Simple hyperplasia
Adenomatous hyperplasia	Complex hyperplasia (adenomatous hyperplasia without cytologic atypia)
Atypical adenomatous hyperplasia	Atypical hyperplasia (adenomatous hyperplasia with cytologic atypia)
Architectural atypia (mild, moderate, severe)	
Cytologic atypia (mild, moderate, severe)	

elements and stromal cell elements prolifer-ate excessively. Histologically, glands that are simple tubules demonstrate marked variation in size, from small to enlarged, cystically dilated glands (the hallmark of this hyperplasia). Cystic glandular hyper-plasia should not be confused with a normal postmenopausal variant—cystic involution of the endometrium—which is histologi-cally not a hyperplastic condition.

ADENOMATOUS HYPERPLASIA (COMPLEX HYPERPLASIA)

Endometrial adenomatous hyperplasia represents an *abnormal proliferation of primarily glandular elements without concomitant proliferation of stromal elements.* This increased gland:stroma ratio gives the endometrium a "crowded" picture, frequently with glands appearing almost back to back. As the severity of the hyperplasia increases, the glands become more crowded and more structurally bizarre. It is thought that adenomatous hyperplasia represents a true intraepithelial neoplastic process, and it is occasionally found coexisting with areas of endometrial adenocarcinoma; however, it may also be found microscopically in small areas within normal proliferative endometrium.

ATYPICAL ADENOMATOUS HYPERPLASIA (ATYPICAL HYPERPLASIA WITH CYTOLOGIC ATYPIA)

Adenomatous hyperplasia, which *contains significant numbers of glandular elements that exhibit cytologic atypia and disordered maturation (loss of cellular polarity, nuclear enlargement with increased nucleus-to-cytoplasmic ratio, dense chromatin, and prominent nucleoli),* is considered particularly important as a precursor lesion to endometrial carcinoma. This so-called *carcinoma in situ of the endometrium* has at least a 20% to 30% risk for malignant transformation.

Estrogen-Independent Endometrial Carcinoma

Endometrial carcinoma develops in postmenopausal women from seemingly atrophic endometrial, *estrogen-independent endometrial carcinoma.* This variety of endometrial carcinoma, which is more common in older, postmenopausal, thin women, especially of African-American and Asian heritage, is often more poorly differentiated than estrogen-dependent endometrial carcinoma and has a corresponding poorer overall prognosis.

Evaluation

The diagnosis of endometrial hyperplasia and carcinoma can be made by taking a sample of the endometrium for histologic evaluation. This is most easily accomplished by any of a number of different atraumatic aspiration devices available for office use (e.g., Pipelle, Vabra). The diagnostic accuracy of these office aspiration sampling techniques is 90%–98% when compared with subsequent findings of dilation and curettage (D&C) or hysterectomy. The routine *Pap smear is not reliable* in diagnosing endometrial hyperplasia or cancer as only 30%–40% of patients with endometrial carcinoma, for example, have abnormal Pap test results; however, this diagnosis must be considered when atypical endometrial cells are found on the Pap smear and an appropriate evaluation undertaken. The most common *indication for endometrial sampling is abnormal bleeding,* with liberal consideration given to obtaining a specimen *in patients older than 35 years of age who present with abnormal uterine bleeding.* After ruling out pregnancy by simple urine pregnancy testing in premenopausal women, patients can be adequately sampled with relatively little discomfort. Further management is usually dictated by the results of the biopsy specimen. D&C or hysteroscopy with directed endometrial biopsy may be undertaken when outpatient sampling is not possible (e.g., a stenotic cervical os or a patient unable to tolerate the outpatient procedure) or on occasion when the outpatient sampling has been nondiagnostic and the clinical circumstances warrant further evaluation.

Sometimes the office endometrial biopsy will be reported as "insufficient tissue for diagnosis." In a postmenopausal woman not on estrogen replacement, these data may be sufficient, because they are compatible with the suspected atrophic condition of the endometrium. In other cases, the clinical suspicion of a possible hyperplastic endometrial process may be high enough to warrant hysteroscopic evaluation with directed sampling, which allows more complete evaluation of the endometrium as well as direct diagnosis of polyps, myomas, and structural abnormalities. Although somewhat more expensive and inconvenient for the patient, it offers some theoretical advantages over a blind biopsy, especially because traditional endometrial biopsy techniques sample only a small part of the surface area of the endometrial cavity. Although office endometrial biopsy is considered a sufficient technique for endometrial sampling, clinical judgment as to its interpretation must be applied in each situation.

Transvaginal ultrasound (with or without the installation of fluid for contrast, *ultrasonohysterography*) is used as an adjunctive means of evaluation for endometrial hyperplasia as well as polyps, myomas, and structural abnormalities of the uterus. An endometrial thickness of greater than 5 mm, a polypoid mass, or fluid collection is often considered indication for further evaluation to obtain histologic samples. It is also useful to help determine if, for patients with multiple medical problems, the risks of endometrial sampling are less than the risk of not sampling. However, an endometrial stripe of less than 5 mm, while consistent with menopause and endometrial atrophy, does not exclude the possibility of a nonestrogen-dependent carcinoma of the atrophic endometrium.

The best approach to the monitoring of women whose breast cancer regimen includes the use of tamoxifen (which acts as a weak estrogen and is associated with increased risk of endometrial hyperplasias and carcinoma) is unclear. Certainly endometrial biopsy is indicated if there is abnormal bleeding, but it is not unreasonable to consider regular endometrial sampling, perhaps yearly, in those patients at increased risk.

Management

If *simple hyperplasia, cystic hyperplasia, or adenomatous hyperplasia* of the simple variety has been diagnosed by tissue sample, medical treatment is usually offered because the therapy has low risk and some of these hyperplasias will progress to cancer (an esti-

mated 1% of patients with simple hyperplasia, 3% of patients with complex hyperplasia, and 30% of those with atypical hyperplasias). It is also suggested that the mean duration of progression from endometrial hyperplasia to carcinoma in those that do progress is relatively long, perhaps 10 years for those without atypia and 4 years for those with atypia. In most cases, *medical treatment* involves the administration of a form of synthetic progesterone (progestin) in doses that inhibit and eventually reverse the hyperplastic response evoked by estrogen stimulation. Probably the most common regimen is Provera (medroxyprogesterone acetate), 10–20 mg/day for 10–14 days each month, although a continuous regimen using megestrol acetate (Megace) 20–40 mg daily is also often used and likewise effective. Progestin therapy works to alter the enzymatic pathways, which eventually convert endogenous estradiol to weaker estrogens, as well as to decrease the number of estrogen receptors in the endometrial glandular cells. Progestins have a net effect of decreasing endometrial glandular proliferation, and, when administered for sufficient periods of time or in high enough doses, actually render the endometrium atrophic. In addition, with progestin withdrawal, the endometrium is sloughed, analogous to corpus luteum progesterone withdrawal in a normal menstrual cycle (the so-called chemical D&C).

Atypical adenomatous hyperplasia is usually treated surgically by hysterectomy because it is this variant that is much more likely to become endometrial carcinoma. This treatment decision is usually fairly clear, because most patients with this disorder are in their late reproductive or perimenopausal years. In selected patients (e.g., younger women who may wish to become pregnant), longer-term progestin management after thorough endometrial curettage may be used to avoid a hysterectomy. Typical regimens might include depo-medroxyprogesterone acetate (Depo-Provera), 1000 mg/week intramuscularly for 4 weeks, followed by 5 months of monthly therapy with 400 mg/month, or megestrol acetate (Megace), 80 mg/day for 6 to 12 weeks. Patients who are treated medically for atypical adenomatous hyperplasia should also be followed with periodic endometrial sampling (3 months after therapy and then once to twice per year) so that treatment response can be gauged.

ENDOMETRIAL POLYPS

Most endometrial polyps represent focal accentuated benign hyperplastic processes. Their histologic architecture is characteristic and may commonly be found in association with other types of endometrial hyperplasia or even carcinoma. Polyps occur most frequently in perimenopausal or immediately postmenopausal women, when the ovary is characterized by unopposed estrogen production because of chronic anovulation. The most common presenting symptom is abnormal bleeding. Small polyps often may be incidentally found as part of endometrial aspiration or curettage done for evaluation of the bleeding problem. Rarely, a large polyp may begin to protrude through the cervical canal, and the patient presents not only with bleeding irregularities but also with low, dull, midline pain as the cervix is slowly dilated and effaced. The appearance of these on speculum examination is quite striking. In these cases, surgical removal is necessary to reduce the amount of bleeding and to prevent infection from the exposed endometrial surface. *Less than 5% of polyps show malignant change,* and when they do, they may represent any endometrial histologic variant. Polyps in postmenopausal women are more likely to be associated with endometrial carcinoma than are those found in reproductive age women.

ENDOMETRIAL CARCINOMA

Endometrial carcinoma is typically a disease of the postmenopausal woman. Approximately 75% of patients with endometrial carcinoma are postmenopausal, whereas 15% to 20% are perimenopausal and only 5% to 10% are premenopausal. Between 15% and 25% of postmenopausal women with bleeding have uterine malignancy.

Most primary endometrial carcinomas are adenocarcinomas and are described according to their histologic and glandular architecture. Because squamous epithelium appears to coexist with the glandular elements in an adenocarcinoma, descriptive terms that include the squamous element may be used, depending on the amount of squamous tissue present in the histologic specimen. In cases where the squamous element makes up >10% of the histologic picture, and it appears benign, the term *adenoacanthoma* is used. Uncommonly, the squamous element may appear malignant on histologic assessment, and this is referred to as *adenosquamous carcinoma.* Other descriptions such as clear cell carcinoma and papillary serous adenocarcinoma may be applied, depending on the histologic architecture. Knowledge of these unusual subtypes is less important than an overall appreciation of the fact that all of these carcinomas are considered under the general category of adenocarcinoma of the endometrium.

The diagnosis of endometrial cancer is most frequently made by endometrial sampling after a patient presents with abnormal uterine bleeding. Indeed, vaginal bleeding or discharge is the only presenting complaint in 80%–90% of women with endometrial carcinoma. In some, often older patients, cervical stenosis may sequester the blood in the uterus with the presentation being hematometra or pyometra and a purulent vaginal discharge. In more advanced disease, pelvic discomfort or an associated sensation of pressure caused by uterine enlargement or extrauterine disease spread may accompany the complaint of vaginal bleeding or even be the presenting complaint. Less than 5% of women found to have endometrial carcimoma are actually asymptomatic. Thus, special consideration should be given to the patient who presents with postmenopausal bleeding (i.e., bleeding that occurs after 6 months of amenorrhea in a patient who has been diagnosed as menopausal). In this group of patients, it is mandatory to assess the endometrium histologically because the chance of having an endometrial carcinoma is approximately 10%–15%, although other causes are more common (Table 46.4). Other gynecologic assessments should also be made, including careful physical and pelvic examination as well as a screening Pap smear.

Because of the current International Federation of Gynecology and Obstetrics (FIGO) staging of endometrial carcinoma (Table 46.5), which is surgical rather than clinical, differential sampling of the endocervical canal and endometrial cavity before therapy is less important now than with previous staging criteria. Fractional curettage should, however, be kept in mind for patients who are not surgical candidates because of other risk factors, such as patients whose primary treatment is radiation therapy.

TABLE 46.4. Causes of Postmenopausal Uterine Bleeding

Cause	Frequency (%)
Atrophy of the endometrium	60–80
Hormone replacement therapy	15–25
Endometrial carcinoma	10–15
Endometrial polyps	2–12
Endometrial hyperplasia	5–10

Route of Spread and Histologic Types of Endometrial Carcinoma

Knowledge of the route of spread of endometrial cancer guides the surgeon toward thorough surgical assessment of potentially involved tissues and serves as the basis for the FIGO staging system. Endometrial carcinoma usually spreads throughout the endometrial cavity first and then begins to invade the myometrium, endocervical canal and, eventually, lymphatics. Hematogenous spread occurs with endometrial carcinoma more readily than in cervical

TABLE 46.5. FIGO Surgical Staging of Endometrial Carcinoma (1988)

Stage	Description
IB G123	Invasion to less than one half of the myometrium
IC G123	Invasion to more than one half of the myometrium
IIA G123	Endocervical glandular involvement only
IIB G123	Cervical stromal invasion
IIIA G123	Tumor invading serosa, adnexa, or both and/or positive peritoneal cytology
IIIB G123	Vaginal metastases
IIIC G123	Metastases to pelvic and/or periaortic lymph nodes
IVA G123	Tumor invades bladder, bowel mucosa, or both
IVB	Distant metastases, including intra-abdominal and/or inguinal lymph node

Rules related to staging
1. Because corpus cancer is now surgically staged, procedures previously used for differentiation of stages are no longer applicable (e.g., the findings of dilation and curettage to differentiate between stage I and stage II). It is appreciated that there may be a small number of patients with corpus cancer who are treated primarily with radiation therapy. If that is the case, the clinical staging adopted by FIGO in 1971 would still apply, but use of that staging system would be noted.
2. Ideally, the width of the myometrium is measured along with the width of tumor invasion.

cancer or ovarian cancer. Invasion of adnexal structures may occur through lymphatics or direct implantation through the fallopian tubes. Once there is extrauterine spread to the peritoneal cavity, cancer cells have access to the entire abdominal pelvic cavity and may spread in a fashion similar to that of ovarian cancer.

Unusual histologic subtypes, including *papillary serous adenocarcinoma and clear cell adenocarcinoma* of the endometrium, tend to be more aggressive in abdominopelvic spread than the more common adenocarcinoma of the endometrium (Table 46.6). Microscopic spread may also be present despite the absence of gross abdominal

TABLE 46.6. Histologic Types of Endometrial Carcinoma

Histologic Type	Discussion	Percentage of Endometrial Carcinomas
Endometrioid	Composed of glands that *resemble* normal endometrial glands but which contain more solid areas, less glandular formation, and more cytologic atypia as they become less well differentiated	80–85
Endometrial carcinoma with squamous differentiation	Encompasses tumors with benign-appearing squamous areas (also called adenoacanthomas) and those with malignant looking squamous elements (also called adenosquamous carcinomas)	15–25
Villoglandular	Endometrial cells with characteristics of endometrioid cells, arranged in papillary fibrovascular stalks, always well differentiated	2
Secretory endometrial carcinoma		1
Mucinous	50% of cells have intracytoplasmic mucin; most behave like well-differentiated endometrioid carcinoma; good prognosis	5
Papillary serous	Endometrial carcinoma that resembles serous carcinoma of the ovary and fallopian tube; very aggressive, poorer prognosis	3–4
Clear cell	Mixed histologic pattern; more common in older women; very aggressive, poor prognosis	<5
Squamous	Generally pure cell type, some with glands; associated with older women and cervical stenosis; very poor prognosis	<1
Mixed carcinomas		<1

pelvic lesions. Accordingly, cytologic assessment of peritoneal washings is important at the outset of surgical treatment for endometrial carcinoma. The current FIGO guidelines for the staging of endometrial carcinoma emphasize the need for thorough surgical assessment of the abdominopelvic cavity, including sampling of both periaortic and pelvic lymph nodes when depths of invasion are more than one third of the myometrial thickness and in cases where there are obvious peritoneal foci of tumor.

Prognostic Factors

The single most important prognostic factor for endometrial carcinoma is histologic grade. Histologically, poorly differentiated or undifferentiated tumors are associated with a considerably poorer prognosis because of the likelihood of extrauterine spread through adjacent lymphatics and peritoneal fluid. This is true even of relatively limited lesions. Therefore, this finding is important in the initial surgical management of the patient and is of significance in deciding on adjunctive therapy with radiation or chemotherapy.

The grading system of the *FIGO adopted in 1988 lists three grades of endometrial carcinoma:* G1 is highly differentiated adenomatous carcinoma (less than 5% of the tumor shows a solid growth pattern), G2 is moderately differentiated adenomatous carcinoma with partly solid areas (6%–50% of the tumor shows a solid growth pattern), and G3 is predominantly solid or entirely undifferentiated carcinoma (more than 50% of the tumor shows a solid growth pattern). Most patients with endometrial carcinoma have G1 or G2 lesions by this classification, with 15% to 20% having undifferentiated or poorly differentiated G3 lesions.

Depth of myometrial invasion is the second most important prognostic factor. When the tumor has invaded greater than one third of the thickness of the myometrium, the prognosis is markedly worsened. Worsening grade of tumor closely parallels depth of myometrial invasion and lymph node metastasis. Other factors that have prognostic value include the original tumor volume both within the uterus and defined by extrauterine spread, lymphatic involvement, and hematogenous spread.

Survival rates vary widely, depending on the grade of tumor and depth of penetration into the myometrium. A patient with a G1 tumor that does not invade the myometrium has a 95% 5-year survival rate, whereas a patient with a poorly differentiated (G3) tumor with deep myometrial invasion may have a 5-year survival rate of only 20%.

Treatment

Because endometrial carcinoma is a surgically staged disease, *primary surgical treatment is the cornerstone of management.* After opening the abdomen, peritoneal washings are obtained. The abdominopelvic cavity is manually and visually explored, and then a *total abdominal hysterectomy with bilateral salpingo-oophorectomy* is performed. The decision to include pelvic and/or periaortic nodes is determined by the depth of myometrial invasion. *Vaginal hysterectomy* has been used successfully in the treatment of stage I disease in selected patients, and may be especially useful in patients for whom the stress of abdominal surgery may be problematic. There is a 5% to 10% incidence of *vaginal apex recurrence* after simple hysterectomy for endometrial carcinoma, probably because of paravaginal lymphatic involvement in most cases. This incidence of apex recurrence is reduced by one half with the use of preoperative radiation, although the 5-year survival rates for those receiving preoperative radiation and those who do not are not different.

Many gynecologic oncologists advise routine *sampling of the common iliac nodes* regardless of depth of penetration or histologic grade, citing as their reason the inherent inaccuracies of gross myometrial inspection and frozen-section assessment of the histologic grade and depth of penetration. In addition, they cite the incidence of pelvic nodal metastasis as between 2% and 10% for all stage I lesions, G1–3.

Adjunctive therapy after hysterectomy, which may include external-beam radiation, has been shown to reduce significantly the risk of pelvic and vaginal recurrence. *Postoperative radiation* therapy may be especially valuable in patients with deeply invasive cancers, those with cervical involvement, and those with poorly differentiated tumors. *Preoperative radiation* may be useful to those patients with obvious endocervical involvement and/or may be important in reducing a bulky endometrial tumor.

RECURRENT ENDOMETRIAL CARCINOMA

Recurrent endometrial carcinoma occurs in about one fourth of patients treated for early disease, one half of these within 2 years and three fourths within 3–4 years. In general, those with recurrent vaginal disease have a better prognosis than those with pelvic recurrence, who in turn fare better than those with distant metastatic disease (lung, abdomen, lymph nodes, liver, brain, and bone).

The first line of *treatment for recurrent disease* is *progestin preparations* given in high doses (Depo-Provera, 400 mg/week for at least 12 weeks; if there is a positive response, progestin at a lower dosage is recommended for life). Approximately one third of these patients have a short-term (< 5 years) response, and approximately 15% have a long-term response (> 5 years). A major advantage of high-dose progestin therapy is its minimal complication rate. *Chemotherapy* with drugs, including Adriamycin (doxorubicin) and cisplatin, produces occasional favorable short-term results, but long-term remissions with these therapies are rare.

HORMONE REPLACEMENT THERAPY AFTER TREATMENT FOR ENDOMETRIAL CARCINOMA

The use of *estrogen replacement therapy* in patients previously treated for endometrial carcinoma is controversial, although there is growing agreement that the benefits of hormone replacement therapy (HRT; decreasing the morbidity and mortality from heart disease, strokes, and osteoporosis as well as addressing the discomfort of vasomotor instability) may outweigh the possible risk of the activation of occult or indolent metastatic or residual endometrial carcinoma. For example, women treated for well-differentiated, minimally invasive endometrial carcinoma may well benefit from HRT. Whether or not to include progestational agents is not clear from present data, although intuitively it would seem appropriate to do so. Cautious individualized assessment of risks and benefits should be accorded on a case-by-case basis.

CASE STUDIES

Case 46A

A 62-year-old woman whose last normal menstrual period was 7 years ago presents with a 2-month history of intermittent vaginal bleeding. She has had two children (ages 39 and 40 years) and is in generally good health and currently taking no medications. Physical examination reveals a patient of average height and weight and normal blood pressure. Pelvic examination shows some atrophy of the vaginal mucosa with a small and smooth cervix without evidence of blood. Bimanual examination demonstrates a small, firm, anteflexed uterus of normal size with an unremarkable adnexal examination. Rectovaginal examination is negative and the stool is guaiac negative.

(Continued)

Question Case 46A

Having performed a Pap smear, including samples of both the exocervix and cervical canal, your next diagnostic assessment should be to

A. Await results of Pap smear before further assessment
B. Obtain vaginal maturation index for estrogen production
C. Obtain pelvic ultrasound
D. Perform endometrial biopsy
E. Schedule for dilation and curettage

Answer: D

This case illustrates a high-risk history for endometrial carcinoma: new-onset postmenopausal bleeding. Despite having normal physical and pelvic examinations, this patient has approximately a 15% risk of endometrial carcinoma. The Pap smear is unreliable in detecting this neoplasm, and it is mandatory to obtain endometrial sampling. The preferable technique for this is by office biopsy. D&C is reserved for patients in whom the clinician encounters technical difficulty or there is an inadequate office sample.

The Pap smear is satisfactory and negative. The Pipelle endometrial biopsy is reported as insufficient tissue for pathologic diagnosis. Your management should now entail

A. Progestin therapy: medroxyprogesterone 10 mg po qd for 10 days
B. Estrogen therapy: premarin 0.625 mg po qd and medroxyprogesterone 2.5 mg po qd
C. Schedule for dilation and curettage
D. Pelvic ultrasound
E. Repeat Pipelle endometrial biopsy

Answer: B

This postmenopausal woman is estrogen deficient, and her bleeding is from the scant endometrium left. A lack of tissue is expected; no further sampling is required at this time. Progestin therapy will not help and, indeed, may worsen the bleeding. Hormone replacement therapy should stop the bleeding and benefit the patient in other ways, including beneficial effects on her risk of cardiovascular disease and osteoporosis.

Case 46B

A 27-year-old patient comes in with a 3-year history of progressively infrequent menstrual periods. Her menarche was age 17 years, she has never had "monthly periods" but has always had six or seven periods per year. In the last 3 years, she has had only two or three menstrual periods per year. She has also been unable to become pregnant. Her last bleeding episode was 2 months ago. Physical examination reveals a woman 5 feet, 4 inches tall, weighing 210 pounds, with a normal pelvic examination. After a negative pregnancy test, an endometrial biopsy performed as part of her infertility assessment reveals adenomatous hyperplasia.

Question Case 46B

The most efficacious treatment for this patient would be

A. Pharmacologic ovulation induction
B. Intermittent short-term progestin therapy
C. Oral contraceptives
D. Dilation and curettage
E. Artificial insemination

Answer: A

This patient has chronic anovulation with resultant hyperplasia of the endometrium. Because she is also infertile, the optimal treatment of ovulation induction may help enable her to become pregnant, also reversing the hyperplasia by the production of progesterone. Other therapy such as intermittent progestin use and/or oral contraceptive use may treat the endometrial hyperplasia problem but would not address the infertility concern. Adenomatous hyperplasia without atypia carries a low risk for malignancy. Therefore, aggressive surgical treatment such as D&C is not warranted. Likewise, D&C is no better a diagnostic tool than office sampling. Artificial insemination is of no value in a chronically anovulatory patient. For completeness, other etiology for oligomenorrhea in the patient should also be assessed (e.g., pituitary or thyroid dysfunction).

Case 46C

A 32-year-old G3 P3003 who had a postpartum tubal ligation with her last pregnancy presents with irregular vaginal bleeding for 6 months. She has had a recent significant weight gain, and now weighs 245 pounds. Her pelvic examination reveals a normal cervix, a normal-sized, mid-position uterus, no adnexal masses, and a negative rectovaginal examination with negative guaiac. A Pap smear and cultures were performed. Because of her history of irregular bleeding, a Pipelle endometrial biopsy is also performed.

The Pap smear is reported as satisfactory and negative. The endometrial biopsy is reported as adenomatous hyperplasia with marked atypia.

Question Case 46C

You should now recommend

A. Dilation and curettage
B. Hysteroscopy
C. Progestin therapy
D. Hormone-replacement therapy
E. Hysterectomy

Answer: E

Adenomatous hyperplasia with marked atypia is also called "endometrial carcinoma in situ," because it carries a high risk of becoming endometrial carcinoma. Because this patient has completed her childbearing, hysterectomy, with adjuvant therapy as indicated by the pathology specimen results, is the best management. If this patient had wanted more children or wished to avoid hysterectomy if possible, progestin therapy could be attempted, but with close monitoring of her endometrium to document efficacious results.

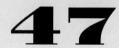
OVARIAN AND ADNEXAL DISEASE

This chapter deals primarily with APGO Objective(s):

OBJECTIVE 59   Ovarian Neoplasms

A. Describe the approach to the adnexal mass and how factors such as age and mass characteristics affect the evaluation.

B. Describe the symptoms/physical findings, risk factors, diagnostic methods and FIGO staging, and histological classifications of functional and benign ovarian neoplasia and ovarian carcinoma.

The structures occupying the area between the lateral pelvic wall and the cornu of the uterus medially are referred to as the *adnexa*. These include the ovaries, fallopian tubes, the upper portion of the broad ligament and mesosalpinx, and remnants of the embryonic müllerian duct. Of these, the organs most commonly affected by disease processes are the ovaries and fallopian tubes.

This chapter describes the physiologic variations of the ovary and fallopian tubes that can mimic disease as well as the benign and malignant ovarian and fallopian tube neoplasms. It also illustrates how nongynecologic structures in the region, such as the bowel and bladder, may produce symptoms that can be confused with "gynecologic" adnexal disease. Pelvic infection, ectopic pregnancy, and endometriosis are discussed in separate chapters.

ADNEXAL SPACE AND ASSOCIATED NONGYNECOLOGIC DISEASE

In addition to the reproductive organs, parts of the urinary and gastrointestinal tracts are located near the adnexal space. The most common urologic disorders are upper and lower *urinary tract infection,* and the less common, *renal and ureteral calculi.* Even rarer are anatomic abnormalities such as a *ptotic kidney,* which may present as a solid pelvic mass. An isolated pelvic kidney may likewise present as an asymptomatic, solid, cul-de-sac mass. Right adnexal signs and symptoms are associated with acute *appendicitis,* which should be considered in the differential diagnosis of acute right lower quadrant pain, usually preceded by anorexia. Less commonly, symptoms in the right adnexa may be related to intrinsic *inflammatory bowel disease* involving the ileocecal junction. Left-sided bowel disease involving the rectosigmoid is seen more often in older patients, as in acute or chronic diverticular disease. Because of the age of these patients and the proximity of the left ovary to the sigmoid, *sigmoid diver-*

ticular disease is included in the differential diagnosis of a left-sided adnexal mass. Finally, left-sided pelvic pain or a mass may be related to *rectosigmoid carcinoma.*

THE OVARIES

Pelvic examination is central in evaluation of the ovary. Symptoms that may arise from physiologic and pathologic processes of the ovary must be correlated with physical examination findings. Also, because some ovarian conditions are asymptomatic, incidental physical examination findings may be the only information available when an evaluation begins. Interpretation of examination findings requires knowledge of the physical characteristics of the ovary during the stages of the life cycle.

In the *premenarchal age group,* the ovary *should not be palpable.* If it is, a pathologic condition is presumed and further evaluation is necessary.

In the *reproductive age group,* the normal *ovary is palpable about half of the time.* Important considerations include ovarian size, shape, consistency (firm or cystic), and mobility. In reproductive-age women taking oral contraceptives, the ovaries are palpable less frequently and are smaller and more symmetric than in women who are not using contraceptives.

In the *postmenopausal* patient, the ovaries are functionally different because they are less responsive to gonadotropin secretion, and therefore their surface follicular activity diminishes over time, disappearing in most women within 3 years of the onset of natural menopause. Women who are close to the natural menopause are more likely to have residual functional cysts. In general, palpable ovarian enlargement in a postmenopausal patient should be assessed more critically than in a younger woman, because the incidence of ovarian malignant neoplasm is increased in this group.

One quarter of all ovarian tumors in postmenopausal women are malignant, whereas in reproductive-age women only about 10% of ovarian tumors are malignant.

Indeed, this risk was considered so great in the past that the presence of any ovarian enlargement in a postmenopausal woman was an indication for surgical investigation, the so-called palpable postmenopausal ovary (PPO) syndrome. With the advent of more sensitive pelvic imaging techniques to assist in diagnosis, routine removal of minimally enlarged postmenopausal ovaries is no longer recommended. If the patient is within 3 years of natural menopause, and transvaginal ultrasonography confirms the presence of a simple, unilocular cyst of less than 5 cm in diameter, the management may be serial pelvic and transvaginal ultrasound examinations. Masses that are larger or appear complex on ultrasonography are best managed surgically.

Functional Ovarian Cysts

Functional ovarian cysts are not neoplasms but rather anatomic variations, arising as a result of normal ovarian function. They may present as an asymptomatic adnexal mass or become symptomatic, requiring evaluation and possibly treatment.

When an ovarian follicle fails to rupture during follicular maturation, ovulation does not occur and a *follicular cyst* may develop. This, by definition, involves a lengthening of the follicular phase of the cycle with resultant secondary amenorrhea. Follicular cysts are lined by normal granulosa cells and the fluid contained in them is rich in estrogen.

A follicular cyst becomes clinically significant if it is large enough to cause pain or if it persists beyond one menstrual interval. For poorly understood reasons, the granulosa cells lining the follicular cyst persist through the time when ovulation should have occurred and continue to enlarge through the second half of the cycle. A cyst may enlarge beyond 5 cm and continue to fill with estrogen-rich follicular fluid from the thickened granulosa cell layer. Symptoms associated with a follicular cyst may include mild to moderate unilateral lower abdominal pain and alteration of the menstrual interval. The latter may be the result

of both failed subsequent ovulation and bleeding stimulated by the large amount of estradiol produced in the follicle. This estrogen-rich environment along with the lack of ovulation over stimulates the endometrium and causes irregular bleeding. Pelvic examination findings may include unilateral tenderness with a palpable, mobile, cystic adnexal mass.

Given a patient with these findings, the physician must decide whether further diagnostic assessment and treatment are necessary. Pelvic ultrasonography is occasionally warranted in reproductive-age patients who have cysts larger than 5 cm in diameter. Ultrasound characteristics include a unilocular simple cyst without evidence of blood or soft tissue elements and without evidence of external excrescences. For most patients, however, ultrasound confirmation is not required. Instead, the patient may be reassured and followed with a repeat pelvic examination in about 6 to 8 weeks, once pregnancy has been ruled out.

Most follicular cysts spontaneously resolve during this time. Alternatively, an estrogen- and progesterone-containing oral contraceptive may be given to suppress gonadotropin stimulation of the cyst. Although this practice has not been shown to "shrink" the existing follicle cyst, it may suppress the development of a new cyst and permit resolution of the existing problem. If the cyst persists despite expectant management, the presence of another type of cyst or neoplasm should be suspected, and further evaluated by imaging studies and/or surgery. The role of transvaginal sonography with directed-needle aspiration of such cysts is controversial but under investigation in prospective studies.

On occasion, *rupture of a follicular cyst* may cause acute pelvic pain. Because release of follicular fluid into the peritoneum produces only transient symptoms, surgical intervention is rarely necessary.

A *corpus luteum cyst* is the other common type of functional ovarian cyst, designated a cyst rather than simply a corpus luteum when its diameter exceeds about 3 cm. It is related to the postovulatory (i.e., luteal-dominant) phase of the menstrual cycle. Two variations of corpus luteum cysts are encountered. The first is a slightly enlarged corpus luteum, which may continue to produce progesterone for longer than the usual 14 days. Menstruation is delayed from a few days to several weeks, although it usually occurs within 2 weeks of the missed period. Persistent corpus luteum cysts are often associated with dull lower quadrant pain. This pain and a missed menstrual period are the most common complaints associated with *persistent corpus luteum cysts.* Pelvic examination usually discloses an enlarged, tender, cystic or solid adnexal mass. Because of the triad of missed menstrual period, unilateral lower quadrant pain, and adnexal enlargement, ectopic pregnancy is often considered in the differential diagnosis. A negative pregnancy test eliminates this possibility, whereas a positive pregnancy test mandates further evaluation as to the location of the pregnancy. Patients with recurrent persistent corpus luteum cysts may benefit from cyclic oral contraceptive therapy. The second common type of corpus luteum cyst is the rapidly enlarging luteal-phase cyst into which there is spontaneous hemorrhage. Sometimes called the *corpus hemorrhagicum,* this hemorrhagic cyst may rupture late in the luteal phase, resulting in the following clinical picture: a patient not using oral contraceptives, with regular periods, who presents with acute pain late in the luteal phase. Some patients present with evidence of hemoperitoneum as well as hypovolemia and require surgical resection of the bleeding cyst. In others, the acute pain and blood loss are self-limited. These patients may be managed with mild analgesics and reassurance.

The least common functional cyst is the *theca lutein cyst,* associated with pregnancy and usually bilateral. They are more common in multiple gestation, trophoblastic disease, and also with ovulation induction with clomiphene and human menopausal gonadotropin/human chorionic gonadotropin. They may become quite large and are multicystic, but also regress spontaneously in most cases without intervention.

Benign Ovarian Neoplasms

Although most ovarian enlargements in the reproductive age group are functional cysts, about 25% prove to be nonfunctional ovarian neoplasms. In the reproductive age group, 90% of these neoplasms are benign, whereas the risk of malignancy rises to approximately 25% when postmenopausal patients are also included. Thus, ovarian masses in older patients and in reproductive patients where there is no response to oral contraceptives are of special concern. Unfortunately, unless the mass is particularly large or becomes symptomatic, these masses may remain undetected for some time. Many ovarian neoplasms are first discovered at the time of routine pelvic examination.

Ovarian neoplasms are usually categorized by the cell type of origin: (a) epithelial cell tumors, the largest class of ovarian neoplasm; *(b) germ cell tumors,* which include the most common ovarian neoplasm in reproductive-age women, the benign cystic teratoma or dermoid; and *(c) stromal cell tumors.* The classification of ovarian tumors by cell line of origin is presented in Table 47.1.

BENIGN EPITHELIAL CELL NEOPLASMS

The exact cell source for the development of epithelial cell tumors of the ovary is unclear; however, the cells are characteristic of typical glandular epithelial cells. They contain microscopic glandular and secretory apparatus, they secrete into a luminal surface, and they are separated from underlying stroma by a basement membrane. Evidence exists to suggest that these cells are derived from mesothelial cells lining the peritoneal cavity. Because the müllerian duct-derived tissue becomes the female genital tract by differentiation of the mesothelium from the gonadal ridge, it is hypothesized that these tissues are also capable of differentiating into glandular tissue. Accordingly, the more common epithelial tumors of the ovary are grouped into serous, mucinous, and endometrial neoplasms, as shown in Table 47.2.

TABLE 47.1. Histogenic Classification of All Ovarian Neoplasms

From coelomic epithelium (epithelial)
  Serous
  Mucinous
  Endometrioid
  Brenner
From gonadal stroma
  Granulosa theca
  Sertoli-Leydig (arrhenoblastoma)
  Lipid cell fibroma
From germ cell
  Dysgerminoma
  Teratoma
  Endodermal sinus (yolk sac)
  Choriocarcinoma
Miscellaneous cell line sources
  Lymphoma
  Sarcoma
  Metastatic
    Colorectal
    Breast
    Endometrial

The most common epithelial cell neoplasm is the *serous cystadenoma*. Seventy percent of serous tumors are benign; approximately 10% have intraepithelial cellular characteristics, which suggest that they are of low malignant potential; and the remaining 20% are frankly malignant by both histologic criteria and clinical behavior. Benign tumors usually present clinically as cystic adnexal masses, which may be bilateral about 15% of the time. Typically, they are larger than functional ovarian cysts and may cause perceptible increasing abdominal girth. These tumors may occur in any age group, although they are more common in the perimenopausal and postmenopausal patient. On ultrasonography, these cysts tend to appear multilocular, especially if they are large. The *treatment of serous tumors* is surgical because of the relatively high rate of malignancy. In the younger patient with smaller tumors, an attempt can be made to perform an ovarian cystectomy to try to minimize the amount of ovarian tissue removed. For large, unilateral serous tumors in young patients, unilateral oophorectomy with preservation of the

TABLE 47.2. Histologic Classification of the Common Epithelial Tumors of the Ovary

Serous tumors
  Serous cystadenomas
  Serous cystadenomas with proliferating activity of the epithelial cells and nuclear abnormalities but with no infiltrative destructive growth (low potential malignancy)
  Serous cystadenocarcinoma
Mucinous tumors
  Mucinous cystadenomas
  Mucinous cystadenomas with proliferating activity of the epithelial cells and nuclear abnormalities but with no infiltrative destructive growth (low potential malignancy)
  Mucinous cystadenocarcinoma

Endometrioid tumors (similar to adenocarcinomas in the endometrium)
  Endometrioid benign cysts
  Endometrioid tumors with proliferating activity of the epithelial cells and nuclear abnormalities but with no infiltrative destructive growth (low potential malignancy)
  Adenocarcinoma
Brenner tumor
Unclassified carcinoma

contralateral ovary is indicated to maintain fertility. In patients past the reproductive age, bilateral oophorectomy along with hysterectomy may be indicated, not only because of the chance of future malignancy but because of the increased risk of a similar occurrence in the contralateral ovary.

Mucinous tumors are also of epithelial (mesothelial) cell origin. The *mucinous cystadenoma* is the second most common epithelial cell tumor of the ovary. The malignancy rate of 15% is lower than that for serous tumor, as is the 5% rate of bilaterality. These cystic tumors can become very large, sometimes filling the entire pelvis and extending into the abdominal cavity. In fact, when enormous cystic adnexal masses are found, mucinous cystadenomas should be suspected. Ultrasound assessment shows multilocular septation. Surgery is the treatment of choice.

A third type of benign epithelial neoplasm is the *endometrioid tumor*. Most benign endometrioid tumors take the form of endometriomas, which are cysts lined by well-differentiated, endometrial-like glandular tissue. There is further discussion of this neoplasm in "Malignant Ovarian Neoplasms," later.

The *Brenner cell tumor* is an uncommon benign epithelial cell tumor of the ovary. This tumor is usually described as a solid ovarian tumor because of the large amount of stroma and fibrotic tissue that surrounds the epithelial cells. It is more common in older women and occasionally occurs in association with mucinous tumors of the ovary. When discovered as an isolated tumor of the ovary, it is relatively small compared with the large size often attained by the serous and especially by the mucinous cystadenomas. It is rarely malignant.

BENIGN GERM CELL NEOPLASMS

Germ cell tumors are derived from the primary germ cells. The tumors arise in the ovary and may contain relatively differentiated structures such as hair or bone. The most common tumor found in women of all ages is the *benign cystic teratoma*, also called a *dermoid cyst* or *dermoid*. Eighty percent occur during the reproductive years, with a median age of occurrence of 30 years. However, in children and adolescents, mature cystic teratomas account for about one half of benign ovarian neoplasms. Dermoids may contain differentiated tissue from all three embryonic germ layers (ectoderm, mesoderm, and endoderm). The most common elements found are of ectodermal origin, primarily squamous cell tissue such as skin appendages (sweat, sebaceous glands) with associated hair follicles and sebum. It is because of this predominance of dermoid derivatives that the term *dermoid* is used. Other constituents of dermoids include central nervous system tissue, cartilage, bone, teeth, and intestinal glandular elements, most of which are found in well-differentiated form. One unusual variant is the *struma ovarii*, in which functioning thyroid tissue is found.

A dermoid cyst is frequently encountered as an asymptomatic, unilateral cystic adnexal mass that is mobile, nontender, and often felt anterior to the broad ligament (i.e., just under the abdominal examining fingers rather than deep in the pelvis). This "floating" position may be because of the high fat content of most dermoid cysts and may explain the relatively high risk of 15% of torsion of dermoid cysts. The diagnosis can be confirmed by ultrasound, because of the peculiar pattern of echogenicity from inside the cyst caused by its contents.

Treatment of benign cystic teratomas is necessarily surgical, even though the rate of malignancy is less than 1%. Surgical removal is required because of the possibility of ovarian torsion and rupture, resulting in intense chemical peritonitis and a potential surgical emergency. Between 10% and 20% of these cysts are bilateral, underscoring the need for examination of the contralateral ovary at the time of surgery.

BENIGN STROMAL CELL NEOPLASMS

Stromal cell tumors of the ovary are usually considered solid tumors and are derived from specialized sex cord stroma of the developing gonad. These tumors may develop along a primarily female cell type into *granulosa theca cell tumors* or into a primarily male gonadal type of tissue, known as *Sertoli-Leydig cell tumors*. Both of these tumors are referred to as functioning tumors because of their hormone production. *Granulosa theca cell tumors primarily produce estrogenic components* and may be manifest in patients through feminizing characteristics, and *Sertoli-Leydig cell tumors produce androgenic components*, which may contribute to hirsutism or virilizing symptoms. These neoplasms occur with approximately equal frequency in all age groups, including pediatric patients. When the granulosa cell tumor occurs in the pediatric age group, it may contribute to signs and symptoms of precocious puberty, including precocious thelarche and vaginal bleeding. Vaginal bleeding may also occur when this tumor develops in the postmenopausal years. Both the granulosa cell tumor and the Sertoli-Leydig cell tumor have malignant potential, as discussed later.

The *ovarian fibroma* occurs in approximately 10% of patients with ovarian neoplasms, but is unlike the other stromal cell tumors in that it does not secrete sex steroids. It is usually a small, solid tumor with a smooth surface and occasionally is clinically misleading because of the presence of ascites. The combination of benign ovarian fibroma coupled with ascites and right unilateral hydrothorax has historically been referred to as *Meigs syndrome*.

In summary, the following points regarding benign ovarian neoplasms can be made: (a) they are more common than malignant tumors of the ovary in all age groups, *(b)* the chance for malignant transformation increases with increasing age, *(c)* they warrant surgical treatment because of their potential for malignancy, *(d)* preoperative assessment may be assisted by the use of pelvic imaging techniques such as ultrasound, and *(e)* surgical treatment may be conservative for benign tumors, especially if future reproduction is desired.

Malignant Ovarian Neoplasms

Ovarian cancer is the *fifth most common of all cancers in women* in the United States and the *third most common gynecologic malignancy*, having a frequency of approximately one fourth that of endometrial carcinoma. Yet the *mortality rate of this disease is the highest of all the gynecologic malignancies*, primarily because early detection of the disease before widespread dissemination is difficult. Ovarian neoplasms are rarely symptomatic in early stages of disease, becoming symptomatic only after extensive metastasis. As yet, there is no effective screening test for ovarian cancer similar to the Pap smear for cervical cancer, so that approximately two thirds of the patients with ovarian cancer have advanced disease at the time of diagnosis. Of the 25,000 to 30,000 new cases of ovarian cancer yearly, some 60% will die within 5 years. The most important demographic observation regarding ovarian cancer is that it *presents most commonly in the fifth and sixth decade of life*. There is a higher incidence of ovarian cancer in Western European countries and in the United States, with a five- to sevenfold greater incidence than age-matched populations in East Asia. Whites are 50% more likely to contract ovarian cancer than blacks living in the United States.

A woman's risk for development of ovarian cancer during her lifetime is approximately 1%. The risk increases with age until approximately 70 years, at which time it declines modestly. The certain epidemiologic factors associated with development of ovarian cancer include low parity, decreased fertility, and delayed childbearing. Some investigators have suggested a possible carcinogenic source introduced into the lower genital tract by way of the vagina that eventually reaches the ovary. Inert agents such as asbestos and talc can be found in the peritoneal mesothelial cells, although the role of these and other potentially carcinogenic agents is unclear. An association with viral exposure, in particular with prior infection with mumps virus, has been suggested.

Recently, demonstration of the genetic inheritance of ovarian cancer has revealed important information regarding the possible etiology of the disease. The *BRCA1* gene has been found to be associated with ovarian cancers in approximately 5% of cases. Although this observation has been confirmed by repeated experiments, the expression of this gene in *BRCA1* carriers is unpredictable. Therefore, routine testing for this gene has limited value at this time. Similarly, mutations in the tumor suppressor gene, *P53*, have been shown to be associated with a high proportion of epithelial cell carcinomas. Investigators are working to elucidate further the role of inheritance and genetics in the development of ovarian cancer, thus providing hope for future screening techniques as well as gene specific therapies.

Long-term suppression of ovulation may protect against the development of ovarian cancer, at least for epithelial cell tumors. It has been suggested that so-called incessant ovulation may predispose to neoplastic transformation of the epithelial cell surfaces of the ovary. Oral contraceptives that cause anovulation appear to provide significant protection against the occurrence of ovarian cancer. Five years' cumulative use of oral contraceptives decreases the lifetime risk by one half. No evidence exists to implicate the use of postmenopausal hormone replacement therapy in the development of ovarian cancer.

PATHOGENESIS AND DIAGNOSIS

Malignant ovarian epithelial cell tumors spread primarily by direct extension within the peritoneal cavity because of direct cell sloughing from the ovarian surface. This process explains the observation that there is often widespread peritoneal dissemination of these cancers at the time of diagnosis, even with relatively small primary ovarian lesions. Although epithelial cell ovarian cancers also spread by lymphatic and blood-borne routes, it is the direct extension into the virtually unlimited space of the peritoneal cavity that contributes to their late clinical presentation.

The early diagnosis of ovarian cancer is also made difficult by the *lack of effective screening tests.* Approximately 60% of patients have advanced disease at the time of diagnosis. Refined imaging techniques (especially transvaginal ultrasonography) and serum tumor markers—such as the monoclonal antibody OC125, which recognizes the antigen Ca125 (which is present in serous ovarian tumors but not in mucinous or nonepithelial ovarian tumors)—offer promise for the future. Much work remains, however, before these or similar tests are considered accurate or cost effective. Serum tumor markers have been shown to be useful in the follow-up of previously treated epithelial cell neoplasms of the ovary but not for detection. Until these techniques are shown to be efficacious, detection is limited by the physician's index of suspicion and skill in the assessment of women who present with persistent but vague abdominopelvic symptoms or findings. The clinician is cautioned against the application of seemingly exacting technology while abandoning the exercise of sound clinical judgment. Further study of imaging techniques and serum tumor markers is ongoing in hopes of enabling earlier diagnosis of these tumors.

HISTOLOGIC CLASSIFICATION

Malignant ovarian neoplasms are usually categorized by the cell type of origin, similar to their benign counterparts: *(a) malignant epithelial cell tumors,* which are the most common type; *(b) malignant germ cell tumors;* and *(c) malignant stromal cell tumors* (see Table 47.1). Most malignant ovarian tumors have histologically similar but benign counterparts. The relationship between a benign ovarian neoplasm and its malignant counterpart is clinically important. If the benign counterpart is found in a patient, removal of both ovaries is strongly considered, because of the possibility of future malignant transformation in the remaining ovary. The decision as to removal of one or both ovaries, however, must be individualized based on age, type of tumor,

TABLE 47.3. FIGO Staging for Primary Carcinoma of the Ovary

Stage	Description
I	Growth limited to the ovaries
Ia	Growth limited to one ovary; no ascites containing malignant cells; no tumor on the external surface; capsule intact
Ib	Growth limited to both ovaries; no ascites containing malignant cells; no tumor on the external surface; capsule intact
Ic	Tumor either stage Ia or Ib but with tumor on the surface of one or both ovaries; or with capsule ruptured, or with ascites present containing malignant cells, or with positive peritoneal washings
II	Growth involving one or both ovaries with pelvic extension
IIa	Extension and/or metastases to the uterus and/or tubes
IIb	Extension to other pelvic tissues
IIc	Tumor either stage IIa or IIb but with tumor on the surface of one or both ovaries; or with capsule(s) ruptured, or with ascites present containing malignant cells, or with positive peritoneal washings
III	Tumor involving one or both ovaries with peritoneal implants outside the pelvic and/or positive retroperitoneal or inguinal nodes; superficial liver metastasis equals stage III; tumor is limited to the true pelvis, but histologically proven malignant extension is to small bowel or omentum
IIIa	Tumor grossly limited to the true pelvis with negative nodes but with histologically confirmed microscopic seeding of abdominal peritoneal surfaces
IIIb	Tumor of one or both ovaries with histologically confirmed implants of abdominal peritoneal surface; none exceeding 2 cm in diameter; nodes negative
IIIc	Abdominal implants > 2 cm in diameter and/or positive retroperitoneal or inguinal nodes
IV	Growth involving one or both ovaries with distant metastasis; if pleural effusion is present, there must be positive cytologic test results to deem a case stage IV; parenchymal liver metastasis equals stage IV

and future risks. For example, it has been shown that *approximately 10% of seemingly benign epithelial cell tumors may contain histologic evidence of intraepithelial neoplasia, commonly referred to as borderline malignancies, or "tumors of low malignant potential."* These tumors of low malignant potential usually remain confined to the ovary, are more common in premenopausal women (between 30 and 50 years of age as compared to invasive ovarian carcinomas, which are more common in women between 50 and 70 years of age), and have generally good prognoses. However, it should be noted that about one fifth of such tumors show spread beyond the ovary.

STAGING

The staging of ovarian carcinoma is based on extent of spread of tumor and histologic evaluation of the tumor. The International Federation of Gynecology and Obstetrics (FIGO) classification of ovarian cancer is presented in Table 47.3.

BORDERLINE OVARIAN TUMORS

Borderline ovarian tumors (tumors of low malignant potential) require carefully individualized therapy following the initial surgical resection of the primary tumor. If frozen section pathology or later permanent pathology demonstrates borderline histology, unilateral oophorectomy and follow-up are appropriate when a woman wishes to retain ovarian function and understands the risks of such conservative management.

EPITHELIAL CELL OVARIAN CARCINOMA

Approximately 90% of all ovarian malignancies are of the epithelial cell type. These are thought to represent abnormalities in the differentiation of the pluripotential mesothelial cells (which were derived embryologically from the gonadal ridge) that occupy parts of the visceral peritoneum. The ovary contains these cells as part of an ovarian capsule just overlying the actual stroma of the ovary. When these mesothelial cell elements are situated over developing follicles, they go through metaplastic transformation whenever ovulation occurs. Repeated ovulation is, therefore, associated with the histologic change in these cells derived from coelomic epithelium.

Malignant epithelial serous tumors (serous cystadenocarcinoma) are the most common malignant epithelial cell tumors. Approximately 50% of these cancers are thought to be derived from their benign precursors (serous cystadenoma), and as many as 30% of these tumors are bilateral at the time of clinical presentation. They are typically multiloculated and often have external excrescences on an otherwise smooth capsular surface. Calcified, laminated structures, *psammona bodies,* are found in more than one half of serous carcinomas.

Another epithelial cell variant, which contains cells reminiscent of endocervical glandular mucous secreting cells, is the *malignant mucinous epithelial tumor (the mucinous cystadenocarcinoma).* These tumors have a lower rate of bilaterality (10%–15%) and can be among the largest of ovarian tumors, often measuring greater than 20 cm. They may be associated with widespread peritoneal extension with thick, mucinous ascites, termed *pseudomyxomatous peritonei.*

While most epithelial carcinomas occur sporadically, a small percentage (< 5%) occur in familial or hereditary patterns. *Site-specific familial ovarian cancer* risk depends on the number of first- or second-degree relatives with a history of epithelial ovarian cancer. For example, in families where two first-degree relatives (i.e., mother, sister, daughter) have epithelial carcinoma, the risk that a female first-degree relative will have an affected gene may be as high as 50%. Such hereditary ovarian cancers generally occur earlier than non-hereditary tumors. *Breast/ovarian familial cancer syndrome,* a combination of epithelial ovarian and breast cancers in first- and second-degree family members, are at 2–3 times the risk of these cancers as the general population. Women with this syndrome have an increased risk of bilaterality of breast cancer and developing ovarian tumors at a younger age. This syndrome has been associated with the BRCA1 gene, a locus on the 17q chromosome. Women with this gene mutation have a cumulative lifetime risk of 85%–90% for breast cancer and 50% for ovarian cancer. Women of Ashkenazi Jewish extraction have a 1% chance of carrying this gene, a 10-fold risk over the general population. *Lynch II syndrome* occurs in families with first- and second-degree members with combinations of colon, ovarian, endometrial, and breast cancers. Women in families with this syndrome may have a three-fold increased risk of cancer over the general population. Women in families with these syndromes should have more frequent screening tests and may benefit from prophylactic surgery in some cases.

Endometrioid Tumors

Endometrioid epithelial cell tumors are the second most common type of epithelial cell malignancy of the ovary, constituting approximately 20% of all ovarian cancers. These tumors contain histologic features similar to those of endometrial carcinoma. Endometrioid tumors may arise in association with a primary endometrial carcinoma, making it difficult to determine whether they are primary to the ovary or metastatic from the endometrium. Only approximately 10% of these tumors are found in association with endometriosis, and even fewer are known to have progressed from benign endometriotic precursors.

Other Epithelial Cell Ovarian Carcinomas

Of the remaining epithelial cell carcinomas of the ovary, *clear cell carcinomas* are thought to arise from mesonephric elements and Brenner tumors are thought to arise uncommonly (< 5%) from their benign counterpart. Interestingly, Brenner tumors occur approximately 10% of the time in the same ovary that contains mucinous cystadenoma; the reason for this is unclear.

GERM CELL TUMORS

Germ cell tumors constitute less than 5% of all ovarian malignancies. However, they are the *most common ovarian cancers in women younger than 20 years of age,* making up 60% of the malignant tumors discovered in this age group. Germ cell tumors may be functional, producing human chorionic gonadotropin (hCG) or α-fetoprotein (AFP), both of which can be used as tumor markers. The most common germ cell malignancies are *dysgerminoma* and *immature teratoma*. Other tumors are recognized as *mixed germ cell tumors, endodermal sinus tumors, and embryonal tumors*. There has been remarkable progress in treatment of this group of tumors in the last 10 years. Improved chemotherapeutic and radiation protocols have resulted in greatly improved 5-year survival rates.

Dysgerminomas are unilateral in approximately 90% of patients. They are the *most common type of germ cell tumor seen in patients with gonadal dysgenesis*. These tumors often arise in benign counterparts called the gonadoblastoma. The tumors are particularly *radiosensitive*, rendering adjunctive therapy efficacious.

Because of the young age of patients with dysgerminomas, removal of only the involved ovary with preservation of the uterus and contralateral tube and ovary may be considered if the tumor is less than approximately 10 cm and if there is no evidence of extraovarian spread. Unlike the epithelial cell tumors, these malignancies are more likely to spread by lymphatic channels, and therefore the pelvic and periaortic lymph nodes must be assessed carefully at the time of surgery. If disease has spread outside the ovaries, conventional hysterectomy and bilateral salpingo-oophorectomy are necessary, usually followed by postoperative radiation to the abdomen and pelvis. Chemotherapy is usually reserved for primary treatment failures. The prognosis of these tumors is generally excellent. The overall 5-year survival rate for patients with dysgerminoma is 90% to 95% when the disease is limited to one ovary that is less than 10 cm in size.

Immature teratomas are the malignant counterpart of benign cystic teratomas (dermoids). These are the *second most common germ cell cancer and are most often found in women younger than 25 years of age*. They are usually unilateral, although on occasion a benign counterpart may be found in the contralateral ovary. Because these tumors are rapidly growing, they may produce painful symptomatology relatively early, because of hemorrhage and necrosis during the rapid growth process. As a result, the diagnosis is made when the disease is limited to one ovary in two thirds of these young women. As with dysgerminoma, if an immature teratoma is limited to one ovary, unilateral oophorectomy is sufficient. Dramatic progress has been made in the treatment of these tumors in the past 15 years, with a 5-year survival rate greater than 80% for patients with well-differentiated tumors.

RARE GERM CELL TUMORS

Endodermal sinus tumors and embryonal cell carcinomas are uncommon malignant ovarian tumors for which there has been a remarkable improvement in cure rate. Before about 10 years ago, these tumors were almost uniformly fatal. New chemotherapeutic protocols have resulted in an overall 5-year survival rate of greater than 60%. These tumors typically occur in childhood and adolescence, with the primary treatment being surgical resection of the involved ovary followed by combination chemotherapy. The endodermal sinus tumor produces α-fetoprotein, whereas the embryonal cell carcinoma produces both α-fetoprotein and β-hCG.

GONADAL STROMAL CELL TUMORS

The gonadal stromal cell tumors make up an unusual group of tumors characterized by hormone production; hence, these tumors are called *functioning tumors.* The hormonal output from these tumors is usually in the form of female or male sex steroids, or, on occasion, adrenal steroid hormones.

The *granulosa cell tumor* is the *most common in this group.* These tumors occur in all ages, although in older patients they are more likely to be benign. Granulosa cell tumors may *secrete large amounts of estrogen, which in 15% to 20% of older women may cause endometrial hyperplasia or endometrial carcinoma.* Thus, endometrial sampling is especially important when ovarian tumors such as the granulosa tumor are estrogen producing. Measurement of estrogen levels as a reflection of tumor dissemination has not been found useful, nor has follow-up of estrogen production been suggested as a useful tumor marker. The survival of patients with this neoplasm is contingent on factors similar to those for other tumors, in particular, whether the tumor has ruptured at the time of surgical exploration.

Surgical treatment should include extirpation of the uterus and both ovaries in postmenopausal women as well as in women of reproductive age who no longer wish to remain fertile. In a young woman with the lesions limited to one ovary with an intact capsule, unilateral oophorectomy with careful surgical staging may be adequate. This tumor may demonstrate recurrences up to 10 years later. This is especially true with large tumors, which have a 20% to 30% chance of late recurrence.

Sertoli-Leydig cell tumors (arrhenoblastoma) are the rare, testosterone-secreting counterparts to granulosa cell tumors. They usually occur in older patients and should be suspected in the differential diagnosis of perimenopausal or postmenopausal patients with hirsutism or virilization and an adnexal mass. Treatment of these tumors is similar to that for other ovarian malignancies in this age group and is based on extirpation of uterus and ovaries.

Other stromal cell tumors include *fibromas* and *thecomas,* which very rarely demonstrate malignant counterparts, the *fibrosarcoma* and *malignant thecoma.*

Other Ovarian Malignancies

Very rarely, the ovary may be the site of initial manifestation of *lymphoma.* These are usually found in association with lymphoma elsewhere, although there have been case reports of primary ovarian lymphoma. Once the diagnosis has been made, management is similar to that for lymphoma of other origin.

Malignant mesodermal sarcomas are another rare type of ovarian tumor, which usually show aggressive behavior and are diagnosed at late stages. The survival rate is poor and clinical experience with these tumors is limited.

Cancer Metastatic to the Ovary

Classically, the term *Krukenberg tumor* describes an ovarian tumor that is metastatic from other sites such as the gastrointestinal tract (80% from stomach, remainder from colon), breast, and endometrium. They account for 30%–40% of cancers metastatic to the ovary. Most of these tumors are characterized as infiltrative, mucinous carcinoma of predominantly signet-ring cell type and as bilateral and associated with widespread metastatic disease. On occasion, these tumors are associated with abnormal uterine bleeding or virilization, leading to the supposition that some may produce estrogens or androgens. Breast cancer metastatic to the ovary is common, with autopsy data suggesting ovarian metastasis in one quarter of cases.

In 10% of patients with cancer metastatic to the ovary, an extraovarian primary site cannot be demonstrated. In this regard, it is important to consider ovarian preservation versus "prophylactic" oophorectomy at the time of hysterectomy in patients who have a strong family history (first-degree relatives) of epithelial ovarian cancer, primary gastrointestinal tract cancer, or breast cancer. In patients previously treated for cancer or gastrointestinal cancer, consideration should be given to the incidental removal of the ovaries at the time of hysterectomy, because these patients have a high predilection for development of ovarian cancer. The prognosis for most patients with carcinoma metastatic to the ovary is dismal, with 5% to 10% 5-year survival rates being quoted.

FALLOPIAN TUBES

Normal fallopian tubes cannot be palpated and usually are not considered in the differential diagnosis of adnexal disease *in the asymptomatic patient.* There are common problems involving the fallopian tubes, including ectopic pregnancy, salpingitis/ hydrosalpinx/tuboovarian abscess, and endometriosis (which can present as masses or be symptomatic). These conditions are discussed in other chapters.

Benign Disease of the Fallopian Tube and Mesosalpinx

Paraovarian cysts develop in the mesosalpinx from vestigial wolffian structures, tubal epithelium, and peritoneum inclusions. These are differentiated from *paratubal cysts,* which are found near the fimbriated end of the fallopian tube, are common, and are called *hydatids of Morgagni.* Both are usually small and symptomatic, although rarely they can reach large proportions.

Carcinoma of the Fallopian Tube

Primary fallopian tube carcinoma is usually an adenocarcinoma, although other cell types, including adenosquamous carcinoma and sarcoma, are rarely reported. About two thirds of patients with this rare gynecologic malignancy (< 1% of gynecologic malignancies) are postmenopausal. Grossly, these tumors are often rather large, resembling a hydrosalpinx, with a normal contralateral tube in 95% of cases. Microscopically, most are typical papillary serous cystadenocarcinomas of the ovary. The symptoms of this tumor are so slight that the tumor is often advanced before recognition of a problem. The most common complaint associated with fallopian tube carcinoma is postmenopausal bleeding followed by abnormal vaginal discharge. If such a discharge is profuse and serosanguineous, it is termed *hydrotubae profluens,* sometimes considered diagnostic of this tumor. However, the classic triad of symptoms associated with fallopian tube carcinoma (watery vaginal discharge, pain, and pelvic mass) is noted in less than 15% of cases. Staging is surgical, *similar to that for ovarian carcinoma* (Table 47.4); progression is similar to that of ovarian carcinoma, with intraperitoneal metastases and ascites. However, the fallopian tubes are richly permeated with lymphatic channels so that para-aortic and pelvic lymph node spread is common, the former in perhaps one third of all cases. Treatment is total abdominal hysterectomy with bilateral removal of the adnexa; careful exploration of the diaphragm, liver, pericolic gutters, omentum, and bowel; and sampling for biopsy of the omentum and retroperitoneal nodes. The overall 5-year survival rate is 35% to 45%, with stage I having the best rate, approaching 70%. There are too few data to ascertain whether adjunctive therapy is useful, and this management must be made on a case-by-case basis.

Carcinoma metastatic to the fallopian tube is far more common than primary fallopian tube carcinoma, including uterine and ovarian tumors. A few cases of *other, very rare tumors of the fallopian tube are reported,* including malignant mixed müllerian tumors, primary choriocarcinoma, fibroma, and adenomatoid tumors.

TABLE 47.4.   Surgical Staging for Primary Tubal Carcinoma

Stage	Description
I	
IA	Disease confined to one tube with no ascites
IB	Disease confined to both tubes with no ascites
IC	Disease confined to one or both tubes but ascites present with malignant cells in the fluid
II	
IIA	Extension to the uterus or ovaries or both
IIB	Extension to the uterus or ovaries and to other intraperitoneal organs or tissues beyond the true pelvis
III	Extension to the uterus or ovaries and to other intraperitoneal organs and tissues beyond the true pelvis
IV	Metastases present in organs or tissues outside the peritoneal cavity

GENERAL PRINCIPLES IN THE SURGICAL MANAGEMENT OF OVARIAN AND FALLOPIAN TUBE MALIGNANCY

Primary surgical therapy is indicated in most of the ovarian malignancies, regardless of stage. This surgery is based on the principle of *cytoreductive surgery, or "tumor debulking."* The rationale for cytoreductive surgery is that adjunctive radiation therapy and chemotherapy are more effective when all tumor masses are reduced to less than 1 cm in size (see Chapter 41). Because direct peritoneal seeding is the primary method of intraperitoneal spread, multiple adjacent structures commonly contain tumor, resulting in cytoreductive procedures that are often quite extensive. Each procedure includes the following.

1. Peritoneal cytology is obtained; this is used to assess microscopic spread of tumor. Samples are taken immediately after entering the abdomen before extensive surgery has been undertaken. Gross ascites is aspirated and submitted for cytologic analysis. If there is no gross ascites, saline irrigation is used to "wash" the peritoneal cavity in an attempt to find microscopic disease. The wash is then submitted for cytologic assessment.
2. To determine visually and by palpation the extent of disease, thorough inspection and palpation are done, including the uterus, fallopian tubes and ovaries, surfaces of the pelvis, right and left pericolic gutters, omentum, upper abdominal, viscera including the surface of the liver and spleen, and undersurface of the diaphragm.
3. Partial omentectomy is usually performed, with or without evidence of tumor involvement.
4. Sampling of the pelvic and periaortic lymph nodes is done in earlier-stage disease of stromal cell and germ cell tumors, which have a higher likelihood of lymphatic spread. In the absence of gross disease, biopsies are obtained from the pelvic peritoneum and peritoneum of the right and left upper and lower pericolic gutters.

Because most ovarian cancer presents at an advanced stage, *adjunctive treatment* using chemotherapy or, on occasion, radiation therapy, is usually necessary. First-line chemotherapy is with *paclitaxel (Taxol)* combined with *cisplatin* or *carboplatin.* This is usually accomplished in three to six courses of chemotherapy, although the exact dosages and regimen are still under study.

With *recurrence of disease,* other chemotherapeutic agents may be used, including ifosfamide, hexamethylmelamine, and tamoxifen. Recently, the Food and Drug Administration approved topotecan for second-line therapy in ovarian cancer based on excellent results in preliminary studies.

There is only a limited role for *radiation therapy* in the management of ovarian cancer, and it is usually not used in other than investigational settings. Whole-abdomen radiation has diminished in popularity. Occasional patients with earlier-staged disease (stage 1 or 2) may benefit from intraperitoneal use of phosphorus-32 isotope.

Follow-up consists of clinical history and examination; various imaging studies, such as ultrasound and/or computed tomography; and in epithelial cell tumors, the use of serum tumor markers such as Ca125. One other area of special consideration for ovarian cancer patients is the *second-look laparotomy.* This procedure is reserved for patients who have no clinically evident disease after the completion of primary surgical therapy and a standard course of adjunctive chemotherapy. If the patient has been rendered clear of gross disease at the time of surgery and if she has undergone a course of standard chemotherapy for presumed microscopic residual disease, it is often difficult to know whether residual disease remains. Therefore, many ovarian cancer treatment protocols include second-look laparotomy to ascertain whether residual disease remains.

CASE STUDIES

Case 47A

A 23-year-old G1 P1001 describes a new, crampy pain in her right pelvis over the last 3 days. Her last menstrual period was 3 weeks ago and was normal. She uses a diaphragm for contraception and her urine pregnancy test is negative. On pelvic examination a 3 × 4 cm tender cystic mass is found in the right adnexa. The remainder of her examination is negative.

Questions Case 47A

The best management at this time would be to schedule

A. A return visit in 1 week
B. A return visit to the office in 2 months
C. A return visit to the office in 1 year
D. A diagnostic laparoscopy
E. An exploratory laparotomy

Answer: B

Although the differential diagnosis includes various tumors and benign gynecologic disease, the most likely diagnosis is a "functional" ovarian cyst (i.e., a follicular or corpus luteum cyst). A return visit is necessary because a functional cyst will resolve, whereas other lesions will not; 2 months is a reasonable time, but 1 year is too long. Surgical intervention is far too aggressive a measure at this time. Transvaginal or transabdominal ultrasound provides additional information as to size and consistency of the mass and should be ordered on a case-by-case basis.

Which medications are appropriate for this patient at this time?

A. Oral contraceptives
B. Oral progesterone
C. Oral estrogen

D. Gonadotropin-releasing hormone (GnRH) agonist
E. Oral doxycycline

Answer: A

Gonadotropin suppression with oral contraceptives can be used in a patient with a functional ovarian cyst, although this is not a "required" management. It would be particularly appropriate if the patient were to express a desire to switch to oral contraceptives for birth control purposes also. Indeed, no medication (i.e., watchful expectation) would also be an acceptable management. Progesterone and estrogen would not aid in cyst resolution. No evidence of infection was given, hence antibiotic therapy is not indicated. GnRH agonist would eliminate gonadotropin stimulation of the ovary but would be overtreating this clinical situation.

The mass persists after 2 months of oral contraceptive therapy; in fact, it is now 2 cm larger. Ultrasound examination confirms a cystic mass. Ca125 is within normal ranges, as are all other laboratory evaluations. At exploratory laparotomy, a cystic mass is found without any other pelvic abnormalities. An ovarian cystectomy is performed. The final pathology report is serous cystadenoma. What options should be presented to the patient at this time?

A. Total abdominal hysterectomy and bilateral salpingo-oophorectomy
B. Unilateral salpingo-oophorectomy
C. Radiation therapy
D. Chemotherapy
E. Observation

Answer: E

This benign ovarian neoplasm requires no specific follow-up, although yearly examinations are important in this young woman who has had a benign ovarian neoplasm.

Case 47B

A 53-year-old woman notices increased facial and body hair and a deepening tone of voice. On physical examination, the patient has considerable coarse facial hair and a 3 × 4 cm, firm, left adnexal mass.

Questions Case 47B

The serum concentration of which of the following hormones would most likely be elevated?

A. hCG
B. Progesterone
C. Estradiol
D. Testosterone

Answer: D

The history and physical examination are most consistent with a Sertoli-Leydig cell tumor, the rare testosterone-secreting counterpart to the granulosa cell tumor.

The best management at this time would be to schedule

A. A transvaginal pelvic ultrasound examination
B. A return visit to the office in 2 months
C. A return visit to the office in 1 year
D. A diagnostic laparoscopy
E. An exploratory laparotomy

Answer: E

Exploratory laparotomy and total abdominal hysterectomy with bilateral salpingo-oophorectomy are indicated. Temporizing with a probable ovarian malignancy in a postmenopausal patient is not appropriate. Ultrasound evaluation might offer more information about the characteristics of the adnexal mass but would not alter the surgical management.

(Continued)

Case 47C

A 17-year-old G0 complains of a painful full sensation in her right lower quadrant. She has had regular menstrual periods since age 14 years and uses a low-dose oral contraceptive. She has no history of sexually transmitted diseases, admits to one sexual partner, and has had serial negative cultures as part of her annual examinations. She had a negative pelvic examination with satisfactory, negative Pap smear 9 months before her visit with this complaint. On physical examination you find a nervous young woman weighing 105 pounds with a normal general physical examination and pelvic examination except for a 5 × 5 cm, firm, mobile mass in the right adnexa. Her urine pregnancy test is negative.

Questions Case 47C

Your immediate evaluation should include

A. Repeat Pap smear
B. Endometrial biopsy
C. Pelvic ultrasound
D. Carcinoembryonic antigen (CEA)
E. β-hCG

Answer: C

Repeat Pap smear and endometrial biopsy are not consistent with this complaint and finding. Hormonal markers are likewise of little value. The mass feels solid, and ultrasound will help establish its internal structure.

The ultrasound confirms a 5 × 5 cm right adnexal mass that is described as composed of mixed cystic and solid components, some of which are calcified. There is no evidence of ascites, and the left adnexa appears unremarkable. Your management suggestion should now be

A. Observation, because there is no evidence of ascites, hence malignancy
B. Observation, because malignancy is uncommon in this age group and the risks of intervention are not warranted
C. Observation with serial ultrasound examinations, because adnexal masses are common in young women and resolve spontaneously in most cases
D. Diagnostic laparoscopy
E. Exploratory laparotomy or operative laparoscopy

Answer: E

This is a new and symptomatic mass, solid in nature, so that benign follicular tumor is unlikely. Further observation is not appropriate because an adnexal accident may occur (e.g., torsion), and the tumor may be malignant, however unlikely. Diagnostic laparoscopy is not indicated because removal of the mass is required. Either exploratory laparotomy or operative laparoscopy may be used to remove the mass, depending on the operator's skills and training.

At exploratory laparotomy, a unilateral cystic mass is discovered. When opened at the operating table, it contained mature structures such as hair and teeth. Subsequently, the pathology report was benign cystic teratoma.

UNIT VI

Human Sexuality

CHAPTER

48

HUMAN SEXUALITY

OBJECTIVE 62   Physician Sexuality

A. Demonstrate awareness of the influence of the physician's behaviors and attitudes on interactions with patients.
B. Describe the behavioral patterns of seductive patients.
C. Describe appropriate boundaries of physician behavior.

An estimated 60% of women, 40% of men, and over 50% of couples experience sexual problems. One in three women has difficulty achieving orgasm and one in 10 never does. Illness, medical and surgical treatment, initiation of sexual activity in the teen years before maturity sufficient to appropriately deal with this powerful life experience, and stress increase the frequency and often severity of these problems as well as engendering new ones. Physicians must be able to identify these problems and know whether to offer treatment or make referral to a specialist.

The first problem faced by the physician is to determine if there is a sexual problem and to specifically identify it. By demonstrating a supportive and nonjudgmental attitude, the physician creates a sense that it is permissible to discuss sexual matters and problems. To create this kind of comfortable environment, each physician must explore his or her own attitudes about the range of sexual expressions that may be encountered, his or her own sexuality, and how to address both in a manner conducive to good patient care.

DEVELOPMENT OF SEXUALITY

Human sexuality begins with the distribution of Y chromosomes, but thereafter the paths to an individual's present sexual status are complex. Various endocrinologic factors determine the expression of genetic sexual assignment. Overlaying this are the learned behaviors, first from parents, then siblings and peers, then by the individual's maturing evaluation of her own character.

Most individuals are ultimately comfortable with a heterosexual identity, but others may follow gay/lesbian, bisexual, or asexual lifestyles. Further, these sexual identities may change during the course of an individual's life. In addition, there are the *paraphilias*, intense sexual experiences with three basic characteristics (being intense, recurrent, and involving fantasy, urges, or behaviors; focusing on specific objects, such as animals, children, the dead; resulting in distress and other psychosocial dysfunction). Whether any or all of the paraphilias in Table 48.1

TABLE 48.1.   The Paraphilias

Paraphilia	Description
Voyeurism	Surreptitious observation of others unclothed or engaged in sex
Exhibitionism	Exposure of genitals to others
Fetishism	Sexual focus on objects (e.g., undergarments)
Masochism	Sexual excitement resulting from one's own humiliation, suffering, or pain
Sadism	Behaviors from fantasy of dominance to physical attack or sexual assault
Pedophilia	Sexual victimization of children; a criminal behavior

are considered "normal" is often as much a political, legal, and theological question as it is a medical one. Some, however, are clearly dangerous criminal behaviors (e.g., pedophilia) that must be reported so that the patient and potential victims may be protected.

HUMAN SEXUAL RESPONSE

Unlike the cycle-dependent estrus of lower animals, *the human sexual response is functionally volitional* and dependent on a complex interplay of emotional and physiologic factors. This variability allows considerable variety in the kinds of human sexual response and opportunity for sexual dysfunction. Whatever the kind of sexual response possible for an individual, it is dependent on two factors: first, an emotional and physical system that is sufficiently functional to allow a sexual response of some kind; second, *a sustained and sufficient sexual stimulation* to initiate the cascade of responses comprising the human sexual response. *Sustained* in this context means a stimulation that occurs over a long enough interval to effect arousal. *Sufficient* stimulation is physically correct and comfortable stimulation and stimulation effective enough to initiate and sustain the human sexual response. Many of the sexual

TABLE 48.2. Physiologic Reactions of Women During the Sexual Response Cycle

Phase	Sex-Organ Response	General Body Response
Excitement	Vaginal lubrication Thickening of vaginal walls and labia Expansion of inner vagina Elevation of cervix and corpus Tumescence of clitoris	Nipple erection Sex-tension flush
Plateau	Orgasmic platform in outer vagina Full expansion of inner vagina Secretion of mucus by Bartholin's gland Withdrawal of clitoris	Sex-tension flush Carpopedal spasm Generalized skeletal muscle tension Hyperventilation Tachycardia
Orgasm	Contractions of uterus from fundus toward lower uterine segment Contractions of orgasmic platform at 0.8-sec intervals External rectal sphincter contractions at 0.8-sec intervals External urethral sphincter contractions at irregular intervals	Specific skeletal muscle contractions Hyperventilation Tachycardia
Resolution	Ready return to orgasm with retarded loss of pelvic vasocongestion Return of normal color and orgasmic platform in primary (rapid) stage Loss of clitoral tumescence and return to position	Sweating reaction Hyperventilation Tachycardia

difficulties presenting to the clinician involve unsustained or insufficient stimulation.

With effective and sustained stimulation, the *human sexual response* may be initiated. Masters and Johnson, Kaplan, and others have demonstrated the value of considering the continuum of events comprising the human sexual response as consisting of "phases." Masters and Johnson have described four phases (excitement, plateau, orgasm, and resolution), whereas Kaplan has suggested a modification, combining the excitement and plateau phases and adding a desire phase at the start of the sexual response cycle. Both classifications are understood to be artificial in the sense that they describe highly variable components of

a continuum of emotional and physiologic events.

The *physiologic components of the female sexual response* (Table 48.2) are mediated primarily by changes in muscle tone (myotonic activity) and changes in blood flow (vasocongestion). Figures 48.1 through 48.4 demonstrate some of the physiologic changes seen in these phases. The duration of each phase varies with each individual and for a given individual at different times in her life. The human sexual response is a continuum of events with no clear boundaries between the described "phases." The value of these classifications lies in their use to understand the events comprising the human sexual response and

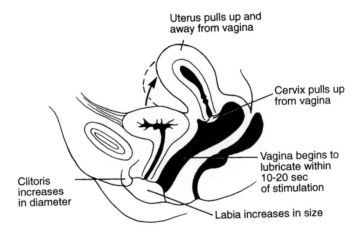

Uterus pulls up and away from vagina

Cervix pulls up from vagina

Vagina begins to lubricate within 10-20 sec of stimulation

Clitoris increases in diameter

Labia increases in size

FIGURE 48.1.   Excitement stage.

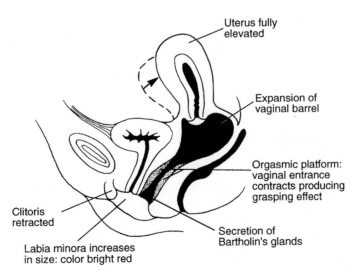

Uterus fully elevated

Expansion of vaginal barrel

Orgasmic platform: vaginal entrance contracts producing grasping effect

Clitoris retracted

Secretion of Bartholin's glands

Labia minora increases in size: color bright red

FIGURE 48.2.   Plateau stage.

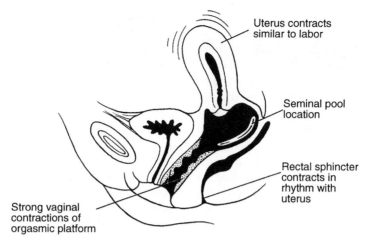

FIGURE 48.3. Orgasm stage.

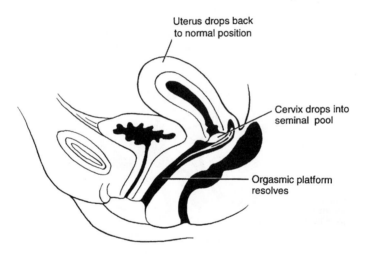

FIGURE 48.4. Resolution stage.

to assist in the clinical classification of sexual problems and dysfunctions.

EVALUATING SEXUAL CONCERNS

Sexual History and Physical Examination

Some patients present with a complaint involving a sexual issue or of a specific sexual dysfunction. Relatively detailed and focused questions are appropriate early on in the history taking, because these patients, by raising their issues, have indicated a willingness to discuss them. Other patients have a medical problem or have or have had a medical or surgical therapy that is known to be associated with sexual issues or problems (Table 48.3). Still other patients neither express a sexually related complaint nor have a medical problem with a commonly associated sexual issue. Introductory, nonobtrusive screening questions are useful to facilitate these communications. Three simple questions will help discern most sexual problems: "Are you sexually active?" "Are you satisfied with your sexual life?" "Do you have any sexual problems or questions?"

TABLE 48.3. Medical Conditions, Personal Behaviors, or Medications and Drugs Associated with Sexual Problems

Item	Sexual Problem
Medical problem or personal behavior	
Diabetes	Impotence
Hypertension	Impotence
Smoking	Erectile dysfunction
Substance abuse	Loss of libido, personal dysfunction, and altered interpersonal relationships
Depression	Decreased libido and sexual interest; altered interpersonal relationships
Hypotestosteronemia	Female: decreased libido, orgasmic dysfunction
	Male: erectile dysfunction, decreased libido
Menopause	Vaginal dryness, decreased libido
Medications and drugs (primary use)	
Aldomet (alpha-methyldopa; hypertension)	Erectile dysfunction, decreased libido in some
Amitriptyline (depression; Elavil)	Loss of desire, impotence, ejaculatory dysfunction
Barbiturates (depression; seizure disorders)	Increased libido at low doses, but with higher doses CNS depression and decreased libido
Benzodiazepines (depression; Lorazepam, Ativan, Librium)	CNS depression, decreased libido in higher doses and especially if mixed with alcohol
Carbamazepine (seizures; Tegretol)	Impotence
Chlorthalidone (hypertension; Hygroton)	Decreased desire, impotence
Cimetidine (peptic ulcer)	Erectile dysfunction, some libido effect
Clonidine (hypertension; Catapres)	Erectile dysfunction, some libido effect
Digoxin (heart failure, atrial fibrillation)	Decreased libido, impotence
Hydralazine (hypertension; Apresoline)	Impotence, priapism
Lithium (manic-depressive psychosis)	Decreased libido, impotence
Metoclopramide (gastroesophageal reflux, emesis; Reglan)	Decreased libido, erectile dysfunction
Metoprolol (hypertension; Lopressor)	Impotence
Monoamine oxidase inhibitors (depression)	Decreased libido, anorgasmia, retrograde ejaculation, erectile dysfunction
Nifedipine (hypertension)	Erectile dysfunction
Nortriptyline (Aventyl, Pamelor)	Impotence, decreased libido
Paroxetine (depression, panic disorder; Paxil)	Decreased libido, delayed or no orgasm
Phenothiazines (psychosis)	Decreased libido, erectile and ejaculatory dysfunction

The sexual history taken by the sex therapist is detailed and highly focused. For most clinicians, however, its purposes are less ambitious. First, it should convey to the patient a sense of comfort and trust that the physician regards sexuality and related issues as a legitimate part of health care. This is facilitated by the physician's general behavior, but also more specifically by care to listen carefully for hints of sexually related issues followed by nonobtrusive questions that give the patient "permission" to discuss her problems. If a patient perceives the physician as harboring prejudice toward her sexual values, communication is doomed to failure. Second, the physician should obtain enough information to determine if a sexual problem exists and whether it is appropriate to treat the patient or to refer her for more specialized care.

Physical examination for patients with sexual concerns is based on a thorough basic gynecologic examination. For example, dyspareunia in a young woman might be associated with extensive endometriosis or adhesions following pelvic inflammatory disease (PID) and, in an older woman not on hormone replacement therapy (HRT), with atrophic vaginitis. Detailed "sexological" examinations involving sexual evaluation, education, and counseling are appropriately reserved for sex therapists.

Barriers to Evaluating Sexual Problems

There are many barriers between the patient with a sexuality-related problem and effective care. One of the less discussed but potentially difficult barriers occurs *when the physician is uncomfortable with his or her own sexuality and/or sexual issues,* conveying this discomfort to the patient so that she, in turn, is unable to discuss her problems. A task for each physician is to review his or her own attitudes and feelings about sexual matters, seeking help when needed to resolve them at least within the context of the professional relationship.

A related barrier occurs *when the physician feels inadequately prepared in knowledge or skills or has insufficient time* to deal appropriately with a sexual problem. In this situation, the physician may directly or indirectly avoid identification of such problems. This barrier can be overcome by obtaining sufficient information and evaluation/management skills to identify a sexual problem, then treating the small number of problems amenable to limited care by a primary physician and referring the majority of problems to those with special training in sexual therapy.

Managing Sexual Problems

Some sexual problems can be managed by the primary physician, whereas others are best referred to a sex therapist. In general, single disorders of less than 1 year's duration in the context of a stable relationship are more likely to be amenable to simple interventions by a primary physician. Conversely, those patients with one or more problems that are comprised of multiple disorders, are of greater than 1 year's duration, and/or are in the context of an unstable or problematic relationship are usually best referred to a sex therapist. In addition, it is useful to determine whether a sexual problem is primary (present throughout the patient's lifetime) or secondary (began after an interval of satisfactory sexuality) and whether it is constant (occurs in all situations, with all partners) or situational (occurs in some situations, with some partners). In general, problems that are secondary and/or situational are more easily and successfully treated than those that are primary and/or constant. The former often involve simple problems causing sexual stimulation to not be effective or sustained enough. Careful history taking to determine the problem and corrective counseling often relieve the barrier to effective, sustained stimulation and return the couple to satisfactory sexuality.

Sexual dysfunctions are often categorized into the arousal and orgasmic disorders, the disorders of desire, and the paraphilias that have been discussed previously. *Arousal disorders* involve the inability or difficulty in becoming sexually excited, whereas *orgasmic disorders* involve the inability to obtain orgasm. Both categories of disorders may be caused by failure to have sustained effective sexual stimulation, may have physical causes (see Table 48.3), or may have emotional causes. If masturbation is possible, physical causes are unlikely although inadequate sexual stimulation remains a possible cause. In any case, these dysfunctions are often longstanding so that frustration and fear may engender confusion with disorders of desire. Patients with arousal or orgasmic disorders, it is noted, are generally interested in re-establishing satisfactory sexual function. *Disorders of desire* may be expressed as a part of other complaints, such as depression or marital conflict, or as a chief complaint. Two such disorders are *hypoactive sexual desire disorder,* a deficiency or absence of sexual fantasies or desire, and *sexual aversion disorder,* an aversion to or avoidance of genital sexual contact. Both cause interpersonal distress as well as dysfunction. Patients with such complex problems are usually best referred to a qualified sex therapist.

The PLISSIT model for treatment of sexual problems is useful for the physician who chooses to treat a sexual problem along the guidelines noted. *P is permission,* giving the patient explicit or implicit permission to deal with sexual issues or problems. It also includes permission for normal behavior such as the normal exploration of sexuality via masturbation during the teen years. *LI is limited information,* providing the patient with pertinent limited amounts of useful information. In this example, learning that limited masturbation is normal and not harmful facilitates the permission. *SS is specific suggestion,* giving the patient one or two specific suggestions for action. For example, following childbirth some couples have less satisfaction with coitus because the woman's vaginal walls are less elastic or the muscles looser than previously. Teaching the patient Kegel exercises to strengthen these muscles may alleviate this complaint. *IT is intensive therapy,* which in the context of the primary care physician means referral to a specialist in sexual therapy. Examples would be therapy for orgasmic dysfunction, male sexual dysfunction, and dyspareunia.

CASE STUDIES

For each of the following situations, imagine yourself a primary care physician in a rural practice. You have been presented or discovered a sexual problem and taken a brief but reasonably complete history of the problem and a general sexual history. You must now decide whether to treat the patient yourself (A), perhaps using the PLISSIT model, or refer the patient to a specialist in the treatment of sexual problems (B). For each case, choose one answer.
  A. Treat
  B. Refer

Case 48A

Your patient has been married for 6 months after a courtship of 2 years. At first, her marriage was fine, but now, with two new jobs and a new home, she and her husband just are not enjoying sex like they did before marriage. They are worried that something is wrong with them or that perhaps they made a mistake in getting married.

Answer: A

It is reasonable to treat this couple using the PLISSIT model. The most likely problems are inappropriate expectations of each other and of marriage, exhaustion, and coping with new and worrisome responsibilities. For example, giving "permission" to feel as they do may remove some underlying guilt that may be present. Providing "limited information"

(Continued)

about the effects of their life on their sexual relationship may help explain their feelings. Making "specific suggestions" about how to set aside time for each other may aid the therapeutic process. If these steps are ineffective, referral would then be appropriate.

Case 48B

After 6 years of marriage to her policeman husband, your patient is worried about her femininity (i.e., whether she is normal). Despite a vigorous and previously quite satisfactory sex life, she is unable to have multiple orgasms with her husband during intercourse. Both she and her husband are worried. Their relationship is strained; sex is now a feared chore.

Answer: A

Limited information within the framework of the PLISSIT model will help this couple understand that multiple orgasm is a possibility but not a requirement for all people for every sexual encounter. Permission to continue their previously satisfactory sex life should be helpful.

Case 48C

Your patient has been at college for a year now, but has been unable to enjoy herself on a date, just as throughout high school. She "knows" that at her age she should enjoy sex, but it is simply repulsive to think about being touched by a man. She is afraid of her future, afraid she may actually be a lesbian, although she is aware of no more positive feelings about women then she has for men.

Answer: B

Whatever problems this young woman has, they are of long duration and by definition complex. The PLISSIT model helps in this case by allowing you to give her permission to be afraid, limited information that she can receive help, and referral for therapy.

UNIT VII

Violence Against Women

C H A P T E R

49

SEXUAL ASSAULT AND DOMESTIC VIOLENCE

CHAPTER OBJECTIVES

This chapter deals primarily with APGO Objective(s):

OBJECTIVE 63   Sexual Assault

A. Describe the evaluation and treatment of victims of child and adult sexual assault.

B. Describe the rape trauma syndrome and the long-term physical and psychological adjustments of sexual assault victims.

OBJECTIVE 64   Domestic Violence

Describe the prevalence and incidence, assessment, and management options (including short- and long-term safety plans, appropriate social agency referral) for violence against women, older women, and children.

Sexual assault and domestic violence are the experience of far too many women and girls in the United States. They pose obvious immediate health and emotional risks, but in addition are associated with long-term effects on the mental and physical health of the victim and her family. The compassionate and thoughtful care of victims and their families is an important goal of everyone involved in the health care of women and girls.

SEXUAL ASSAULT

Sexual assault is the nonconsensual performance of acts, which in a consensual setting would be sexual or perceived as sexual, or which involve the body in such a manner that the victim perceives a sexual intrusion. An estimated one of every four women and children in the United States are sexual assault victims. Because of the stigmata associated with sexual assault, only 1 of 10 victims seeks help. Unfortunately, those victims who do seek help are often as traumatized by those from whom they seek help as by those who assaulted them. Because of the complex problems caused by sexual assault, treatment by a *multidisciplinary team* using prepared protocols is best. The health care team has three tasks: *(a) care for the victim's emotional needs, (b) evaluate and treat medically, and (c) collect forensic specimens.*

CARING FOR THE ADULT SEXUAL ASSAULT VICTIM

Rape Trauma Syndrome

During sexual assault, the victim realizes that she cannot escape the situation and has lost control. This *loss of control,* which is the most serious emotional problem faced by the victim, is based in fact, because *threatened or actual violence is always an integral part of sexual assault.* Victims of sexual assault may react to the experience in various ways. One recognized aftermath is the *rape trauma syndrome.* This syndrome has three phases. The *acute phase of rape trauma syndrome* begins with the assault, but may not be fully manifest until the time of initial disclosure, when the victim first tells someone of the assault. In this emotionally volatile time, the victim may appear calm, may be tearful and agitated, or may move from one extreme to another. *An inability to think clearly or remember things such as her past medical history, termed "cognitive dysfunction," is a particularly distressing aspect of the syndrome.* The involuntary loss of cognition may raise fears of "being crazy" or of being perceived as "crazy" by others. It is also frustrating for the health team unless it realizes that this is an involuntary reaction to the assault and not a willful action.

After the assault and before seeking care, the victim may have performed routine tasks such as shopping or cleaning the house. This *retreat to routine activities* is an emotional attempt to regain control, the presence or absence of which is not related to the severity of the assault. *Safety and regaining control are the victim's main emotional needs during this time.* The patient should be reassured about her immediate safety and offered as much control over events as is reasonable for her clinical situation. Discussing the sexual assault within a supportive environment facilitates a sense of control, even if the topics of discussion are themselves unpleasant.

During the *middle or "readjustment" phase,* the patient appears to resolve most issues about the assault. This resolution involves a rationalization that she should or could have prevented the assault, coupled with unrealistic plans to avoid another assault. The plans of this phase ultimately break down in the *late or "reorganization" phase,* as the victim begins to deal with the reality of her victimization.

The late phase, which may be quite lengthy, is a difficult and very painful time, often characterized by drastic changes in lifestyle, friends, and work. Ongoing counseling is important if the victim is to recover fully from the emotional traumas of the assault.

Initial Care

A team member should remain with the patient to help provide a sense of safety and security. The patient should be encouraged, in a supportive, nonjudgmental manner, to talk about the assault and her feelings. This starts the patient's emotional care and also provides historical data. Treatment for life-threatening trauma is, of course, begun immediately. Fortunately, such trauma is uncommon, although minor trauma is seen in one fourth of victims. Even in life-threatening situations, any sense of control that can be given the patient is helpful. Obtaining consents for treatment is not only a legal requirement but also an important aspect of the emotional care of the victim. Although patients are often reticent to do so, they should be gently encouraged to work with the police, because such cooperation is clearly associated with improved emotional outcomes for victims.

History taking about a sexual assault is uncomfortable for victims and health care providers alike. History taking is not, however, an additional trauma. Instead, it is both a necessary activity to gain medical and forensic information and an important therapeutic activity. Recalling the details of the assault in the supportive environment of the health care setting allows the victim to begin to gain an understanding of what has happened and to see that she and others can deal with the events. Victims of sexual assault characteristically perceive themselves as guilty of causing the assault, especially in situations in which they used poor judgment (e.g., hitchhiking). To say that any activity was acceptable when it involved poor judgment is a falsehood that destroys the patient's ultimate trust and the care provider's credibility. Reminding the patient that *"poor judgment is not a rapable offense"* helps the patient begin to place blame where it truly belongs: on the rapist.

Victims of sexual assault should be given a *complete general physical examination,* including a pelvic examination. Forensic specimens should be collected, and cultures for sexually transmitted diseases should be obtained. When collecting *forensic specimens,* it is critical that the clinician follow the directions on the forensic specimens kit. These specimens are kept in a health professional's possession or control

until turned over to an appropriate legal representative. This "protective custody" of the specimens ensures that the correct specimen reaches the forensic laboratory, and is called the "chain of evidence."

Initial *laboratory tests* should include cultures from the vagina, the anus, and, usually, the pharynx for gonorrhea and *Chlamydia,* rapid plasma reagin (RPR) for syphilis, hepatitis antigens, human immunodeficiency virus (HIV) if indicated (usually), urinalysis (UA) and culture and sensitivity (C&S), and a pregnancy test for menstrual-aged women (regardless of contraceptive status).

Antibiotic prophylaxis should be offered to all adult victims. The risk of infection is unknown, but it is clearly higher than for a consensual sexual experience. Recommended regimens include oral *doxycycline* (100 mg orally twice daily for 7 days) or oral *amoxicillin* (3 g orally once) plus *probenecid* (1 g orally once), followed by oral *erythromycin* base (500 mg orally twice daily for 7 days) for pregnant victims or those allergic to tetracyclines. In areas with a prevalence rate greater than 1% for antibiotic-resistant strains of *Neisseria gonorrhoeae,* ceftriaxone [Rocephin; 250 mg intramuscularly (IM)] followed by oral doxycycline (100 mg orally twice daily for 7 days) is recommended. *Tetanus toxoid* should be administered if indicated.

Ovral (0.05 mg ethinyl estradiol and 0.5 mg norgestrel), two tablets orally followed by two tablets 12 hours later, may be given as *postcoital contraceptive medication.* Other regimens are listed in Chapter 25. If a postcoital contraception is chosen, the patient should be reminded that these medications may be teratogenic, so that a therapeutic abortion is offered if pregnancy does occur despite their use.

Within 24 to 48 hours, victims should be contacted by phone or seen for an *immediate posttreatment evaluation.* At this time, emotional or physical problems are managed and follow-up appointments arranged for 1 and 6 weeks. Potentially serious problems such as suicidal ideation, rectal bleeding, or evidence of pelvic infection may go unrecognized by the victim during this time because of fear or continued cognitive dysfunction. Gently stated but specific questions must be asked to ensure that such problems have not arisen.

Subsequent Care

At the 1-week visit, a general review of the patient's progress is made and any specific new problems addressed. The next routine visit is at 6 weeks, when a complete evaluation, including physical examination, repeat cultures for sexually transmitted diseases, and a repeat RPR, is performed. Another visit at 12 to 18 weeks may be indicated for repeat HIV titers, although the current understanding of HIV infection does not allow an estimate of the risk of exposure for sexual assault victims. Each victim should receive as much counseling and support as is necessary, with referral to a long-term counseling program if needed.

CARING FOR THE CHILD SEXUAL ASSAULT VICTIM

A total of 90% of child victimization is by parents, family members, or family friends; "stranger rape" is relatively uncommon in children. The assailants play on the child's need for love and her dependency on family. To get past this conflict, it is best to interview child victims apart from parents and other family members, if possible by interviewers skilled in child interview techniques. Although such interviewing and the interpretation of information gained are difficult, in general, a child who displays a knowledge of sexual matters, anatomy, or function beyond that expected for her years is very likely a victim of sexual abuse. Expert interviewers may use such specialized techniques as anatomically correct doll play and drawing interpretation to facilitate the process.

The physical examination of a small child requires patience and much experience. Sedation should be avoided, because it cannot be done sufficiently to allay anxiety in an outpatient setting. Instead, it usually adds to the child's fear and sense of helplessness. Examination under anesthesia may be required, although nonobtrusive techniques have been developed to avoid this procedure.

Prophylactic antibiotic therapy should be offered children if there is evidence that the assailant is infected, if follow-up compliance is unlikely, or if the assailant is a stranger. Otherwise, prophylactic antibiotic therapy usually is not indicated. Of course, any diagnosed infection in the child is treated as appropriate. Recommended regimens include amoxicillin (50 mg/kg body weight once) plus probenecid (25 mg/kg body weight to a maximum dose of 1 g). For penicillin-allergic children or in geographic areas with a high prevalence of penicillinase-producing gonococci, spectinomycin (40 mg/kg body weight IM) or ceftriaxone (125 mg IM once) followed by erythromycin (50 mg/kg body weight orally for 7 days) can be given.

It is the responsibility of the care team to determine if the child may safely return home or if the risk of ongoing abuse requires foster home placement or hospitalization. *Because suspected child sexual abuse must be reported to police and child welfare authorities,* these agencies may officially help in this decision, although responsibility rests with the care team at the time of the initial disclosure.

DOMESTIC VIOLENCE

Domestic violence is experienced by an estimated 25%–50% of women during their life and is suggested as a significant source of illness and injury to women. Consider that one in five women who present to an emergency room has been injured by her partner; in approximately 90% of domestic homicides there is a history of a police call for domestic violence within the year; about 10% of adolescents are battered by a parent; and an estimated three-fourths of women indicate that they have been victims of domestic violence and would have discussed the situation with their physician if they had been asked.

TABLE 49.1.   Indicators of Physical Abuse in Domestic Violence

Area of Injury	Descriptions
Head and neck	Bruises, abrasions, strangle marks, black eye, broken nose, orbital ridge, or jaw, pulled hair, permanent hearing loss, facial lacerations
Trunk	Evidence of blunt trauma, including bruises (especially breasts and abdomen), fractured collarbones and ribs
Skin	Multiple lesions in various stages of healing, "rug rash" abrasions, burns (cigarette, lighter, liquid splash), bites
Extremities	Evidence of restraint, including muscle strains, spiral fractures, rope or restraint burns, "crescent moon" shape fingernail marks or bruises in the shape of a hand or blunt instrument

What is domestic violence, and how is it recognized? *Domestic violence* may involve one or more of three presentations. *Physical abuse* such as hitting, slapping, kicking, and choking is the most obvious presentation. It is suspected when there is evidence of trauma, especially to the head and neck or trunk associated with a history of violence, or when an explanation of the trauma doesn't seem appropriate (Table 49.1). Unfortunately, pregnancy appears to be a period of greater risk for such episodes. *Sexual abuse* is another presentation of domestic violence. The third presentation is *emotional* or *psychological abuse* and is often very traumatic. Examples include undermining of self worth, deprivation of sleep or emotional support, repetitive unpredictability of response to life situations, threats, destruction of personal property or the killing of pets, lies, manipulation of friends, and interference in the workplace. Domestic violence is usually cyclic and repetitive, with periods of calm alternating with periods of rapidly increasing tensions or violence, the latter often increasing in severity with each iteration of the cycle.

Recognition is the first, most important, and most often missed issue. When domestic violence is suspected, compassionate and thoughtful discussion with the possible victim as well as attention to any physical injury is requisite. Indeed, all patients should be asked about the presence of violence in their lives as part of the routine health history.

When addressing this issue with a patient, the acronym *SAFE* is easy to remember and addresses the basic issues:

S   Does the patient feel safe? At home? At school? In the workplace? If not, who or what does she fear, and why?

A   Has the patient felt abused in a relationship? In her present relationship? How? When someone is angry in the patient's home, what is it like and what is likely to happen?

F   Are there friends or family, or clergy, who can help? Who can the patient turn to for support?

E   Does the patient have a plan, or idea, of what she would do in an emergency? If she has children, do they know where to go for and how to get help?

Clearly, no simple rule will suffice to deal with these complex and emotionally charged situations. Each must be dealt with according to its specifics and the wishes of the patient. As in the evaluation and treatment of the sexual assault victim, the patient's consent for each stage of care is needed and facilitates the process. Similarly, if there is evidence of immediate risk to the patient or to her children or someone else, law enforcement contact is required.

Just listening and being supportive is in itself helpful. Follow-up may include refer- ral to a battered women's hotline, shelter, or counseling center. Therefore, familiarity with these resources in the practice area is important.

CASE STUDIES

Case 49A

A 15-year-old G2 P2 presents to the emergency room accompanied by police, to whom she has reported a sexual assault. She is quiet but seems disoriented, dressed in a see-through blouse and tight stretch pants. She tells the nurses that she was raped by a "friend." The police ask that you speed your evaluation, because they have other calls and need to be on their way.

Questions Case 49A

Which of the following should guide your initial evaluation of this patient?

A. Rapid conclusion of the evaluation to cooperate with the police
B. Dismissing the claim of rape because it was a friend, hence clearly consensual sex rather than rape
C. Concern that the historical information is incomplete, requiring a full evaluation regardless of pressure to proceed more rapidly
D. Because she is a minor, calling her parents to get permission to see the patient and obtain further information

Answer: C

Your primary responsibilities are emotional and physical health care of the patient. Cooperation with police is important, especially in the initial phase to provide immediate information for pursuit of the assailant. Thereafter, police action is best left until after health care is completed. Knowing that sexual abuse in children is often performed by family members, you may contact parents, but plan to pay special attention to the child's history. The patient's attire is irrelevant unless it is torn, stained, or otherwise presents information about what has happened.

Your sexual assault team completes its evaluation, and you discover that your patient lives with her mother and stepfather. She is afraid to tell your team about details of what has happened, but does indicate it has been going on for some time. She is frightened to return home. Her physical examination is unremarkable except that her uterus is about 14 weeks' size and soft. What laboratory tests are indicated?

A. UA
B. Urine human chorionic gonadotropin (hCG)
C. Urine drug screen
D. Papanicolaou smear
E. Hepatitis screen

Answer: B

By history and examination, pregnancy is likely and a pregnancy test is appropriate. The other tests listed may be useful in general, but do not address the specific issue: Who is abusing this child?

(Continued)

Case 49B

A 35-year-old mother of three and wife of a heavy-equipment operator presents, complaining that her husband raped her earlier in the day after she refused him "his sex." She says he threatened to beat her if she did not "lie down and take it," so she did. Physical examination reveals only motile sperm in the vagina. The patient has had a postpartum tubal ligation. She says she wishes medical care but does not want the police notified because they will "cause too much trouble." Her husband arrives and demands that you "get out of his business" and let his wife go so that she can fix dinner.

Question Case 49B

Your appropriate response(s) to this situation include

A. Tell the patient to go home, that how and when she and her husband have sex is their business and not yours

B. Complete a sexual assault workup

C. Notify the police

D. Call psychiatry because the patient is clearly not demonstrating an appropriate response to a sexual assault

Answers: B, C

In some states, a husband cannot by law rape his wife (in effect, she is in the eyes of the law his sexual property), whereas in other states, rape is defined as a nonconsensual experience. In either case, this legal decision is not properly made by you, but by the police, who should be notified. You may support the patient's decision not to talk to the police—although you should encourage her to do so—but you must call the police because a violent crime has been reported and because you do not know what the situation is at home, especially in relation to the safety of the children.

STUDY QUESTIONS

INSTRUCTIONS FOR STUDY QUESTIONS

The study questions are designed to help you test how well you learned the content of each chapter, and to maximize the usefulness of the questions you should:

1. Read the chapter through completely at least once.
2. Answer all of the study questions (do not check your answer after each question).
3. Reread the parts of the chapter related to the questions you answered incorrectly.

The correct answer to each question is contained in the chapter. Questions do not necessarily follow the order that the information is presented in the chapter.

The questions are in multiple choice and matching format. For the matching questions, more than one option may be correct. Read the questions carefully and read instructions for the different item formats.

Questions and Answers Chapter 1:
Health Care for Women

1.1 The last menstrual period is dated from the
   a. first day of the last normal period
   b. last day of the last normal period
   c. first day of the last bleeding episode
   d. last day of the last bleeding episode

1.2 Postmenopausal bleeding is defined as
   a. bleeding beginning 6 months after cessation of menses
   b. irregular bleeding continuing for 6 months after cessation of regular menses
   c. bleeding beginning 12 months after cessation of menses
   d. irregular bleeding continuing for 12 months after cessation of regular menses

ANSWERS (1.1–1.2)

1.1   a   1.2   a

1.3 The passage of clots during menstruation
a. is always abnormal
b. may be either normal or abnormal
c. is always normal

Instructions for items 1.4 to 1.8: Match the abbreviation in the obstetric history with its appropriate definition. An option may be used once, more than once, or not at all.

G [4] P [5][6][7][8]

1.4 [4] stands for

1.5 [5] stands for

1.6 [6] stands for

1.7 [7] stands for

1.8 [8] stands for
a. Number of living children
b. Number of pregnancies
c. Number of term pregnancies
d. Number of preterm pregnancies
e. Number of abortions

1.9 Inquiry concerning adult and child history of sexual abuse and assault should be included in the sexual history
a. only for a patient with whom the physician has a long-standing rapport
b. only if a specific indication is noted
c. always, even for a new patient
d. sometimes, if the length of the visit permits

1.10 Tanner's classification with respect to the breast relates to changes in
a. the breast before and after lactation
b. the breast associated with malignancy
c. the breast associated with maturation
d. breast configuration associated with galactorrhea

1.11 Breast examination is done in the
a. supine position
b. sitting position
c. both
d. neither

1.12 Peau d'orange change in the breast is associated with
a. edema of the lymphatics
b. jaundice
c. too vigorous breast-feeding
d. galactorrhea

1.13 Which kind of speculum is often most suitable for examination of the nulliparous patient?
a. Graves speculum
b. Pederson speculum
c. Mogans speculum
d. Ling speculum

1.14 During the speculum examination, vaginal lubricant does NOT interfere with
a. cervical cytology
b. cervical cultures
c. wet preparation
d. cervical visualization

1.15 Which uterine configuration is most difficult to assess for size, shape, configuration, and mobility?
a. Anteverted
b. Anteverted, anteflexed
c. Midposition
d. Retroverted
e. Retroverted, retroflexed

1.16 Pap smears should be fixed no more than how many second(s) after preparation?
a. 1
b. 10
c. 20
d. 30

ANSWERS (1.3–1.16)					
1.3 b	1.6 d	1.9 c	1.11 c	1.13 b	1.15 e
1.4 b	1.7 e	1.10 c	1.12 a	1.14 d	1.16 b
1.5 c	1.8 a				

1.17 The rectovaginal examination should be performed
  a. only when there are symptoms of pelvic relaxation or fecal incontinence
  b. only at the initial patient visit, except when symptoms are present
  c. at the initial patient visit and all annual visits

Instructions for items 1.18 to 1.22: Match the condition and the test to detect it with the appropriate screening examination recommendation. An option may be used once, more than once, or not at all.

1.18 Thyroid disease, thyroid-stimulating hormone

1.19 Cervical dysplasia, Pap smear

1.20 Hypercholesterolemia, cholesterol/lipid profile

1.21 Breast cancer, mammography

1.22 Bowel cancer, sigmoidoscopy
  a. Every 5 years from age 19, every 3–4 years after age 65
  b. Every other year from age 40, yearly after age 50
  c. Every 3–5 years after age 65
  d. Annually from puberty or at onset of sexual activity
  e. Every 3–5 years after age 40

Instructions for items 1.23 to 1.26: Match the immunization with the appropriate recommendation for its timing. An option may be used once, more than once, or not at all.

1.23 Tetanus–diphtheria booster

1.24 Influenza vaccine

1.25 Pneumococcal vaccine

1.26 Hepatitis B vaccine
  a. Every 10 years from age 19–64 when at risk
  b. Once between ages 14 and 16
  c. For at risk groups
  d. Every 10 years between ages 19–64 when at risk; yearly after age 65

1.27 Obstetrician–gynecologists provide primary as well as specialty care for about what percent of women in the United States?
  a. 25%
  b. 50%
  c. 75%
  d. 100%

Instructions for items 1.28 to 1.31: For women in each of the following age categories, select the significant causes(s) of morbidity. An option may be used once, more than once, or not at all.

1.28 12–18 years of age

1.29 19–39 years of age

1.30 40–64 years of age

1.31 More than 65 years of age
  a. Head, ears, eyes, nose, and throat (HEENT) conditions
  b. Upper respiratory infections
  c. Infection (viral, parasites, bacterial)
  d. Sexual abuse
  e. Accidental injury
  f. Digestive tract conditions
  g. Acute urinary conditions
  h. Osteoporosis/arthritis
  i. Hypertension
  j. Orthopedic conditions
  k. Heart disease
  l. Hearing and vision impairment
  m. Urinary incontinence

ANSWERS (1.17–1.31)

1.17 c	1.21 b	1.25 a	1.28 a, b, c, d, e, f, g	1.30 a, b, h, i, j, k, l
1.18 c	1.22 e	1.26 c		
1.19 d	1.23 b	1.27 b	1.29 a, b, c, e, g	1.31 a, b, e, h, i, k, l, m
1.20 a	1.24 d			

Instructions for items 1.32 to 1.35: For women in the following age categories, select the significant cause(s) of death from the list of conditions/situations. An option may be used once, more than once, or not at all.

1.32 12–18 years of age

1.33 19–39 years of age

1.34 40–64 years of age

1.35 More than 65 years of age
   a. Motor vehicle accidents
   b. Homicide
   c. Suicide
   d. Leukemia
   e. Cardiovascular disease
   f. Coronary artery disease
   g. Acquired immune deficiency syndrome
   h. Breast cancer
   i. Uterine cancer
   j. Lung cancer
   k. Cerebrovascular accident
   l. Colorectal cancer
   m. Obstructive lung disease
   n. Ovarian cancer
   o. Pneumonia/influenza
   p. Accidents

Instructions for items 1.36 to 1.42: Match the risk factor or condition with the recommended screening test or intervention. An option may be used once, more than once, or not at all.

1.36 Cervical dysplasia

1.37 Skin cancer

1.38 Anemia

1.39 Hypercholesterolemia, coronary artery disease

1.40 Breast cancer

1.41 Colorectal cancer

1.42 Thyroid disease
   a. Sickle-cell preparation
   b. Cholesterol/lipid profile
   c. Yearly physician examination
   d. Self-examination
   e. Screening mammography
   f. Hemogram
   g. Physical examination of suspicious lesions
   h. Fecal occult blood test
   i. Thyroid-stimulating hormone
   j. Sigmoidoscopy
   k. Pap smear

1.43 Which of the following is NOT usually a task for the physician at the time of the initial patient evaluation?
   a. Establishing and developing a professional relationship of mutual trust and respect with the patient
   b. Gathering historical information
   c. Gathering physical information
   d. Making a differential diagnosis
   e. Making a definitive diagnosis
   f. Identifying issues involving health maintenance and disease prevention

1.44 If a patient becomes uncomfortable with a topic during a history-taking session, the best response of the physician is to
   a. ignore the discomfort and proceed with questioning
   b. discontinue discussion of the topic to avoid further patient discomfort and damage to the patient–physician relationship
   c. address the patient's discomfort in a positive and supportive manner
   d. make a joke about the patient's evident discomfort to relieve tension

ANSWERS (1.32–1.44)

1.32 a, b, d	1.35 e, f, h, j,	1.36 k	1.39 b	1.42 i
1.33 a, b, e, f,	k, l, m,	1.37 g	1.40 c, d, e	1.43 e
g, h, i, m	o, p	1.38 a, f	1.41 h, j	1.44 c
1.34 e, f, h, j,				
k, l, m, n				

1.45 When recording the chief complaint in the medical record, the physician should always
   a. record the complaint as a direct quote
   b. summarize the complaint so as to be efficient
   c. take care not to obscure the patient's meaning with medical jargon

1.46 Inquiry about pelvic pain, which interferes with daily activities or requires more analgesia than provided by plain aspirin or acetaminophen, should include questions about
   a. the duration and quality of pain
   b. the timing of the pain in relation to menses
   c. the radiation of pain to areas outside of the pelvis
   d. the association of pain with body position
   e. all of the above items

1.47 Which of the following is not typically included in an inquiry about menses?
   a. An estimation of the menstrual flow in milliliters
   b. The number of pads or tampons used during the heavy part of menstrual flow
   c. Whether pads or tampons are soaked at the time of removal
   d. The presence and size of clots
   e. The presence of intermenstrual bleeding

1.48 In the gynecologic history, it is often possible to distinguish between vaginitis and pelvic inflammatory disease by inquiring about
   a. the route of medical therapy used (topical or oral/parenteral)
   b. the symptoms present (fever/chills, itching)
   c. the presence and character of vaginal discharge
   d. all of the above

1.49 Which of the following should be included in the history of a patient with infertility?
   a. Previous fertility
   b. Previous disease in the male partner
   c. Sexual practices
   d. All of the above

1.50 The most cost-effective and reliable means of early detection of breast cancer is
   a. a yearly mammogram alone
   b. a yearly breast examination alone
   c. a yearly breast examination, combined with appropriately scheduled mammography
   d. a yearly breast examination and instruction in self breast examination, combined with appropriately scheduled mammography

1.51 Which of the following statements about the steps in the breast examination is correct?
   a. Palpation is done first
   b. Inspection is done first
   c. Palpation and inspection are done simultaneously

ANSWERS (1.45–1.51)

| 1.45 c | 1.47 a | 1.48 d | 1.49 d | 1.50 d | 1.51 b |
| 1.46 e | | | | | |

1.52 Elevating the head of the examining table approximately 30 degrees facilitates
a. the ability of the patient to comfortably look around to distract her from the examination
b. the contraction of the abdominal wall muscle groups making examination easier
c. the observation of the patient's responses
d. the physician not being distracted by eye contact with the patient

1.53 Which statement about use of gloves during the routine pelvic examination is correct?
a. Gloves are only needed if there is a history of sexually transmitted disease
b. A glove is only needed on the right (dominant) hand
c. Gloves should be worn on both hands

1.54 The presence of dissymmetry of the external genitalia
a. is usually normal and needs no follow-up
b. may be caused by disease and should be evaluated
c. should only be followed-up if there is accompanying pain or pressure sensation

Instructions for items 1.55 to 1.56: Match the type of speculum with the indications for its more common use. An option may be used once, more than once, or not at all.

1.55 Graves speculum

1.56 Pederson speculum
a. Parous menstrual woman
b. Prepubertal girl

1.57 Which of the following statements about the bimanual examination is INCORRECT?
a. A partially filled bladder generally facilitates bimanual identification of the adnexa
b. Pressure with the abdominal hand should be applied with the flat and not the tips of the fingers
c. The uterus should be evaluated for size, shape, consistency, configuration, and mobility
d. An anteverted cervix is usually associated with a retroverted uterus
e. Sharp flexion of the uterus may alter the expected relations between the cervix and uterus

1.58 Normal ovaries are palpable in the menstrual-aged woman what percent of the time?
a. 30%
b. 40%
c. 50%
d. 60%
e. 70%

ANSWERS (1.52–1.58)

1.52 c	1.54 b	1.55 a	1.56 b	1.57 a	1.58 c
1.53 c					

Instructions for items 1.59 to 1.65: Match the breast finding with the condition with which it is most commonly associated. An option may be used once, more than once, or not at all.

1.59 Mobile lump

1.60 Axillary involvement

1.61 Lump is well circumcised in examination

1.62 Lump with limited mobility

1.63 Nipple discharge

1.64 Rubbery feel

1.65 Multiple lumps
   a. Fibrocystic disorder
   b. Fibroadenoma
   c. Carcinoma of the breast

Instructions for items 1.66 to 1.67: Match the item with the description with which it is best associated. An option may be used once, more than once, or not at all.

1.66 Consultation

1.67 Referral
   a. Clinical opinion
   b. Clinical care

ANSWERS (1.59–1.67)

1.59 a, b	1.61 a, b	1.63 c	1.65 a	1.66 a	1.67 b
1.60 c	1.62 c	1.64 b			

Questions and Answers Chapter 2:
Ethics in Obstetrics and Gynecology

2.1 A 32-year-old patient has delivered at 25 weeks of gestation, three days after premature rupture of the membranes. She has discussed the circumstances with her obstetrician and requests that no attempts at resuscitation should be made. At delivery there are rare gasping breathing movements. The pediatrician demands that intubation be done. The individual with the clearest primary responsibility for this decision is the:
   a. mother
   b. pediatrician
   c. obstetrician
   d. hospital attorney

2.2 Which of the following is NOT among the main domains of ethical concern in medical care?
   a. Justice issues
   b. Patient preference issues
   c. Legal issues
   d. Medical indications or benefit issues
   e. Quality of life issues

2.3 Quality of life issues primarily concern the:
   a. physician's estimate of outcome
   b. patient's experience of outcome
   c. population-based evaluation of outcome
   d. patient's choice of outcome

2.4 Respect for patient wishes (autonomy) requires that there be assessment of all of the following EXCEPT the:
   a. patient's ability to consider information
   b. severity of the illness and the potential success of the proposed therapy
   c. impact of the patient's choice on her family
   d. cost of the proposed treatment

2.5 A 62-year-old woman with newly diagnosed stage III ovarian cancer refuses chemotherapy. She wants to "go home to die." The next step in evaluating this patient is to:
   a. assess the patient's comprehension and look for evidence of depression
   b. accept the patient's wishes and discharge her from the hospital
   c. call the hospital attorney to assess risk of malpractice
   d. call the family for a conference

2.6 A 90-year-old woman is found to have a 20-centimeter pelvic/abdominal mass. Her Ca125 is 90. Your recommendation for care should be based in the ethical area of:
   a. beneficence–non-maleficence
   b. statutory law
   c. autonomy
   d. justice
   e. quality of life
   f. conflict of interest
   g. futility
   h. surrogate decision making
   i. advance directives

ANSWERS (2.1–2.6)

| 2.1 | a | 2.2 | c | 2.3 | b | 2.4 | a | 2.5 | a | 2.6 | a |

2.7 A 33-year-old physician sees a 21-year-old primigravid woman in the emergency room for a urinary tract infection (UTI). She discovers the patient is going to give the child up for adoption and gives the patient her lawyer's phone number. She states she has been looking for a child to adopt and goes over all the advantages she can offer the child. Her actions fall into the ethical area of:
a. beneficence–non-maleficence
b. statutory law
c. autonomy
d. justice
e. quality of life
f. conflict of interest
g. futility
h. surrogate decision making
i. advance directives

2.8 A 60-year-old woman is admitted semicomatose with fever and a white blood count of 1000, 10 days after chemotherapy for breast cancer. She has an advance directive on record and her husband accompanies her. The decision to treat is made based on the ethical area of:
a. beneficence–non-maleficence
b. statutory law
c. autonomy
d. justice
e. quality of life
f. conflict of interest
g. futility
h. surrogate decision making
i. advance directives

2.9 A 28-year-old woman with metastatic breast cancer wants to try a bone marrow transplant-supported treatment. Her insurance company refuses. The ethical area involved is:
a. beneficence–non-maleficence
b. statutory law
c. autonomy
d. justice
e. quality of life
f. conflict of interest
g. futility
h. surrogate decision making
i. advance directives

Instructions for items 2.10 to 2.13: Match the issue with the corresponding illustrative questions. An option may be used once, more than once, or not at all.

2.10 Medical indication

2.11 Patient preference

2.12 Quality of life

2.13 Contextual issues
a. What does the patient want?
b. What are the needs of society?
c. What impact will the proposed treatment or lack of it have on the patient's life?
d. What is the best treatment? Best alternatives?

Instructions for items 2.14 to 2.17: Match the issue with the corresponding ethical principle. An option may be used once, more than once, or not at all.

2.14 Medical indication

2.15 Patient preference

2.16 Quality of life

2.17 Contextual issues
   a. Beneficence
   b. Non-maleficence
   c. Autonomy
   d. Justice

Instructions for items 2.18 to 2.21: Match the ethical principle with the appropriate definition. An option may be used once, more than once, or not at all.

2.18 Beneficence

2.19 Non-maleficence

2.20 Autonomy

2.21 Justice
   a. The patient should be given what is "due."
   b. There should be respect for the patient's right to self-determination.
   c. There is a duty not to inflict harm or injury.
   d. There is a duty to promote the good of the patient.

Questions and Answers Chapter 3: Embryology, Anatomy, and Reproductive Genetics

3.1   The genital system develops from embryonic
 a. ectoderm
 b. mesoderm
 c. endoderm

3.2   The urogenital ridges give rise to elements of the
 a. cardiovascular system
 b. reproductive system
 c. muscular system
 d. skeletal system

3.3   What part of the ovary comes to contain the developing follicles?
 a. Cortex
 b. Medulla

3.4   The first indication of the sex of the embryo is the
 a. entry of primordial germ cells
 b. formation of the tunica albuginea
 c. formation of primordial follicles
 d. degeneration of the genital ducts

3.5   The primordial germ cells can be identified during the fourth week of development in the
 a. yolk sac
 b. gonadal ridge
 c. urogenital sinus
 d. cortical cords

3.6   In the female, which of the following persists to form the major parts of the reproductive tract?
 a. Paramesonephric (müllerian) ducts
 b. Mesonephric (wolffian) ducts

3.7   The formation of the uterus and fallopian tubes
 a. is dependent on the presence of ovaries
 b. is not dependent on the presence of ovaries

3.8   Absence of the ovaries
 a. is the most common anomaly of the female reproductive tract
 b. typically occurs in association with other anomalies
 c. arises from the failure of the paramesonephric ducts to fuse

Instructions for items 3.9 to 3.10: Match the developmental abnormality of the uterus with the underlying cause. An option may be used once, more than once, or not at all.

3.9   Absence of uterus

3.10   Double uterus (uterus didelphys)
 a. Inferior parts of the paramesonephric ducts do not fuse
 b. Paramesonephric ducts degenerate

Instructions for items 3.11 to 3.12: Match the developmental abnormality of the vagina with the underlying cause. An option may be used once, more than once, or not at all.

3.11   Absence of the vagina

3.12   Vaginal atresia
 a. Vaginal plate does not canalize
 b. Vaginal plate does not develop

ANSWERS (3.1–3.12)

3.1 b	3.3 a	3.5 a	3.7 b	3.9 b	3.11 b
3.2 b	3.4 b	3.6 a	3.8 b	3.10 a	3.12 a

3.13 Which of the following does NOT form from the urogenital sinus?
a. Urethra
b. Hymen
c. Epithelium of the urinary bladder
d. Rectum

3.14 Which of the following passes through an indifferent (undifferentiated) stage during development?
a. Genital ducts
b. Gonads
c. External genitalia
d. All of the above

3.15 The labia minora develop from the
a. genital tubercle
b. urogenital folds
c. labioscrotal swellings
d. urogenital sinus

3.16 The labia majora develop from the
a. genital tubercle
b. urogenital folds
c. labioscrotal swellings
d. urogenital sinus

3.17 The clitoris develops from the
a. genital tubercle
b. urogenital folds
c. labioscrotal swellings
d. urogenital sinus

3.18 The fallopian tube is derived from the
a. wolffian (mesonephric) ducts
b. metanephric ducts
c. müllerian (paramesonephric) ducts
d. urogenital sinus

3.19 The vagina originates from the
a. urogenital sinus and müllerian ducts
b. müllerian ducts and wolffian ducts
c. mesonephric ducts and metanephric ducts
d. urogenital sinus and wolffian ducts

3.20 In the female, the embryologic homolog of the penis is the
a. labia majora
b. frenulum
c. clitoris

3.21 Which of the following is NOT a component of the innominate bones?
a. Ilium
b. Tibia
c. Ischium
d. Pubis

3.22 The false pelvis and true pelvis are separated by the
a. acetabulum
b. sacrospinous ligament
c. linea terminalis
d. obturator membrane
e. obturator foramen

3.23 The dimensions of which pelvis must be adequate to permit passage of the fetus during labor?
a. True pelvis
b. False pelvis

3.24 The false pelvis is separated from the true pelvis by the plane of the
a. pelvic inlet
b. greatest diameter
c. least diameter
d. pelvic outlet

ANSWERS (3.13–3.24)

3.13 d	3.15 b	3.17 a	3.19 a	3.21 b	3.23 a
3.14 d	3.16 c	3.18 c	3.20 c	3.22 c	3.24 a

3.25 Arrest of fetal descent occurs most commonly at the plane of the
a. pelvic inlet
b. greatest diameter
c. least diameter
d. pelvic outlet

Instructions for items 3.26 to 3.29: Match the pelvic plane diameter with the appropriate value. An option may be used once, more than once, or not at all.

3.26 Obstetric conjugate

3.27 Transverse diameter of inlet

3.28 Bispinous diameter of midplane

3.29 Transverse diameter of greatest diameter
a. 10.0–11.0
b. 10.0
c. 12.5
d. 13.5

3.30 Based on the Caldwell and Moloy classification, the most common pelvic type is the
a. gynecoid
b. android
c. anthropoid
d. platypelloid

Instructions for items 3.31 to 3.32: Match the component of the vulva with the structures that it contains. An option may be used once, more than once, or not at all.

3.31 Labia majora

3.32 Labia minora
a. Sebaceous glands
b. Sweat glands
c. Hair follicles

Instructions for items 3.33 to 3.37: Match the structure with the type of epithelium that lines it. An option may be used once, more than once, or not at all.

3.33 Bartholin's duct

3.34 Skene's duct

3.35 Urethra

3.36 Vagina

3.37 Endocervical canal
a. Squamous
b. Columnar
c. Transitional

3.38 Compared with the posterior wall, the anterior wall of the vagina is
a. longer
b. the same length
c. shorter

3.39 The uterine (fallopian) tubes enter into which part of the uterus?
a. Fundus
b. Cornu
c. Mesosalpinx
d. Cardinal ligament
e. Lower uterine segment

3.40 The two main anatomic divisions of the uterus are the
a. corpus and fundus
b. cornu and fundus
c. corpus and cervix
d. cervix and isthmus

3.41 Which of the following vessels does NOT supply the uterus?
a. Ovarian artery
b. Uterine artery
c. Vaginal artery

ANSWERS (3.25–3.41)					
3.25 c	3.28 b	3.31 a, b, c	3.34 c	3.37 b	3.40 c
3.26 a	3.29 c	3.32 a, b	3.35 c	3.38 c	3.41 c
3.27 d	3.30 a	3.33 c	3.36 a	3.39 b	

3.42 The uterine veins enter the
  a. common iliac veins
  b. internal iliac veins
  c. inferior vena cava
  d. femoral veins
  e. external iliac veins

3.43 The portion of the fallopian tube that borders the ovary is the
  a. isthmus
  b. ampulla
  c. infundibulum

3.44 Which of the following ligaments does NOT support the uterus?
  a. Uterosacral ligaments
  b. Cardinal ligaments
  c. Round ligaments
  d. Broad ligaments
  e. Ovarian ligaments

3.45 Before puberty, the ratio of the length of the body of the uterus to the length of the cervix is approximately
  a. 1:1
  b. 2:1
  c. 3:1
  d. 4:1

3.46 Which of the following statements about the uterine artery is INCORRECT?
  a. It is a branch of the hypogastric artery
  b. It anastomoses with the ovarian vessels
  c. It anastomoses with the vaginal vessels
  d. It penetrates the uterus at the level of the internal cervical os after passing under the ureter

3.47 The portion of the broad ligament between the ovaries and the fallopian tube is called the
  a. round ligament
  b. ligament of Jacobs
  c. cardinal ligament
  d. mesosalpinx

3.48 The uterosacral ligaments
  a. arise from the lateral wall of the uterus
  b. attach to the sacrum at S3-4
  c. prevent prolapse of the uterus into the vagina
  d. exert tension on the cervix ventrally

3.49 Which of the following statements about the attachment of the ovary is INCORRECT?
  a. The ovary is attached to the broad ligament by the mesovarium
  b. The ovary is attached to the uterus by the ovarian ligament
  c. The ovary is attached to the side of the pelvis by the infundibulopelvic ligament
  d. The ovary is attached to the fallopian tube by the ovarian ligament

3.50 Hilus cells are found in the
  a. ovarian cortex
  b. ovarian medulla
  c. mesovarium
  d. graafian follicles

3.51 The streak ovary is associated with
  a. Klinefelter's syndrome
  b. Asherman's syndrome
  c. osteogenesis imperfecta
  d. embryonic gonadal death

3.52 The blood supply to the fallopian tubes is from
  a. the ovarian arteries only
  b. the uterine arteries only
  c. both the ovarian and uterine arteries

3.53 Compared with the reproductive years, the size of the ovary of a menopausal woman is
  a. increased
  b. unchanged
  c. decreased

ANSWERS (3.42–3.53)

3.42 b	3.44 e	3.46 d	3.48 c	3.50 b	3.52 c
3.43 c	3.45 a	3.47 d	3.49 d	3.51 d	3.53 c

3.54 The diploid number of chromosomes in humans is
   a. 23
   b. 32
   c. 46
   d. 48
   e. 92

3.55 Which of the following statements about human chromosomes is INCORRECT?
   a. Genes are located along the length of a chromosome in a linear fashion
   b. Genes are lengths of DNA that encode a specific peptide sequence
   c. Chromosomes are composed of DNA associated with histones
   d. Human chromosomes are formed in 23 heterologous pairs
   e. The normal human chromosome complement is 44 autosomes and two sex chromosomes

3.56 Which of the following should NOT be part of standard genetic counseling?
   a. Obtaining information from patients
   b. Reviewing appropriate diagnostic modalities
   c. Assessing risk in future pregnancies
   d. Guiding the patient to the most appropriate management option
   e. Providing empathetic support for a patient's decision

3.57 Which of the following chromosome abnormalities is the most common among live-born infants?
   a. Trisomy 21
   b. Trisomy 18
   c. Trisomy 13
   d. Turner's syndrome (monosomy X)
   e. Cri du chat (del 5p) syndrome

3.58 Chorionic villus sampling can be used for the detection of
   a. neural tube defects
   b. fetal omphalocele
   c. trisomy 18
   d. achondroplasia
   e. Marfan's syndrome

3.59 The most common chromosomal abnormality reliably diagnosed by amniocentesis is
   a. trisomy 13
   b. 21/22 translocation
   c. 13–15/21 translocation
   d. trisomy 18
   e. trisomy 21

3.60 Which of the following statements about cri du chat syndrome is INCORRECT?
   a. It is caused by deletion of part of the short arm of chromosome 5
   b. The infants typically are macrosomic
   c. Individuals with the syndrome have low-set ears and a moonlike face
   d. There is no relation to parental age
   e. Female infants are affected more often than males

3.61 Which of the following statements about autosomal dominant inheritance is incorrect?
   a. The inheritance is usually independent of sex
   b. Both sexes are equally affected
   c. The inheritance is a result of a pair of mutant genes situated on an autosomal chromosome
   d. One half of the children born to an affected person are affected
   e. One half of the siblings of an affected person are affected

ANSWERS (3.54–3.61)

3.54 c	3.56 d	3.58 c	3.59 e	3.60 b	3.61 c
3.55 d	3.57 a				

3.62 If there is complete failure of testicular development following the formation of an XY zygote,
   a. the individual will develop as a female with uterus, tubes, vagina, and vulva
   b. the individual will develop as a male with undescended testes and hypospadias
   c. the external genitalia will be normal
   d. the external genitalia will be ambiguous and there will be an absence of vagina, uterus, and tubes
   e. the individual will become a transsexual

3.63 Which of the following is a mendelian dominant hereditary bleeding disorder that affects both sexes?
   a. Hemophilia
   b. Christmas disease
   c. Von Willebrand's disease
   d. Down syndrome

3.64 The level of α-fetoprotein is normal in amniotic fluid in which of the following conditions?
   a. Spina bifida
   b. Anencephaly
   c. Esophageal atresia
   d. Rh isoimmunization
   e. Postmaturity

3.65 In which of the following will an afflicted individual typically live to at least 10 years of age?
   a. Trisomy 21
   b. Trisomy 18
   c. Trisomy 16
   d. Trisomy 13
   e. All of the above

3.66 Advanced maternal age as a screening test question fails to detect pregnancies with Down syndrome in what percent of cases?
   a. 20%
   b. 40%
   c. 60%
   d. 80%

3.67 Triple screen detects about what percent of Down syndrome pregnancies?
   a. 20%
   b. 40%
   c. 60%
   d. 80%

3.68 Finding a fetal cardiac malformation on antepartum obstetric ultrasound examinations is associated with what percent chance of the fetus having a chromosomal abnormality?
   a. 20%
   b. 40%
   c. 60%
   d. 80%

3.69 The most commonly used maternal serum screening test involves measurement of
   a. maternal α-fetoprotein, human chorionic gonadotropin, and unconjugated estriol
   b. maternal progesterone, human chorionic gonadotropin, and unconjugated estriol
   c. maternal α-fetoprotein, human chorionic gonadotropin, and maternal progesterone
   d. maternal α-fetoprotein, maternal progesterone, and unconjugated estriol

ANSWERS (3.62–3.69)

3.62 a	3.64 e	3.66 d	3.67 d	3.68 b	3.69 a
3.63 c	3.65 a			

3.70 Direct genetic tests for the associated mutation are available for all the following diseases EXCEPT
  a. cystic fibrosis
  b. α-thalassemia
  c. β-thalassemia
  d. Duchenne's muscular dystrophy

3.71 The most common genetic cause of mental retardation is
  a. fragile-X
  b. Down syndrome
  c. intrauterine growth restriction
  d. cystic fibrosis

3.72 In a woman who has a child with a neural tube defect, in subsequent pregnancies she should take a prenatal vitamin that contains how much folic acid?
  a. 0.04 mg
  b. 0.4 mg
  c. 4 mg
  d. 40 mg

3.73 Prenatal ingestion of an appropriate dose of folic acid daily acts to prevent
  a. the occurrence of neural tube defects
  b. the recurrence of neural tube defects
  c. both the occurrence and recurrence of neural tube defects
  d. neither the occurrence nor the recurrence of neural tube defects

Instructions for items 3.74 to 3.76: Match the organ/organ system precursor with its time of maximum susceptibility to teratogens. An option may be used once, more than once, or not at all.

3.74 Brain

3.75 Neural tube

3.76 Heart
  a. 3 to 6 weeks
  b. 3 to 16 weeks
  c. 2 to 4 weeks

Instructions for items 3.77 to 3.81: Match the medication with the teratogenic effect with which it is best associated. An option may be used once, more than once, or not at all.

3.77 Alcohol

3.78 Phenytoin

3.79 Valproate

3.80 Warfarin

3.81 Accutane
  a. Neural tube defects, craniofascial abnormalities
  b. Cardiac defects, mental retardation (50-80IA), microcephaly, facial anomalies
  c. Broad nasal bridge, cleft lip and palate, microcephaly, decreased IQ
  d. Depressed nasal bridge, stippled epiphysis, seizures, developmental delay
  e. Hydrocephalus, microcephaly, microtia, cleft lip and palate, cardiac defects

ANSWERS (3.70–3.81)

| 3.70 c | 3.72 b | 3.74 b | 3.76 a | 3.78 c | 3.80 d |
| 3.71 a | 3.73 c | 3.75 c | 3.77 b | 3.79 a | 3.81 e |

Questions and Answers Chapter 4: Maternal–Fetal Physiology

4.1 Which of the following statements about dental care during pregnancy is correct?
   a. Dental care is not advisable throughout pregnancy, except in situations where the mother's health is placed in extreme risk by delaying care
   b. Dental care is permissible in the second and third, but not first, trimesters
   c. Dental care is permissible in pregnancy, but anesthesia and x-ray must be avoided due to fetal risks
   d. Dental care is permissible during pregnancy

4.2 In pregnancy, the incidence of dental caries
   a. increases
   b. remains the same
   e. decreases

4.3 In pregnancy, the incidence of gingival disease
   a. increases
   b. remains the same
   c. decreases

Instructions for items 4.4 to 4.6: Match the molecule with the mechanism(s) by which it crosses the placenta. An option may be used once, more than once, or not at all.

4.4 Oxygen

4.5 Glucose

4.6 Amino acids
   a. Simple diffusion
   b. Facilitated diffusion
   c. Active transport
   d. Pinocytosis

Instructions for items 4.7 to 4.12: Match the gastrointestinal tract activity with the change that is expected in pregnancy. An option may be used once, more than once, or not at all.

4.7 Appetite

4.8 Gastric motility

4.9 Intestinal transit time

4.10 Bile composition

4.11 Liver enzyme levels

4.12 Gastric reflux
   a. Increases
   b. Decreases
   c. Remains the same
   d. Unpredictable

4.13 "Morning sickness" typically begins during which weeks of pregnancy?
   a. 1–3
   b. 4–8
   c. 10–12
   d. 14–18

4.14 Treatment of morning sickness includes all of the following EXCEPT
   a. reassurance
   b. frequent small meals
   c. three large meals with antacids
   d. inclusion of bland foods

4.15 Ptyalism is caused by
   a. excess production of saliva
   b. excess production of gastric acid
   c. inability of the patient to swallow normal amounts of saliva
   d. allergic reactions to various foods during pregnancy

Answers (4.1–4.15)					
4.1 d	4.4 a	4.7 a	4.10 c	4.12 a	4.14 c
4.2 b	4.5 b	4.8 b	4.11 a	4.13 b	4.15 c
4.3 a	4.6 c	4.9 a			

4.16 Decreased gastrointestinal motility during pregnancy is related to increased levels of
a. progesterone
b. human chorionic gonadotropin
c. estrogen
d. androstenedione
e. thyrotropin-releasing factor

4.17 The recommended dietary allowance in pregnancy is how many additional calories per day?
a. 100
b. 300
c. 500
d. 700
e. 900

4.18 Transit time in the stomach and small bowel increase by what percent in the second and third trimesters of pregnancy?
a. 1%–15%
b. 15%–30%
c. 30%–45%
d. 45%–60%

4.19 During pregnancy the tone of the sphincter at the gastroesophageal junction
a. increases
b. is unchanged
c. decreases
d. varies with gestational age

4.20 Which of the following is NOT related to constipation in pregnancy?
a. Mechanical obstruction of the colon by the enlarging bowel
b. Reduced motility of the colon
c. Increased gastrointestinal motility elsewhere than the colon
d. Increased water absorption

4.21 Pica can include craving for which of the following?
a. Ice
b. Laundry starch
c. Clay
d. All of the above

4.22 Epulis is a pregnancy-related vascular swelling of the
a. gums
b. nares
c. epiglottis
d. nail beds
e. larynx

4.23 Of the following pulmonary measurements, which is decreased in pregnancy?
a. Oxygen requirement
b. Carbon dioxide pressure
c. Oxygen pressure
d. Tidal volume

4.24 Which of the following measures of pulmonary function decreases in late pregnancy?
a. Functional reserve capacity
b. Tidal volume
c. Respiratory rate
d. Inspiratory capacity

4.25 Which of the following pulmonary measurements is increased in pregnancy?
a. Inspiratory capacity
b. Vital capacity
c. Minute volume
d. All of the above

4.26 The increased nasal stuffiness and perception of increased nasal secretions during pregnancy are associated with
a. mucosal hyperemia
b. increased immunoglobulin production
c. increased interluminal production of mast cell toxins
d. all of the above

ANSWERS (4.16–4.26)

| 4.16 a | 4.18 b | 4.20 c | 4.22 a | 4.24 a | 4.26 a |
| 4.17 b | 4.19 c | 4.21 d | 4.23 b | 4.25 d | |

4.27 The acid–base status in pregnancy is characterized by
   a. mild respiratory alkalosis
   b. mild metabolic alkalosis
   c. mild respiratory acidosis
   d. mild metabolic acidosis

4.28 The tidal volume in pregnancy increases by what percent?
   a. 10%–20%
   b. 30%–40%
   c. 50%–60%
   d. 70%–80%

4.29 In a normal singleton pregnancy, maternal blood volume
   a. increases by 10%–15%
   b. increases by 45%
   c. decreases by 10%–15%
   d. decreases by 45%

4.30 Which of the following is NOT characteristic of a normal pregnancy?
   a. The cardiac volume increases by 10%
   b. The electrocardiogram shows deviation to the left
   c. Arterial blood pressure and vascular resistance increase
   d. The rest pulse rate increases by approximately 10–15 beats per minute
   e. The heart is displaced upward and to the left

4.31 Maternal arterial pH during pregnancy
   a. is increased from normal prepregnancy levels
   b. is maintained at normal prepregnancy levels
   c. is decreased from normal prepregnancy levels

4.32 Measured blood pressure in a pregnant woman is highest when she is
   a. seated
   b. supine
   c. supine on her side

4.33 In the lateral recumbant position, maternal blood pressure in the inferior arm is
   a. higher than in the superior arm
   b. the same as in the superior arm
   c. lower than in the superior arm

4.34 Pregnancy associated systolic ejection murmurs are best heard
   a. over the left upper sternal border
   b. over the left midclavicular line
   c. over the cardiac apex
   d. over the inferior aspect of the sternum

4.35 Compensation for the occlusion of the inferior vena cava by the pregnant uterus is accomplished by shunting blood through
   a. the uterine venous plexus
   b. the sacral plexus
   c. the paraverterbral collateral circulation
   d. the renal venous plexus

4.36 Blood flow to which of the following organs is NOT increased during pregnancy?
   a. Kidney
   b. Breast
   c. Skin
   d. Brain

ANSWERS (4.27–4.36)

4.27 a	4.29 b	4.31 b	4.33 a	4.35 c	4.36 d
4.28 b	4.30 c	4.32 a	4.34 a		

4.37 Inferior vena cava syndrome is caused by
  a. baroreceptor changes in cardiac function associated with changes in position
  b. transient release of epinephrine associated with uterine displacement caused by fetal movement
  c. transient cardiac arrhythmias secondary to positional changes in the mother
  d. spasm of the inferior vena cava secondary to fetal movement
  e. compression of the inferior vena cava by the gravid uterine corpus

4.38 The peripheral vascular resistance decreases during pregnancy because of increased levels of
  a. estrogen
  b. progesterone
  c. androstenedione
  d. estrone

4.39 Which of the following normal physical findings during pregnancy is a result of a hyperdynamic state of the cardiovascular system?
  a. Distended neck veins
  b. Low grade systolic ejection murmur
  c. Diastolic murmurs
  d. All of the above

4.40 On chest x-ray, the heart appears to demonstrate cardiomegaly during pregnancy because it is displaced
  a. upward and to the left
  b. upward and to the right
  c. downward and to the left
  d. downward and to the right

4.41 Plasma volume begins to increase at the sixth week of pregnancy and reaches its maximum at approximately
  a. 20–24 weeks
  b. 25–29 weeks
  c. 30–34 weeks
  d. 35–39 weeks
  e. term

4.42 Which of the following hematologic parameters is decreased in pregnancy?
  a. Mean cell volume
  b. Total erythrocyte volume
  c. Hematocrit
  d. All of the above

4.43 Which of the following hematologic parameters is increased during pregnancy?
  a. Serum iron
  b. Total iron-binding capacity
  c. Hemoglobin concentration
  d. All of the above

4.44 During pregnancy, the risk for thromboembolism
  a. increases
  b. decreases
  c. remains the same
  d. increases for the first month, then decreases toward term

4.45 A lack of maternal iron ingestion during pregnancy results in
  a. fetal anemia
  b. fetal anomalies
  c. maternal anemia
  d. all of the above

4.46 Which of the following renal parameters is increased during pregnancy?
  a. Renal plasma flow
  b. Glomerular filtration rate
  c. Renin
  d. All of the above

ANSWERS (4.37–4.46)

4.37 e	4.39 b	4.41 c	4.43 b	4.45 c	4.46 d
4.38 b	4.40 a	4.42 c	4.44 a		

4.47 Which of the following renal parameters is NOT increased in pregnancy?
a. Angiotensin I
b. Angiotensin II
c. Renin substrate
d. 24-hour protein excretion

4.48 What is the normal effect of progesterone on ureters in pregnancy?
a. There is more dilation of the left ureter than of the right
b. There is more dilation of the right ureter than of the left
c. Both ureters dilate equally
d. Both ureters constrict equally

4.49 The decreased bladder tone in pregnancy caused by progesterone is associated with which of the following?
a. Increased residual volume
b. Dilated collecting systems
c. Urinary stasis
d. All of the above

4.50 In normal pregnancy, which of the following renal parameters is decreased?
a. Creatinine
b. Uric acid
c. Blood urea nitrogen
d. All of the above

4.51 Striae gravidarum in which anatomic sites are affected by weight control?
a. Abdominal wall
b. Breasts
c. Thighs
d. None of the above

4.52 Chloasma is the
a. increased hair growth seen in early pregnancy
b. loss of hair that occurs soon after delivery
c. physiologic nipple discharge of late pregnancy
d. change in facial pigmentation of pregnancy
e. transient depression encountered after delivery

4.53 Which of the following statements accurately reflects the description of the normal effects of pregnancy on bone?
a. Bone density decreases as pregnancy progresses
b. Bone density increases as pregnancy progresses
c. The rate of bone turnover increases during pregnancy
d. Bone turnover is inversely proportional to calcium intake

4.54 Blurred vision during pregnancy is a result of
a. swelling of the lens
b. aging of the patient
c. reduced blood flow to the eye
d. increased retinal glucose metabolism

4.55 What percent of total cardiac output is channeled to the uterus at term?
a. 5%
b. 10%
c. 20%
d. 30%
e. 40%

4.56 Which of the following is characteristic of normal pregnancy?
a. Hyperglycemia
b. Hypoinsulinemia
c. Hypotriglyceridemia
d. All of the above

ANSWERS (4.47–4.56)

4.47 d	4.49 d	4.51 d	4.53 c	4.55 c	4.56 a
4.48 b	4.50 d	4.52 d	4.54 a		

4.57 The "hemorrhoids" that develop in late pregnancy are caused by
a. a response to infection
b. increased pelvic venous outflow
c. loose stools
d. irritation from increased vaginal secretions
e. elevated pelvic venous pressure

4.58 The net effects of the normal thyroid changes of pregnancy will result in patients typically being
a. moderately hypothyroid
b. mildly hypothyroid
c. euthyroid
d. mildly hyperthyroid
e. moderately hyperthyroid

4.59 Diastasis recti is the
a. dilation of the rectum
b. constipation of pregnancy
c. linear stretch marks found on the abdomen
d. midline separation of the rectus muscles
e. fatigue syndrome of early pregnancy

4.60 In the later half of pregnancy, the CO_2 gradient between fetus and mother
a. increases
b. remains the same
c. decreases

4.61 The blood urea nitrogen falls about what percent in the first trimester of pregnancy?
a. 10%
b. 25%
c. 40%
d. 55%

4.62 Urinary protein loss in pregnancy is approximately
a. 0–200 mg/24 hours
b. 100–300 mg/24 hours
c. 200–400 mg/24 hours
d. 300–500 mg/24 hours

4.63 The hair loss commonly encountered in the 2nd to 4th month postpartum will return to the prepregnant state approximately how many months after delivery?
a. 3–6 months
b. 6–12 months
c. 12–18 months
d. 18–24 months

4.64 The breast enlargement associated with pregnancy typically is seen starting in which trimester?
a. First
b. Second
c. Third

4.65 The vision changes in pregnancy associated with increased thickness of the cornea typically regress within the first
a. few days postpartum
b. 1–3 weeks postpartum
c. 6–8 weeks postpartum
d. 6 months postpartum
e. year postpartum

4.66 The common practice of giving supplemental vitamin K to newborns is a result of
a. the relative deficiency of maternal vitamin K
b. maternal liver dysfunction in pregnancy
c. fetal liver immaturity in the immediate newborn period
d. lack of vitamin K absorption

4.67 As compared to nonpregnant normal values, serum bicarbonate levels in normal pregnancy are
a. significantly lower
b. somewhat lower
c. equivalent to
d. somewhat higher
e. significantly higher

ANSWERS (4.57–4.67)

4.57 e	4.59 d	4.61 b	4.63 b	4.65 c	4.67 a
4.58 c	4.60 a	4.62 b	4.64 a	4.66 c	

Questions and Answers Chapter 5:
Antepartum Care

5.1 Which of the following is NOT an early sign of pregnancy?
a. Fatigue
b. Urinary retention
c. Nausea
d. Breast tenderness
e. Bloating

5.2 Quickening is generally first felt by how many weeks of gestation?
a. 12
b. 16
c. 20
d. 24

5.3 A positive pregnancy test may be associated with
a. spontaneous abortion
b. intrauterine pregnancy
c. ectopic pregnancy
d. trophoblastic disease
e. all of the above

5.4 Congestion and a bluish color of the vagina is called
a. Chadwick's sign
b. Hegar's sign
c. Newman's sign
d. Smith's sign
e. Stoppard's sign

5.5 A softening of the cervix on physical examination is referred to as
a. Chadwick's sign
b. Hegar's sign
c. Newman's sign
d. Smith's sign
e. Stoppard's sign

5.6 Fetal heart tones in a normal, viable pregnancy may routinely be heard by simple auscultation at or beyond how many weeks' gestational age?
a. 12–14
b. 15–17
c. 18–20
d. 21–23

5.7 Commonly used electronic Doppler devices will detect fetal heart tones at approximately how many weeks of gestation?
a. 8
b. 10
c. 12
d. 14
e. 16

5.8 Home urine pregnancy tests become positive approximately how many weeks following the first day of the last normal menstrual period?
a. 3
b. 4
c. 5
d. 6
e. 8

5.9 A serum progesterone level of greater than 25 ng/ml is usually consistent with
a. incomplete abortion
b. nonviable intrauterine pregnancy
c. ectopic pregnancy
d. viable intrauterine pregnancy

5.10 Intrauterine pregnancy is generally detectable by transvaginal ultrasonography when the β-human chorionic gonadotropin concentration is greater than
a. 500–750 mIU/ml
b. 1000–2000 mIU/ml
c. 3000–4000 mIU/ml
d. 5000–6000 mIU/ml

Answers (5.1–5.10)

5.1	b	5.3	e	5.5	b	5.7	c	5.9	d	5.10	b
5.2	c	5.4	a	5.6	c	5.8	b				

5.11 Which of the following tests is done as part of routine prenatal care?
a. Blood group/Rh
b. Antibody screen
c. Complete blood count
d. All of the above

5.12 In approximately what percent of pregnant women is the rubella titer positive?
a. 55%
b. 65%
c. 75%
d. 85%
e. 95%

5.13 Specific screening for treponema is required following a positive
a. sickle-cell test
b. rubella titer
c. hepatitis B surface antigen
d. rapid plasma reagin
e. maternal serum α-fetoprotein

5.14 Maternal serum α-fetoprotein testing is best done at
a. 7–10 weeks
b. 11–14 weeks
c. 15–18 weeks
d. 19–22 weeks

5.15 "Normal" pregnancy lasts 40 weeks from the first day of the last menstrual period with a margin of error of how many weeks?
a. 1
b. 2
c. 3
d. 4

5.16 The fertilization age or conception age is how many weeks less than the menstrual or gestational age?
a. 1
b. 2
c. 3
d. 4

5.17 Data from which of the following is not used in the final determination of the expected date of delivery?
a. Determination of last menstrual period
b. Date of quickening
c. Maternal α-protein level
d. Date when fundus is at the level of the umbilicus

5.18 In a normal singleton pregnancy, from approximately 16 to 18 weeks' gestation until approximately 36 weeks' gestation, the fundal height in centimeters is roughly equal to
a. one half the number of weeks gestational age
b. the number of weeks gestational age
c. the number of weeks gestational age minus 5
d. twice the number of weeks gestational age

5.19 The generally prescribed recommendation for weight gain during pregnancy is
a. 15–20 pounds
b. 25–30 pounds
c. 40–45 pounds
d. 50–55 pounds

5.20 Which of the following is a direct result of "lightening?"
a. Rupture of the membranes
b. Expulsion of cervical mucous plug
c. Urinary retention
d. Decreased fundal height
e. Appearance of bloody show

ANSWERS (5.11–5.20)

5.11 d	5.13 d	5.15 b	5.17 c	5.19 b	5.20 d
5.12 d	5.14 c	5.16 b	5.18 b		

Instructions for items 5.21 to 5.23: Match the fetal presentation with the estimated incidence of its occurrence. An option may be used once, more than once, or not at all.

5.21 Cephalic presentation

5.22 Breech presentation

5.23 Shoulder presentation
   a. 95%
   b. 1%
   c. 3.5%
   d. 15%

5.24 Estimation of gestational age by ultrasound is least accurate at which of the following times during pregnancy?
   a. 4–6 weeks
   b. 16–18 weeks
   c. 26–28 weeks
   d. 36–38 weeks

5.25 The normal fetal heart rate at term is
   a. 50–75 beats per minute (bpm)
   b. 80–100 bpm
   c. 120–160 bpm
   d. 175–190 bpm

5.26 A reactive nonstress test is characterized by a fetal heart rate increase of how many beats per minute?
   a. 50
   b. 25
   c. 15
   d. 5

5.27 Which of the following statements correctly describes an abnormal contraction stress test?
   a. Fetal heart rate decreases in response to a uterine contraction
   b. Fetal heart rate increases in response to fetal movement
   c. Maternal heart rate decreases in response to a uterine contraction
   d. Maternal blood pressure increases in response to fetal movement

5.28 The number of contractions in a 10-minute window that must occur for a contraction stress test to be measurable is
   a. 1
   b. 2
   c. 3
   d. 4
   e. 5

5.29 A biophysical profile in which there is one or more episodes of fetal breathing in 30 minutes, three or more discrete movements in 30 minutes, opening/closing of the fetal hand, a nonreactive nonstress test, and no pockets of amniotic fluid greater than 1 cm would have a total score of
   a. 2
   b. 4
   c. 6
   d. 8

5.30 Exclusive of the fetal heart rate reactivity, which of the following elements of the biophysical profile is generally considered most important?
   a. Fetal breathing
   b. Gross body movement
   c. Fetal tone
   d. Qualitative amniotic fluid volume

Answers (5.21–5.30)					
5.21 a	5.23 b	5.25 c	5.27 a	5.29 c	5.30 d
5.22 c	5.24 d	5.26 c	5.28 c		

5.31 Repetitive decelerations following each contraction when three contractions occur in a 10-minute window is generally an indication of
a. increased placental blood flow
b. nonreassuring fetal status
c. reduced amniotic fluid
d. fetal well-being

5.32 Further evaluation of fetal well-being should follow which answer to the question, "Is your baby moving more, less, or the same this week compared to last week?"
a. Moving more
b. Moving the same
c. Moving less

5.33 Tests of fetal lung maturity are generally used when delivery of a fetus is contemplated at a gestational age of less than how many weeks?
a. 30
b. 32
c. 34
d. 36
e. 38

5.34 At how many weeks' gestational age does phospholipid production increase, resulting in a positive phosphatidylglycerol test?
a. 27–29
b. 30–31
c. 32–33
d. 34–35
e. 36–37

5.35 What percent of correctly performed positive tests of fetal lung maturity are associated with a subsequent development of respiratory distress syndrome?
a. 0%
b. 2%
c. 4%
d. 6%
e. 8%

5.36 Which of the following activities is CONTRAINDICATED during pregnancy?
a. Regular, non-weight bearing activity on a three-times per week schedule
b. Supine exercises
c. Bathtub bathing
d. Air travel after 28 weeks

5.37 During a normal pregnancy, the patient should be encouraged to engage in non-weight bearing activity at least how many times per week?
a. Once
b. Three times
c. Daily
d. Not at all

5.38 Which of the following information is not included in antepartum infant feeding (breast-feeding, bottle-feeding) counseling?
a. Breast-feeding may contribute to a "natural child spacing"
b. Breast-feeding promotes more rapid uterine involution postpartum
c. Breast-feeding is not inferior in nutritional value to other methods
d. Breast-feeding helps provide immunologic protection for the infant in the immediate newborn period

5.39 Which of the following is NOT included in the list of "high risk" situations for which sexual activity is generally proscribed?
a. Uterine leiomyoma
b. History of preterm labor and/or delivery
c. Placenta previa
d. Premature rupture of the membranes

ANSWERS (5.31–5.39)

| 5.31 b | 5.33 d | 5.35 b | 5.37 a, b | 5.38 c | 5.39 a |
| 5.32 c | 5.34 c | 5.36 b | | | |

5.40 "Physiologic" constipation in pregnancy is NOT associated with
a. increased transit time
b. increased water absorption
c. decreased blood flow to the gut
d. decreased bulk in the maternal diet

5.41 Which of the following statements about low back pain in pregnancy is INCORRECT?
a. Low back pain is associated with an altered center of gravity
b. Platform shoes can readjust the center of gravity reducing the severity of low back pain
c. Maternity girdles can readjust the center of gravity reducing the severity of low back pain
d. Heat and focused massage can reduce the severity of low back pain

5.42 In pregnancy, *psyllium hydrophilic mucilloid* is useful in the management of
a. heartburn
b. constipation
c. low back pain
d. headache

5.43 Due to the position of the fetus, round ligament pain is often more pronounced
a. on the right side
b. in the center
c. on the left side
d. in the fundus

5.44 The neonatal mortality rate is
a. synonymous with the stillbirth rate
b. the number of neonatal deaths per 1000 births
c. the number of neonatal deaths per 1000 live births
d. the number of neonatal deaths per 1000 population
e. the number of neonatal deaths in the first 7 days of life

5.45 The maternal mortality rate is
a. the number of deaths in pregnant women per 1000 population
b. the number of deaths in pregnant women
c. the number of deaths in pregnant women per 100,000 live births

ANSWERS (5.40–5.45)

| 5.40 c | 5.41 b | 5.42 b | 5.43 a | 5.44 c | 5.45 c |

Instructions for items 5.46 to 5.50: Match the pregnancy risk factor (PRF) for medications in pregnancy with the item or items with which it best corresponds. An option may be used once, more than once, or not at all.

5.46 PRF A

5.47 PRF B

5.48 PRF C

5.49 PRF D

5.50 PRF X

a. Controlled human studies demonstrate no evidence of risk in pregnancy in any trimester
b. Animal-reproduction studies have not demonstrated fetal risk and there are no controlled human studies
c. Animal-reproduction studies have demonstrated an adverse fetal effect and there are no controlled human studies
d. Positive evidence of human fetal risk exists
e. Animal-reproduction and human studies demonstrate fetal abnormalities such that the risk of use of drugs in this PRF in pregnant women clearly outweighs any possible benefit
f. The possibility of fetal harm appears remote
g. Animal-reproduction studies have demonstrated an adverse effect that was not confirmed in controlled human studies in the first trimester, and there is no evidence of a risk in later trimesters

h. Drugs in this category should be given only if the potential benefits justify the potential risk to the fetus
i. Animal-reproduction and human studies are not available
j. Use of drugs in this PRF category may be acceptable despite the fetal risk if the drug is needed in a life-threatening situation, or for a serious disease for which safer drugs cannot be used or are ineffective

5.51 Factors to be considered in the selection of medications during pregnancy include
a. whether the drug is contraindicated in pregnancy
b. drug interactions
c. physiological parameters such as renal or hepatic function
d. serious or uncomfortable side effects and their frequency
e. all the above

5.52 Which pregnancy risk factor category is characterized by the presence of animal or human studies that do not demonstrate fetal risk in pregnancy?
a. A
b. B
c. C
d. D
e. X

ANSWERS (5.46–5.52)

5.46 a, f	5.48 c, h, i	5.49 d, j	5.50 e	5.51 e	5.52 b
5.47 b, g					

Questions and Answers Chapter 6: Intrapartum Care

6.1 Which of the following is NOT required for a diagnosis of true labor?
a. Rhythmic contractions
b. Cervical dilatation
c. Cervical effacement
d. Bloody show

6.2 Bloody show is associated at term with
a. marginal placental separation as labor ensues
b. spiral artery breakdown under labor-associated progesterone influence
c. extrusion of endocervical gland mucus
d. altered maternal coagulation mechanisms at term

Instructions for items 6.3 to 6.9: Match each statement about labor with whether it is characteristic of active labor or false labor.

6.3 Commonly associated with low back pain

6.4 Uterine contractions of increasing intensity

6.5 Spontaneous onset of uterine activity

6.6 Progressive cervical dilation

6.7 Lower abdomen and groin pain

6.8 Intensity of uterine contractions waxes and wanes

6.9 Progressive cervical effacement
a. Active labor
b. False labor

6.10 Which of the following is characteristic of "Braxton Hicks" contractions?
a. Rhythmic contractions
b. No cervical change on serial examinations
c. Lower abdominal discomfort
d. All of the above

6.11 Late in pregnancy, the fetal head descends into the pelvis and the contour of the abdomen changes. This is referred to as
a. false descent
b. lightening
c. Braxton Hicks labor
d. effacement

6.12 Frequent urination found in late pregnancy is due to
a. increased clearance of free water
b. fluid shifts from diminishing amniotic fluid volume
c. decreased pressure on the maternal diaphragm
d. compression of the bladder caused by descent of the fetal head

6.13 With lightening, a patient may notice
a. increased urinary frequency
b. increased ease of respiratory effort
c. a flatter abdomen
d. all of the above

Answers (6.1–6.13)					
6.1 d	6.4 a	6.6 a	6.8 b	6.10 d	6.12 d
6.2 c	6.5 a, b	6.7 b	6.9 a	6.11 b	6.13 d
6.3 a, b					

6.14 Which of the following is NOT an indication that a patient in late pregnancy should come to the hospital for evaluation?
  a. Regular contractions 15–20 minutes apart
  b. Sudden gush of fluid
  c. Continuing gradual leakage of fluid
  d. Vaginal bleeding
  e. Decreased fetal movement

Instructions for items 6.15 to 6.17: Match the terms related to fetal location with the appropriate description(s). An option may be used once, more than once, or not at all.

6.15 Lie

6.16 Presentation

6.17 Position
  a. Relationship of the fetal presenting part to the right and left side of the maternal pelvis
  b. Relationship of the long axis of the fetus with the maternal long axis
  c. Portion of the fetus lowest in the birth canal
  d. Part of the fetus that is most easily palpable on abdominal examination

6.18 Leopold's maneuvers are used to establish all of the following EXCEPT
  a. fetal gender
  b. fetal lie
  c. fetal presentation
  d. fetal position

Instructions for items 6.19 to 6.22: Match the description with the appropriate maneuver of Leopold. An option may be used once, more than once, or not at all.

6.19 Identifying descent of the presenting part

6.20 Determining location of small parts

6.21 Determining what occupies the fundus

6.22 Identifying the cephalic prominence
  a. First maneuver
  b. Second maneuver
  c. Third maneuver
  d. Fourth maneuver

6.23 The most common fetal lie found during early labor is
  a. oblique
  b. transverse
  c. vertex
  d. longitudinal

6.24 The most common fetal presentation found in early labor is
  a. oblique
  b. transverse
  c. vertex
  d. longitudinal

6.25 Vaginal examination of a patient in early labor finds the cervix to be approximately 1 cm in length and 1 cm dilated. The effacement is
  a. 10%
  b. 25%
  c. 50%
  d. 75%
  e. 100%

6.26 The turning of the fetal head toward the sacrum is termed
  a. transverse lie
  b. anterior asynclitism
  c. left side position
  d. occipital presentation

ANSWERS (6.14–6.26)

6.14 a	6.17 a	6.19 c	6.21 a	6.23 d	6.25 c
6.15 b	6.18 a	6.20 b	6.22 d	6.24 c	6.26 b
6.16 c					

6.27 Vaginal examination of a patient in early labor finds the presenting part (vertex) to be at the level of the ischial spines. The station is reported as
a. +2
b. +1
c. 0
d. –1
e. –2

6.28 At 0 station, where is the biparietal diameter of the fetal head in relation to the pelvic inlet?
a. It has not yet reached it
b. It is at the pelvic inlet
c. It has passed below the pelvic inlet

6.29 The clinical significance of the fetal head presenting at 0 station is that the biparietal diameter of the fetal head, the greatest transverse diameter of the fetal skull, has negotiated the
a. pelvic inlet
b. pelvic midplane
c. pelvic outlet

6.30 Cervical effacement relates to
a. how far the cervix is opened
b. the degree of cervical thinning
c. the relation of the presenting part to the cervix
d. the softness of the cervix

Instructions for items 6.31 to 6.34: Match the stage of labor with the appropriate description(s). An option may be used once, more than once, or not at all.

6.31 First stage

6.32 Second stage

6.33 Third stage

6.34 Fourth stage
a. Complete dilation of the cervix to delivery of the infant
b. Delivery of infant to the delivery of the placenta
c. Onset of labor to full cervical dilation
d. Period extending up to 2 hours after delivery of the placenta

6.35 The active phase of the first stage of labor is generally defined to begin at what dilation of the cervix?
a. 2 cm
b. 3 cm
c. 4 cm
d. 5 cm
e. 6 cm

6.36 The vertex presentation occurs in approximately what percent of term labors?
a. 65%
b. 75%
c. 85%
d. 95%

Instructions for items 6.37 to 6.40: Match the movements of the fetus during labor with the appropriate description(s). An option may be used once, more than once, or not at all.

6.37 External rotation

6.38 Extension

6.39 Flexion

6.40 Descent
a. Movement of the presenting part through the birth canal
b. Allows the smaller diameter of the head to present to the maternal pelvis
c. Occurs when the head reaches the introitus
d. Occurs after the delivery of the head

Answers (6.27–6.40)

6.27 c	6.30 b	6.33 b	6.35 c	6.37 d	6.39 b
6.28 c	6.31 c	6.34 d	6.36 d	6.38 c	6.40 a
6.29 a	6.32 a				

Instructions for items 6.41 to 6.46: Select the mean duration of the latent and active phases of the first stage of labor and the second stage of labor for nulliparas and multiparas. An option may be used once, more than once, or not at all.

6.41 Latent phase of stage one, nulliparas

6.42 Active phase of stage one, nulliparas

6.43 Second stage, nulliparas

6.44 Latent phase of stage one, multiparas

6.45 Active phase of stage one, multiparas

6.46 Second stage, multiparas
    a. 0.5 hrs
    b. 1.0 hrs
    c. 2.5 hrs
    d. 4.5 hrs
    e. 5.0 hrs
    f. 6.5 hrs

6.47 All of the following should occur after spontaneous rupture of the membranes EXCEPT
    a. examination of the fluid for blood
    b. examination of the fluid for meconium
    c. auscultation or measurement of the fetal heart rate
    d. measurement of the pH of the fluid

6.48 During the active phase of labor, if electronic fetal monitoring is not used, the fetal heart rate should be auscultated every
    a. 5 minutes
    b. 10 minutes
    c. 15 minutes
    d. 20 minutes
    e. 25 minutes

6.49 During the second stage of labor in the absence of electronic fetal monitoring, fetal heart rate auscultation should be performed after
    a. each uterine contraction
    b. every other uterine contraction
    c. every third uterine contraction
    d. every contraction generating more than 15–20 mm Hg pressure

6.50 An external tocodynamometer provides information about
    a. contraction frequency
    b. fetal heart rate variability
    c. contraction strength
    d. baseline uterine pressure

6.51 The sensory nerves from the lower birth canal and perineum enter the spinal cord at
    a. T1–T2
    b. T6–T8
    c. T9
    d. L1–L3
    e. S2–S4

Instructions for items 6.52 to 6.54: Match the obstetric anesthetic technique with the use with which it is best associated. An option may be used once, more than once, or not at all.

6.52 Epidural anesthesia

6.53 Spinal anesthesia

6.54 Pudendal anesthesia or block
    a. Provides perineal anesthesia for vaginal delivery
    b. Anesthesia for the active phase of labor and delivery
    c. Short-term anesthesia for vaginal or abdominal delivery
    d. Anesthesia for latent phase of labor

ANSWERS (6.41–6.54)

6.41 f	6.44 e	6.47 d	6.49 a	6.51 e	6.53 c
6.42 d	6.45 c	6.48 c	6.50 a	6.52 b	6.54 a
6.43 b	6.46 a				

6.55 Which of the following anesthetic techniques is associated with maternal aspiration?
a. General anesthesia
b. Spinal anesthesia
c. Epidural anesthesia
d. Pudendal anesthesia

6.56 Which of the following is an associated maternal risk when spinal anesthesia is used?
a. Hypotension
b. Loss of desire to push
c. Headache
d. All of the above

6.57 Maternal aspiration syndrome is a particularly significant risk of general anesthesia in obstetric cases because of
a. high alkaline content of the maternal gut during pregnancy
b. decreased gastrointestinal function during labor
c. pica-like eating habits of women just before labor
d. most general anesthetics causing reflex spasm of the stomach

6.58 The major cause of maternal mortality from obstetrical anesthesia is
a. cardiac arrest
b. aspiration of vomitus
c. hemorrhage and shock
d. fatal reaction to local anesthetic
e. excessive concentration causing respiratory failure

6.59 The most common outcome of compression of the fetal head during labor is
a. mental retardation
b. epilepsy
c. cerebral palsy
d. cleft lip
e. molding

Instructions for items 6.60 to 6.62: Match the type of forceps delivery with the appropriate description(s). An option may be used once, more than once, or not at all.

6.60 Outlet forceps

6.61 Low forceps

6.62 Midforceps
a. Head engaged, leading edge of skull above +2 station
b. Fetal skull at perineal floor, scalp visible, anteroposterior (AP), right occiput anterior (ROA) to left occiput anterior (LOA) [45°]
c. Leading edge of skull beyond +2 station
d. Complete breech presentation

6.63 Forceps may be used to
a. rotate the fetal head
b. augment maternal voluntary pushing efforts
c. control delivery of fetal head
d. all of the above

6.64 The usual postpartum blood loss at vaginal delivery is
a. 100 ml
b. 300 ml
c. 500 ml
d. 700 ml
e. 900 ml

6.65 What percent of patients will undergo spontaneous labor and delivery between 37 and 42 weeks?
a. 80%
b. 85%
c. 90%
d. 95%
e. +99%

Instructions for items 6.66 to 6.69: Match the category of obstetric laceration with the appropriate description(s). An option may be used once, more than once, or not at all.

6.66 First degree

6.67 Second degree

6.68 Third degree

6.69 Fourth degree
   a. Involves underlying fascia or muscle but not rectal sphincter or rectal mucosa
   b. Extends through the rectal sphincter but not into the rectum
   c. Extends into the rectal mucosa
   d. Involves the vaginal mucosa and perineal skin

6.70 Compared with mediolateral episiotomy, what is the risk of extension of a midline episiotomy?
   a. Greater risk
   b. Same risk
   c. Less risk

6.71 During delivery of the fetal head, the likelihood of laceration or extension of episiotomy is decreased by performance of
   a. Spinelli's maneuver
   b. Leopold's maneuver
   c. Ritgen's maneuver
   d. Marceaus' maneuver

6.72 Which of the following is NOT a sign of placental separation?
   a. The uterus rises in abdomen to become globular in shape
   b. There is a decreased sensation of pressure
   c. There is a gush of blood
   d. There is an apparent "lengthening" of the umbilical cord

6.73 It is customary to wait approximately how many minutes for spontaneous extrusion of the placenta?
   a. 10
   b. 20
   c. 30
   d. 40
   e. 50

6.74 Obstetric cervical lacerations are most commonly discovered at what "o-clock" during postpartum cervical inspection?
   a. 12
   b. 12 & 6
   c. 3 & 9
   d. 6

6.75 The maternal mortality rate associated with cesarean delivery is how many times that of a vaginal birth?
   a. One to two
   b. Two to four
   c. Four to eight
   d. Eight to twelve

6.76 Postpartum uterine hemorrhage occurs in approximately what percent of patients?
   a. 1%
   b. 3%
   c. 5%
   d. 7%

ANSWERS (6.66–6.76)

6.66 d	6.68 b	6.70 a	6.72 b	6.74 c	6.76 a
6.67 a	6.69 c	6.71 c	6.73 c	6.75 b	

Questions and Answers Chapter 7:
Abnormal Labor

7.1   Which of the following statements about prolapse of the umbilical cord is INCORRECT?
   a. It occurs in approximately 0.5% of patients
   b. It occurs more frequently in patients of high parity
   c. It most frequently occurs in breech presentation, twins, and in the presence of polyhydramnios
   d. It is associated with an increased perinatal mortality
   e. Manual replacement of the cord is indicated when the presenting part is not engaged in the pelvis

7.2   Which of the following is NOT associated with uterine rupture?
   a. Amniocentesis
   b. Previous cesarean section
   c. Myomectomy
   d. Administration of oxytocin
   e. Difficult forceps delivery

7.3   Older gravidas have an increased incidence of
   a. uterine inertia
   b. malpresentation
   c. hypertension
   d. all of the above

7.4   The breech hydrocephalus is best managed by
   a. cesarean section
   b. destructive procedure
   c. decompression of the head transvaginally
   d. decompression of the head transabdominally

7.5   Abnormal labor, or dystocia, can result from
   a. anatomic anomalies of the fetus
   b. anatomic anomalies of the maternal bony pelvis
   c. anatomic anomalies of the uterus
   d. functional abnormalities of the uterus
   e. all of the above

Instructions for items 7.6 to 7.8: Match the abnormal pattern of labor with the appropriate description(s). An option may be used once, more than once, or not at all.

7.6   Prolonged latent phase

7.7   Protraction disorder

7.8   Arrest disorder
   a. No progress from latent to active phase of labor
   b. Secondary arrest of dilatation
   c. Prolonged active phase of labor

7.9   Cervical dilation that proceeds at less than 1.2 cm/hr (for a nulligravida) would be classified as
   a. a prolonged latent phase
   b. a protraction disorder
   c. an arrest disorder
   d. a normal labor

7.10 A situation where there has been no descent of the presenting part for over 1 hour during the second stage of labor would be classified as
   a. a prolonged latent phase
   b. a protraction disorder
   c. an arrest disorder
   d. a normal labor

Answers (7.1–7.10)

7.1	e	7.3	d	7.5	e	7.7	c	7.9	b	7.10	c
7.2	a	7.4	a	7.6	a	7.8	b				

7.11 Which of the following provides a quantitative measurement of the strength of uterine contractions?
a. Manual palpation of maternal abdomen
b. Intrauterine pressure catheter
c. "Indentation" of uterus on palpation during contraction
d. Tocodynamometer

7.12 For a labor pattern to be considered optimal, contractions must generate a maximum intrauterine pressure of approximately how many mm Hg?
a. 10–20
b. 30–40
c. 50–60
d. 70–80

7.13 The incidence of shoulder dystocia and the need for cesarean delivery increase markedly if the fetus has an estimated weight of at least
a. 2500 grams
b. 3500 grams
c. 4500 grams
d. 5500 grams

7.14 Which of the following typically converts to either a vertex or face presentation?
a. Brow
b. Compound
c. Breech
d. Shoulder

7.15 What is the frequency of brow presentation?
a. 1 in 30
b. 1 in 300
c. 1 in 3000
d. 1 in 30,000

7.16 What is the frequency of face presentation?
a. 1 in 60
b. 1 in 600
c. 1 in 6000
d. 1 in 10,000

7.17 Which of the following usually resolves spontaneously as labor continues?
a. Compound presentation
b. Breech presentation
c. Shoulder presentation
d. Vertex presentation

7.18 Causes of dystocia may include
a. contracted bony maternal pelvis
b. distended bladder or colon
c. adnexal mass
d. uterine leiomyomata
e. all of the above

7.19 Which of the following is appropriate to use for the augmentation of labor?
a. Oxytocin
b. Prostaglandin gel
c. Laminaria
d. All of the above

7.20 In a primigravid patient, the active phase of labor is defined as prolonged if it lasts longer than
a. 10 hours
b. 12 hours
c. 14 hours
d. 16 hours
e. 18 hours

7.21 In multiparous patients, the active phase is defined as prolonged if it lasts more than
a. 2 hours
b. 4 hours
c. 6 hours
d. 8 hours
e. 10 hours

Answers (7.11–7.21)

7.11 b	7.13 c	7.15 c	7.17 a	7.19 a	7.21 c
7.12 c	7.14 a	7.16 b	7.18 e	7.20 b	

7.22 There has been secondary arrest of dilatation when cervical dilatation during the active phase of labor stops for at least
a. 1 hour
b. 2 hours
c. 3 hours
d. 4 hours

7.23 If pelvic examination shows a dilation of 1–2 cm, 60% effacement, a cephalic part of –1 station, and a soft cervix that is midposition, the Bishop's score would be
a. 9
b. 7
c. 5
d. 3

7.24 There is a significant likelihood that induction has failed if the Bishop's score falls below how many points?
a. 2
b. 4
c. 6
d. 8
e. 10

7.25 The prolonged latent phase in labor may be managed by
a. rest
b. augmentation with Pitocin
c. amniotomy
d. all of the above

7.26 Which of the following is NOT a risk to the fetus from prolonged labor?
a. Sepsis
b. Subdural hematoma
c. Delivery associated trauma
d. Hemorrhage

7.27 Meconium aspiration syndrome is associated with
a. prolonged labor
b. postdates pregnancy
c. intrauterine growth restriction
d. chronic maternal hypertension
e. all of the above

7.28 What percent of singleton term deliveries are breech presentations?
a. 1%
b. 3%
c. 5%
d. 7%
e. 9%

7.29 Vaginal delivery of the term breech is generally avoided when the fetus weighs less than
a. 1000 grams
b. 1500 grams
c. 2000 grams
d. 2500 grams
e. 3000 grams

7.30 Which of the following is NOT a selection criterion for external cephalic version?
a. Normal fetus
b. Reassuring fetal heart rate tracing
c. No uterine surgical scars
d. Presenting part in the pelvis
e. Adequate amniotic fluid

7.31 All of the following are risks of external cephalic version EXCEPT
a. uterine rupture
b. sepsis
c. cord accident
d. placental abruption
e. premature rupture of the membranes

7.32 Cesarean delivery is required in what percent of term breeches because of hyperextension of the fetal head?
a. 5%
b. 10%
c. 15%
d. 20%
e. 25%

ANSWERS (7.22–7.32)

| 7.22 b | 7.24 b | 7.26 d | 7.28 b | 7.30 d | 7.32 a |
| 7.23 b | 7.25 d | 7.27 e | 7.29 c | 7.31 b | |

Instructions for 7.33 to 7.35: Match the forceps classification with the appropriate station of the leading edge of the fetal skull.

7.33 Outlet forceps

7.34 Low forceps

7.35 Mid forceps
   a. At +2
   b. At the perineum
   c. Above +2

Instructions for 7.36 to 7.39: Match the statements about uterine contractions with the designation of true or false labor.

7.36 Uterine contractions at irregular intervals

7.37 Sedation provides relief from discomfort of uterine contractions

7.38 Uterine contractions of unchanging intensity

7.39 Abdominal but not back discomfort with contractions
   a. True labor
   b. False labor

Instructions for 7.40 to 7.47: Match the description of clinical obstetric situations or conditions to whether it is an indication for or contraindication to the induction of labor.

7.40 Vasa previa

7.41 Prior classical uterine incision

7.42 Premature rupture of membranes

7.43 Intrauterine fetal demise

7.44 Cord presentation

7.45 Abnormal fetal lie

7.46 Chorioamnionitis

7.47 Active genital herpes infection
   a. Indication for induction of labor
   b. Contraindication to induction of labor

7.48 Which of the following is NOT a criterion for a vaginal breech delivery?
   a. A normal labor curve
   b. Estimated fetal weight between 1500 and 4500 g
   c. A reassuring fetal heart tracing
   d. An adequate maternal pelvis by clinical pelvimetry
   e. A normally flexed fetal head

7.49 The delivery of the fetal head in the assisted breach delivery is often facilitated with what type of forceps?
   a. Simpson
   b. Piper
   c. Kielland
   d. Vacuum

ANSWERS (7.33–7.49)

7.33 b	7.36 b	7.39 b	7.42 a	7.45 b	7.48 b
7.34 a	7.37 b	7.40 b	7.43 a	7.46 a	7.49 b
7.35 c	7.38 b	7.41 b	7.44 b	7.47 b	

Questions and Answers Chapter 8:
Intrapartum Fetal Surveillance

8.1 Nonreassuring fetal status during labor occurs in approximately what percent of pregnancies?
 a. Less than 1%
 b. 5%–10%
 c. 15%–20%
 d. 25%–30%

8.2 Which of the following is NOT a criterion for the diagnosis of fetal asphyxia?
 a. Metabolic or mixed acidemia
 b. Persistent Apgar scores of 3 or below
 c. Evidence of neonatal neurologic sequelae
 d. Heart rate acceleration

8.3 If a fetus experiences progressive and sustained hypoxia, the mixed metabolic and respiratory acidosis that may ensue is especially associated with
 a. aerobic glycolysis
 b. anaerobic glycolysis
 c. aerobic gluconeogenesis
 d. anaerobic gluconeogenesis

8.4 The one-minute Apgar for a newborn with a heart rate of less than 100, slow respiratory rate, flaccid muscle tone, a grimace, and blue color is
 a. 1
 b. 2
 c. 3
 d. 4
 e. 5

8.5 The one-minute Apgar for a newborn with a heart rate of more than 100, good respiratory effort, active muscular activity, a good grimace, and pink color is
 a. 6
 b. 7
 c. 8
 d. 9
 e. 10

8.6 Intermittent fetal heart rate auscultation to monitor fetal well-being should be employed at least how often in the active phase of labor?
 a. Every 1 minute
 b. Every 5 minutes
 c. Every 10 minutes
 d. Every 15 minutes
 e. Every 20 minutes

8.7 Intermittent fetal hart rate auscultation to monitor fetal well-being should be employed at least how often in the second stage of labor?
 a. Every 1 minute
 b. Every 5 minutes
 c. Every 10 minutes
 d. Every 15 minutes
 e. Every 20 minutes

8.8 Baseline fetal tachycardia is defined as a heart rate greater than how many beats per minute?
 a. 150
 b. 160
 c. 170
 d. 180
 e. 190

ANSWERS (8.1–8.8)

8.1	b	8.3	b	8.5	d	8.6	d	8.7	b	8.8	b
8.2	d	8.4	c								

8.9   The common cause of fetal tachycardia is
a. fetal anemia
b. maternal anemia
c. maternal hypothermia
d. maternal hyperthermia

8.10 Baseline fetal bradycardia is defined as a heart rate of less than how many beats per minute?
a. 90
b. 100
c. 110
d. 120
e. 130

8.11 A sinusoidal fetal heart rate pattern is frequently associated with
a. Rh isoimmunization
b. umbilical cord prolapse
c. placental abruption
d. preeclampsia

8.12 Fetal arrhythmias are seen in what percent of monitored labors?
a. Less than 1%
b. 5%
c. 10%
d. 15%

8.13 Fetal sleep is associated with what change in fetal heart rate variability?
a. Increased
b. Unchanged
c. Decreased

8.14 Which of the following is characteristic of short-term variability?
a. Variation in amplitude seen on a beat-to-beat basis
b. Amplitude of 3–8 beats per minute
c. Normally encountered after approximately 28 weeks' gestation
d. All of the above

8.15 Long-term variability is associated with an amplitude of
a. 1–3 beats per minute
b. 5–15 beats per minute
c. 15–20 beats per minute
d. 60–80 beats per minute

8.16 Accelerations of the fetal heart rate (FHR) are defined as an increase in the FHR above the baseline of at least how many bpm, usually of 15- to 20-second duration?
a. 5
b. 10
c. 15
d. 20
e. 25

8.17 Accelerations of the fetal heart rate are associated with an intact fetal mechanism that is
a. mildly stressed by hypoxia and acidemia
b. moderately stressed by hypoxia and acidemia
c. severely stressed by hypoxia and acidemia
d. unstressed by hypoxia and acidemia

8.18 If an observed fetal heart rate pattern is a mixture of two more patterns and variations of baseline values, it is usually prudent to manage the obstetric situation based on
a. the most reassuring pattern present
b. an equal weighting of both patterns observed
c. the most substantially nonreassuring pattern
d. fetal scalp sampling for pH

ANSWERS (8.9–8.18)

8.9 d	8.11 a	8.13 c	8.15 b	8.17 d	8.18 c
8.10 d	8.12 a	8.14 d	8.16 c		

8.19 Fetal tachycardia is associated with all of the following EXCEPT
 a. maternal fever and infection
 b. maternal treatment with β-blockers
 c. fetal immaturity
 d. fetal hypoxia

8.20 Which of the following is a cause of fetal tachycardia?
 a. Maternal thyrotoxicosis
 b. Fetal anemia
 c. Fetal infection
 d. All of the above

8.21 All the following are associated with fetal bradycardia EXCEPT
 a. maternal treatment with β-blockers
 b. maternal treatment with atropine
 c. fetal anoxia
 d. fetal congenital heart block

Instructions for items 8.22 to 8.24: Match the type of fetal heart rate deceleration with the appropriate description(s). An option may be used once, more than once, or not at all.

8.22 Early deceleration

8.23 Variable deceleration

8.24 Late deceleration
 a. Associated with umbilical cord compression
 b. Associated with pressure on the fetal head
 c. Associated with uteroplacental insufficiency

8.25 The presence of persistent late decelerations and decreased beat-to-beat variability should lead to which of the following?
 a. Direct measurement of fetal acid–base status
 b. Monitoring the frequency of fetal movement
 c. Measurement of maternal blood pressure
 d. Measurement of amniotic volume

8.26 Which of the following describes a late fetal heart rate deceleration?
 a. Deceleration starts after uterine contraction begins, nadir after peak of uterine contraction, resolves to baseline after uterine contraction is over
 b. Deceleration begins with uterine contraction, nadir at peak of uterine contraction, returns to baseline at end of uterine contraction
 c. Deceleration may start before or after the start of the uterine contraction

8.27 Repetitive late fetal heart rate (FHR) decelerations are considered particularly ominous with respect to fetal well-being if associated with
 a. variable decelerations
 b. early decelerations
 c. increased FHR variability
 d. decreased FHR variability

Answers (8.19–8.27)					
8.19 b	8.21 b	8.23 a	8.25 a	8.26 a	8.27 d
8.20 d	8.22 b	8.24 c			

8.28 In the face of evidence of intrauterine fetal compromise, which drug may relax uterine tone and slow contraction rate?
a. Atropine
b. Meperidine
c. Terbutaline
d. Succinylcholine
e. Morphine

8.29 The single most reliable indicator of fetal status using electronic fetal monitoring is
a. variability
b. baseline
c. accelerations
d. periodic decelerations

8.30 Uteroplacental insufficiency should be suspected with
a. maternal hypertension
b. diabetes mellitus
c. toxemia
d. all of the above

8.31 A normal fetal scalp blood gas pH is in the range of
a. 6.80–6.95
b. 7.00–7.15
c. 7.25–7.40
d. 7.50–7.65

8.32 Fetal compromise is strongly expected with a scalp pH less than
a. 7.26
b. 7.24
c. 7.22
d. 7.20
e. 7.18

8.33 The normal range for fetal scalp oxygen for a term fetus during labor is thought to be
a. 10%–50%
b. 20%–60%
c. 30%–70%
d. 40%–80%
e. 50%–90%

8.34 Fetal scalp oxygen values for a term fetus during labor that trend below 30% are thought to be associated with a predicted fetal scalp pH value of less than
a. 7.30
b. 7.25
c. 7.20
d. 7.15
e. 7.10

Answers (8.28–8.34)

8.28 c	8.30 d	8.31 c	8.32 d	8.33 c	8.34 c
8.29 a					

Questions and Answers Chapter 9:
Immediate Care of the Newborn

9.1 Which of the following clinical circumstances has a higher than usual risk of the need for neonatal resuscitation such that the provision for personnel highly skilled in these procedures may be advisable before delivery?
a. Cesarean delivery
b. Suspected fetal anomaly
c. Maternal fever
d. Multiple gestation
e. All of the above

9.2 Approximately what percent of cesarean deliveries may require the need for neonatal resuscitation personnel?
a. Less than 1%
b. 5%
c. 10%
d. 50%

9.3 In what position is the infant placed in the warming unit?
a. Supine, with the head lowered, turned to one side
b. Supine, with the head up
c. In the sitting position
d. In the prone position with the head lowered

9.4 Which of the following are examples of mild stimulation to the newborn?
a. Suctioning
b. Rubbing the back
c. Slapping the feet
d. All of the above

9.5 Which of the following statements regarding the Apgar score is an accurate reflection of its proper use?
a. It is used to define birth asphyxia
b. It indicates the cause of the newborn's depression
c. The 1-minute Apgar score identifies newborns requiring special attention
d. The 5-minute Apgar score predicts neurologic injury

9.6 Mild to moderate depression of the newborn is defined as Apgar scores of
a. less than 2
b. 2–4
c. 4–7
d. 8–9

9.7 Causes of neonatal asphyxia may include
a. trauma
b. severe maternal disease
c. decreased uteroplacental blood flow
d. all of the above

9.8 Scalp hair that is coarse suggests an estimated gestational age greater than how many weeks?
a. 33
b. 35
c. 37
d. 39

ANSWERS (9.1–9.8)

9.1	e	9.3	a	9.5	c	9.6	c	9.7	d	9.8	d
9.2	b	9.4	d								

9.9 A neonate's ear lobe that lacks cartilage suggests a gestational age below how many weeks?
   a. 34
   b. 36
   c. 38
   d. 40

9.10 At 37–38 weeks' gestation, a neonate's breast nodule is expected to be how many millimeters?
   a. 2
   b. 4
   c. 6
   d. 8

9.11 In a neonate estimated to be 39 weeks, which of the following accurately describes the sole creases on its feet?
   a. There are no sole creases
   b. There is a single anterior transverse crease
   c. Creases cover two thirds of the foot
   d. There are extensive creases covering the entire sole

9.12 Which of the following is the correct management of the umbilical cord stump in a newborn?
   a. Keep it covered with Vaseline
   b. Apply antiseptic solution daily
   c. Keep uncovered to expose it to air
   d. Excise it after 24 hours of life

9.13 What percent of newborns will pass stool within the first 24 hours of life?
   a. 60%
   b. 70%
   c. 80%
   d. 90%

9.14 Which of the following are characteristics of normal stool in the first 2–3 days of life?
   a. Greenish-brown in color
   b. Sterile
   c. Odorless
   d. All of the above

9.15 Which of the following statements regarding newborn weight loss is correct?
   a. Preterm newborns lose relatively more weight than their term counterparts
   b. Preterm newborns regain their weight faster than their term counterparts
   c. Term infants do not lose weight in the newborn period until one week of life
   d. Newborn weight loss in preterm newborns is regained in the first 4 days of life

9.16 Application of silver nitrate is designed to prevent
   a. conjunctivitis
   b. optic neuritis
   c. corneal scarring
   d. all of the above

9.17 Physiologic jaundice of the newborn occurs in what proportion of all newborns?
   a. 1:10
   b. 1:3
   c. 1:2
   d. 2:3

9.18 Jaundice becomes clinically apparent in the newborn when bilirubin levels reach what level?
   a. 1 mg/dl
   b. 3 mg/dl
   c. 5 mg/dl
   d. 10 mg/dl

ANSWERS (9.9–9.18)

| 9.9 b | 9.11 d | 9.13 d | 9.15 a | 9.17 b | 9.18 c |
| 9.10 b | 9.12 c | 9.14 d | 9.16 a | | |

9.19. Meconium stained amniotic fluid is encountered in ( ) percent of gestations?
   a. 0–5
   b. 10–15
   c. 20–25
   d. 30–35
   e. 40–45

9.20. The most meaningful assessment of metabolic status of the baby at the time of delivery is through analysis of _____ blood gases
   a. umbilical artery
   b. umbilical vein
   c. twice the umbilical artery plus the umbilical vein pH divided by three
   d. twice the umbilical vein plus the umbilical artery pH divided by three

9.21. About ( ) of infants born with meconium in the amniotic fluid will have meconium in the lungs.
   a. ⅓
   b. ⅔
   c. all

9.22. About ( ) of infants born with meconium in the amniotic fluid will develop significant respiratory distress.
   a. ¹⁄₁₀
   b. ³⁄₁₀
   c. ½
   d. ⁷⁄₁₀

9.23. Immediate intubation and suctioning should be performed _____ when there is thin meconium stained amniotic fluid.
   a. at all times
   b. at all times if a neonatologist is present at delivery
   c. at all times for post-dates neonates
   d. at all times when warranted by the clinical judgement of the delivering clinician or physician and/or pediatrician attending the delivery.

9.24. The scrotum of newborn males of greater than 39 weeks gestational age is characterized by
   a. Few rugae
   b. Intermediate rugae
   c. Extensive rugae

9.25. In the fetal circulation, the highest PO_2 is contained in the
   a. umbilical vein
   b. umbilical arteries
   c. fetal aorta
   d. fetal pulmonary artery
   e. pulmonary vena cava

9.26. Fetal cord blood gases most closely represent the baby at the time of
   a. the end of the first stage of labor
   b. the end of the second stage of labor
   c. the first minute of extra-uterine life
   d. the fifth minute of extra-uterine life

ANSWERS (9.19–9.26)

9.19 b	9.21 a	9.23 d	9.24 e	9.25 a	9.26 b
9.20 a	9.22 a				

9.27. Which of the following is the most useful initial arterial cord blood value to manage the acidotic newborn?
   a. pH
   b. PCO_2
   c. PO_2
   d. base deficit

9.28. The gastrointestinal tract of the newborn is colorized by normal bacterial flora at approximately
   a. in labor after rupture of membranes
   b. the time of delivery
   c. one hour of life
   d. 12 hours of life
   e. 72 hours of life

9.29. Currently, the most effective newborn prophylaxis to prevent ophthalmia neonatorum is
   a. penicillin
   b. erythromycin
   c. tetracycline
   d. silver nitrate
   e. cephalosporin

9.30. Ioterus neonatorum is most often caused by
   a. temporary hepatic obstruction
   b. billary atresis
   c. reabsorption of free bilirubin from the fetal intestine
   d. increased erythrocyte destruction of fetal hemoglobin

ANSWERS (9.27–9.30)
   9.27 d   9.28 d   9.29 d   9.30 c

Questions and Answers Chapter 10: Postpartum Care

10.1 The puerperium, which is the period following birth during which the reproductive tract returns to its normal, nonpregnant state, lasts approximately
a. 4 weeks
b. 6 weeks
c. 8 weeks
d. 10 weeks
e. 12 weeks

10.2 Uterine involution is a result of a decrease in the
a. number of cells in the uterine myometrium
b. size of cells in the uterine myometrium
c. size of the intercellular spaces in the uterine myometrium
d. number of intercellular spaces in the uterine myometrium

10.3 How many weeks does it take for the uterus to return to its prepregnancy position in the true pelvis?
a. 1
b. 2
c. 3
d. 4
e. 5

10.4 How many weeks does it take for the uterus to return to its prepregnancy size?
a. 2
b. 3
c. 4
d. 5
e. 6

10.5 Immediate postpartum uterine hemostasis is maintained by
a. primary clotting of blood in the uterine artery
b. contraction of the uterine smooth muscle
c. scar formation within the uterine cavity
d. tamponade effect of clots

10.6 The remnants of the hymen in the postpartum woman appear as fleshy tags at the introitus that are called
a. the hymenal ring
b. myrtiform caruncles
c. inclusion bodies
d. hyperplastic nodes of Smith

10.7 The mean time to ovulation in the nonlactating postpartum woman is approximately
a. 2 weeks
b. 4 weeks
c. 6 weeks
d. 8 weeks
e. 10 weeks

10.8 Fifty percent of women ovulate within how many days of delivery?
a. 30
b. 60
c. 90
d. 120
e. 150

10.9 The elevated pulse rate characteristic of pregnancy
a. decreases at the end of the third stage of labor
b. decreases approximately one hour after delivery
c. persists for approximately 3 weeks postpartum
d. is a reflection of the fetal heart rate

ANSWERS (10.1–10.9)

| 10.1 | b | 10.3 | b | 10.5 | b | 10.7 | e | 10.8 | c | 10.9 | b |
| 10.2 | b | 10.4 | b | 10.6 | b | | | | | | |

10.10   Transitory urinary retention in the postpartum period following vaginal delivery is primarily related to
a. sympathomimetic discharge
b. peripartum cystitis
c. periurethral edema
d. progesterone-associated loss of bladder contractility

10.11   Immediately after delivery, how much does a normal uterus weigh?
a. 500 g
b. 1000 g
c. 1500 g
d. 2000 g

10.12   Postpartum uterine contractile pain is greater in breast-feeding women because suckling releases
a. progesterone
b. prostaglandins
c. oxytocin
d. estrogen

10.13   Breast engorgement in non–breast-feeding women typically occurs how many days postpartum?
a. 1
b. 3
c. 5
d. 7
e. 9

10.14   Postpartum breast engorgement usually resolves within how many days if the patient is not breast-feeding?
a. 1
b. 3
c. 5
d. 7
e. 9

10.15   Which of the following best describes breast engorgement?
a. Unilateral location, localized swelling, intense localized pain, patient generally feels ill
b. Unilateral location, localized swelling, localized pain, patient generally feels well
c. Bilateral location, generalized swelling, generalized pain, patient generally feels well
d. Associated with fever

10.16   Which of the following best describes a plugged duct?
a. Unilateral location, localized swelling, intense localized pain, patient generally feels ill
b. Unilateral location, localized swelling, localized pain, patient generally feels well
c. Bilateral location, generalized swelling, generalized pain, patient generally feels well
d. Associated with fever

10.17   Approximately what percent of the total dosage of any medication is seen in breast milk?
a. 1%
b. 4%
c. 7%
d. 10%
e. 13%

10.18   All of the following medications are contraindications to breast-feeding EXCEPT
a. lithium carbonate
b. tetracycline
c. bromocriptine
d. methotrexate
e. dicloxacillin

ANSWERS (10.10–10.18)

| 10.10 c | 10.12 c | 10.14 b | 10.16 b | 10.17 a | 10.18 e |
| 10.11 b | 10.13 b | 10.15 c | | | |

10.19 On approximately what postpartum day does milk production begin?
   a. First
   b. Third
   c. Fifth
   d. Seventh
   e. Ninth

10.20 When after delivery is the endometrium reestablished in most patients?
   a. First week
   b. Second week
   c. Third week
   d. Fourth week
   e. Fifth week

10.21 The silvery stripes seen on the abdomen skin postpartum are called
   a. diastasis recti
   b. tunica albuginea
   c. striae
   d. myrtiform caruncles

10.22 In a normal patient immediately after delivery, loss of fluid through diuresis and loss of extravascular fluid is approximately
   a. 1 kg
   b. 3 kg
   c. 5 kg
   d. 7 kg
   e. 9 kg

10.23 Infection of episiotomy sites occurs in what percent of patients?
   a. 0.1%
   b. 1%
   c. 10%
   d. 25%

10.24 Which vitamin is not found in human breast milk?
   a. A
   b. D
   c. C
   d. K
   e. E

10.25 Suicidal ideation is associated with postpartum depression in approximately one in how many pregnancies?
   a. 500
   b. 1000
   c. 1500
   d. 2000
   e. 2500

10.26 Which of the following statements about colostrum is INCORRECT?
   a. The immunoglobulin A content of colostrum may help protect the newborn infant from enteric infection
   b. The secretion of colostrum persists for at least 2 weeks
   c. Antibodies are readily demonstrable in colostrum
   d. Colostrum contains more protein and minerals than breast milk
   e. Colostrum contains less sugar and fat than breast milk

10.27 Which of the following is NOT involved in stimulating milk production and secretion?
   a. Thyroid-stimulating hormone
   b. Progesterone and estrogen
   c. Human placental lactogen
   d. Prolactin
   e. Cortisol and insulin

10.28 During the first 5 months of pregnancy, breast development occurs because of
   a. increased fat deposition
   b. increased cardiac output
   c. slowed venous return from the breasts
   d. capillary dilation
   e. synergistic hormone action

ANSWERS (10.19–10.28)

10.19 b	10.21 c	10.23 a	10.25 d	10.27 a	10.28 e
10.20 c	10.22 c	10.24 d	10.26 b		

10.29 Breast-feeding in the postpartum period
   a. markedly diminishes blood loss
   b. slightly diminishes blood loss
   c. does not affect the amount of blood loss
   d. slightly increases blood loss
   e. markedly increases blood loss

10.30 Mastitis followed by breast abscess is most frequently due to
   a. bacterial vaginosis
   b. *Pneumococcus*
   c. *Escherichia coli*
   d. *Streptococcus pyogenes*
   e. *Staphylococcus aureus*

10.31 The return of normal tone to the pelvic floor muscles postpartum may be enhanced by
   a. exogenous estrogen supplementation
   b. exogenous progesterone supplementation
   c. Kegel exercises
   d. avoiding coitus for 3–6 months

10.32 Heavy postpartum bleeding associated with separation and passage of the placental escar most commonly begins between __ and __ days postpartum.
   a. 2 and 8
   b. 5 and 11
   c. 8 and 14
   d. 11 and 17
   e. 14 and 20

10.33 The diagnosis of delayed postpartum hemorrhage comprises what percent of patients where postpartum bleeding is excessive?
   a. 1
   b. 3
   c. 5
   d. 7
   e. 9

10.34 The heavier postpartum bleeding associated with placental escar passage is best managed by
   a. suction curettage
   b. oxytocic administration
   c. hysteroscopic surgery
   d. reassurance
   e. hypogastric artery ligation

10.35 Delayed postpartum hemorrhage is associated with retained placental tissues in about what percent of cases?
   a. 10
   b. 30
   c. 50
   d. 70
   e. 90

10.36 Surgical management of postpartum hemorrhoids may be considered how soon postpartum?
   a. Immediately
   b. 3 months
   c. 6 months
   d. 9 months
   e. 12 months

10.37 What is the expulsion rate for intrauterine devices inserted immediately postpartum?
   a. 0%–10%
   b. 10%–20%
   c. 20%–30%
   d. 30%–40%
   e. 40%–50%

ANSWERS (10.29–10.37)

| 10.29 c | 10.31 c | 10.33 a | 10.35 b | 10.36 c | 10.37 b |
| 10.30 e | 10.32 c | 10.34 d | | | |

10.38 Which of the following statements about postpartum contraception is INCORRECT?

a. Basal body temperature methods are not reliable until regular menses are established

b. Cervical mucus methods are not reliable until regular menses are established

c. Progestin contraceptives may inhibit lactation slightly

d. Combined estrogen-progestin oral contraceptives may inhibit lactation slightly

e. Intrauterine device insertion is acceptable in appropriately selected patients

Answer (10.38)

10.38 c

Questions and Answers Chapter 11:
Isoimmunization

11.1 When the father is homozygous Rh+ and the mother is Rh−, what is the probability that the fetus will be Rh+?
   a. 25%
   b. 50%
   c. 75%
   d. 100%

11.2 Which of the following statements about isoimmunization is INCORRECT?
   a. It involves the development of fetal antibodies in response to maternal red blood cells
   b. The antibodies involved in isoimmunization cross the placental barrier
   c. The ability of the fetus to produce red blood cells can to some degree counter the isoimmunization process
   d. The father must be Rh+ and the mother Rh− for Rh isoimmunization to occur

11.3 The major class of antibody responsible for Rh isoimmunization is
   a. immunoglobulin G (IgG)
   b. IgM
   c. IgE
   d. IgA

11.4 In the case of an Rh+ fetus and an Rh− mother, complications will usually first appear in which pregnancy?
   a. First
   b. Second
   c. Third
   d. Fourth

11.5 Pregnancies with severely affected Rh-immunized fetuses may be complicated by
   a. polyhydramnios
   b. fetal hydrops
   c. fetal cardiac failure
   d. fetal anemia
   e. all of the above

11.6 Hydrops fetalis is associated with
   a. severe fluid retention due to renal failure in the fetus
   b. irreversible carbohydrate metabolic failure
   c. decreased fetal aldosterone secretion
   d. the ability of the fetal hematopoietic tissue to compensate for anemia resulting from red cell destruction

11.7 Which of the following is NOT associated with hydrops fetalis?
   a. Fetal ascites
   b. Low output cardiac failure
   c. Anemia
   d. Decreased oncotic pressure in the fetal intravascular space

Instructions for items 11.8 to 11.12: Match the event with the risk of sensitization. An option may be used once, more than once, or not at all.

11.8 Mismatched blood transfusion

11.9 Spontaneous abortion

11.10 Ectopic pregnancy

11.11 Full-term delivery

ANSWERS (11.1–11.11)									
11.1	d	11.3	a	11.5	e	11.7	b	11.9	b	11.11	d
11.2	a	11.4	b	11.6	d	11.8	e	11.10	a		

11.12 Induced abortion
a. Less than 1%
b. 3%–4%
c. 5%–6%
d. 15%
e. 90%

11.13 In cases of fetal Rh isoimmunization, which statement reflects the relationship between the degree of fetal hypoproteinemia and fetal hepatic red cell production?
a. They are positively correlated
b. They are negatively correlated
c. They are unrelated

11.14 Antibody development will occur in approximately what percent of cases of an Rh– mother and an Rh+ fetus?
a. 5%
b. 15%
c. 25%
d. 35%
e. 45%

11.15 The Liley curve is based on the measurement of amniotic fluid
a. whole red blood cells
b. hemoglobin
c. Rh-D antigen
d. bilirubin
e. albumin

11.16 The major cause of fetal erythrocytes entering the maternal circulation is
a. labor and delivery
b. normal placental circulation
c. spontaneous abortion
d. premature rupture of membranes
e. low level placental abruption

11.17 Rh immune globulin is effective against which antigen of the Rh system?
a. A
b. B
c. C
d. D
e. E

11.18 Rh immune globulin (RhoGAM) should be administered to an Rh– patient at all of the following times EXCEPT
a. at 28 weeks' gestation
b. within 3 days of delivery of an Rh+ infant
c. at the time of amniocentesis
d. at the onset of labor

11.19 When is administration of Rh immune globulin (RhoGAM) appropriate for an Rh– patient?
a. After an ectopic pregnancy
b. After a spontaneous abortion
c. After an elective abortion
d. In all of the above circumstances

11.20 Human Rh immune globulin (RhoGAM)
a. prevents the transfer of incompatible fetal cells to the mother
b. attaches to the fetal Rh+ cells in the maternal circulation and obscures the antigen sites
c. prevents antibody production in the maternal hematopoietic system
d. destroys fetal Rh+ cells in the maternal circulation

11.21 The administration of a 300 mg dose of Rh immune globulin (RhoGAM) to Rh– patients at 28 weeks' gestation is found to reduce the risk of sensitization to approximately
a. 0.2%
b. 0.5%
c. 1.0%
d. 5.0%
e. 10.0%

ANSWERS (11.12–11.21)

11.12 c	11.14 b	11.16 a	11.18 d	11.20 b	11.21 a
11.13 a	11.15 d	11.17 d	11.19 d		

11.22 The standard 300 mg dose of Rh immune globulin (RhoGAM) will effectively neutralize how many milliliters of fetal red blood cells?
a. 5
b. 10
c. 15
d. 20
e. 25

11.23 Direct fetal transfusion into the umbilical cord under ultrasound guidance carries with it a risk of fetal death of up to
a. 1%
b. 3%
c. 5%
d. 7%
e. 15%

11.24 The volume of fetal red cells required to elicit an antibody response is estimated to be
a. 0.001 ml
b. 0.01 ml
c. 0.1 ml
d. 1.0 ml
e. 10.0 ml

11.25 Which of the following statements about the Kleihauer-Betke test is INCORRECT?
a. It is used to detect fetomaternal hemorrhage
b. A negative result is an indication to administer Rh immune globulin
c. It identifies fetal cells in the maternal circulation
d. The ratio of fetal to maternal cells are assessed microscopically

11.26 The relative proportion of patients with ABO hemolytic disease and non-Rh D/non-ABO hemolytic disease, as compared to patients with Rh isoimmunization has
a. increased
b. remained the same
c. decreased

11.27 Which of the following statements about ABO hemolytic disease is INCORRECT?
a. It results in milder fetal kernicterus than Rh hemolytic disease
b. It is rarely associated with hydrops fetalis
c. The disease severity is probably related to the relatively smaller number of A and B antigenic sites on fetal red blood cells
d. It usually occurs in the second trimester

Instructions for items 11.28 to 11.34: For patients with positive antibody screens for the following irregular antibodies, select the appropriate next management step. An option may be used once, more than once, or not at all.

11.28 Kell – K

11.29 Duffy – Fy^b

11.30 Lutheran – Lu^a, Lu^b

11.31 Kidd – Jk^a, Jk^b

11.32 Non-D Rh-c, C, e, E

11.32 I, P

11.33 Duffy – Fy^a

11.34 Lewis – Le^a, Le^b
a. Test father for presence of antigen
b. No further management is required
c. Perform amniocentesis

ANSWERS (11.22–11.34)

11.22 c	11.25 b	11.27 d	11.29 b	11.31 a	11.33 a
11.23 b	11.26 a	11.28 a	11.30 b	11.32 a	11.34 b
11.24 b					

Questions and Answers Chapter 12: Postpartum Hemorrhage

12.1 The traditional definition of postpartum hemorrhage is blood loss in excess of
a. 250 ml
b. 500 ml
c. 750 ml
d. 1000 ml

12.2 The most common cause of postpartum hemorrhage is
a. uterine laceration
b. uterine atony
c. cervical laceration
d. retained uterine tissue
e. vaginal laceration

12.3 Excessive postpartum bleeding from the placental implantation site is primarily prevented by
a. muscular contraction of the uterus
b. coagulation of the uterine vascular bed
c. mechanical obstruction of vessels
d. sludging effect of the postpartum state

12.4 Which of the following characteristics of labor is associated with uterine atony?
a. Prolonged labor
b. Augmentation of labor
c. Precipitous delivery
d. All of the above

12.5 Which of the following medications may interfere with uterine contractility resulting in uterine atony?
a. Magnesium sulfate
b. Ampicillin
c. Demerol
d. All of the above

12.6 Intravenous administration of undiluted oxytocin can lead to
a. hypotension
b. hypertension
c. seizures
d. blindness
e. liver failure

12.7 Which of the following is appropriate for the initial treatment of uterine atony?
a. Rapid infusion of oxytocin
b. Uterine massage
c. Administration of methergine
d. Administration of prostaglandin
e. All of the above are appropriate

12.8 Persistent uterine atony is treated with which of the following invasive modalities?
a. Uterine artery ligation
b. Hypogastric artery ligation
c. Hysterectomy
d. Selective arterial embolization
e. All of the above

12.9 Which of the following is NOT a predisposing factor to lower genital tract laceration?
a. Forceps delivery
b. Breech delivery
c. Delivery of a macrosomic infant
d. Precipitous delivery
e. Premature rupture of the membranes

ANSWERS (12.1–12.9)									
12.1	b	12.3	a	12.5	a	12.7	e	12.8	e
12.2	b	12.4	d	12.6	a				

(12.9 e)

12.10 Which of the following statements about vulvar hematomas is INCORRECT?
    a. They usually are associated with exquisite pain
    b. They usually are associated with shock
    c. If less than 5 cm and stable in size, they may be managed expectantly
    d. If the size is increasing, surgical management usually is required

12.11 The site of postpartum hematoma associated with the greatest morbidity is the
    a. vulva
    b. lower vagina
    c. upper vagina
    d. cervix

Instructions for items 12.12 to 12.14: Match the type of placental penetration into the uterus with the appropriate description(s). An option may be used once, more than once, or not at all.

12.12 Placenta accreta

12.13 Placenta increta

12.14 Placenta percreta
    a. Penetration into the uterine muscle
    b. Penetration into the superficial lining of the uterus
    c. Penetration involving the full thickness of the muscular uterine wall

12.15 Which of the following is NOT a predisposing factor to retention of parts of the placenta?
    a. Uterine leiomyomas
    b. Previous cesarean delivery
    c. Multiple gestation
    d. Prior uterine curettage
    e. Succenturiate lobe

12.16 Patients treated intrapartum and postpartum with intravenous magnesium sulfate are predisposed to
    a. uterine atony
    b. retained placenta
    c. uterine inversion
    d. placental infarction

12.17 The presence of retained placental tissue can be identified by
    a. external palpation of the abdomen
    b. ultrasound examination of the uterus
    c. measurement of progesterone levels
    d. hysteroscopy

12.18 The most common cause of death in amniotic fluid embolism is
    a. cardiorespiratory collapse
    b. afibrinogenemia
    c. massive hemorrhage
    d. acute renal failure
    e. cerebral infarction

ANSWERS (12.10–12.18)

| 12.10 b | 12.12 b | 12.14 c | 12.16 a | 12.17 b | 12.18 a |
| 12.11 c | 12.13 a | 12.15 c | | | |

12.19 Which laceration can be directly related to the postpartum placement of a Foley catheter?
   a. Second degree vaginal
   b. Third degree vaginal
   c. Fourth degree vaginal
   d. Periurethral
   e. Cervical

Instructions for items 12.20 to 12.24: Match the finding associated with amniotic fluid embolism with its most common order of occurrence.

12.20 Respiratory distress

12.21 Cardiovascular collapse

12.22 Cyanosis

12.23 Hemorrhage

12.24 Coma
   a. Occurs first
   b. Occurs second
   c. Occurs third
   d. Occurs fourth
   e. Occurs fifth

12.25 What is the maternal mortality in amniotic fluid embolism?
   a. 10%–30%
   b. 30%–50%
   c. 50%–70%
   d. 70%–90%

ANSWERS (12.19–12.25)

12.19 d	12.21 c	12.22 b	12.23 d	12.24 e	12.25 b
12.20 a					

Questions and Answers Chapter 13:
Postpartum Infection

13.1 The definition of puerperal febrile morbidity includes a temperature greater than
a. 37.5°C
b. 38°C
c. 38.5°C
d. 39°C

13.2 Which of the following factors does NOT predispose to postpartum infection?
a. Maternal obesity
b. Anemia
c. Prolonged labor
d. Postdates pregnancy
e. Premature rupture of the membranes

Instructions for items 13.3 to 13.6: Match the postpartum day with the site(s) where infection is most likely to appear. An option may be used once, more than once, or not at all.

13.3 Day 1

13.4 Day 2

13.5 Day 3

13.6 Day 4
a. Urinary tract (cystitis, pyelonephritis)
b. Lungs (atelectasis, pneumonia)
c. Wound (superficial infection, necrotizing fascitis)
d. Extremities (thrombophlebitis)

13.7 The most common infection following cesarean delivery is
a. metritis
b. pneumonia
c. pyelonephritis
d. pelvic abscess
e. wound infection

13.8 The cause of postpartum pelvic infection is most commonly
a. gram-positive aerobes
b. gram-negative aerobes
c. gram-positive anaerobes
d. gram-negative anaerobes
e. polymicrobial

13.9 All of the following are gram-positive aerobes EXCEPT
a. *Enterococcus*
b. *Staphylococcus*
c. *Streptococcus*
d. *Peptostreptococcus*

13.10 All of the following are gram-negative aerobes EXCEPT
a. *Proteus*
b. *Escherichia coli*
c. *Klebsiella*
d. *Clostridium*

13.11 Which of the following is a gram-negative anaerobe?
a. *Bacteroides*
b. *Clostridium*
c. *Klebsiella*
d. *Proteus*

13.12 Which of the following is NOT a feature that can be present with metritis?
a. Fever
b. Uterine tenderness
c. Diminished or absent bowel sounds
d. Leukocytosis in the range of 15,000–30,000 cells/mL
e. Calf tenderness

ANSWERS (13.1–13.12)

13.1 b	13.3 b	13.5 c	13.7 a	13.9 d	13.11 a
13.2 d	13.4 a	13.6 d	13.8 e	13.10 d	13.12 e

13.13 Intravenous antibiotic therapy for metritis is continued until the patient
   a. is asymptomatic
   b. has normal bowel function
   c. is afebrile for at least 24 hours
   d. is all of the above

13.14 It is customary to provide additional antibiotic therapy in a patient being treated for postpartum metritis if there has been no response to the initial therapy within
   a. 12–24 hours
   b. 24–36 hours
   c. 36–48 hours
   d. 48–72 hours
   e. 72–96 hours

13.15 A postpartum pseudomass associated with fever is most commonly due to postcesarean
   a. phlegmon
   b. pelvic abscess
   c. hematoma
   d. urinoma

13.16 All of the following are characteristics of a pelvic abscess as a complication of postpartum metritis EXCEPT
   a. persistent fever
   b. paradoxical sense of well-being
   c. delayed return to gastrointestinal function
   d. localized pain or tenderness on abdominal examination
   e. evidence of pelvic mass on imaging

13.17 Which of the following statements about the management of a pelvic abscess complicating postpartum metritis is INCORRECT?
   a. Ultrasound, computed tomography, and/or magnetic resonance imaging are often useful in diagnosis
   b. Initial therapy should include broad spectrum antibiotics
   c. Initial therapy should include drainage of the abscess
   d. Rupture may be associated with shock and constitutes a surgical emergency

13.18 As compared with cesarean delivery, postpartum urinary tract infections after vaginal delivery are
   a. less common
   b. as common
   c. more common

13.19 Which of the following is useful in identifying the presence of postpartum urinary tract infection?
   a. Dysuria
   b. Frequency of urination
   c. Costovertebral tenderness
   d. Urinary hesitancy

13.20 Which of the following statements concerning infection of the incision site following cesarean delivery is INCORRECT?
   a. The incision should be probed to determine the extent of infection
   b. Broad spectrum antibiotic therapy often is used
   c. Culture of the wound is not usually required
   d. Drainage of the wound is required

Answers (13.13–13.20)

13.13 d	13.15 a	13.17 c	13.18 a	13.19 c	13.20 c
13.14 d	13.16 b				

13.21 The initial treatment for an episiotomy site infection includes
   a. suture removal
   b. drainage
   c. sitz bath
   d. all of the above

13.22 Which of the following statements concerning necrotizing fascitis is correct?
   a. It is a rare postpartum infection
   b. It is especially virulent, involving the adjacent fascial, muscle, and subcutaneous tissue
   c. It is frequently fatal
   d. It requires surgical debridement in all cases
   e. All of the above statements are correct

13.23 Mastitis most often first appears
   a. at the onset of nursing
   b. in the first week postpartum
   c. about one month postpartum
   d. about six months postpartum

13.24 Which of the following statements about respiratory complications following delivery is correct?
   a. Complications characteristically present in the first postpartum day
   b. Complications are often associated with atelectasis
   c. Pneumonia may occur, especially in patients with predelivery respiratory disease
   d. Complications are more common if general anesthesia was used
   e. All of the above statements are correct

13.25 Which of the following statements about septic pelvic thrombophlebitis is INCORRECT?
   a. It is a sequela of postpartum pelvic infection
   b. It is associated with venous stasis and bacterial colonization
   c. It may be complicated by microembolization to the lungs and other organs by way of the inferior vena cava
   d. It usually presents as residual fever and tachycardia during treatment for metritis
   e. The patient typically experiences severe uterine tenderness and absent bowel sounds

13.26 The standard treatment for septic pelvic thrombophlebitis in the postpartum period is
   a. a switch from double- to triple-antibiotic therapy
   b. placement of an inferior vena cava sieve
   c. empiric treatment with heparin
   d. administration of fever-reducing drugs and rest

13.27 In a case of necrotizing fascitis, which organism is most likely to contribute to the appearance of subcutaneous gas on x-ray or computed tomography?
   a. *Bacteriodes* species
   b. *Escherichia coli*
   c. *Pseudomonas*
   d. *Clostridium*
   e. *Staphylococcus aureus*

ANSWERS (13.21–13.27)

13.21 d	13.23 c	13.24 e	13.25 e	13.26 c	13.27 d
13.22 e					

13.28 Puerperal mastitis is most often caused by
a. *Staphylococcus aureus*
b. Beta-hemolytic streptococcus
c. Alpha-hemolytic streptococcus
d. *Proteus* species

13.29 In cases of mastitis, the breast is colonized by a pathogen that comes from
a. infected lochia
b. infected skin
c. the newborn's oral pharynx
d. the maternal oral pharynx

13.30 Which of the following organisms is most likely to produce fulminant maternal sepsis from metritis within 24 hours following delivery?
a. Beta-hemolytic streptococcus
b. *Escherichia coli*
c. *Clostridium* species
d. *Pseudomonas*
e. *Bacteroides* species

13.31. The timing of prophylactic antibiotics at the time of cesarean delivery is based on providing maximal protection
a. of the surgical wound
b. from maternal pulmonary complications
c. for the newborn
d. for the upper urinary tract

ANSWERS (13.28–13.31)

13.28 a   13.29 c   13.30 a   13.31 c

Questions and Answers Chapter 14: Abortion

14.1 Abortion is generally defined as termination of pregnancy before what gestational age?
a. 12 weeks
b. 15 weeks
c. 20 weeks
d. 25 weeks

14.2 Abortion is generally defined as a pregnancy loss in which the fetus weighs less than
a. 100 grams
b. 200 grams
c. 500 grams
d. 1000 grams

14.3 Approximately 80% of spontaneous abortions occur by what gestational age?
a. 6 weeks
b. 8 weeks
c. 10 weeks
d. 12 weeks

14.4 What is the incidence of clinically recognized spontaneous abortion?
a. 5%–10%
b. 15%–25%
c. 30%–40%
d. 50%–60%

14.5 What is the most common chromosomal anomaly associated with early spontaneous abortion?
a. Trisomy
b. Monosomy
c. Triploidy
d. Tetraploidy

14.6 Trisomy accounts for what percent of chromosomal abnormalities identified in early spontaneous abortion?
a. 20%–30%
b. 30%–40%
c. 40%–50%
d. 50%–60%
e. 60%–70%

14.7 Recurrent abortion is associated with what chance that one parent is an asymptomatic carrier of a chromosomal abnormality?
a. 1%
b. 3%
c. 5%
d. 7%

14.8 A 34-year-old patient reports that her first pregnancy ended in the spontaneous abortion of a chromosomally abnormal fetus at 10 weeks of gestation. Her risk of having another such event is
a. increased compared with her first pregnancy
b. decreased compared with her first pregnancy
c. the same as in her first pregnancy
d. indeterminate

14.9 All of the following are risk factors for spontaneous abortion EXCEPT
a. increasing maternal age
b. increasing paternal age
c. increasing parity
d. increasing maternal weight

ANSWERS (14.1–14.9)					
14.1 c	14.3 d	14.5 a	14.7 b	14.8 a	14.9 d
14.2 c	14.4 b	14.6 c			

14.10 A spontaneous abortion at which of the following gestational ages is most likely to be chromosomally abnormal?
a. 6 weeks
b. 10 weeks
c. 14 weeks
d. 20 weeks

14.11 Which of the following is the least likely cause for a second trimester spontaneous abortion?
a. Abnormal placentation
b. Chromosomal abnormality
c. Maternal systemic disease
d. Uterine anomaly

14.12 Which of the following maternal infections has been associated with spontaneous abortion?
a. *Chlamydia trachomatis*
b. *Neisseria gonorrhoeae*
c. *Ureaplasma urealyticum*
d. *Herpes zoster*

14.13 How is luteal phase defect best diagnosed?
a. Timed serum progesterone
b. Timed endometrial biopsy
c. Timed serum estradiol
d. Timed serum luteinizing hormone
e. Hysterosalpingogram

14.14 Which of the following drugs is used to manage luteal phase defect?
a. Bromocriptine
b. Thyroxine
c. Estrogen
d. Clomiphene citrate

14.15 What is the effect on the rate of spontaneous abortion if the mother smokes more than one pack of cigarettes per day?
a. No effect on the rate
b. Twofold increase
c. Fourfold increase
d. Undetermined effect

14.16 Which location of leiomyomata is most associated with spontaneous abortion?
a. Subserosal
b. Submucosal
c. Intramural
d. Pedunculated

14.17 Pregnancies complicated by first trimester bleeding are at higher risk for which of the following?
a. Preeclampsia
b. Preterm delivery
c. Fetal macrosomia
d. Intrauterine infection

14.18 The combination of which two tests is most valuable in the evaluation of threatened abortion?
a. Ultrasound and complete blood count (CBC)
b. Human chorionic gonadotropin (hCG) and CBC
c. Ultrasound and hCG
d. hCG and progesterone

14.19 Transabdominal ultrasonography can identify an intact gestational sac if the β-human chorionic gonadotropin level is at least
a. 1500 mIU/ml
b. 2500 mIU/ml
c. 5000 mIU/ml
d. 7500 mIU/ml

14.20 What is the appropriate therapy for a missed abortion at 10 weeks of gestation?
a. Hysterotomy
b. Suction curettage
c. Administration of Methergine (methylergonovine maleate)
d. Dilatation and evacuation

ANSWERS (14.10–14.20)

14.10 a	14.12 c	14.14 d	14.16 b	14.18 c	14.20 b
14.11 b	14.13 b	14.15 b	14.17 b	14.19 c	

14.21 Approximately what percentage of threatened abortions proceed to spontaneous abortion?
a. 10%
b. 25%
c. 50%
d. 75%

14.22 The characteristic history of incompetent cervix includes
a. pain but no bleeding
b. no pain or bleeding
c. no pain but with bleeding
d. both pain and bleeding

14.23 Cervical incompetence is characterized by the expulsion of a normal sac and fetus between what weeks of gestation?
a. 6th and 20th
b. 12th and 26th
c. 18th and 32nd
d. 24th and 38th

14.24 Ultrasonographic findings associated with cervical incompetence include cervical funneling and
a. cervical shortening
b. cervical blunting
c. cervical lengthening

14.25 What is the appropriate time for placement of a McDonald cerclage?
a. Before pregnancy
b. Early in pregnancy, before dilatation occurs
c. Early in pregnancy, after dilation has reached 3 cm
d. Immediately after an abortion

14.26 The Shirodkar cerclage is characterized by what placement of the suture?
a. Through and through
b. Submucosal

14.27 The presence of Asherman's syndrome is confirmed by which of the following?
a. History
b. Physical examination
c. Hysteroscopy
d. Ultrasound

14.28 Treatment of Asherman's syndrome involves lysis of the adhesions and treatment with
a. estrogen
b. progesterone
c. steroids
d. clomiphene citrate
e. oral contraceptives

14.29 All of the following are techniques for second trimester pregnancy termination EXCEPT
a. dilatation and evacuation
b. prostaglandin vaginal suppository
c. intra-amniotic infusion of hypertonic saline
d. suction curettage

14.30 Which of the following may be present in cases of septic abortion?
a. Sepsis
b. Shock
c. Renal failure
d. Hemorrhage
e. All of the above

14.31 All of the following should be included in the management of septic abortion EXCEPT
a. intravenous fluids
b. antibiotics
c. evacuation of the uterus
d. prostaglandins

ANSWERS (14.21–14.31)

| 14.21 c | 14.23 c | 14.25 b | 14.27 c | 14.29 d | 14.31 d |
| 14.22 b | 14.24 a | 14.26 b | 14.28 a | 14.30 e | |

14.32 What percent of women with septate uteri have problems with fetal wastage?
a. 5%
b. 15%
c. 25%
d. 35%

14.33 The differential diagnosis of threatened abortion should include all the following EXCEPT
a. placental abruption
b. friable cervix
c. cervical polyp
d. ectopic pregnancy

14.34 All of the following medical conditions are associated with an increased risk of first trimester spontaneous abortion EXCEPT
a. diabetes
b. luteal phase inadequacy
c. hypothyroidism
d. hyperthyroidism

14.35 Postabortal syndrome following elective pregnancy termination results from
a. retained fetal tissue
b. uterine atony
c. inadequate surgical technique
d. the presence of a combined pregnancy

Answers (14.32–14.35)

| 14.32 b | 14.33 a | 14.34 c | 14.35 b |

Questions and Answers Chapter 15:
Ectopic Pregnancy

15.1 Approximately what percent of patients with a prior ectopic pregnancy will have a subsequent full term birth?
a. 30%
b. 50%
c. 70%
d. 90%

15.2 Currently, the ratio of ectopic to intrauterine pregnancies in the United States is approximately
a. 1:25
b. 1:50
c. 1:100
d. 1:200

15.3 Which of the following is associated with the greatest increased risk of ectopic pregnancy?
a. Use of oral contraceptives
b. Intrauterine contraceptive device use
c. Previous elective abortion
d. Previous ectopic pregnancy

15.4 At what gestational age do women with tubal ectopic pregnancies first experience clinical symptoms?
a. 2 weeks
b. 4 weeks
c. 6 weeks
d. 8 weeks
e. Varies with location of the tubal pregnancy

15.5 Which of the following symptoms is NOT associated with ectopic pregnancy?
a. Acute pelvic pain
b. Lower abdominal pain
c. Vaginal bleeding
d. Acute nausea and vomiting
e. Amenorrhea

15.6 Which of the following physical findings can be compatible with the diagnosis of ectopic pregnancy?
a. Abdominal tenderness
b. Adnexal mass
c. Uterine enlargement
d. Normal blood pressure
e. All of the above

15.7 What is the etiology for vaginal bleeding in cases of ectopic pregnancy?
a. Coagulopathy
b. Sloughing of decidua
c. Bleeding from the fallopian tube
d. Progesterone excess

15.8 Absence of villi on uterine curettage rules out which of the following diagnoses?
a. Combined pregnancy
b. Heterotropic pregnancy
c. Tubal pregnancy
d. None of the above diagnoses is ruled out

15.9 The great majority of ectopic pregnancies implant in the
a. ovary
b. cervix
c. peritoneal cavity
d. fallopian tube

15.10 Of tubal ectopic pregnancies, approximately 80% implant in the
a. isthmus
b. fimbriae
c. ampulla
d. corneau

ANSWERS (15.1–15.10)									
15.1	b	15.3	d	15.5	d	15.7	b	15.9	d	15.10	c
15.2	b	15.4	e	15.6	e	15.8	d				

15.11 Which of the following laboratory and radiologic findings are consistent with the diagnosis of ectopic pregnancy?
   a. Empty uterine cavity on ultrasound
   b. A white blood count of 16,500
   c. A hematocrit of 37%
   d. Serum progesterone of 25 ng/ml
   e. All of the above

15.12 In the diagnosis of ectopic pregnancy, a culdocentesis that obtains 3 ml of straw-colored fluid would be considered
   a. negative
   b. positive
   c. nondiagnostic
   d. unsatisfactory

15.13 Implantation in which of the following sites is likely to reach term?
   a. Abdomen
   b. Ovary
   c. Cervix
   d. Fallopian tube
   e. Implantation in none of the above sites is likely to reach term

15.14 A heterotropic pregnancy is defined as
   a. an ectopic pregnancy outside the fallopian tube
   b. a twin ectopic pregnancy in the same site
   c. coexistent intrauterine and ectopic pregnancies
   d. ectopic pregnancy in two different sites outside the uterus

15.15 All of the following are included in Spiegelberg's criteria for ovarian pregnancy EXCEPT
   a. an intact fallopian tube
   b. an ovary in the normal position
   c. ovarian tissue in the wall of the gestational sac
   d. a fallopian tube connected to the uterus by the ovarian ligament

15.16 In the management of ectopic pregnancy, methotrexate may be administered
   a. orally
   b. intramuscularly
   c. by direct injection into the ectopic gestational sac
   d. through all of the above routes

15.17 All of the following are useful in the diagnosis of an ectopic pregnancy EXCEPT
   a. observation of the Arias-Stella reaction on histologic examination
   b. the presence of a gestational sac visualized on ultrasound examination of the fallopian tube
   c. observation of an empty uterus on ultrasound accompanied by human chorionic gonadotropin level of 8500 mIU/ml
   d. the laparoscopic visualization of 3-cm mass in the fallopian tube

15.18 The incidence of tubal ectopic pregnancy has been steadily rising in the United States, primarily because of increased
   a. use of oral contraceptives
   b. incidence of elective abortion
   c. incidence of pelvic inflammatory disease
   d. delay in the onset of sexual activity in couples

ANSWERS (15.11–15.18)

15.11 e	15.13 e	15.15 d	15.16 d	15.17 a	15.18 c
15.12 a	15.14 c				

15.19 The mortality rate associated with ectopic pregnancy has decreased from 3.5 maternal deaths per 1000 cases to less than 1 death per 1000 cases primarily because of
   a. earlier detection of the ectopic pregnancy
   b. greater availability of blood for transfusion
   c. modern intensive care technology to combat shock and blood loss
   d. increased use of sophisticated laparoscopic surgical techniques

15.20 About what percentage of women who have had an ectopic pregnancy are subsequently successful in having a full term live birth?
   a. 10%
   b. 25%
   c. 50%
   d. 75%

15.21 Which of the following is the most significant risk factor for ectopic pregnancy?
   a. Oral contraceptive use
   b. Current intrauterine device use
   c. Prior history of salpingitis
   d. Young maternal age

15.22 Compared with women 15–23 years of age, women in the 35–44 years of age bracket have
   a. a decreased risk of ectopic pregnancy
   b. an equal risk of ectopic pregnancy
   c. an increased risk of ectopic pregnancy

15.23 Over one half of all ectopic pregnancies occur in women who have had at least
   a. 2 pregnancies
   b. 3 pregnancies
   c. 4 pregnancies
   d. 5 pregnancies

15.24 Hemoperitoneum associated with ruptured ectopic pregnancy may result in irritation of the diaphragm and pain referred to the
   a. flank
   b. shoulder
   c. mid-chest
   d. arm

15.25 Which of the following statements concerning ectopic gestation is correct?
   a. Ectopic pregnancies are symptomatic from the early stages
   b. Abdominal pain, amenorrhea, and vaginal bleeding are noted in virtually all cases of ectopic pregnancy
   c. The patient feels pain on the side of the ectopic pregnancy in virtually all cases
   d. Ectopic pregnancy is more likely to be symptomatic if implantation is in the proximal portion of the tube

15.26 Syncope is reported in what proportion of patients with ruptured tubal ectopic pregnancies and hemoperitoneum?
   a. 1:6
   b. 1:3
   c. 2:3
   d. All

Answers (15.19–15.26)

| 15.19 a | 15.21 c | 15.23 b | 15.24 b | 15.25 d | 15.26 b |
| 15.20 c | 15.22 c | | | | |

15.27 Approximately what percent of patients with tubal ectopic pregnancy present with hypovolemic shock?
a. 5%
b. 15%
c. 25%
d. 35%

15.28 In cases of ectopic pregnancy, how often are urinary pregnancy tests found to be positive?
a. 90%
b. 80%
c. 70%
d. 60%

15.29 Early in pregnancy, quantitative β-human chorionic gonadotropin levels should increase by what percent in 48 hours?
a. 90%
b. 75%
c. 66%
d. 50%

15.30 Transvaginal pelvic ultrasonography should be able to identify an intrauterine pregnancy by the time the serum β-human chorionic gonadotropin level reaches what level?
a. 500 mIU/ml
b. 1500 mIU/ml
c. 2500 mIU/ml
d. 3500 mIU/ml

15.31 As a clinical cut-off, a serum progesterone below what level suggests a non-viable pregnancy?
a. 1 ng/ml
b. 5 ng/ml
c. 10 ng/ml
d. 15 ng/ml

15.32 What percent of all abnormal pregnancies, ectopic or intrauterine, are associated with serum progesterone levels of greater than 25 ng/ml?
a. 0.5%
b. 2.5%
c. 4.5%
d. 6.5%
e. 7.5%

15.33 Survival of the intrauterine twin of a combined pregnancy has been reported in approximately what percentage of cases?
a. 20%
b. 33%
c. 50%
d. 75%

15.34 Rubin's criteria for cervical pregnancy include all of the following EXCEPT
a. cervical glands opposite the placental attachment
b. chorionic villi in the cervical canal
c. chorionic villi in the corpus uteri
d. internal cervical os closed, external cervical os open or closed

15.35 The use of assisted reproductive technology has what effect on the incidence of combined (heterotropic) pregnancy?
a. No effect on the incidence
b. A decrease in the incidence
c. An increase in the incidence

15.36 As compared to pregnancy following a "normal cycle," a combined pregnancy following the use of assisted reproductive technology is
a. more likely
b. as likely
c. less likely

ANSWERS (15.27–15.36)

15.27 a	15.29 c	15.31 b	15.33 b	15.35 c	15.36 a
15.28 a	15.30 b	15.32 b	15.34 c		

Instructions for items 15.37 to 15.39:
Match the type of ectopic pregnancy following a normal menstrual cycle with its incidence. An option may be used once, more than once, or not at all.

15.37 Cervical

15.38 Abdominal

15.39 Ovarian
   a. 1:3000–4000
   b. 1:7000–50,000
   c. 1:10,000–20,000
   d. 1:18,000–25,000

15.40 Which of the following statements about the pelvic pain associated with tubal ectopic pregnancy is INCORRECT?
   a. The pain may be caused by peritoneal irritation from blood
   b. The pain usually is colicky
   c. The patient always feels the pain on the same side as the ectopic pregnancy
   d. The pain may be caused by distention of the fallopian tube

15.41 Which of the following situations associated with tubal ectopic pregnancy is LEAST COMMON?
   a. Tubal rupture with intraperitoneal hemorrhage
   b. Tubal abortion with or without intraperitoneal hemorrhage
   c. Tubal abortion with subsequent implantation on an intraperitoneal structure

15.42 A serum progesterone of less than 5.0 ng/ml strongly suggests a nonviable pregnancy that is
   a. intrauterine in location
   b. extrauterine in location
   c. either intrauterine or extrauterine in location

Instructions for items 15.43 to 15.46:
Match the type of ectopic pregnancy following a normal menstrual cycle with its incidence. An option may be used once, more than once, or not at all.

15.43 Cornueal

15.44 Fimbrial

15.45 Isthmic

15.46 Ampullary
   a. 2%
   b. 6%
   c. 12%
   d. 80%

15.47 What is the most common kind of tubal ectopic pregnancy?
   a. Ampullary
   b. Isthmic
   c. Fimbrial
   d. Cornueal

15.48 Cervical pregnancy is ___ times more likely after cycles following the use of assisted reproductive technology.
   a. two
   b. four
   c. six
   d. eight
   e. ten

ANSWERS (15.37–15.48)					
15.37 b	15.39 c	15.41 c	15.43 a	15.45 c	15.47 a
15.38 a	15.40 c	15.42 c	15.44 b	15.46 d	15.48 a

Questions and Answers Chapter 16: Medical and Surgical Conditions of Pregnancy

16.1 Anemia in pregnancy is generally defined as a hemoglobin level of less than:
a. 6 g/dl
b. 8 g/dl
c. 10 g/dl
d. 12 g/dl

16.2 The most frequent type of anemia in pregnancy is:
a. iron-deficiency anemia
b. folate-deficiency anemia
c. sickle-cell anemia
d. vitamin B_{12}-deficiency anemia
e. thalassemia anemia

16.3 During pregnancy, the serum iron usually is:
a. increased
b. unchanged
c. decreased

16.4 During pregnancy, the total iron-binding capacity is:
a. increased
b. unchanged
c. decreased

16.5 Which of the following statements accurately reflects iron-deficiency anemia in pregnancy?
a. One pregnancy can cause anemia in the next pregnancy.
b. Adequate treatment is 100 mg ferrous gluconate daily.
c. With absent iron stores, a patient with iron-deficiency anemia can be treated with 60 mg of elemental iron daily.
d. All of the above are accurate.

16.6 Women with sickle-cell trait (HbSA disease) have increased:
a. incidence of spontaneous abortion
b. perinatal mortality
c. incidence of urinary tract infections
d. incidence of preterm births
e. incidence of low-birth weight babies

16.7 Patients with sickle cell disease are more likely to have:
a. asymptomatic bacteria
b. urinary tract infections
c. nephrolithiasis
d. cholelithiasis
e. all the above

16.8 Which of the following is NOT characteristic of von Willebrand's disease?
a. Decreased factor VII
b. Decreased factor VIII
c. Family history of the disease
d. Prolonged bleeding time

16.9 When iron therapy is initiated during a normal pregnancy, the response is first seen as an increase in the reticulocyte count within:
a. 24 hours
b. 48 hours
c. 96 hours
d. 1 week

16.10 Anemia associated with folate deficiency is found in:
a. multiple gestation
b. patients with a high alcohol intake
c. patients taking Dilantin
d. patients eating the normal adult intake of folate
e. all of the above

ANSWERS (16.1–16.10)

16.1	c	16.3	c	16.5	a	16.7	e	16.9	d	16.10 e
16.2	a	16.4	a	16.6	c	16.8	b			

16.11 Vitamin B_{12} deficiency is associated with which of the following diseases?
   a. Chronic malabsorption syndrome
   b. Pancreatic disease
   c. Crohn's disease
   d. Ulcerative colitis
   e. All of the above

16.12 A mixed iron and folate deficiency is characterized by:
   a. normocytic and normochromic anemia
   b. microcytic and normochromic anemia
   c. microcytic and megaloblastic anemia
   d. normocytic and megaloblastic anemia

16.13 Which of the following anemias presents as microcytic and hypochromic but with a normal serum iron and total iron-binding capacity?
   a. Iron-deficiency anemia
   b. Thalassemia trait
   c. Sickle-cell anemia
   d. Sickle-cell trait

16.14 The pH of urine in pregnancy, as compared with a nonpregnant state, is:
   a. increased
   b. the same
   c. decreased
   d. dependent on gestational age

16.15 The appropriate management for a pregnant patient with asymptomatic bacteriuria is:
   a. no treatment
   b. antibiotics
   c. dietary alterations
   d. changes of sexual behavior
   e. urinary alkalization

16.16 What percent of patients with asymptomatic bacteriuria during pregnancy will develop symptomatic urinary tract infections?
   a. 25%
   b. 50%
   c. 75%
   d. 100%

16.17 If a pregnant patient with pyelonephritis does not improve on appropriate intravenous antibiotic therapy within 48–72 hours, consideration would be given to:
   a. the possibility of urinary tract obstruction
   b. reevaluation of the antibiotic used for treatment
   c. the use of single-shot intravenous pyelogram or ultrasonography
   d. all of the above

16.18 The most common organism cultured from the urine of pregnant patients with urinary tract symptoms is:
   a. *Pseudomonas*
   b. *Escherichia coli*
   c. *Proteus*
   d. *Neisseria gonorrhoeae*

16.19 In pregnancy, the glomerular filtration rate increases by:
   a. 25%
   b. 50%
   c. 75%
   d. 100%

16.20 Which of the following is NOT related to the increased incidence of symptomatic urinary tract infection in pregnancy?
   a. decreased ureteral tone
   b. compression of the ureters at the pelvic brim
   c. decreased pH of the urine
   d. pregnancy associated mild glycosuria
   e. bladder compression

ANSWERS (16.11–16.20)

16.11 e	16.13 b	16.15 b	16.17 d	16.19 b	16.20 c
16.12 a	16.14 a	16.16 a	16.18 b		

16.21 Provided other complications are absent in patients with mild renal impairment, individuals with serum creatinine levels below what figure generally have uneventful pregnancies?
a. 0.6 mg/dl
b. 1.0 mg/dl
c. 1.4 mg/dl
d. 1.8 mg/dl
e. 2.2 mg/dl

16.22 What factor in association with preexisting renal disease results in a particularly poor prognosis for baby and mother?
a. Retinopathy
b. Hypertension
c. Atrophic skin changes
d. Obesity
e. Anemia

16.23 Bronchial asthma is encountered in approximately what percent of pregnant patients?
a. 0.01%
b. 0.1%
c. 1.0%
d. 10%

16.24 Pregnant patients who smoke have an increased risk of:
a. spontaneous abortion
b. ectopic pregnancy
c. preterm labor and delivery
d. all of the above

16.25 Pneumonia occurs in approximately what percent of all pregnancies?
a. 0.01–0.1%
b. 0.1–1.0%
c. 1.0–5.0%
d. 5.0–10.0%
e. 25%

16.26 The most common bacterial pneumonia is associated with what organism?
a. *Streptococcus pneumoniae*
b. *Haemophilus influenza*
c. *Klebsiella pneumoniae*
d. *Staphylococcus aureus*
e. *Mycoplasma pneumoniae*

16.27 Pneumonia in pregnancy is associated with an overall mortality rate of:
a. 1–2%
b. 3–4%
c. 5–6%
d. 7–8%
e. 9–10%

Instructions for items 16.28 to 16.34. Match the signs, symptoms, and laboratory findings listed with either bacterial or mycoplasma pneumonia in pregnancy.

16.28 Acute febrile illness

16.29 Low grade fever

16.30 Substantial leukocytosis

16.31 Acute febrile illness

16.32 Lobar chest X-ray pattern

16.33 Nonproductive cough

16.34 Productive cough
a. bacterial pneumonia in pregnancy
b. mycoplasma pneumonia in pregnancy

16.35 Influenza pneumonia in pregnancy is usually self limited, with spontaneous resolution in:
a. 1–2 days
b. 3–4 days
c. 5–6 days
d. 7–8 days
e. 9–10 days

ANSWERS (16.21–16.35)					
16.21 c	16.24 d	16.27 b	16.30 a	16.32 a	16.34 a
16.22 b	16.25 b	16.28 a	16.31 a	16.33 b	16.35 b
16.23 c	16.26 a	16.29 b			

16.36 *Varicella* pneumonia occurs in up to what percent of women with *varicella* infection (chicken pox) in pregnancy?
a. 10%
b. 20%
c. 30%
d. 40%
e. 50%

16.37 *Varicella* pneumonia is associated with a maternal mortality of:
a. 5–15%
b. 15–25%
c. 25–35%
d. 35–45%
e. 45–55%

16.38 *Varicella* pneumonia in pregnancy is usually appropriately treated with:
a. outpatient supportive therapy
b. outpatient acyclovir oral therapy
c. inpatient parenteral acyclovir therapy
d. inpatient parenteral amoxicillin therapy

16.39 What percentage of pregnant women experience no change in their asthma or worsening of symptoms?
a. 10%
b. 20%
c. 30%
d. 40%
e. 50%

16.40 What percent of pregnant women experience an improvement of their asthma symptoms?
a. 10%
b. 20%
c. 30%
d. 40%
e. 50%

16.41 The peak expiratory flow rate (PEFR):
a. doubles in pregnancy
b. remains unchanged in pregnancy
c. halves in pregnancy
d. changes in pregnancy in proportion to the BMR

16.42 Which finding on sputum gram stain of a pregnant patient with an acute asthma attack is most consistent with an allergic response?
a. eosinophils
b. neutrophils
c. platelets
d. erythrocytes
e. hyphae

16.43 A peak flow less than approximately what percent of the predicted value in a pregnant patient with an acute asthmatic attack should engender therapy?
a. 80–90%
b. 60–70%
c. 50–60%
d. 40–50%

16.44 Treatment for an acute asthma attack in pregnancy is centered in beta$_2$ agonist therapy, with bronchodilation starting within:
a. 1–3 minutes
b. 3–5 minutes
c. 5–10 minutes
d. 10–15 minutes
e. 15–30 minutes

16.45 The management of an acute asthmatic exacerbation in pregnancy includes administration of oxygen sufficient to maintain a PO$_2$ of over:
a. 98mmHg
b. 90mmHg
c. 80mmHg
d. 70mmHg
e. 60mmHg

Answers (16.36–16.45)

16.36 b	16.38 c	16.40 b	16.42 a	16.44 c	16.45 d
16.37 c	16.39 d	16.41 b	16.43 b		

16.46 In chronic mild asthma in pregnancy, serial peak flow measurements are expected to remain in the range of:
a. 90–100%
b. 80–90%
c. 70–80%
d. 60–70%
e. 50–60%

16.47 Symptoms occurring up to how many times per week are consistent with, although not entirely diagnostic of, mild chronic asthma in pregnancy?
a. 2
b. 3
c. 4
d. 5
e. 6

16.48 Intravenous hydrocortisone (100 mg every 8 hours) is indicated for asthmatic patients in labor who:
a. are classified as mild asthmatics
b. are classified as moderate asthmatics
c. are classified as severe asthmatics
d. have been taking two agents during pregnancy
e. have been taking steroids during pregnancy

Instructions for items 16.49 to 16.52. Match the classification of medication used for asthma in pregnancy with the drugs listed.

16.49 Albuterol

16.50 Hydrocortisone

16.51 Terbutaline

16.52 Cromolyn sodium
a. Beta-Agonist
b. Steroid
c. Anti-inflammatory

16.53 Newborns of women taking tuberculosis therapy should receive a PPD at birth and again at how many months of age?
a. 1
b. 3
c. 6
d. 12
e. 18

Instructions for items 16.54 to 16.56. Match the indication for tuberculosis management in pregnancy with the appropriate regimen.

16.54 Conversion of PPD within 2 years and negative a chest X-ray

16.55 Conversion of PPD unknown and under 35 years of age

16.56 Active tuberculosis in pregnancy
a. Isoniazid, 300 mg/d for 6–9 months postpartum
b. Isoniazid, 300 mg/d, after 1st trimester, for 6–9 months thereafter
c. Isoniazid and Rifampin for 9 months

16.57 Pyridoxine (Vitamin B_6) therapy is indicated for pregnant patients taking isoniazid to combat:
a. retinopathy
b. nephropathy
c. neuropathy
d. cardiomyopathy
e. dermatitis

16.58 Most pregnant patients with tuberculosis:
a. are asymptomatic
b. have night sweats
c. have low grade fevers
d. have leukocytosis on blood count
e. have hemoptysis

ANSWERS (16.46–16.58)

16.46 b	16.49 a	16.52 c	16.54 c	16.56 a	16.58 a
16.47 a	16.50 b	16.53 b	16.55 b	16.57 c	
16.48 e	16.51 a				

16.59 Pregnant smokers or their infants are at increased risk of all of the following EXCEPT:
a. placenta previa
b. abruptio placenta
c. decreased birth weight
d. intrauterine growth restriction
e. long-term neurologic abnormalities

16.60 During pregnancy, the incidence and severity of the common cold [upper respiratory infection (URI)] are:
a. increased
b. unchanged
c. decreased

16.61 Patients with which of the following cardiac diseases are best advised not to become pregnant?
a. Primary pulmonary hypertension
b. Uncorrected tetralogy of Fallot
c. Eisenmenger syndrome
d. All of the above

16.62 In normal patients, cardiac output in pregnancy increases approximately:
a. 20%
b. 40%
c. 60%
d. 80%
e. 100%

Instructions for items 16.63 to 16.66: Match the New York Heart Association class with its appropriate symptoms. An option may be used once, more than once, or not at all.

16.63 Class I

16.64 Class II

16.65 Class III

16.66 Class IV
a. No symptoms of cardiac decompensation at rest, marked limitation of physical activity
b. No cardiac decompensation or limitation of physical activity
c. No symptoms of cardiac decompensation at rest, minor limitations of physical activity
d. Symptoms of cardiac decompensation at rest, increased discomfort with any physical activity

16.67 The fetuses of patients with functionally significant cardiac disease are at increased risk for:
a. low-birth weight
b. sepsis
c. congenital heart defects
d. neural tube defects

16.68 The majority of obstetric patients with severe cardiac disease who die, do so during the:
a. second trimester
b. third trimester
c. intrapartum period
d. postpartum period

16.69 Which of the following is characteristic of patients at increased risk for peripartum cardiomyopathy?
a. Asian heritage
b. History of preeclampsia
c. Under 25 years of age
d. First pregnancy

16.70 What percent of the offspring of pregnant patients with Marfan's syndrome will inherit the disease?
a. Less than 3%
b. 25%
c. 50%
d. 100%

ANSWERS (16.59–16.70)					
16.59 a	16.61 b	16.63 b	16.65 a	16.67 a	16.69 b
16.60 b	16.62 b	16.64 c	16.66 d	16.68 d	16.70 c

Instructions for items 16.71 to 16.73: Match the American Diabetic Association (ADA) classification with the appropriate description. An option may be used once, more than once, or not at all.

16.71 Type I diabetes

16.72 Type II diabetes

16.73 Gestational diabetes
   a. Adult-onset glucose intolerance
   b. Glucose intolerance diagnosed in childhood
   c. Glucose intolerance identified during pregnancy

16.74 In pregnancy, human placental lactogen results in all of the following EXCEPT:
   a. increased levels of free fatty acids
   b. increased gluconeogenesis
   c. decreased glucose uptake
   d. increased lipolysis

Instructions for items 16.75 to 16.82: Match the White classification of diabetes with the appropriate description. An option may be used once, more than once, or not at all.

16.75 A

16.76 B

16.77 C

16.78 D

16.79 E

16.80 F

16.81 R

16.82 T
   a. Onset between ages 10 and 13, duration 10–19 years, no vascular disease
   b. Pelvic arteriosclerosis by X-ray
   c. Onset under age 10, duration greater than 20 years, some vascular disease
   d. Onset after 2 years of age, duration less than 10 years, no vascular disease
   e. Transplantation
   f. Proliferative retinopathy
   g. Vascular nephritis
   h. Gestational diabetes, onset in pregnancy

16.83 During normal pregnancy, how many milligrams of glucose are spilled per day in the urine?
   a. 10
   b. 100
   c. 300
   d. 500
   e. 700

16.84 Infants of diabetic mothers are at an increased risk for which of the following congenital anomalies?
   a. Cardiac deformities
   b. Craniofacial deformities
   c. Reproductive tract deformities
   d. Situs inversus

16.85 Infants born to mothers with insulin-dependent diabetes are at higher risk for:
   a. neonatal hyperbilirubinemia
   b. neonatal hypoglycemia
   c. hypocalcemia
   d. polycythemia
   e. all of the above

ANSWERS (16.71–16.85)

16.71 b	16.74 b	16.77 a	16.80 g	16.82 e	16.84 a
16.72 a	16.75 h	16.78 c	16.81 f	16.83 c	16.85 e
16.73 c	16.76 d	16.79 b			

16.86 Which of the following are known risk factors for gestational diabetes?
a. History of giving birth to an infant weighing more than 4000 g
b. History of repeated spontaneous abortion
c. History of unexplained stillbirth
d. Family history of diabetes
e. All of the above

16.87 Beginning at approximately 30–32 weeks' gestation in pregnant diabetics, which of the following measures of fetal well-being is commonly employed?
a. Daily fetal kick counts
b. Serial nonstress testing
c. Serial biophysical profile testing
d. Serial ultrasonography
e. All of the above

16.88 Most pregnant diabetics are maintained on a daily calorie intake of approximately:
a. 1600–1700
b. 2300–2400
c. 2800–2900
d. 3300–3400

16.89 For a diabetic patient taking a mixed regimen of NPH and regular insulin in the morning and evening, the fasting glucose reflects the:
a. regular insulin given in the morning
b. NPH insulin given in the morning
c. NPH insulin given the previous evening
d. regular insulin given in the evening

16.90 In the well-controlled diabetic with no complications, induction of labor is often undertaken at how many weeks' gestation?
a. 40–42
b. 38–40
c. 36–38
d. 34–36
e. 32–34

16.91 What percent of gestational diabetics return to a normal glucose status postpartum?
a. Over 95%
b. 85%–95%
c. 75%–85%
d. 65%–75%
e. 55%–65%

16.92 What is the currently recognized upper normal limit for the 1-hour 50 g glucose challenge test?
a. 120 mg/dl
b. 140 mg/dl
c. 160 mg/dl
d. 180 mg/dl
e. 200 mg/dl

16.93 Of the patients screened by the 1-hour 50 g glucose challenge test between 24 and 28 weeks' gestation, approximately 15% will be found to have an abnormal glucose value. Of these, approximately how many will be found to have gestational diabetes using a 3-hour glucose tolerance test?
a. 5%
b. 15%
c. 30%
d. 45%
e. 60%

ANSWERS (16.86–16.93)

16.86 e	16.88 b	16.90 b	16.91 a	16.92 b	16.93 b
16.87 e	16.89 c				

16.94 "Ideal" control for a pregnant diabetic would be maintaining a fasting plasma glucose measurement in the range of
a. 60–70 mg/ml
b. 90–100 mg/ml
c. 100–110 mg/ml
d. 110–120 mg/ml

16.95 What percent of pregnancies are complicated by hyperthyroidism?
a. .2%
b. 2%
c. 5%
d. 10%

16.96 Which of the following is a symptom of hyperthyroidism in pregnancy?
a. Weakness
b. Palpitations
c. Tremor
d. Heat intolerance
e. All of the above

16.97 Which of the following is a potential side effect of propylthiouracil (PTU) when used as treatment for hyperthyroidism during pregnancy?
a. Neonatal hypothyroidism
b. Neonatal hyperbilirubinemia
c. Neonatal seizures
d. Placental abruption
e. Intrauterine growth restriction

16.98 How many weeks does it take for thyroid-stimulating hormone (TSH) levels to return to normal after initiation of appropriate therapy for hypothyroidism?
a. 2
b. 4
c. 6
d. 8
e. 10

Instructions for items 16.99–16.104. Match the thyroid function test with the effect of pregnancy on its normal value.

16.99 Total thyroxine (T_4)

16.100 $3,5,3^1$-triiodothyronine (T_3)

16.101 T_3 Resin uptake (T_3RU)

16.102 Thyroxine binding globin (TBG)

16.103 Free T_4

16.104 Free T_3
a. elevated
b. lowered
c. unchanged

16.105 To avoid toxoplasma infection, pregnant women should be advised to:
a. eat only well-cooked meat
b. avoid exposure to cats
c. avoid exposure to cat feces
d. all of the above

16.106 Microcephaly, chorioretinitis, deafness, and mental retardation are the characteristic results of which intrauterine infection?
a. Cytomegalovirus
b. Coxsackie B
c. Mumps
d. Rubeola
e. Rubella

16.107 Which of the following antibiotics, when given to a mother during pregnancy, may produce enamel defects and yellowing of the teeth in her infant?
a. Cephaloridine
b. Colistimethate sodium
c. Penicillin
d. Tetracycline
e. Chloramphenicol

ANSWERS (16.94–16.107)

16.94 b	16.97 a	16.100 a	16.102 a	16.104 c	16.106 a
16.95 a	16.98 d	16.101 b	16.103 c	16.105 d	16.107 d
16.96 e	16.99 a				

16.108 T_4 and T_3 serum concentrations are lowered during pregnancy primarily because of:
a. estrogen-induced alterations of thyroid gland production
b. progesterone-induced alterations of thyroid gland production
c. estrogen-induced increases in thyroxin-binding globulin
d. progesterone-induced increases in thyroxin-binding globulin

16.109 Approximately what percent of pregnant women have asymptomatic cervical colonization by β-hemolytic streptococci?
a. 10%
b. 30%
c. 50%
d. 70%
e. 90%

16.110 Hutchinson's teeth, mulberry molars, saddle nose, and saber shins are characteristic of congenital:
a. rubella
b. syphilis
c. toxoplasmosis
d. bacterial vaginosis

16.111 *Treponema pallidum* reaches the fetus by:
a. direct contact through the chorion
b. transplacental circulation
c. the amniotic fluid
d. lymphatics

16.112 Which of the following is associated with congenital syphilis?
a. Cutaneous lesions
b. Osteochondritis of the long bones
c. Pseudoparalysis
d. Hepatosplenomegaly
e. All of the above

16.113 What increase in the serologic titer for syphilis indicates either inadequate treatment or reinfection and is an indication for further therapy?
a. 2-fold
b. 4-fold
c. 6-fold
d. 8-fold
e. 10-fold

16.114 Which of the following is successful in preventing neonatal gonococcal ophthalmia in the newborn of a woman with *Neisseria gonorrhoeae* infection?
a. Penicillin
b. Tetracycline
c. Ampicillin
d. All of the above

16.115 Bacterial vaginosis in the antepartum period has been associated with an increased incidence of:
a. postpartum metritis
b. premature rupture of membranes
c. amniotic fluid infection
d. preterm labor
e. all of the above

16.116 Approximately what percent of women with bacterial vaginosis in pregnancy are asymptomatic?
a. 10%
b. 25%
c. 50%
d. 75%
e. 100%

ANSWERS (16.108–16.116)

16.108 c	16.110 b	16.112 e	16.114 b	16.115 e	16.116 c
16.109 b	16.111 b	16.113 b			

16.117 Clue cells are the single most reliable diagnostic criterion for bacterial vaginosis when they account for greater than what percent of the cells seen?
a. 10%
b. 20%
c. 30%
d. 40%
e. 50%

16.118 Delivery of an infant through a birth canal with primary herpes infection is associated with a neonatal infection rate of:
a. 10%
b. 20%
c. 30%
d. 40%
e. 50%

16.119 The risk of congenital rubella syndrome is greatest if the woman contracts the infection during which trimester?
a. First trimester
b. Second trimester
c. Third trimester

16.120 Congenital rubella syndrome following vaccination during an undiagnosed pregnancy:
a. occurs about 1% of cases
b. occurs about 0.5% of cases
c. occurs about 0.1% of cases
d. occurs about 0.01% of cases
e. has not been reported

16.121 Which of the following is NOT a neonatal abnormality associated with congenital rubella infection?
a. Cataracts and/or retinopathy
b. Patent ductus arteriosus or pulmonary artery hyperplasia
c. Musculoskeletal anomalies, including phocomelia
d. Deafness or impaired hearing
e. Hepatosplenomegaly

16.122 The most classic eye finding in fetal congenital rubella is:
a. retinopathy
b. cataracts
c. glaucoma
d. microphthalmia
e. myopia

16.123 Approximately what percent of Americans infected with the HIV virus are women?
a. 20%
b. 40%
c. 60%
d. 80%

16.124 What percent of pediatric human immunodeficiency virus (HIV) infection is due to vertical transmission from mother to fetus?
a. 20%
b. 40%
c. 60%
d. 80%
e. 100%

16.125 The sensitivity and specificity of the combined use of enzyme-linked immunoabsorbent assay (ELISA) and Western blot tests for human immunodeficiency virus (HIV) infection is:
a. 59%
b. 69%
c. 79%
d. 89%
e. 99%

ANSWERS (16.117–16.125)

16.117 b	16.119 a	16.121 c	16.123 a	16.124 d	16.125 e
16.118 e	16.120 e	16.122 b			

16.126 The management of labor for a human immunodeficiency virus (HIV) infected woman should include all the following EXCEPT:
a. avoiding the use of fetal scalp electrodes
b. avoiding fetal scalp blood sampling
c. intrapartum administration of zidovudine as part of an intrapartum–antepartum–postpartum regime
d. cesarean section to avoid infection

16.127 The risk of deep vein thrombosis during pregnancy as compared with the immediate postpartum period is:
a. higher
b. the same
c. lower
d. unpredictable

16.128 The goal of heparin anticoagulation for deep thrombophlebitis during pregnancy is to maintain a partial thromboplastin time (PTT) that is how many times greater than baseline?
a. 2-fold
b. 3-fold
c. 4-fold
d. 5-fold

16.129 Recurrent pulmonary embolization from pelvic thrombophlebitis is best treated with:
a. anticoagulation
b. ligation of femoral veins
c. ligation of inferior vena cava
d. paravertebral block of sympathetic chain

16.130 What is the increased risk of bearing children with congenital anomalies for pregnant women with epilepsy?
a. 2-fold
b. 4-fold
c. 6-fold
d. 8-fold

16.131 During an epileptic seizure, the immediate risk to the fetus includes:
a. abruptio placentae
b. placenta previa
c. vasa previa
d. all of the above

16.132 Because of concerns about teratogenesis, which is the most commonly used anticonvulsant drug during pregnancy?
a. Phenytoin
b. Dilantin
c. Carbamazepine
d. Phenobarbital

16.133 Hyperemesis gravidarum is characterized by all of the following EXCEPT:
a. weight loss
b. increased appetite
c. dehydration
d. ketosis

16.134 Which of the following is a cause of gastroesophageal reflux in pregnancy?
a. Decrease of intra-abdominal space
b. Increased pressure from the enlarging uterus
c. Progesterone effect decreasing esophageal sphincter tone
d. All of the above

ANSWERS (16.126–16.134)

| 16.126 d | 16.128 a | 16.130 b | 16.132 c | 16.133 b | 16.134 d |
| 16.127 c | 16.129 c | 16.131 a | | | |

16.135 The most common perinatal complication associated with appendicitis in pregnancy is:
a. premature rupture of membranes
b. premature labor
c. placenta previa
d. abruptio placentae

16.136 The morbidity of regional enteritis in pregnancy is primarily related to:
a. intestinal obstruction
b. toxic megacolon
c. colonic perforation
d. colonic stricture

Instructions for items 16.137 to 16.141: Match the type of hepatitis with the appropriate description(s). An option may be used once, more than once, or not at all.

16.137 Hepatitis A

16.138 Hepatitis B

16.139 Hepatitis C

16.140 Hepatitis D

16.141 Hepatitis E
a. Often associated with fulminant hepatitis
b. Represents 50% of cases of hepatitis in pregnancy
c. Spread by water, food, or fecal contamination
d. Spread primarily by blood or blood product transfusion
e. Associated with unexpected high maternal mortality

16.142 Acute fatty liver of pregnancy is associated with a fetal mortality rate of:
a. 90%
b. 75%
c. 60%
d. 45%
e. 30%

16.143 Patients with cholestasis of pregnancy present with which of the following?
a. Pruritus
b. Fatigue
c. Jaundice
d. All of the above

16.144 Cholelithiasis and cholecystitis complicate about what percent of pregnancies?
a. 1%
b. 3%
c. 5%
d. 7%
e. 9%

16.145 Cholecystectomy during pregnancy is associated with a fetal loss rate of:
a. 1%
b. 3%
c. 5%
d. 7%
e. 9%

16.146 The fetal loss rate approaches what percent if pancreatitis is present at the time of cholecystectomy during pregnancy?
a. 50%
b. 60%
c. 70%
d. 80%
e. 90%

16.147 The most important obstetric consideration involving blunt abdominal trauma to the abdomen is:
a. uterine perforation
b. abruptio placentae
c. premature rupture of the membranes
d. uterine rupture

ANSWERS (16.135–16.147)

16.135 b	16.138 b	16.140 a	16.142 c	16.144 b	16.146 b
16.136 a	16.139 d	16.141 e	16.143 d	16.145 c	16.147 b
16.137 c					

16.148 Newborn narcotic withdrawal syndrome is seen in up to what proportion of infants born to opiate users?
a. 1/6
b. 1/3
c. 2/3
d. 3/4
e. 9/10

16.149 At least how many beers, glasses of wine, or standard mixed drinks daily during pregnancy is highly associated with fetal alcohol syndrome in the newborn?
a. 2
b. 4
c. 6
d. 8
e. 10

16.150 Fetal alcohol syndrome is associated with:
a. mental retardation
b. prenatal and postnatal growth deficiency
c. cardiovascular and central nervous system anomalies
d. craniofacial anomalies
e. all of the above

16.151 Segmental intestinal atresia, limb-reduction defects, disruptive brain anomalies, congenital heart defects, and prune-belly syndrome are associated with the ingestion of:
a. marijuana
b. cocaine
c. alcohol
d. caffeine

16.152 In a woman with immune thrombocytopenic purpura (ITP), a platelet count of less than what level on percutaneous umbilical sampling may be considered an indication for cesarean birth?
a. 10,000/mm^3
b. 50,000/mm^3
c. 100,000/mm^3
d. 150,000/mm^3
e. 200,000/mm^3

16.153 Immune thrombocytopenic purpura (ITP) occurs in what proportion of pregnancies?
a. 8–10 per 1000
b. 6–7 per 1000
c. 4–5 per 1000
d. 1–2 per 1000

16.154 Thrombocytopenia-associated spontaneous bleeding during pregnancy usually occurs with a platelet concentration of less than:
a. 100,000/mm^3
b. 80,000/mm^3
c. 60,000/mm^3
d. 40,000/mm^3
e. 20,000/mm^3

16.155 The initial treatment of immune thrombocytopenic purpura in pregnancy is:
a. administration of g-globulin
b. splenectomy
c. administration of corticosteroids
d. transfusion of platelets

16.156 Patients with lupus anticoagulant have a rate of reproductive wastage in excess of:
a. 30%
b. 50%
c. 70%
d. 90%

ANSWERS (16.148–16.156)

16.148 c	16.150 e	16.152 b	16.154 e	16.155 c	16.156 d
16.149 b	16.151 b	16.153 d			

16.157 Other than genetic causes, what is the most common cause of mental retardation?
a. Cocaine use in pregnancy
b. Marijuana use in pregnancy
c. Alcohol use in pregnancy
d. Opiate use during labor
e. Fetal asphyxia during labor

16.158 The stage-for-stage survival rates for breast cancer in pregnancy is:
a. one-half that when unassociated with pregnancy
b. one-quarter that when unassociated with pregnancy
c. the same as when unassociated with pregnancy
d. twice that when unassociated with pregnancy

16.159 Colorectal carcinoma is encountered in what proportion of pregnancies?
a. 1 in 1,000
b. 1 in 10,000
c. 1 in 100,000
d. 1 in 1,000,000

Questions and Answers for Chapter 17:
Hypertension in Pregnancy

17.1 Hypertension in pregnancy is defined as a sustained systolic blood pressure at or above
   a. 130 mm Hg
   b. 140 mm Hg
   c. 150 mm Hg
   d. 160 mm Hg

17.2 Hypertension in pregnancy is defined as a sustained diastolic blood pressure at or above
   a. 90 mm Hg
   b. 100 mm Hg
   c. 110 mm Hg
   d. 120 mm Hg

17.3 A rise in the diastolic blood pressure of how many mm Hg is used to define hypertension in pregnancy?
   a. 5 mm Hg
   b. 10 mm Hg
   c. 15 mm Hg
   d. 20 mm Hg

17.4 A rise in how many mm Hg of the systolic blood pressure is needed to define hypertension in pregnancy?
   a. 10 mm Hg
   b. 20 mm Hg
   c. 30 mm Hg
   d. 40 mm Hg

17.5 The blood pressure is lowest if measured when the patient is
   a. lying in the lateral position
   b. standing
   c. sitting
   d. lying in the prone position

17.6 During normal pregnancy, blood pressure follows which of the following patterns?
   a. Increases slightly during the second trimester
   b. Decreases slightly in the second trimester
   c. Fluctuates irregularly
   d. Increases gradually toward term

17.7 Pregnancy-induced hypertension develops in what percent of pregnancies that proceed beyond the first trimester?
   a. Less than 5%
   b. 5%–10%
   c. 11%–15%
   d. 16%–20%
   e. 21%–25%

17.8 Which of the following is characteristic of preeclampsia?
   a. Hypertension
   b. Proteinuria
   c. Edema
   d. All of the above

17.9 What is the most likely diagnosis of a patient who presents with hypertension in the twelfth week of pregnancy?
   a. Preeclampsia
   b. Eclampsia
   c. Chronic hypertension
   d. Hyperthyroidism

17.10 Approximately what percent of women with chronic hypertension develop superimposed preeclampsia or eclampsia?
   a. 25%
   b. 50%
   c. 75%
   d. 100%

ANSWERS (17.1–17.10)

17.1	b	17.3	c	17.5	a	17.7	b	17.9	c	17.10	c
17.2	a	17.4	c	17.6	c	17.8	d				

17.11 The intrauterine growth restriction often associated with hypertensive disease in pregnancy is most likely related to
a. chronic uteroplacental insufficiency
b. congenital anomalies of the fetus
c. anomalies of placental structure
d. associated placental abruption

17.12 In the patient with preeclampsia, visual disturbances such as scotomata and persistent severe headache are usually due to
a. infarct
b. vasospasm
c. partial embolic occlusion
d. demyelinization of nerves

17.13 The right upper quadrant pain seen in preeclampsia arises from
a. hepatic infarction
b. hepatic capsule distention
c. hepatic rupture
d. cholecystitis
e. cholelithiasis

17.14 In a patient with preeclampsia, which of the following indicates a worsening disease process?
a. Decreasing hematocrit
b. Increasing hematocrit
c. Increasing white blood cell count
d. Increasing platelet count

17.15 All of the following are included in the definition of severe preeclampsia EXCEPT
a. oliguria (500 ml or less in 24 hours) and a rising plasma creatinine level
b. severe thrombocytopenia or overt intravascular hemolysis
c. the development of convulsions in the absence of neurologic disease
d. proteinuria of 5 g or more in 24 hours
e. a persistent systolic blood pressure of at least 160 mm Hg or a diastolic blood pressure of at least 110 mm Hg

17.16 In general, antihypertensive therapy is indicated in preeclampsia when the diastolic blood pressure is repeatedly above
a. 90 mm Hg
b. 100 mm Hg
c. 110 mm Hg
d. 120 mm Hg
e. 130 mm Hg

17.17 All of the following should be part of the management of a patient with mild preeclampsia who is being cared for at home EXCEPT
a. bed rest
b. recording of daily fetal movement
c. daily dosing with magnesium sulfate
d. daily weighing

17.18 Intravenous magnesium sulfate is used in the management of preeclampsia to
a. prevent convulsions
b. treat active convulsions
c. lower blood pressure
d. stabilize renal function

Answers (17.11–17.18)

| 17.11 a | 17.13 b | 17.15 c | 17.16 c | 17.17 c | 17.18 a |
| 17.12 b | 17.14 b | | | | |

17.19 Muscular paralysis and respiratory difficulty occur when the serum concentration of magnesium is at least
a. 4–7 mg/dl
b. 8–12 mg/dl
c. 15–17 mg/dl

17.20 Magnesium sulfate toxicity is treated with the slow intravenous administration of
a. insulin
b. calcium gluconate
c. potassium hydroxide
d. magnesium gluconate

Instructions for items 17.21 to 17.27: Match the antihypertensive medication with its mechanism of action. An option may be used once, more than once, or not at all.

17.21 Thiazide

17.22 Methyldopa

17.23 Hydralazine

17.24 Propranolol

17.25 Labetalol

17.26 Nifedipine

17.27 Prazosin
a. Calcium channel blocker
b. β-Adrenergic blocker
c. α- and β-Adrenergic blockers
d. Direct vasodilation, cardiac effects
e. Decreased plasma volume and cardiac output
f. False neurotransmission, central nervous system effects
g. Direct peripheral vasodilation

17.28 Magnesium sulfate given intravenously in a large dose for eclampsia may be associated with all of the following EXCEPT
a. transient loss of beat-to-beat variation
b. bone deposition of magnesium
c. hypermagnesia in the fetus
d. reduction in the glomerular filtration rate
e. diminished patellar reflex

17.29 In the postpartum period, reversal of the vasospastic process associated with preeclampsia is manifested by
a. decreased deep tendon reflexes
b. a rapid fall in blood pressure
c. brisk diuresis
d. continued weight gain

17.30 In a patient with hypertension, midepigastric pain in the last trimester is suggestive of
a. ruptured splenic aneurysm
b. impending eclampsia
c. Crohn's disease
d. hepatic hemorrhage
e. abruptio placentae

17.31 All of the following are elements of the HELLP syndrome EXCEPT
a. seizures
b. hemolysis
c. hepatic dysfunction
d. low platelet count

17.32 Platelet transfusion for the HELLP syndrome is usually indicated when the platelet count falls below
a. $10,000/mm^3$
b. $20,000/mm^3$
c. $30,000/mm^3$
d. $40,000/mm^3$
e. $50,000/mm^3$

ANSWERS (17.19–17.32)					
17.19 c	17.22 f	17.25 c	17.27 d	17.29 c	17.31 a
17.20 b	17.23 g	17.26 a	17.28 d	17.30 b	17.32 b
17.21 e	17.24 b				

17.33 For a 17-year-old patient at 32 weeks' gestation who presents to the hospital having an eclamptic seizure, the most appropriate management is
a. an immediate vaginal delivery
b. an immediate cesarean delivery
c. administration of magnesium
d. administration of Pitocin

17.34 Preeclampsia occurs in approximately what percent of deliveries?
a. 3%
b. 7%
c. 10%
d. 14%

17.35 Which of the following events is NOT characteristic of patients with chronic hypertension/preeclampsia?
a. Fetal macrosomia
b. Intrauterine growth restriction
c. Oligohydramnios
d. Dysmaturity

17.36 Which of the following is an appropriate fetal evaluation in patients suspected of having hypertension in pregnancy?
a. Biophysical profile
b. Amniotic fluid volume
c. Fetal weight and growth evaluation
d. All of the above

17.37 In patients with hypertension in pregnancy, which of the following tests is useful in evaluating a patient with suspected coagulopathy?
a. Complete blood count
b. Platelet count
c. Fibrin split products
d. Prothrombin time/partial thromboplastin time
e. All of the above

17.38 Eclampsia occurs in what percent of deliveries?
a. 0.01 to 0.1%
b. 0.5 to 4%
c. 4.5 to 6 %
d. 6.5 to 8%

17.39 Perinatal mortality associated with preeclampsia increases progressively with increasing mean arterial pressure, primarily associated with uteroplacental insufficiency and
a. disseminated intravascular coagulation
b. renal failure
c. abruptio placentae
d. cardiomyopathy
e. hepatoma

Instructions for items 17.40 to 17.43: Match the diagnosis with the statement[s] with which they are best associated. An answer may be used once, more than once, or not at all.

17.40 Transient hypertension of pregnancy

17.41 Preeclampsia

17.42 Severe preeclampsia

17.43 Eclampsia
a. Systolic blood pressure > 140 mm or diastolic blood pressure > 90 mm Hg
b. Systolic blood pressure > 140 mm or diastolic blood pressure > 90 mm Hg and significant proteinuria or edema
c. Systolic blood pressure > 140 mm or diastolic blood pressure > 90 mm Hg and oliguria
d. Systolic blood pressure > 140 mm or diastolic blood pressure > 90 mm Hg and significant proteinuria or edema and convulsions

ANSWERS (17.33–17.43)

17.33 c	17.35 a	17.37 e	17.39 c	17.41 b	17.43 d
17.34 b	17.36 d	17.38 b	17.40 a	17.42 c, d	

Questions and Answers Chapter 18:
Multifetal Gestation

Instructions for items 18.1 to 18.4: Match the clinical situation with the appropriate incidence in the general population. An option may be used once, more than once, or not at all.

18.1   Monozygotic twins

18.2   Dizygotic twins

18.3   Twinning after clomiphene citrate induction of ovulation

18.4   Twinning with in vitro fertilization using several fertilized ova
    a. 1 in 3 pregnancies
    b. 1 in 12 pregnancies
    c. 1 in 90 pregnancies
    d. 1 in 250 pregnancies
    e. 1 in 500 pregnancies

18.5   The overall incidence of recognized twins in the United States is almost:
    a. 1%
    b. 3%
    c. 5%
    d. 7%
    e. 9%

18.6   The rate of twinning is:
    a. increasing
    b. stable
    c. decreasing

Instructions for items 18.7 to 18.11. Match the statement with the type of twinning with which it best corresponds. An option may be used once, more than once, or not at all.

18.7   Two separate ova fertilized by two separate sperm.

18.8   Incidence fairly constant around the world.

18.9   Division of a fertilized ovum after conception.

18.10   Incidence quite variable around the world.

18.11   Incidence approximately 1 in 250 pregnancies.
    a. dizygotic twinning
    b. monozygotic twinning

Instructions for items 18.12 to 18.15: Match the time of division of the conceptus (twinning) with the corresponding organization of fetal membranes. An option may be used once, more than once, or not at all.

18.12   Twinning within 3 days of fertilization

18.13   Twinning between 4 and 8 days of fertilization

18.14   Twinning between 9 and 12 days of fertilization

18.15   Twinning 12 days or more after fertilization
    a. Conjoined twins
    b. Monoamniotic/monochorionic
    c. Diamniotic/dichorionic
    d. Diamniotic/monochorionic

18.16   Approximately what percent of twin pregnancies detected in the first trimester result in delivery of viable twins?
    a. 30%
    b. 50%
    c. 70%
    d. 90%

18.17   All of the following are more commonly associated with multiple pregnancy EXCEPT:
    a. megaloblastic anemia
    b. fetal macrosomia
    c. vasa previa
    d. congenital anomalies
    e. polyhydramnios

ANSWERS (18.1–18.17)									
18.1	d	18.4	a	18.7	a	18.10	a	18.13	d	18.16	b
18.2	c	18.5	b	18.8	b	18.11	b	18.14	b	18.17	b
18.3	b	18.6	a	18.9	b	18.12	c	18.15	a		

18.18 Multifetal pregnancy is associated with an increased incidence of all of the following EXCEPT:
   a. perinatal morbidity
   b. fetomaternal hemorrhage
   c. intrauterine growth restriction
   d. umbilical cord prolapse
   e. postpartum hemorrhage

18.19 Patients with multiple gestations are at increased risk for all of the following EXCEPT:
   a. preeclampsia
   b. congenital anomalies
   c. oligohydramnios
   d. intrauterine growth restriction

18.20 The perinatal morbidity in twin gestation is increased how many times that for a comparable singleton pregnancy?
   a. 1–2 times
   b. 3–4 times
   c. 4–5 times
   d. 5–6 times
   e. 7–8 times

18.21 In monozygotic twins, oligohydramnios and anemia of one twin and hydramnios with polycythemia of the other twin are caused by:
   a. congenital anomalies of the fetus
   b. vascular anastomoses between the fetuses
   c. umbilical cord compression
   d. maternal diabetes

18.22 A familial factor is present in twinning that follows the:
   a. maternal lineage
   b. paternal lineage
   c. both maternal and paternal lineages

Instructions for items 18.23 to 18.26: Match the number of fetuses with the average time of delivery. An option may be used once, more than once, or not at all.

18.23 Singleton pregnancy

18.24 Twin pregnancy

18.25 Triplet pregnancy

18.26 Quadruplet pregnancy
   a. 25 weeks
   b. 29 weeks
   c. 33 weeks
   d. 37 weeks
   e. 40 weeks

18.27 A twin pregnancy in which one twin is characterized by impaired growth, anemia, and hypovolemia and the other twin by hypervolemia, hypertension, polycythemia, and congestive heart failure is suffering from:
   a. conjoined twin syndrome
   b. twin–twin transfusion syndrome
   c. single umbilical artery syndrome
   d. congenital rubella syndrome
   e. twin–twin isoimmunization

18.28 Multifetal pregnancy is associated with an increased risk of all of the following EXCEPT:
   a. maternal diabetes
   b. preeclampsia
   c. preterm labor
   d. preterm delivery

18.29 The differential diagnosis for multifetal gestation at 34 weeks gestational age by dates includes all of the following EXCEPT:
   a. twins
   b. polyhydramnios
   c. hydatiform mole
   d. uterine leiomyoma
   e. ovarian mass

ANSWERS (18.18–18.29)					
18.18 b	18.20 b	18.22 a	18.24 d	18.26 b	18.28 a
18.19 c	18.21 b	18.23 e	18.25 c	18.27 b	18.29 c

18.30 Diagnosis of multiple gestation is usually made by:
a. ultrasound
b. Leopold's maneuvers
c. pelvic examination
d. fundal height measurement
e. amniography

18.31 When should women carrying multifetal pregnancies begin to limit their activities to avoid premature labor?
a. 18–20 weeks
b. 21–23 weeks
c. 24–26 weeks
d. 27–29 weeks

18.32 What is the chief antenatal assessment to evaluate the progress of twin pregnancy?
a. periodic fundal height measurements
b. serial ultrasonography
c. periodic pelvic examination
d. serial urinary estriols

18.33 Periodic ultrasonography is done approximately every 4 weeks beginning at:
a. 16 weeks
b. 20 weeks
c. 24 weeks
d. 28 weeks
e. 32 weeks

18.34 What percent difference in weight between the larger and smaller fetus defines discordant growth?
a. 10%
b. 20%
c. 30%
d. 40%

18.35 Antenatal concerns in twin pregnancies include all of the following EXCEPT:
a. adequate nutrition
b. pregnancy-induced hypertension
c. postterm morbidity
d. inadequate fetal growth

18.36 Intrapartum management of twin pregnancies at term is usually determined by:
a. gestational age
b. presentation of the twins
c. local custom
d. size of the twins

18.37 Which of the following statements about multifetal pregnancy is incorrect?
a. There is a familial tendency to multifetal pregnancy along paternal lines.
b. There is an increased incidence of multifetal pregnancy with the use of fertility agents.
c. With each additional fetus in a multifetal pregnancy the length of gestation decreases approximately 4 weeks.
d. Ovum division within 3 days after fertilization is associated with diamniotic dichorionic pregnancy.
e. The incidence of spontaneous miscarriage and congenital anomalies both increased with multifetal pregnancy.

18.38 A single umbilical artery is seen in approximately what percent of twins?
a. 1–2%
b. 3–4%
c. 5–6%
d. 7–8%
e. 9–10%

ANSWERS (18.30–18.38)

| 18.30 a | 18.32 b | 18.34 b | 18.36 b | 18.37 a | 18.38 b |
| 18.31 c | 18.33 b | 18.35 c | | | |

Questions and Answers Chapter 19: Fetal Growth Abnormalities

19.1 Intrauterine growth restriction (IUGR) is defined as a fetus whose weight is at or below what percentile of the normal population?
a. 5th
b. 10th
c. 15th
d. 20th

19.2 Intrauterine growth restriction (IUGR) is based on weight for a:
a. given parity
b. specific gestational age
c. specific population
d. gender

19.3 About what proportion of stillborn infants are growth-restricted?
a. 1/6
b. 1/3
c. 2/3
d. 5/6

19.4 The normal fetus grows throughout pregnancy, but the rate of growth falls off after what gestational age?
a. 39 weeks
b. 37 weeks
c. 35 weeks
d. 33 weeks
e. 31 weeks

19.5 The placenta grows early and rapidly compared to the fetus, reaching a maximum surface area at about how many weeks gestational age?
a. 39 weeks
b. 37 weeks
c. 35 weeks
d. 33 weeks
e. 31 weeks

19.6 After the placenta has reached maximal surface area, there is a slow but steady decline primarily because of:
a. decreased distribution of cardiac output to the uterus at term
b. increased fetal vascular resistance
c. resorption of the placental collagen matrix
d. microinfarctions of the placental vascular system

19.7 A fetus with intrauterine growth restriction (IUGR) is at higher risk for all the following EXCEPT:
a. neonatal death
b. meconium aspiration
c. hyperglycemia
d. asphyxia during labor

19.8 Early onset intrauterine growth restriction (IUGR) is associated with all the following EXCEPT:
a. irreversible reduction in organ size
b. reversible decrease in cell size
c. genetic factors
d. immunologic abnormalities

19.9 Delayed onset intrauterine growth restriction (IUGR) is associated with:
a. uteroplacental insufficiency
b. irreversible reduction in organ size
c. genetic factors
d. immunologic abnormalities

19.10 All of the following are causes of intrauterine growth restriction (IUGR) EXCEPT:
a. recent onset maternal diabetes
b. smoking
c. hypertension
d. fetal rubella

Answers (19.1–19.10)					
19.1 b	19.3 b	19.5 b	19.7 c	19.9 a	19.10 a
19.2 b	19.4 b	19.6 d	19.8 b		

19.11 The most common maternal factor associated with intrauterine growth restriction (IUGR) is:
   a. hypertensive disease
   b. inadequate nutrition
   c. alcohol use
   d. drug use
   e. smoking

19.12 Congenital anomalies account for what percent of all cases of intrauterine growth restriction (IUGR)?
   a. 5%
   b. 10%
   c. 15%
   d. 35%
   e. 45%

Instructions for items 19.13 to 19.18. Match the ultrasound findings with the type of intrauterine growth restriction with which it is best associated.

19.13 Biparietal diameter appropriate for dates

19.14 Normal or low amniotic fluid volume

19.15 Head to abdominal circumference ratio (HC/AC ratio) greater than 95th percentile

19.16 Biparietal diameter may be smaller than expected for dates

19.17 Low amniotic fluid volume

19.18 Head to abdominal circumference ratio (HA/AC ratio) in normal range
   a. asymmetric IUGR
   b. symmetric IUGR

19.19 Asymmetrical intrauterine growth restriction (IUGR) is associated with:
   a. unequal decrease in the size of structures
   b. severe nutritional deficiencies
   c. hypertension
   d. all of the above

19.20 Symmetrical intrauterine growth restriction (IUGR) is associated with:
   a. equal decrease in the size of structures
   b. congenital anomalies
   c. early intrauterine infection
   d. all of the above

19.21 Compared with asymmetrical intrauterine growth restriction (IUGR), morbidity with symmetrical IUGR is:
   a. greater
   b. the same
   c. less

19.22 An efficient screening procedure for intrauterine growth restriction (IUGR) is:
   a. clinical estimations of fetal weight
   b. serial fundal height measurements
   c. maternal weight gain
   d. maternal blood pressure measurements

19.23 The most useful initial evaluation of intrauterine growth restriction is serial:
   a. obstetric ultrasound
   b. maternal weight measurement
   c. fundal height measurement
   d. nonstress testing
   e. biophysical profile testing

ANSWERS (19.11–19.23)

19.11 a	19.14 b	19.16 b	19.18 b	19.20 d	19.22 b
19.12 b	19.15 a	19.17 a	19.19 d	19.21 a	19.23 c
19.13 a					

19.24 To monitor the extent of growth restriction, ultrasound evaluation should be carried out every:
a. 1–2 weeks
b. 2–3 weeks
c. 3–4 weeks
d. 4–5 weeks
e. 5–6 weeks

19.25 In patients with suspected intrauterine growth restriction (IUGR) and uncertain dates, what ultrasonographic measurement may be useful in establishing gestational age?
a. Biparietal diameter
b. Intraorbital diameter
c. Cerebrum diameter
d. Cerebellum diameter
e. Femur length

19.26 Compared with intrauterine growth restriction (IUGR) alone, a case of IUGR with oligohydramnios is likely to have what type of outcome?
a. Worse
b. Unchanged
c. Improved

19.27 Amniocentesis allows which of the following direct studies to be accomplished?
a. Chromosomal analysis
b. Viral cultures
c. Immunoglobulin studies
d. Acid-base studies

19.28 Percutaneous umbilical blood sampling (PUBS) allows for all of the following direct fetal studies EXCEPT:
a. chromosomal analysis
b. viral cultures
c. evaluation of free floating fibroblasts
d. immunoglobulin studies
e. oxygenation and acid-base studies

19.29 Chorionic villus sampling allows for which of the following direct fetal studies?
a. Chromosomal analysis
b. Viral culture
c. Oxygenation studies
d. Acid-base studies

19.30 Bed rest is often recommended for patients with intrauterine growth restriction (IUGR) in order to:
a. regulate fetal heart rate
b. increase uteroplacental blood flow
c. decrease maternal metabolic activity
d. decrease maternal catecholamine release

19.31 Which of the following may be used to evaluate fetal well-being in cases of intrauterine growth restriction (IUGR)?
a. Fetal "kick-counts"
b. Nonstress test
c. Biophysical profile
d. Doppler ultrasound of blood flow through the umbilical cord
e. All of the above

19.32 Hyperviscosity syndrome associated with intrauterine growth restriction is defined as a fetal hematocrit of more than:
a. 35%
b. 45%
c. 55%
d. 65%
e. 75%

19.33 Hyperviscosity syndrome in intrauterine growth restriction is associated with all of the following EXCEPT:
a. a lower-than-normal fetal hematocrit
b. multiorgan thrombosis
c. heart failure
d. hyperbilirubinemia

ANSWERS (19.24–19.33)

19.24 c	19.26 a	19.28 c	19.30 b	19.32 d	19.33 a
19.25 d	19.27 a	19.29 a	19.31 e		

19.34 Which of the following is useful in the treatment of fetal heart rate deceleration in a patient with intrauterine growth restriction (IUGR) and oligohydramnios?
a. Pitocin augmentation
b. Amnioinfusion
c. Intravenous fluids
d. Blood transfusion

19.35 Growth restricted newborns have difficulty maintaining euglycemia because they:
a. have less fat deposition in late pregnancy
b. have relative hyperthyroid status
c. have a low hematocrit
d. have hyperbilirubinemia

19.36 Fetal macrosomia is defined as weight greater than how many grams?
a. 3000
b. 4000
c. 5000

19.37 A definition of macrosomia is a fetal weight above what percentile for gestational age?
a. 70th
b. 80th
c. 90th

19.38 All of the following can be consequences of fetal macrosomia EXCEPT:
a. prolonged second stage of labor
b. hypothermia
c. shoulder dystocia
d. intrapartum fetal injury

19.39 Which of the following should be included in the differential diagnosis of a larger than expected uterine size?
a. Large but normal fetus
b. Polyhydramnios
c. Uterine leiomyomata
d. Multiple pregnancy
e. All of the above

19.40 Recommended weight gain in pregnancy is approximately how many pounds?
a. 20–30
b. 25–35
c. 30–40
d. 35–45
e. 40–50

19.41 In a diabetic mother, the development of fetal macrosomia is thought to be caused by transfer of:
a. glucose from mother to fetus
b. insulin from fetus to mother
c. growth hormone from mother to fetus
d. insulin from mother to fetus

ANSWERS (19.34–19.41)

| 19.34 b | 19.36 b | 19.38 b | 19.39 e | 19.40 b | 19.41 b |
| 19.35 a | 19.37 c | | | | |

Questions and Answers Chapter 20: Third-Trimester Bleeding

20.1 Approximately what percent of women will experience bleeding at some time during the second and third trimesters of pregnancy?
a. 5%
b. 10%
c. 15%
d. 20%
e. 25%

20.2 Bleeding in the second half of pregnancy can come from which of the following sources?
a. Vaginal tears or lacerations
b. Cervical carcinoma
c. Cervicitis
d. All of the above

20.3 An 18-year-old primigravida at term, not in labor, has sudden onset of severe continuous lower abdominal pain with a rapid pulse, low blood pressure, fetal bradycardia, and a tender abdomen. Which of the following is the most likely diagnosis?
a. Abruptio placentae
b. Placenta previa
c. Uterine rupture
d. Amniotic fluid embolus
e. Supine hypotensive syndrome

20.4 A primigravida at term has profuse vaginal bleeding. Fetal heart tones are normal. The cervix is 2–3 cm dilated with an edge of placenta palpable. Which of the following is the most appropriate treatment?
a. Voorhees' bag
b. Braxton-Hicks version
c. Cesarean delivery
d. Rupture of the fetal membranes to stimulate delivery
e. Replace blood loss and await vaginal delivery

20.5 All of the following are associated with massive placental abruption EXCEPT:
a. painless vaginal bleeding
b. uterine rigidity
c. uterine pain
d. maternal cardiovascular collapse
e. absent fetal heart sounds

20.6 Vasa previa diagnosed in early labor is best treated with:
a. Voorhees' bag
b. forceps delivery
c. spontaneous delivery
d. cesarean section
e. Willett clamp

Instructions for items 20.7 to 20.10: Match the type of placenta previa with the appropriate description. An option may be used once, more than once, or not at all.

20.7 Complete or total placenta previa

20.8 Partial placenta previa

20.9 Marginal placenta previa

20.10 Low-lying placenta previa
a. The margin of the placenta extends across part but not all of the internal os.
b. The entire cervical os is covered by the placenta.
c. The placenta is located near but not directly adjacent to the internal os.
d. The edge of the placenta lies adjacent to the internal os.

ANSWERS (20.1–20.10)

20.1	a	20.3	a	20.5	a	20.7	b	20.9	d
20.2	d	20.4	c	20.6	d	20.8	a		

20.10 c

20.11 All of the following factors are associated with placenta previa EXCEPT:
   a. increasing maternal age
   b. increasing parity
   c. previous cesarean section
   d. presence of a twin pregnancy
   e. maternal hypertension

20.12 What is the frequency of placenta previa?
   a. 1 in 100
   b. 1 in 250
   c. 1 in 500
   d. 1 in 1000
   e. 1 in 1500

20.13 Compared with multiparas, what is the incidence of placenta previa in nulliparas?
   a. lower
   b. the same
   c. greater

20.14 In placenta previa, the first bleeding episode occurs most commonly at what gestational age?
   a. 23–24 weeks
   b. 25–26 weeks
   c. 27–28 weeks
   d. 29–30 weeks
   e. 31–32 weeks

20.15 Placenta previa is coincident with abruptio placentae in approximately what percent of cases?
   a. Less than 5%
   b. 10%
   c. 20%
   d. 40%

20.16 Transvaginal ultrasonography is especially useful in the diagnosis of what type of placenta previa?
   a. Anterior
   b. Lateral
   c. Posterior
   d. All types of placenta previa

20.17 The initial management of a patient with placenta previa and a bleeding episode always includes which of the following?
   a. Hospitalization
   b. Immediate cesarean section
   c. Immediate Pitocin induction of labor
   d. Blood transfusion

20.18 Which of the following are criteria for outpatient care of a patient with known placenta previa?
   a. Highly motivated patient
   b. Evidence of understanding of and compliance with instructions
   c. Immediate access to the hospital
   d. All of the above

20.19 What is the current perinatal morality rate associated with placenta previa?
   a. less than 10%
   b. 15%
   c. 20%
   d. 30%
   e. 40%

20.20 Vaginal delivery with known placenta previa may be indicated if:
a. the fetus is dead
b. there are major fetal malformations, leading to likely fetal demise
c. the pregnancy is clearly previable
d. the placental location and stage of labor are such that it is anticipated that vaginal delivery can be accomplished with a relatively small blood loss
e. all of the above

20.21 Compared with that of all pregnancies, what is the incidence of congenital anomalies in cases of placenta previa?
a. the same
b. twice as high
c. three times as high
d. four times as high

20.22 In placenta previa accreta, the trophoblastic tissue invades the:
a. cervix
b. lower uterine segment
c. vaginal wall
d. mesosalpinx

20.23 Which of the following are common to both placenta previa and abruptio placentae?
a. Vaginal bleeding
b. Abdominal discomfort
c. Painful uterine contractions
d. Presence of a normal fetal heart rate

20.24 Placental abruption is defined as:
a. abnormal position of the placenta
b. abnormal separation of the normally implanted placenta
c. abnormal morphology of the placenta

20.25 Placental abruption is associated with:
a. maternal hypertension
b. polyhydramnios
c. maternal trauma
d. maternal cocaine use
e. all of the above

20.26 Couvelaire uterus is associated with:
a. placenta previa
b. abruptio placentae
c. vasa previa
d. all of the above

20.27 The diagnosis of placental abruption is made primarily by:
a. clinical presentation and evaluation
b. ultrasound
c. amniocentesis
d. laboratory evaluation

Instructions for items 20.28 to 20.31: Match the blood component with the factors that are present. An option may be used once, more than once, or not at all.

20.28 Packed red blood cells (RBCs)

20.29 Fresh frozen plasma

20.30 Cryoprecipitate

20.31 Fresh whole blood
a. Fibrinogen, factors VII and XIII
b. RBCs only
c. All procoagulants, no platelets
d. RBCs and all procoagulants

20.32 All of the following are included in the "classic clinical presentation" of abruptio placentae EXCEPT:
a. vaginal bleeding
b. tender uterus
c. frequent painful uterine contractions
d. normal fetal heart rate

ANSWERS (20.20–20.32)

20.20 e	20.23 a	20.25 e	20.27 a	20.29 c	20.31 d
20.21 b	20.24 b	20.26 b	20.28 b	20.30 a	20.32 d
20.22 b					

20.33 In vasa previa, the umbilical cord inserts into the:
a. central mass of the placenta
b. membranes of the placenta
c. internal os
d. endocervix

20.34 Which of the following tests is useful in differentiating maternal blood from fetal blood?
a. Kleihauer-Betke
b. Coombs'
c. Venereal Disease Research Laboratory (VDRL)
d. Lee-White

20.35 What is the appropriate treatment for ruptured vasa previa?
a. augmentation of labor
b. tocolysis
c. immediate cesarean delivery
d. periumbilical artery transfusion

20.36 In the absence of massive blood loss, coagulation defects are most common in which of the following?
a. Abruptio placentae
b. Placenta previa
c. Vasa previa
d. Routine labor

Instructions for items 20.37 to 20.42: Match the type of uterine wall separation with the sign, symptom or finding with which it is often associated. An option may be used once, more than once, or not at all.

20.37 Involves only the muscular wall

20.38 Separation of the placenta

20.39 Minimal bleeding

20.40 Fetus remains in utero

20.41 Fetal bradycardia

20.42 Nonreassuring fetal status
a. uterine scar dehiscence
b. uterine rupture

20.43 Uterine rupture is associated with nonreassuring fetal status in about what percent of cases?
a. 1–25%
b. 25–50%
c. 50–75%
d. 75–100%

20.44 Because of the risk of uterine rupture in a woman with a previous uterine rupture involving the upper uterine segment, repeat cesarean section is usually recommended at a gestational age of:
a. 30–31 weeks
b. 33–34 weeks
c. 36–37 weeks
d. 39–40 weeks

20.45 What is the overall incidence of uterine rupture in a woman with a previous uncomplicated lower segment transverse cesarean section?
a. 0.5%
b. 2.5%
c. 4.5%
d. 6.5%

Answers (20.33–20.45)

20.33 b	20.36 a	20.38 b	20.40 a	20.42 b	20.44 c
20.34 a	20.37 a	20.39 a	20.41 b	20.43 c	20.45 a
20.35 c					

Questions and Answers Chapter 21:
Postterm Pregnancy

21.1 A normal pregnancy is defined to last from 38 weeks to how many weeks?
a. 40
b. 41
c. 42
d. 43
e. 44

21.2 A patient is considered postterm if she has not delivered by the end of what week from the first day of the last menstrual period?
a. 40
b. 41
c. 42
d. 43
e. 44

21.3 If a patient's due date is November 11, she is said to be postterm on
a. November 18
b. November 25
c. November 12
d. December 2

21.4 Postterm pregnancy occurs in what percent of pregnancies?
a. 8%–10%
b. 11%–13%
c. 14%–16%
d. 17%–19%
e. 20%–22%

21.5 Approximately what percent of patients having one postterm pregnancy will have a prolonged pregnancy with their next gestation?
a. 0%
b. 25%
c. 50%
d. 75%
e. 100%

21.6 What is the most common "cause" of postterm pregnancy?
a. Anencephaly
b. Placental sulfatase deficiency
c. Inaccurate date
d. Extrauterine pregnancy

21.7 Which of the following "causes" of postterm pregnancy is associated with altered estrogen production?
a. Inaccurate dates
b. Anencephaly
c. Extrauterine pregnancy

21.8 Which of the following statements about the dysmaturity (postmaturity) syndrome is incorrect?
a. It occurs in approximately one-fifth of true postterm pregnancies.
b. It is associated with fetal growth restriction.
c. Integumentary changes (scaling epidermis, meconium staining) are seen.
d. Increased amounts of subcutaneous fat are common.

21.9 In macrosomia associated with postterm pregnancy, all of the following are likely to be present EXCEPT:
a. hyperglycemia
b. hyperbilirubinemia
c. shoulder dystocia
d. fetopelvic disproportion

ANSWERS (21.1–21.9)

21.1	c	21.3	b	21.5	c	21.7	b	21.8	d	21.9	a
21.2	c	21.4	a	21.6	c						

21.10 Postterm pregnancy may be associated with:
a. increased incidence of fetal compromise
b. placental dysfunction
c. meconium aspiration
d. oligohydramnios
e. all of the above

21.11 Dysmature newborns may demonstrate altered glucose and bilirubin metabolism and are at risk for:
a. hyperglycemia and hypobilirubinemia
b. hyperglycemia and hyperbilirubinemia
c. hypoglycemia and hypobilirubinemia
d. hypoglycemia and hyperbilirubinemia

21.12 If, after rupture of membranes, meconium stained amniotic fluid is discovered in the intrapartum patient, the next management step should be:
a. immediate cesarean section
b. periumbilical blood gas measurement
c. amnioinfusion
d. fetal scalp blood sampling
e. close electronic monitoring of fetal status

21.13 In utero meconium passage is seen in about what percent of term pregnancies?
a. 15%
b. 25%
c. 35%
d. 45%
e. 55%

21.14 An amnionic fluid index (AFI) of less than what value is usually considered consistent with oligohydramnios?
a. 2
b. 5
c. 8
d. 11

21.15 Brachial plexus injury is reported in what proportion of term deliveries?
a. 1 in 250
b. 1 in 500
c. 1 in 750
d. 1 in 1000

21.16 Approximately what percent of placentas from postterm pregnancies demonstrate anatomic changes consistent with decreased functional capability?
a. 20%
b. 40%
c. 60%
d. 80%
e. 100%

21.17 What percent of placentas from postterm pregnancies demonstrate placental infarcts, calcifications, and fibrosis?
a. 20%
b. 40%
c. 60%
d. 80%

21.18 The management options of inducing labor or continuing to monitor fetal well-being should be considered once the patient approaches how many weeks of gestation?
a. 38
b. 39
c. 40
d. 41
e. 42

Answers (21.10–21.18)

| 21.10 e | 21.12 e | 21.14 b | 21.16 b | 21.17 b | 21.18 d |
| 21.11 d | 21.13 a | 21.15 b | | | |

21.19 All of the following may be used to assess fetal well-being during a postterm pregnancy EXCEPT:
   a. daily fetal movement counts
   b. biweekly nonstress testing
   c. biweekly biophysical profile testing
   d. weekly oxytocin challenge testing
   e. ultrasound for biparietal diameter

21.20 Cesarean birth should be considered when the estimated fetal weight exceeds how many grams?
   a. 3500–4000
   b. 4000–4500
   c. 4500–5000
   d. 5000–5500

21.21 Which of the following can be used to induce labor in the postterm pregnancy?
   a. Oxytocin
   b. Prostaglandin vaginal suppository
   c. Laminaria
   d. All of the above

21.22 Erb palsy results in paralysis of which of the following muscles?
   a. Deltoid
   b. Infraspinatus
   c. Flexor muscles of the forearm
   d. All of the above

21.23 Paralysis of the hand is also termed:
   a. Erb palsy
   b. Duchenne palsy
   c. Bell palsy
   d. Klumpke's paralysis

ANSWERS (21.19–21.23)

21.19 e   21.20 c   21.21 d   21.22 d   21.23 d

Questions and Answers Chapter 22: Preterm Labor

22.1   Labor occurring prior to the completion of how many weeks of gestation (counted from the LMP) is considered preterm labor?
a. 35
b. 36
c. 37
d. 38
e. 39

22.2   Of neonatal deaths that are not due to congenital malformations, what percent are associated with premature labor and birth?
a. 25
b. 50
c. 75
d. 100

22.3   All of the following are predisposing factors for respiratory distress syndrome EXCEPT:
a. short gestation
b. cesarean section
c. prenatal asphyxia
d. maternal diabetes
e. grand multiparity

22.4   The 10% of babies born prematurely in the United States account for what percent of all perinatal morbidity and mortality?
a. 30–45%
b. 45–60%
c. 60–75%
d. 75–90%

22.5   An infant born at 30 weeks of gestation and weighing 2600 g would be defined as:
a. low-birth weight
b. preterm
c. both low-birth weight and preterm
d. neither low-birth weight nor preterm

22.6   Preterm labor (PTL) is functionally defined as the presence of regular uterine contractions, between 20 and 36 weeks' gestation, occurring with a frequency of:
a. 5 minutes or less and lasting at least 30 seconds
b. 5 minutes or less and lasting at least 60 seconds
c. 10 minutes or less and lasting at least 30 seconds
d. 10 minutes or less and lasting at least 60 seconds

22.7   Premature birth is associated with all of the following perinatal complications EXCEPT:
a. respiratory distress syndrome
b. intraventricular hemorrhage
c. skeletal abnormalities
d. sepsis
e. seizures

22.8   All of the following factors have been associated with preterm birth EXCEPT:
a. maternal infections
b. maternal age
c. uterine distortion
d. placental abnormalities
e. substance abuse

22.9   About what percent of preterm births are in multiple gestations?
a. 10%
b. 20%
c. 30%
d. 40%

22.10 If a patient's first pregnancy ends in preterm labor and delivery, her risk in a subsequent pregnancy is increased:
a. 2-fold
b. 4-fold
c. 6-fold
d. 8-fold

ANSWERS (22.1–22.10)					
22.1 c	22.3 e	22.5 b	22.7 c	22.9 a	22.10 a
22.2 c	22.4 c	22.6 c	22.8 b		

22.11 All of the following indicators often precede preterm birth EXCEPT:
   a. increased uterine irritability
   b. increased frequency of contractions
   c. rapid weight gain
   d. feeling of pelvic pressure

22.12 Which of the following are recognized signs and symptoms associated with preterm labor?
   a. Low, dull backache
   b. Pelvic pressure
   c. Abdominal cramps
   d. Change in vaginal discharge
   e. All of the above

22.13 All of the following should be included in the evaluation of suspected preterm labor EXCEPT:
   a. status of the cervix
   b. computed axial tomography (CAT) scan for gestational age
   c. electronic fetal monitor for frequency of contractions
   d. abdominal palpation for strength of contractions

22.14 Which of the following laboratory studies is useful in the evaluation of a patient at risk for preterm labor?
   a. Urinalysis and urine culture
   b. Culture for β-streptococcus
   c. Culture for *Neisseria gonorrhoeae*
   d. Wet preparation for bacterial vaginosis
   e. All of the above

22.15 Which of the following statements about fetal fibronectin (fFN) is incorrect?
   a. It has been associated with preterm labor.
   b. It is an extracellular glycoprotein normally found in the amniotic fluid in early pregnancy and then again near term.
   c. A rise in the concentration of fFN may be associated with the impending onset of preterm labor.
   d. Its absence is uncommonly associated with a patient who delivers in the 7 days after the sample is taken.

Instructions for items 22.16 to 22.19: Match the class of tocolytic agent with its proposed mode of action. An option may be used once, more than once, or not at all.

22.16 Magnesium sulfate

22.17 β-adrenergic agents (ritodrine or terbutaline)

22.18 Prostaglandin-synthetase inhibitors (indomethacin)

22.19 Calcium-channel blockers (nifedipine)
   a. Increases cyclic AMP in cells, which decreases free calcium
   b. Competes with calcium for entry into cells
   c. Prevents calcium entry into muscle cells
   d. Decreases prostaglandin production

ANSWERS (22.11–22.19)

22.11 c	22.13 b	22.15 b	22.17 a	22.18 d	22.19 c
22.12 e	22.14 e	22.16 b			

Instructions for items 22.20 to 22.23: Match the tocolytic agent with its possible complications. An option may be used once, more than once, or not at all.

22.20 Magnesium sulfate

22.21 β-adrenergic agents (ritodrine or terbutaline)

22.22 Prostaglandin-synthetase inhibitors (indomethacin)

22.23 Calcium-channel blockers
   a. Maternal hypertension, tachycardia, anxiety, chest tightening, and electrocardiogram (ECG) changes
   b. Premature constriction of ductus arteriosus, especially after 34 weeks' gestation
   c. Maternal flushing and headache, respiratory depression at high doses
   d. Possible decrease in uteroplacental blood flow with fetal hypoxia and hypercarbia

22.24 It is customary to stop tocolytic therapy at:
   a. 30 weeks
   b. 32 weeks
   c. 34 weeks
   d. 36 weeks
   e. 38 weeks

22.25 All of the following are contraindications to tocolysis EXCEPT:
   a. mature fetus
   b. anomalous fetus
   c. intrauterine infection
   d. maternal age greater than 35 years
   e. presence of advanced labor

22.26 With regard to preterm labor, what is the tocolytic agent generally considered to have the highest degree of safety?
   a. terbutaline
   b. indomethacin
   c. magnesium sulfate
   d. nifedipine

22.27 In patients with preterm labor before 32 weeks' gestation, corticosteroids are often given to:
   a. decrease uterine activity
   b. stabilize vascular membranes
   c. enhance fetal lung maturity
   d. prevent infection

22.28 What is the most common cause of perinatal morbidity and mortality?
   a. Preterm birth resulting from preterm labor
   b. Multiple gestation
   c. Intrapartum asphyxia
   d. Inadequate neonatal resuscitation

22.29 All of the following are surgically correctable causes of preterm birth EXCEPT:
   a. incompetent cervix
   b. uterine leiomyomas
   c. septate uterus
   d. vaginal stenosis

22.30 Maternal smoking is strongly associated with:
   a. preterm labor
   b. large for gestational age infants
   c. fetal anemia
   d. neonatal hypercalcemia

22.31 All of the following are related to excessive uterine enlargement that may lead to preterm birth EXCEPT:
   a. multiple gestation
   b. leiomyomata uteri
   c. hydramnios
   d. incorrect menstrual dates

ANSWERS (22.20–22.31)					
22.20 c	22.22 b	22.24 d	22.26 c	22.28 a	22.30 a
22.21 a	22.23 d	22.25 d	22.27 c	22.29 d	22.31 d

22.32 Which of the following are factors associated with preterm birth?
a. Placental abnormalities
b. Uterine distortion
c. Excessive uterine enlargement
d. All of the above

22.33 A routine pelvic examination is often performed at what gestational age to determine whether or not asymptomatic dilation and effacement of the cervix is occurring?
a. 12–14 weeks
b. 18–20 weeks
c. 24–28 weeks
d. 34–36 weeks

22.34 Which of the following statements about betamethasone therapy in preterm labor is incorrect?
a. It generally is administered when preterm delivery is expected within 7 days.
b. It generally is administered between 24 and 37 weeks of gestation.
c. It generally is administered as two 12 mg doses given 24 hours apart.
d. The benefits of administration include increased pulmonary volume and surfactant pool.

Instructions for Items 22.35 to 22.39. Indicate whether each of the following statements is an indication or contraindication to tocolysis.

22.35 Regular uterine contractions and cervical effacement and dilation at 30 weeks gestational age

22.36 Chorioamnionitis

22.37 Regular uterine contractions and cervical effacement and dilation at 37 weeks gestational age

22.38 Multiple fetal anomalies

22.39 Evidence of fetal maturity
a. Indication
b. Contraindication

ANSWERS (22.32–22.39)

22.32 d	22.34 a	22.36 b	22.37 b	22.38 b	22.39 b
22.33 c	22.35 a				

Questions and Answers Chapter 23: Premature Rupture of Membranes

23.1 Amniotic fluid serves to protect against
a. infection of the fetus
b. fetal trauma
c. umbilical cord compression
d. all of the above

23.2 Premature rupture of membranes is defined as rupture of the chorioamniotic membrane
a. before the onset of labor
b. at the onset of labor
c. during the active phase of labor
d. before complete effacement

23.3 Premature rupture of membranes occurs in what percent of all pregnancies?
a. Less than 2%
b. 2%–5%
c. 10%–15%
d. 20%–25%

23.4 Premature rupture of membranes is associated with about what percent of term pregnancies (37 weeks' gestational age or more)?
a. 10%
b. 30%
c. 50%
d. 70%

23.5 Premature rupture of membranes is associated with about what percent of preterm deliveries?
a. 15%
b. 30%
c. 45%
d. 60%
e. 75%

23.6 Mid-trimester preterm premature rupture of membranes (between 16 and 26 weeks' gestational age) complicates about what percent of all pregnancies?
a. 0.01%
b. 0.1%
c. 1.0%
d. 10%

23.7 The most serious primary risk resulting from preterm premature rupture of membranes is
a. chorioamnionitis
b. cord compression
c. preterm delivery
d. abruptio placentae

23.8 Risk factors for premature spontaneous rupture of membranes (PSROM) include
a. prior PSROM
b. prior preterm delivery
c. smoking
d. bleeding in early pregnancy
e. all of the above

23.9 Which of the following can cause a false-negative nitrazine test?
a. Basic urine
b. Presence of cervical mucus
c. Blood contamination
d. Earlier premature rupture of the membranes with no residual fluid
e. All of the above

23.10 Which of the following are circumstances associated with a false-positive nitrazine test?
a. *Trichomonas vaginalis*
b. Presence of semen
c. Blood contamination
d. All of the above

ANSWERS (23.1–23.10)

23.1	d	23.3	c	23.5	b	23.7	c	23.9	d	23.10 d
23.2	a	23.4	a	23.6	c	23.8	e			

23.11 The most common situation that can be confused at term with premature rupture of membranes is
a. bloody show
b. passage of cervical mucus
c. intermittent urinary leakage
d. yeast vaginitis

23.12 The nitrazine test is used to assess for premature rupture of membranes based on the fact that amniotic fluid is
a. acid pH
b. alkaline pH
c. neutral pH
d. of higher specific gravity than water
e. of lower specific gravity than water

23.13 Of the following, which is the best predictor of intrauterine infection?
a. Presence of bacteria on Gram stain of amniotic fluid
b. Presence of white cells in amniotic fluid
c. Decelerations of fetal heart tones
d. Onset of uterine contractions

23.14 Which of the following factors should be considered in developing a management plan for a patient with premature rupture of the membranes?
a. The gestational age at the time of rupture
b. The presence of uterine contractions
c. The amount of amniotic fluid around the fetus
d. All of the above

23.15 Premature rupture of the membranes presents the risks of pulmonary hypoplasia and amniotic band syndrome before what gestational age?
a. 25 weeks
b. 27 weeks
c. 29 weeks
d. 31 weeks

23.16 The expectant management of premature rupture of membranes in a fetus that is significantly preterm usually includes all of the following EXCEPT
a. daily white blood cell counts for the first few days
b. frequent ultrasound assessment for amniotic fluid volume
c. serial cervical digital examinations to detect the onset of labor
d. daily fetal movement monitoring
e. intermittent electronic monitoring

23.17 The diagnosis of rupture of membranes may be based on all of the following EXCEPT
a. nitrazine test
b. patient history
c. white blood cell count
d. ultrasound findings

23.18 Which of the following mechanisms does NOT contribute to amniotic fluid production?
a. Fetal urine production
b. Fetal bowel movements
c. Fetal pulmonary effluent
d. Passage of fluid across the fetal membranes
e. Passage of fluid across the fetal skin

ANSWERS (23.11–23.18)

23.11 c	23.13 a	23.15 a	23.16 c	23.17 b	23.18 b
23.12 b	23.14 d				

23.19 What percent of patients with premature spontaneous rupture of membranes will have a preterm birth?
a. 1%
b. 5%
c. 10%
d. 15%
e. 20%

23.20 Between 28 weeks' gestational age and term, about what percent of patients with premature spontaneous rupture of membranes labor within 24 hours?
a. 40%
b. 50%
c. 60%
d. 70%
e. 80%

23.21 Between 28 weeks' gestational age and term, about what percent of patients with premature spontaneous rupture of membranes labor within one week?
a. 40%
b. 50%
c. 60%
d. 70%
e. 80%

23.22 Between 24 and 28 weeks' gestational age, about what percent of patients with premature spontaneous rupture of membranes labor within one week?
a. 40%
b. 50%
c. 60%
d. 70%
e. 80%

23.23 Preterm labor and delivery occurs within one week in about what percent of all patients with premature spontaneous rupture of membranes before 37 weeks' gestational age?
a. 25%
b. 50%
c. 75%
d. 95%

23.24 Which of the following statements regarding premature rupture of membranes (PROM) and intrauterine infections is incorrect?
a. Intact membranes with normal amniotic fluid volume fully protect the fetus from infection
b. Subclinical intra-amniotic infection may play a role in PROM
c. Metabolites from intrauterine infection may weaken the amniotic membranes
d. Metabolites from intrauterine infection may initiate uterine contractions through stimulation of prostaglandin synthesis

23.25 Which of the following statements about premature rupture of membranes and chorioamnionitis is INCORRECT?
a. Purulent discharge often precedes fever and uterine tenderness by several hours
b. This situation often leads to tumultuous, spontaneous labor
c. Fever greater than 100.5°F is common
d. This situation is often associated with fetal tachycardia
e. Treatment consists of antibiotic therapy and prompt delivery

23.26 The differential diagnosis of premature rupture of the membranes includes
a. urinary incontinence
b. increased vaginal secretions in pregnancy
c. vaginal discharge associated with vaginitis
d. vesicovaginal fistula
e. all of the above

23.27 Betamethasone therapy to enhance fetal lung maturity is generally recommended in preterm premature spontaneous rupture of membranes until approximately how many weeks gestational age?
a. 37 weeks
b. 36 weeks
c. 34 weeks
d. 32 weeks
e. 30 weeks

ANSWERS (23.26–23.27)
23.26 e   23.27 d

Questions and Answers Chapter 24:
Obstetric Procedures

24.1 Chorionic villus sampling is generally associated with what risk of fetal loss?
a. 0.5%
b. 1.5%
c. 2.5%
d. 3.5%

24.2 What is the role of obstetric forceps?
a. Augment the expulsive forces of the second stage of labor
b. Replace the expulsive forces of the second stage of labor
c. Augment the contractions of the first stage of labor
d. Overcome uterine inertia in the first stage of labor

24.3 Which type of forceps delivery is not practiced because it presents an unacceptable risk to mother and fetus?
a. Outlet forceps
b. Low forceps
c. Low forceps rotation
d. Midforceps rotation
e. High forceps

24.4 Which type of uterine incision at the time of cesarean section is generally accepted to require cesarean section with subsequent pregnancies?
a. Low transverse
b. Low vertical
c. Classical

24.5 The primary indication for circumcision of the male infant is
a. reduction of the prevalence of penile carcinoma
b. improved penile hygiene
c. social–religious considerations

24.6 Which of the following tests may be performed by means of percutaneous umbilical blood sampling?
a. Fetal blood count
b. Fetal genetic status
c. Fetal blood chemistries
d. All of the above

24.7 Which type of obstetrical forceps is especially suited for a rotation of the fetal head?
a. Piper
b. Simpson
c. Kielland
d. All of the above

24.8 Pregnancy termination during the first trimester is usually performed by
a. hysterectomy
b. hysteroscopy
c. suction curettage
d. hysterotomy

Instructions for items 24.9 to 24.14: Match the type of incision with the item with which it is best associated.

24.9 Lower segment transverse

24.10 Low vertical

24.11 Midline

24.12 Pfannensteil

24.13 Maylard

24.14 Classical
a. Abdominal incision
b. Uterine incision

Answers (24.1–24.14)				
24.1 a	24.4 c	24.7 c	24.9 b	24.11 a	24.13 a
24.2 a	24.5 c	24.8 c	24.10 b	24.12 a	24.14 b
24.3 e	24.6 d				

24.15 Cesarean sections are generally classified by
a. the indication
b. the type of abdominal incision
c. the type of uterine incision
d. the stage of fetal maturity

24.16 When performed by an experienced, skilled operator, external cephalic version is successful about what percent of the time?
a. 1%–25%
b. 25%–50%
c. 50%–75%
d. 75%–100%

Answers (24.15–24.16)

24.15 c   24.16 c

Questions and Answers Chapter 25: Contraception

25.1   In assessing the effectiveness of various contraceptive methods, the "method failure rate" reflects the rate of failure when the method is
a. used by a random sample of women
b. tested in the laboratory
c. used correctly 100% of the time
d. compared with the use of no contraception at all

Instructions for items 25.2 to 25.4: Match the mechanism of contraceptive action with the relevant contraceptive(s). An option may be used once, more than once, or not at all.

25.2   Inhibit the development and release of the egg

25.3   Impose a barrier between the sperm and egg

25.4   Alter the ability of the fertilized egg to implant and grow
a. Intrauterine device
b. Foam
c. Oral contraceptive
d. Long-acting progesterone injection
e. Diaphragm

25.5   Which of the following contraceptive methods does NOT provide some measure of protection from sexually transmitted diseases?
a. Male condom
b. Diaphragm
c. Spermicidal jelly
d. Female condom
e. Intrauterine contraceptive device

25.6   The most common method of contraception among younger women in the United States is
a. spermicidal foam
b. male condom
c. long-acting hormone (rod or injection)
d. oral contraceptive
e. intrauterine device

25.7   The synthetic estrogen most frequently found in oral contraceptives is
a. ethinyl estradiol
b. β-estradiol
c. mestranol
d. levonorgestrel
e. norethindrone

25.8   The hormone used in implantable contraceptive rods (Norplant) is
a. ethinyl estradiol
b. β-estradiol
c. mestranol
d. levonorgestrel
e. norethindrone

25.9   Ethinyl estradiol is approximately how many times as potent as the same weight of mestranol?
a. 0.5
b. 1.0
c. 1.3
d. 1.7
e. 2.3

25.10 Which of the following progestins used in oral contraceptives has the LEAST biologic potency?
a. Norethindrone acetate
b. Norgestrel
c. Ethynodiol acetate
d. Norethindrone
e. Norethynodrel

ANSWERS (25.1–25.10)

25.1 c	25.3 b, e	25.5 e	25.7 a	25.9 d	25.10 d
25.2 c, d	25.4 a	25.6 d	25.8 d		

25.11 Progesterone-only oral contraceptive agents are less widely used by younger women because they
a. cost more than monophasic oral contraceptives
b. cause breast tenderness
c. have a higher failure rate
d. raise serum high-density lipoprotein levels

25.12 Combination oral contraceptive pills mainly act to prevent pregnancy through
a. altering cervical mucus
b. inducing endometrial atrophy
c. causing elevated endometrial prostaglandin formation
d. suppressing follicle-stimulating hormone and luteinizing hormone release
e. altering tubal motility

25.13 The progestins used in most oral contraceptives tend to
a. increase the occurrence of acne
b. increase smooth muscle tone
c. decrease sebum production
d. decrease hair growth

25.14 Which of the following occurs in users of multiphasic (low dose) oral contraceptives at a higher rate than it occurs in the general population?
a. Ovarian cancer
b. Intermenstrual bleeding
c. Ectopic pregnancy
d. Anemia
e. Dysmenorrhea

25.15 A 20-year-old G0P0 moderately obese patient consults you about the use of oral contraceptives. Her menarche was at age 15 and her period comes every 30 to 45 days and lasts 2–4 days. If this patient were to use an oral contraceptive agent, she would be at greater risk for
a. "post-pill amenorrhea"
b. endometrial cancer
c. ectopic pregnancy
d. acne

25.16 When taken concurrently, which of the following will reduce the efficacy of oral contraceptives?
a. Insulin
b. Tricyclic antidepressants
c. Oral penicillin
d. Methyldopa
e. Aspirin

25.17 The most common side effect of injectable or implantable contraceptive steroids is
a. involuntary weight loss
b. dysmenorrhea
c. vaginal dryness
d. random vaginal bleeding

25.18 Which of the following is NOT an attribute of long-acting injectable and implantable progestins?
a. Good compliance
b. Patient controlled reversibility
c. Low failure rate
d. Low incidence of major side effects

25.19 A couple wishes to use "natural family planning" for contraception. Her periods are regular, coming every 28 ± 3 days. This patient's "fertile" period would be days
a. 7–14
b. 7–17
c. 7–20
d. 10–17
e. 10–20

Instructions for items 25.20 to 25.22: A couple is using natural family planning for contraception. The chart shows the basal temperature graph made for the previous month. Using the chart, match the letter with the appropriate description.

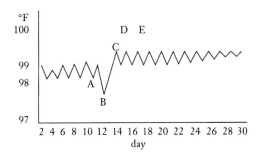

25.20 The time of ovulation

25.21 The time when unprotected intercourse may resume

25.22 The time when thin, "stretchy" cervical mucus would be found
a. Letter A
b. Letter B
c. Letter C
d. Letter D
e. Letter E

25.23 Following unprotected coitus, it is recommended that high-dose estrogen preparations be given within a maximum of
a. 1 day
b. 2 days
c. 3 days
d. 4 days
e. 5 days

Instructions for items 25.24 to 25.39: Match the contraceptive method with its corresponding typical pregnancy rate in the first year of use. An option may be used once, more than once, or not at all.

25.24 No method of contraception

25.25 Combination pill

25.26 Progestin pill

25.27 Norplant

25.28 Depo-Provera

25.29 Spermicides

25.30 Condom

25.31 Sponge, parous woman

25.32 Sponge, nulliparous woman

25.33 Cervical cap

25.34 Diaphragm and spermicide

25.35 Intrauterine device

25.36 Withdrawal

25.37 Postcoital douche

25.38 Periodic abstinence

ANSWERS (25.19–25.38)					
25.19 c	25.23 d	25.27 a	25.30 f	25.33 g	25.36 g
25.20 c	25.24 l	25.28 b	25.31 j	25.34 g	25.37 k
25.21 e	25.25 e	25.29 h	25.32 g	25.35 e	25.38 h
25.22 c	25.26 e				

25.39 Yuzpe Method
   a. 0.2
   b. 0.3
   c. < 1
   d. < 2
   e. 3
   f. 12
   g. 18
   h. 20
   i. 25
   j. 28
   k. 40
   l. 85

Instructions for items 25.40 to 25.46: Match the symptom occurring in a patient using an oral contraceptive with the action that should be taken. An option may be used once, more than once, or not at all.

25.40 Diplopia

25.41 Hemoptysis

25.42 Hepatic mass

25.43 Slurring of speech

25.44 Severe headache

25.45 Severe chest/neck pain

25.46 Severe leg pain, tenderness
   a. Continue oral contraceptive but evaluate immediately
   b. Discontinue oral contraceptive and evaluate immediately, start nonhormonal contraceptive method

25.47 The failure of oral contraceptives usually is related to
   a. an inherent problem in the estrogen to progesterone ratio
   b. interference by other medications that the patient is taking
   c. missed doses of the oral contraceptive
   d. altered gastrointestinal absorption of the oral contraceptive due to hormonal influences

25.48 The estrogenic components of oral contraceptives preferentially inhibit
   a. follicle-stimulating hormone (FSH) and are dose dependent
   b. FSH and are not dose dependent
   c. luteinizing hormone (LH) and are dose dependent
   d. LH and are not dose dependent

25.49 Hormonal agents in oral contraceptives make cervical mucus
   a. thicker
   b. thinner

25.50 The use of oral contraceptives offers some protection against all of the following EXCEPT
   a. endometrial carcinoma
   b. asthma
   c. benign breast disease
   d. ovarian carcinoma
   e. ectopic pregnancy

25.51 Compared with low-dose oral contraceptives, high-dose oral contraceptives have a
   a. higher incidence of breakthrough bleeding
   b. similar incidence of breakthrough bleeding
   c. lower incidence of breakthrough bleeding

ANSWERS (25.39–25.51)

25.39 i	25.42 b	25.44 a	25.46 b	25.48 a	25.50 b
25.40 b	25.43 b	25.45 b	25.47 c	25.49 a	25.51 c
25.41 b					

25.52 Approximately what percent of patients will experience post-pill amenorrhea when discontinuing oral contraceptives after long-term use?
a. 1%
b. 3%
c. 5%
d. 7%
e. 9%

25.53 Post-pill amenorrhea is more likely to be experienced by
a. older women
b. younger women
c. smokers
d. nonsmokers
e. women with regular menses

25.54 What is the dosage of Depo-Provera that is given every three months for the purpose of contraception?
a. 50 mg
b. 100 mg
c. 150 mg
d. 200 mg
e. 250 mg

25.55 Most women who discontinue Depo-Provera injections will not become fertile for how many months?
a. 1–2
b. 2–3
c. 3–4
d. 4–5
e. 5–6

25.56 Norplant is effective for how many years after insertion?
a. 1
b. 2
c. 3
d. 4
e. 5
f. 6

25.57 Injectable and implantable progestin contraceptive methods cause all of the following EXCEPT
a. suppressed ovulation
b. thickened cervical mucus
c. thinned cervical mucus
d. impeded sperm transport

25.58 Which of the following is NOT a positive attribute of barrier contraceptives?
a. Requirement for good patient compliance
b. Patient controlled reversibility
c. Low failure rate
d. Low incidence of major side effects
e. Low cost per month

25.59 In addition to the failure rate, which of the following is the most common problem associated with the use of condoms?
a. Premature ejaculation
b. Increased risk of vaginal yeast infection
c. Contact dermatitis
d. Urinary retention

25.60 When used for contraception, a diaphragm must be left in place following intercourse for at least
a. 1 hour
b. 2–3 hours
c. 6–8 hours
d. 12–18 hours
e. 24 or more hours

ANSWERS (25.52–25.60)

25.52 b	25.54 c	25.56 e	25.58 a	25.59 c	25.60 c
25.53 b	25.55 d	25.57 c			

25.61 If a diaphragm is in place following intercourse (during the "waiting time" before diaphragm removal), what should be done before additional intercourse?
a. Delay intercourse until the waiting time has expired
b. Remove the diaphragm, reapply the contraceptive jelly, and restart the waiting time
c. Insert additional jelly without disturbing the diaphragm and restart the waiting time
d. Remove the diaphragm, reapply the contraceptive jelly, and remove the diaphragm at the end of the original waiting time
e. Remove the diaphragm and use an alternate method of contraception

25.62 When correctly fitted and worn, a contraceptive diaphragm should
a. completely cover the posterior vaginal wall
b. have its apex in the posterior fornix
c. rest firmly against the posterior fourchette
d. sit 1–2 cm below the symphysis

25.63 Susceptibility to urinary tract infections by women who use diaphragms is
a. slightly higher
b. about the same
c. slightly lower

25.64 Following intercourse using contraceptive foam, douching should be avoided for at least
a. 30–60 minutes
b. 1–2 hours
c. 4–6 hours
d. 8–10 hours
e. 12 or more hours

25.65 Spermicidal foam provides protection for
a. a single act of intercourse
b. 1–3 hours
c. 4–6 hours
d. 10–12 hours
e. up to 24 hours

25.66 How does the presence of a reservoir tip in a condom affect the likelihood of breakage during use?
a. Increases the likelihood
b. Does not affect the likelihood
c. Decreases the likelihood

25.67 The vaginal sponge acts as a contraceptive primarily by
a. acting as a barrier to sperm
b. delivering spermicide
c. irritating the vaginal wall

25.68 Following unprotected intercourse, an intrauterine contraceptive device may prevent pregnancy if it is inserted within
a. 12 hours
b. 24 hours
c. 36 hours
d. 72 hours
e. 5 days

25.69 The main contraceptive action of intrauterine contraceptive devices as a class is to
a. inhibit ovulation
b. cause cervical mucus thickening
c. alter tubal motility
d. prevent implantation
e. cause heavy metal poisoning of sperm

Answers (25.61–25.69)

25.61 c	25.63 a	25.65 a	25.67 b	25.68 e	25.69 d
25.62 b	25.64 d	25.66 c			

25.70 The most important factor in selection of patients for intrauterine device use is
a. age
b. parity
c. risk of sexually transmitted diseases
d. history of dysmenorrhea

25.71 The relative ratio of extrauterine pregnancy to intrauterine pregnancy in an intrauterine device user compared to an oral contraceptive user is
a. greater
b. the same
c. less

25.72 The overall risk of ectopic pregnancy in users of intrauterine devices is
a. increased
b. unchanged
c. decreased

25.73 The spontaneous expulsion rate of intrauterine devices in the first year following insertion is
a. 5%
b. 10%
c. 15%
d. 20%
e. 25%

25.74 What is the best time for insertion of an intrauterine device?
a. At the time of ovulation
b. In the time between the menstrual period and ovulation
c. In the time between ovulation and the menstrual period
d. At the time of the menstrual period

25.75 Increased vaginal bleeding and menstrual pain is experienced in what percent of women using an intrauterine device?
a. 1%–5%
b. 5%–10%
c. 10%–15%
d. 15%–20%
e. 20%–25%

25.76 The increased vaginal bleeding and menstrual pain sometimes associated with intratuterine device (IUD) use may be lessened in some women by the use of what adjunctive regimen in the first few months of IUD use?
a. Oral contraceptives
b. Lupron
c. Nonsteroidal anti-inflammatory drugs
d. Doxycycline

Instructions for items 25.77 to 25.79: Match the type of intrauterine device (IUD) with the best description. An option may be used once, more than once, or not at all.

25.77 ParaGard IUD

25.78 Progestasert IUD

25.79 Lippes Loop IUD
a. Medicated
b. Unmedicated

25.80 For a women with mild dysmenorrhea, which intrauterine device may offer advantages in addition to contraception?
a. ParaGard
b. Progestasert
c. Lippes Loop

25.81 The copper from copper-containing intrauterine devices may exert all the following additional contraceptive effects EXCEPT
a. endometrial decidualization
b. enhanced endometrial inflammatory response
c. enhanced spermidical effect in cervical mucus

25.82 Which of the following patients should not use intrauterine devices for contraception?
a. Adolescents
b. Nulliparas
c. Immunosuppressed individuals
d. Individuals with uterine fibroids

25.83 The management of an asymptomatic woman with a positive cervical culture for gonorrhea and an intrauterine device (IUD) is
a. removal of the IUD and treatment of the infection by standard protocol
b. treatment of the infection without IUD removal and careful observation

Instructions for items 25.84 to 25.85: Match the antibiotic regimen with the type of intrauterine device-associated pelvic infection it is used to prevent or treat. An option may be used once, more than once, or not at all.

25.84 Insertional infection (occurs within 6–8 weeks of insertion)

25.85 Delayed infection (occurs 3 or more months after insertion)
a. Doxycycline 200 mg po before insertion
b. Ceftriaxone 25 mg IM and doxycycline 100 mg po bid × 7 days

25.86 Women who are breast-feeding and are given an intrauterine device generally have a
a. greater incidence of post-insertional discomfort/bleeding
b. unchanged incidence of post-insertional discomfort/bleeding
c. decreased incidence of post-insertional discomfort/bleeding

25.87 What percent of patients will spontaneously abort if they become pregnant while using an intrauterine device?
a. 20%–30%
b. 40%–50%
c. 60%–70%
d. 80%–90%

25.88 Removal of an intrauterine device in the first trimester of a pregnancy is associated with a spontaneous abortion rate of
a. 10%
b. 30%
c. 50%
d. 70%
e. 90%

25.89 If an intrauterine device is left *in situ* during pregnancy, there is an increased incidence of
a. congenital facial anomalies in the fetus
b. congenital trunk anomalies in the fetus
c. placental implantation problems
d. preterm labor and delivery
e. intrauterine growth restriction

ANSWERS (25.81–25.89)

25.81 a	25.83 b	25.85 b	25.87 b	25.88 b	25.89 d
25.82 c	25.84 a	25.86 c			

25.90 Which of the following is an effective postcoital antifertility method?
a. Yuzpe method
b. Postcoital douche
c. Immediate uterine curettage
d. Carbonic anhydrase
e. Hydroxyzine hydrochloride

25.91 The two types of estrogen compounds present in oral contraceptives are
a. estrone and mestranol
b. ethinyl estradiol and mestranol
c. estradiol and estrone
d. estriol and mestranol

25.92 Which of the following has been implicated as the causative agent of thromboembolism in women using oral contraceptives?
a. Estrogen
b. Progesterone

25.93 Which of the following statements about the progestin-only mini-pill is INCORRECT?
a. It is more effective in younger women
b. It does not alter the quality of breast milk
c. It does not alter the quantity of breast milk
d. It may be started immediately postpartum
e. It must be taken at the same time every day

25.94 Which of the following is NOT a mechanism of action of the progestin-only mini-pill?
a. It makes the endometrium resistant to implantation

b. It has a synergistic effect with lactation-associated prolactin effects
c. It suppresses ovulation
d. It causes a thickening of the cervical mucus

25.95 The failure rate of the Yuzpe method of postcoital contraception is approximately
a. 5%
b. 15%
c. 25%
d. 35%
e. 45%

Instructions for items 25.96 to 25.99: Match the oral contraceptive preparation with its appropriate dosage schedule in the Yuzpe method of postcoital contraception. An option may be used once, more than once, or not at all.

25.96 Lo-Ovral

25.97 Ovral

25.98 Nordette

25.99 Triphasil (yellow pills)
a. 2 tablets followed by 2 tablets in 12 hours, administered within 72 hours of the unprotected coital event
b. 4 tablets followed by 4 tablets in 12 hours, administered within 72 hours of the unprotected coital event

25.100 About what percent of women who successfully use the Yuzpe method of emergency contraception will have a menstrual period within 3 weeks?
a. 100%
b. 75%
c. 50%
d. 25%

Answers (25.90–25.100)					
25.90 a	25.92 a	25.94 c	25.96 b	25.98 b	25.100 a
25.91 b	25.93 a	25.95 c	25.97 a	25.99 b	

Instructions for items 25.101 to 25.117: Indicate whether the condition is a relative or absolute contraindication to the use of biphasic oral contraceptive therapy. An option may be used once, more than once, or not at all.

25.101 Migraine headache

25.102 Thrombophlebitis, thromboembolic disease

25.103 Cervical vascular disease

25.104 Coronary occlusion

25.105 Impaired liver function

25.106 Known or suspected breast cancer

25.107 Undiagnosed abnormal vaginal bleeding

25.108 Known or suspected pregnancy

25.109 Hypertension and under the age of 35

25.110 Diabetes mellitus

25.111 Gallbladder disease

25.112 Obstructive jaundice in previous pregnancy

25.113 Epilepsy

25.114 Severe obesity

25.115 Smoker over the age of 35

25.116 Congenital hyperlipidemia

25.117 Hepatic neoplasm
   a. Relative contraindication
   b. Absolute contraindication

25.118 Which of the following is NOT common in individuals using the Depo-Provera and Norplant systems?
   a. Thickening of the cervical mucus
   b. Decidualization of the endometrium
   c. Inhibition of ovulation

25.119 What percent of women using Depo-Provera will resume normal menses within 6 months?
   a. 25%
   b. 50%
   c. 75%
   d. 100%

25.120 In which of the following cases should biphasic oral contraceptives be discontinued?
   a. Amenorrhea
   b. Galactorrhea
   c. Right upper quadrant pain
   d. Hepatic mass with tenderness

25.121 Injectable medroxyprogesterone and estradiol cyprionate are given how often for the purpose of contraception?
   a. Every month
   b. Every 2 months
   c. Every 6 months
   d. Every year
   e. Every 5 years

25.122 As compared to the Yuzpe method, Plan B emergency contraception has
   a. an increased incidence of nausea
   b. a similar incidence of nausea
   c. a decreased incidence of nausea

25.123 The Yuzpe or Plan B contraceptive regimens are best used for all the following indications EXCEPT
   a. intrauterine device expulsion
   b. unintended unprotected intercourse
   c. interval contraception
   d. sexual assault when no contraceptive method is in use

ANSWERS (25.101–25.123)

25.101 a	25.105 b	25.109 a	25.113 a	25.117 b	25.121 a
25.102 b	25.106 b	25.110 a	25.114 a	25.118 c	25.122 c
25.103 b	25.107 b	25.111 a	25.115 b	25.119 b	25.123 c
25.104 b	25.108 b	25.112 a	25.116 b	25.120 d	

Questions and Answers Chapter 26:
Sterilization

26.1   Among the methods used to control
        fertility in the United States,
        sterilization is the
        a. most frequently used
        b. second most frequently used
        c. third most frequently used
        d. least frequently used

26.2   Roughly what proportion of
        married couples in the United States
        use sterilization for contraception?
        a. 1 in 8
        b. 1 in 5
        c. 1 in 3
        d. 1 in 2

26.3   Despite careful counseling, what
        percent of patients will request
        sterilization reversal?
        a. 1%
        b. 3%
        c. 5%
        d. 8%
        e. 12%

26.4   Successful reversal of sterilization is
        possible in approximately what
        percent of cases?
        a. 5%–10%
        b. 20%–30%
        c. 40%–60%
        d. 70%–80%
        e. 90%–95%

26.5   Vasectomy accounts for
        approximately what percent of all
        sterilization procedures?
        a. 10%–15%
        b. 20%–25%
        c. 30%–35%
        d. 40%–45%
        e. 50%–55%

26.6   Antibodies against sperm are found
        in what proportion of men who
        have undergone vasectomy?
        a. 10%–15%
        b. 20%–25%
        c. 30%–35%
        d. 40%–45%
        e. 50%–55%

26.7   When compared with female
        sterilization, which of the following
        is NOT an advantage of
        vasectomy?
        a. Lower incidence of postoperative
           depression
        b. Greater reversibility
        c. Lower cost
        d. Lower operative complication
           rate
        e. The possibility of routine
           postoperative verification

26.8   Which of the following is the
        LEAST likely complication
        associated with vasectomy?
        a. Hematoma formation
        b. Wound infection
        c. Femoral nerve damage
        d. Continued bleeding at the
           operative site

26.9   The most common reason for
        pregnancy following a vasectomy is
        a. recanalization
        b. sexual activity too soon after
           surgery
        c. ligation of the tunica albicans
        d. operative hematoma formation

26.10 Sterilization after vasectomy usually
        is complete by
        a. 24–36 hours
        b. 3–5 days
        c. 2–3 weeks
        d. 4–6 weeks
        e. 8–10 weeks

ANSWERS (26.1–26.10)					
26.1 d	26.3 a	26.5 c	26.7 a	26.9 b	26.10 d
26.2 c	26.4 c	26.6 e	26.8 c		

26.11 Which of the following anesthetic methods is NOT used for laparoscopic sterilization procedures?
  a. Local
  b. General
  c. Epidural
  d. Spinal
  e. Saddle

26.12 Which of the following female sterilization methods is most likely to result in future ectopic pregnancy?
  a. Hulka clip
  b. Falope ring
  c. Electrocautery
  d. Pomeroy tubal ligation
  e. Kroener fimbriectomy

26.13 Which of the following female sterilization methods is most likely to be successfully reversed?
  a. Hulka clip
  b. Falope ring
  c. Electrocautery
  d. Pomeroy tubal ligation
  e. Kroener fimbriectomy

26.14 Which of the following female sterilization methods is most likely to result in operative complications?
  a. Hulka clip
  b. Falope ring
  c. Electrocautery
  d. Pomeroy tubal ligation
  e. Kroener fimbriectomy

26.15 Which of the following female sterilization methods is most likely to result in postoperative pain requiring strong analgesics?
  a. Hulka clip
  b. Falope ring
  c. Electrocautery
  d. Pomeroy tubal ligation
  e. Kroener fimbriectomy

Instructions for items 26.16 to 26.21: Match the tubal ligation technique with the appropriate description of the procedure. An option may be used once, more than once, or not at all.

26.16 Madlener

26.17 Pomeroy

26.18 Irving

26.19 Cook

26.20 Kroener

26.21 Aldridge
  a. Fimbriated end of tube excised
  b. Fimbriated end of tube buried in broad ligament
  c. Tube divided, proximal stump buried in uterine wall, distal stump buried in leaves of broad ligament
  d. Tube divided, proximal stump buried in round ligament, distal stump buried in leaves of broad ligament
  e. Tube elevated, base crushed in clamp, crushed area ligated with nonabsorbable suture
  f. Loop of tube from middle third of tube elevated, ligated with plain gut and excised

26.22 Compared with electrocautery, the Hulka clip has a
  a. higher failure rate
  b. similar failure rate
  c. lower failure rate

26.23 Which of the following is NOT required as part of vaginal tubal sterilization procedures?
  a. Specialized equipment
  b. Prophylactic antibiotics
  c. Restrictions on intercourse
  d. Restrictions on douching

ANSWERS (26.11–26.23)

26.11 e	26.14 c	26.16 e	26.18 c	26.20 a	26.22 a
26.12 c	26.15 b	26.17 f	26.19 d	26.21 b	26.23 a
26.13 a					

26.24 The term "interval sterilization" refers to procedures that
   a. remove a segment of the fallopian tube
   b. destroy a portion of the fallopian tube
   c. are performed after the immediate postpartum period
   d. are performed during the immediate postpartum period

26.25 Compared with tubal ligation, vasectomy is
   a. more easily reversed
   b. as easily reversed
   c. less easily reversed

26.26 A women who becomes pregnant three months after tubal ligation most likely has
   a. an ectopic pregnancy
   b. an intrauterine pregnancy
   c. a combined pregnancy

26.27 A patient who has undergone reversal of a tubal ligation and then exhibits signs of pregnancy should initially be presumed to have
   a. a normal intrauterine pregnancy
   b. an abnormal intrauterine pregnancy
   c. an ectopic pregnancy
   d. a false pregnancy

26.28 Which of the following statements about surgical sterilization is INCORRECT?
   a. There is an approximately 1% chance of pregnancy after female tubal sterilization
   b. The rate of permanent surgical sterilization has steadily risen in recent years
   c. Approximately equal numbers of men and women request surgical sterilization

26.29 Postoperative complications of vasectomy such as bleeding, hematoma formation, and local skin infection occur in about what percent of cases?
   a. < 1%
   b. 3%–5%
   c. 7%–9%
   d. 12%–15%

26.30 Post-tubal ligation syndrome is considered to include
   a. menstrual dysfunction
   b. dysmenorrhea
   c. disruption of blood flow in the area of the fallopian tubes
   d. all of the above

26.31 What is the failure rate in the Pomeroy method of tubal ligation?
   a. 1 in 100
   b. 1 in 200
   c. 1 in 300
   d. 1 in 400
   e. 1 in 500

26.32 The fatality rate in women from sterilization is what percent of the rate from childbearing?
   a. 1%
   b. 2%
   c. 5%
   d. 10%

26.33 Compared to countries with a low vasectomy rate, the incidence of prostate cancer in countries where there is a high rate of vasectomy is
   a. higher
   b. the same
   c. lower

ANSWERS (26.24–26.33)

| 26.24 c | 26.26 b | 26.28 c | 26.30 d | 26.32 d | 26.33 b |
| 26.25 a | 26.27 c | 26.29 b | 26.31 e | | |

Questions and Answers Chapter 27: Vulvitis and Vaginitis

27.1 Complaints of vulvar irritation account for approximately what percent of gynecologic office visits?
a. 3%
b. 5%
c. 10%
d. 15%
e. 25%

27.2 Which of the following characterizes a physiologic discharge?
a. Few white blood cells with multiple, flat, polygonal small nuclei on microscopic examination
b. Positive whiff test
c. Vaginal pH of 5.5
d. Motile protozoa on microscopic examination

27.3 Which of the following is characteristic of bacterial vaginosis?
a. Vaginal pH less than 4.5
b. Curdy consistency
c. Greenish tinge
d. Fishy odor

27.4 Vaginal candidiasis is characterized by
a. White cells
b. Foul odor
c. Thin, homogeneous consistency
d. Intense itching

27.5 Which of the following characterizes vaginal trichomoniasis?
a. Cervical ectropion
b. Vaginal dryness
c. Motile protozoa on microscopic examination
d. White discharge

27.6 What types of cells are characteristic of atrophic vaginitis?
a. Columnar cells
b. Parabasal cells
c. Ciliated cells
d. White cells

27.7 Vulvar ulceration characterizes which of the following?
a. condyloma acuminatum
b. psoriasis
c. scabies
d. herpes simplex

27.8 Most of the liquid portion of physiologic vaginal secretions in a woman of reproductive age comes from
a. the cervix
b. vaginal transudate
c. the Bartholin's glands
d. the Skene's glands

27.9 The creamy white portion of physiologic vaginal secretions in a woman of reproductive age comes from
a. cervical mucus
b. vaginal epithelium
c. the Bartholin's glands
d. vaginal white blood cells

27.10 The average amount of vaginal secretion produced in 24 hours by a woman of reproductive age is approximately
a. 0.1 g
b. 0.5 g
c. 1.5 g
d. 3.0 g
e. 5.0 g

ANSWERS (27.1–27.10)

27.1 c	27.3 d	27.5 c	27.7 d	27.9 b	27.10 c
27.2 a	27.4 d	27.6 b	27.8 a		

27.11 The normal pH of vaginal secretions of reproductive aged women is
a. 3.5-4.5
b. 5.0-6.0
c. 6.5-7.5
d. 8.0-9.0

27.12 The normal pH of the vagina after the menopause but without estrogen replacement therapy is
a. 2.0-3.0
b. 3.5-5.5
c. 6.0-8.0
d. 9.0-11.0

27.13 The most common symptom associated with a vaginal infection is
a. fever
b. pain
c. pruritus
d. discharge

27.14 The most common cause of persistently increased vaginal secretions is
a. sexual arousal
b. microbiologic infection
c. contact vulvitis
d. hormonal variation

27.15 The most common cause of increased vaginal discharge is
a. candidiasis
b. trichomoniasis
c. bacterial vaginosis
d. human papillomavirus

27.16 A 25 year old patient complains of vaginal discharge. The diagnosis is established by
a. odor
b. microscopic examination
c. symptoms
d. color of the discharge

27.17 A 30 year old patient with bacterial vaginosis complains of a foul odor after intercourse. She should be told that it is caused by
a. the alkaline pH of semen
b. colonization of the vagina by penile microorganisms
c. bacterial digestion of seminal proteins
d. liberation of prostaglandins from sperm

27.18 Which of the following best describes a "whiff test?"
a. mixing of vaginal secretions with 10% potassium hydroxide to liberate amines
b. testing for odor of undiluted secretions from the vaginal apex
c. mixing of vaginal secretions with normal saline to determine color
d. passing of the speculum under the nose to detect odor

27.19 Which of the following best describes a "clue cell?"
a. clumped white blood cells
b. immature vaginal epithelial cells
c. keratinized vaginal epithelial cells with adherent white blood cells
d. vaginal epithelial cells with adherent bacteria

27.20 *Trichomonas vaginalis* is a flagellate protozoan that can live in the
a. vagina
b. oropharynx
c. anus
d. bladder

ANSWERS (27.11–27.20)

27.11 a	27.13 d	27.15 c	27.17 a	27.19 d	27.20 a
27.12 c	27.14 b	27.16 b	27.18 a		

27.21 Approximately what percent of sexual partners of women with *Trichomonas* infections also have the infections?
   a. < 10%
   b. 20%-30%
   c. 40%-50%
   d. > 60%

27.22 Approximately what percent of women with a *Trichomonas* infection of the vagina are symptomatic?
   a. 10%
   b. 25%
   c. 50%
   d. 75%
   e. 90%

27.23 Which of the following characterizes the microscopic appearance of *Trichomonas*?
   a. multiple pseudopods
   b. circular shape
   c. slightly larger than a white blood cell
   d. fine stippling

27.24 Characteristic petechia, or strawberry patches, are found in the upper vagina or on the cervix of patients with *Trichomonas vaginalis* in approximately what percent of cases?
   a. 10%
   b. 30%
   c. 50%
   d. 70%
   e. 90%

27.25 A standard treatment for *Trichomonas* vaginal infection is
   a. metronidazole 2 g orally in one dose
   b. metronidazole 250 mg orally every day for 14 days
   c. clindamycin 1 g orally in one dose
   d. ampicillin 500 mg orally four times a day for 10 days

27.26 The standard treatment for *Trichomonas vaginalis* will generally give a cure rate of
   a. 100%
   b. 90%
   c. 80%
   d. 70%
   e. 60%

27.27 What percent of patients with *Trichomonas vaginalis* will also have bacterial vaginosis?
   a. 0%
   b. 25%
   c. 50%
   d. 75%
   e. 100%

27.28 When prescribing metronidazole for the treatment of *Trichomonas* infections, it is important to advise the patient to avoid alcohol intake because alcohol
   a. diminishes gastric uptake of metronidazole
   b. induces metronidazole resistance in *Trichomonas*
   c. decreases tissue levels of metronidazole
   d. may cause severe nausea and vomiting

Answers (27.21–27.28)

| 27.21 d | 27.23 c | 27.25 a | 27.26 b | 27.27 b | 27.28 d |
| 27.22 c | 27.24 a | | | | |

27.29 The most common source of monilial infections of the vagina is from
   a. sexual contact with an infected partner
   b. airborne colonization
   c. contaminated clothing
   d. bath water retained in the vagina following bathing

27.30 Roughly 90% of vaginal "yeast" infections are caused by
   a. *Candida albicans*
   b. *Candida tropicalis*
   c. *Candida glabrata*
   d. *Torulopsis glabrata*

27.31 Which of the following is thought to increase the risk of vaginal "yeast" infection?
   a. nulliparity
   b. vitamin ingestion
   c. urinary tract infection
   d. use of spermicidal foam
   e. immunosuppression

27.32 Approximately what percent of women with vaginal "yeast" infections are symptomatic?
   a. 10%
   b. 25%
   c. 40%
   d. 60%
   e. 80%

27.33 The normal pH of vaginal secretions found in women with vaginal "yeast" infections is
   a. 4.0-4.5
   b. 5.5-6.0
   c. 6.5-7.0
   d. 8.0-9.0

27.34 The most common presenting complaint in women with vaginal "yeast" infections is
   a. thick discharge
   b. vulvar burning
   c. dysuria
   d. intense itching

27.35 A 10% potassium hydroxide (KOH) solution is used for a wet prep when "yeast" infection is suspected because this solution
   a. renders *Candida albicans* noninfective
   b. causes lysis of white blood cells
   c. liberates amines from solution
   d. immobilizes *Trichomonas* organisms

27.36 Despite compliant therapy with an appropriate medication, the recurrence rate for vaginal yeast infections is
   a. 5%
   b. 10%
   c. 25%
   d. 40%
   e. 60%

27.37 The primary treatment of candidal vaginitis is
   a. topical synthetic imidazoles
   b. systemic corticosteroids
   c. topical cephalosporins
   d. systemic penicillin

27.38 An appropriate treatment of *Pthirus pubis* (crab louse) is
   a. ampicillin
   b. gentamicin
   c. sulfamethoxazole
   d. clindamycin
   e. gamma-Benzene hexachloride

27.39 The presence of "clue" cells is usually diagnostic of
   a. tinea cruris
   b. bacterial vaginosis
   c. diabetic vulvitis
   d. scabies

ANSWERS (27.29–27.39)

27.29 b	27.31 e	27.33 a	27.35 b	27.37 a	27.39 b
27.30 a	27.32 e	27.34 d	27.36 c	27.38 e	

27.40 Which of the following accurately describes the vagina?
 a. Apocrine glands
 b. Sweat glands
 c. Hair follicles
 d. Sebaceous glands
 e. Nonkeratinized squamous epithelium

27.41 Which of the following is characteristic of the vagina?
 a. vulnerability to contact with external irritants
 b. mucus-secreting epithelium
 c. keratinized epithelium
 d. sweat glands

27.42 Vulvitis in children is associated with
 a. constipation
 b. urinary retention
 c. puberty
 d. sexual abuse

27.43 In a patient with recurrent yeast infections, what concurrent disease should be suspected?
 a. Systemic lupus erythematosus (SLE)
 b. Diabetes mellitus
 c. Syphilis
 d. Cushing's syndrome

27.44 Which of the following accurately describes contact dermatitis?
 a. Pale
 b. Ulcerated
 c. Hemorrhagic
 d. Edematous

27.45 Which of the following conditions affects up to 3% of women and seems to have a familial pattern?
 a. Contact dermatitis
 b. Psoriasis
 c. Seborrheic dermatitis
 d. Hidradenitis suppurativa

27.46 Which of the following conditions often presents with deep painful scars, foul discharge, and may require wide surgical excision?
 a. Hidradenitis suppurativa
 b. Seborrheic dermatitis
 c. Contact dermatitis
 d. Psoriasis
 e. Yeast vulvitis

27.47 Which bacteria in the lower genital tract of normal women break down glycogen to lactic acid?
 a. *Gardnerella*
 b. *Streptococcus*
 c. *Trichomonas*
 d. *Lactobacillus*

27.48 A wet prep showing clumps of epithelial cells with adherent bacteria is associated with
 a. *Trichomonas vaginalis*
 b. Candidal vaginitis
 c. Bacterial vaginosis
 d. Cervical dysplasia

27.49 When does cytolytic vaginitis worsen?
 a. Follicular phase
 b. Puberty
 c. Menopause
 d. Luteal phase

27.50 Which of the following is suggestive of desquamative inflammatory vaginitis?
 a. Clear discharge
 b. Vesicles
 c. Overgrowth of gram negative bacilli
 d. Purulent discharge

Answers (27.40–27.50)

27.40 e	27.42 d	27.44 d	27.46 a	27.48 c	27.50 d
27.41 a	27.43 b	27.45 b	27.47 d	27.49 d	

Questions and Answers, Chapter 28:
Sexually Transmitted Diseases

28.1 Approximately what percent of patients with a sexually transmitted disease (STD) have more than one STD?
a. Less than 3%
b. 5%–10%
c. 20%–50%
d. 60%–80%
e. 95%–100%

28.2 In approximately what percent of cases will a single sexual contact with a patient with an active herpes infection result in transmission of the infection?
a. Less than 3%
b. 5%–10%
c. 20%–50%
d. 60%–80%
e. 95%–100%

28.3 The normal progression of symptoms in primary herpes infections is a prodromal phase followed by
a. ulcer, vesicle, crusting, resolution
b. ulcer, crusting, vesicle, resolution
c. crusting, vesicle, ulcer, resolution
d. vesicle, ulcer, crusting, resolution
e. vesicle, crusting, ulcer, resolution

28.4 What percent of genital herpes lesions are caused by the herpes simplex virus type II?
a. 95%
b. 85%
c. 75%
d. 65%
e. 55%

28.5 Approximately what percent of patients with an initial herpes genitalis infection will require hospitalization for pain control or management of urinary complications?
a. 10%
b. 20%
c. 30%
d. 40%
e. 50%

28.6 Primary herpes genitalis infections are characterized by malaise, low grade fever, and inguinal adenopathy in approximately what percent of patients?
a. 20%
b. 40%
c. 60%
d. 80%

28.7 Recurrent herpes genitalis lesions occur in approximately what percent of patients?
a. 10%
b. 30%
c. 50%
d. 70%

28.8 Compared with primary genital lesions, recurrent herpes lesions are
a. longer in duration
b. more severe
c. milder
d. more systemic

ANSWERS (28.1–28.8)

| 28.1 | c | 28.3 | d | 28.5 | a | 28.6 | b | 28.7 | b | 28.8 | c |
| 28.2 | d | 28.4 | b | | | | | | | | |

28.9 A pregnant patient at term presents in active labor. Membranes are intact. She has active herpetic lesions in the vagina. If vaginal delivery occurs, what is the likelihood that the newborn will be infected?
   a. 25%
   b. 50%
   c. 75%
   d. 100%

28.10 Neonatal herpes infection acquired at the time of delivery is associated with a mortality rate of approximately
   a. 100%
   b. 80%
   c. 60%
   d. 40%
   e. 20%

28.11 An 18-year-old patient presents with a 5-day history of very painful vulvar ulcers that began as small "blisters." She is now complaining of a low grade fever, headache, and meningismus. Large, painful vulvar and perineal ulcers and inguinal adenopathy are found on examination. The most likely diagnosis is
   a. disseminated gonococcal infection
   b. primary herpes vulvitis
   c. secondary syphilis
   d. lymphogranuloma venereum
   e. molluscum contagiosum

28.12 A 23-year-old G3 P2001 patient presents at term in early labor with an active herpes infection of the labia that has been present for the past 3 days. Membranes are intact. Contractions are regular at 3-minute intervals and have been present for the last 3 hours. Her last term labor was 3 years ago and lasted 12 hours, ending in a vaginal delivery of a normal 7-pound infant. Which of the following is the best management of this patient?
   a. Anticipate normal labor and delivery
   b. Anticipate normal labor and delivery, plan acyclovir prophylaxis for the infant
   c. Anticipate rapid labor and delivery but avoid episiotomy
   d. Tocolysis and intravenous acyclovir (200 mg)
   e. Immediate cesarean delivery

28.13 All of the following are caused by infection by *Chlamydia* species EXCEPT
   a. cervicitis
   b. pelvic inflammatory disease
   c. lymphogranuloma venereum
   d. granuloma inguinale

28.14 *Chlamydia* infections are frequently associated with co-infections by
   a. herpes simplex
   b. *Neisseria gonorrhoeae*
   c. human papillomavirus
   d. *Treponema pallidum*

28.15 Antibodies to *Chlamydia* are found in approximately what percent of sexually active women?
   a. 1%–5%
   b. 10%–15%
   c. 20%–40%
   d. 60%–80%
   e. Greater than 90%

Answers (28.9–28.15)

| 28.9 | b | 28.11 | b | 28.12 | e | 28.13 | d | 28.14 | b | 28.15 | c |
| 28.10 | b | | | | | | | | | | |

28.16   How long does it take to confirm the diagnosis of *Chlamydia* using the culture technique?
    a. 12–24 hours
    b. 24–48 hours
    c. 48–72 hours
    d. 96 hours

28.17   The outpatient treatment with doxycycline or erythromycin for suspected or confirmed *Chlamydia* infection is associated with a cure rate of
    a. 95%
    b. 80%
    c. 65%
    d. 50%

28.18   A common sequela of infection by *Chlamydia trachomatis* is
    a. recurrent vulvar growths
    b. cyclic, migratory arthralgia
    c. involuntary infertility
    d. vaginismus

28.19   *Neisseria gonorrhoeae* is a
    a. gram-negative intracellular diplococcus
    b. gram-negative extracellular diplococcus
    c. gram-positive intracellular diplococcus
    d. gram-positive extracellular diplococcus

28.20   Infection of the pharynx is found in what percent of heterosexual women with confirmed *Neisseria gonorrhoeae* infections?
    a. 1%–10%
    b. 10%–20%
    c. 20%–30%
    d. 30%–40%
    e. 40%–50%

28.21   For women, a single encounter with a partner infected with *Neisseria gonorrhoeae* is estimated to lead to infection in what percent of cases?
    a. 20%–30%
    b. 40%–50%
    c. 60%–70%
    d. 80%–90%
    e. 100%

28.22   Following initial infection by *Neiseria gonorrhoeae*, symptoms first appear in
    a. 1–2 days
    b. 3–5 days
    c. 1–2 weeks
    d. 3–5 weeks

28.23   A 22-year-old G0P0 patient has just been successfully treated for *Neisseria gonorrhoeae* salpingitis and asks about her chances of infertility. Based on this single infection, her chances of involuntary infertility are approximately
    a. less than 1%
    b. 3%–5%
    c. 8%–10%
    d. 15%–20%

28.24   A 22-year-old G0P0 patient has just been successfully treated for her third episode of *Neisseria gonorrhoeae* salpingitis and asks about her chances of infertility. Based on these infections, her chances of involuntary infertility are approximately
    a. less than 10%
    b. 20%–25%
    c. 40%–50%
    d. 70%–80%

ANSWERS (28.16–28.24)

| 28.16 | c | 28.18 | c | 28.20 | b | 28.22 | b | 28.23 | d | 28.24 | d |
| 28.17 | a | 28.19 | a | 28.21 | d | | | | | | |

28.25 Lower genital tract infections by *Neisseria gonorrhoeae* are usually characterized by
a. malodorous, purulent vaginal or urethral discharge
b. firm, painless vulvar ulcer
c. inguinal adenopathy
d. fever, malaise, and labial swelling bilaterally

28.26 The most frequent site of infection with gonorrhea in women is the
a. Bartholin's glands
b. Skene's glands
c. cervix
d. urethra
e. rectal crypts

28.27 Which of the following criteria is necessary in order to make a diagnosis of acute salpingitis?
a. fever greater than 38 degrees C
b. adnexal tenderness
c. mass on ultrasound
d. pus obtained via culdocentesis

28.28 All of the following are criteria for the hospitalization of patients with pelvic inflammatory disease EXCEPT
a. coexisting pregnancy
b. significant gastrointestinal symptoms
c. patient less than 20 years of age
d. white blood count greater than 20,000
e. nulliparity

28.29 The initiation of treatment for presumed pelvic inflammatory disease is based on
a. clinical suspicion
b. cervical gram stain
c. anaerobic culture
d. white blood cell count less than 8000
e. rebound tenderness

28.30 The development of cervical cancer is associated with
a. *Chlamydia trachomatis* infections
b. herpes simplex type II infections
c. human papillomavirus (HPV) infections
d. herpes zoster infections

28.31 In approximately what percent of cases will a single sexual contact with an individual with a human papillomavirus (HPV) infection result in transmission of the infection?
a. Less than 3%
b. 5%–10%
c. 30%–40%
d. 60%–70%
e. 95%–100%

28.32 Lesions caused by human papillomavirus (HPV) may be confused with those of
a. early herpes simplex type II infections
b. late lymphogranuloma venereum
c. granuloma inguinale
d. secondary syphilis

28.33 Human papillomavirus (HPV) infection is associated with
a. condyloma lata
b. cyst formation
c. deep ulcers
d. kissing lesions
e. tender vesicles

28.34 The human papillomavirus (HPV) is found in approximately what percent of women?
a. 2.5%–4%
b. 6.5%–7%
c. 8.5%–10%
d. 12%–15%

ANSWERS (28.25–28.34)

28.25 a	28.27 b	28.29 a	28.31 d	28.33 d	28.34 a
28.26 c	28.28 c	28.30 c	28.32 d		

28.35 All of the following modalities are used to treat simple condylomata acuminata EXCEPT
a. podophyllin in tincture of benzoin
b. trichloracetic acid
c. 5-fluorouracil
d. acyclovir

28.36 All of the following patient descriptions make a patient more resistant to therapy for condylomata acuminata EXCEPT
a. pregnant
b. immunosuppressed
c. smoker
d. overweight

28.37 Vaginal delivery of a patient with extensive condylomata acuminata of the vulva may result in
a. infant herpes encephalopathy
b. maternal hemorrhage
c. maternal febrile morbidity
d. infant laryngeal papillomas

28.38 Transplacental spread of *Treponema pallidum* can occur
a. only during the first trimester of pregnancy
b. only during the third trimester of pregnancy
c. at any time during pregnancy
d. only after rupture of membranes

28.39 The chancre of primary syphilis will
a. spontaneously heal in 3–9 weeks
b. coalesce to form running sores
c. transform into raised fleshy growths that persist indefinitely
d. result in regional adenopathy and abscess formation within 2 weeks

28.40 Which of the following is characteristic of primary syphilis?
a. Chancre appears 3–5 days after infection
b. Chancre is often asymptomatic
c. Serologic testing usually is positive
d. Accompanying low grade fever and anorexia are common

28.41 The most contagious stage of syphilis is
a. primary
b. secondary
c. tertiary
d. latent

28.42 The mucous patches of secondary syphilis will
a. spontaneously heal in 2–6 weeks
b. progress to coalesced running sores
c. progress to raised fleshy growths that persist indefinitely
d. progress with regional adenopathy and abscess formation

28.43 Which of the following is a non-treponemal test?
a. Rapid plasma reagin (RPR)
b. Venereal Disease Research Laboratory (VDRL)
c. Automated reagin test (ART)
d. All of the above

ANSWERS (28.35–28.43)

28.35	d	28.37	d	28.39	a	28.41	b	28.42	a	28.43	d
28.36	d	28.38	c	28.40	b						

Instructions for items 28.44 to 28.47:
Match the test for syphilis with its approximate sensitivity in detecting primary syphilis. An option may be used once, more than once, or not at all.

28.44 Venereal Disease Research Laboratory (VDRL)

28.45 Rapid plasma reagin (RPR)

28.46 Fluorescent treponemal antibody absorption (FTA-ABS)

28.47 Microhemagglutination assay-*Treponema pallidum* (MHA-TP)
a. 45%
b. 55%
c. 65%
d. 75%
e. 85%

28.48 Which of the following serologic tests for syphilis has a sensitivity of approximately 100% for secondary syphilis?
a. Venereal Disease Research Laboratory (VDRL)
b. Rapid plasma reagin (RPR)
c. Fluorescent treponemal antibody absorption (FTA-ABS)
d. Microhemagglutination assay-*Treponema pallidum* (MHA-TP)
e. All of the above

28.49 A false-positive Venereal Disease Research Laboratory (VDRL) or rapid plasma reagin (RPR) test may be associated with all of the following EXCEPT
a. gonorrhea
b. malaria
c. systemic lupus erythematosus
d. connective tissue disease

28.50 Which of the following is characteristic of secondary syphilis?
a. Asymptomatic chancre that is often missed
b. Non-infectious mucous patches
c. Low grade fever, headache, malaise, sore throat, anorexia, and generalized lymphadenopathy
d. Serologic testing for syphilis generally negative

28.51 Without intervention, the risk of transmission of the human immunodeficiency virus (HIV) to a fetus is approximately
a. 25%
b. 50%
c. 75%
d. 100%

28.52 The diagnosis of human immunodeficiency virus (HIV) infection is established on the basis of
a. serum immunoassay
b. Western blot testing
c. CD_4 white blood cell counts
d. presence of clinical symptoms

28.53 Painless ulcerated vulvar lesions are characteristic of infections with
a. herpes simplex, type II
b. *Chlamydia trachomatis*
c. *Treponema pallidum*
d. *Haemophilus ducreyi*

28.54 Which of the following conditions has an incubation period (from infection to clinical symptoms) of greater than 1 month?
a. Genital herpes
b. Condyloma acuminata
c. Chancroid
d. Lymphogranuloma venereum

ANSWERS (28.44–28.54)										
28.44	d	28.46	e	28.48	e	28.50	c	28.52	b	28.54	b
28.45	e	28.47	d	28.49	a	28.51	b	28.53	c		

28.55   Multiple vulvar vesicles are typical of which of the following infections?
a. Genital herpes
b. Condyloma acuminata
c. Chancroid
d. Lymphogranuloma venereum

Instructions for items 28.56 to 28.58: Match the sexually transmitted disease (STD) with its incubation period. An option may be used once, more than once, or not at all.

28.56   Herpes

28.57   Genital warts

28.58   Syphilis
a. 3–7 days
b. 1–8 months
c. 10–60 days
d. 1–4 weeks
e. 8–12 weeks

Instructions for items 28.59 to 28.63: Match the sexually transmitted disease (STD) with the causative organism. An option may be used once, more than once, or not at all.

28.59   Genital wart

28.60   Syphilis

28.61   Chancroid

28.62   Lymphogranuloma venereum

28.63   Granuloma inguinale
a. Human papillomavirus (HPV)
b. *Haemophilus ducreyi*
c. *Calymmatobacterium granulomatis*
d. *Chlamydia trachomatis*
e. *Treponema pallidum*

28.64   All of the following sexually transmitted diseases (STDs) are generally associated with lymphadenopathy EXCEPT
a. herpes
b. genital warts
c. syphilis
d. chancroid
e. lymphogranuloma venereum

8.65   Which of the following sexually transmitted diseases (STDs) is associated with a purulent, hemorrhagic secretion?
a. Granuloma inguinale
b. Lymphogranuloma venereum
c. Chancroid
d. Syphilis
e. Genital warts

28.66   Which of the following sexually transmitted diseases (STDs) is characteristically associated with multiple vesicular lesions that often coalesce?
a. Herpes
b. Genital warts
c. Syphilis
d. Chancroid
e. Lymphogranuloma venereum

28.67   True statements concerning acute cervicitis include all of the following EXCEPT
a. there is polymorphonuclear infiltration of the mucosa
b. the presenting symptom is often leukorrhea
c. it may be caused by acute *Neisseria gonorrhoeae* infection
d. treatment in the acute phase is surgical
e. patients may have associated acute salpingitis

ANSWERS (28.55–28.67)					
28.55 a	28.58 c	28.60 e	28.62 d	28.64 b	28.66 a
28.56 a	28.59 a	28.61 b	28.63 c	28.65 c	28.67 d
28.57 b					

28.68 What percent of normal women with *Neisseria gonorrhoeae* cervicitis will develop acute pelvic inflammatory disease?
a. 5%
b. 15%
c. 25%
d. 35%
e. 45%

28.69 A Word catheter being used to drain a Batholin gland abscess should be left in place for a minimum of :
a. 24 hours
b. 48 hours
c. 3 days
d. 1 week

28.70 Condyloma acuminata that exceed 2 cm in size are best treated with
a. Podofilox
b. Trichloroacetic acid
c. Laser therapy
d. Interferon injections

28.71 What proportion of patients is infected with HIV?
a. 1 in 3
b. 1 in 30
c. 1 in 300
d. 1 in 3000
e. 1 in 30,000

28.72 A false positive screening test for AIDS is more likely in what women?
a. Caucasian
b. Age over 30
c. Taking oral contraceptives
d. History of syphilis

28.73 Measures to prevent HIV include use of latex condoms containing
a. Nonoxynol 9
b. Doxycycline
c. Azithromycin
d. HAART

28.74 When neurosyphilis is clinically suspected, a VDRL should be obtained on what fluid?
a. Peritoneal fluid
b. Cerebrospinal fluid
c. Serum
d. Urine
e. Gastric secretions

28.75 What is the additional risk for ectopic pregnancy in patients with a history of salpingitis?
a. 2 fold
b. 4 fold
c. 8 fold
d. 20 fold

ANSWERS (28.68–28.75)

28.68	b	28.70	c	28.72	c	28.73	a	28.74	b	28.75	c
28.69	d	28.71	c								

Questions and Answers Chapter 29:
Pelvic Relaxation, Urinary Incontinence, and UTI

29.1 Which of the following is NOT a characteristic symptom of pelvic relaxation?
a. Pelvic pressure
b. Dyspareunia
c. Stress incontinence (urinary)
d. Intermittent diarrhea

29.2 What percent of women will have loss of urine during coughing, laughing, or other stress at some time in their lives?
a. 5%
b. 20%
c. 50%
d. 70%
e. 90%

29.3 Approximately what percent of women suffer significant, recurrent urinary incontinence in the presence of increased intra-abdominal pressure?
a. < 5%
b. 10%–15%
c. 20%–25%
d. 30%–35%
e. 40%–45%

29.4 Which of the following structures does NOT provide direct support to the pelvic organs?
a. Pelvic floor muscles
b. Fascia
c. Bony pelvis
d. Ligaments

29.5 In a patient with enterocele, there is a descent or herniation of the
a. uterus
b. apex of the vagina
c. bladder
d. urethra
e. rectum

Instructions for items 29.6 to 29.9: Match the clinical situation with the appropriate definition. An option may be used once, more than once, or not at all.

29.6 A 45-year-old patient complains of frequent loss of urine when she coughs, laughs, or strains. The volume lost is small, but it occurs frequently. She does not report any dysuria.

29.7 A 45-year-old diabetic patient complains of frequent loss of urine. The volume lost is small, but it occurs almost continuously. She does not report any sense of fullness, urgency, or dysuria. She voids frequently but in small amounts. She does not ever feel "full" but also never has the sense that she has completely emptied her bladder.

29.8 A 22-year-old patient complains of occasional loss of urine. The volume lost is large when it occurs. She reports a sense of intense fullness and urgency just before the urine is lost. She voids infrequently but in large amounts. She does not ever feel that she "gets enough warning" to get to the bathroom.

ANSWERS (29.1–29.8)

| 29.1 | d | 29.3 | b | 29.5 | b | 29.6 | a | 29.7 | c | 29.8 | b |
| 29.2 | c | 29.4 | c | | | | | | | | | |

29.9 A 22-year-old patient complains of occasional loss of urine. The volume lost is large when it occurs. She reports that the loss occurs primarily when she changes position (e.g., rising from a chair) or when she is around running water.
   a. Stress incontinence
   b. Urgency incontinence
   c. Overflow incontinence
   d. Behavioral incontinence
   e. Enuresis

29.10 A symptomatic rectocele is often characterized by
   a. loss of urine during stress
   b. urinary retention
   c. intermittent diarrhea
   d. difficulty passing stools

29.11 A cystocele may best be demonstrated clinically by
   a. a Valsalva maneuver with the patient supine
   b. use of a Sims speculum to retract the anterior vaginal wall
   c. gentle traction on the cervix
   d. observing posterior rotation of the anterior vaginal wall in response to change in position

29.12 What condition is most likely in a patient who needs to press on the back of her vagina with her fingers to facilitate having a bowel movement?
   a. Rectocele
   b. Cystocele
   c. Urethral prolapse (urethrocele)
   d. Enterocele

29.13 A patient who loses urine when she coughs or sneezes most likely has a(n)
   a. rectocele
   b. cystocele
   c. urethral prolapse (urethrocele)
   d. enterocele

29.14 Small bowel herniation is found in
   a. rectocele
   b. cystocele
   c. urethral prolapse (urethrocele)
   d. enterocele

29.15 Which of the following is lined with peritoneum, making it a true hernia?
   a. Rectocele
   b. Cystocele
   c. Urethral prolapse (urethrocele)
   d. Enterocele

29.16 Which of the following is NOT a manifestation of pelvic relaxation?
   a. Uterine prolapse
   b. Procidentia
   c. Vaginal vault prolapse
   d. Uterine retroversion

29.17 A cough causes genuine stress incontinence when the bladder pressure is
   a. less than the urethral pressure
   b. the same as the urethral pressure
   c. greater than the urethral pressure

29.18 Which of the following conditions is associated with urinary incontinence?
   a. Bladder atony
   b. Bladder spasm
   c. Psychosis
   d. Fistulous tract
   e. All of the above

ANSWERS (29.9–29.18)

29.9 b	29.11 a	29.13 c	29.15 d	29.17 c	29.18 e
29.10 d	29.12 a	29.14 d	29.16 d		

Instructions for items 29.19 to 29.21:
Match the clinical situation with the type of prolapse. An option may be used once, more than once, or not at all.

29.19 The structure (e.g., the cervix) is noted to descend to the upper third of the vagina

29.20 The structure is noted to descend to the vaginal introitus

29.21 The structure is noted to descend to outside the vaginal opening
  a. First degree prolapse
  b. Second degree prolapse
  c. Third degree prolapse
  d. Procidentia

29.22 A "Q-tip test" is used to evaluate the
  a. presence of residual urine
  b. support for the posterior vaginal wall
  c. degree of cervical descent down the vaginal canal
  d. amount of urethral mobility
  e. degree of urethral sensitivity

29.23 When performing a "Q-tip test," incontinence is generally associated with upward rotation of
  a. less than 5 degrees
  b. 10 degrees
  c. 20 degrees
  d. 30 degrees

29.24 The key anatomic abnormality in stress incontinence is
  a. a urethrovesical angle of less than 90 degrees

  b. the urethra prolapsing at times of increased intra-abdominal pressure
  c. the pressure of bladder herniation
  d. the urethra dropping outside the influence of intra-abdominal pressure whereas the bladder remains within

29.25 Which of the following may result from the vaginal mucosa prolapsing beyond the introitus?
  a. Bleeding
  b. Ulceration
  c. Infection
  d. All of the above

29.26 Pelvic relaxation is best demonstrated with the patient
  a. at rest, supine
  b. at rest, upright
  c. straining
  d. under anesthesia

29.27 While a speculum is retracting the posterior vaginal wall, a 51-year-old patient is asked to strain down. There is a bulge from the anterior vaginal wall. This is most likely
  a. a rectocele
  b. a cystocele
  c. an enterocele
  d. a vaginal vault prolapse

29.28 Which of the following is associated with procidentia?
  a. Fecal incontinence
  b. Constipation
  c. Ureteral obstruction
  d. Bladder atony

ANSWERS (29.19–29.28)

29.19 a	29.21 c	29.23 d	29.25 d	29.27 b	29.28 c
29.20 b	29.22 d	29.24 d	29.26 c		

Instructions for items 29.29 to 29.31: Match the category of drug used to treat incontinence with examples of drugs from that category. An option may be used once, more than once, or not at all.

29.29 Anticholinergic

29.30 Musculotropic

29.31 Antidepressant
  a. Oxybutynin chloride (Ditropan)
  b. Metaproterenol sulfate (Alupent)
  c. Flavoxate hydrochloride (Urispas)
  d. Diazepam (Valium)
  e. Imipramine hydrochloride (Tofranil)

29.32 Which of the following is the LEAST effective treatment for urgency incontinence?
  a. Biofeedback
  b. Surgery
  c. Bladder training
  d. Medical therapy

29.33 Bladder training programs have which of the following goals?
  a. Increasing the amount of time between voiding
  b. Decreasing the duration of urine flow
  c. Decreasing bladder volume
  d. Increasing midstream urine flow

29.34 The purpose of Kegel exercises is to
  a. strengthen pelvic floor muscles
  b. improve bladder capacity and control
  c. tighten uterine ligaments
  d. increase bladder awareness

29.35 Kegel exercises may be useful in a patient with
  a. second degree prolapse of the uterus
  b. symptomatic rectocele
  c. mild stress incontinence
  d. dyspareunia

29.36 The main function of pessaries is to
  a. obstruct the urethra
  b. provide mechanical support to the vagina
  c. focus intra-abdominal pressure toward the introitus
  d. decrease bladder capacity

Instructions for items 29.37 to 29.40: Match the procedure with the pelvic defect it is designed to correct. An option may be used once, more than once, or not at all.

29.37 Hysterectomy

29.38 Colpocleisis

29.39 Posterior colporrhaphy

29.40 Paravaginal repair
  a. Vaginal vault prolapse
  b. Stress incontinence
  c. Uterine prolapse
  d. Rectocele

Instructions for items 29.41 to 29.44: Match the statement with the surgical procedure that it best describes. An option may be used once, more than once, or not at all.

29.41 Does not require an abdominal incision

29.42 Obliterates the vaginal canal

29.43 Provides a sling for the vagina

29.44 Decreases the possibility of future enterocele formation
  a. Marshall-Marchetti-Krantz
  b. Burch
  c. Pereyra
  d. LeFort
  e. Moskowitz

ANSWERS (29.29–29.44)					
29.29 a	29.32 b	29.35 c	29.38 a	29.41 d	29.43 c
29.30 c	29.33 a	29.36 b	29.39 d	29.42 d	29.44 e
29.31 e	29.34 a	29.37 c	29.40 b		

29.45 The first step in the treatment of a vesicovaginal fistula first noted 4 days after an abdominal hysterectomy is
a. catheter drainage of the bladder
b. insertion of a vaginal pessary
c. surgical dissection of the fistulous tract
d. irradiation to create scarring

29.46 Approximately what percent of women will suffer a urinary tract infection at some point in their lives?
a. Less than 5%
b. 10%–15%
c. 20%–25%
d. 30%–35%
e. 40%–45%

29.47 The relative prevalence of urinary tract infections in men and women (M:F) is
a. 10:1
b. 5:1
c. 1:1
d. 1:5
e. 1:10

29.48 In women, most urinary tract infections occur through
a. hematogenous seeding
b. lymphatic spread
c. ascending contamination from the urethra
d. retained urine

29.49 Which of the following factors is associated with a higher risk of bladder infection in women as compared with men?
a. Relatively shorter urethra in women
b. Estrogen effects
c. Sexual activity
d. Trauma
e. All of the above

29.50 Asymptomatic bacteriuria is found in approximately what percent of postmenopausal women?
a. Less than 5%
b. 10%–15%
c. 20%–25%
d. 30%–35%
e. 40%–45%

29.51 First urinary tract infections in women are most commonly caused by
a. β-streptococcus
b. *Proteus mirabilis*
c. *Escherichia coli*
d. *Clostridium perfringes*

29.52 Irritation of the trigone (trigonitis) causes which of the following symptoms?
a. Frequency
b. Urgency
c. Nocturia
d. All of the above

29.53 A single drop of uncentrifuged urine is examined under the microscope and 2 white blood cells per high-power field are found. What is the likelihood that this patient has a bladder infection?
a. 15%
b. 30%
c. 50%
d. 70%
e. 90%

29.54 The culture of a urine sample is reported to show greater than 100,000 colonies of "mixed flora." This is most likely indicative of
a. infection of the proximal urethra
b. trigonitis
c. upper urinary tract infection
d. a contaminated specimen

ANSWERS (29.45–29.54)

29.45 a	29.47 e	29.49 e	29.51 c	29.53 e	29.54 d
29.46 b	29.48 c	29.50 b	29.52 d		

29.55 In a symptomatic patient, which of the following is indicative of lower urinary tract infection?
a. 10,000 colonies of *Escherichia coli*
b. 10,000 colonies of *Staphylococcus aureus*
c. > 100,000 colonies of mixed flora
d. 1000 colonies of *Bacteroides* species

29.56 When treating an uncomplicated first episode of lower urinary tract infection, which of the following is most likely to precipitate a concomitant vaginal yeast infection?
a. Ascorbic acid
b. Phenazopyridine hydrochloride (Pyridium)
c. Nitrofurantoin (Macrodantin)
d. Ampicillin

29.57 Which is the LEAST likely finding in a patient with cystitis?
a. Frequency
b. Dysuria
c. Fever
d. Suprapubic tenderness

29.58 Which of the following provides urinary analgesia?
a. Ascorbic acid
b. Phenazopyridine hydrochloride (Pyridium)
c. Nitrofurantoin (Macrodantin)
d. Ampicillin

29.59 In the region where the urethra joins the bladder, the urethra is surrounded by circular smooth muscle fibers called
a. the pubovesicocervical neck
b. the external sphincter
c. Retzius' angle
d. the internal sphincter

Instructions for items 29.60 to 29.63: Match the anatomic defect with its best description. An option may be used once, more than once, or not at all.

29.60 Urethrocele

29.61 Cystocele

29.62 Rectocele

29.63 Enterocele
a. Herniation of top of vagina
b. Descent or prolapse of urethra
c. Descent or prolapse of rectum
d. Descent or prolapse of bladder

29.64 Procidentia describes uterine descent beyond the
a. plane of the pelvic inlet
b. level of the uterine artery
c. vaginal introitus
d. vulva

Answers (29.55–29.64)					
29.55 a	29.57 c	29.59 d	29.61 d	29.63 a	29.64 d
29.56 d	29.58 b	29.60 b	29.62 c		

Questions and Answers Chapter 30: Endometriosis

30.1   All of the following symptoms are associated with endometriosis EXCEPT:
a. infertility
b. dysmenorrhea
c. incontinence
d. dyspareunia
e. chronic pelvic pain

30.2   The diagnosis of endometriosis is suspected on the basis of:
a. culture and sensitivity
b. histology
c. typical history
d. family history

30.3   The diagnosis of endometriosis is confirmed on the basis of:
a. culture and sensitivity
b. histology
c. typical history
d. pelvic examination
e. family history

30.4   Which of the following is thought to be associated with an increased risk of endometriosis?
a. Early menopause
b. Multiparity
c. First degree relative with endometriosis
d. Middle to upper income socioeconomic status

30.5   About what percent of women in the general population have endometriosis?
a. 1–2%
b. 4–5%
c. 7–8%
d. 10–11%
e. 13–14%

30.6   About what percent of infertile women have endometriosis?
a. 10–30%
b. 30–50%
c. 50–70%
d. 80–90%

30.7   A first-degree relative of a woman with endometriosis has an approximately what percent chance of being similarly affected?
a. 3%
b. 7%
c. 11%
d. 15%
e. 19%

30.8   Sampson's theory of the development of endometriosis is based on the occurrence of:
a. retrograde menstruation
b. multipotent coelomic cells
c. vascular and lymphatic dissemination
d. a viral DNA vector

30.9   The occurrence of distant implants of endometriosis (such as in the pleural cavity or kidney) supports the theory of endometriosis development based on:
a. retrograde menstruation
b. multipotent coelomic cells
c. vascular and lymphatic dissemination
d. a viral DNA vector

30.10 Which of the following is the most common site in which endometriosis is found?
a. Posterior cul-de-sac
b. Uterosacral ligaments
c. Ovary
d. Fallopian tube

ANSWERS (30.1–30.10)

| 30.1 | c | 30.3 | b | 30.5 | a | 30.7 | b | 30.9 | c | 30.10 | c |
| 30.2 | c | 30.4 | c | 30.6 | b | 30.8 | a | | | | |

30.11 All of the following findings at the time of laparoscopy are consistent with the diagnosis of mild endometriosis EXCEPT:
a. 1-mm vascular hemorrhagic area in the posterior cul-de-sac
b. multiple rust-colored spots on the peritoneal surfaces, 1–2 mm in diameter
c. small puckered white lesions on the uterosacral ligaments
d. small, firm, yellow nodules on the anterior surface of the uterus

30.12 What percent of women with endometriosis have ovarian involvement?
a. 10%
b. 20%
c. 40%
d. 60%
e. 80%

30.13 The term endometrioma refers to:
a. an isolated collection of endometriosis involving an ovary and creating a tumor
b. any endometrial implant greater than 5 mm
c. endometrial tissue found deep within the wall of the uterus
d. endometrial implants that are symptomatic

30.14 The histologic diagnosis of endometriosis requires the presence of all the following findings EXCEPT:
a. glands
b. stroma
c. decidual reaction
d. hemosiderin-laden macrophages

30.15 What percent of cases with a clinical diagnosis of endometriosis can be supported by histologic findings?
a. 95%
b. 85%
c. 70%
d. 50%

30.16 The presence of endometrial glands and stroma within the wall of the uterus is termed:
a. endometriosis
b. adenomyosis
c. endometrial hyperplasia
d. endometrioma

30.17 It is estimated that approximately what percent of women with adenomyosis are asymptomatic?
a. 5%
b. 15%
c. 40%
d. 60%
e. 85%

30.18 All of the following symptoms are consistent with the clinical diagnosis of endometriosis EXCEPT:
a. cyclic pelvic pain
b. "deep thrust" dyspareunia
c. vaginal bleeding between periods
d. intermittent fever
e. painful bowel movements

30.19 What is the most common cause for infertility in patients with endometriosis?
a. pelvic scarring
b. persistent anovulation
c. elevated levels of follicle-stimulating hormone (FSH)
d. increased macrophage activity

ANSWERS (30.11–30.19)

30.11 d	30.13 a	30.15 c	30.17 c	30.18 d	30.19 a
30.12 d	30.14 c	30.16 b			

30.20 What is the estimated overall incidence of endometriosis in women in the general population?
   a. 0.1%
   b. 1%
   c. 10%
   d. 20%
   e. 35%

30.21 The prevalence of endometriosis in infertile women is approximately:
   a. 5%
   b. 10%–15%
   c. 20%–25%
   d. 35%–40%
   e. 60%–65%

30.22 In which age group is endometriosis most likely to be diagnosed?
   a. Prepubertal (less than 12 years of age)
   b. Adolescent (13–17 years)
   c. 20–35 years
   d. Perimenopausal (45–52 years)
   e. Postmenopausal (63–68 years)

30.23 Endometriosis is discovered in about what proportion of teenagers undergoing laparoscopy for evaluation of chronic pelvic pain or dysmenorrhea?
   a. 1/4
   b. 1/2
   c. 3/4
   d. almost all

30.24 Intermenstrual bleeding occurs in approximately what proportion of women with endometriosis?
   a. 1/6
   b. 1/3
   c. 2/3
   d. 3/4

30.25 Vaginal bleeding between periods occurs in approximately what percent of women with endometriosis?
   a. Less than 5%
   b. 10%–15%
   c. 20%–25%
   d. 30%–35%
   e. 40%–45%

30.26 What is the dysmenorrhea associated with endometriosis?
   a. not necessarily proportional to the extent of the disease
   b. due to a fixed, retroverted uterus
   c. a result of uterosacral involvement
   d. worse in patients who are infertile
   e. indicative of ovarian involvement

30.27 What is a typical finding on pelvic examination of patients with adenomyosis?
   a. retroversion of the uterus
   b. reduced mobility of the uterus
   c. adnexal thickening
   d. nodularity of the cul-de-sac
   e. firm, symmetrical enlargements of the uterus

30.28 All of the following physical findings are consistent with a clinical diagnosis of endometriosis EXCEPT:
   a. retroversion of the uterus
   b. reduced mobility of the uterus
   c. adnexal thickening
   d. nodularity of the cul-de-sac
   e. firm, symmetrical enlargements of the uterus

ANSWERS (30.20–30.28)

30.20 b	30.22 c	30.24 b	30.26 a	30.27 e	30.28 e
30.21 d	30.23 b	30.25 d			

30.29 According to the American Fertility Society classification of endometriosis, a patient with complete obliteration of the cul-de-sac by adhesions has:
a. minimal disease
b. mild disease
c. moderate disease
d. severe disease

30.30 According to the American Fertility Society classification of endometriosis, a patient with extensive ovarian adhesions enclosing two-thirds of both ovaries but no other signs of disease has:
a. minimal disease
b. mild disease
c. moderate disease
d. severe disease

30.31 Infertility in the presence of minimal endometriosis is caused by:
a. adhesions
b. tubal obstruction
c. autoantibodies
d. prostaglandin overproduction
e. unknown causes

30.32 What type of abnormal bleeding is associated with endometriosis?
a. Menorrhagia
b. Intermenstrual bleeding
c. Amenorrhea
d. Hypermenorrhea

30.33 A 25-year-old patient is found to have minimal endometriosis at the time of laparoscopy for infertility. What is appropriate treatment for this patient?
a. administration of oral contraceptives
b. administration of a gonadotropin-releasing hormone (GnRH) agonist
c. laser surgery
d. expectant management

30.34 In a patient that has undergone total abdominal hysterectomy and bilateral salpingo-oophorectomy for endometriosis, estrogen-replacement therapy should be:
a. begun immediately
b. begun after follow-up laparoscopy 1 year later
c. begun only after 5 symptom-free years
d. avoided indefinitely

30.35 Continuous administration of combination oral contraceptives is effective in treating endometriosis because they:
a. lower follicle-stimulating hormone (FSH) and luteinizing hormone (LH) levels
b. induce anovulation
c. reduce endometrial prostaglandin production
d. induce a decidual reaction in the endometrial implants

30.36 Medical therapy for endometriosis can be expected to accomplish all of the following EXCEPT:
a. improvement of dyspareunia
b. reduction of adhesions
c. reduction of cyclic pain
d. reduction of menstrual flow

Instructions for items 30.37 to 30.38: Match the appropriate description with the drug(s) used to treat endometriosis. An option may be used once, more than once, or not at all.

30.37 Induces "pseudopregnancy"

30.38 Side effects include hot flashes and alterations of lipoprotein metabolism
a. Oral contraceptives
b. Danazol (17α-ethinyl testosterone derivative)
c. Gonadotropin-releasing hormone (GnRH) agonist
d. Medroxyprogesterone acetate

ANSWERS (30.29–30.38)					
30.29 d	30.31 e	30.33 d	30.35 d	30.37 a	30.38 b
30.30 c	30.32 b	30.34 a	30.36 b		

30.39 Gonadotropin-releasing hormone (GnRH) agonists act by:
a. suppression of endometrial responsiveness
b. down-regulation of the pituitary gland
c. hyperstimulation of the ovary
d. stimulation of the metabolism of progesterone

30.40 Definitive surgical therapy for endometriosis includes:
a. total abdominal hysterectomy
b. bilateral salpingo-oophorectomy
c. lysis of adhesions
d. removal of endometriotic implants
e. all of the above

30.41 After conservative surgical therapy, what is the pregnancy rate possible for patients who have had severe endometriosis?
a. 80%
b. 60%
c. 40%
d. 20%

30.42 In danazol induced pseudomenopause, which of the following statements about FSH and LH levels is correct?
a. Both are suppressed.
b. Both are elevated.
c. FSH is elevated and LH is suppressed.
d. FSH is suppressed and LH is elevated.

ANSWERS (30.39–30.42)

30.39 b   30.40 e   30.41 c   30.42 a

Questions and Answers Chapter 31: Dysmenorrhea and Chronic Pelvic Pain

31.1 What is the most common cause of dysmenorrhea in a 19-year-old?
   a. anovulation
   b. excess prostaglandin production
   c. adenomyosis
   d. endometriosis
   e. pelvic congestion syndrome

31.2 Which of the following is NOT a physiologic mechanism responsible for the generation of a neurologic signal that is perceived as pain?
   a. Ischemia
   b. Stretch
   c. Inflammation
   d. Spasm
   e. Perforation

31.3 It is uncommon for primary dysmenorrhea to occur:
   a. after the birth of a child
   b. after tubal ligation
   c. during breast feeding
   d. during the first 3–6 menstrual cycles of reproductive life

31.4 Childbearing affects:
   a. both the occurrence of primary and secondary dysmenorrhea
   b. neither the occurrence of primary nor secondary dysmenorrhea
   c. the occurrence of primary but not secondary dysmenorrhea
   d. the occurrence of secondary but not primary dysmenorrhea

31.5 What is the agent thought to be responsible for causing primary dysmenorrhea?
   a. estrogen
   b. progesterone
   c. prostaglandin E_2.
   d. prostaglandin F_{2a}.

31.6 Prostaglandin production in the uterus associated with dysmenorrhea normally increases under the influence of:
   a. progesterone only
   b. both estrogen and progesterone
   c. estrogen only
   d. prolactin

31.7 Primary and secondary dysmenorrhea cause significant disability for approximately what percent of women?
   a. 1%–2%
   b. 5%–8%
   c. 10%–15%
   d. 20%–25%
   e. 30%–35%

31.8 During primary dysmenorrhea, intrauterine pressures may reach a maximum of:
   a. 50 mm Hg
   b. 80 mm Hg
   c. 125 mm Hg
   d. 250 mm Hg
   e. 4000 mm Hg

31.9 The uterine contractions associated with primary dysmenorrhea result in baseline intrauterine pressures in excess of
   a. 30 mm Hg
   b. 50 mm Hg
   c. 80 mm Hg
   d. 110 mm Hg
   e. 140 mm Hg

ANSWERS (31.1–31.9)

31.1 b	31.3 d	31.5 d	31.7 c	31.8 e	31.9 c
31.2 d	31.4 b	31.6 a			

31.10 Which of the following would establish a diagnosis of secondary dysmenorrhea?
  a. Crampy, episodic pain
  b. Pain that begins on the first day of menstrual flow
  c. Patient began to experience pain at age 20
  d. Presence of an abnormal pelvic examination
  e. Presence of a heavy menstrual flow

31.11 A patient is referred for evaluation of possible primary dysmenorrhea. Which of the following would cause suspicion of secondary dysmenorrhea?
  a. Dyspareunia
  b. Presence of blood clots in menstrual flow
  c. Nausea and vomiting during period
  d. Irregular periods

31.12 Compared with primary dysmenorrhea, secondary dysmenorrhea tends to be:
  a. more common in older women
  b. as common in older women
  c. less common in older women

31.13 In secondary dysmenorrhea, intrauterine resting pressure is typically:
  a. decreased
  b. unchanged
  c. increased

31.14 Which of the following is an action of prostaglandin F_{2a}?
  a. Vasodilation
  b. Hyperemia
  c. Smooth muscle contraction
  d. Hypomotility of the intestines

Instructions for items 31.15 to 31.16: Use the following case history when answering. A 23-year-old G0P0 patient complains of increasing pelvic heaviness and cyclic lower abdominal pain that begins 1 day before her menstrual flow and lasts for 3 days. Periods are regular, but are heavy with clots. She has been attempting pregnancy for the past 3 years.

31.15 Which of the following is NOT a likely diagnosis for this patient?
  a. Primary dysmenorrhea
  b. Adenomyosis
  c. Uterine myomas
  d. Endometriosis

31.16 Pelvic examination is normal except for painful nodules posterior to the cervix. Which of the following is the most likely diagnosis for this patient?
  a. Primary dysmenorrhea
  b. Adenomyosis
  c. Uterine myomas
  d. Endometriosis

Instructions for items 31.17 to 31.18: Use the following case history when answering. An 18-year-old G0P0 patient complains of cyclic, sharp, crampy, lower abdominal pain that begins on the day of her menstrual flow and lasts for 2–3 days. Periods are regular and heavy, with clots. She has been attempting pregnancy for the past year. Pelvic examination is normal.

31.17 Which of the following is the most likely diagnosis for this patient?
  a. Primary dysmenorrhea
  b. Adenomyosis
  c. Uterine myomas
  d. Endometriosis

Answers (31.10–31.17)

31.10 d	31.12 a	31.14 c	31.15 a	31.16 d	31.17 a
31.11 a	31.13 b				

31.18 The most appropriate therapy for this patient would be:
   a. low dose, monophasic oral contraceptive pills
   b. an acetaminophen/codeine combination
   c. a nonsteroidal anti-inflammatory agent
   d. an injectable progestin contraceptive agent

31.19 An identifiable cause is found in what percent of patients who undergo diagnostic laparoscopy for pelvic pain?
   a. 10%–15%
   b. 30%–40%
   c. about 50%
   d. 60%–70%
   e. 90%–95%

31.20 Thickening in the adnexae is consistent with:
   a. pelvic inflammatory disease
   b. leiomyoma uteri
   c. endometritis
   d. adenomyosis uteri

31.21 The term chronic pelvic pain is applied to pain that has been present for:
   a. three consecutive menstrual periods
   b. at least 6 months
   c. three or more of a woman's first six menstrual cycles
   d. more than 21 days in a given month

31.22 The term chronic pelvic pain is generally applied to pelvic discomfort:
   a. not solely associated with menstruation and that lasts of more than 6 months
   b. solely associated with menstruation and that lasts more than 6 months
   c. not solely associated with menstruation and that lasts more than 12 months
   d. solely associated with menstruation and that lasts more than 12 months

31.23 The Rome criteria for the diagnosis of irritable bowel syndrome include the presence of abdominopelvic pain in the past 12 months that cannot be explained by known disease and which persists for how many weeks (not necessarily consecutive)?
   a. 3
   b. 6
   c. 9
   d. 12

31.24 For purposes of treatment, irritable bowel syndrome often is subcategorized using all of he following predominant complaints EXCEPT:
   a. pain
   b. blood in the stool
   c. diarrhea
   d. constipation
   e. alternating constipation and diarrhea

ANSWERS (31.18–31.24)

31.18 c	31.20 a	31.21 b	31.22 a	31.23 d	31.24 b
31.19 d					

31.25 Which of the following would not contribute to a diagnosis of irritable bowel syndrome?
   a. Pain relieved by defecation
   b. Change in the frequency of bowel movements
   c. Change in appetite
   d. Change in the form of stool

31.26 The pathophysiology of irritable bowel syndrome may include all of the following EXCEPT:
   a. altered bowel mobility
   b. visceral insensitivity
   c. psychosocial factors (especially stress)
   d. an imbalance of neurotransmitters (especially serotonin)
   e. infection (often indolent or subclinical)

31.27 Which of the following statements about the diagnosis of irritable bowel syndrome is incorrect?
   a. The diagnosis relies heavily on the history.
   b. The diagnosis relies on colonoscopy plus barium enema in women under about 50 years of age.
   c. The diagnosis relies on flexible sigmoidoscopy in women under about 50 years of age.
   d. The diagnosis relies on biopsy of the mucosae of the descending colon when diarrhea is a predominant symptom.

31.28 Which of the following would not be part of the management of a patient whose irritable bowel syndrome has constipation as the predominant sympton?
   a. Keeping a food diary
   b. Fiber
   c. Lactulose
   d. Loperamide

31.29 Depending on the patient's situation, which of the following is an appropriate goal in the management of chronic pelvic pain?
   a. Alleviation of the cause of the pain
   b. Management of pain symptoms
   c. Both a and b above

31.30 In the treatment of chronic pelvic pain, analgesics are best administered on:
   a. a fixed time schedule that is independent of symptoms
   b. a fixed schedule that is dependent on symptoms
   c. an as needed schedule that is independent of symptoms
   d. an as needed schedule that is dependent on symptoms

Instructions for items 31.31 to 31.38: Match the nonsteroidal anti-inflammatory drug with the initial and subsequent dosage (in mg) and regimen. An option may be used once, more than once, or not at all.

31.31 Diclofenac potassium (Cataflam)

31.32 Diclofenac sodium (Voltaren)

31.33 Fenoprofen calcium (Fenoprofen)

31.34 Ibuprofen (Motrin, Nuprin)

31.35 Ketoprofen (Orudis, Ketoprofen)

31.36 Mefenamic acid (Ponstel)

31.37 Naproxen (Naprosyn, Naproxen)

31.38 Naproxen sodium (Anaprox)
   a. 100 mg; 100 mg every 4–6 hours
   b. 400 mg; 400 mg every 4 hours
   c. 500 mg; 250 mg every 4–6 hours
   d. 75 mg; 75 mg three times a day
   e. 50–100 mg; 50 mg twice a day
   f. 75–150 mg; 75 mg twice a day
   g. 200 mg; 200 mg every 4–6 hours

ANSWERS (31.25–31.38)

31.25 c	31.28 d	31.31 e	31.33 a	31.35 d	31.37 c
31.26 b	31.29 c	31.32 f	31.34 b	31.36 c	31.38 g
31.27 b	31.30 a				

Questions and Answers Chapter 32: Disorders of the Breast

32.1 What is the blood supply of the breast?
a. sparse
b. rich

32.2 As a malignancy in women, breast cancer ranks where in frequency?
a. First
b. Second
c. Third
d. Fourth
e. Fifth

32.3 Collecting ducts arising from breast lobes terminate (drain) at the:
a. areola
b. nipple
c. Montgomery's ducts
d. chest wall lymphatics

32.4 What is the most common benign breast condition?
a. ductal ectasia
b. fibroadenoma
c. fibrocystic change
d. intraductal papilloma
e. galactocele

32.5 What is the benign breast condition most commonly mistaken for cancer?
a. fat necrosis
b. fibrocystic change
c. ductal ectasia
d. intraductal papilloma

32.6 What is the most common presenting complaint of women with fibrocystic breast change?
a. solitary breast mass
b. localized breast tenderness
c. bilateral, cyclic pain
d. nipple discharge
e. multiple breast masses

32.7 What is the usual sequence of events in the development of fibrocystic breast change?
a. obstruction of ducts, cyst formation, fibrosis
b. fibrosis, ductal expansion, cyclic breast pain
c. ductal atrophy, fibrosis, cyst formation
d. proliferation of stroma, adenosis, cyst formation

32.8 A 23-year-old patient presents with a 2–3 cm firm, painless, freely movable mass in her left breast. She reports that the mass does not change during her menstrual cycle and has grown slowly over the past year. The patient found the mass during breast self-examination. What is the most likely diagnosis?
a. intraductal carcinoma
b. fibroadenoma
c. ductal ectasia
d. fibrocystic change

32.9 Multiple fibroadenomas develop in approximately what percent of patients?
a. Less than 5%
b. 5%–10%
c. 15%–20%
d. 25%–30%
e. 35%–40%

ANSWERS (32.1–32.9)

32.1	b	32.3	b	32.5	a	32.7	d	32.8	b	32.9	c
32.2	c	32.4	c	32.6	c						

32.10 A 34-year-old patient complains of cyclic breast tenderness and diffuse nodularity on monthly breast self-examination. Your examination finds multiple firm, mobile masses, predominately in the upper outer quadrants of each breast. You aspirate one of these masses and obtain clear, straw colored fluid. What is the best initial management of this condition?
a. mechanical support of the breast
b. danazol sodium therapy
c. progesterone-only oral contraceptives
d. gonadotropin-releasing hormone (GnRH) agonist therapy
e. excisional biopsy

32.11 When atypia are found in hyperplastic ducts or in apocrine cells in a histologic specimen of a woman with fibrocystic breast disorder, her risk of future carcinoma is increased:
a. 5-fold
b. 10-fold
c. 15-fold
d. 20-fold

32.12 Fibroadenomas occur in about what percent of all women?
a. 1–2%
b. 10–20%
c. 30–40%
d. 50–60%

32.13 Which of the following statements about the management of suspected fibroadenomas is incorrect?
a. Ultrasound is not useful in distinguishing fibroadenomas from breast cysts.
b. Surgical excision is indicated if the breast mass is painful.
c. Surgical indication is indicated if the breast mass is rapidly growing.
d. Fine needle aspiration may provide sufficient information to allow management by frequent examination and mammographic evaluation.

32.14 Breast self-examination should be performed:
a. following menstruation
b. at 2-week intervals, on the same day of the week
c. weekly, on the same day of the week
d. 3–5 days before menstruation

32.15 Approximately what percent of breast cancers are found by the patient herself?
a. 10%
b. 30%
c. 50%
d. 70%
e. 90%

32.16 Currently, a woman living in the United States has what lifetime risk of developing breast cancer?
a. 1 in 2
b. 1 in 4
c. 1 in 6
d. 1 in 8
e. 1 in 10

ANSWERS (32.10–32.16)

32.10 a	32.12 b	32.13 a	32.14 a	32.15 e	32.16 d
32.11 b					

32.17 What is the risk of developing breast cancer for a woman over the age of 60?
   a. 1 in 120
   b. 1 in 90
   c. 1 in 60
   d. 1 in 30
   e. 1 in 3

Instructions for items 32.18 to 32.34. Match the risk factor for developing breast cancer in women with its relative risk.

32.18 Menarche at less than 12 years of age

32.19 One first-degree relative with breast cancer (pre- or postmenopausal, unilateral disease)

32.20 Personal history of cancer of major salivary glands

32.21 Personal history of cancer of the endometrium, ovary, or colon

32.22 Menarche at greater than 17 years of age

32.23 Menopause before age 45

32.24 Term pregnancy before age 35

32.25 Premenopausal first degree relative with bilateral breast cancer

32.26 Age greater than 65 years

32.27 Inherited genetic mutations for breast cancer

32.28 Personal history of breast cancer

32.29 Never breast fed a child

32.30 No full-term pregnancies (for cancer diagnosed after age 40)

32.31 First full-term pregnancy after age 35 years

32.32 Menopause after age 55

32.33 Atypical hyperplasia on breast biopsy

32.34 Two or more first-degree relatives with breast cancer
   a. 0–1.0
   b. 1.1–2.0
   c. 2.1–4.0
   d. >4
   e. >8

Instructions for items 32.35 to 32.39: Match the risk factor for breast cancer with the appropriate relative risk. An option may be used once, more than once, or not at all.

32.35 First degree relative, sister or mother, with breast cancer

32.36 Oral contraceptive use

32.37 Estrogen replacement therapy

32.38 Contralateral breast cancer

32.39 Atypical hyperplasia on breast biopsy
   a. No effect
   b. 1.2–3.0
   c. 4.0–6.0
   d. 5.0

32.40 Historical risk factors identify what percent of breast cancer patients?
   a. 10%
   b. 25%
   c. 40%
   d. 55%
   e. 70%

32.41 What proportion of patients 30–54 years of age with breast cancer are identified by specific risk factors?
   a. 1:5
   b. 2:5
   c. 3:5
   d. 4:5

ANSWERS (32.17–32.41)

32.17 d	32.22 a	32.26 d	32.30 b	32.34 d	32.38 d
32.18 b	32.23 a	32.27 d	32.31 b	32.35 b	32.39 c
32.19 c	32.24 a	32.28 d	32.32 b	32.36 a	32.40 b
32.20 c	32.25 e	32.29 b	32.33 c	32.37 a	32.41 a
32.21 d					

32.42 What percent of all breast cancer occurs after the age of 40?
a. 95%
b. 85%
c. 75%
d. 65%

32.43 Breast pain is a presenting symptom in approximately what percent of patients with breast cancer?
a. 10%
b. 30%
c. 50%
d. 70%
e. 90%

32.44 What is the average doubling time of breast cancer cells?
a. 35 days
b. 100 days
c. 175 days
d. 300 days
e. 450 days

32.45 Mutations or alterations in the breast cancer susceptibility genes (such as BRCA1 and BRCA2) appear in what percent of the general population?
a. Less than 1 %
b. About 5%
c. About 10%
d. About 25%
e. About 40%

32.46 What is the most common form of breast cancer?
a. cystosarcoma phylloides
b. infiltrating intraductal carcinoma
c. noninfiltrating intraductal carcinoma
d. lobular carcinoma
e. Paget's disease

32.47 Paget's disease accounts for approximately what percent of breast cancers?
a. 1%
b. 10%
c. 15%
d. 20%
e. 35%

32.48 Compared with detection of breast cancer by self-examination, breast cancer may be detected by mammography:
a. significantly earlier
b. at about the same time
c. significantly later

32.49 Approximately what percent of breast cancers present as a mass?
a. 20%
b. 40%
c. 60%
d. 80%
e. 100%

32.50 A 30-year-old patient with a family history of breast cancer undergoes a needle aspiration of a cystic breast mass. The fluid obtained is clear. Your next step in the management of this patient would be to:
a. send the fluid for cytology
b. obtain a mammogram
c. check the site for recurrence of the mass
d. perform a needle biopsy of the cyst wall

32.51 The advantage of mammography is that it can:
a. identify suspicious lesions 2 or more years before they are palpable
b. assess the degree of spread of malignancy
c. differentiate between benign and malignant conditions
d. provide reassurance about suspicious masses

ANSWERS (32.42–32.51)

32.42 b	32.44 b	32.46 b	32.48 a	32.50 c	32.51 a
32.43 a	32.45 a	32.47 a	32.49 d		

32.52 The accuracy of mammography in diagnosing breast cancer is approximately:
a. 45%
b. 65%
c. 85%
d. 100%

32.53 The current use of mammography has been credited with reducing the overall mortality rate of breast cancer by:
a. 5%
b. 15%
c. 30%
d. 45%
e. 60%

32.54 Current mammography techniques result in radiation exposure that approximates:
a. 0.5–1 rad
b. 3–5 rad
c. 8–10 rad
d. 12–15 rad

Instructions for items 32.55 to 32.60. Match the BI-RADS Classification for Screening Mammography with the description with which it is best associated.

32.55 Category 0

32.56 Category 1

32.57 Category 2

32.58 Category 3

32.59 Category 4

32.60 Category 5
a. Negative
b. Benign finding
c. Additional imaging evaluation needed
d. Probably benign finding
e. Suspicious abnormality
f. Highly suggestive of malignancy

Instructions for items 32.61 to 32.66. Match the BI-RADS Classification for Screening Mammography with the description with which it is best associated.

32.61 Category 0

32.62 Category 1

32.63 Category 2

32.64 Category 3

32.65 Category 4

32.66 Category 5
a. Lesions are noted which do not have the characteristic morphologies of breast cancer but have a definite probability of being malignant.
b. The finding has a high probability of being benign, but the mammographer would prefer to establish its mammographic stability over a short interval.
c. A finding is noted which warrants further imaging.
d. Breasts are symmetrical and masses, architectural disturbances, or suspicious calcifications are not noted.
e. A mammographer wishes to describe a finding while concluding that there is no mammographic evidence of malignancy.

32.67 The recurrence rate of fibroadenomas of the breast is approximately:
a. 1%–3%
b. 5%–8%
c. 12%–15%
d. 18%–20%
e. 30%–33%

ANSWERS (32.52–32.67)

32.52 c	32.55 c	32.58 d	32.61 c	32.64 b	32.66 f
32.53 c	32.56 a	32.59 e	32.62 d	32.65 a	32.67 d
32.54 a	32.57 b	32.60 f	32.63 e		

32.68 A 42-year-old woman presents with a firm, non-tender mass in her right breast. You perform fine needle aspiration, which is reported as "negative for malignancy." The next step in the management of this patient should be:
a. open biopsy
b. immediate mammography
c. repeat fine needle aspiration
d. mammography in 6 months
e. reassurance and mammography as per routine

32.69 What is the most common presenting complaint of patients with intraductal papillomas of the breast?
a. unilateral bloody nipple discharge
b. unilateral cyclic pain
c. sub-areolar palpable mass
d. bilateral milky discharge

32.70 Nipple discharge associated with burning, itching, or nipple discomfort in older patients is suggestive of:
a. intraductal papilloma
b. fibroadenoma
c. ductal ectasia
d. papillary carcinoma

32.71 Cytologic evaluation of nipple discharge is associated with a false-negative rate of approximately:
a. 3%
b. 8%
c. 12%
d. 20%

ANSWERS (32.68–32.71)

32.68 a	32.69 a	32.70 c	32.71 d

Questions and Answers Chapter 33: Gynecologic Procedures

33.1 Which of the following statements about ultrasonography is INCORRECT?
   a. The technique uses high energy sound waves to directly image organs
   b. It should not be used to replace the pelvic examination
   c. There may be interference from substances such as bowel gas
   d. In Doppler mode, it may be useful in evaluating blood flow patterns

33.2 Which of the following is NOT an appropriate use for ultrasonography?
   a. To differentiate solid from cystic mass
   b. To routinely confirm findings from the pelvic examination
   c. To measure size of uterine fibroids
   d. To identify possible cause of pelvic pain

33.3 Which of the following statements about magnetic resonance imaging is INCORRECT?
   a. The technology is based on the magnetic characteristics of the atoms and molecules composing various bodily tissues
   b. It is most useful in the imaging of bony structures
   c. It may be of value in the staging of cervical malignancy
   d. It may be of value in the evaluation of breast lesions

33.4 Which of the following statements about hysterosalpingography is INCORRECT?
   a. It is useful to determine the size and shape of the uterine cavity
   b. It is useful to visualize the configuration of the uterine cavity
   c. It is useful to determine fallopian tube patency
   d. It is not useful to visualize fallopian tube anatomy

Instructions for Items 33.5 to 33.8: Match the type of genital tract biopsy with the terms or phrases with which it is best associated. An answer may be used once, more than once, or not at all.

33.5 Vulvar biopsy

33.6 Vaginal biopsy

33.7 Cervical biopsy

33.8 Endometrial biopsy
   a. Usually performed in the office setting
   b. Uses Keyes biopsy instrument
   c. Uses Pipelle biopsy instrument
   d. Uses biopsy forceps
   e. Usually done with local anesthetic

33.9 A profuse watery vaginal discharge is most commonly associated with which therapy for cervical dysplasia?
   a. Colposcopy
   b. Cryotherapy
   c. Laser therapy
   d. Conization

ANSWERS (33.1–33.9)					
33.1 a	33.3 a	33.5 a, b, e	33.7 a, d	33.8 a, c	33.9 b
33.2 b	33.4 d	33.6 a, d			

33.10 Which of the following are indications for cervical conization?
   a. A two-step discrepancy between Pap smear and colposcopically directed biopsy
   b. A colposcopy where the squamocolumnar junction cannot be visualized
   c. Therapy for cervical dysplasia
   d. All of the above are indications

33.11 Total abdominal hysterectomy refers to the removal of the
   a. uterus
   b. ovaries
   c. fallopian tubes
   d. bladder

33.12 Which term refers to the surgical removal of the uterine corpus?
   a. Total hysterectomy
   b. Subtotal hysterectomy
   c. Radical hysterectomy

33.13 Which of the following is an advantage of abdominal hysterectomy over vaginal hysterectomy?
   a. Ability to visualize associated pelvic pathology
   b. Shorter recovery period
   c. Repair of rectocele more readily accessible
   d. Fewer incisional complications

33.14 Hysteroscopy can be used for which of the following?
   a. Polypectomy
   b. Endometrial ablation
   c. Evaluation of bleeding
   d. All of the above

33.15 Biopsy of what organ is usually performed with an aspiration technique?
   a. Vulva
   b. Vagina
   c. Cervix
   d. Endometrium

33.16 In the initial evaluation of a possible adnexal mass, the most appropriate imaging technique is
   a. computed axial tomography scanning
   b. magnetic resonance imaging
   c. ultrasound
   d. flat plate of the abdomen

33.17 Colposcopy is most commonly used to evaluate an abnormality of what organ?
   a. Cervix
   b. Breast
   c. Endometrium
   d. Ovary

Answers (33.10–33.17)

33.10 d	33.12 b	33.14 d	33.15 d	33.16 c	33.17 a
33.11 a	33.13 a				

Questions and Answers Chapter 34: Reproductive Cycle

34.1 At what average age is a regular, predictable reproductive cycle established in women?
a. 11 years
b. 13 years
c. 15 years
d. 17 years

34.2 At what average age does the female reproductive cycle become inefficient?
a. 30 years
b. 35 years
c. 40 years
d. 45 years

34.3 A woman's optimal reproductive time occupies approximately how many years?
a. 10
b. 15
c. 20
d. 30

34.4 On average, how many times during the year will a healthy, non-pregnant woman ovulate?
a. 6–8 times
b. 10–12 times
c. 13–14 times
d. 16–18 times

34.5 What is the average length of the female reproductive cycle?
a. 26 days
b. 28 days
c. 30 days
d. 32 days

34.6 What is the name of the pulse generator that secretes gonadotropin-releasing hormone?
a. Arcuate nucleus of the anterior hypothalamus
b. Anterior lobe of the pituitary gland
c. Posterior lobe of the pituitary gland
d. Third ventricle

34.7 Gonadotropin-releasing hormone flows from the hypothalamus to the anterior pituitary gland through the
a. cerebrospinal fluid
b. lymphatic system
c. pituitary portal venous plexus
d. cerebral venous drainage

34.8 What is the pulse frequency of hypothalamic gonadotropin-releasing hormone secretion?
a. Every 50–60 minutes
b. Every 70–90 minutes
c. Every 100–120 minutes
d. Every 6–8 hours
e. Every 2–3 days

34.9 Given a woman with the inability to secrete gonadotropin-releasing hormone (GnRH; Kallmann's syndrome), at what pulse frequency should an external GnRH pump be set?
a. Every 50–60 minutes
b. Every 70–90 minutes
c. Every 100–120 minutes
d. Every 6–8 hours
e. Every 2–3 days

ANSWERS (34.1–34.9)

34.1	c	34.3	d	34.5	b	34.7	c	34.8	b	34.9	b
34.2	d	34.4	c	34.6	a						

Instructions for items 34.10 to 34.21: For each item, select the most appropriate reproductive hormone. An option may be used once, more than once, or not at all.

34.10 The hormone that stimulates the granulosa cells of the primary ovarian follicle

34.11 The hormone that triggers ovulation

34.12 The principal sex steroid secreted by the granulosa cells of the ovarian follicle

34.13 The hormone that stimulates the pregranulosa cells of the primordial follicle to become granulosa cells

34.14 The hormone that facilitates preparation of the endometrium for implantation of the blastocyst following fertilization

34.15 The hormone that has the greatest effect on the hypothalamic thermoregulatory center

34.16 The hormone that is associated with the development of the secretory endometrium

34.17 The hormone that stimulates the ductal elements of the breast (nipples, areolae, and ducts)

34.18 The hormone that stimulates the acinar elements of the breast (milk producing glands)

34.19 The hormone associated with the development of a proliferative endometrium

34.20 The hormone that reflects the activity of the arcuate nucleus

34.21 The hormone that is most heavily secreted in response to a perceived estrogen deficiency
  a. Estradiol
  b. Estrone
  c. Estriol
  d. Progesterone
  e. Testosterone
  f. Androstenedione
  g. Follicle-stimulating hormone
  h. Luteinizing hormone
  i. Gonadotropin-releasing hormone
  j. Thyroid-stimulating hormone
  k. Melanocyte-stimulating hormone

34.22 Which is the principal sex steroid hormone secreted by the theca lutein cells?
  a. Estradiol
  b. Testosterone
  c. Progesterone
  d. Estriol

34.23 Which of the following is secreted by the theca lutein cells during the follicular phase of the cycle and acts as a precursor in the synthesis of sex steroid hormone by granulosa cells?
  a. Androgens
  b. Prostaglandins
  c. Estrogens
  d. Endorphins

34.24 The oocyte in the primordial follicle is arrested in what stage of division?
  a. Prophase of meiosis
  b. Metaphase of meiosis
  c. Prophase of mitosis
  d. Metaphase of mitosis

ANSWERS (34.10–34.24)

34.10 g	34.13 g	34.16 d	34.19 a	34.21 g	34.23 a
34.11 h	34.14 d	34.17 a	34.20 i	34.22 c	34.24 a
34.12 a	34.15 d	34.18 d			

34.25 Which of the following stimulates the arrested oocyte to complete maturation?
a. A critical level of follicle-stimulating hormone (FSH)
b. The luteinizing hormone (LH) surge
c. An FSH:LH ratio of 3:1
d. A critical level of estradiol

34.26 What endocrine event initiates the onset of menstruation?
a. Luteinizing hormone (LH) surge
b. Estradiol peak
c. Involution of the corpus luteum
d. A follicle-stimulating hormone (FSH):LH ratio of 3:1

34.27 What is the average volume of blood lost each menstrual cycle?
a. 10–25 ml
b. 30–50 ml
c. 70–90 ml
d. 120–150 ml

34.28 Where do the prostaglandins that initiate uterine contractions during menstruation originate?
a. Ovary
b. Endocervix
c. Uterine musculature
d. Endometrium
e. Pituitary

34.29 What is the clinical condition associated with symptomatic uterine contractions during menstruation?
a. Primary dysmenorrhea
b. Secondary dysmenorrhea
c. Dyspareunia
d. Dyschezia
e. Menorrhagia

34.30 What is the preferred form of treatment for women who suffer from menstrual pain?
a. β-blockers
b. Calcium-channel blockers
c. Prostaglandin synthetase inhibitors
d. Narcotics

34.31 The pituitary gland begins to secrete follicle-stimulating hormone to initiate a new reproductive cycle
a. just before ovulation
b. just after ovulation
c. 24 to 48 hours before the onset of menstruation
d. 24 to 48 hours after the onset of menstruation

34.32 What is the consequence of an androgen to estrogen ratio of greater than one in a follicle that is undergoing stimulation?
a. Multiple gestation
b. Atretic follicle
c. Chromosomal abnormalities
d. Spontaneous abortion

34.33 What is the presumed chemical stimulus for extrusion of the oocyte from the follicle at the time of ovulation?
a. Metabolism of endorphins
b. Release of progesterone
c. Synthesis of prostaglandins
d. Liberation of intrafollicular prostaglandins

34.34 What is the consequence if prostaglandin synthetase inhibitors are administered at the expected time of ovulation?
a. The oocyte will be retained in the follicle
b. Mittelschmerz is intensified
c. Progesterone synthesis is enhanced
d. The corpus luteum is ruptured

Answers (34.25–34.34)

34.25 b	34.27 b	34.29 a	34.31 c	34.33 d	34.34 a
34.26 c	34.28 d	34.30 c	34.32 b		

34.35 What term is given to the pain associated with ovulation?
a. Premenstrual syndrome
b. Dysmenorrhea
c. Dyspareunia
d. Mittelschmerz

34.36 The clinical term for insufficient progesterone production by the corpus luteum is
a. secondary dysmenorrhea
b. primary dysmenorrhea
c. inadequate luteal phase
d. premenstrual syndrome
e. spontaneous abortion

34.37 Which hormone is necessary to sustain the corpus luteum beyond 14 days?
a. Progesterone
b. Human chorionic gonadotropin
c. Estradiol
d. Human chorionic somatomammotropin

34.38 At approximately what age will a woman begin to notice changes in her reproductive cycle associated with perimenopause?
a. 30–32 years
b. 34–36 years
c. 38–42 years
d. 45–48 years
e. 50–52 years

34.39 What is the first evidence of diminished reproductive efficiency in a woman?
a. A change in the length of the reproductive cycle
b. Hot flushes
c. Vaginal atrophy
d. Premenstrual mood changes

34.40 What is the clinical condition when the few remaining ovarian follicles are resistant to stimulation by follicle-stimulating hormone?
a. Polycystic ovarian disease
b. Menopause
c. Kallmann's syndrome
d. Premenstrual syndrome

34.41 What procedure is used for endometrial dating, to diagnose inadequate luteal phase?
a. Transvaginal ultrasound
b. Hysteroscopy
c. Endometrial biopsy
d. Hysterosalpingogram
e. Serum estrogen measurement

34.42 What is the common condition characterized by breast tenderness, mood changes, fluid retention, abdominal bloating, and weight gain?
a. Primary dysmenorrhea
b. Secondary dysmenorrhea
c. Premenstrual syndrome
d. Perimenopause

ANSWERS (34.35–34.42)

34.35 d	34.37 b	34.39 a	34.40 b	34.41 c	34.42 c
34.36 c	34.38 c				

Questions and Answers Chapter 35: Puberty

35.1 The event that triggers puberty is
a. achieving a critical body weight
b. unknown
c. reaching a critical height
d. having a specific body surface area

35.2 The hypothalamic-pituitary axis is first known to function
a. in utero
b. at birth
c. at 1 year of age
d. at 13 years of age

35.3 What is the first endocrine event associated with secondary sexual maturation?
a. Secretion of dehydroepiandrosterone by the adrenal glands
b. Ovarian hormone secretion
c. Pituitary development
d. Hypothalamus down-regulation

35.4 What is the usual length of time from the first physical signs of secondary sexual maturation until sexual maturation is complete?
a. 1 year
b. 2 years
c. 3 years
d. 4 years
e. 5 years

35.5 What is the expected sequence of secondary sexual development in girls?
a. Adrenarche, growth spurt, thelarche, menarche, ovulation
b. Menarche, growth spurt, thelarche, adrenarche, ovulation
c. Growth spurt, menarche, adrenarche, thelarche, ovulation
d. Thelarche, adrenarche, growth spurt, menarche, ovulation

35.6 Which of the following is required for timely secondary sexual maturation?
a. Sufficient body fat
b. Sufficient sleep
c. Sufficient height
d. Exposure to adequate levels of light
e. Sufficient body fat AND sleep AND light

35.7 What is the baseline percentage of body fat needed to sustain female reproductive function?
a. 6%
b. 12%
c. 24%
d. 36%

35.8 What is the earliest sign of delayed puberty in girls?
a. Failure of growth spurt by age 10
b. Failure of menarche by age 12
c. Failure of breast budding by age 13
d. Failure of ovulation by age 17

35.9 When adrenarche occurs first, what is the expected interval to the onset of thelarche?
a. 4–5 months
b. 6–9 months
c. 12–15 months
d. 24 months

35.10 Which of the following does NOT typically cause premature ovarian failure in adolescent girls?
a. Turner's syndrome (45X karyotype)
b. Deletion of the long arm of the X chromosome
c. Mature teratoma
d. Alkylating chemotherapy

ANSWERS (35.1–35.10)

35.1	b	35.3	a	35.5	d	35.7	c	35.9	b	35.10	c
35.2	a	35.4	d	35.6	e	35.8	c				

35.11 What is the most common genital tract cause of primary amenorrhea?
a. Congenital absence of the uterus
b. Imperforate hymen
c. Asherman's syndrome
d. Premature ovarian failure

35.12 Which of the following is a method for treating vaginal agenesis?
a. Vaginal vault suspension
b. Vulvectomy
c. Vulvar flap
d. Vaginal marsupialization
e. Pressure dilation of the vaginal space

35.13 What is the simple, definitive treatment for imperforate hymen?
a. Hymenectomy
b. Hymenotomy
c. Vaginal reconstruction
d. Administration of a gonadotropin-releasing hormone (GnRH) agonist
e. Topical estrogen therapy

35.14 What is the definitive chemical evidence of ovarian failure?
a. Depressed estradiol
b. Elevated prolactin
c. Elevated follicle-stimulating hormone (FSH)
d. Depressed testosterone
e. Absent gonadotropin-releasing hormone (GnRH)

35.15 Genetic information that regulates the rate of ovarian follicular atresia is located on
a. the short arm of the X chromosome
b. the long arm of the X chromosome
c. chromosome 21
d. chromosome 18

35.16 Genetic information that determines height and somatic characteristics is located on
a. the short arm of the X chromosome
b. the long arm of the X chromosome
c. chromosome 21
d. chromosome 18

35.17 Which of the following hormones must be replaced in girls with premature ovarian failure?
a. Prolactin
b. Progesterone
c. Estradiol-17β
d. Testosterone
e. Gonadotropin-releasing hormone (GnRH)

35.18 What is the risk of administering excessive estradiol-17β (or other estrogens) in girls with pubertal failure?
a. Endometrial cancer
b. Short stature
c. Hirsutism
d. Vaginal agenesis
e. Amenorrhea

35.19 What is the risk of delaying administration of estradiol-17β in girls with pubertal failure?
a. Short stature
b. Mental retardation
c. Osteoporosis
d. Clinical depression
e. Endometrial cancer

35.20 Alteration of the gonadotropin-releasing hormone (GnRH) pulse frequency in adolescent girls will result in
a. ovarian hyperstimulation
b. ovarian atrophy
c. ovarian neoplasm
d. no pituitary stimulation of the ovary

ANSWERS (35.11–35.20)

| 35.11 | b | 35.13 | b | 35.15 | b | 35.17 | c | 35.19 | c | 35.20 | d |
| 35.12 | e | 35.14 | c | 35.16 | a | 35.18 | b | | | | |

35.21 What condition is associated with olfactory tract hypoplasia and failure of gonadotropin-releasing hormone (GnRH) secretion?
a. Turner's syndrome
b. Cushing's syndrome
c. Kallmann's syndrome
d. Swyer's syndrome

35.22 What condition is associated with failure to establish secondary sexual development, a webbed neck, and short stature?
a. Turner's syndrome
b. Cushing's syndrome
c. Kallmann's syndrome
d. Swyer's syndrome

35.23 During clinical evaluation, how can Kallmann's syndrome be recognized?
a. Serum estradiol levels
b. Visual field evaluation
c. Serum follicle-stimulating hormone (FSH)
d. Olfactory challenge

35.24 How would a patient with Kallmann's syndrome be treated to help her conceive?
a. Artificial insemination
b. Pulsatile administration of gonadotropin-releasing hormone (GnRH)
c. Administration of clomiphene citrate
d. Administration of sequential estrogen and progesterone

35.25 In adolescents, what would be evidence of incomplete puberty that is caused by marijuana use?
a. Elevated estradiol
b. Elevated testosterone
c. Suppressed gonadotropins [follicle-stimulating hormone (FSH) and luteinizing hormone (LH)]
d. Suppressed prolactin

35.26 What is the prognosis for adolescent girls who have delayed puberty or secondary amenorrhea due to participation in competitive athletics?
a. Increased incidence of congenital anomalies in offspring can be anticipated
b. Infertility can be anticipated
c. Normal secondary sexual development can be anticipated
d. Reduced reproductive capacity can be anticipated
e. Early menopause can be anticipated

35.27 Isosexual precocious puberty is defined as
a. premature sexual maturation following the normal sequence
b. premature sexual maturation following an abnormal sequence
c. sexual maturation on time but following an abnormal sequence
d. sexual maturation on time but following a prolonged sequence

35.28 What is the most common cause of inappropriate hormone secretion leading to precocious puberty in girls?
a. Cushing's syndrome
b. Addison's syndrome
c. Adrenal hyperplasia, 21-hydroxylase type
d. Adrenal hyperplasia, 11-hydroxylase type

35.29 What is the treatment of choice for children with isosexual precocious puberty?
a. Steroids
b. Estrogen alone
c. Gonadotropin-releasing hormone (GnRH) agonist
d. Oral contraceptives

ANSWERS (35.21–35.29)

| 35.21 | c | 35.23 | d | 35.25 | c | 35.27 | a | 35.28 | c | 35.29 | c |
| 35.22 | a | 35.24 | b | 35.26 | c | | | | | | |

35.30 Isosexual precocious puberty generally results in
a. infertility
b. secondary menorrhea
c. obesity
d. short stature
e. disordered pubertal (developmental) sequence

35.31 A woman with uterine and vaginal agenesis can have her own genetic child through
a. sequential administration of estrogen and progesterone for three reproductive cycles
b. tonic administration of estrogen alone
c. pelvic reconstructive surgery
d. ovum donation
e. insemination with donor sperm

35.32 Premature ovarian failure is characterized by
a. Lower estrogen level, lower gonadotropin levels
b. Elevated estrogen level, lower gonadotropin levels
c. Lower estrogen level, elevated gonadotropin levels
d. Elevated estrogen level, elevated gonadotropin levels

35.33 In patients with premature ovarian failure, the daily dose of conjugated estrogen to initiate secondary sexual maturation is
a. 0.3 mg
b. 1.25 mg
c. 2.5 mg
d. 5.0 mg

35.34 In patients with premature ovarian failure, the daily dose of conjugated estrogen to induce menarche is
a. 0.3 mg
b. 0.625 mg
c. 1.25 mg
d. 2.5 mg

35.35 In patients with premature ovarian failure, induction of cyclic bleeding is accomplished with the cyclic administration of
a. estrogen
b. progestin
c. GnRH
d. testosterone

ANSWERS (35.30–35.35)
35.30 d   35.31 d   35.32 c   35.33 a   35.34 c   35.35 b

Questions and Answers Chapter 36: Amenorrhea and Dysfunctional Uterine Bleeding

36.1 At what average chronological age is a regular, predictable reproductive cycle established?
a. 9 years
b. 11 years
c. 13 years
d. 15 years

36.2 Dysfunctional uterine bleeding is defined as
a. failure ever to menstruate
b. failure to menstruate due to anatomic obstruction
c. irregular menstruation without anatomic lesions of the uterus
d. failure to menstruate within 6 months of a previous menstrual cycle

36.3 Which of the following do amenorrhea and dysfunctional uterine bleeding have in common?
a. Both are associated with endometriosis
b. Both can result from anovulation
c. Both have similar levels of testosterone
d. Both have similar amounts of bleeding
e. Both carry a risk of cancer

36.4 What is the most common cause of secondary amenorrhea?
a. Ovarian failure
b. Cervical stenosis
c. Pregnancy
d. Vaginal agenesis
e. Outflow obstruction

36.5 What is the most common cause of pathologic amenorrhea?
a. Outflow obstruction
b. Disruption of the hypothalamic–pituitary axis
c. Asherman's syndrome
d. Kallmann's syndrome
e. Turner's syndrome

36.6 Which of the following distinguishes secondary from primary amenorrhea?
a. Absence of anatomic defects
b. History of prior menses
c. Chance of future fertility
d. Amount of bleeding at times other than menses
e. Follicle-stimulating hormone (FSH) levels

36.7 Disruption of the pulsatile secretion of gonadotropin-releasing hormone (GnRH) directly interferes with the secretion of
a. follicle-stimulating hormone (FSH)
b. estradiol
c. catecholamines
d. prolactin
e. adrenocorticotropic hormone (ACTH)

36.8 What tests can help differentiate hypothalamic–pituitary amenorrhea from ovarian failure?
a. Measurement of follicle-stimulating hormone (FSH) levels
b. Measurement of serum estradiol
c. Pregnancy test
d. Measurement of testosterone

Answers (36.1–36.8)											
36.1	c	36.3	b	36.5	b	36.6	b	36.7	a	36.8	a
36.2	c	36.4	c								

36.9　Ovarian failure is associated with
a. oligomenorrhea
b. hypomenorrhea
c. menorrhagia
d. amenorrhea
e. dysmenorrhea

36.10　What is the most common cause of
secondary amenorrhea that results
from anatomic abnormalities of the
genital outflow tract?
a. Cervical stenosis
b. Vaginal septum
c. Asherman's syndrome
d. Intact hymen
e. Labial adhesions

36.11　What is the typical cause of the
endometrial scarring that
characterizes Asherman's syndrome?
a. Infection
b. Previous dilation and curettage
c. Previous intrauterine device
(IUD) use
d. Previous hysterosalpingogram

36.12　Which of the following patients
would be classified as having
oligomenorrhea?
a. A 16 year old who has never
menstruated
b. A 22 year old with periods that
occur every 35 days and last 5
days
c. A 26 year old with periods that
occur every 28 days and last 2
days
d. A 45 year old with periods that
occur every 45 days and last
8–10 days
e. A 36 year old with periods that
occur every 8–10 months and
last 3–5 days

36.13　Estrogen is the primary therapy for
which of the following conditions?
a. Dysfunctional uterine bleeding
b. Menopausal vaginal atrophy
c. Precocious puberty
d. Oligomenorrhea
e. Secondary amenorrhea

36.14　What is the endocrine environment
that leads to dysfunctional uterine
bleeding?
a. Falling prolactin
b. Chronic progesterone effect
c. Chronic estrus
d. Fluctuating testosterone

36.15　What causes irregular bleeding in
women with dysfunctional uterine
bleeding?
a. Subclinical infection
b. Progesterone withdrawal
c. Noncyclical stimulation of
endometrial polyps
d. Endometrium outgrows its
blood supply
e. Secretory changes

36.16　What is the medical treatment of
choice for immediate management
of dysfunctional uterine bleeding?
a. Daily oral contraceptives
b. Progestin for 10 days
c. Progesterone in oil for 1 month
d. Gonadotropin-releasing
hormone (GnRH) agonist

36.17　What is the medical treatment of
choice for long-term management
of dysfunctional uterine bleeding?
a. Daily oral contraceptives
b. Progestin for 10 days
c. Progesterone in oil for 1 month
d. Gonadotropin-releasing
hormone (GnRH) agonist

36.18　In luteal phase defect, the
endometrium is not maintained
because there is insufficient
a. estrogen
b. progesterone
c. prolactin
d. follicle-stimulating hormone
(FSH)
e. luteinizing hormone (LH)

ANSWERS (36.9–36.18)

| 36.9 | d | 36.11 | b | 36.13 | b | 36.15 | d | 36.17 | a | 36.18 | b |
| 36.10 | c | 36.12 | d | 36.14 | c | 36.16 | b | | | | |

36.19 In evaluating the patient with amenorrhea, in what condition is serum prolactin elevated?
a. Pituitary adenoma
b. Weight loss
c. Obesity
d. Anorexia nervosa

36.20 In patients with hypothalamic amenorrhea, what is the typical pattern of FSH and LH?
a. FSH high, LH high
b. FSH low, LH low
c. FSH high, LH low
d. FSH low, LH high

36.21 In mild cases of intrauterine scarring, the best treatment is
a. Systemic estrogen administration
b. D and C
c. Vaginal estrogen administration
d. Laparoscopy

36.22 In cases of Asherman syndrome, the regeneration of endometrium in previously denuded areas is stimulated by what hormone?
a. Estrogen
b. Progesterone
c. Testosterone
d. Androstenedione

36.23 Hyperprolactinemia associated with some pituitary adenomas is associated with amenorrhea and
a. Hirsutism
b. Vaginal atrophy
c. Hot flushes
d. Galactorrhea

36.24 What percent of pituitary tumors secrete prolactin?
a. 5%
b. 20%
c. 50%
d. 80%

36.25 Which of the following conditions is commonly associated with chronic anovulation, also termed dysfunctional uterine bleeding?
a. Obesity
b. Anorexia nervosa
c. Leiomyomata uteri
d. Cervicitis

36.26 What type of bleeding pattern is characteristic of polycystic ovarian disease (aka polycystic ovarian syndrome)?
a. Menorrhagia
b. Amenorrhea
c. Hypomenorrhea
d. Chronic anovulation/ dysfunctional uterine bleeding

36.27 In patients with dysfunctional uterine bleeding, the lack of predictable ovulation results in the lack of the cyclic effect of what luteal phase hormone?
a. Estrogen
b. Prolactin
c. Progesterone
d. Testosterone

36.28 What phenomenon do amenorrhea and dysfunctional uterine bleeding share?
a. Anovulation
b. Pain
c. Vaginal discharge
d. Molimina

36.29 Which of the following is an example of dysfunctional uterine bleeding in the presence of ovulation?
a. Midcycle spotting
b. Postcoital spotting
c. Metrorrhagia
d. Postmenopausal bleeding

ANSWERS (36.19–36.29)

36.19 a	36.21 b	36.23 d	36.25 a	36.27 c	36.29 a
36.20 b	36.22 a	36.24 d	36.26 d	36.28 a	

36.30 A patient with luteal phase defect would typically complain of
a. Irregular periods
b. Shortened interval between periods
c. Unpredictable spotting
d. Postcoital bleeding

36.31 All of the following premenstrual symptoms are suggestive of ovulation EXCEPT
a. Abdominal bloating
b. Urinary frequency
c. Breast fullness
d. Mood changes
e. Edema

36.32. In which condition are cycles totally unpredictable?
a. Leiomyomata Uteri
b. Cervical Cancer
c. Dysfunctional uterine bleeding
d. Endometritis

36.33. What is a likely finding on endometrial biopsy of a patient with dysfunctional uterine bleeding (chronic anovulation)?
a. Secretory endometrium
b. Atrophic endometrium
c. Endometritis
d. Endometrial hyperplasia

36.34 A patient with dysfunctional uterine bleeding is at greater risk for developing what type of cancer?
a. Vaginal
b. Cervical
c. Endometrial
d. Ovarian
e. Gestational trophoblastic disease

36.35 Which of the following mimics the physiologic hormonal event that induces normal menstrual bleeding?
a. Administering estrogen
b. Administering progestin
c. Discontinuing estrogen
d. Discontinuing progestin

Questions and Answers Chapter 37: Hirsutism and Virilization

37.1   Which of the following is a common cause of hirsutism and virilization?
a. Hilus cell tumor
b. Polycystic ovarian disorder
c. Sertoli-Leydig tumor
d. Exogenous testosterone administration

37.2   Hirsutism and virilization are characterized as
a. estrogen excess disorders
b. androgen excess disorders
c. progesterone excess disorders
d. prolactin excess disorders

37.3   Which of the following is a major function of androgens in women?
a. Control of blood pressure
b. Determinant of adult weight
c. Precursor for estrogen biosynthesis
d. Modulator of anxiety disorders

37.4   The treatment for androgen excess disorders is directed at
a. suppression of source of androgen
b. stimulation of production of feminizing hormones
c. induction of estrogen receptors
d. reduction of hair growth

37.5   What histologic structure is characteristic of the hilus cell tumor?
a. Signet cell
b. Clue cell
c. Reinke crystalloid
d. Donovan body

37.6   Hirsutism is associated with
a. increased circulating testosterone
b. temporal balding
c. development of acne
d. enlargement of the clitoris
e. remodeling of the limb–shoulder girdle

37.7   Which is the first event usually associated with virilization?
a. Involution of the breasts
b. Deepening of the voice
c. Enlargement of the clitoris
d. Terminal hair growth
e. Temporal balding

37.8   In adipose tissue, there is extraglandular production of testosterone from
a. dehydroepiandrosterone
b. androstenedione
c. estrone
d. estriol

37.9   In hair follicles, dihydrotestosterone is produced by the local action of 5α-reductase on
a. dehydroepiandrosterone
b. testosterone
c. estrone
d. prolactin

37.10   What percent of testosterone is not bound to sex hormone–binding globulin (SHBG)?
a. 1% to 3%
b. 5% to 7%
c. 10% to 15%
d. 20% to 25%

37.11   The hepatic production of sex hormone–binding globulin (SHBG) is stimulated by
a. testosterone
b. dihydrotestosterone
c. estrogen
d. adrenocorticotropic hormone (ACTH)

ANSWERS (37.1–37.11)

37.1 b	37.3 c	37.5 c	37.7 c	37.9 b	37.11 c
37.2 b	37.4 a	37.6 c	37.8 b	37.10 a	

37.12 In women, the most common cause of hirsutism associated with androgen excess is
a. luteinizing hormone excess
b. genetic predisposition
c. obesity
d. polycystic ovarian disease

37.13 All of the following are characteristic symptoms of polycystic ovarian disease EXCEPT
a. oligomenorrhea
b. amenorrhea
c. anovulation
d. acne
e. virilization

37.14 Which of the following is a characteristic finding in women with polycystic ovarian disease?
a. Decreased luteinizing hormone:follicle-stimulating hormone (LH:FSH) ratio
b. Estradiol in greater concentration than estrone
c. Androstenedione at the upper limits of normal or increased
d. Testosterone at or below normal limits

37.15 All of the following result from treatment of polycystic ovarian disease with oral contraceptives EXCEPT
a. suppressed luteinizing hormone (LH) production
b. decreased production of androstenedione
c. decreased production of testosterone
d. increased ovarian contribution to total androgen pool
e. decreased incidence of endometrial hyperplasia

37.16 Virilization associated with polycystic ovarian disease is seen in
a. hyperthecosis
b. androgen insensitivity syndrome
c. hyperandrogenic syndrome
d. acanthosis nigricans

37.17 Sertoli-Leydig cell tumors are characterized by which of the following?
a. The tumors secrete testosterone
b. They are a common form of ovarian tumor
c. They typically occur in women who are between the ages of 50 and 60
d. They are usually bilateral

37.18 Patients with Sertoli-Leydig cell tumors typically have
a. an increased level of follicle-stimulating hormone (FSH)
b. an increased level of luteinizing hormone (LH)
c. a high plasma androstenedione level
d. an elevated level of testosterone

37.19 Following the surgical removal of a unilateral Sertoli-Leydig cell tumor
a. ovulatory cycles return spontaneously in most patients
b. hirsutism is reversed in most patients
c. the clitoris reverts to its pretreatment dimensions
d. the 10-year survival rate is approximately 50%–55%

Instructions for items 37.20 to 37.21: Match the virilizing–masculinizing ovarian tumor with the appropriate descriptions. An option may be used once, more than once, or not at all.

37.20 Gynandroblastoma

37.21 Lipid (lipoid) cell tumors
   a. Overgrowth of mature hilus cells or from the ovarian mesenchyme
   b. Small tumor containing sheets of round, clear, pale staining cells
   c. Granulosa cell and arrhenoblastoma components
   d. Contain Reinke crystalloids
   e. Unilateral and usually benign

37.22 Following medical treatment of adrenal hyperplasia with prednisone
   a. facial acne usually persists
   b. ovulation is usually restored
   c. new terminal hair growth accelerates
   d. hirsutism resolves quickly

37.23 Which of the following is characteristic of 11β-hydroxylase deficiency?
   a. Severe hypertension
   b. Severe hirsutism
   c. Increased serum desoxycorticosterone
   d. Reduced conversion of progesterone to cortisol

37.24 Women with constitutional hirsutism
   a. do not ovulate
   b. have greater activity of 5α-reductase
   c. have abnormal estrogen levels
   d. have severe acne

37.25 The potent metabolite of testosterone that is produced in genital skin and hair follicles is
   a. dehydroepiandrosterone
   b. dihydrotestosterone
   c. androstenedione

37.26 Which of the following is associated with hirsutism?
   a. Excess body hair
   b. Involution of the breasts
   c. Deepening voice
   d. Remodeling of limb-shoulder girdle

37.27 An elevated 24-hour free cortisol is suggestive of what condition?
   a. Cushing's disease
   b. Polycystic ovarian disease
   c. Sarcoidosis
   d. Porphyria

Questions and Answers Chapter 38: Menopause

38.1 The climacteric is defined as the:
a. time of the last menstrual flow
b. time when the symptoms of menopause first begin
c. transition from the reproductive to the nonreproductive years
d. last five regular menstrual cycles

38.2 The average age of menopause is approximately:
a. 40 years
b. 45 years
c. 50 years
d. 55 years
e. 60 years

38.3 Ovarian function ceases by 55 years of age in what percent of women?
a. 80%
b. 85%
c. 90%
d. 95%
e. 99%

38.4 Between infancy and the time of menopause, the number of oocytes in the ovary:
a. steadily increases
b. increases and then decreases
c. steadily decreases
d. remains constant

38.5 Approximately how many oocytes will a woman ovulate during her reproductive years?
a. 100
b. 200
c. 300
d. 400
e. 500

38.6 Approximately how many oocytes does a woman have at the time of puberty?
a. 4000
b. 40,000
c. 400,000
d. 4 million

38.7 As a woman approaches menopause, there is:
a. increased sensitivity of granulosa cells to testosterone
b. reduced sensitivity of oocytes to follicle-stimulating hormone (FSH)
c. increased sensitivity of theca luteal cells to estrogen
d. reduced sensitivity of ovarian stromal cells to gonadotropin-releasing hormone (GnRH)

38.8 Which hormone is the major product of the postmenopausal ovary?
a. Luteinizing hormone (LH)
b. Estradiol-17β
c. Testosterone
d. Estrone

38.9 The plasma concentration of follicle-stimulating hormone (FSH) begins to increase:
a. approximately 10 years before menopause
b. approximately 3 years before menopause
c. at the time of menopause
d. approximately 3 years after menopause
e. approximately 10 years after menopause

ANSWERS (38.1–38.9)					
38.1 c	38.3 d	38.5 d	38.7 b	38.8 c	38.9 b
38.2 c	38.4 c	38.6 c			

Instructions for items 38.10 to 38.13: Match the life stage with the corresponding follicle-stimulating hormone (FSH) level that normally would be expected. An option may be used once, more than once, or not at all.

38.10 Childhood

38.11 Prime reproductive years

38.12 Perimenopause

38.13 Menopause
  a. >30 mIU/ml
  b. 14–24 mIU/ml
  c. 6–10 mIU/ml
  d. <4 mIU/ml

38.14 Which of the following is generally the first physical manifestation of ovarian failure?
  a. Sleep disturbance
  b. Vaginal dryness
  c. Hot flushes
  d. Mood changes
  e. Skin thickening

38.15 Decrease in the level of which of the following hormones is responsible for the vasomotor symptoms of menopause?
  a. Progesterone
  b. Estrogen
  c. Testosterone
  d. Follicle-stimulating hormone (FSH)
  e. Androstenedione

38.16 Which of the following statements about hot flushes is INCORRECT?
  a. Over 95% of perimenopausal and menopausal women experience hot flushes (vasomotor instability).
  b. As a woman approaches menopause, the frequency and intensity of hot flushes increases.
  c. Hot flushes may be associated with disabling diaphoresis.
  d. If a menopausal woman does not receive estrogen replacement therapy, hot flushes will resolve within 6–9 months.

38.17 What is the effect of decreasing estrogen on the sleep cycle?
  a. Latent phase shortened, sleep period shortened
  b. Latent phase shortened, sleep period lengthened
  c. Latent phase lengthened, sleep period shortened
  d. Latent phase lengthened, sleep period lengthened

38.18 Which of the following statements about vaginal atrophy associated with menopause is INCORRECT?
  a. The vaginal epithelium becomes thin.
  b. Cervical secretions increase in quantity.
  c. Many patients experience dyspareunia.
  d. Vaginal tissue is more likely to become infected by local flora.

38.19 Which of the following is an effect of estrogen deficiency on paravaginal tissue?
  a. Bladder prolapse
  b. Uterine retroversion
  c. Urinary retention
  d. Vaginal vault prolapse

ANSWERS (38.10–38.19)

38.10 d	38.12 b	38.14 c	38.16 d	38.18 b	38.19 a
38.11 c	38.13 a	38.15 b	38.17 c		

38.20 Which of the following is NOT a consequence of estrogen deficiency?
a. Acne
b. Thinning of the skin
c. Brittle nails
d. Synchronous hair shedding

38.21 Which of the following is not a sign or symptom common to menopausal women not taking estrogen replacement therapy?
a. Dyspareunia
b. Urinary frequency and urgency
c. Increased breast size
d. Altered libido
e. Vasomotor symptoms

38.22 About what percent of women experience vasomotor symptoms (hot flushes) in the perimenopausal and menopausal period?
a. 35%
b. 55%
c. 75%
d. 95%

38.23 Increased facial hair in menopausal women results from:
a. increased testosterone production
b. increased dihydrotestosterone production
c. increased dehydroepiandrosterone sulfate (DHEAS) production
d. reduced sex hormone-binding globulin

38.24 What is the expected rate of bone loss in perimenopausal women?
a. 0.1% per year
b. 0.5% per year
c. 1% per year
d. 5% per year

38.25 What is the expected rate of bone loss in postmenopausal women who are not receiving estrogen?
a. 0.1%–0.2% per year
b. 0.5% per year
c. 1%–2% per year
d. 5% per year

38.26 Which of the following is NOT a risk factor for osteoporosis?
a. Reduced height for weight
b. Family history of osteoporosis
c. Late menopause
d. Low calcium intake
e. Cigarette smoking
f. Nulliparity
g. High alcohol intake
h. High caffeine intake

38.27 Which of the following is most effective in reducing postmenopausal bone loss?
a. Weight-bearing exercise
b. Calcium supplementation
c. Estrogen replacement therapy
d. Vitamin D supplementation
e. Calcitonin therapy

38.28 Compared with normal women, What is the number of ovarian follicles in women with Savage's syndrome?
a. increased
b. unchanged
c. reduced

38.29 Cigarette smoking has what effect on the timing of menopause?
a. Smokers experience menopause 3–5 years earlier than nonsmokers.
b. Smokers experience menopause at about the same time as nonsmokers.
c. Smokers experience menopause 3–5 years later than nonsmokers.
d. Smokers experience a longer period of menopausal symptoms.

ANSWERS (38.20–38.29)

38.20 a	38.22 d	38.24 b	38.26 c	38.28 b	38.29 a
38.21 c	38.23 d	38.25 c	38.27 c		

38.30 Individuals who smoke:
   a. do not respond as well as nonsmokers to estrogen replacement therapy
   b. respond equally as well as nonsmokers to estrogen replacement therapy
   c. respond better than nonsmokers to estrogen replacement therapy

38.31 Approximately what percent of women will experience menopause before the age of 40?
   a. 1%
   b. 5%
   c. 10%
   d. 15%

38.32 Which of the following has not been found to be a factor in premature menopause?
   a. Chromosomal abnormalities
   b. Follicle resistance to follicle-stimulating hormone (FSH)
   c. Production of autoantibodies
   d. Obesity

Instructions for items 38.33 to 38.39: Match the commercial preparation listed below with the reproductive hormone that it contains. An option may be used once, more than once, or not at all.

38.33 Climara/Estraderm patch

38.34 Ogen

38.35 Premarin

38.36 Estrace

38.37 Depo-Provera

38.38 Provera (oral)

38.39 Norlutate
   a. Estradiol-17β
   b. Conjugated estrogens
   c. Esterified estrogen
   d. Estropipate (piperazine estrone sulfate)
   e. Ethinyl estradiol
   f. Medroxyprogesterone acetate
   g. Micronized estradiol
   h. Norethindrone acetate

38.40 Women with a history of thromboembolic disease:
   a. should not receive estrogen replacement therapy
   b. may receive oral or injectable estrogen replacement therapy
   c. may receive transdermal estrogen replacement therapy

38.41 Which of the following is a known risk of unopposed estrogen replacement therapy?
   a. Endometrial hyperplasia
   b. Leiomyoma uteri
   c. Endocervical adenocarcinoma
   d. Squamous cell carcinoma of the cervix

38.42 If estrogen is administered alone for menopausal hormone replacement therapy because of unacceptable side effects of progestins, then the patient should specifically be counseled as to the need for which if the following tests?
   a. Yearly PAP smear
   b. Yearly endometrial biopsy
   c. Yearly complete blood count
   d. Yearly fecal occult blood test

Answers (38.30–38.42)					
38.30 a	38.33 a	38.35 b	38.37 f	38.39 h	38.41 a
38.31 a	38.34 d	38.36 g	38.38 f	38.40 c	38.42 b
38.32 d					

**Questions and Answers Chapter 39:
Infertility**

39.1   Approximately what percent of
       couples will conceive within one
       year?
       a. 50%
       b. 60%
       c. 70%
       d. 80%
       e. 90%

39.2   Infertility is defined as a couple's
       failure to conceive following
       unprotected sexual intercourse for
       a. 6 months
       b. 1 year
       c. 2 years
       d. 3 years
       e. 4 years

39.3   Infertility affects what percent of
       reproductive age couples in the
       United States?
       a. 1%
       b. 5%
       c. 10%
       d. 15%
       e. 25%

39.4   What percent of couples with a
       clinical diagnosis of infertility may
       expect to have a child with
       appropriate specific diagnosis and
       treatment?
       a. 55%
       b. 65%
       c. 75%
       d. 85%
       e. 95%

39.5   Fertility is decreased by about how
       much between about the 37th and
       45th year of a woman's life?
       a. 25%
       b. 50%
       c. 75%
       d. 90%

39.6   Anovulation, anatomic defects of
       the female genital tract, and
       abnormal spermatogenesis together
       account for what percent of
       reproductive dysfunction?
       a. 65%
       b. 75%
       c. 85%
       d. 95%

39.7   The characteristic biphasic
       temperature shift associated with
       ovulation occurs in what percent of
       ovulating women?
       a. 60%
       b. 70%
       c. 80%
       d. 90%
       e. 99%

39.8   A rise in basal body temperature
       typically occurs
       a. 2–3 days before ovulation
       b. at the time of ovulation
       c. 2–3 days after ovulation
       d. immediately before menstruation

39.9   If a woman does not conceive, how
       many days after ovulation will her
       basal body temperature return to
       pre-ovulatory levels?
       a. 8
       b. 10
       c. 14
       d. 18
       e. 22

39.10 There is a strong possibility of
       pregnancy if basal body
       temperature remains elevated at
       least
       a. 10 days
       b. 14 days
       c. 16 days
       d. 20 days
       e. 24 days

ANSWERS (39.1–39.10)

| 39.1 | e | 39.3 | d | 39.5 | b | 39.7 | d | 39.9 | c | 39.10 | c |
| 39.2 | b | 39.4 | d | 39.6 | d | 39.8 | b | | | | |

39.11 What portion of an ejaculate contains the greatest density of sperm?
   a. First quarter
   b. Second quarter
   c. Third quarter
   d. Last quarter

39.12 After a semen specimen is collected, semen analysis should be performed within
   a. 1 hour
   b. 2 hours
   c. 4 hours
   d. 6 hours
   e. 8 hours

39.13 In a normal semen specimen, abnormal sperm forms constitute less than what percent of the total?
   a. 10%
   b. 15%
   c. 20%
   d. 25%
   e. 30%

39.14 A normal semen analysis contains at least what percent of motile sperm?
   a. 40%
   b. 50%
   c. 60%
   d. 70%
   e. 80%

39.15 A normal semen analysis excludes a male cause for infertility in what percent of cases?
   a. 50%
   b. 60%
   c. 70%
   d. 80%
   e. 90%
   f. 100%

39.16 A normal semen analysis is characterized by full liquefaction within
   a. 15 minutes
   b. 60 minutes
   c. 90 minutes
   d. 120 minutes

39.17 In detecting abnormalities of the genital tract, a hysterosalpingogram has a diagnostic accuracy of approximately
   a. 30%
   b. 50%
   c. 70%
   d. 90%

39.18 On average, the menstrual cycle of a healthy woman between the ages of 18 and 36 is characterized by
   a. ovulation 13 to 14 times per year
   b. ovulation occurring on the tenth day
   c. menstruation beginning on the thirtieth day
   d. menstruation lasting approximately 3 days

39.19 Following ovulation, the basal body temperature
   a. increases by 0.6°F
   b. increases by 0.2°F
   c. does not change
   d. decreases by 0.2°F
   e. decreases by 0.6°F

39.20 Which of the following is typical of the luteal phase of the menstrual cycle?
   a. Improvement of mood
   b. Presence of a proliferative endometrium
   c. Appearance of sticky cervical mucus
   d. Proliferation of the breast ducts

ANSWERS (39.11–39.20)

39.11 a	39.13 d	39.15 e	39.17 c	39.19 a	39.20 c
39.12 b	39.14 c	39.16 b	39.18 a		

39.21 Which of the following is NOT associated with abnormal sperm morphology?
a. Varicocele
b. Infection
c. Immunologic factors, including antisperm antibodies
d. Stress

39.22 Capacitation of sperm occurs in the
a. fallopian tube
b. endometrial cavity
c. endocervix
d. vagina

39.23 The generation time of sperm is approximately
a. 33 days
b. 53 days
c. 73 days
d. 93 days
e. 113 days

39.24 Normal sperm production typically occurs at a temperature that is approximately
a. 3°F above body temperature
b. 1°F above body temperature
c. at body temperature
d. 1°F below body temperature
e. 3°F below body temperature

39.25 Which of the following does NOT result in decreased sperm production resulting from thermal shock?
a. Spending excessive time in hot tubs or hot baths
b. Sitting on the testicles for long periods of time with poor heat dispersion
c. Wearing tight clothing
d. Living in a climate where the temperature exceeds 90°F for long periods

Instructions for items 39.26 to 39.31: For each case of infertility described below, select the most appropriate initial test or procedure. An option may be used once, more than once, or not at all.

39.26 A 32-year-old G2P2002 who has recently married a 35-year-old man with no children

39.27 A 21-year-old G1P0010 who has had amenorrhea since an elective abortion that was followed by infection

39.28 A 28-year-old G1P1001 who wishes to increase her chance of pregnancy by the timing of intercourse

39.29 A 32-year-old G0 with a history of chronic pelvic pain and dysmenorrhea whose partner has a normal semen analysis

39.30 A 26-year-old G0 with a history of irregular periods, who works several jobs, and has unpredictable sleeping patterns

39.31 A couple undergoing infertility evaluation who demonstrate clumping of sperm on the Hunter-Sims test
a. Antisperm antibodies
b. Basal body temperature record
c. Diagnostic laparoscopy
d. Endometrial biopsy
e. Hysterosalpingogram
f. Hysteroscopy
g. Luteal phase progesterone
h. Postcoital test
i. Semen analysis
j. Urinary luteinizing hormone detection kit

ANSWERS (39.21–39.31)

39.21 c	39.23 c	39.25 d	39.27 e	39.29 c	39.31 a
39.22 c	39.24 d	39.26 i	39.28 b	39.30 g	

39.32 Clomiphene citrate
  a. acts by stimulating estrogen production and binding
  b. should be administered in conjunction with progesterone
  c. results in an increase in the release of follicle-stimulating hormone from the pituitary
  d. dosage should not exceed 50 mg/day

39.33 What is the success rate of clomiphene citrate in inducing spermatogenesis?
  a. 5%
  b. 10%
  c. 15%
  d. 20%
  e. 25%

39.34 The expected success rate of in vitro fertilization in properly selected couples is approximately
  a. 13% to 17% per cycle
  b. 18% to 22% per cycle
  c. 23% to 27% per cycle
  d. 28% to 32% per cycle
  e. 33% to 37% per cycle

39.35 How many days after the completion of therapy with clomiphene citrate do presumptive signs of ovulation occur?
  a. 1–3 days
  b. 4–6 days
  c. 7–11 days
  d. 12–14 days
  e. 15–17 days

39.36 "Spinnbarkeit" is a term that means
  a. mucus secretion of the cervix
  b. thinning of the cervical mucus
  c. threading of cervical mucus
  d. crystallization of the cervical mucus

39.37 Luteal phase failure as a cause of infertility is treated by
  a. thyroid hormone
  b. estrogens and progestins combined
  c. progestins alone
  d. Pergonal

39.38 A serum progesterone level above what level is 80% accurate in distinguishing a normal from an abnormal cycle?
  a. 15 ng/ml
  b. 25 ng/ml
  c. 35 ng/ml
  d. 45 ng/ml

39.39 A serum progesterone level below what level is rarely associated with normal cycles?
  a. 40 ng/ml
  b. 30 ng/ml
  c. 20 ng/ml
  d. 10 ng/ml

ANSWERS (39.32–39.39)

39.32 c	39.34 b	39.36 c	39.37 c	39.38 a	39.39 d
39.33 d	39.35 c				

Questions and Answers Chapter 40: Premenstrual Syndrome

40.1   Which of the following statements about premenstrual syndrome (PMS) is INCORRECT?
a. PMS occurs in a regular, cyclical relationship to the luteal phase of the menstrual cycle
b. The signs and symptoms of PMS can resemble certain psychiatric conditions
c. It has been suggested that PMS is more than a single clinical entity
d. The signs and symptoms of PMS tend to increase in severity over time

40.2   The symptoms of premenstrual syndrome typically resolve
a. near the onset of menses
b. midway through menses
c. near the end of menses
d. about 2 weeks after menses

40.3   In premenstrual syndrome, there is a symptom-free interval of at least
a. 1 week
b. 2 weeks
c. 3 weeks

40.4   What percent of women have some physical or emotional premenstrual symptoms?
a. 30%
b. 50%
c. 70%
d. 90%

40.5   Premenstrual syndrome that is severe and debilitating occurs in what percent of women?
a. 10%
b. 20%
c. 30%
d. 40%

40.6   Premenstrual syndrome tends to be more common in women in which of the following age groups?
a. Teens and 20s
b. 20s and 30s
c. 30s and 40s
d. 40s and 50s

40.7   In making the diagnosis of premenstrual syndrome, the characteristic that is most important is the
a. severity of symptoms
b. duration of symptoms
c. cyclic occurrence of symptoms
d. degree of disability in the patient
e. association with exogenous therapy

Instructions for items 40.8 to 40.12: Match the theoretical etiology of premenstrual syndrome with the appropriate supporting evidence. An option may be used once, more than once, or not at all.

40.8   Psychiatric basis

40.9   Endocrinologic basis

40.10 Dietary basis

40.11 Endorphin basis

40.12 Serotonin basis
a. Occurrence of premenstrual hypoglycemic episodes
b. Production of this substance declines during the luteal phase
c. Presence of abnormal luteal phase steroid levels
d. Lower premenstrual levels than in comparable control patients, associated with depression
e. Cyclic manifestation of underlying pathology

ANSWERS (40.1–40.12)					
40.1 d	40.3 a	40.5 a	40.7 c	40.9 c	40.11 b
40.2 c	40.4 c	40.6 c	40.8 e	40.10 a	40.12 d

40.13 Data supporting the endorphin basis of premenstrual syndrome comes from patients who report alleviation of symptoms with
a. aspirin consumption
b. exercise
c. caffeine consumption
d. bed rest
e. sexual arousal

40.14 The most useful diagnostic tool with respect to premenstrual syndrome is
a. serial progesterone levels
b. serial blood glucose determinations
c. a menstrual diary
d. cyclic vaginal wall cytology
e. a symptom list

40.15 Buspirone (BuSpar) has been found to have effect in premenstrual syndrome patients after approximately how many weeks of therapy?
a. 1 week
b. 2 weeks
c. 3 weeks
d. 4 weeks
e. 5 weeks

40.16 Which of the following is NOT a component of dietary therapy for premenstrual syndrome?
a. Increased intake of fresh fruits and vegetables
b. Decreased intake of refined sugars
c. Intake of three substantial meals a day with no between meal snacking
d. Decreased intake of salt
e. Decreased intake of caffeine

40.17 Which of the following may be useful in the long-term treatment of premenstrual syndrome-associated mastodynia?
a. Tetracycline
b. Premarin
c. Bromocriptine
d. Gonadotropin-releasing hormone agonist
e. Prostaglandin $F_{2\alpha}$

40.18 Which of the following is useful to confirm the diagnosis of premenstrual syndrome?
a. Tetracycline
b. Premarin
c. Bromocriptine
d. Gonadotropin-releasing hormone agonist
e. Prostaglandin $F_{2\alpha}$

Answers (40.13–40.18)

| 40.13 b | 40.14 c | 40.15 b | 40.16 c | 40.17 c | 40.18 d |

Questions and Answers Chapter 41: Cell Biology and Principles of Cancer Therapy

41.1 Cells are especially vulnerable to anticancer therapies during what portion of the cell cycle?
   a. The portion of the cycle when cells are dividing.
   b. The portion of time when cells are in the resting stage.
   c. Both the dividing and resting stages

Instructions for items 41.2 to 41.6: Match the phase of the cell cycle with the major event occurring during the phase. An option may be used once, more than once, or not at all.

41.2 G_0

41.3 G_1

41.4 G_2

41.5 S

41.6 M
   a. Synthesis of RNA and protein in preparation for DNA synthesis
   b. DNA synthesis
   c. Additional RNA, protein, and specialized DNA synthesis
   d. Cell division occurs
   e. Resting phase

41.7 Anticancer therapies specifically designed to affect cells engaged in synthetic activities are LEAST effective during which stage of the cell cycle?
   a. G_0
   b. G_1
   c. G_2
   d. S

41.8 What is the phase of the cell cycle that is the most variable in length?
   a. G_1
   b. S
   c. G_2
   d. M

41.9 The growth fraction is the number of cells in a tumor that are NOT in the:
   a. G_0 phase
   b. S phase
   c. G_1 phase
   d. G_2 phase

41.10 As a tumor enlarges in size, the growth fraction:
   a. increases
   b. remains the same
   c. decreases

41.11 Cytoreductive debulking surgery has what effect on the remaining tumor cells?
   a. Causes tumor cells to enter the G_0 phase
   b. Causes tumor cells to leave the G_0 phase
   c. Causes the growth fraction of tumor cells to decrease
   d. The surgery has no effect on the remaining tumor cells

Instructions for items 41.12 to 41.15: Match the class of antineoplastic drug with its major characteristic/action(s). An option may be used once, more than once, or not at all.

41.12 Alkylating agents

41.13 Antitumor antibiotics

41.14 Antimetabolites

ANSWERS (41.1–41.14)

41.1	a	41.4	c	41.7	a	41.9	a	41.11	b	41.13	c
41.2	e	41.5	b	41.8	a	41.10	c	41.12	d	41.14	b
41.3	a	41.6	d								

41.15 Plant alkaloids
  a. Affects assembly of microtubules
  b. Structural analogs of normal molecules necessary for cell function
  c. Inhibits DNA directed RNA synthesis
  d. Interferes with base pairs, producing cross links, causing single- and double-strand breaks

Instructions for items 41.16 to 41.19: Match the class of antineoplastic drug with the phase of the cell cycle in which the drug is active. An option may be used once, more than once, or not at all.

41.16 Alkylating agents

41.17 Antitumor antibiotics

41.18 Antimetabolites

41.19 Plant alkaloids
  a. G_1
  b. S
  c. G_2
  d. M
  e. Phase nonspecific

41.20 Suppression of blood cell formation is a common side effect of:
  a. alkylating agents
  b. antitumor antibiotics
  c. plant alkaloids
  d. antimetabolites
  e. all of the above

41.21 Impaired renal function is most often associated with the use of which antineoplastic drug?
  a. Methotrexate
  b. Cisplatin
  c. Busulfan
  d. Hydroxyurea

Instructions for items 41.22 to 41.25: Match the class of antineoplastic drug with examples of drugs from that class. An option may be used once, more than once, or not at all.

41.22 Alkylating agents

41.23 Antitumor antibiotics

41.24 Antimetabolites

41.25 Plant alkaloids
  a. Busulfan (Myleran)
  b. Chlorambucil (Leukeran)
  c. Bleomycin (Blenoxane)
  d. Actinomycin D
  e. Methotrexate
  f. 6-Mercaptopurine
  g. 5-Fluorouracil
  h. Hydroxyurea
  i. Mitoxantrone
  j. Nitrogen mustard
  k. Cyclophosphamide
  l. Doxorubicin
  m. Melphalan
  n. Ifosfamide
  o. Vinblastine
  p. Vincristine
  q. Cisplatin

41.26 Which of the following is NOT a criterion that must be met in order for antineoplastic drugs to be used in combination?
  a. They must be effective when used singularly.
  b. They must have different mechanisms of action.
  c. They must be additive in action.
  d. They must not lead to drug resistance.

ANSWERS (41.15–41.26)

41.15 a	41.18 b	41.21 b	41.23 c, d, i, l	41.25 o, p
41.16 a, b	41.19 d	41.22 a, b, j, k, m, n	41.24 e, f, g, h	41.26 d
41.17 e	41.20 e			

Instructions for items 41.27 to 41.29: Match the type of interaction between antineoplastic drugs with the appropriate definition. An option may be used once, more than once, or not at all.

41.27 Additive

41.28 Antagonistic

41.29 Synergistic
   a. Improved antitumor activity or decreased toxicity compared with each agent alone
   b. Enhanced antitumor activity equal to the sum of each of the individual agents
   c. Less antitumor activity than each individual agent

41.30 In sequential blockade combination chemotherapy, the drugs:
   a. interfere with different steps in the synthesis of DNA or RNA
   b. attack parallel biochemical pathways leading to the same end product
   c. block enzymes in a single biochemical pathway

Instructions for items 41.31 to 41.33: Match the type of chemotherapy regimen with its definition and therapeutic goal. An option may be used once, more than once, or not at all.

41.31 Adjuvant chemotherapy

41.32 Induction chemotherapy

41.33 Maintenance chemotherapy
   a. A short course of combination chemotherapy given in high doses for the purpose of eliminating residual cancer cells
   b. Long-term and low-dose therapy designed to keep a patient in remission by inhibiting the growth of remaining cancer cells
   c. High-dose combination chemotherapy with the goal of causing remission

41.34 Radiation therapy kills cells according to:
   a. zero order kinetics
   b. first order kinetics
   c. second order kinetics

41.35 Compared with fractionated small doses, a single, large focused dose of radiation is:
   a. more likely to be effective in destroying a tumor
   b. as likely to be effective in destroying a tumor
   c. less likely to be effective in destroying a tumor

41.36 How does the presence of oxygen affect tumor cells' vulnerability to radiation?
   a. Oxygen increases vulnerability
   b. Oxygen does not affect vulnerability
   c. Oxygen decreases vulnerability

41.37 Local irradiation of tumor cells is termed:
   a. teletherapy
   b. brachytherapy
   c. maintenance therapy

Answers (41.27–41.37)

41.27 b	41.29 a	41.31 a	41.33 b	41.35 c	41.37 b
41.28 c	41.30 c	41.32 c	41.34 b	41.36 a	

41.38 One gray equals:
a. 1 rad
b. 10 rads
c. 100 rads
d. 1000 rads

41.39 One gray is defined as one joule per:
a. kilogram
b. meter^2
c. meter
d. rad

41.40 Tamoxifen acts as a competitive inhibitor of:
a. progesterone binding
b. estrogen binding
c. prolactin binding
d. follicle-stimulating hormone (FSH) binding

**Questions and Answers Chapter 42:
Gestational Trophoblastic Disease**

42.1   Approximately what percent of
patients with gestational
trophoblastic disease will develop
persistent or malignant disease?
a. 10%
b. 20%
c. 30%
d. 40%
e. 60%

42.2   The incidence of gestational
trophoblastic disease in the United
States is approximately one in how
many pregnancies?
a. 500
b. 1000
c. 1500
d. 2000
e. 2500
f. 3000

42.3   Genetically, complete moles are of:
a. paternal origin only
b. maternal origin only
c. mixed paternal and maternal
origin

42.4   Approximately what percent of
molar pregnancies are of the
complete mole type?
a. 50%
b. 60%
c. 70%
d. 80%
e. 90%

**Instructions for items 42.5 to 42.6: Match
the type of molar pregnancy with its appropriate characteristics. An option may be
used once, more than once, or not at all.**

42.5   Complete molar pregnancy

42.6   Incomplete molar pregnancy
a. Karyotype commonly 69,XXY
b. Karyotype commonly 46,XX
c. Fetal membranes absent
d. Chromosomally abnormal fetus
present
e. Proliferation of the
syncytiotrophoblast
f. Proliferation from the
cytotrophoblast
g. All villi edematous

42.7   Compared with a partial mole,
what is the potential for malignant
transformation in a complete mole?
a. higher
b. the same
c. lower

42.8   Abnormal bleeding during a
complete molar pregnancy most
commonly occurs early in which
trimester?
a. First
b. Second
c. Third

42.9   A discrepancy between the uterine
size and the gestational age is seen
in approximately what percent of
patients with complete molar
pregnancy?
a. 30%
b. 50%
c. 70%
d. 90%

42.10   Which of the following is NOT a
sign or symptom commonly seen in
molar pregnancy?
a. Pregnancy-induced hypertension
b. Severe nausea
c. Bradycardia
d. Visual disturbances

ANSWERS (42.1–42.10)

42.1 a	42.3 a	42.5 b, c, e, g	42.7 a	42.9 c	42.10 c
42.2 d	42.4 e	42.6 a, d, f	42.8 b		

42.11 Which of the following statements about invasive mole is incorrect?
   a. It is a complete mole invading the myometrium without any intervening endometrial stroma.
   b. It often is diagnosed months after evacuation of a complete mole following evaluation for hCG levels which do not fall appropriately.
   c. It may be diagnosed on curettage at the time of initial molar evacuation.
   d. Its natural course includes local invasion and, on occasion, vascular invasion and metastasis.
   e. It follows after 35–45% of complete hydatidiform moles.

42.12 A molar pregnancy is confirmed through:
   a. serial measurement of human chorionic gonadotropin (hCG) levels
   b. use of ultrasound imaging
   c. bimanual pelvic examination

42.13 Compared with patients with complete molar pregnancy, patients with partial molar pregnancy typically present at:
   a. an earlier gestational age
   b. the same gestational age
   c. a later gestational age

42.14 The determination of human chorionic gonadotropin (hCG) titers associated with molar pregnancy is NOT useful for:
   a. classifying the risk category for the tumor
   b. serving as a tumor marker in follow-up of therapy
   c. ascertaining whether the pregnancy is a partial or complete mole

42.15 Which of the following is NOT characteristic of high-risk gestational trophoblastic disease?
   a. Uterus greater than 16-week size
   b. Presence of a large theca lutein cyst
   c. Marked trophoblastic proliferation and/or anaplasia
   d. Hyperthyroidism
   e. 46,XX karyotype

42.16 What is the basic treatment of molar pregnancy?
   a. evacuation of the uterine contents
   b. abdominal hysterectomy
   c. abdominal hysterectomy with bilateral salpingo-oophorectomy
   d. radiation therapy
   e. chemotherapy

42.17 In the follow-up of a molar pregnancy, serum human chorionic gonadotropin (hCG) levels should be obtained monthly for how many months?
   a. 6 months
   b. 12 months
   c. 18 months
   d. 24 months

42.18 Following molar pregnancy, what is the incidence of placental accreta?
   a. increased
   b. unchanged
   c. decreased

42.19 In the United States, what is the incidence of choriocarcinoma?
   a. 1 in 40 normal pregnancies
   b. 1 in 5000 normal pregnancies
   c. 1 in 15,000 normal pregnancies
   d. 1 in 150,000 normal pregnancies

ANSWERS (42.11–42.19)

42.11 e	42.13 c	42.15 e	42.17 b	42.18 a	42.19 d
42.12 b	42.14 c	42.16 a			

42.20 In the United States, choriocarcinoma is associated with approximately one in how many moles?
a. 1 in 40
b. 1 in 5000
c. 1 in 15,000
d. 1 in 150,000

42.21 In the United States, choriocarcinoma is associated with approximately one in how many abortions?
a. 1 in 40
b. 1 in 5000
c. 1 in 15,000
d. 1 in 150,000

42.22 In the United States, choriocarcinoma is associated with approximately one in how many ectopic pregnancies?
a. 1 in 40
b. 1 in 5000
c. 1 in 15,000
d. 1 in 150,000

42.23 Which of the following is not an indication for chemotherapy in trophoblastic disease?
a. Histologic diagnosis of choriocarcinoma
b. Evidence of metastatic disease
c. Plateaued or rising human chorionic gonadotropin (hCG) titers after evacuation
d. β-hCG titer that has returned to normal after 12 weeks' post evacuation
e. Increased β-hCG titer after a normal level has been obtained, exclusive of a normal pregnancy

42.24 The recurrence rate for gestational trophoblastic disease is approximately:
a. 2%
b. 4%
c. 6%
d. 8%

42.25 The treatment of a patient with a hydatidiform mole could include all of the following EXCEPT:
a. period assays of serum β-human chorionic gonadotropin (β-hCG)
b. periodic clinical examinations for the detection of malignant changes
c. radiotherapy
d. prophylactic chemotherapy
e. evacuation of the uterus.

42.26 Eclampsia in the first trimester is most frequently associated with:
a. abruptio placenta
b. acute glomerulonephritis
c. molar degeneration
d. pregnancy-induced hypertension
e. berry aneurysm

42.27 What is a serious complication of choriocarcinoma?
a. intestinal obstruction
b. uterine perforation and massive bleeding
c. cardiac arrhythmia
d. multifocal seizures

42.28 Which of the following statements about placental site tumors is incorrect?
a. The tumor is comprised of monomorphic populations of intermediate cytotrophoblast cells which are locally invasive at the site of placental implantation.
b. The tumor secretes placental lactogen.
c. The tumor is rarely metastatic.
d. The tumor is very sensitive to standard chemotherapy.

ANSWERS (42.20–42.28)

42.20 a	42.22 b	42.24 a	42.26 c	42.27 b	42.28 d
42.21 c	42.23 d	42.25 c			

Questions and Answers Chapter 43:
Vulvar and Vaginal Disease and Neoplasia

Instructions for items 43.1 to 43.4: Match the common vulvar dermatosis with the appropriate description. An option may be used once, more than once, or not at all.

43.1 Lichen simplex chronicus (LSC)

43.2 Lichen planus

43.3 Psoriasis

43.4 Seborrheic dermatitis
 a. Lesions are pale to red to yellow–pink and may be covered by an oily-appearing, scaly crust
 b. Lesions are typically slightly raised, round, or ovoid patches with a silver scale appearance atop an erythematous base
 c. Areas of whitish lacy bands of keratosis near reddish ulcerated-like lesions
 d. Diffusely reddened areas with occasional hyperplastic or hyperpigmented plaques of red to reddish-brown

Instructions for items 43.5 to 43.8: Match the common vulvar dermatosis with its treatment. An option may be used once, more than once, or not at all.

43.5 Lichen simplex chronicus (LSC)

43.6 Lichen planus

43.7 Psoriasis

43.8 Seborrheic dermatitis
 a. Antipruritic to inhibit nighttime itching and topical steroid creams
 b. Topical steroid preparations, but stronger fluorinated steroid preparations may be used in the presence of hyperkeratosis
 c. Topical cold tar preparations, followed by exposure to ultraviolet light
 d. Burrow's solution soaks, followed by topical corticosteroid lotions or creams

43.9 Which of the following statements about vulvar vestibulitis is INCORRECT?
 a. Vulvar vestibulitis involves the vestibular glands located just inside the vaginal introitus near the hymenal ring.
 b. Most commonly, patients report a progressive worsening of the condition over 3–4 months.
 c. Light touch of a moistened cotton tip applicator to the proper anatomic areas will duplicate the pain of the complaint.
 d. The affected areas often appear as small, reddened patches.
 e. Treatment with hydrocortisone ointments and topical Xylocaine jelly is uniformly successful.

43.10 New onset insertional dyspareunia is especially associated with:
 a. chronic cervicitis
 b. vulvar dysplasia
 c. vestibulitis
 d. Bartholin's abscess

ANSWERS (43.1–43.10)

43.1 d	43.3 b	43.5 a	43.7 c	43.9 e	43.10 c
43.2 c	43.4 a	43.6 b	43.8 d		

Instructions for items 43.11 to 43.15: Match the benign vulvar lesion with the appropriate descriptive statement. An option may be used once, more than once, or not at all.

43.11 Inclusion cyst

43.12 Hydrocele

43.13 Fibroma

43.14 Hidradenoma

43.15 Nevi
   a. Usually small, although occasionally may become large and pedunculated
   b. Cyst of the canal of Nuck
   c. Small smooth nodular masses containing cheesy material
   d. Almost always benign and arises from the sweat glands on the inner surface of the labia majora
   e. Pigmented lesions that must be distinguished from a common malignant lesion, which may occur on the external genitalia

43.16 Which of the following conditions may be associated with high urinary oxalic acid concentrations?
   a. Hidradenoma
   b. Seborrheic dermatitis
   c. Lichen simplex chronicus
   d. Vestibulitis
   e. Psoriasis

43.17 Lichen sclerosis and hyperplastic dystrophy without atypia carry what estimated risk of vulvar carcinoma?
   a. 0%–1%
   b. 2%–3%
   c. 4%–5%
   d. 6%–7%
   e. 8%–9%

43.18 Mixed dystrophy—lichen sclerosis admixed with areas of hyperplastic dystrophy—is treated by:
   a. corticosteroid cream alone
   b. testosterone appropionate cream alone
   c. corticosteroid cream for 2–3 weeks, then topical testosterone appropionate
   d. topical testosterone appropionate for 2–3 weeks, then corticosteroid cream
   e. laser ablation

Instructions for items 43.19 to 43.20: Match the chronic vulvar disease with the appropriate statement(s) about its identification and clinical course. An option may be used once, more than once, or not at all.

43.19 Hyperplastic dystrophy

43.20 Lichen sclerosis
   a. The lesion is unlikely to totally resolve, requiring intermittent treatment for an indefinite period
   b. The lesion usually resolves completely by 6 months of therapy
   c. The vulva is characteristically diffusely involved with very thin whitish epithelium often termed "onion skinned" epithelium
   d. There is obviously hyperkeratotic skin with secondary excoriation

Instructions for items 43.21 to 43.24: Match the vulvar lesion with the appropriate statement(s) about its identification and progression. An option may be used once, more than once, or not at all.

43.21 Vulvar intraepithelial neoplasia I and II (VIN I and VIN II)

43.22 Vulvar intraepithelial neoplasia III (VIN III, carcinoma in situ)

Answers (43.11–43.22)

| 43.11 c | 43.13 a | 43.15 e | 43.17 b | 43.19 b, d | 43.21 c, e, f, g |
| 43.12 b | 43.14 d | 43.16 d | 43.18 c | 43.20 a, c | 43.22 d, e, g |

43.23 Paget's disease

43.24 Melanoma
   a. May be associated with carcinoma of the skin
   b. Associated with a higher incidence of underlying internal carcinoma, particularly colon and breast
   c. Human papillomavirus (HPV) changes occasionally seen in these lesions
   d. Full thickness loss of maturation
   e. Raised gross lesions
   f. High predilection for progression to severe intraepithelial lesions and eventually carcinoma
   g. Associated with vulvar pruritus and chronic irritation
   h. Raised, irritated, pruritic pigmented lesion

43.25 When vulvar melanoma invades to the depth of the subcutaneous tissue, survival is generally:
   a. 0–20%
   b. 20–40%
   c. 40–60%
   d. 60–80%

43.26 Extended vulvar intraepithelial neoplasia I and II (VIN I and VIN II) lesions are best treated by:
   a. cryocautery
   b. electrodesiccation
   c. laser cautery, using local anesthetic
   d. laser ablation, using general anesthetic

43.27 Vulvar carcinoma accounts for approximately what percent of all gynecologic malignancies?
   a. 4%
   b. 8%
   c. 12%
   d. 20%

43.28 What percent of all squamous vulvar malignancies are found in women less than 40-years-old?
   a. <1%
   b. 5%
   c. 10%
   d. 15%
   e. 20%

43.29 What percent of vulvar carcinomas are of the squamous cell type?
   a. 30%
   b. 50%
   c. 70%
   d. 90%

43.30 In patients with vulvar carcinoma, what is the most common presenting complaint?
   a. an exophytic ulcerative lesion on a labium majus
   b. vulvar pruritus
   c. dysuria
   d. dyspareunia

43.31 Which of the following statements concerning squamous cell carcinoma of the vulva is INCORRECT?
   a. In most cases, the disease remains localized for a relatively long period of time.
   b. Spread of the disease is usually unpredictable, along many routes.
   c. Lesions greater than 2 centimeters in diameter and 0.5 centimeter in depth have an increased incidence of nodal metastasis.
   d. Lesions rising in the anterior third of the vulva may spread directly to the deep pelvic nodes.

ANSWERS (43.23–43.31)					
43.23 a, b	43.25 a	43.27 a	43.29 d	43.30 b	43.31 b
43.24 h	43.26 d	43.28 c			

43.32 The overall incidence of lymph node metastasis in squamous cell carcinoma of the vulva is approximately:
  a. 10%
  b. 20%
  c. 30%
  d. 40%

43.33 For patients with negative inguinal and femoral lymph nodes, the 5 year survival rate for patients with vulvar carcinoma is approximately:
  a. 30%
  b. 50%
  c. 70%
  d. 90%

43.34 Which of the following statements about carcinoma of Bartholin's gland is INCORRECT?
  a. It arises either from the squamous epithelium of the ducts or the glandular epithelium of the greater vestibular glands.
  b. It is most common in the fifth decade or later.
  c. Treatment is radical vulvectomy and bilateral lymphotomy with radiation therapy, in most cases.
  d. The 5 year overall survival rate is 85%–95%.

Instructions for items 43.35 to 43.36: Match the benign vaginal mass with the appropriate description(s). An option may be used once, more than once, or not at all.

43.35 Gartner duct cyst

43.36 Inclusion cyst
  a. Arises from vestigial remnants of the Wolffian or mesonephric system
  b. Arises from imperfect alignment of childbirth lacerations or episiotomy
  c. Lined with stratified squamous epithelium and filled with "cheesy" material
  d. Found along outer aspect of vaginal canal
  e. Should be excised if symptomatic

43.37 Which of the following does NOT increase the likelihood of vaginal carcinoma in situ?
  a. A preexisting lower genital tract neoplasia
  b. Previous hysterectomy for cervical carcinoma in situ
  c. Radiation therapy for another gynecologic malignancy
  d. Exposure to diethylstilbestrol (DES) in utero

43.38 Invasive vaginal cancer accounts for approximately what percent of gynecologic malignancies?
  a. 1%–2%
  b. 3%–4%
  c. 5%–6%
  d. 7%–8%
  e. 9%–10%

43.39 Squamous cell carcinoma accounts for what percent of vaginal carcinoma?
  a. 35%
  b. 55%
  c. 75%
  d. 95%

ANSWERS (43.32–43.39)

43.32 c	43.34 d	43.36 b, c, e	43.37 d	43.38 a	43.39 d
43.33 d	43.35 a, d, e				

Instructions for items 43.40 to 43.44: Match the stage of vaginal carcinoma with the appropriate description. An option may be used once, more than once, or not at all.

43.40 Stage 0

43.41 Stage 1

43.42 Stage 2

43.43 Stage 3

43.44 Stage 4
   a. Carcinoma involving the subvaginal tissue but not extending onto the pelvic wall
   b. Carcinoma extending onto the pelvic side wall
   c. Carcinoma limited to the vaginal mucosa
   d. Carcinoma in situ
   e. Carcinoma extending into the bladder mucosa or distant metastases

43.45 Approximately what fraction of patients with vaginal carcinoma in situ will have an antecedent or coexistent neoplasm of the lower genital tract?
   a. 1/5–1/3
   b. 1/3–1/2
   c. 1/2–2/3
   d. 3/4–4/5

43.46 Which of the following statements about sarcoma botryoides is INCORRECT?
   a. Presents as a mass of polyps protruding from the introitus of very young girls and infants.
   b. Arises from the undifferentiated mesenchyme of the lamina propria of the anterior vaginal wall.
   c. Often associated with a bloody discharge
   d. Treated in almost all cases by radical pelvic exenteration.

43.47 Screening for the recognition of potential malignancy of the cervix is best accomplished by:
   a. self-investigation of the vagina
   b. Papanicolaou (Pap) smear
   c. cervical canal curettage
   d. aspiration of endocervical mucus
   e. posterior fornix aspiration

43.48 Diethylstilbestrol administered to a pregnant woman is associated with which condition in the female offspring?
   a. Clear cell adenocarcinoma of the vagina
   b. Endometrial carcinoma
   c. Hidradenitis
   d. Carcinoma in situ of the vagina
   e. Embryonal rhabdomyosarcoma

43.49 What is the recommended procedure for the evaluation of a chronic vulvar ulcer?
   a. darkfield examination
   b. biopsy
   c. Pap smear
   d. culture of lesion
   e. lymphangiography

43.50 The most common cause of the delay in diagnosing vulva carcinoma is the:
   a. unreliability of a Pap smear of the vulva
   b. equivocal histology of early lesions
   c. failure to biopsy lesions
   d. lack of visibility of most lesions

Answers (43.40–43.50)

43.40 d	43.42 a	43.44 e	43.46 d	43.48 a	43.50 c
43.41 c	43.43 b	43.45 b	43.47 b	43.49 b	

Questions and Answers Chapter 44:
Cervical Neoplasia and Carcinoma

44.1 Which of the following is a risk factor associated with cervical neoplasia?
a. Multiple sexual partners
b. Low socioeconomic status
c. Previous venereal infection
d. Cigarette smoking
e. All of the above

44.2 Which of the following statements best describes cervical "erosion?"
a. Cervical tissue exposed to *Trichomonas vaginalis*
b. Exocervical tissue undergoing squamous metaplasia
c. Normal endocervical tissue that has moved to the cervical surface
d. Endocervical tissue undergoing squamous metaplasia
e. Endocervical tissue associated with mechanical abrasion

44.3 The transformation zone develops:
a. before puberty
b. during puberty and adolescence
c. during pregnancy
d. at the time of menopause

44.4 In the menopausal years, the location of the squamocolumnar junction shifts:
a. into the endocervical canal
b. to just outside the external os
c. onto the cervical surface

44.5 What percent of squamous intraepithelial neoplasia and cervical cancer arise from within the transformation zone?
a. 55%
b. 65%
c. 75%
d. 85%
e. 95%

44.6 Which of the following statements about human papillomavirus is correct?
a. The human papillomavirus is a direct cervical carcinogen.
b. The human papillomavirus may serve as a cofactor in the abnormal maturation and division of epithelial cells.
c. The great majority of women who harbor the human papillomavirus have accompanying abnormal cytologic changes.

44.7 Which of the following types of human papillomavirus is LEAST associated with a high risk of squamous intraepithelial neoplasia?
a. 16
b. 18
c. 21
d. 31

44.8 The current recommendation of the American College of Obstetricians and Gynecologists with respect to Pap smear screening is to obtain the first Pap smear at the time a woman becomes sexually active or reaches the age of:
a. 14
b. 16
c. 18
d. 20

44.9 According to the American College of Obstetricians and Gynecologists, Pap smears should be obtained:
a. yearly
b. every 2 years
c. every 3 years
d. at no set interval

ANSWERS (44.1–44.9)

44.1	e	44.3	b	44.5	e	44.7	c	44.8	c	44.9	a
44.2	c	44.4	a	44.6	b						

Instructions for items 44.10 to 44.14: Match the Pap smear class system classification with the appropriate description(s). An option may be used once, more than once, or not at all.

44.10 Class I

44.11 Class II

44.12 Class III

44.13 Class IV

44.14 Class V
  a. Carcinoma in situ (CIS)
  b. Severe dysplasia
  c. Moderate dysplasia
  d. Mild dysplasia
  e. Inflammation
  f. Normal
  g. Squamous cell cancer

Instructions for items 44.15 to 44.18: Match the Bethesda system of Pap smear classification with the appropriate description(s). An option may be used once, more than once, or not at all.

44.15 Within normal limits

44.16 Low-grade squamous intraepithelial lesion (LGSIL)

44.17 High-grade SIL (HGSIL)

44.18 Squamous cell cancer
  a. Carcinoma in situ (CIS)
  b. Severe dysplasia
  c. Moderate dysplasia
  d. Mild dysplasia
  e. Inflammation
  f. Normal
  g. Squamous cell cancer

44.19 Carcinoma in situ of the cervix becomes classified as invasive cervical cancer when the dysplastic cells traverse the:
  a. transformation zone
  b. squamocolumnar junction
  c. basement membrane
  d. endocervical canal
  e. canal of Nuck

44.20 What percent of all cases of mild dysplasia of the cervix [low-grade squamous intraepithelial lesion (LGSIL)] will spontaneously regress?
  a. 25%
  b. 35%
  c. 45%
  d. 55%
  e. 65%

44.21 What percent of all cases of mild dysplasia of the cervix [low-grade squamous intraepithelial lesion (LGSIL)] will progress to worsening disease?
  a. 5%
  b. 15%
  c. 25%
  d. 30%
  e. 45%

Instructions for items 44.22 to 44.25: Match the Bethesda system classification of cervical cytology with the appropriate follow-up. An option may be used once, more than once, or not at all.

44.22 Atypical squamous cells of undetermined significance (ASCUS)

44.23 Low-grade squamous intraepithelial lesions (LGSIL)

44.24 High-grade SIL (HGSIL)

ANSWERS (44.10–44.24)					
44.10 f	44.13 a, b	44.16 d	44.19 c	44.21 b	44.23 a, b
44.11 e	44.14 g	44.17 a, b, c	44.20 e	44.22 a, c, d	44.24 b
44.12 c, d	44.15 e, f	44.18 g			

44.25 Atypical glandular cells of undetermined significance (AGCUS)
   a. Repeat Pap every 4–6 months for 2 years until there are 3 consecutive negative smears; if second abnormal Pap, colposcopy should be considered
   b. Colposcopy with endocervical curettage and directed biopsies as indicated
   c. If Pap report is qualified by severe inflammation, any specific infection should be treated and the Pap repeated in 2–3 months
   d. In postmenopausal patient, repeat Pap smear following course of vaginal estrogen therapy; if still abnormal, colposcopy should be considered
   e. Options including repeat Pap with endocervical brush, endometrial biopsy, and/or cone biopsy

44.26 A colposcopy is considered to be satisfactory when the entire:
   a. squamocolumnar junction is visualized
   b. external cervical os is visualized
   c. internal cervical os is visualized
   d. vesicouterine reflection is visualized
   e. erosive zone is visualized

44.27 Which of the following is NOT an indication for conization of the cervix?
   a. Unsatisfactory colposcopy
   b. Atypical squamous cells of undetermined significance (ASCUS)
   c. Positive endocervical curettage
   d. Two-step discrepancy between Pap smear and cervical biopsy results

44.28 The acetic acid solution used to wash the cervix before colposcopy functions as a:
   a. stain
   b. emulsifier
   c. desiccant
   d. antiseptic

44.29 The endocervical curettage will be positive for dysplasia in what percent of women with a dysplastic Pap smear?
   a. Less than 5%
   b. 5%–10%
   c. 11%–15%
   d. 16%–20%
   e. 21%–25%

44.30 Approximately what percent of colposcopically directed biopsies and endocervical curettages will demonstrate a significant discrepancy between the screening Pap smear and the histologic data?
   a. 1%
   b. 5%
   c. 10%
   d. 15%
   e. 20%

44.31 To ensure adequate evaluation of a cervix from which an abnormal Pap smear has been obtained, biopsies should be taken from what location(s) at the time of colposcopy?
   a. At lease two quadrants of the cervix
   b. At least three quadrants of the cervix
   c. From areas of colposcopic abnormality and at least one other quadrant of the cervix
   d. From areas of colposcopic abnormality

ANSWERS (44.25–44.31)

44.25 e   44.27 b   44.28 c   44.29 b   44.30 c   44.31 d
44.26 a

44.32 For a conization specimen to be considered satisfactory, it is NOT necessary that the specimen encompass:
   a. the entire cervix
   b. the entire squamocolumnar junction
   c. the entire extent of identified lesions
   d. a portion of the endocervical canal

44.33 Which of the following techniques is NOT commonly used for conization of the cervix?
   a. Scalpel and scissors
   b. Heated electric wire
   c. Super-cooled electric probe
   d. Laser

44.34 Which of the following is NOT a risk factor for a woman undergoing conization of the cervix who desires future childbearing?
   a. Incompetent cervical os
   b. Abnormal cervical contours impeding coitus
   c. Reduced cervical capacity to facilitate sperm transport
   d. Loss of uterus secondary to hysterectomy associated with hemorrhage

Instructions for items 44.35 to 44.38: Match the methods of treatment of cervical intra-epithelial neoplasia with the appropriate descriptions. An option may be used once, more than once, or not at all.

44.35 Cryocautery

44.36 Laser therapy

44.37 Cervical conization

44.38 Excisional biopsy
   a. May be considered for the treatment of specific focal areas of abnormality
   b. May involve the use of a hot wire loop
   c. May involve the use of "mushroom-tip" stainless steel probe, super-cooled with circulating liquid nitrogen or carbon dioxide
   d. Permits precise control of depth of ablation
   e. Popular method for the treatment of low-grade cervical intraepithelial neoplasia (CIN)
   f. Procedure is routinely considered both therapeutic and diagnostic
   g. Procedure is associated postoperatively with profuse watery discharge admixed with necrotic cellular debris
   h. May be used for the treatment of high-grade intraepithelial lesions

44.39 The average age of diagnosis of invasive cervical carcinoma is approximately:
   a. 20 years
   b. 30 years
   c. 40 years
   d. 50 years
   e. 60 years

44.40 Advanced cervical intraepithelial neoplasia is thought to precede the occurrence of invasive cervical carcinoma by an average of:
   a. 1 year
   b. 5 years
   c. 10 years
   d. 15 years
   e. 20 years

ANSWERS (44.32–44.40)

44.32 a	44.34 b	44.36 d, h	44.38 a	44.39 d	44.40 c
44.33 c	44.35 c, e, g	44.37 b, f			

44.41 What percent of cervical cancer is of the squamous cell variety?
   a. 45%
   b. 55%
   c. 65%
   d. 75%
   e. 85%
   f. 95%

44.42 Approximately what percent of cervical carcinoma is adenocarcinoma arising from the cervical glands?
   a. 5%
   b. 15%
   c. 25%
   d. 35%
   e. 45%
   f. 55%

44.43 Clear cell carcinoma of the cervix is associated with intrauterine exposure to
   a. progesterone
   b. estrone
   c. dehydroepiandrosterone
   d. diethylstilbestrol
   e. cigarette smoke

Instructions for items 44.44 to 49.47: Match the stage of cervical carcinoma with the approximate 5-year survival rate. An option may be used once, more than once, or not at all.

44.44 Stage 1

44.45 Stage IIA

44.46 Stage IIIA

44.47 Stage IV
   a. 5%
   b. 14%
   c. 25%
   d. 45%
   e. 64%
   f. 83%
   g. 91%

44.48 Which of the following is present in all patients with invasive cervical cancer?
   a. Postcoital bleeding
   b. Pain
   c. Abnormal uterine bleeding
   d. None of the above

Instructions for items 44.49 to 44.57: Match the clinical staging of carcinoma of the cervix [International Federation of Gynecology and Obstetrics (FIGO)] with the appropriate description(s). An option may be used once, more than once, or not at all.

44.49 Stage I AI

44.50 Stage I AII

44.51 Stage IB

44.52 Stage IIA

44.53 Stage IIB

44.54 Stage IIIA

44.55 Stage IIIB

44.56 Stage IVA

ANSWERS (44.41–44.56)

44.41 e	44.44 g	44.47 b	44.50 e	44.53 f	44.55 g
44.42 b	44.45 f	44.48 d	44.51 c	44.54 a	44.56 h
44.43 d	44.46 d	44.49 d	44.52 b		

44.57 Stage IVB
  a. Carcinoma involves the lower third of the vagina, but there is no extension to the pelvic wall
  b. Carcinoma extends beyond the cervix but not to the pelvic wall; there is no obvious parametrial involvement
  c. All cases of stage I cancer not included in other classifications or divisions
  d. Minimal evidence of stromal invasion on microscopic examination
  e. Microscopic lesion(s) no more than 5 millimeters in depth measured from base of epithelial surface or glandular surface from which it originates, and horizontal spread not to exceed 7 millimeters
  f. Carcinoma extends beyond cervix with obvious parametrial involvement
  g. Carcinoma extends to pelvic side wall
  h. Carcinoma has spread to adjacent pelvic organs
  i. Carcinoma has spread to distant organs

44.58 All patients with cervical carcinoma with hydronephrosis or a nonfunctioning kidney should be included in at least stage:
  a. I
  b. II
  c. III
  d. IV

44.59 In general, surgical therapy for cervical carcinoma is indicated for most patients with:
  a. stage I
  b. stage II
  c. stage III
  d. stage IV

44.60 Which of the following is a complication noted after radiation therapy for cervical carcinoma?
  a. Radiation cystitis
  b. Radiation proctitis
  c. Dyspareunia
  d. Fistulae
  e. All of the above

44.61 A 31-year-old female who has three living children and has had a tubal ligation has a Pap smear reported as high-grade squamous intraepithelial lesion (HGSIL). There are no macroscopic lesions. The management should involve which of the following?
  a. Hysterectomy
  b. Radiotherapy
  c. Local chemotherapy
  d. Colposcopically directed cervical biopsies
  e. Systemic chemotherapy

44.62 What are the primary lymph nodes involved in the spread of cervical carcinoma?
  a. paracervical and obturator
  b. sacral and inguinal
  c. common iliac and aortic
  d. perineal
  e. femoral

44.63 Metastatic cervical carcinoma can cause:
  a. hydronephrosis
  b. paraplegia
  c. hematemesis
  d. colon obstruction
  e. all of the above

ANSWERS (44.57–44.63)

44.57 i	44.59 a	44.60 e	44.61 d	44.62 a	44.63 e
44.58 c					

44.64 The healing process after cervical cryotherapy usually is complete after:
a. 1 month
b. 2 months
c. 3 months
d. 4 months

44.65 Repeat Pap smears after ablative surgical therapy of the cervix are usually started after:
a. 4 weeks
b. 8 weeks
c. 12 weeks
d. 16 weeks

44.66 Serotyping of HPV found on the cervix is:
a. recommended for all patients less than age 30
b. recommended for patients with low grade lesions on Pap smear
c. recommended for patients with high grade lesions on Pap smear
d. recommended for patients with recurrent abnormal Pap smears
e. not recommended

ANSWERS (44.64–44.66)
44.64 b   44.65 c   44.66 e

Questions and Answers Chapter 45:
Uterine Leiomyoma and Neoplasia

45.1 Which of the following statements about leiomyoma uteri is INCORRECT?
a. About 70% of American women have these benign tumors.
b. The majority of women with leiomyoma do not require hysterectomy.
c. Leiomyoma is an indication in approximately one-third of hysterectomies performed.
d. Histologically, leiomyomas are benign tumors with localized proliferation of smooth muscle cells surrounded by a pseudocapsule.
e. Leiomyomas grow in response to estrogen.

45.2 All of the following are common symptoms or clinical manifestations of uterine fibroids EXCEPT:
a. pain
b. pressure
c. anemia
d. bleeding
e. constipation

45.3 Estrogen may cause leiomyoma growth by stimulation of the production of:
a. progesterone receptors in the myometrium, where progesterone binding to these sites stimulates the production of several growth factors causing the growth of myomas
b. estrogen receptors in the myometrium, where estrogen binding to these sites stimulates the production of several growth factors causing the growth of myomas
c. estrogen receptors in the myometrium, where estrogen binding to these sites directly stimulates myometrial cell growth
d. prolatcin receptors in the myometrium, where prolactin binding to these sites stimulates the production of several growth factors causing the growth of myomas

45.4 Sensitive DNS studies suggest that each myoma arises from a:
a. single smooth muscle cell
b. single vascular endothelial cell
c. single connective tissue cell
d. dormant leiomyoma cell present at birth

ANSWERS (45.1–45.4)

45.1 a   45.2 c   45.3 a   45.4 a

45.5   Which of the following statements about leiomyoma is incorrect?
a. Pelvic examination is the most cost effective means of identification and evaluation of uterine myomas.
b. Cystic appearing areas in an image consistent with a leiomyoma are commonly associated with areas of degeneration.
c. Endometrial sampling usually does not provide additional information towards making the diagnosis of leiomyoma of the uterus.
d. Irregular uterine bleeding in a woman with known uterine myomas does not require endometrial sampling.

45.6   Leiomyosarcomas occur in what percent of leiomyoma?
a. 0.01%
b. 0.1%
c. 1.0%
d. 10%

45.7   Which of the following statements about leiomyosarcoma is correct?
a. Leiomyosarcoma arises from degeneration of a normal fibroid.
b. This malignancy is more common in patients under the age of 40.
c. Patients typically present with a rapidly enlarging uterine mass, unusual vaginal discharge, and pelvic pain.
d. Leiomyosarcoma consists of a cell type found only in the uterus.

Instructions for items 45.8 to 45.10: Match the type of benign uterine myoma with the appropriate description(s). An option may be used once, more than once, or not at all.

45.8   Intravenous leiomyomatosis

45.9   Benign metastasizing leiomyoma

45.10   Leiomyomatosis peritonealis disseminata
a. Has been found in cardiac, pulmonary, and lymphatic nodules
b. Has been found in pelvic veins and the vena cava
c. Implants on peritoneal surfaces

45.11   Postmenopausal patients who present with rapidly enlarging uterine masses should be considered at high risk for:
a. uterine leiomyoma
b. uterine leiomyosarcoma
c. intravenous leiomyomatosis
d. benign metastasizing leiomyoma
e. leiomyomatosis peritonealis disseminata

45.12   What is the most common change occurring in myomas during pregnancy?
a. red degeneration
b. calcification
c. liquefaction
d. hyalinization
e. parasitic growth

45.13   Red degeneration of uterine leiomyoma refers to:
a. hyalinization of the smooth muscle elements
b. calcification of the smooth muscle stroma
c. hemorrhagic changes in the myometrium associated with rapid growth
d. inflammatory changes in the surrounding smooth muscle stroma

ANSWERS (45.5–45.13)

45.5 d	45.7 c	45.9 a	45.11 b	45.12 a	45.13 c
45.6 b	45.8 b	45.10 c			

45.14 Menorrhagia associated with uterine leiomyoma is characterized by an increased:
  a. amount of menstrual flow only
  b. duration of menstrual flow only
  c. amount and duration of menstrual flow
  d. amount and frequency of menstrual flow
  e. frequency of menstrual flow

45.15 Menorrhagia associated with uterine leiomyoma is defined as menstrual blood loss of greater than:
  a. 40 ml
  b. 80 ml
  c. 120 ml
  d. 160 ml
  e. 200 ml

45.16 Which of the following is NOT a generally accepted mechanism to explain the increased bleeding associated with uterine fibroids?
  a. Alteration of normal myometrial contractile function in the small arteries and the arteriolar blood supply underlying the endometrium.
  b. Inability of the overlying endometrium to respond to the normal estrogen–progesterone menstrual phases.
  c. Pressure necrosis of the overlying endometrial bed exposing vascular surfaces that bleed excessively with endometrial sloughing.
  d. Increased proliferation of small blood vessels in the endometrium under the influence of hormonal stimulation.

45.17 What is the type of leiomyoma most commonly associated with abnormal uterine bleeding?
  a. subserosal
  b. intramural
  c. submucosal
  d. parasitic
  e. disseminated

45.18 Which of the following is an uncommon clinical complication of large uterine leiomyoma?
  a. Hydroureter
  b. Hydronephrosis
  c. Costovertebral angle (CVA) tenderness
  d. Colon or rectal obstruction
  e. All of the above

45.19 Which of the following statements about the physical examination and physical diagnosis of uterine fibroids is incorrect?
  a. There is characteristic presence of a large midline mobile mass with an irregular contour.
  b. The mass usually has a "hard-feel" or solid quality.
  c. Subserosal pedunculated myomas are easily distinguishable from solid adnexal masses.
  d. Uterine fibroids are usually appreciable on abdominal examination when they are greater than 14–16 weeks' equivalent gestational size.

45.20 Which of the following has the highest cost-benefit for diagnosing uterine myomas?
  a. Magnetic resonance imaging
  b. Computerized axial tomography
  c. Ultrasound
  d. Pelvic examination

ANSWERS (45.14–45.20)

45.14 c	45.16 d	45.17 c	45.18 e	45.19 c	45.20 d
45.15 b					

45.21 Which of the following statements about the ultrasound evaluation of presumed uterine leiomyoma is INCORRECT?
   a. Ultrasound is commonly used for confirmation of uterine myomas.
   b. Ultrasound can usually demonstrate hypoechogenicity amid otherwise normal myometrial patterns.
   c. Ultrasound can usually resolve the presence of a distorted endometrial stripe.
   d. Ultrasound cannot usually distinguish a myoma from a solid adnexal mass.

45.22 According to current data, what percent of patients undergoing hysteroscopic removal of submucous leiomyoma will require additional therapy within 10 years?
   a. 10%
   b. 20%
   c. 30%
   d. 40%
   e. 50%

45.23 Which of the following statements about the management of patients with uterine fibroids is INCORRECT?
   a. The majority of patients with uterine leiomyoma do not require surgical treatment.
   b. Assessment of uterine growth requires regular computerized axial tomography (CAT) scans.
   c. Uterine bleeding may be minimized by intermittent progestin supplementation if significant endometrial cavity distortion is not present.
   d. Myomectomy may be warranted in young patients whose fertility is being compromised by intracavitary distortion.
   e. Periodic physical examination generally provides adequate follow-up.

45.24 Which of the following statements about the use of gonadotropin-releasing hormone agonists (GnRH analogs) is correct?
   a. They may be used as follow-up treatment (3–6 months) after surgery.
   b. They may be used for relatively long-term therapy (12–36 months) to bring about major reduction in large tumor size.
   c. Treatment is often associated with reduction in uterine masses by as much as 40%–60%.
   d. Treatment will permanently reduce the size of myomas.

ANSWERS (45.21–45.24)

| 45.21 d | 45.22 b | 45.23 b | 45.24 c |

45.25 Which of the following statements about pregnancy associated with leiomyoma uteri is INCORRECT?
a. The overall course of pregnancy is usually unremarkable.
b. There is usually a normal labor and delivery.
c. Myomas typically shrink during pregnancy.
d. Pregnancy is sometimes associated with red or carneous degeneration of myomas.

45.26 Which of the following statements about the relationship of leiomyomas and pregnancy is incorrect?
a. Leiomyomas are a significant cause of infertility.
b. Pregnancy with leiomyomas is usually unremarkable.
c. Bed rest and analgesia usually suffices in the management of carneous degeneration.
d. Myomas located in the lower uterine segment are a rare cause of soft tissue dystocia.

45.27 Adenomyosis is found in coexistence with leiomyoma in approximately what percent of hysterectomy specimens?
a. 10%
b. 20%
c. 30%
d. 40%
e. 50%

45.28 What is a common treatment for adenomyosis of the uterus?
a. therapy with estrogens
b. therapy of gonadotropin-releasing hormone (GnRH) agonists
c. "watchful waiting"
d. hysterectomy

45.29 Leiomyosarcoma accounts for approximately what percent of cancers involving the body of the uterus?
a. 1%
b. 3%
c. 6%
d. 9%
e. 12%

45.30 Which of the following statements about uterine sarcomas is incorrect?
a. Uterine sarcoma should be suspected with the enlargement of a previously-known myomatous uterus in a postmenopausal woman.
b. Postmenopausal bleeding is associated with uterine adenocarcinoma, not uterine sarcomas.
c. The virulence of uterine sarcoma is directly related to the number of mitotic figures and cellular proliferation as defined histologically.
d. Uterine sarcoma is more likely to spread hematogenously than is endometrial adenocarcinoma.

45.31 Which of the following is not related to the virulence of uterine sarcomas?
a. The number of mitotic figures.
b. The degree of cellular proliferation.
c. The association of the sarcoma with leiomyoma.
d. B and C above

45.32 The overall 5-year survival rate for patients with leiomyosarcoma is approximately:
a. 30%
b. 50%
c. 70%
d. 90%

ANSWERS (45.25–45.32)

45.25 c	45.27 c	45.29 b	45.30 b	45.31 c	45.32 b
45.26 a	45.28 d				

45.33 What is the most reliable method for the diagnosis of leiomyosarcoma?
   a. Pap smear
   b. endocervical curretage
   c. pipelle endometrial biopsy
   d. dilation and curettage (D&C)
   e. histology of a hysterectomy specimen

45.34 Which of the following statements about the management of uterine sarcomas is incorrect?
   a. The staging for uterine sarcoma is surgical and identical to that for endometrial adenocarcinoma.
   b. The overall rate of survival for patients with uterine sarcoma is essentially equivalent stage for stage to that for endometrial adenocarcinoma.
   c. Adjunctive radiation therapy and chemotherapy provide little additional benefit as primary adjuvant therapy or as therapy for recurrent disease.
   d. Unlike endometrial adenocarcinoma, uterine sarcomas are not responsive to hormonal treatment with high-dose progestins.

45.35 Indications and actions prior to myomectomy for infertility patients should include:
   a. the presence of leiomyoma of sufficient size or location to be a probable factor in infertility
   b. the absence of a more likely explanation for the failure to conceive
   c. evidence of normal ovarian function
   d. evidence of normal fallopian tube function
   e. all of the above

45.36 Which of the following would be a criterion for hysterectomy for leiomyoma?
   a. The presence of asymptomatic leiomyoma that are palpable abdominally.
   b. The presence of uterine bleeding that is uncomfortable for the patient, but without anemia.
   c. The presence of acute or severe pelvic discomfort caused by myoma.
   d. Patient concern in the presence of asymptomatic leiomyoma.

45.37 Which of the following actions is NOT necessary before hysterectomy for leiomyoma uteri?
   a. Confirmation of the absence of cervical malignancy
   b. Elimination of anovulation or other causes of abnormal bleeding
   c. Confirmation of the absence of endometrial malignancy by endometrial biopsy in all patients over the age of 25
   d. Assessment of surgical risk from anemia and the need for presurgical treatment
   e. Consideration of psychological risk associated with hysterectomy

45.38 Which of the following is NOT a sign or symptom of uterine myomata?
   a. Bladder irritability with urinary frequency
   b. Heavy periods
   c. Amenorrhea
   d. Pressure on the rectum with pain on defecation
   e. A palpable pelvic mass

ANSWERS (45.33–45.38)

| 45.33 e | 45.34 b | 45.35 e | 45.36 c | 45.37 c | 45.38 c |

45.39 Adenomyosis is characterized by:
   a. invasion of the myometrium with benign endometrial cells
   b. infiltration of the myometrium with lymphocytes secondary to endometritis
   c. invasion of the myometrium with endometrial adenocarcinoma
   d. invasion of pelvic tissues with endometrial adenocarcinoma
   e. invasion of the myometrium with squamous cell carcinoma of the cervix

45.40 Uterine sarcomas may originate from all of the following tissues EXCEPT:
   a. blood vessels
   b. uterine fibroids (myomata)
   c. endometrium
   d. nerve fibers
   e. myometrium

45.41 What is the most common malignant nonepithelial tumor of the uterus?
   a. leiomyosarcoma
   b. hemangiopericytoma
   c. fibrosarcoma
   d. endometrial sarcoma
   e. mixed mesodermal tumor

ANSWERS (45.39–45.41)
45.39 a   45.40 d   45.41 a

Questions and Answers Chapter 46: Endometrial Hyperplasia and Cancer

46.1 Among female genital tract malignancies, endometrial carcinoma ranks where in frequency?
a. First
b. Second
c. Third
d. Fourth
e. Fifth

46.2 Endometrial carcinoma ranks where in frequency among all cancers?
a. Second
b. Third
c. Fourth
d. Fifth
e. Sixth

46.3 About what percent of all women will develop endometrial carcinoma?
a. 1–2%
b. 2–3%
c. 3–4%
d. 4–5%
e. 5–6%

46.4 What percent of endometrial carcinoma is found in women who are perimenopausal?
a. 1–5%
b. 5–10%
c. 10–15%
d. 15–20%
e. 20–25%

46.5 Approximately what percent of patients with endometrial carcinoma are diagnosed in the postmenopausal years?
a. 25%
b. 50%
c. 75%
d. 100%

46.6 What percent of endometrial carcinoma is found in women who are premenopausal?
a. 1–5%
b. 5–10%
c. 10–15%
d. 15–20%
e. 20–25%

Questions 46.7 to 46.9: Match the type of endometrial hyperplasia with the estimated risk of its progression to endometrial carcinoma. An option may be used once, more than once, or not at all.

46.7 Complex hyperplasia

46.8 Simple hyperplasia

46.9 Atypical hyperplasia
a. 1%
b. 3%
c. 30%
d. 50%

46.10 Endometrial hyperplasia and endometrial carcinoma are often overgrowths of the endometrium in response to:
a. progesterone
b. estrogen
c. prolactin
d. prostaglandin
e. testosterone

Answers (46.1–46.10)

46.1	a	46.3	b	46.5	c	46.7	b	46.9	c	46.10	b
46.2	c	46.4	d	46.6	b	46.8	a				

46.11 Conversion of androstenedione to estrogen occurs mainly in:
   a. peripheral tissue stroma
   b. peripheral muscular tissue
   c. peripheral fat tissue
   d. centers of bone marrow activity

46.12 Endometrial hyperplasia is defined as abnormal proliferation of:
   a. both glandular and stromal elements, with altered histologic architecture
   b. only glandular elements, with altered histologic architecture
   c. only stromal elements, with altered histologic architecture
   d. both glandular and stromal elements, with normal histologic architecture

Instructions for items 46.13 to 46.15: Match the traditional histologic classifications of endometrial hyperplasia with the appropriate International Society of Gynecologic Pathologist classification. An option may be used once, more than once, or not at all.

46.13 Cystic hyperplasia

46.14 Adenomatous hyperplasia

46.15 Atypical adenomatous hyperplasia
   a. Complex hyperplasia
   b. Atypical hyperplasia
   c. Simple hyperplasia
   d. Adenomatous hyperplasia without cytologic atypia
   e. Adenomatous hyperplasia with cytologic atypia

46.16 If no clinical intervention occurs, which of the following histologic variations of endometrial hyperplasia will uniformly become endometrial carcinoma?
   a. Cystic glandular hyperplasia
   b. Adenomatous hyperplasia
   c. Atypical adenomatous hyperplasia
   d. None of the above

46.17 If no clinical intervention occurs, which of the following histologic variations of endometrial hyperplasia presents the highest risk for the development of endometrial carcinoma?
   a. Cystic glandular hyperplasia
   b. Adenomatous hyperplasia
   c. Atypical adenomatous hyperplasia
   d. None of the above

Instructions for items 46.18 to 46.19: Match the kind of endometrial carcinoma with its most relevant characteristics.

46.18 Estrogen dependent endometrial carcinoma

46.19 Estrogen independent endometrial carcinoma
   a. Arises from atrophic endometrium
   b. Less well differentiated
   c. Generally well differentiated
   d. Slender postmenopausal women
   e. Perimenopausal (younger) women
   f. Better prognosis
   g. Poorer prognosis

ANSWERS (46.11–46.19)					
46.11 c	46.13 c	46.15 b,e	46.17 c	46.18 c,e,f	46.19 a,b,d,g
46.12 a	46.14 a,d	46.16 d			

46.20 Which of the following patient groups is NOT at increased risk for endometrial hyperplasia?
   a. Patients only exposed to exogenous estrogen
   b. Patients who have a history of regular ovulation and associated regular estrogen stimulation
   c. Obese postmenopausal women
   d. Women with menopause at more than 55 years of age

Instructions for items 46.21 to 46.23: Match the type of endometrial hyperplasia with the appropriate statement(s) about its morphology. An option may be used once, more than once, or not at all.

46.21 Cystic endometrial hyperplasia (simple hyperplasia)

46.22 Adenomatous hyperplasia (complex hyperplasia)

46.23 Atypical adenomatous hyperplasia (atypical hyperplasia with cytologic atypia)
   a. Significant numbers of glandular elements exhibiting cytologic atypia
   b. Increased gland: stroma ratio giving a "crowded" or "back-to-back" appearance
   c. Simple tubules, with marked variation in size from small to enlarged, cystic dilated glands
   d. Carcinoma in situ of the endometrium
   e. A significant amount of disordered maturation
   f. Abnormal proliferation of primarily glandular elements without substantial proliferation of stromal elements
   g. Both glandular and stromal elements proliferate excessively

Instructions for items 46.24 to 46.29: Match the risk factor for endometrial hyperplasia and carcinoma with the relative risk with which it is best associated. An answer may be used once, more than once, or not at all.

46.24 Menopause

46.25 Unopposed estrogen therapy

46.26 Nulliparity

46.27 Obesity

46.28 Tamoxifen therapy

46.29 Diabetes mellitus
   a. 3–10
   b. 2–3
   c. 4–8
   d. 3

46.30 Which of the following has an approximately 20–30% risk for malignant transformation?
   a. Cystic endometrial hyperplasia
   b. Adenomatous hyperplasia
   c. Atypical adenomatous hyperplasia

46.31 If a woman is more than 50 pounds over her ideal weight, what is her relative risk of developing endometrial carcinoma?
   a. 2
   b. 5
   c. 10
   d. 15
   e. 25

46.32 The relative risk for developing endometrial carcinoma is 2.4 times higher when a woman goes through menopause:
   a. before age 49
   b. between ages 49 and 52
   c. after age 52

ANSWERS (46.20–46.32)

46.20 b	46.23 a,d,e	46.25 c	46.27 a	46.29 d	46.31 c
46.21 c,g	46.24 b	46.26 b	46.28 b	46.30 c	46.32 c
46.22 b,f					

46.33 Tamoxifen increases the relative risk of developing endometrial carcinoma because it acts like:
a. progestin
b. estrogen
c. prolactin
d. insulinase
e. testosterone

46.34 The mean length of time for progression from endometrial hyperplasia without atypia to endometrial carcinoma is estimated to be:
a. 2 years
b. 4 years
c. 6 years
d. 8 years
e. 10 years

46.35 When compared with the findings of dilation and curettage or hysterectomy, what is the diagnostic accuracy of office endometrial sampling techniques?
a. 90–98%
b. 80–89%
c. 70–79%
d. 60–69%
e. 50–59%

46.36 What is the main theoretical disadvantage of the "office endometrial biopsy" technique?
a. significant patient discomfort
b. associated cost
c. need for cervical dilation and instrumentation to perform this procedure
d. small part of the endometrial surface that is sampled

46.37 About what percent of patients with endometrial carcinoma may be expected to have abnormal PAP smear results?
a. 10–20%
b. 30–40%
c. 50–60%
d. 70–80%
e. 90-100%

46.38 Abnormal vaginal bleeding or discharge is the only presenting complaint in what percent of women with endometrial carcinoma?
a. 80–90%
b. 60–70%
c. 40–50%
d. 20–30%

46.39 About what percent of women found to have endometrial carcinoma were asymptomatic prior to diagnosis?
a. 5%
b. 15%
c. 25%
d. 35%
e. 45%

46.40 The endometrial biopsy of a healthy, thin postmenopausal woman not on estrogen replacement therapy and without medical problems or substantial risk factors for endometrial carcinoma is reported as "insufficient tissue for diagnosis." What should be the follow-up testing for this patient?
a. Dilation and curettage (D&C)
b. Hysteroscopic evaluation
c. No follow-up testing needed

ANSWERS (46.33–46.40)

| 46.33 b | 46.35 a | 46.37 b | 46.38 a | 46.39 a | 46.40 c |
| 46.34 e | 46.36 d | | | | |

Instructions for items 46.41 to 46.44: Match the type of endometrial hyperplasia with the appropriate medical therapy. An option may be used once, more than once, or not at all.

46.41 Simple endometrial hyperplasia

46.42 Atypical adenomatous hyperplasia

46.43 Cystic endometrial hyperplasia

46.44 Adenomatous endometrial hyperplasia
    a. Cyclic oral medroxyprogesterone acetate (Provera)
    b. High dose intramuscular medroxyprogesterone acetate (Depo-Provera)
    c. Continuous oral megestrol acetate (Megace)

46.45 Patients with endometrial polyps most commonly present with:
    a. abrupt onset pelvic pain
    b. abnormal bleeding
    c. abnormal vaginal discharge
    d. pelvic pressure

46.46 Approximately what percent of endometrial polyps show malignant change?
    a. 5%
    b. 10%
    c. 20%
    d. 30%
    e. 40%

46.47 Compared with polyps in menstrual-aged women, those in postmenopausal women are:
    a. more likely to be associated with endometrial carcinoma
    b. as likely to be associated with endometrial carcinoma
    c. less likely to be associated with endometrial carcinoma

46.48 Approximately what percent of postmenopausal women with bleeding have uterine malignancy?
    a. 5–15%
    b. 15–25%
    c. 30–40%
    d. 50–60%

Instructions for items 46.49 to 46.53: Match the condition with the frequency of its association with postmenopausal uterine bleeding. An option may be used once, more than once, or not at all.

46.49 Atrophy of the endometrium

46.50 Hormone replacement therapy

46.51 Endometrial carcinoma

46.52 Endometrial polyps

46.53 Endometrial hyperplasia
    a. 2–12
    b. 5–10
    c. 10–15
    d. 15–25
    e. 60–80

Instructions for items 46.54 to 46.59: Match the type of endometrial carcinoma with the percentage it represents of all endometrial carcinomas.

46.54 Endometrioid

46.55 Mucinous

46.56 Papillary serous

46.57 Clear Cell

46.58 Squamous

46.59 Mixed
    a. <1%
    b. 3–4%
    c. 5%
    d. 80–85%

ANSWERS (46.41–46.59)

46.41 a,c	46.45 b	46.48 b	46.51 c	46.54 d	46.57 c
46.42 b,c	46.46 a	46.49 e	46.52 a	46.55 c	46.58 a
46.43 a,c	46.47 a	46.50 d	46.53 b	46.56 b	46.59 a
46.44 a					

Instructions for items 46.60 to 46.63: Match the statement with the type of endometrial carcinoma with which it is best associated.

46.60 Benign—appearing squamous areas

46.61 Intracytoplasmic mucin

46.62 Resembles an ovarian and fallopian tube carcinoma

46.63 Fibrovascular papillary stalks
   a. Mucinous
   b. Adenoacanthoma
   c. Villoglandular
   d. Papillary Serous

46.64 Which grade of endometrial carcinoma is characterized by more than 50% of the tumor showing solid growth?
   a. G1
   b. G2
   c. G3

Instructions for items 46.65 to 46.74: Match the International Federation of Gynecology and Obstetrics (FIGO) surgical staging of endometrial carcinoma with the appropriate descriptions about its spread. An option may be used once, more than once, or not at all.

46.65 Stage IA

46.66 Stage IB

46.67 Stage IC

46.68 Stage IIA

46.69 Stage IIB

46.70 Stage IIIA

46.71 Stage IIIB

46.72 Stage IIIC

46.73 Stage IVA

46.74 Stage IVB
   a. Vaginal metastases
   b. Cervical stromal invasion
   c. Endocervical glandular involvement only
   d. Invasion to more than one-half of the myometrium
   e. Tumor invades serosa, adnexa, or both; and/or positive peritoneal cytology
   f. Metastases to pelvic and/or periaortic lymph nodes
   g. Tumor invades bladder, bowel mucosa, or both
   h. Invasion to less than one-half of the myometrium
   i. Tumor limited to the endometrium
   j. Distant metastases including intra-abdominal and/or inguinal lymph nodes

46.75 The term adenoacanthoma refers to the situation in which the squamous element of the tumor comprises more than what percent of the histologic image?
   a. 5%
   b. 10%
   c. 15%
   d. 20%
   e. 25%

46.76 The diagnosis of endometrial carcinoma is most frequently made by:
   a. Pap smear
   b. endometrial sampling
   c. laparoscopy

ANSWERS (46.60–46.76)

46.60 b	46.64 c	46.68 c	46.71 a	46.74 j
46.61 a	46.65 i	46.69 b	46.72 f	46.75 b
46.62 c	46.66 h	46.70 e	46.73 g	46.76 b
46.63 d	46.67 d			

46.77 Special consideration should be given to endometrial sampling in patients who present with abnormal uterine bleeding and who are over the age of:
a. 25
b. 35
c. 45
d. 55

46.78 One indication for endometrial sampling is an endometrial thickness of more than how many millimeters on transvaginal ultrasound?
a. 3 mm
b. 5 mm
c. 7 mm
d. 9 mm
e. 11 mm

46.79 An endometrial thickness of less than how many millimeters excludes the possibility of endometrial carcinoma?
a. 3 mm
b. 5 mm
c. 7 mm
d. 9 mm
e. No thickness excludes the possibility of endometrial carcinoma

46.80 Compared with cervical or ovarian carcinoma, hematogenous spread in endometrial carcinoma occurs:
a. more frequently
b. as frequently
c. less frequently

46.81 Compared with adenocarcinoma of the endometrium, papillary serous adenocarcinoma tends to be:
a. more aggressive in abdominal pelvic spread
b. equally aggressive in abdominal pelvic spread
c. less aggressive in abdominal pelvic spread

46.82 What is the most important prognostic factor for endometrial carcinoma?
a. the depth of invasion of the myometrium
b. the cytologic grade of the carcinoma
c. the patient's age at the time of diagnosis

46.83 The International Federation of Gynecology and Obstetrics (FIGO) guidelines for cervical staging of endometrial carcinoma suggests the need for sampling of the periaortic and pelvic lymph nodes when the depth of invasion of the myometrium is:
a. more than one-third of the myometrial thickness
b. more than two-thirds of the myometrial thickness
c. the total myometrial thickness

Instructions for items 46.84 to 46.86: Match the grading using the International Federation of Gynecology and Obstetrics system for endometrial carcinoma with the best description of tumor type. An option may be used once, more than once, or not at all.

46.84 G1

46.85 G2

46.86 G3
a. Predominantly solid or entire undifferentiated carcinoma
b. Mildly differentiated adenomatous carcinoma with partly solid areas
c. Highly differentiated adenomatous carcinoma

ANSWERS (46.77–46.86)

46.77 b	46.79 e	46.81 a	46.83 a	46.85 b	46.86 c
46.78 b	46.80 a	46.82 b	46.84 a		

46.87 The 5–year survival rate for grade 1 tumors of the endometrium is approximately:
a. 95%
b. 85%
c. 75%
d. 65%
e. 55%

46.88 What is the incidence of vaginal apex recurrence when simple hysterectomy is used for the treatment of endometrial carcinoma?
a. Less than 5%
b. 5–10%
c. 15–20%
d. 25–30%

46.89 What is the primary surgical treatment of endometrial carcinoma?
a. total abdominal hysterectomy alone
b. total abdominal hysterectomy with bilateral salpingo-oophorectomy
c. vaginal hysterectomy
d. radical hysterectomy
e. pelvic exenteration

46.90 What is the first line of treatment for recurrent endometrial carcinoma?
a. debulking surgery
b. hormonal therapy, usually progestins
c. radiation therapy
d. chemotherapy

46.91 Endometrial carcinoma is often associated with:
a. chronic pelvic inflammatory disease
b. feminizing ovarian neoplasms
c. endometriosis
d. mesonephroma

46.92 Endometrial carcinoma is most closely associated with which ovarian tumor?
a. Serous cystadenoma
b. Sertoli-Leydig cell
c. Mucinous cystadenoma
d. Granulosa-theca cell
e. Arrhenoblastoma

46.93 About what percent of recurrent endometrial carcinoma appears within 3–4 years of initial treatment?
a. 25%
b. 50%
c. 75%
d. 100%

ANSWERS (46.87–46.93)

46.87 a   46.89 b   46.90 b   46.91 b   46.92 d   46.93 c
46.88 b

Questions and Answers Chapter 47:
Ovarian and Adnexal Disease

Instructions for items 47.1 to 47.4: Match the tissue type with the specific ovarian neoplasm(s) arising from it. An item may be used once, more than once, or not at all.

47.1   Coelomic epithelium (epithelial)

47.2   Gonadal stroma

47.3   Germ cells

47.4   Miscellaneous cell line sources
    a. Sertoli-Leydig cell tumor
    b. Teratoma
    c. Lymphoma
    d. Brenner tumor
    e. Endometrioid
    f. Granulosa-theca
    g. Metastatic tumor from colon, breast, and endometrium
    h. Dysgerminoma
    i. Choriocarcinoma
    j. Sarcoma
    k. Serous epithelial tumor
    l. Mucinous tumor
    m. Lipid cell fibroma
    n. Endodermal sinus tumor

Instructions for items 47.5 to 47.7: Match the histologic classification of common epithelial tumors of the ovary with the appropriate specific example(s). An option may be used once, more than once, or not at all.

47.5   Serous tumors

47.6   Mucinous tumors

47.7   Endometrioid tumors
    a. Mucinous, cystadenoma
    b. Serous cystadenomas with low malignant potential
    c. Mucinous cystadenocarcinoma
    d. Serous cystadenomas
    e. Endometrioid benign cysts
    f. Adenocarcinoma
    g. Serous cystadenocarcinoma
    h. Endometrioid tumors of low malignant potential
    i. Mucinous cystadenoma of low malignant potential

Instructions for items 47.8 to 47.11: Match the Independent Federation of Gynecology and Obstetrics (FIGO) staging for primary carcinoma of the ovary with the degree of tumor spread. An option may be used once, more than once, or not at all.

47.8   Stage 1

47.9   Stage 2

47.10   Stage 3

47.11   Stage 4
    a. Growth involving one or both ovaries with pelvic extension
    b. Tumor involving one or both ovaries with peritoneal implants outside the pelvis and/or positive retroperitoneal or inguinal nodes
    c. Growth limited to the ovaries
    d. Growth involving one or both ovaries with distant metastasis

47.12   Which of the following structures is not contained within the adnexae?
    a. Fallopian tubes
    b. Appendix
    c. Ovaries
    d. Upper portion of the broad ligament
    e. Mesosalpinx

ANSWERS (47.1–47.12)					
47.1 d,e,k,l	47.3 b,h,i,n	47.5 b,d,g	47.7 e,f,h	47.9 a	47.11 d
47.2 a,f,m	47.4 c,g,j	47.6 a,c,i	47.8 c	47.10 b	47.12 b

47.13 Which structure in the genitourinary (GU) system may mimic a solid adnexal mass?
   a. Bladder
   b. Pelvic kidney
   c. Ureter
   d. Urethra
   e. Renal pelvis

47.14 In which age group of women is it most likely that the ovaries will be palpable?
   a. Premenarchal
   b. Reproductive
   c. Postmenopausal

47.15 Compared with reproductive age patients, palpable ovarian enlargement in the postmenopausal patient is:
   a. more likely to be the result of a malignancy
   b. as likely to be the result of a malignancy
   c. less likely to be the result of a malignancy

47.16 The use of oral contraceptives makes the ovaries:
   a. more likely to be palpable
   b. as likely to be palpable
   c. less likely to be palpable

47.17 A small, unilocular ovarian mass in a patient within 3 years of natural menopause is managed by:
   a. surgical removal of the mass
   b. observation through serial transvaginal ultrasound examinations

47.18 Functional ovarian cysts are:
   a. neoplasms
   b. anatomic variations
   c. malignant tumors

47.19 Which of the following statements about ovarian follicular cysts is INCORRECT?
   a. They arise from the failure of an ovarian follicle to rupture.
   b. They are associated with a shortening of the follicular phase.
   c. They are lined with normal granulosa cells.
   d. They are filled with estrogen-rich fluid.

47.20 Alterations in the menstrual cycle associated with follicular cysts can be due to:
   a. mechanical pressure by the enlarged cyst
   b. stimulation by the large amount of estradiol produced by the granulosa cells within the follicle
   c. large concentrations of progesterone produced by the ovary in response to cyst growth

47.21 Follicular cysts usually are followed for how many weeks, with or without accompanying oral contraceptive treatment, before surgical evaluation is considered?
   a. 2–4
   b. 6–8
   c. 10–12
   d. 14–16

47.22 A patient not using oral contraceptives, with regular periods, presents with acute pain late in the luteal phase. This clinical picture is most consistent with:
   a. serous cystadenoma
   b. mucinous cystadenoma
   c. corpus hemorrhagicum
   d. dermoid cyst
   e. follicular cyst

ANSWERS (47.13–47.22)

47.13 b	47.15 a	47.17 b	47.19 b	47.21 b	47.22 c
47.14 b	47.16 c	47.18 b	47.20 b		

47.23 Corpus luteum cysts are often associated with a delay in menstruation for 1–2 weeks and dull lower quadrant pain. Which of the following must be measured before consideration of conservative management of this situation?
   a. Progesterone
   b. Estrogen
   c. Estradiol
   d. β-human chorionic gonadotropin (β-hCG)
   e. Follicle-stimulating hormone (FSH)

Instructions for items 47.24 to 47.26: Match the site of origin with the resulting ovarian neoplasm. An option may be used once, more than once, or not at all.

47.24 Coelomic epithelium

47.25 Gonadal stroma

47.26 Germ cells
   a. Teratoma
   b. Granulosa-theca
   c. Serous
   d. Mucinous
   e. Choriocarcinoma

47.27 Approximately what percent of serous cystadenomas are benign?
   a. 10%
   b. 30%
   c. 50%
   d. 70%
   e. 90%

Instructions for items 47.28 to 47.31: Match the epithelial tumor of the ovary with its corresponding characteristics. An option may be used once, more than once, or not at all.

47.28 Serous cystadenoma

47.29 Mucinous cystadenoma

47.30 Endometrioid tumor

47.31 Brenner cell tumor
   a. Potentially the largest type of cystic tumor
   b. The most common epithelial cell neoplasm
   c. Bilateral approximately 15% of the time
   d. Bilateral 5% of the time
   e. Most common in peri- and postmenopausal women
   f. Large amount of stroma and fibrotic tissue surrounds the epithelial cells
   g. Cyst lined by well-differentiated endometrial-like glandular tissue

47.32 Hyperthyroidism is associated with what ovarian neoplasm?
   a. Mucinous cystadenoma
   b. Serous cystadenoma
   c. Stroma ovarii
   d. Benign cystic teratoma

47.33 Which of the following is not characteristic of benign cystic teratomas?
   a. They contain derivatives from all of the embryonic germ layers.
   b. The most common elements are mesodermal in origin.
   c. 10–20% are bilateral
   d. Diagnosis can be confirmed on ultrasound.
   e. They often are felt anterior to the broad ligament on physical examination.

ANSWERS (47.23–47.33)

47.23 d	47.25 b	47.27 d	47.29 a,d	47.31 f	47.33 b
47.24 c,d	47.26 a,e	47.28 b,c,e	47.30 g	47.32 c	

Instructions for items 47.34 to 47.36:
Match the stromal cell tumor of the ovary
with its characteristics. An option may be
used once, more than once, or not at all.

47.34 Granulosa-theca cell tumor

47.35 Sertoli-Leydig cell tumor

47.36 Ovarian fibroma
   a. Produces hormones
   b. May contribute to precocious
      puberty
   c. Produces androgenic components
   d. Produces estrogenic components
   e. May contribute to hirsutism or
      virilizing symptoms
   f. May result in feminization
   g. May be associated with ascites

47.37 Compared with malignant tumors,
   for women of all ages benign
   ovarian neoplasms are:
   a. more common
   b. as common
   c. less common

47.38 A woman's risk of developing
   ovarian cancer during her lifetime is
   approximately:
   a. 1%
   b. 3%
   c. 5%
   d. 7%
   e. 9%

47.39 Ovarian cancer presents most
   commonly in which decades of life?
   a. 30s and 40s
   b. 50s and 60s
   c. 70s and 80s

47.40 Approximately what percent of
   patients with ovarian cancer have
   metastatic disease at the time of
   diagnosis?
   a. 20%
   b. 30%
   c. 40%
   d. 50%
   e. 60%

47.41 Which ovarian tumor has the
   highest malignant potential?
   a. Cystadenofibroma
   b. Brenner tumor
   c. Mucinous cystadenoma
   d. Serous cystadenoma
   e. Dermoid

47.42 Which of the following has not
   been associated with a risk of
   developing ovarian cancer?
   a. Use of hormone replacement
      therapy
   b. Low parity
   c. Delayed childbearing
   d. Familial predisposition

47.43 Malignant ovarian epithelial cell
   tumors spread primarily by:
   a. direct extension within the
      peritoneal cavity
   b. lymphatic dissemination
   c. hematogenous dissemination

47.44 The combination of benign ovarian
   fibroma and ascites and right
   unilateral hydrothorax is termed:
   a. Sertoli-Leydig syndrome
   b. familial cancer syndrome
   c. Meigs syndrome
   d. hydro-tubae profluens

47.45 What percent of all ovarian
   malignancies are of the epithelial
   cell type?
   a. 90%
   b. 70%
   c. 50%
   d. 30%

ANSWERS (47.34–47.45)					
47.34 a,b,d,f	47.36 g	47.38 a	47.40 e	47.42 a	47.44 c
47.35 a,c,e	47.37 a	47.39 b	47.41 d	47.43 a	47.45 a

Instructions for items 47.46 to 47.48: Match the epithelial cell ovarian carcinoma with the appropriate description(s). An option may be used once, more than once, or not at all.

47.46 Malignant serous epithelial tumors

47.47 Malignant mucinous epithelial tumors

47.48 Malignant endometrioid tumors
   a. Associated with pseudo myxomatous peritonei
   b. Most common malignant epithelial cell tumors
   c. 10%–15% bilateral
   d. 30% bilateral
   e. Typically multiloculated
   f. Contain histologic features similar to endometrial carcinoma
   g. May be associated with widespread peritoneal extensions

47.49 What is the most common ovarian cancer in women under the age of 20?
   a. malignant serous cystadenocarcinoma
   b. malignant mucinous cystadenocarcinoma
   c. clear cell carcinoma
   d. germ cell tumor

47.50 What is the primary surgical approach involved in the treatment of ovarian carcinoma?
   a. total abdominal hysterectomy
   b. cytoreductive surgery or "tumor debulking"
   c. radical hysterectomy
   d. laparoscopically assisted vaginal hysterectomy

47.51 Which of the following statements about dysgerminomas is correct?
   a. They are most commonly bilateral.
   b. They are less likely than epithelial cell tumors to spread via lymphatic channels.
   c. The tumors are radiosensitive.
   d. The survival rate for patients with small, unilateral tumors is approximately 50%.

47.52 Which of the following statements about treatment of dysgerminomas is INCORRECT?
   a. If tumor size is less than 10 cm and there is no evidence of extra-ovarian spread, treatment may include only the removal of the affected ovary.
   b. Pelvic and periaortic nodes must be assessed at the time of surgery.
   c. In all cases, there should be postoperative irradiation to the abdomen and pelvis.
   d. Chemotherapy usually is reserved for primary treatment failures.

Instructions for items 47.53 to 47.54: Match the gonadal stromal cell tumor with its appropriate characteristics. An option may be used once, more than once, or not at all.

47.53 Granulosa cell tumor

47.54 Sertoli-Leydig cell tumor
   a. Secretes testosterone
   b. Secretes estrogen
   c. May result in endometrial hyperplasia
   d. Occurs in patients of all ages
   e. More common in older patients

ANSWERS (47.46–47.54)						
47.46 b,d,e	47.48 f	47.50 b	47.52 c	47.53 b,c,d		47.54 a,e
47.47 a,c,g	47.49 d	47.51 c				

47.55 Which of the following tumors is metastatic to the ovary from other sites?
a. Krukenberg tumors
b. Malignant mesodermal sarcomas
c. Fibrosarcomas

47.56 What is the rarest carcinoma of the female genital tract?
a. carcinoma of the fallopian tube
b. Bartholin's gland carcinoma
c. vulvar carcinoma
d. leiomyosarcoma

47.57 Which of the following statements about fallopian tube carcinoma is INCORRECT?
a. The most common primary fallopian tube carcinomas are adenosquamous carcinoma and sarcoma.
b. Primary fallopian tube carcinoma may be associated with a profuse serosanguineous discharge, hydro-tubae profluens.
c. Overall 5–year survival rate for primary fallopian tube carcinoma is 35–45%.
d. Carcinoma metastatic to the fallopian tube is more common than primary fallopian tube carcinoma.

47.58 What is a "pathognomonic sign" of tubal carcinoma?
a. secondary amenorrhea coupled with intermittent pelvic pain
b. a pelvic mass
c. profuse serosanguineous vaginal discharge
d. colicky abdominal pain

47.59 Which of the following is appropriate when clinically palpable ovarian enlargement is detected in a postmenopausal woman?
a. Take a Pap smear and review in 6 weeks
b. Treat with parenteral progestins
c. X-ray to evaluate osteoporosis and collect urine for 24–hour total estrogen excretion
d. Take a Pap smear and review in 6 months
e. Take a sonogram of pelvis and consider surgical evaluation

47.60 Which of the following is not a complication of functional ovarian cysts (follicular or luteal)?
a. Hemorrhage into the cyst
b. Rupture with hemoperitoneum
c. Rupture with brief acute pelvic pain
d. Pseudomyxoma peritonei
e. Torsion

47.61 Granulosa-theca cell ovarian tumors are seen most frequently:
a. before puberty
b. during the childbearing years
c. postmenopausal

47.62 Abnormal uterine bleeding due to an ovarian neoplasm is secondary to:
a. pressure
b. increased vascularity
c. metastasis
d. biologic activity of the hormones produced

47.63 Physiologic enlargement of the ovaries can be due to:
a. follicle cysts
b. corpus luteum cysts
c. theca lutein cysts
d. all of the above

ANSWERS (47.55–47.63)

47.55 a	47.57 a	47.59 e	47.61 c	47.62 d	47.63 d
47.56 a	47.58 c	47.60 d			

47.64 Which of the following is the most common masculinizing ovarian tumor?
a. Arrhenoblastoma
b. Gynandroblastoma
c. Adrenal rest tumor
d. Leydig cell tumor

47.65 What is the hormone responsible for the findings in arrhenoblastoma?
a. androstenedione
b. androsterone
c. testosterone
d. estriol

47.66 What is the treatment of Brenner tumors of the ovary?
a. simple excision
b. excision and exploration of the other ovary
c. excision and hysterectomy

47.67 The presence of a signet-ring cell type in ovarian tumors is most characteristic of:
a. hilus cell tumors
b. adrenal rest tumors
c. Brenner tumors
d. Krukenberg tumors
e. serous adenoma

47.68 In autopsy data, breast cancer metastatic to the ovary is found in what proportion of cases?
a. 1/4
b. 1/2
c. 3/4
d. Most

47.69 Krukenberg tumors account for what percent of cancers metastatic to the ovary?
a. 10–20%
b. 30–40%
c. 50–60%
d. 70–80%

47.70 Approximately what percent of epithelial ovarian carcinomas occur in familial or hereditary patterns?
a. 5%
b. 15%
c. 25%
d. 35%
e. 45%

Instructions for items 47.71 to 47.73: Match the hereditary ovarian cancer syndrome with the statements with which it is best associated. An option may be used once, more than once, or not at all.

47.71 Site-Specific Familial Ovarian Cancer

47.72 Breast/Ovarian Familial Cancer Syndrome

47.73 Lynch II Syndrome
a. There is an increased risk of bilaterality of breast cancer and of developing ovarian tumors at a younger age.
b. The risk depends on the number of first- or second-degree relatives with a history of epithelial ovarian cancer.
c. The condition is associated with the BRCA1 gene, a locus on the 17q chromosome.
d. The condition occurs in families with first- and second-degree members with combinations of colon, ovarian, endometrial, and breast cancers.

47.74 Women with the BRAC1 gene mutation have a cumulative lifetime risk for ovarian cancer of:
a. 10%
b. 30%
c. 50%
d. 70%
e. 90%

ANSWERS (47.64–47.74)

47.64 a	47.66 a	47.68 a	47.70 a	47.72 a,c	47.74 a
47.65 c	47.67 d	47.69 b	47.71 b	47.73 d	

47.75 Compared to the general population, what is the increased risk of women of Ashkenazi Jewish extraction for carrying the BRAC1 gene?
   a. 2–fold
   b. 5–fold
   c. 10–fold
   d. 15–fold
   e. 20–fold

47.76 Of the new cases of ovarian cancer yearly, what percent will die within 5 years?
   a. 20
   b. 40
   c. 60
   d. 80

47.77 The classic triad of symptoms associated with fallopian tube carcinoma (watery vaginal discharge, pain, and pelvic mass) is noted in less than what percent of cases?
   a. 15%
   b. 25%
   c. 35%
   d. 45%

47.78 Para-aortic lymph node spread occurs in what proportion of fallopian tube cancers?
   a. ⅕
   b. ¼
   c. ⅓
   d. ½

47.79 Which of the following statements about tumors of low malignant potential is INCORRECT?
   a. They usually remain confined to the ovary.
   b. They are about equally common in premenopausal and menopausal women.
   c. About ⅕ show spread beyond the ovary.
   d. They may be managed by unilateral oophorectomy if histologic and surgical criteria for borderline tumors are met.

47.80 The risk of torsion for mature cystic teratomas is approximately:
   a. 5%
   b. 15%
   c. 25%
   d. 35%
   e. 45%

47.81 Which of the following statements about theca lutein cysts is INCORRECT?
   a. They are the least common functional cysts.
   b. They are more commonly unilateral.
   c. They are usually multicystic.
   d. They are more common with multiple gestation.

47.82 A corpus luteum greater than how many centimeters in diameter is usually designated a corpus luteum cyst?
   a. 1 cm
   b. 3 cm
   c. 5 cm
   d. 7 cm
   e. 9 cm

47.83 In children and adolescents, mature cystic teratomas account for what proportion of benign ovarian neoplasms?
   a. ¼
   b. ½
   c. ¾
   d. Most

Answers (47.75–47.83)					
47.75 c	47.77 a	47.79 b	47.81 b	47.82 b	47.83 b
47.76 c	47.78 c	47.80 b			

Questions and Answers Chapter 48: Human Sexuality

48.1 What percent of couples are estimated to have sexual problems at some time during their relationship?
a. 10%
b. 30%
c. 50%
d. 70%
e. 90%

48.2 During an individual's life, sexual identity:
a. may change
b. remains constant

48.3 The human sexual response is:
a. functionally volitional
b. cycle dependent

48.4 The human sexual response is dependent on:
a. a physical and emotional system sufficiently functional to allow the sexual response
b. a sustained and sufficient sexual stimulation
c. both a and b
d. neither a nor b

48.5 Which of the following does not mediate the physiologic components of the human sexual response?
a. Hormone levels
b. Muscle tone (myotonic activity)
c. Blood flow (vasocongestion)

48.6 Sexual practices and attitudes may be classified as normal or abnormal based on:
a. standard psychological indices
b. physiologic criteria
c. physical criteria
d. none of the above

Instructions for items 48.7 to 48.10: Match the stages of the human sexual response according to Masters and Johnson with the appropriate description. An option may be used once, more than once, or not at all.

48.7 First stage

48.8 Second stage

48.9 Third stage

48.10 Fourth stage
a. Orgasmic phase
b. Plateau phase
c. Resolution phase
d. Excitement phase

48.11 The clinical and behavioral boundaries marking the different stages of the human sexual response are:
a. clear and well defined
b. unclear and poorly defined

48.12 Across different individuals, the duration of the phases of the human sexual response is:
a. variable
b. constant

48.13 The orgasmic platform develops in the:
a. introitus
b. vagina
c. cervix
d. uterus

48.14 Sexual flush, which occurs in the face and anterior aspect of the thorax, is primarily mediated through:
a. myotonic activity
b. vasocongestive activity

ANSWERS (48.1–48.14)										
48.1	c	48.4	c	48.7	d	48.9	a	48.11	b	48.13	b
48.2	a	48.5	a	48.8	b	48.10	c	48.12	a	48.14	b
48.3	a	48.6	d								

Instructions for items 48.15 to 48.18:
Match the stage of the human sexual response according to Masters and Johnson with the corresponding description(s) of events occurring during the stage. An option may be used once, more than once, or not at all.

48.15 Excitement stage

48.16 Plateau stage

48.17 Orgasm stage

48.18 Resolution stage
   a. Vagina begins to lubricate
   b. Uterus contracts similar to labor
   c. Orgasmic platform resolves
   d. Uterus fully elevated
   e. Expansion of vaginal barrel
   f. Strong vaginal contractions of orgasmic platform
   g. Uterus drops back into normal position
   h. Clitoris increases in diameter

48.19 Which of the following is the initial determinant in the development of human sexuality?
   a. Distribution of the Y chromosome
   b. Learned behaviors from siblings and peers
   c. Learned behaviors from parents
   d. Endocrinologic development
   e. Mature adult evaluation of own character

48.20 Introital muscle spasm that interferes with intercourse is termed:
   a. lack of libido
   b. frigidity
   c. orgasmic dysfunction
   d. vaginismus
   e. dyspareunia

48.21 Which of the following is not required of the physician when dealing with patient sexual issues?
   a. Exploring his or her own attitudes about the range of human sexual expression
   b. Exploring his or her own sexuality
   c. Accepting that the entire range of sexual expression is normal and non-pathological
   d. Attempting to address sexual issues in a supportive and nonjudgmental manner

48.22 Which of the following can likely be managed by the patient's primary physician?
   a. Single disorders of less than one year's duration
   b. Disorders in the context of an unstable relationship
   c. Multiple disorders
   d. All of the above

48.23 Physician comfort with his/her own sexuality and/or with sexual issues is:
   a. independent of the physician's ability to appropriately and completely deal with patients' sexual issues
   b. required for the physician's ability to appropriately and completely deal with patients' sexual issues

Instructions for items 48.24 to 48.27:
Match the components of the PLISSIT model for the treatment of sexual problems with the appropriate description(s). An option may be used once, more than once, or not at all.

48.24 P

48.25 LI

ANSWERS (48.15–48.25)					
48.15 a,h	48.17 b,f	48.19 a	48.21 c	48.23 b	48.25 c
48.16 d,e	48.18 c,g	48.20 d	48.22 a	48.24 d	

48.26 SS

48.27 IT
  a. Providing suggestions for action
  b. Referring to a specialist for intensive therapy
  c. Providing pertinent information
  d. Giving the patient permission to deal with sexual issues/problems

48.28 Which of the following statements about the management of sexual problems is INCORRECT?
  a. In general, single disorders lasting less than 1 year in the context of a stable relationship are more likely to be amenable to simple interventions.
  b. Sexual problems lasting longer than 1 year and/or with multiple dysfunctions are best referred to a sex therapist.
  c. Sexual problems usually arise independent from medical problems and are best evaluated and treated separately.

48.29 Which of the following is not characteristic of the paraphilias?
  a. Focusing on specific objects
  b. Being intense and recurrent
  c. Engendering emotional distress
  d. Falling uniformly outside legal behaviors

Instructions for items 48.30 to 48.35:
Match the paraphilia with the best description. An option may be used once, more than once, or not at all.

48.30 Voyeurism

48.31 Exhibitionism

48.32 Fetishism

48.33 Masochism

48.34 Sadism

48.35 Pedophilia
  a. Sexual victimization of children (a criminal behavior)
  b. Sexual focus on objects (e.g. undergarments)
  c. Surreptitious observation of others unclothed or engaged in sex
  d. Behaviors from a fantasy of dominance to physical attack or sexual assault.
  e. Sexual excitement resulting from one's own humiliation, suffering, or pain
  f. Exposure of genitals

Instructions for items 48.36 to 48.40:
Match the effect on sexual function with the medication(s) which cause the effect. An option may be used once, more than once, or not at all.

48.36 Erectile dysfunction

48.37 Decreased libido

48.38 Impotence

48.39 Ejaculatory dysfunction

48.40 Orgasmic dysfunction
  a. Aldomet
  b. Amitriptyline
  c. Barbiturates
  d. Benzodiazepines
  e. Carbamazepine
  f. Chlorathidone
  g. Cimetidine
  h. Clonidine
  i. Digoxin
  j. Hydralazine
  k. Lithium
  l. Metoclopramide
  m. Metoprolol
  n. Monoamine oxidase inhibitors
  o. Nifedipine
  p. Nortriptyline
  q. Paroxetine
  r. Phenothiazine

ANSWERS (48.26–48.37)					
48.26 a	48.29 d	48.32 b	48.34 d	48.36 a,g,h,l,	48.37 a,b,c,d,f,g,h,
48.27 b	48.30 c	48.33 e	48.35 a	n,o,r	i,k,l,n,p,q,r
48.28 c	48.31 f				

48.41 About what proportion of women have difficulty achieving orgasm?
 a. One in three
 b. Two in three
 c. All

48.42 About what percent of women never achieve orgasm?
 a. 1%
 b. 10%
 c. 20%
 d. 30%
 e. 40%

48.43 Patients with arousal or orgasmic disorders are interested in re-establishing satisfactory sexual function:
 a. always
 b. generally
 c. rarely
 d. never

Instructions for items 48.44 to 48.47: Match the sexual dysfunction with the phrase with which it is best associated. An item may be used once, more than once, or not at all.

48.44 Arousal disorder

48.45 Orgasmic disorder

48.46 Hypoactive sexual desire disorder

48.47 Sexual aversion disorder
 a. Inability or difficulty in becoming sexually excited
 b. avoidance of genital sexual contact
 c. inability to obtain orgasm
 d. deficiency or absence of sexual fantasies

48.48 Which of the following statements about the sexual dysfunctions is INCORRECT?
 a. Arousal disorders may be of physical or emotional etiology.
 b. Hypoactive sexual desire disorder may include a deficiency of sexual fantasy.
 c. Masturbation is consistent with sexual dysfunction of physical etiology.
 d. Disorders of desire are often confused with arousal disorders.
 e. Disorders of desire are often confused with orgasmic disorders.

ANSWERS (48.38–48.48)					
48.38 b,e,f,i, j,k,m,p	48.39 b 48.40 n,q	48.41 a 48.42 b	48.43 b 48.44 a	48.45 c 48.46 d	48.47 b 48.48 c

Questions and Answers Chapter 49:
Sexual Assault and Domestic Violence

49.1   What percent of women and children in the United States are victims of sexual assault?
  a. Less than 1%
  b. 5%
  c. 15%
  d. 25%

49.2   What percent of victims of sexual assault seek help of any kind?
  a. 50%
  b. 25%
  c. 10%
  d. 5%
  e. Less than 1%

49.3   In caring for a victim of sexual assault, which of the following is not a direct responsibility of the health care team?
  a. Care of the victim's emotional needs
  b. Identification of the perpetrator
  c. Collection of forensic specimens
  d. All of the above

49.4   What is the most serious emotional problem faced by the sexual assault victim?
  a. gender identity conflict
  b. fear of infection
  c. loss of control
  d. uncontrolled anger

49.5   Threatened or actual violence is an integral part of sexual assault:
  a. always
  b. sometimes
  c. never

Instructions for items 49.6 to 49.8: Match the stage of the rape trauma syndrome with the statements that best describes it. An option may be used once, more than once, or not at all.

49.6   Acute phase

49.7   Middle phase

49.8   Late phase
  a. Unrealistic plans to avoid further sexual assault
  b. Readjustment
  c. Rationalization that the victim should or could have prevented the assault
  d. Begins with the assault
  e. May not be fully manifested until time of initial disclosure
  f. May be associated with cognitive dysfunction
  g. Safety and regaining control are the victim's main emotional needs during this time
  h. Reorganization
  i. Retreat to routine activities
  j. Emotionally volatile time
  k. May be associated with drastic changes in life-style, friends, and work

49.9   A woman's retreat to routine activities after a rape is misinterpreted by health care team members and police as evidence that a sexual assault did not actually occur:
  a. always
  b. often
  c. sometimes
  d. never

Answers (49.1–49.9)							
49.1 d	49.3 b	49.5 a		49.7 a,b,c	49.8 h,k	49.9 b
49.2 c	49.4 c	49.6 d,e,f,g,i,j				

49.10 The rape trauma syndrome:
   a. has a common presentation in all victims
   b. has a predictable onset
   c. is involuntary in nature
   d. is typically of short duration

49.11 The presence or absence of retreat to routine activities is directly related to:
   a. the severity of the victim's assault experience
   b. the timing of the sexual assault
   c. the identity of the attacker
   d. none of the above

49.12 The inability of the patient to think clearly after an assault is:
   a. a manifestation of an underlying psychosis
   b. not usually recognized by the patient
   c. involuntary in nature
   d. relatively rare in occurrence

49.13 Which of the following is not part of the initial care of the sexual assault victim?
   a. The provision of a safe environment.
   b. The treatment of serious or life-threatening trauma.
   c. The avoidance of discussion of the details of the assault.
   d. A gentle encouragement to work with the police.

49.14 Minor trauma is seen in approximately what percent of sexual assault victims?
   a. 1%
   b. 10%
   c. 25%
   d. 50%

49.15 Victims of sexual assault perceive themselves as guilty and responsible for their assault:
   a. often
   b. sometimes
   c. never

49.16 Which of the following statements about the physical examination of a sexual assault victim is INCORRECT?
   a. A general complete physical examination is not required as it would be too traumatic for the patient.
   b. Forensic specimens should be collected and cultures sent to test for sexually transmitted disease.
   c. Forensic specimens should be kept in the health professional's possession or control until turned over to an appropriate representative of the police laboratory.
   d. Genital and rectal evaluations are mandatory in the evaluation of a sexual assault victim.

49.17 Antibiotic prophylaxis for sexually transmitted disease should be offered to child victims of sexual assault:
   a. if there is evidence that the assailant is infected
   b. if follow-up compliance is unlikely
   c. if the assailant is a stranger
   d. in all of the above situations

49.18 Which of the following is routinely required as part of laboratory testing following sexual assault?
   a. Complete blood count
   b. Liver function tests
   c. Renal function tests
   d. Hepatitis screen

ANSWERS (49.10–49.18)

| 49.10 c | 49.12 c | 49.14 c | 49.16 a | 49.17 d | 49.18 d |
| 49.11 b | 49.13 c | 49.15 a | | | |

49.19 If diethylstilbestrol (DES) is used as a postcoital contraceptive method following sexual assault, it should be combined with an antiemetic such as Compazine (prochlorperazine):
a. always
b. sometimes
c. never

49.20 If a female victim of sexual assault of menstrual age is using an effective method of contraception, a pregnancy test should be included as part of the sexual assault evaluation:
a. always
b. sometimes
c. never

49.21 Which of the following antibiotics is appropriate to administer prophylactically following sexual assault?
a. Penicillin
b. Doxycycline
c. Cephalexin
d. Cipro Floxin

49.22 Under what circumstances should ceftriaxone (Rocephin) be offered to victims of sexual assault?
a. For all patients whose culture is positive for *Neisseria gonorrhoeae*
b. If the patient is penicillin allergic
c. When the prevalence rate of antibiotic resistant strains of *N. gonorrhoeae* exceeds 1%
d. If the victim is pregnant

49.23 What is the appropriate dose of diethylstilbestrol (DES) for postcoital contraception?
a. 2 tablets twice a day for 3 days
b. 2 tablets every day for 3 days
c. 2 tablets twice a day for 5 days
d. 2 tablets every day for 5 days

49.24 Which of the following statements about child sexual victimization is correct?
a. Victimization is most commonly by parents, family members, or family friends.
b. Rape by a stranger is relatively uncommon in children.
c. It is best to interview child victims apart from parents and other family members.
d. The use of anatomically correct dolls is a useful routine adjunct to history taking in young children.
e. All of the above are correct.

49.25 In examination of a small child, sedation should be used:
a. always
b. sometimes
c. rarely

49.26 Suspected child sexual abuse should be reported to the authorities:
a. always
b. sometimes
c. rarely

49.27 Whose responsibility is it to determine if a child may safely return home after evaluation of sexual assault or if the risk of ongoing abuse requires foster home placement or hospitalization?
a. Health care team
b. Department of Social Work
c. Police
d. State's Attorney General

ANSWERS (49.19–49.27)

49.19 a	49.21 b	49.23 a	49.25 c	49.26 b	49.27 a
49.20 a	49.22 c	49.24 e			

49.28 A child who displays knowledge of sexual matters, anatomy, or function beyond that expected for her years:
   a. is always is a victim of sexual abuse
   b. may be a victim of sexual abuse
   c. rarely is a victim of sexual abuse

49.29 Domestic violence is experienced by about what percent of women during their lives?
   a. 1-25%
   b. 25-50%
   c. 50-75%
   d. 75-99%

49.30 Approximately what proportion of women presenting to an emergency room have been injured by their partners?
   a. One in five
   b. Two in five
   c. Three in five
   d. Four in five

49.31 Which of the following is NOT one of the common presentations of domestic violence?
   a. Substance abuse
   b. Physical abuse
   c. Sexual assault
   d. Emotional abuse

Instructions for items 49.32 to 49.35: Match the statements which best fit the acronym SAFE as applied to the evaluation of domestic violence.

49.32 s

49.33 a

49.34 f

49.35 e

   a. Has the patient felt abused in a relationship? In her present relationship? How? When someone is angry in the patient's home, what is it like and what is likely to happen?
   b. Are there friends or family, or clergy, who can help? Who can the patient turn to for support?
   c. Does the patient have a plan, or idea, of what she would do in an emergency? If she has children, do they know where to go for and how to get help?
   d. Does the patient feel safe? At home? At school? In the workplace? If not, who or what does she fear, and why?

ANSWERS (49.28–49.35)

49.28 b	49.30 a	49.32 d	49.33 a	49.34 b	49.35 c
49.29 b	49.31 a				

INDEX

Note: Page numbers in *italics* indicate figures; page numbers followed by (t) indicate tables; and page numbers in **boldface** type indicate case studies.

Abdomen, gravid, trauma to, **257–258**
Abdominal pregnancy, 211–212
Abdominal surgical conditions, in
      pregnancy, 251
Abdominal trauma
  to gravid abdomen, **257–258**
  in pregnancy, 251–252
Abdominal wall
  physiologic changes in, during pregnancy, 70
  postpartum changes in, 154
Abnormal labor, 115–127, **128–130**
  active phase of labor, management of, 123
  APGO objectives, 115–116
  arrest disorders, 116
  artificial rupture of membranes in, 122
  augmentation of, 121
  breech presentation, 124–127, *125, 126*
  causes of, 116–119, *117, 119*
  "cephalopelvic disproportion," 116
  cervical status in, Bishop score for, 122(t)
  described, 116
  evaluation of, 119–120
  "failure to progress," 116
  false labor, 122, 123(t)
  forceps delivery, indications for, 127, 127(t)
  induction of, 121, 121(t), 122(t)
    contraindications to, 122(t)
    indications for, 122(t)

laminaria in, 122, *123*
management of, 121–124, 121(t)-123(t), *123*
misoprostol in, 122
operative delivery in, indications for,
    127, 127(t)
"passage" in, evaluation of, 118–119
"passenger" in, evaluation of, 118, *119*
patterns of, 116, *116,* 116(t), 120–121, *120*
  prolonged active phase, *116,* 120, *120*
  prolonged latent phase, *116,* 120, *120*
  secondary arrest of dilation, *116,*
    120–121, *120*
pelvic examination in, 119
"power" in, evaluation of, 116–118, *117*
prolonged
  of first stage of, 121, 122(t)
  of latent phase, management of, 122
  risk factors for, 124
  of second stage, management of, 123–124
prostaglandin E$_2$ gel in, 121–122
situations associated with, *119*
Abnormal obstetrics. *See* Obstetric(s), abnormal
ABO hemolytic disease, 170
Abortion, 191–198, **198–201**
  APGO objectives, 191–192
  complete, 195
  incomplete, 195, **200–201**
  induced, 197–198

Abortion (continued)
  inevitable, 194–195
  missed, 195
  recurrent, 195–196, *196*
  septic, 198
  spontaneous, 192–197
    causes of, 192, 194(t)
    diabetes mellitus and, 232, 232(t)
    differential diagnosis of, 194–196, *196*
    environmental factors in, 193
    ethical issues related to, **38**
    fetal factors in, 193
    immunologic factors in, 193–194
    incidence of, 192
    infectious factors in, 192
    maternal factors in, 192–193
    paternal factors in, 193
    systemic factors in, 193
    treatment of, 196–197
    uterine factors in, 193
  threatened, 194
Abruptio placentae, 289–291, *289*, 290(t)
Abscess(es), Bartholin's, surgical treatment of,
    372, *372*
Abuse
  alcohol
    in pregnancy, 252–253, 253(t)
  cocaine, during pregnancy, ethical issues
      related to, **37–38**
  heroin, during pregnancy, 254
  opiate, in pregnancy, 254
  physical, in domestic violence, indicators of,
      618, 618(t)
  substance, 252–254, 253(t). *See also*
      Substance abuse, in pregnancy
Acoustic stimulation, 137
Acquired immune deficiency syndrome (AIDS),
    378–379
  in pregnancy, 243–244, 244(t)
ACTH (adrenocorticotropic hormone), in
      androgen production regulation, 474
Acute cystitis, in pregnancy, 221
Acute fatty liver of pregnancy, 251
Acute salpingitis, 500
  diagnosis of, 373(t)
Adenocanthoma(s), 579
Adenocarcinoma
  clear cell, 581, 581(t)
  papillary serous, 581, 581(t)
Adenoma(s), adrenal, hirsutism due to, 479
Adenomatous hyperplasia, 576(t), 577,
    584–585
  atypical, 576(t), 577
Adenomyosis, 409–410
  defined, 397
Adenosquamous carcinoma, 579

Adnexa
  bimanual examination of, 24, *24*
  composition of, 587
  defined, 587
Adnexal space, nongynecologic disease in, 587
Adrenal adenoma, hirsutism due to, 479
Adrenal androgen excess disorders, 478–479
Adrenal function, during pregnancy, 71(t), 72
Adrenal hyperplasia
  congenital, 478–479
  late onset, **481**
  treatment of, 479
Adrenal neoplasms, 479
Adrenarche, 456, 456(t), *457*
β-Adrenergic agents, in preterm labor, 308(t)
Adrenocorticotropic hormone (ACTH), in
      androgen production regulation, 474
Adriamycin (doxorubicin), for recurrent
      endometrial carcinoma, 583
Age
  as factor in breast cancer, 421–422,
      421(t), 422(t)
  as factor in cancer mortality rates in United
      States, 6
  as factor in cervical cancer mortality rates,
      548, *548*
  as factor in infertility, 495
  as factor in ovarian carcinoma, 592
  as factor in vulvar cancer, 540
  gestational. *See* Gestational age
  maternal, advanced, prenatal cytogenetic
      analysis for, 50–51, 51(t)
  at menopause, and female life expectancy,
      483, *483*
AIDS, 378–379. *See also* Human
      immunodeficiency virus (HIV) infection
  in pregnancy, 243–244, 244(t)
  STDs and, 367
Alcohol abuse, in pregnancy, 252–253, 253(t)
Alkylating agents, in cancer therapy, *519*,
    520, 520(t)
Allergy(ies), vulvitis due to, 358
Alprazolam (Xanax), for PMS, 514
Amenorrhea, 464–468, **470–471**. *See also*
      Dysfunctional uterine bleeding
  APGO objectives, 464
  defined, 465
  differential diagnosis of, **493**
  with dysfunctional uterine bleeding, 468
  estrogen deficiency in, 468
  evaluation of, pregnancy in, 465
  in hypthalamic-pituitary dysfunction,
      465–466, 466(t)
  in obstruction of genital outflow tract, 467
  oral contraceptives and, 333
  in ovarian failure, 466–467, 466(t)

Amenorrhea (continued)
   pituitary prolactinoma in, **493**
   postpill, 334
   prevalence of, 465
   primary
      differential diagnosis of, **463**
      müllerian agenesis in, **470–471**
   primary *vs.* secondary, 465
   treatment of, 467–468
American Fertility Society Revised Classification
      of Endometriosis, *401–402*
Amniocentesis, 320–321, *320*
   defined, 320
   in prenatal diagnosis of chromosome
      abnormalities, 57
   with ultrasound guidance, *320*
Amnioinfusion, 124, 148
Amniotic fluid, assessment of, in
      isoimmunization, 167–169, *168*
Amniotic fluid embolism, postpartum
      hemorrhage due to, 178–179
Analgesia, postpartum, 155
Anamnestic response, 166
Anatomy, of reproductive system, 42–49. *See
      also specific site and* Reproductive
      system
Androblastoma(s), 477–478
Androgen(s)
   action of, 473–475, 474(t), *475*
   in female reproductive cycle, 446–447, *446*
   production of, 473–475, 474(t), *475*
      ovarian, 474
      regulation of, 474
      sites of, in evaluating and treating hirsutism
         and virilization, 473, 474(t)
Androgen excess
   adrenal causes of, 478–479
      adrenal neoplasms, 479
      congenital adrenal hyperplasia, 478–479
      Cushing syndrome, 479
   iatrogenic, 480
   obesity and, 475–476
   ovarian, conditions caused by, 475–478
      hyperthecosis, 477
      polycystic ovarian syndrome, 475–476,
         476, 477
      Sertoli-Leydig cell tumors, 477–478
      uncommon virilizing and masculinizing
         ovarian tumors, 478, *478*
   treatment of, 473
Androgen excess disorders, 478–479
   hirsutism and virilization and, 473
Androstenedione, in hirsutism and virilization
      analysis, 474, 474(t)
Anemia(s)
   folate deficiency, 218–219

iron-deficiency, 217–218
megaloblastic
   macrocytic, 219
   in pregnancy, 218–219
in pregnancy, 217–220, 218(t), 220(t)
   folate deficiency, 218–219
   macrocytic megaloblastic, 219
   sickle-cell diseases, 219, 220(t)
   thalassemias, 219, 220(t)
Anemia(s)3, iron-deficiency. *See* Iron-deficiency
   anemia
Anesthesia/anesthetics, in labor, 106–107
   epidural block, 107
   general, 107
   local block, 107
   pudendal block, 107, *108*
   spinal block, 107
Anorectal canal, 41
Anovulation
   amenorrhea due to, 468
   infertility due to, 499–500, **506**
      treatment of, 503–504
   symptoms of, 500
Antepartum care, 78–96, **96–97**. *See also*
      Pregnancy
   APGO objectives, 78–79
   breast-feeding education, 93
   fetal assessment, 86–91
      fetal growth, 86–87
      fetal maturity, 89–91, 90(t)
      fetal well-being, 87–89, *88,* 89(t)
   management plans, 91, *91*
   maternal assessment
      diagnosis of pregnancy in, 80–81, *81*
      initial evaluation, 81–82, 82(t)-83(t)
      of gestational age, 82–84, *84, 85*
      subsequent evaluation, 84–86, *85*
   patient education, 91, *91*
   purpose of, 79
Antibiotic(s), antitumor, in cancer therapy, *519,*
      520, 520(t)
Antibody(ies)
   antisperm, 503
   irregular, management of, 170, *171*
Anticholinergic drugs, for urinary
      incontinence, 389
Antidepressant(s), for PMS, 514
Antiemetic(s), in pregnancy, 247–248, 247(t)
Antihypertensive(s), for preeclampsia,
      265–266, 266(t)
Anti-inflammatory drugs, nonsteroidal
   for dysmenorrhea, 410, 411(t), 412(t)
   for PMS, 514
Anti-Kell, **172**
Antimetabolite(s), in cancer therapy, *519,*
      520, 520(t)

Antineoplastic drugs
  in cancer therapy, 519–521, *519,*
      520(t), 521(t)
    alkylating agents, *519, 520,* 520(t)
    antimetabolites, *519, 520,* 520(t)
    antitumor antibiotics, *519, 520,* 520(t)
    classes of, *519, 520,* 520(t)
    plant (vinca) alkaloids, *519, 520,* 521(t)
    side effects of, 521(t)
    toxicity of, 520–521
  within cell cycle, actions of, 519–521, *519,*
      520(t), 521(t)
Antisperm antibodies, 503
Antithrombin III deficiency, in pregnancy, 256
Antitumor antibiotics, in cancer therapy, *519,*
      520, 520(t)
Anxiety, in postpartum period, 159–161, 160(t)
Anxiolytic(s), for PMS, 514
Apgar score, 133–134, 133(t), **150**
  described, 146–147, 146(t)
  indications for, 146–147, 146(t)
Appendicitis
  in pregnancy, 248
  vs. ovarian carcinoma, 587
Aqueous crystalline penicillin, in syphilis, 379(t)
Arachidonic acid, biosynthetic pathways of,
      448, *448*
Arrest disorder, 116
Arrhenoblastoma(s) (Sertoli-Leydig cell tumors),
      477–478, 590(t), 592, 596
  management of, **600–601**
Arrhythmia(s)
  fetal, 136
  maternal, in pregnancy, 230
Artificial insemination, techniques of, 504,
      504, 505(t)
Artificial insemination using donor sperm
      (AID), for spermatogenesis-related
      abnormalities, 504, *504,* 505(t)
Artificial rupture of membranes, 107
  intrauterine pressure catheter insertion
      with, **128**
Asherman's syndrome, 193, 195–196, 467, 500
Asphyxia
  fetal, diagnosis of, criteria for, 132, 132(t)
  neonatal, 148
Aspiration, breast cyst, in breast cancer
      screening, 426–427, *426*
Aspiration pneumonia, 186
Asthma, in pregnancy, 223–226, 224(t), 225(t)
  acute exacerbations of, 224–225, 225(t)
  chronic asthma, 225
  labor and delivery issues, 226, 226(t)
  medications for, 224–225, 225(t)
Asynclitism, 101, *102*
Atelectasis, 186

Atypical hyperplasia with cytologic atypia,
      576(t), 577
Autoimmune disorders, premature ovarian
      failure in, 489
Automated reagin test (ART), in syphilis
      detection, 378, 378(t)
Autonomy, 35

Bacillus(i), Doderlein's, 360
Back pain, during pregnancy, 94–95
Bacterial endocarditis, genitourinary
      procedures and, American Heart
      Association (AHA) recommendations
      related to, 228, 228(t)
Bacterial vaginosis, 360–361, *361,* 361(t)
  causes of, 360–361, 361(t)
  clinical aspects of physiologic vaginal
      secretions in, 357(t)
  in pregnancy, 239–240, *240,* 240(t)
  symptoms of, 361, *361,* **365**
  treatment of, 361
Balanced reciprocal translocations, 53–54
Barrier contraceptives, 336–340, *338, 339. See*
      also Contraceptive(s), barrier
Bartholin's gland, 45
  abscess of, surgical treatment of, 372, *372*
  carcinoma of, 543
  palpation of, 19, *20*
Basal body temperature measurement, in
      ovulation evaluation, 495–497, *496,*
      497, **506**
Baseline fetal bradycardia, defined, 134
Benign cystic teratoma, 590(t), 591, **602**
Benzathine penicillin G, in syphilis, 379(t)
Bilateral salpingo-oophorectomy, with
      hysterectomy, **523**
  total abdominal, for endometrial carcinoma,
      582–583
Biofeedback, for urinary incontinence, 389
Biophysical profile, 88, 89(t), **97**
BI-RADS (Breast Imaging Reporting and Data
      System) classification, of screening
      mammograms, 425(t)
Birth rate, 96
Bishop score, for cervical status, 122(t)
Bladder training programs, for urinary
      incontinence, 389
Bleeding. *See also* Hemorrhage
  breakthrough, oral contraceptives
      and, 333
  intermenstrual, endometriosis and, 399
  irregular, causes of, 469, 469(t)
  postmenopausal
    defined, 10
    treatment of, **29–30**
  rectal, endometriosis and, 399

Bleeding (continued)
  third-trimester, 285–292, **292–295.** *See also*
    Third-trimester bleeding
  vaginal
    management of, **181**
    in second half of gestation, 292
Bleeding disorders, evaluation of, **75–76**
Bleeding time, during pregnancy, 68
Blood replacement products, 290(t)
Bloody show, 99
Body fat, as factor in secondary sexual
    maturation, 456
Body temperature, basal, in infertility
    evaluation, 495–497, *496, 497*
Body weight
  as factor in secondary sexual maturation,
    456, 460
  low, premature ovarian failure due to, 489
Bone demineralization, 487–488, 487(t)
Bony pelvis, anatomy of, 42–44, *43, 44,* 44(t)
Bowel movements, postpartum, 156
Brachial plexus injury, postterm pregnancy
    and, 298
Brachycardia, fetal, baseline, defined, 134
Brachytherapy, 522
Braxton Hicks contractions, 99, 123(t)
BRCA1 gene, in ovarian carcinoma, 593
Breast(s)
  blocked duct in, **162**
  clinical anatomy of and examination schema
    for, 12, 14, *14*
  development of, 456, 456(t), *457*
    delayed, estrogen for, 459
  disorders of, 417–430, **430–431**
    APGO objectives, 417
    benign, 420–421
      fat necrosis, 421
      fibroadenoma, 420–421, **430**
      fibrocystic changes, 420, **431**
      galactoceles, 421
      intraductal papilloma, 421
      lipomas, 421
      mammary duct ectasia, 421
    malignant, 421–430. *See also* Breast cancer
  examination of, 12–17. *See also* Breast
    examination
  lymphatic drainage of, 418, *419*
  palpation of, 16, *16*
  physiologic changes in, during pregnancy, 69
  postpartum, 158, 158(t)
  reproductive cycle changes in, 453
  self-examination of, 16–17, *18*
  sexual maturity of, Tanner's classification of, *15*
  structure of, 418, *418*
  tissue of, 418–419, *419*
  weight of, 418

Breast cancer, 421–430, **430–431**
  age and, 421–422, 421(t), 422(t)
  clinical detection of, 423, *423*
  clinical staging in, 429, 429(t)
  demographics of, 421–422, 421(t), 422(t)
  differential diagnosis of, by complaint of
    finding, 427–428
  estrogen replacement therapy and, 492, **492–493**
  evaluation of, 424–427
    breast cyst aspiration in, 426–427, *426*
    fine-needle aspiration in, 427, *427*
    imaging in, 424–426, 425(t), *426*
    mammography in, 424–426, 425(t), *426*
    open biopsy in, 427, *428*
    stereotactic core needle biopsy in, 427
    ultrasonography in, 426–427, *426*
  mammography in, 423, *423*
  mortality due to, 419
  in patient evaluation, 12
  patient history in, 424
  physical examination in, 424
  in pregnancy, 256
  prevalence of, 419
  simplified classification of, 423(t)
  survival from, determinants of, 423
  symptoms of, 424
  treatment of, 429–430, 429(t)
    follow-up care, 429–430
    refusal of, ethical issues related to, **38**
    selection of therapy, 429, 429(t)
  types of, 422–423, *423,* 423(t)
Breast care, postpartum, 155
Breast cyst aspiration, in breast cancer
    screening, 426–427, *426*
Breast disease, in patient evaluation, 12
Breast engorgement, 155
Breast examination, in patient evaluation,
    12–17, 13(t), *14–16,* 17(t), *18*
  inspection, 14, *15*
  self-examination, 16–17, *18*
Breast lumps, characteristics of, 16, 17(t)
Breast mass, mammographic and clinical
    detection of, 423, *423*
Breast-feeding
  patient education concerning, 93
  postpartum, 157–158, *158,* 159(t)
Breast/ovarian familial cancer syndrome, 595
Breech extraction, *274, 275*
Breech presentation, 124–127, *125, 126*
  cord prolapse in, 125–126
  morbidity and mortality rates associated
    with, 125
  Piper forceps in, 322, *322*
  prevalence of, 124
  types of, 124–125, *125*
  vaginal delivery, 125–126, *125, 126*(t)

Brenner cell tumors, 590(t), 591, 596
Bromocriptine (Parlodel), for amenorrhea, 467
Brow presentation, 118
Burrow's solution soaks, 536
BuSpar (buspirone), for PMS, 514
Buspirone (BuSpar), for PMS, 514

Cabergoline, for amenorrhea, 467
Calcium-channel blockers, in preterm labor, 308(t), 309(t)
Calculus
 renal and ureteral, *vs.* ovarian carcinoma, 587(t)
 urinary, in pregnancy, 222
Cancer. *See also Tumor(s); specific types and sites and* Neoplasia
 death due to, age-adjusted, in United States, 6
 ovarian. *See* Ovarian neoplasia, malignant
 in pregnancy, 256
 vulvar, 540–543. *See also* Vulva, cancer of
Cancer therapy
 cell biology related to, 518–523, **523**
 cell cycle and, 519–520, *519*
 chemotherapy, *519,* 520–521, 520(t)
  adjuvant, 521
  alkylating cancer chemotherapy, premature ovarian failure due to, 489
  antineoplastic agents, 519–521, *519,* 520(t), 521(t). *See also* Antineoplastic drugs, in cancer therapy
  cell-cycle (phase) nonspecific, 520
  cell-cycle (phase) specific, 520
  combination therapy, 521
  for gestational trophoblastic disease, 530(t), 531(t)
  induction, 521
  maintenance, 521
  for ovarian carcinoma, 599–600
  for recurrent endometrial carcinoma, 583
  regimens in, 521
 estrogen receptors in, 522–523
 gene therapy, 523
 hormonal therapy, 522–523
 principles of, 518–523, **523**
 progestin receptors in, 523
 radiation therapy, 521–522
Candida (monilial) vaginitis, 362–363, 363(t)
Candidiasis, clinical aspects of physiologic vaginal secretions in, 357(t)
Caput succedaneum, 108
Carbohydrate metabolism, during pregnancy, 70–71, 71(t)
Carboplatin, for ovarian carcinoma, 599
Carcinoma. *See specific types and sites*
Cardiac disease
 New York Heart Association functional classification of, 227, 227(t)

 in pregnancy, 226–230, 227(t)-229(t)
  cardioactive drugs and, 229(t)
  Marfan's syndrome, 230
  maternal cardiac arrhythmias, 230
  mitral valve prolapse, 230
  peripartum cardiomyopathy, 230
  rheumatic heart disease, 230
Cardinal movements of labor, 103–104, *104, 105*
Cardiomyopathy(ies), peripartum, in pregnancy, 230
Cardiovascular examination, during pregnancy, 67
Cardiovascular system
 physiologic changes in, during pregnancy, 66–67, 66(t)
 postpartum changes in, 154
Catecholestrogen(s), 489
Catheter(s), intrauterine pressure, in abnormal labor, 117, *117*
Cefixime, in gonorrhea/PID, 375(t)
Cefotetan, in gonorrhea/PID, 375(t)
Cefoxitin, in gonorrhea/PID, 375(t)
Ceftriaxone, in gonorrhea/PID, 375(t)
Cell cycle
 antineoplastic drugs within, actions of, 519–521, *519,* 520(t), 521(t)
 phases of, 519–520, *519*
"Cephalopelvic disproportion", 116
Cervical caps, 339
Cervical conization
 after abnormal Pap smear, *555, 557*
 in gynecology, 439–440, *440*
Cervical dilation, 102
Cervical disease and neoplasia, 547–566, **566–567**
 APGO objectives, 547
 carcinoma, 561–566
  age at diagnosis, 561–562
  causes of, 562
  clinical evaluation of, 563, 559(t), *564*
  management of, 563–565, *565,* 566(t), **567**
   follow-up care, 565, 566(t)
   pelvic lymphadenectomy in, 563
   radiation therapy in, 563, *565,* **567**
   radical surgical excision in, *565,* **567**
  prevalence of, 561
  recurrent, management of, 565
  survival rates for, 563
  types of, 562
 epidemiologic factors in, 548, 549(t)
 intraepithelial neoplasia, 549–557
  Pap smear in, 551–557
   abnormal, histologic evaluation of, 555, *555, 557*–558
   in screening, 551–552, 553–554(t), *554,* 555–556(t), **566–567**

Cervical disease and neoplasia (continued)
    intraepithelial neoplasia (continued)
        of squamocolumnar junction, 549–551, *550*
        treatment of, 560–561
            follow-up care, 561
    mortality rates due to, age-adjusted, 548, *548*
Cervical intraepithelial neoplasia (CIN) system,
    in screening for cervical intraepithelial
    neoplasia, 549–551, 549(t), *560*
Cervical mucus, hormonal contraceptives in
    alteration of, 333
Cervical pregnancy, 212, 212(t)
Cervix, 46
    postpartum physiology of, 153
Cesarean delivery (cesarean section), 112, **114,**
    129, 143–144, 322, 323, *323*
    classical, 322, *323*
    complications of, 112–113
    defined, 322
    incisions at, *323*
    indications for, 112
    lower uterine segment, 322, *323*
    prevalence of, 112
    vaginal birth after, 112, 322
Chancre, of vulva, 377, *377*
Chancroid, 380(t)
    genital lesions in, 381(t)
Chemotherapy. *See* Antineoplastic drugs;
    Cancer therapy, chemotherapy
Chief complaint, in patient evaluation,
    9–10, 13(t)
Children, sexual assault to, caring for, 617
Chlamydia trachomatis, 370–371, *371*
    chronic vaginitis due to, 364
Chloasma, during pregnancy, 69
Cholecystitis, in pregnancy, 250–251
Cholelithiasis, in pregnancy, 250–251
Cholestasis, in pregnancy, 250
Chorioadenoma destruens, 527
Choriocarcinoma, 529
Chorionic villus sampling (CVS), 320–321, *320*
    in prenatal diagnosis of chromosome
        abnormalities, 57
Chromosome abnormalities, prenatal diagnosis
    for, 50, 51(t), *52*
Chronic hypertension, **267–268**
    defined, 262
CIN system. *See* Cervical intraepithelial
    neoplasia (CIN) system
Ciprofloxacin, in gonorrhea/PID, 375(t)
Circulation, fetal, 72–73, *73–74*
Circumcision, 324
Cisplatin
    for ovarian carcinoma, 599
    for recurrent endometrial carcinoma, 583
Clear cell adenocarcinoma, 581, 581(t)

Clear cell carcinomas, ovarian, 596
Cleocin (clindamycin)
    for bacterial vaginosis, 361
    for gonorrhea/PID, 375(t)
Climacteric, defined, 10
Clindamycin (Cleocin), for bacterial
        vaginosis, 361
Clindamycin (Cleomycin), for
        gonorrhea/PID, 375(t)
Clinical ethical decision making, functional
        scheme for, 33, 34(t)
Clinical ethics, 33, 34(t)
Clinical pelvimetry, 118
Clitoris, 42, *42*
Clomiphene citrate, for anovulation, 503, 506
Clotting time, during pregnancy, 68
Clue cells, in bacterial vaginosis, 361, *361*
CMV infection (cytomegalovirus (CMV)
        infection), in pregnancy, 241
Coagulation defects, postpartum hemorrhage
        due to, 178
Coagulation disorders, in pregnancy,
        254–256, 255(t)
    hereditary coagulation defects, 256
    thrombocytopenia, 254–256, 255(t)
Cocaine abuse, during pregnancy, 253–254
    ethical issues related to, **37–38**
Colitis, ulcerative, in pregnancy, 249
Colorectal cancer, in pregnancy, 256
Colposcopy
    after abnormal Pap smear, 557–558
    in gynecology, 438
Colpotomy, sterilization by, 351–352
Combined pregnancy, 210–211
Complaint, chief, in patient evaluation, 9–10
Complex hyperplasia, 576(t), 577, **584–585**
Comprehensive health planning, and patient
        management, 25
Computed tomography (CT), in gynecology,
        435, *435*
Condom(s), 337–338, *338*
    female, 338, *338*
    Reality, 338
    Women's Choice, 338
Condyloma acuminata, 376, *376*, **382–383**
Condyloma lata, of vulva, 377, *377*
Congenital adrenal hyperplasia, 478–479
    treatment of, 461–462, *461*
Conjunctivitis, in newborns, 149
Constipation, during pregnancy, 65, 94
Consultation, in patient evaluation, 26–27
Contact dermatitis, vulvar, 359
Contextual issues, 34, 35–36
Contraception, 327–344, **344–346.** *See also*
        Contraceptive(s)
    APGO objectives, 327

Contraception (continued)
  counseling related to, **344–345, 346**
  ethical issues related to, **38**
  folklore-based techniques of, 344
  hormonal, 329–336, *330,* 332(t), 334(t),
      335(t), *336,* 337(t), *338*
  methods of
    factors affecting choice of, 329, *330*
    failure in, 328
    ineffective, 344
    pregnancy rates with, 328, 328(t)
  natural family planning in, 342–343
  patient failure in, 328
  postcoital/emergency, 343–344
  postpartum, 156
  pregnancy rates with, 328, 328(t)
Contraceptive(s). *See also specific methods and
      devices and* Contraception
  barrier, 336–340, *338, 339*
    condoms, 337–338, *338*
    diaphragms and cervical caps, 338–339, *339*
    spermicides, 339–340
  factors affecting choice of, 329, *330*
  hormonal
    in altering cervical mucus, 333
    beneficial effects of, 333
    biochemistry and methods of action of,
        331–333, 332(t)
    blocking ovulation in, 331, 332
    in changing endometrium, 333
    complications of, 333–334, 334(t)
    Depo-Provera (medroxyprogesterone
        acetate), *330,* 335–336, *336,*
        337(t), **345**
    effects of, 333–334, 334(t)
    injectable and implantable, *330,* 335–336,
        336, **345**
    nonreproductive system effects of,
        333–334, 334(t)
    Norplant contraceptive system, 336, *338*
    patient evaluation for use of, 334–335,
        335(t), **344–345**
    in reversible pregnancy prevention,
        329, 331
  IUCDs (IUDs), 340–342, *340, 342,*
      344–345
  mode of action of, 329
  oral. *See* Oral contraceptives
  patient evaluation in use of, 12, 13(t)
  progestin-only, 331
Contraction(s)
  Braxton Hicks, 99
  uterine. *See* Uterine contractions
Cord accidents, postterm pregnancy and, 298
Cord prolapse, 125–126
Cornu, 46
Corpus hemorrhagicum, 589

Corpus luteum
  cysts of, 588–589
  in female reproductive cycle, 447, *447*
  in menstrual cycle, 450, *451*
Counseling
  contraception-related, **344–345, 346**
  genetic, 49–50
  nondirective, 50
  in sterilization, 348, **354–355**
Crab louse (Pthirus pubis), 358, *359*
Cramp(s)
  leg, during pregnancy, 94
  menstrual, prostaglandins and, 448, *448*
  uterine, in menstrual cycle, 448
Creatinine clearance, during pregnancy, 68
Cryocautery, for cervical intraepithelial
      neoplasia, 561, *560*
Cryotherapy, in gynecology, 438, *438*
CT. *See* Computed tomography (CT)
Culdocentesis, 208, *208*
Curettage, defined, 438
Cushing syndrome, 479
Cyclic vulvovaginitis, 364
Cyst(s)
  corpus luteum, 588–589
  inclusion, 537
  ovarian
    dermoid, 590(t), 591
    follicular, 588
    functional, 588–589. *See also* Ovarian cysts,
        functional
    oral contraceptives for, **600–601**
  paraovarian, 598
  paratubal, 598
  sebaceous, 537
  theca lutein, 589
Cystadenocarcinoma
  mucinous, 595
  serous, 595
Cystadenoma(s)
  mucinous, ovarian, 590(t), 591
  serous, ovarian, 590, 590(t)
Cystic teratoma, ovarian, benign, 590(t), 591
Cystitis, acute, in pregnancy, 221
Cystocele(s), pelvic relaxation due to, 385, *386*
Cystourethrocele(s), **395**
Cytogenetic analysis, prenatal, indications for,
      50–54, 51(t)
  advanced maternal age, 50–51, 51(t)
  parental chromosome abnormality, 52–54, *53*
  previous child with chromosome
      abnormality, 52
Cytolytic vaginitis, 364
Cytomegalovirus (CMV) infection, in
      pregnancy, 241
Cytoreductive debulking surgery, 519
  for ovarian carcinoma, 599

Dalkon Shield, 340
Danazol
  for endometriosis, 403–404, 480
  for PMS, 512–513
D&C. *See* Dilation and curettage (D&C)
Death
  female, in United States, causes of, 6(t)
  fetal, during pregnancy, 95
  maternal, during pregnancy, 95
  neonatal, 95–96
  perinatal, 96
Deep venous thrombosis, in pregnancy,
    244, 245(t)
Defeminization, 478
Dehydroepiandrosterone (DHEA), in hirsutism
    and virilization analysis, 474, 474(t)
Dehydrotestosterone (DHT), in hirsutism and
    virilization analysis, 474
del(5p), 51(t)
Delivery, 109–111, *109–111*
  of anterior and posterior shoulders, 111, *111*
  by cesarean section, 112
  crowning of fetal head in, 110, *110*
  dorsal lithotomy position in, 109
  episiotomy in, 109, *109*
  of placenta, 111, *111*
  Ritgen maneuver in, 110, *110*
Demineralization, bone, 487–488, 487(t)
Dental disease, in pregnancy, 249
Dental system, physiologic changes in, during
    pregnancy, 64
Depo-Provera (medroxyprogesterone acetate).
    See Medroxyprogesterone acetate
    (Depo-Provera)
Depression
  in postpartum period, 159–161, 160(t)
  situational, 509, 510(t)
Dermatitis
  contact, vulvar, 359
  seborrheic, 534(t), 535–536
  vulvar, 359–360
Dermoid(s), ovarian, 590(t), 591
Dermoid cyst, ovarian, 590(t), 591
Descent of presenting part, 104
Desquamative inflammatory vaginitis, 364
DHEA. *See* Dehydroepiandrosterone (DHEA)
DHT. *See* Dehydrotestosterone (DHT)
Diabetes mellitus
  classification of, 230–231
  family history of, **257**
  gestational, 233
  in pregnancy, 230–236, 231(t)-233(t)
    complications of, 231–233, 232(t)
    delivery issues, 235–236
    fetal assessment in, 235
    gestational diabetes, 233
    laboratory diagnosis of, 233–234, 233(t)

management of, 234–235
    postpartum management in, 236
    and spontaneous abortion, 232, 232(t)
  and pregnancy, interrelations between,
    231–233, 232(t)
  treatment of, **29–30**
  type 2, polycystic ovarian syndrome
    and, 476
Diabetogenic effect of pregnancy, 70–71
Diagnosis of pregnancy, 80–81, *81*
Diaphoresis, 486
Diaphragm(s), 338–339, *339*
Diastasis recti, during pregnancy, 70
Diclofenac, for dysmenorrhea, 410,
    411(t), 412(t)
Diet, for PMS, 510, 512
Dietary cravings, during pregnancy, 64
Diethylstilbestrol (DES), in patient
    evaluation, 12
Dilation, defined, 438
Dilation and curettage (D&C), in gynecology,
    438–439
Dilation and evacuation (D&E), in
    gynecology, 439
Disseminated intravascular
    coagulopathy (DIC)
  postpartum hemorrhage due to, 178
  in pregnancy, 255
Diuretic(s), for PMS, 514
Doderlein's bacilli, 360
Domestic violence
  APGO objectives, 614
  physical abuse in, indicators of,
    618, 618(t)
  prevalence of, 617–619
Dorsal lithotomy position, 109
Down syndrome (trisomy 21), prenatal
    cytogenetic analysis for, 50–51, 51(t)
Doxorubicin (Adriamycin), for recurrent
    endometrial carcinoma, 583
Doxycycline, in gonorrhea/PID, 375(t)
Drug(s), during pregnancy, 95, 96(t)
Drug-drug interactions, oral contraceptives and,
    334–335
Ductal ectasia, *vs.* breast cancer, 428
Ductus deferens, 41
Dyschezia, endometriosis and, 399
Dysfunctional uterine bleeding, 468–470, **471.**
    See also Amenorrhea
  with amenorrhea, 468
  APGO objectives, 464–465
  causes of, 468
  defined, 468
  diagnosis of, 469, 469(t)
  with ovulation, 468
  treatment of, 469–470, 470(t)
Dysgerminomoma(s), 596

Dysmaturity, postterm pregnancy and, 298
Dysmenorrhea, 407–411, **415–416**
  APGO objectives, 407
  assessment of, 410
  causes of, 408
  clinical evaluation of, 409–410
  endometriosis and, 399
  primary, 408–409, 409(t), **415**
    causes of, 453
    defined, 453
    symptoms of, 453
  secondary, 408, 408(t)
  treatment of, 410–411, 411(t), 412(t), **415**
Dyspnea of pregnancy, 66, **76–77**
Dystocia (abnormal labor), 115–127, **128–130.**
    See also Abnormal labor
Dysuria, 187

Eccrine sweating, during pregnancy, 69
Eclampsia, **269**
  defined, 262
Eclamptic seizures, **269**
  in pregnancy, management of, 267
Ectasia, ductal, *vs.* breast cancer, 428
Ectopic pregnancy, 202–213, **213–215**
  APGO objectives, 202
  causes of, 204
  clinical evaluation of, 204–208, *205*, 205(t),
    206(t), *207, 208*
  combined pregnancy, 210–211
  defined, 203
  diagnostic procedures in, 206–208,
    207, 208
    nonsurgical, 210(t)
  differential diagnosis of, 206
  incidence of, 203–204, *203*
  IUDs and, 341
  management of, 208–212, *209–211,*
    209(t), 212(t)
    linear salpingostomy in, 208–209, *209*
    salpingectomy in, 208–209
    surgical, 208–210, *209*
  nontubal, 211–212, 212(t)
  physical findings in, 205–206, 206(t)
  PID and, 203
  symptoms of, 205(t)
Edwards syndrome (trisomy 18), 51(t)
Effacement, 99, 102, *102*
Ejaculatory ducts, 41
Electrocautery, in laparoscopic sterilization,
    349, *350*, **354–355**
Electronic fetal monitoring, 106
Embolism
  amniotic fluid, postpartum hemorrhage due
    to, 178–179
  pulmonary, in pregnancy, 244–245

Embryology, 40–42, **59–60**
  of genital ducts, 41, *41*
  of ovaries, 40–41
  of urogenital system, 40, *40*
Embryonal cell carcinomas, 596
Emotional issues, in infertility, 495
Employment, during pregnancy, 91
Endocarditis, bacterial, genitourinary
    procedures and, American Heart
    Association (AHA) recommendations
    related to, 228, 228(t)
Endocervix, reproductive cycle changes in, 452
Endocrine disease, in pregnancy,
    236–238, 237(t)
  hyperthyroidism, 236–237
  hypothyroidism, 237–238
  thyroid function studies for, 236–237, 237(t)
Endocrine system
  headaches during, 94
  physiologic changes in, during pregnancy,
    70–72, 71(t)
    adrenal function, 71(t), 72
    carbohydrate metabolism, 70–71, 71(t)
    thyroid function, 71, 71(t)
Endocrinologic issues, in PMS, 509–510
Endodermal sinus tumors, 596
Endometrial biopsy, 437, *437*
Endometrial carcinoma, 579–583
  diagnosis of, 579–580, 580(t)
  estrogen replacement therapy and, 492
  estrogen-independent, 577
  FIGO surgical staging of, 580, 580(t), 582
  histologic types of, 580–581, 581(t)
  prevalence of, 579
  prognostic factors in, 582
  recurrent, treatment of, 583
  route of spread of, 580–581
  treatment of, 582–583
    hormone replacement therapy after, 583
Endometrial cavity tissue sampling, in
    leiomyomas, 568
Endometrial hyperplasia
  adenomatous, 576(t), 577, **584–585**
    atypical hyperplasia with cytologic atypia,
    576(t), 577
  classifications of, 575, 576(t)
  cystic, 575–576, 576(t)
Endometrial hyperplasia/carcinoma, 573–583,
    583–585. *See also* Endometrial carcinoma
  APGO objectives, 573
  cystic endometrial hyperplasia,
    575–576, 576(t)
  estrogen-dependent, 574–577, 575(t),
    576, 576(t)
  evaluation of, 577–578, **584**
  management of, 578–579

Endometrial hyperplasia/carcinoma (continued)
  pathogenesis of, 574
  polyps, 579
  prevalence of, 574
  risk factors for, 574, 575(t)
Endometrial polyps, 579
Endometrioid epithelial cell tumors, 595
Endometrioid tumors, 590(t), 591
Endometrioma(s), defined, 397
Endometriosis, 396–404, **405–406**, 500–501
  APGO objectives, 396
  clinical features of, 397, 399–400, *400*
  clinical impact of, determinants of, 397
  danazol for, 480
  diagnosis of, 400, *401, 402,* **405**
  differential diagnosis of, 400
  dysmenorrhea in, 399
  Halban's theory of, 397
  incidence of, 397
  infertility associated with, 399
  Meyer's theory of, 397–398
  pathogenesis of, 397–398
  pathology of, 398–399, 398(t)
  prevalence of, 397
  prevention of, 402–403
  pseudomenopause in, 403–404
  Sampson's theory of, 397
  signs of, 399–400, *400*
  sites of, 398(t)
  symptoms of, 399
  treatment of, 403–404, **405–406**
    medical, 403–404, **405**
    observation in, 403
    oral contraceptives in, **406**
    surgical, 404
Endometritis, 184–185, *184,* 185(t), *186,* 186(t)
Endometrium
  atrophy of, progesterone-induced, **345**
  hormonal contraceptives in alteration of, 333
  reproductive cycle changes in, 452
Endorphin(s), in PMS, 510
Engagement, defined, 104
Enteric infections, STD-related, 380(t)
Enteritis, regional, in pregnancy, 248–249
Enterocele(s), pelvic relaxation due to, 385, *386*
Environment, as factor in spontaneous
        abortion, 193
Epididymis, 41
Epidural block, 107
Epilepsy, in pregnancy, 245–246
Episiotomy, 109, *109*
Epithelial cell neoplasms, ovarian, benign,
        589–591, 590(t)
Epithelial cell ovarian carcinoma, 595–596
Epulis gravidarum, 64
Erb palsy, postterm pregnancy and, 298

Erythema, palmar, during pregnancy, 69
Estrace (estradiol-17β)
  in delayed breast development, 459
  in menopause, 490, *490*
Estradiol
  in female reproductive cycle, 446, *446*
  in menstural cycle, 449–450
Estradiol-17β (Estrace)
  in delayed breast development, 459
  in menopause, 490, *490*
Estrogen(s)
  in delayed breast development, 459
  endometrial hyperplasia/carcinoma due to,
        574–577, 575(t), *576,* 576(t)
  in menopause, 491
Estrogen deficiency
  in amenorrhea, 468
  ovarian-associated, amenorrhea and,
        466–467, 466(t)
Estrogen receptors, in cancer therapy, 522–523
Estrogen replacement therapy
  after treatment for endometrial
        carcinoma, 583
  breast cancer and, 492, **492–493**
  cautions in use of, 492
  endometrial cancer and, 492
  in menopause, 490–492, 490(t), 491(t)
  in osteoporosis, 487–488, 487(t)
  preparations of, 491
  regimens for, 491
  thromboembolic disease and, 492
Ethical issues, 32–37, **37–38**
  APGO objectives, 32
  autonomy, 35
  clinical decision making, analytical scheme for,
        33, 34(t)
  contextual, 34, 35–36
  nonmaleficence, 35
  in obstetrics and gynecology, 36–37
  quality of life issues, 35
  socioeconomic, 35–36
Ethinyl estradiol, in combination oral
        contraceptive preparations, 331, 332(t)
Evaluation, 9–25. *See also specific components*
  history in, 9–12, 13(t)
  listening in, 9
  physical examination in, 12–25
  physician-patient contract in, 25–27
Excessive fetal growth, 232, 232(t)
Excisional biopsy, for cervical intraepithelial
        neoplasia, 557
Exercise(s)
  Kegel, 153
    for urinary incontinence, 389
  for PMS, 512
  during pregnancy, 91–92

Exhibitionism, defined, 605(t)
Extension of fetal head, 104
External cephalic version, 274–275, *274,*
    323–324, *323*
External rotation, 104
Eye(s), physiologic changes in, during
    pregnancy, 70

Face presentation, 118
"Failure to progress", 116
Fallopian tube(s), 598–599
  anatomy of, 48
  benign disease of, 598
  carcinoma of, 598, 599(t)
Fallopian tube disease, causes of, 500
Falope ring, in laparoscopic sterilization,
    349–351, *350*
False labor, 122, 123(t)
  vs. true labor, 123(t)
Family planning, natural, 342–343
Fasciitis, necrotizing, 187
Fat, body, as factor in secondary sexual
    maturation, 456
Fat necrosis, of breast, 421
Fatigue, during pregnancy, 94
Female condom, 338, *338*
Female genital tract, anatomic disorders of,
    infertility due to, 500–502, *501, 502*
Female reproductive cycle, 444–453, **454**
  breast changes during, 453
  clinical implications of, 453
  cyclical phases of, 446–452, **454**
    luteal phase, 450–451, *451, 454*
    ovulation, 450
    phase I: menstruation and follicular phase,
      447–450, *448, 449*
  described, 445, *445*
  endocervical changes during, 452
  endometrial changes during, 452
  hormonal changes during, clinical
      manifestations of, 452–453
  hypothalamic thermoregulating center changes
      during, 453
  ovarian sex steroid hormone secretion in,
      446–447, *446, 447*
  perimenopause in, 451–452
  pituitary gonadotropin secretion in, 446
  vaginal changes during, 453
Fertile couples, conception rates for, 495, *495*
Fertility rate, 96
Fetal acid—base status, measurement of,
    139, 139(t)
Fetal alcohol syndrome, 253, 253(t)
Fetal arrhythmias, 136
Fetal asphyxia, diagnosis of, criteria for,
    132, 132(t)

Fetal assessment, 86–91
  fetal growth, 86–87
Fetal bradycardia, baseline, defined, 134
Fetal death, during pregnancy, *95*
Fetal distress, 132
Fetal growth
  abnormalities of, 276–282, **282–284**
    APGO objectives, 276
    fetal macrosomia, 282
    intrauterine growth restriction, 277–282
  assessment of, 86–87
Fetal head, crowning of, 110, *110*
Fetal heart rate
  accelerations of, 136–137
  baseline, 135(t)
  defined, 134–136, *135,* 135(t), *136*
  evaluation of, methods in, 134
  patterns of, *135*
    grading of, 138(t)
  periodic changes in, 136–138, 138(t)
  sinusoidal, *136*
  variability in, 136, *137*
Fetal heart rate monitoring, 134–138, *135–137,*
    135(t), 138(t)
Fetal heart tones, in diagnosis of
    pregnancy, 80
Fetal hydantoin syndrome, 245–246
Fetal macrosomia, 282
Fetal maturity, assessment of, 89–91, 90(t)
Fetal oxygen saturation (FS$_p$O$_2$), monitoring of,
    140, *141*
Fetal physiology, 72–73, 73–75
  circulation, 72–73, 73–74
  gonadal differentiation, 74–75
  hemoglobin, 74
  hepatic, 74
  oxygenation, 74
  placental, 74
  renal, 74
  thyroid, 74
Fetal station, 102–103, *103*
Fetal status, nonreassuring, 132, 133(t)
Fetal surveillance
  fetal oxygen saturation (FS$_p$O$_2$), 140, *141*
  intrapartum, 131–142, **142–144**
    acid—base status in, measurement of,
      139, 139(t)
    Apgar score in, 133–134, 133(t)
    APGO objectives, 131
    heart rate, 134–139. *See also* Fetal heart rate
      monitoring of, 134–139, *135–137,* 135(t),
      138(t), 139(t)
  management issues in, 141–142
  scalp pH/blood gas evaluation, 139–140,
      139, 140(t)
Fetal tachycardia, baseline, defined, 134

Fetal well-being, **283**
  assessment of, 87–89, *88, 89*(t)
  biophysical profile in, **97**
Fetishism, defined, 605(t)
Fetus
  movement of, in diagnosis of pregnancy, 80
  palpation of, in diagnosis of pregnancy, 80
Fibroadenoma(s), **430**
  of breast, 420–421, **430**
  vs. breast cancer, 428
Fibrocystic breast changes, 420, **431**
Fibrocystic disease, misnomer of, 420
Fibroid(s), uterine, 564–571, **571–572**. *See also*
      Leiomyoma(s) (uterine fibroids)
Fibroma(s)
  ovarian, 590(t), 592
  vulvar, 537
FIGO staging
  of endometrial carcinoma, 580, 580(t), 582
  of ovarian carcinoma, 594, 594(t)
Fine-needle aspiration, in breast cancer
      screening, 427, *427*
Fitz-Hugh-Curtis syndrome, 370, *371, 372*
Flagyl (metronidazole)
  for bacterial vaginosis, 361
  for *Trichomonas* infections, 362
Flexion of fetal head, 104
Fluid retention, in PMS, 511
Fluorescent tremonemal—antibody absorption
      (FTA—ABS) test, in syphilis detection,
      378, 378(t)
9–α-Fluorocortisone, in precocious puberty
      management, 461, *461*
Fluoxetine (Prozac), for PMS, 514
Folate deficiency anemia, in pregnancy,
      218–219
Follicle(s)
  in menstural cycle, 447–450, *448, 449*
  primordial, 41
    in female reproductive cycle, 446, **454**
Follicle-stimulating hormone (FSH)
  for anovulation, 503
  in female reproductive cycle, 446–452, **454**
Follicular cysts, ovarian, 588
Follicular maturation, 41, 483
Forceps
  classification of, 127, 127(t)
  commonly used, 321–322, *322, 321*
  Kjelland, 321–322, *321*
  Piper, 321–322, *322, 321*
    in breech delivery, 322, *322*
  Simpson, 321–322, *321*
Forceps delivery, 127, 127(t), 321–322, *322, 321*
45,X, 51(t)
47,XXX; 47,XYY; 47,XXY (Klinefelter
      syndrome), 51(t)

Frenulum, 45
Functional ovarian cysts, 588–589. *See also*
      Ovarian cysts, functional
Functioning ovarian tumors, 597
Fundus, 46

Galactocele(s), **431**
  of breast, 421
Gallbladder emptying, during pregnancy, 65
Gamete intrafallopian tube transfer (GIFT),
      504, 505(t)
Gastric reflux, during pregnancy, 65, 94
Gastroesophageal reflux, in pregnancy,
      247–248
Gastrointestinal disease, in pregnancy, 246–249,
      246(t), 247(t)
  appendicitis, 248
  gastroesophageal reflux, 247–248
  inflammatory bowel disease, 248–249
  nausea and vomiting, 246–247, 247(t)
  peptic ulcer disease, 248
  pica, 248
  ptyalism, 248
Gastrointestinal motility, during pregnancy, 65
Gastrointestinal system, physiologic changes in,
      during pregnancy, 64–65, 64(t)
Gene(s), BRCA1, in ovarian carcinoma, 593
Gene therapy, in cancer therapy, 523
Genetic(s), reproductive, 49–58. *See also*
      Reproductive genetics
Genetic factors, in premature ovarian
      failure, 488
Genital ducts, development of, 41, *41*
Genital herpes, in pregnancy, 241
Genital lesions, in STDs, 381(t)
Genital outflow tract obstruction, amenorrhea
      and, 467
Genital tract
  atrophy of, in menopause, 486
  biopsies of, in gynecology, 437, *437*
  female, anatomic disorders of, infertility due
      to, 500–502, *501, 502*
  lower, lacerations of, postpartum hemorrhage
      due to, 176–177, *177*
Genital tubercle, 42, *42*
Genital warts, 381(t)
Genitalia, external, development of, 42, *42*
Genitourinary procedures, American Heart
      Association (AHA) recommendations for
      prevention of bacterial endocarditis in
      patients undergoing, 228, 228(t)
Gentamicin, in gonorrhea/PID, 375(t)
Germ cell(s), primordial, 40
Germ cell tumors, ovarian, 590(t), 591
  malignant, 596
German measles, in pregnancy, 241–242

Gestation, multifetal, 270–274, **275.** *See also*
    Multifetal gestation
Gestational age
  determination of, **96–97, 301–302**
  estimation of, 148, 149(t)
  initial assessment of, 82–84, *84, 85*
Gestational diabetes, 233
Gestational trophoblastic disease, 524–531,
    531–532
  APGO objectives, 524
  causes of, 525
  chemotherapy for, 530(t), 531(t)
  classification of, 525(t)
  clinical features of, 525
  described, 525
  high-risk, conditions defining, 528(t)
  hydatidiform mole (molar pregnancy),
    525–529. *See also* Hydatidiform mole
    (molar pregnancy)
  metastatic/malignant, 529–530, 530(t), 531(t)
  placental site tumors, 531
  recurrent benign, 529
  WHO Prognostic Scoring System for,
    529, 530(t)
GIFT. *See* Gamete intrafallopian tube transfer
    (GIFT)
Gingivitis, pregnancy-associated, 249
Glomerular filtration rate (GFR), during
    pregnancy, 68, 68(t)
Glucose excretion, during pregnancy, 69
Glucose metabolism, effects on pregnancy,
    231–233, 232(t)
Glucose tolerance tests, in pregnancy,
    233–234, 233(t)
GnRH secretion. *See* Gonadotropin-releasing
    hormone (GnRH) secretion
Gonad(s), fetal, 74–75
Gonadal ridge, 40
Gonadal stromal cell tumors, 597
Gonadotropin(s), for amenorrhea, 468
Gonadotropin-releasing hormone (GnRH),
    hypothalamic, dysfunction of,
    465–466, 466(t)
Gonadotropin-releasing hormone (GnRH)
    agonists
  in endometriosis, 404
  for PMS, 512–513, **515**
Gonadotropin-releasing hormone (GnRH)
    secretion, hypothalamic, in female
    reproductive cycle, 445, *445*
Gonadotropin-resistant ovary syndrome
    (Savage's syndrome), premature ovarian
    failure in, 488
Gonococcal salpingitis, **506–507**
Gonorrhea, 371–374, *371, 372,* 373(t)
  damages caused by, 371
  infection potential with, 372

Neisseria gonorrhoeae in, 371–374, *371,
    372,* 373(t)
  described, 371
  PID due to, 372–374, *373,* 373(t), 374(t)
  laboratory diagnosis of, 374
  treatment of, 374, 375(t)
  in pregnancy, 239
  prevalence of, 372
  symptoms of, 372
  treatment of, 375(t)
Granuloma inguinale, 380(t)
  genital lesions in, 381(t)
Granulosa cell(s), in female reproductive cycle,
    446, *447*
Granulosa cell tumors, 597
Granulosa theca cell tumors, 590(t), 592
Graves speculum, 19–20
Gravida, defined, 11(t)
Gravidity, defined, 4
Gray (unit of radiation), 522
Grief, perinatal, 161
Growth fraction, 519
Gynandroblastoma(s), 478
Gynecologic disease, patient evaluation in,
    11–12, 13(t)
Gynecologic procedures, 433–442. *See also*
    specific procedures
  APGO objectives, 433
  cervical conization, 439–440, *440*
  colposcopy, 438
  cryotherapy, 438, *438*
  D&C, 438–439
  dilation and evacuation, 439
  genital tract biopsy, 437, *437*
  historical background of, 5
  hysterectomy, 441–442
  hysteroscopy, 439, *439*
  imaging in, 434–437
    CT, 435, *435*
    hysterosalpingography, 436–437, *436*
    MRI, 435
    screening mammography, 436, *436*
    ultrasonography, 434–435, *434*
  laser vaporization, 438
  pregnancy termination, 439
  subtotal, 441
  suction and curettage, 439

Hair
  changes in
    growth, during pregnancy, 69
    loss, after pregnancy, 76
    in menopause, 487
  terminal, **481**
    defined, 473
HAIRAN syndrome, polycystic ovarian
    syndrome and, 476

Halban's theory of endometriosis, 397
Hallucinogen(s), in pregnancy, 254
HbSC disease, 220(t)
Headache(s), during pregnancy, 94
Health care for women, 2–31
  interventions in, 7(t)
Health screening, inadequate, management of,
    29–30
Heartburn, during pregnancy, 65, 94
HELLP syndrome, in pregnancy, 267
Hematologic changes, during pregnancy,
    67–68, 68(t)
Hematoma(s), postpartum hemorrhage due
    to, 178
Hematopoietic system, postpartum changes
    in, 154
Hematuria, endometriosis and, 399
Hemoglobin, fetal, 74
Hemoglobinopathy(ies), 220(t)
Hemogram, **27–28**
Hemophilia A, in pregnancy, 256
Hemophilia B, in pregnancy, 256
Hemorrhage. *See also* Bleeding
  after delivery, **162–163**
  intraventricular, neonatal, **318**
  postpartum, 173–180, **180–181**. *See also*
    Postpartum hemorrhage
Hemorrhoid(s), during pregnancy, 65, 95
Heparin anticoagulation, for deep vein
    thrombophlebitis, during
    pregnancy, 245(t)
Hepatitis
  hepatitis B vaccine, 8(t)
  in pregnancy, 249–250
Hepatobiliary diseases, in pregnancy, 249–251
  acute fatty liver of pregnancy, 251
  cholelithiasis, 250–251
  cholestasis, 250
  hepatitis, 249–250
Hereditary coagulation defects, in pregnancy, 256
Hernia defects, during pregnancy, 70
Heroin abuse, during pregnancy, 254
Herpes genitalis, 368–369, *368*
  clinical course of, 368, *368*
  diagnosis of, 368–369
  physical examination in, 368
  prevalence of, 368
  treatment of, 369
Herpes simplex virus (HSV) infection
  genital, 368–369, *368*
  genital lesions in, 381(t)
Herpes vulvitis, **382**
Hidradenitis suppurativa, vulvar, 360
Hidradenoma(s), vulvar, 537
High-grade SIL (HGSIL) system, in screening
    for cervical intraepithelial neoplasia,
    556–557, 555(t), 562

Hilus cell tumors, Reinke crystalloid of,
    478, *478*
Hirsutism
  causes of, 473
  constitutional, 479–480
  defined, 473
  idiopathic, constitutional or familial, 473
  polycystic ovarian syndrome and, 475–476,
    476, 477
  and virilization, 472–480, **480–481**
    androgens in, 473–475, 474(t), *475*
    APGO objectives, 472
    danazol for, 480
    oral contraceptives for, 480
HIV infection. *See* Human immunodeficiency
    virus (HIV) infection
Hormonal contraceptives, 329–336. *See also*
    Contraceptive(s), hormonal
Hormonal therapy. *See* Estrogen replacement
    therapy
  in cancer therapy, 522–523
  defined, 10
Hormone replacement therapy. *See* Estrogen
    replacement therapy
Hot flashes. *See* Hot flushes
Hot flushes
  amenorrhea and, differential diagnosis of, **493**
  evaluation for, **28–30**
  in menopause, 485–486
Huhner-Sims test (postcoital test), infertility
    due to, 503
Hulka clip, in laparoscopic sterilization,
    349, *350*
Human chorionic gonadotropin (hCG)
  for anovulation, 503
  in diagnosis of pregnancy, 80, *81*
Human immunodeficiency virus (HIV)
    infection, **258**. *See also* AIDS
  contracting of, methods of, 378–379
  management of, 379
  in pregnancy, 243–244, 244(t)
  prevalence of, 378
  STDs and, 367
Human papillomavirus (HPV), 374, 376, *376*
Human placental lactogen (HPL), 231
Hydatidiform mole (molar pregnancy),
    525–529
  clinical presentation of, 526–527, *527*
  complete, 525, 526(t)
  described, 525
  genetic constitutions of, 525–526, 526(t)
  incomplete, 525, 526(t)
  laboratory assessment of, 527
  postevacuation management of, 528–529,
    528(t), *529*
  posttreatment follow-up for, 528–529,
    528(t), *529*

Hydatidiform mole (molar pregnancy),
  (continued)
  treatment of, 527–528, 528(t)
  villi gross morphology of, 525, 526
Hydatids of Morgagni, 598
Hydralazine, for hypertensive disorders, in
  pregnancy, 266(t)
Hydramnios, 232, 232(t)
Hydrocele(s), 537
Hydrochlorothiazide, for PMS, 514
Hydrops fetalis, 166
Hydrotubae profluens, 598
21–Hydroxylase deficiency, **481**
  in congenital adrenal hyperplasia, 478–479
  in precocious puberty, 461
11β-Hydroxylase deficiency, in congenital
  adrenal hyperplasia, 479
Hyperemesis gravidarum, 64
  in pregnancy, 247
Hyperpigmentation, during pregnancy, 69
Hyperplasia
  adenomatous, 576(t), 577, **584–585**
    atypical, 576(t), 577
  adrenal
    congenital, 478–479
    late onset, **481**
    treatment of, 479
  atypical, with cytologic atypia, 576(t), 577
  complex, 576(t), 577, **584–585**
  congenital adrenal, treatment of, 461–462, *461*
  endometrial. *See* Endometrial hyperplasia;
    Endometrial hyperplasia/carcinoma
  simple, 575–576, 576(t)
  squamous cell, 537–538, 537(t)
Hyperplastic dystrophy (squamous cell
  hyperplasia), 537–538, 537(t)
Hypertension
  chronic, **267–268**
    defined, 262
  during pregnancy, 232, 232(t), 260–267,
    267–269
    APGO objectives, 260
    classification of, 261–262, 262(t)
    defined, 261
    eclamptic seizures, 267
    evaluation of, 263, 264(t)
    HELLP syndrome, 267
    management of, 263
    pathophysiology of, 262–263
    preeclampsia, 263–266, 265(t), 266(t)
Hypertensive disorders, during pregnancy,
    260–269. *See also* Hypertension, in
    pregnancy
Hyperthecosis, 477
Hyperthyroidism, during pregnancy, 236–237
Hypoglycemia, neonatal, 232, 232(t)
Hypomenorrhea, defined, 465

Hypothalamic dysfunction, as factor in
    secondary sexual maturation, 458(t),
    459–460
Hypothalamic thermoregulating center,
    reproductive cycle changes in, 453
Hypothalamic-pituitary dysfunction
  amenorrhea and, 465–466, 466(t)
  causes of, 466(t)
Hypothyroidism
  neonatal, 237
  during pregnancy, 237–238
Hysterectomy
  abdominal, 441
    total, with bilateral salpingo-
      oophorectomy, for endometrial
      carcinoma, 582–583
    uterine fibroids at time of, 566–567
  for adenomatous hyperplasia with marked
    atypia, 585
  with bilateral salpingo-oophorectomy, **523**
  in gynecology, 441–442
  for leiomyomas, 569, 570(t), 572
  premature ovarian failure due to, 489
  prevalence of, 441
  radical, 441
  sterilization by, 352
  supracervical, 441
  total, 441
  vaginal, 441–442
    laparoscopic-assisted, 442
Hysterosalpingography
  in gynecology, 436–437, 436
  in infertility evaluation, 497, 499, 499(t),
    501–502, 502, 501, **506**
Hysteroscopy
  in gynecology, 439, 439
  in leiomyomas, 568

Ibuprofen, for dysmenorrhea, 410,
    411(t), 412(t)
Icterus neonatorum, 149
Immature teratomas, 596
Immediate fixation, 22
Immune thrombocytopenic purpura (ITP), in
    pregnancy, 254–256, 255(t)
Immunization(s). *See also* Vaccine(s)
  postpartum, 155–156
  recommendations for, 8(t)
Immunology of pregnancy, 75
Implantation, of ovum, 500
In vitro fertilization (IVF), 504, 505(t), **506–507**
Inclusion cysts, 537
Incomplete abortion, 195, **200–201**
Incontinence
  overflow, 386
  stress, 386, **395**
  urinary. *See* Urinary incontinence

Infection(s). *See also specific infection*
  intrauterine, **318**
  pelvic
    IUD-related, 341
    pelvic scarring due to, **405**
  postpartum, 182–188, **188–190**. *See also*
      Postpartum infection
Infectious diseases, in pregnancy, 238–243,
      239(t), *240*, 240(t), 244(t)
  AIDS, 243–244, 244(t)
  bacterial vaginosis, 239–240, *240*, 240(t)
  CMV infection, 241
  genital herpes, 241
  gonorrhea, 239
  HIV infection, 243–244, 244(t)
  rubella, 241–242
  syphilis, 238–239, 239(t)
  toxoplasmosis, 242–243
Inferior vena cava syndrome, 66
Infertility, 494–505, **505–507**
  APGO objectives, 494
  causes of, 495, **505–507**
    anatomic abnormalities, treatment of, 504
    anatomic disorders of female genital tract,
        500–502, *501, 502*
    anovulation, 499–500, **506**
      treatment of, 503–504
    spermatogenesis-related abnormalities,
        502–503, 504, *504,* **505–506**
    treatment of, assisted reproductive
        technologies in, 504–505, 505(t)
  defined, 12, 495
  emotional issues in, 495
  endometriosis and, 399
  evaluation of, 495–503
    basal body temperature in, 495–497, *496,*
        497, **506**
    hysterosalpingography in, 497, 499, 499(t),
        501–502, *502, 501,* **506**
    postcoital test (Huhner-Sims test) in, 503
    scheme for, *496*
    semen analysis in, 497, 498(t), **506**
    tests in, 499, 499(t)
  prevalence of, 495, *495*
  reproductive age in, 495
  treatment of, 503–505, *504,* 505(t)
Inflammatory bowel disease
  in pregnancy, 248–249
  vs. ovarian carcinoma, 587
Influenza pneumonia, in pregnancy, 223
Inspection
  in breast examination, 14, *15*
  in pelvic examination, 19
Insulinase, 231
Intermenstrual bleeding, endometriosis
      and, 399
Internal rotation, 104

International Society for the Study of Vulvar
      Disease (ISSVD), 537, 537(t)
Intraductal papillomas
  of breast, 421
  vs. breast cancer, 428
Intrapartum care, 98–113, **113–114**
  APGO objectives, 98
  maternal, 98–114
    case studies, 113–114
    delivery, 109–111, *109–111*
    labor
      analgesic and anesthetic agents in, 106–107
      cesarean section in, 112
      changes before onset of, 99
      electronic fetal monitoring in, 106
      evaluation for, 99–103, *100–103*
      inspection of birth canal in, 112
      management of, 106–109, *107, 108*
      mechanisms of, 103–104, *104, 105*
      molding of head in, 108–109, *108*
      obstetric lacerations in, classification of,
          112, 112(t)
      pelvic examinations in, 107
      position in, 106
      rupture of membranes in, 107
      stages of, 103, *104,* 104(t)
        fourth stage, 113
        second stage, 108–111, *108–111*
        third stage, 111–113, *111,* 112(t)
      vacuum extraction in, 112
Intrapartum clinical situations, **142–143**
Intrapartum fetal surveillance, 131–142,
      142–144. *See also* Fetal surveillance,
      intrapartum
Intrauterine contraceptive devices (IUCDs;
      IUDs), 340–342, *340, 342,* **344–345**
  contraindications to, 341–342
  counseling related to, **344–345,** 346
  and ectopic pregnancy, 341
  effectiveness of, 341
  guidelines for successful use of, 341–342,
      344–345
  insertion procedure for, 342, *342*
  mode of action of, 340–341
  pelvic infection due to, 341
  during pregnancy, 341
  side effects of, 341
  types of, 340, *340*
Intrauterine devices (IUDs). *See* Intrauterine
      contraceptive devices (IUCDs; IUDs)
Intrauterine fetal demise, diabetes mellitus and,
      232, 232(t)
Intrauterine growth restriction, 277–282
  asymmetric, 279
  causes of, 277–278, 278(t)
  delayed-onset, 277
  described, 277

Intrauterine growth restriction (continued)
early-onset, 277
evaluation of, 278–282, *279*, 280(t)
management of, 278–282, 281(t)
symmetric, 279–280
Intrauterine infection, **318**
Intrauterine pressure catheters (IUPCs), in
abnormal labor, 117, *117*
Intrauterine synechiae, 193
Inversion of uterus, 111
Iron-deficiency anemia
laboratory tests for, **75–76**
oxytocin for, **143–144**
in pregnancy, 217–218
Irritable bowel syndrome, 413–414
Isoimmunization, 165–171, **171–172**
amniotic fluid assessment in, 167–169, *168*
APGO objectives, 165
defined, 166
diagnosis of, 167
management of, 167–169, *168*
natural history of, 166–167, 167(t)
nonrhesus blood group, 170–171
in prevention, 169–170, 170(t)
Rh sensitization in, 166–167, 167(t)
transfusions in, 169
ISSVD. *See* International Society for the Study
of Vulvar Disease (ISSVD)
Itch mite (Sarcoptes scabei), 358, *359*
Itching, vulvar, causes of, 359, *359*, **364–365**
IUCDs. *See* Intrauterine contraceptive devices
(IUCDs; IUDs)
IUDs. *See* Intrauterine contraceptive devices
(IUCDs; IUDs)

Jaundice, of newborns, 149

Kallmann syndrome, 458(t), *459*, **463**
Kegel exercises, 153
for urinary incontinence, 389
Kidney(s)
fetal, 74
physiologic changes in, during pregnancy,
68–69, 68(t)
postpartum changes in, 154
ptotic, *vs.* ovarian carcinoma, 587
Kjelland forceps, 321–322, *321*
Klumpke's paralysis, postterm pregnancy
and, 298
KOH test. *See* Saline and potassium hydroxide
(KOH) wet preparations
Krukenberg tumor, 597–598

Labetalol, for hypertensive disorders, in
pregnancy, 266(t)
Labia majora, 42, *42*
Labia minora, 42, *42*

Labor. *See also* Intrapartum care, maternal,
labor; Labor and delivery
abnormal, 115–127, **128–130**. *See also*
Abnormal labor
augmentation of, **128–129**
cardinal movements of, 103–104, *104, 105*
evaluation for, 99–103, *100–103*
cervical dilation in, 102
cervical effacement in, 102
fetal position in, 100–101, *101*
fetal presentation in, 100–101, *101*
fetal station in, 102–103, *103*
Leopold maneuvers in, 100, *100*
physical examination in, 100
prenatal records in, 99
vaginal examination in, 101–102
false, 99, 122, 123(t)
vs. true, 123(t)
induction of, 121, 121(t), 122(t)
management of, 106–109, *107, 108*
maternal changes before onset of, 99, *100*
mechanisms of, 103–104, *104, 105*
monitoring during, continued, **129–130**
premature, **318**
preterm, 304–309, **310–311**. *See also* Preterm
labor
stages of, 103, *104,* 104(t)
true, 99
vs. false labor, 123(t)
Labor and delivery. *See also* Labor
asthma effects on, 226, 226(t)
bleeding after, **162–163**
in diabetic pregnancy, 235–236
Laceration(s), lower genital tract, postpartum
hemorrhage due to, 176–177, *177*
Lactation, postpartum, 157–158, *158,* 159(t)
Laminaria, in abnormal labor, 122, *123*
Laparoscopic-assisted vaginal hysterectomy
(LAVH), 442
Laparoscopy
diagnostic, in pelvic screening due to pelvic
infections, **405, 406**
in gynecology, 440–441, *440*
sterilization by, 349–351, *350*
described, 349
electrocautery-based methods in, 349, *350*
Falope ring in, 349–351, *350*
Hulka clip in, 349, *350*
Laparotomy
second-look, for ovarian carcinoma, 600
sterilization by, 351, *351,* 352(t)
Large loop excision of the transformation zone
(LLETZ), 439–440
after abnormal Pap smear, 560, *560*
Laser therapy, for cervical intraepithelial
neoplasia, 561
Laser vaporization, in gynecology, 438

Last menstrual period (LMP), in patient
     evaluation, 10, 13(t)
LEEP (loop electrosurgical excision
     procedure), 440
  after abnormal Pap smear, 560, 560
Leg cramps, during pregnancy, 94
Leiomyoma(s) (uterine fibroids), 564–571,
     571–572
  APGO objectives, 564
  benign metastasizing, 565
  clinical manifestations of, 565
  diagnosis of, 567–568
  symptoms of, 565–567, 566, 567
  at time of abdominal hysterectomy, 566–567
  treatment of, 568–570, 569(t), 570(t)
  uterine enlargement due to, 565
Leiomyomata uteri, 193
Leiomyomatosis, intravenous, 565
Leiomyomatosis peritonealis disseminata, 565
Leiomyosarcoma, 565, 570–571
Leopold maneuvers, 100, 100
Lesion(s), genital, in STDs, 381(t)
Lichen planus, 534(t), 535
Lichen sclerosus, 537(t), 538
  vulvar, 359
Lichen simplex chronicus, 534–535, 534(t)
Life expectancy, female, age at menopause and,
     483, 483
Lightening, 99
Liley curve, 168
Linear salpingostomy, 208–210, 209
Lipid (lipoid) cell tumors, 478
Lipid changes, in menopause, 488
Lipoma(s)
  of breast, 421
  vulvar, 537
Lippes loop, 340, 340
Listening, in patient evaluation, 9
Liver, fetal, 74
LLETZ (large loop excision of the
     transformation zone), 439–440
  after abnormal Pap smear, 560, 560
Local block, 107
Lochia, 153
Long-term variability, 136
Loop electrosurgical excision procedure
     (LEEP), 440
  after abnormal Pap smear, 560, 560
"Low-grade SIL" system, in screening for
     cervical intraepithelial neoplasia,
     556–557, 555(t), 562
Lupus anticoagulant, in pregnancy, 255
Luteal phase, of reproductive cycle, 450–451,
     451, 454
Luteal phase inadequacy, 193
Luteinizing hormone (LH), in female
     reproductive cycle, 446–452, 454

Luteinizing hormone-releasing hormone (Lh-
     RH) antagonists, in cancer therapy, 523
Lymphadenectomy, pelvic, for cervical
     carcinoma, 563
Lymphogranuloma venereum (LGV), 380(t)
  genital lesions in, 381(t)
Lynch II syndrome, 595

Macrocytic megaloblastic anemia, in
     pregnancy, 219
Macrosomia, 232, 232(t)
  fetal, 282
Magnesium sulfate
  for preeclampsia, 264, 265(t)
  in preterm labor, 308(t), 309(t)
Magnetic resonance imaging (MRI), in
     gynecology, 435
Malignant epithelial serous tumors (serous
     cystadenocarcinoma), 595
Malignant mesodermal sarcomas, 597
Malignant mucinous epithelial tumor (mucinous
     cystadenocarcinoma), 595
Mammary duct ectasia, of breast, 421
Mammography, 59–60
  in breast cancer screening, 423, 423
  in gynecology, 436, 436
  screening, in breast cancer screening,
     424–426, 425(t), 426
     BI-RADS classification of, 425(t)
     guidelines for, 425(t)
Management, 25, 26(t)
Marfan's syndrome, in pregnancy, 230
Marijuana use
  delayed puberty due to, 459–460
  during pregnancy, 254
Masculinization, 478
Masochism, defined, 605(t)
Mastitis, 188–189
  postpartum, 155, 188
Maternal age, advanced, prenatal cytogenetic
     analysis for, 50–51, 51(t)
Maternal cardiac arrhythmias, in
     pregnancy, 230
Maternal death, during pregnancy, 95
Maternal physiology, 64–72. See also
     Pregnancy, physiologic changes in
Maternal-fetal physiology, APGO objectives, 63
Measles
  German, in pregnancy, 241–242
  mumps, rubella (MMR), immunizations for, 8(t)
Meconium aspiration syndrome, 124, 147–148
  postterm pregnancy and, 298
Medroxyprogesterone acetate (Depo-Provera)
  contraindications to, 336, 337(t)
  in delayed breast development, 459
  for dysfunctional uterine bleeding,
     469–470, 470(t)

Medroxyprogesterone acetate (Depo-Provera)
    (continued)
  efficacy of, 335–336
  indications for, 336, 337(t)
  injectable, 330 335–336, 336, 337(t), **345**
  in menopause, 491
  mode of action of, 335, 336
  release of progestin for, 335, 336
Mefenamic acid, for dysmenorrhea, 410,
    411(t), 412(t)
Megaloblastic anemia, in pregnancy, 218–219
Meigs syndrome, 592
Melanoma, vulvar, 540
Melasma, during pregnancy, 69
Mendelian disorders, screening tests for,
    54–56, 55
Menopause, 482–492, **492–493**. *See also*
    Premature ovarian failure
  age at, and female life expectancy, 483, 483
  APGO objectives, 482
  average age at, 484, 484
  cardiovascular lipid changes in, 488
  climacteric relationship to, 483
  defined, 10
  genital tract atrophy in, 486
  hot flushes in, 485–486
  management of, **29–30**, 490–492,
    490(t), 491(t)
  menstruation and, 483–484, 483(t), 485
  mood changes in, 486–487
  osteoporosis in, 487–488, 487(t)
  skin, hair, and nail changes in, 487
  sleep disturbances in, 486
  vaginal dryness in, 486
  vasomotor instability in, 485–486
Menorrhagia, defined, 566
Menstrual cycle
  alterations in, 484–485, 485(t)
  luteal phase of, 499
Menstrual history, in patient evaluation,
    10, 13(t)
Menstruation
  age at first, 465
  age at termination of, 465
  in female reproductive cycle, 447–450,
    448, 449
  and menopause, 483–484, 483(t), 485
Mesonephric ducts, 41
Mesosalpinx, benign disease of, 598
Mestranol, in combination oral contraceptive
    preparations, 331, 332(t)
Methergine, for uterine atony, 175
Methotrexate, in ectopic pregnancy, 209,
    209(t), 210
Methyldopa, for hypertensive disorders, in
    pregnancy, 266(t)

Metritis, **189–190**
  postpartum, 184–185, 184, 185(t), 186, 186(t)
Metronidazole (Flagyl)
  for bacterial vaginosis, 361
  for *Trichomonas* infections, 362
Meyer's theory of endometriosis, 397–398
Microhemagglutination assay for antibodies to
    Treponema palllidum (MHA—TP) test, in
    syphilis detection, 378, 378(t)
Misoprostol, in abnormal labor, 122
Mite(s), itch (sarcoptes scabei), 358, 359
Mitral valve prolapse, in pregnancy, 230
Molar pregnancy. *See* Hydatdidform mole
    (molar pregnancy)
Molding of head, in second stage of labor,
    108–109, 108
Molluscum contagiosum, 380(t)
Monilial infection, in bacterial vagninosis,
    361, 361
Monilial vaginitis, 362–363, 363(t)
Mood changes
  in menopause, 486–487
  during secondary sexual maturation, 457
MRI. *See* Magnetic resonance imaging (MRI)
Mucinous cystadenocarcinoma (malignant
    mucinous epithelial tumor), 595
Mucinous cystadenoma, ovarian, 590(t), 591
Mucinous tumors, ovarian, 590(t), 591
Mucus, cervical, hormonal contraceptives in
    alteration of, 333
Müllerian agenesis (Rokitansky-Küster-Hauser
    syndrome), 460, **463**
  primary amenorrhea in, **470–471**
Multifetal gestation, 270–274, **275**
  APGO objectives, 270
  diagnosis of, 273–274, 273(t)
  incidence of, 271
  intrapartum management of, 274–275, 274
  natural history of, 271–273, 272
Multifocal duct carcinoma, 426, 426
Multigravida, defined, 11(t)
Multipara, defined, 11(t)
Multiple gestation. *See* Multifetal gestation
Musculoskeletal system, physiologic changes in,
    during pregnancy, 70
Myomectomy, for leiomyomas, 568–570,
    569(t), 570(t)
Myrtiform caruncles, 153

Nail changes, in menopause, 487
Natural family planning, 342–343
Nausea and vomiting, during pregnancy, 94,
    246–247, 247(t)
Necrotizing fasciitis, 187
Needle aspiration, in breast cancer screening,
    426–427, 426

Neisseria gonorrhoeae, 371–374, *371, 372,*
    373(t). *See also* Gonorrhea
Neonatal asphyxia, 148
Neonatal death, 95–96
Neonatal hypoglycemia, 232, 232(t)
Neonatal hypothyroidism, 237
Neonatal intraventricular hemorrhage, **318**
Neoplasia, ovarian, 586–600, **600–602.** *See
    also* Ovarian neoplasia
Neoplasm(s), adrenal, 479
Neurectomy, presacral, for dysmenorrhea, 410
Neurologic disease, in pregnancy, 245–246
Nevus(i), vulvar, 537
Newborn(s)
  immediate care of, 145–149, **150**
    APGO objectives, 145
    conjunctivitis, 149
    estimation of gestational age in, 148, 149(t)
    initial assessment in, 146–148, 146(t), 147(t)
    jaundice, 149
    meconium staining of amniotic fluid,
        147–148
    neonatal asphyxia, 148
    normal umbilical cord blood gas values in,
        147, 147(t)
    nutrition, 149
    resuscitation in, 146, 146(t)
    routine care, 148–149, 149(t)
    stool, 148–149
    umbilical cord, 148
    urine, 148–149
  management of, **150**
Nickerson's media, in *Candida* vaginitis
    diagnosis, 363, *365*
Nifedipine
  for hypertensive disorders, in
    pregnancy, 266(t)
  in preterm labor, 308(t), 309(t)
2001 Bethesda system, in screening for cervical
    intraepithelial neoplasia, 552, 557,
    553(t), 555(t)
Nipple care, 158
Nitrazine test, for PROM, 314, 314(t)
Nondirective counseling, 50
Nonmaleficence, 35
Nonreassuring fetal status, 132, 133(t)
  causes of, 133(t)
Non-Rh D/non-ABO hemolytic disease, 171
Norplant contraceptive system, 336, *338*
1,9–Nortestosterone(s), in combination oral
    contraceptive preparations, 331, 332(t)
Nulligravida, defined, 11(t)
Nullipara, defined, 11(t)
Nutrition
  in newborns, 149
  during pregnancy, 92–93

Obesity
  polycystic ovarian syndrome and, 475–476
  treatment of, **29–30**
Obstetric(s)
  abnormal, 165–318. *See also specific topics*
    abortion, 191–198, **198–201**
    ectopic pregnancy, 202–213, **213–215**
    fetal growth abnormalities, 276–282,
        282–284
    hemorrhage, 173–180, **180–181**
    hypertension in pregnancy, 260–267,
        267–269
    medical and surgical conditions of
        pregnancy, 216–256, **257–259**
    multifetal gestation, 270–274, **275**
    postpartum infection, 182–188, **188–190**
    postterm pregnancy, 296–301, **301–303**
    preterm labor, 304–309, **310–311**
    PROM, 312–317, **317–318**
    third-trimester bleeding, 285–292, **292–295**
  historical background of, 5
  patient evaluation in, 10–11, 11(t), 13(t)
Obstetric procedures, 319–324. *See also*
    Obstetric(s)
  aminiocentesis, 320–321, *320*
  APGO objectives, 319
  cesarean delivery, 322, 323, *323*
  chorionic villus sampling, 320–321, *320*
  circumcision, 324
  in determination of gestational age, 84
  external cephalic version, 323–324, *323*
  forceps delivery, 321–322, *322, 321*
  periumbilical artery blood sampling, 321
  vacuum extraction, 322, *322*
Obstetrics and gynecology, historical
    background of, 5
Ofloxacin, in gonorrhea/PID, 375(t)
Oligohydramnios, **283–284**
  postterm pregnancy and, 298
Oligomenorrhea, defined, 465
Oocyte(s), 483
  in fertilization, 500
  premature loss of, causes of, 489(t)
Open biopsy, in breast cancer screening, 427, *428*
Opiate abuse, in pregnancy, 254
Oral contraceptives. *See also* Contraceptive(s),
    hormonal
  beneficial effects of, 333
  breakthrough bleeding due to, 333
  combination therapy, contraindications
    to, 335(t)
  common preparations of, 331, 332(t)
  drug interactions with, 334–335
  for endometriosis, **406**
  ethical issues related to, **38**
  for hirsutism and virilization, 480

Oral contraceptives (continued)
new symptoms in patients using, management
of, 334, 334(t)
nonreproductive system effects of,
333–334, 334(t)
for ovarian cyst, **600–601**
patient evaluation for use of, 334–335, 335(t),
344–345
"phasic" formulations of, 331
for PMS, 512–513
for polycystic ovarian syndrome, 476
prevalence of, 329
Osteoporosis, in menopause, 487–488, 487(t)
Ovarian cysts
functional, 588–589
corpus hemorrhagicum, 589
corpus luteum cysts, 588–589
follicular cysts, 588
theca lutein cysts, 589
oral contraceptives for, **600–601**
Ovarian failure
amenorrhea and, 466–467, 466(t)
causes of, 467, 467(t)
premature, 488–490, 489(t)
signs and symptoms of, 484–488
Ovarian fibroma, 590(t), 592
Ovarian follicles, development of, cyclic
changes in, 447
Ovarian neoplasia, 586–600, **600–602**
APGO objectives, 586
benign, 589–592, 590(t)
epithelial cell, 589–591, 590(t)
Brenner cell tumor, 590(t), 591
endometrioid tumor, 590(t), 591
mucinous cystadenoma, 590(t), 591
mucinous tumors, 590(t), 591
serous cystadenoma, 590, 590(t)
germ cell, 590(t), 591
stromal cell, 590(t), 591–592
treatment of, **600–601**
differential diagnosis of, 587
histogenic classification of, 590(t)
malignant, 592–597
borderline tumors, 594–595
diagnosis of, 593
epithelial cell, 595–596
endometrioid tumors, 595
FIGO staging for, 594, 594(t)
genetic factors in, 593
germ cell tumors, 596
rare, 596
gonadal stromal cell tumors, 597
histologic classification of, 593–594
metastatic to ovary, 597–598
mortality rates due to, 592
pathogenesis of, 593
prevalence of, 592

risk factors for, 592
site-specific familial, 595
surgical management of
follow-up care, 600
general principles in, 599–600
Ovarian pregnancy, 212, 212(t)
Ovarian sex steroid hormone secretion, in
female reproductive cycle, 446–447,
446, 447
Ovarian tumors, borderline, 594–595
Ovary(ies)
anatomy of, 48, 48, 49
development of, 40–41
evaluation of, 587
neoplasia of. See Ovarian neoplasia
palpation of, 587
in postmenopausal patients, 587
postpartum physiology of, 153, 153
tumors of, removal of, **523**
Overflow incontinence, 386
Ovulation
basal body temperature measurement in,
495–497, 496, 497, **506**
blocking of, hormonal contraceptives in,
331, 332
dysfunctional uterine bleeding with, 468
evaluation of, diagnostic studies in, 499–500
features of, 499
in female reproductive cycle, 450
postpartum return of, 153, 153
progesterone in, 499–500
Ovum, implantation of, 500
Oxygenation, fetal, 74
Oxytocin
for induction and augmentation of labor,
121, 121(t)
for iron-deficiency anemia, **143–144**
suckling-induced reduced reflex release of,
somatosensory pathways for, 158
Oxytocin challenge test (OCT), 88

P53, tumor suppressor gene, in ovarian
carcinoma, 593
Paclitaxel (Taxol), for ovarian carcinoma, 599
Paget disease, 540, 540
Pain
back, during pregnancy, 94–95
pelvic, **199–200**. See also Pelvic pain
round ligament, during pregnancy, 95
Painful menstruation (dysmenorrhea), 407–411,
415–416. See also Dysmenorrhea
Palmar erythema, during pregnancy, 69
Palpation
in breast examination, 16, 16
in pelvic examination, 19, 20
Palsy(ies), erb, postterm pregnancy and, 298
Pap smear. See Papanicolaou (Pap) smear

Papanicolaou (Pap) smear, 22, *23, 27–28*
  abnormal
    cervical conization after, 558–560, *560*
    colposcopy after, 558–560
    histologic evaluation of, 558–560, *560*
    in screening for cervical intraepithelial
        neoplasia, 549–557, 553(t), *554,* 555(t),
        566–567
      classification systems of, 549–557, 553(t), *554*
        CIN system, 549–552, 553(t), *554*
        HGSIL system, 549–552, 553(t), *554*
        LGSIL system, 549–552, 553(t), *554*
        SIL system, 549–552, 553(t), *554*
      timing of, 551
Papillary serous adenocarcinoma, 581, 581(t)
Papilloma(s), intraductal
  of breast, 421
  vs. breast cancer, 428
ParaGard, 340, *340*
Paralysis, Klumpe's, postterm pregnancy and, 298
Paramesonephric ducts, 41
Paraovarian cysts, 598
Paraphilia(s), 605–606, 605(t)
Parasite(s), STDs due to, 380(t)
Paratubal cysts, 598
Parental chromosome rearrangements, 53
Parental inversion, 54
Parity, defined, 4
Parlodel (bromocriptine), for amenorrhea, 467
Partial moles, 525
Parturient, defined, 11(t)
"Passage", in abnormal labor, evaluation of,
    118–119
"Passenger", in abnormal labor, evaluation of,
    118, *119*
Patau syndrome (trisomy 13), 51(t)
Patient education
  antepartum, 91, *91*
  postpartum, 157
Patient history, in patient evaluation, 9–12, 13(t)
  chief complaint, 9–10, 13(t)
  contraceptive history, 12, 13(t)
  gynecologic history, 11–12, 13(t)
  menstrual history, 10, 13(t)
  obstetric history, 10–11, 11(t), 13(t)
  sexual history, 12, 13(t)
Patient management, 25, 26(t)
Pederson speculum, 19
Pedophilia, defined, 605(t)
Pelvic examination, 17–25
  bimanual, 23–24, *24*
  in determination of gestational age, 83
  inspection in, 19
  palpation in, 19, *20*
  positioning for, 19
  in pregnancy diagnosis, 80
  preparation for, 17–18

rectovaginal examination in, 24–25, *24*
  speculum examination in, 19–23, *21–23*
  talk before you touch principle in, 17–18
Pelvic infections
  IUD-related, 341
  organisms associated with, 185(t)
  pelvic scarring due to, **405**
Pelvic inflammatory disease (PID),
    369–374
  chlamydial, 370–371, *371*
  ectopic pregnancy due to, 203
  gonorrheal, 371–374, *371, 372,* 373(t)
  hospitalization for patients with, factors
      indicating need for, 373, 373(t)
  misdiagnosis of, correct diagnosis in cases
      of, 374(t)
  pathogenesis of, 369–370
  salpingitis, **383**
  sequelae of, *371*
  symptoms of, frequency of, 373, *373*
  treatment of, 375(t)
Pelvic lymphadenectomy, for cervical
    carcinoma, 560
Pelvic pain, **199–200**
  chronic, 411–414, **416**
    APGO objectives, 407
    assessment of, 412–413
    causes of, 411, 413(t)
    defined, 408
    differential diagnosis of, 412–413
    follow-up for, 414
    patient history in, 411
    prevalence of, 411
    treatment of, 414
  endometriosis and, 399
Pelvic relaxation
  APGO objectives, 384–385
  causes of, 385, *386*
  clinical presentation of, 386–387, 387(t)
  degrees of, 387–388, *388*
  described, 385
  differential diagnosis of, 389, *390*
  evaluation of, 387–388, *388*
  treatment of
    nonsurgical, 389–391, *390*
    surgical, 391–392, 391(t), *392*
  urinary incontinence due to, 385
Pelvic sonography, **59–60**
Pelvic support, loss of, 385, *386. See also* Pelvic
    relaxation
Pelvimetry, clinical, 118
Pelvis
  android, 43–44, *44*
  anthropoid, 44, *44*
  arterial system of, 48, *49*
  bony, anatomy of, 42–44, *43, 44,* 44(t)
  diameter of, 43, *44,* 44(t)

Pelvis (continued)
  gynecoid, 43, *44*
  planes of, 42–43
  platypelloid, 43, *44*
  types of, 43–44, *44*
Pelviscopy, in gynecology, 440–441, *440*
Penicillin(s), aqueous crystalline, in
    syphilis, 379(t)
Penicillin G, in syphilis, 379(t)
Peptic ulcer disease, in pregnancy, 248
Perihepatitis, 370, *371, 372*
Perimenopause, 451–452
Perinatal death, 96
Perinatal grief, 161
Perineum
  anatomy of, 45, *45, 46*
  postpartum care of, 156
Peripartum cardiomyopathy, in pregnancy, 230
Peripheral vascular resistance, during
    pregnancy, 67
Periumbilical artery blood sampling (PUBS), 321
  in prenatal diagnosis of chromosome
    abnormalities, 57
Persistent occiput posterior positions, 118
Pessary(ies), for urinary incontinence,
    389–391, *390*
Phlegmon, postcesarean, 184
Physical abuse, in domestic violence, indicators
    of, 618, 618(t)
Physical examination
  of breasts, 12–25
  of pelvis, 17–25
Physician-patient contract, in patient
    evaluation, 25–27
Pica, 64
  in pregnancy, 248
PID. *See* Pelvic inflammatory disease (PID)
Piper forceps, 321–322, *322, 321*
  in breech delivery, *322, 322*
Pituitary gonadotropin secretion, in female
    reproductive cycle, 446
Pituitary prolactinoma, amenorrhea and, **493**
Placenta
  delivery of, 111, *111*
  during gestation, 74
  retained, postpartum hemorrhage due to,
    177–178
  separation of, 111–112
Placenta accreta, 178
Placenta increta, 178
Placenta percreta, 178
Placenta previa, 286–289, 286(t), *287, 288*
  characteristics of, 286, 286(t)
  defined, 286
  evaluation of, 287–288, *288*
  incidence of, 287
Placenta previa accreta, 288–289

Placental site tumors, 531
"Plan B," in postcoital/emergency
    contraception, 344
Plant (vinca) alkaloids, in cancer therapy, *519,
    520,* 521(t)
Plasma osmolality, during pregnancy, 69
Plasma volume, during pregnancy, 67, 68(t)
Platelet function, abnormal, drugs associated
    with, 255, 255(t)
PLISSIT model, for treatment of sexual
    problems, 611, **611–612**
PMS. *See* Premenstrual syndrome (PMS)
Pneumococcal vaccine, 8(t)
Pneumonia(s)
  aspiration, 186
  influenza, during pregnancy, 223
  postoperative, 186
  during pregnancy, 223
Polycystic ovarian syndrome (PCOS), **480–481**
  androgen excess due to, 475–476, *476,* 477
  mechanism for, 476
  treatment of, 476
Polygenic/multifactorial disorders, screening
    tests for, 56–57
Polyhydramnios, 232, 232(t)
Polymastia, 418
Polyp(s), endometrial, *579*
Polythelia, 418
Ponstel, for dysmenorrhea, **415**
Position, fetal, 101, *101, 102*
Postabortal syndrome, 198, **200–201**
Postcesarean phlegmon, 184
Postcoital test (Huhner-Sims test), infertility due
    to, 503
Postcoital/emergency contraception, 343–344
Postmenopausal bleeding
  defined, 10
  treatment of, 29–30
Postmenopausal women, ovaries in, 587
Postoperative pneumonia, 186
Postpartum care
  maternal, 151–161, 162–163
    of abdominal wall, 154
    anxiety and depression, 159–161, 160(t)
    APGO objectives, 151–152
    of cardiovascular system, 154
    of cervix and vagina, 153
    of hematopoietic system, 154
    in immediate postpartum period, 154–159,
      158, 158(t), 159(t)
      analgesia in, 155
      bowel movement and urination, 156
      breast care, 155
      breast-feeding, 157–158, *158,* 159(t)
      contraception, 156
      hospital stay, 154
      immunizations, 155–156

Postpartum care (continued)
  maternal (continued)
    in immediate postpartum period (continued)
      lactation, 157–158, *158, 159*(t)
      maternal—infant bonding, 154–155
      patient education, 157
      perineum care, 156
      sexual activity, 157
      uterine complications, 155
    involution of uterus in, 152
    lochia in, 153
    ovarian function, 153, *153*
    perinatal grief, 161
    physiology of puerperium in, 152–154, *153*
    postpartum visit, 161
    of renal system, 154
  for maternal sadness, **162**
  maternal—infant bonding and, 154–155
Postpartum hemorrhage, 173–180, **180–181**
  APGO objectives, 173
  causes of, 174–179, **180–181**
    amniotic fluid embolism, 178–179
    coagulation defects, 178
    hematomas, 178
    lower genital tract lacerations, 176–177, *177*
    placenta retention, 177–178
    uterine atony, 174–176, 174(t)
    uterine inversion, 179, *179*
  management of, 176(t), 179, 180(t)
  prevention of, 179, 180(t)
Postpartum infection, 182–188, **188–190**
  evaluation of febrile patients, 183–184
  factors predisposing to, 183, 183(t)
  mastitis, 188
  metritis, 184–185, *184, 185*(t), *186, 186*(t)
  puerperal febrile morbidity, 183
  respiratory, 186
  septic pelvic thrombophlebitis, 187–188
  urinary tract, 186–187
  wound infections, separations, and
    dehiscence, 187
Postpartum mastitis, 155, 188
Postpartum sterilization, 156
Postpartum visit, 161
Postpill amenorrhea, 334
Postterm pregnancy, 296–301, **301–303**
  APGO objectives, 296
  brachial plexus injury due to, 298
  causes of, 297, 297(t)
  cord accidents due to, 298
  defined, 297
  diagnosis of, 299
  effects of, 298–299
  Erb palsy due to, 298
  Klumpke's paralysis due to, 298
  macrosomic infant due to, 298
  management of, 299–301, *300*

meconium aspiration syndrome due to, 298
  oligohydramnios and, 298
  placental dysfunction due to, 298–299
Post-tubal ligation syndrome, 353
"Power", in abnormal labor, evaluation of,
    116–118, *117*
Precocious puberty, 460–462, *461*
  causes of, 460–461
  described, 461–462, *461*
  gender differences in, 460
  21–hydroxylase deficiency in, 461
  isosexual, 460–461
    treatment of, 462
  treatment of, 461–462, *461*
Preconception visit, 79
Preeclampsia, 232, 232(t)
  defined, 261–262
  management of, 263–266, 265(t), 266(t)
  mild, **268–269**
Pregnancy. *See also* Antepartum care
  abdominal, 211–212
  acute fatty liver of, 251
  after tubal ligation, 353
  after vasectomy, 349
  amenorrhea and, 465
  back pain during, 94–95
  cervical, 212, 212(t)
  cocaine abuse during, 253–254
    ethical issues related to, **37–38**
  combined, 210–211
  constipation during, 94
  contraceptive failure and, 328, 328(t)
  diabetes mellitus and, interrelations between,
    231–233, 232(t)
  diabetogenic effect of, 70–71
  diagnosis of, 80–81, *81*
  dietary cravings during, 64
  dyspnea in, **76–77**
  ectopic, 202–213, **213–215**. *See also* Ectopic
    pregnancy
  effects on glucose metabolism,
    231–233, 232(t)
  employment during, 91
  exercise during, 91–92
  failed, **198–199**
  fatigue during, 94
  fetal death during, 95
  gastric reflux during, 94
  glucose tolerance tests in, 233–234, 233(t)
  hair loss after, **76**
  heartburn during, 65, 94
  hematologic laboratory values in, 218(t)
  hemorrhoids during, 95
  hypertension in, 260–267, **267–269**. *See also*
    Hypertension, in pregnancy
  hypertensive disorders in, 260–269. *See also*
    Hypertension, in pregnancy

Pregnancy (continued)
immunology of, 75
IUD use during, 341
leg cramps during, 94
maternal death during, 95
medical and surgical conditions of, 216–256,
257–259. *See also specific condition*
abdominal surgical conditions, 251
abdominal trauma, 251–252
anemias, 217–220, 218(t), 220(t)
APGO objectives, 216–217
cancer, 256
cardiac disease, 226–230, 227(t)-229(t)
coagulation disorders, 254–256, 255(t)
dental disease, 249
diabetes mellitus, 230–236, 231(t)-233(t)
endocrine diseases, 236–238, 237(t)
epilepsy, 245–246
gastrointestinal diseases, 246–249,
246(t), 247(t)
hepatobiliary diseases, 249–251
infectious diseases, 238–243, 239(t), *240*,
240(t), 244(t)
neurologic diseases, 245–246
renal diseases, 222
respiratory diseases, 222–226, *223*, 224(t)-
227(t). *See also* Respiratory diseases, in
pregnancy
substance abuse, 252–254, 253(t)
thromboembolic disorders, 244–245, 245(t)
UTIs, 221–222
medications during, 95, 96(t)
molar. *See* Hydatidiform mole (molar
pregnancy)
nausea and vomiting during, 94
normal, length of, 297
normotensive, 261, *261*
nutrition during, 92–93
ovarian, 212, 212(t)
pelvic examination in, 80
physical examination in, 80
physiologic changes in, 64–72
APGO objectives, 63
breast, 69–70
cardiovascular, 66–67, 66(t)
dental, 64
endocrinologic, 70–72, 71(t)
gastrointestinal, 64–65, 64(t)
hematologic, 67–68, 68(t)
musculoskeletal, 70
ophthalmic, 70
pulmonary, 65–66, 65(t)
renal, 68–69, 68(t)
reproductive tract and abdominal wall, 70
skin, 69
pneumonia in, 223

postterm, 296–301, **301–303**. *See also*
Postterm pregnancy
respiratory changes in, 222–223, *223*
respiratory infections in, 223
round ligament pain during, 95
sexual activity during, 93
smoking during, 93, 226, 227(t)
termination of, 439
thyroid function in, 236
travel during, 93–94
tubal. *See* Ectopic pregnancy
tuberculosis in, 226, 226(t)
ultrasonography during, safety of, 435–436
vaginal secretions during, 95
varicose veins during, 95
weight gain during, 92–93, 92(t), 93(t)
Pregnancy-induced hypertension. *See also*
Hypertension, pregnancy-induced
Pregnancy-induced hypertension (PIH), 232,
232(t), 260–269
Premature labor, **318**
Premature ovarian failure, 458–459, 458(t), *459*,
488–490, 489(t). *See also* Menopause
alkylating cancer chemotherapy and, 489
autoimmune disorders in, 489
genetic factors in, 488
in gonadotropin-resistant ovary syndrome, 488
hysterectomy and, 489
low body weight and, 489
smoking and, 489
Premature rupture of membranes (PROM),
312–317, **317–318**
APGO objectives, 312
causes of, 313–314
defined, 313
diagnosis of, 314–315, *314*, 314(t)
evaluation of, 315–317
fern test in, 314, *314*
management of, 315–317
Premenstrual dysphoric disorder, diagnostic
criteria for, 509, 510(t)
Premenstrual syndrome (PMS), 453, 499,
508–514, **514–525**
APGO objectives, 508
causes of, 509–511
defined, 509
diagnosis of, 511, **514–515**
diet and, 510, 512
differential diagnosis of, 511, 512(t)
endocrinologic basis of, 509–510
endorphin levels and, 510
fluid retention and, 511
incidence of, 509
prostaglandins and, 511
psychiatric basis of, 509
serotonin levels and, 510–511

Premenstrual syndrome (PMS), (continued)
  symptoms of, 509
  treatment of, 511–514, *513, 515*
    algorithm for, *513*
    vitamin deficiency and, 511
    vitamin(s) for, 514
Premphase, in menopause, 491
Prempro, in menopause, 491
Presacral neurectomy, for dysmenorrhea, 410
Presentation, 100–101
Preterm labor, 304–309, **310–311**
  APGO objectives, 304
  causes of, 305–306, 306(t)
  described, 305
  management of, 307–309, 308(t), 309(t)
  prevention of, 305–306
  signs and symptoms of, 305–306, 306(t)
  suspected, evaluation of patient in, 306–307
Primary care, obstetrician-gynecologist role in,
    5–9, *6, 5*(t)-8(t), 6(t)
Primary sex cords, 40
Primigravida, defined, 11(t)
Primipara, defined, 11(t)
Primitive cloaca, 41
Primordial follicles, 41
  in female reproductive cycle, 446, **454**
Primordial germ cells, 40
Probenecid, in gonorrhea/PID, 375(t)
Procidentia, 385
Progestasert, 340, *340*
Progestational therapy, for anovulatory uterine
    bleeding, 469–470, 470(t)
Progesterone
  for anovulation, 503
  in female reproductive cycle, 446–447, *446*
  in menopause, 491
  in menstural cycle, 450–451
  in ovulation, 499–500
  for PMS, 514
Progesterone "challenge" test, in
    amenorrhea, 467
Progesterone-induced endometrial atrophy, **345**
Progestin(s)
  in endometriosis, 403
  in menopause, 491, 491(t)
  in recurrent endometrial carcinoma, 583
Progestin receptors, in cancer therapy, 523
Progestin-containing rods, implantation of,
    bleeding due to, **345**
Progestin-only contraceptives, 331
Prolactinoma(s), pituitary, amenorrhea
    and, **493**
PROM. *See* Premature rupture of membranes
    (PROM)
Propranolol, for hypertensive disorders, in
    pregnancy, 266(t)

Prostaglandin(s)
  menstrual cramps and, biosynthetic pathways
    of, 448, *448*
  menstrual-associated release of, *449*
  in PMS, 511
Prostaglandin E$_2$ gel (dinoprostone), in
    abnormal labor, 121–122
Prostaglandin synthetase inhibitors, in preterm
    labor, 308(t)
Protein loss, 68(t), 69
Provera (medroxyprogesterone acetate). *See*
    Medroxyprogesterone acetate (Depo-
    Provera)
Prozac (fluoxetine), for PMS, 514
Pruritis, vulvar, *Candida* infection and, 358
Psammona bodies, 595
Pseudomenopause, in endometriosis, 403–404
Pseudomyxomatous peritonei, 595
Psoriasis, 534(t), 535
Psychiatric issues, in PMS, 509
Pthirus pubis (crab louse), 358, *359*
Ptotic kidney, *vs.* ovarian carcinoma, 587
Ptyalism, 64–65
  in pregnancy, 248
Puberty, 455–462, **462–463**
  abnormalities of, 457–462
    body weight and, 460
    delayed sexual maturation, 458, 458(t)
    genital tract anomalies, 460
    hypothalamic dysfunction, 458(t), 459–460
    precocious puberty, 460–462, *461*
    premature ovarian failure, 458–459,
      458(t), *459*
  APGO objectives, 455
  defined, 456
  endocrine events in, 456
  marijuana effects on, 459–460
  precocious. *See* Precocious puberty
  secondary sexual maturation in, 456,
    456(t), *457*
    normal sequence of, **462–463**
    Tanner's classification of, *457*
  sleep during, 456–457
Pubic hair
  growth of, in sexual maturation, 456,
    456(t), *457*
  sexual maturity of, Tanner's classification
    of, *15*
PUBS (periumbilical artery blood
    sampling), 321
  in prenatal diagnosis of chromosome
    abnormalities, 57
Pudendal block, 107, *108*
Puerpera, defined, 11(t)
Puerperal febrile morbidity, 183
Puerperium, physiology of, 152–154, *153*

Pulmonary embolism (PE), in pregnancy, 244–245

Pulmonary functions, physiologic changes in, during pregnancy, 66

Pyelonephritis, in pregnancy, 221

Quality of life issues, 35

Radiation, ionizing, effects of, 521–522

Radiation therapy
in cancer therapy, 521–522
for cervical carcinoma, 560, *561*, **563**
complications associated with, 522
delivery modes of, 522
for endometrial carcinoma, 583
measurements in, 522
for ovarian carcinoma, 599–600

Radical surgical excision, for cervical carcinoma, 560, **563**

Radiobiology, "four R's" of, 522

Rape trauma syndrome, 615

Rapid plasma reagin (RPR) test, in syphilis detection, 378, 378(t)

Reality condom, 338

Rectal bleeding, endometriosis and, 399

Rectocele(s), pelvic relaxation due to, 385, *386*

Rectosigmoid carcinoma, *vs.* ovarian carcinoma, 587

Rectovaginal examination, 24–25, *24*

Red cell mass, during pregnancy, 67, 68(t)

Red degeneration, in leiomyomas, 565–566

Referral, in patient evaluation, 27

Regional enteritis, in pregnancy, 248–249

Reinke crystalloid, of hilus cell tumor, 478, *478*

Renal and ureteral calculi, *vs.* ovarian carcinoma, 587

Renal disease, in pregnancy, 222

Renal plasma flow (RPF), during pregnancy, 68, 68(t)

Renal system, physiologic changes in, during pregnancy, 68–69, 68(t)

Reproduction, assisted, abbreviations associated with, 505(t)

Reproductive cycle, 444–453, **454**
female, 444–453, *454. See also* Female reproductive cycle

Reproductive genetics, 49–58
genetic counseling, 49–50
prenatal diagnosis, 50–54, 51(t)
case studies, 59–60
chromosome abnormalities, 50, 51(t), *52*
cytogenetic analysis, indications for, 50–54, 51(t). *See also* Cytogenetic analysis, prenatal, indications for
gynecology/primary care issues, 58
screening tests, 54–58

Reproductive system
anatomy of, 42–49, *48, 49,* **59–60**
bony pelvis, 42–44, *43, 44,* 44(t)
fallopian tubes, 48
perineum, 45, *45*
uterus, 46–47, *47, 48*
vagina, 45–46, *47*
vulva, 45, *45*
anomalies of, 48–49
embryology of, 40–42, *40–42. See also* Embryology
physiologic changes in, during pregnancy, 70

Respiratory diseases, in pregnancy, 222–226, *223,* 224(t)-227(t)
asthma, 223–226, 224(t), 225(t)
respiratory infections, 223

Respiratory distress syndrome, diabetes mellitus and, 233

Respiratory infections, postpartum, 186

Respiratory system, physiologic changes in, during pregnancy, 65–66, 65(t)

Resuscitation, of newborns, 146, 146(t)

Reticulocyte count, in iron-deficiency anemia evaluation, 75–76

Rh immune globulin, 169–170, 170(t)

Rh isoimmunization, 165–171, **171–172.** *See also* Isoimmunization

Rh sensitization, in isoimmunization, 166–167, 167(t)

Rhesus-isoimmunization, 170–171

Rheumatic heart disease, in pregnancy, 230

RhoGAM, **171–172**

Rhythm method, in family planning, 342–343

Ritgen maneuver, 110, *110*

Robertsonian translocations, 53

Rokitansky-Küster-Hauser syndrome (müllerian agenesis), 460, **463**

Rokitansky-Küuster-Hauser syndrome (müllerian agenesis), primary amenorrhea in, **470–471**

Round ligament pain, during pregnancy, 95

Rubella, in pregnancy, 241–242

Rupture of membranes, 107
in abnormal labor, 122

Sabouraud's media, in *Candida* vaginitis diagnosis, 363, *365*

Sadism, defined, 605(t)

SAFE, 618

Saline and potassium hydroxide (KOH) wet preparations test, 357, *358,* **365**

Salpingectomy, 208–209

Salpingitis, **383**
acute, 500
diagnosis of, 373(t)
gonococcal, **506–507**

Salpingo-oophorectomy, bilateral, with
    hysterectomy, **523**
  for endometrial carcinoma, 582–583
Salpingostomy, linear, 208–210, *209*
Sampson's theory of endometriosis, 397
Sarcoma(s), malignant mesodermal, 597
Sarcoma botryoides, 544, *544*
Sarcoptes scabei (itch mite), 358, *359*
Savage's syndrome (gonadotropin-resistant
    ovary syndrome), premature ovarian
    failure in, 488
Scalp pH/blood gas evaluation, fetal, 139–140,
    139, 140(t)
Screening tests
  in prenatal diagnosis of chromosome
      abnormalities, 54–58. *See also specific test*
    amniocentesis, 57
    CVS, 57
    invasive procedures, 57
    mendelian disorders, 54–56, *55*
    polygenic/multifactorial disorders, 56–57
    PUBS, 57
    teratogenesis, 57–58, 58(t)
  for women, 7(t)
Sebaceous cysts, 537
Seborrheic dermatitis, 534(t), 535–536
  vulvar, 359–360
Sebum production, during pregnancy, 69
Second-look laparotomy, for ovarian
    carcinoma, 600
Seizure(s), eclamptic, **269**
  in pregnancy, management of, 267
Semen analysis
  abnoraml, causes of, 498(t)
  in infertility evaluation, 497, 498(t), **506**
  normal, accepted values for, 498(t)
Senile urethritis, 486
Septic pelvic thrombophlebitis, 187–188
  in pregnancy, 245
Serotonin, in PMS, 510–511
Serous cystadenocarcinoma (malignant
    epithelial serous tumors), 595
Serous cystadenoma, ovarian, 590, 590(t)
Sertoli-Leydig cell tumors (androblastoma;
    arrhenoblastoma), 477–478, 590(t),
    592, 596
  management of, **600–601**
Serum Fe/total iron-binding capacity (TIBC), in
    iron-deficiency anemia, **75–76**
Serum pregnancy tests, in pregnancy diagnosis, 80
Sexual abuse, in patient evaluation, 12
Sexual activity, postpartum, 157
Sexual assault, 614–619, **619l**
  adult victim of, caring for, 615–617
    initial, 615–617
    subsequent, 617

APGO objectives, 614
child victim of, caring for, 617
defined, 615
in patient evaluation, 12
rape trauma syndrome, 615
Sexual dysfunction—couple-related, treatment
    of, **29–30**
Sexual history
  concerns related to, 608–610, 609(t)
  in patient evaluation, 12, 13(t)
Sexual intercourse, during pregnancy, 93
Sexual maturation
  delayed, 458, 458(t)
  factors affecting, 456–457
  secondary. *See* Puberty, secondary sexual
      maturation in
  sequence of, in girls, 456, 456(t), *457*
Sexual maturity, Tanner's classification of,
    15, 457
Sexual response, human, 606–608, 606(t),
    608, 607
Sexuality, 604–611, **611–612**
  APGO objectives, 604–605
  changing, and STDs, 367
  development of, 605–606, 605(t)
  human sexual response and, 606–608, 606(t),
      608, 607
    physiologic reactions of women during,
        606(t), 607–608, 608, 607
    stages of, 606(t), 607–608, 608, 607
  sexual concerns related to
    evaluation of, 608–611, 609(t)
      barriers to, 610
      physical examination in, 608–610, 609(t)
      sexual history in, 608–610, 609(t)
    management of, 610–611, **611–612**
      PLISS model in, 611, **611–612**
Sexually transmitted diseases (STDs), **258,**
    366–381, **382–383.** *See also specific*
    disease
  AIDS, 367, 378–379
  APGO objectives, 366–367
  chancroid, 380(t)
  changing sexuality and, 367
  chronic vaginitis, 364
  enteric infections, 380(t)
  genital lesions, 381(t)
  granuloma inguinale, 380(t)
  herpes genitalis, 368–369, *368*
  history and physical examination in,
      367–368
  human papillomavirus, 374, 376, *376*
  lymphogranuloma venereum, 380(t)
  minor, 379, 380(t), 381(t)
  molluscum contagiosum, 380(t)
  parasitic, 380(t)

Sexually transmitted diseases (STDs),
(continued)
in patient evaluation, 11
pelvic tuberculosis, 374
PID, 369–374. See also Pelvic inflammatory
disease (PID)
prevalence of, 367
syphilis, 377–378, *377*, 378(t), 379(t)
types of, 367
vaginitis, 380(t)
Short-term variability, 136
Sickle-cell diseases, in pregnancy, 219, 220(t)
Sickle-cell thalassemia, 220(t)
Sigmoid diverticular disease, *vs.* ovarian
carcinoma, 587
Sigmoidoscopy, **27–28**
SIL system (squamous intraepithelial lesions
(SIL) system), in screening for cervical
intraepithelial neoplasia, 551–553,
552(t), *553*
Simpson forceps, 321–322, *321*
Sinus(es), urogenital, 41
Sinusoidal heart rate pattern, 134–135
Skene's glands, 45
palpation of, 19, *20*
Skin, changes in
in menopause, 487
physiologic, during pregnancy, 69
Sleep, as factor in secondary sexual maturation,
456–457
Sleep disturbances, in menopause, 486
Smoking
during pregnancy, 93, 226, 227(t), 252
premature ovarian failure and, 489
treatment of, **29–30**
Socioeconomic issues, 35–36
Sodium concentration, during pregnancy, 69
Sonography
defined, 435
pelvic, **59–60**
Speculum
insertion of, 21–22, *22*
Pederson, 19
in pelvic examination, 19–23, *21–23*
vaginal, 19–20, *21*
Sperm generation time, 502
Sperm production, 502
Sperm transport, in female genital tract,
disorders related to, 500
Spermatogenesis, abnormalities of, infertility
due to, 502–503, **505–506**
treatment of, 504, *504*
Spermicide(s), 339–340
Spider angiomata, during pregnancy, 69
Spinal anesthetic, 107
Spironolactone, for PMS, 514

Spontaneous abortion, 192–197. *See also*
Abortion, spontaneous
Spontaneous rupture of membranes, 107
Squamocolumnar junction, of cervix,
549–551, *550*
Squamous cell hyperplasia (hyperplastic
dystrophy), 537–538, 537(t)
Squamous intraepithelial lesions (SIL) system, in
screening for cervical intraepithelial
neoplasia, 549–557, 553(t), *554*
STDs. *See* Sexually transmitted diseases (STDs)
Stereotactic core needle biopsy, in breast cancer
screening, 427
Sterilization, 347–354, **354–355**
APGO objectives, 347
counseling related to, 348
decision-making process for, 353–354
described, 348
in men, 348–349, *348*
operative techniques in, changes in, 348
postpartum, 156
prevalence of, 348
reversal of, reasons for, 348
reversal of tubal ligation, 353
in women, 349–353
by colpotomy, 351–352
complications of, 353
by hysterectomy, 352
by laparoscopy, 349–351, *350*
by laparotomy, 351, *351*, 352(t)
by nonsurgical methods, 352
postpartum *vs.* interval, 349
side effects of, 353
Steroid(s), in precocious puberty
management, 461
Stillbirth, 95
diabetes mellitus and, 232, 232(t)
Stool, of newborns, 148–149
Stress incontinence, 386, **395**
Striae gravidarum, during pregnancy, 69
Stromal cell neoplasms, benign, 590(t), 591–592
Struma ovarii, 591
Substance abuse, in pregnancy,
252–254, 253(t)
alcohol abuse, 252–253, 253(t)
cocaine use, 253–254
hallucinogens, 254
marijuana use, 254
opiate abuse, 254
smoking, 252
Suction and curettage (S&C), in gynecology, 439
Sunlight, optic exposure to, as factor in
secondary sexual maturation, 457
Surgical removal of tumor tissue (cytoreductive
debulking surgery), 519
Sweating, eccrine, during pregnancy, 69

Syphilis, 377–378, *377,* 378(t), 379(t)
  clinical presentation of, 377–378, *377*
  course of, 377–378, *377*
  diagnosis of, 378, 378(t)
  genital lesions in, 381(t)
  incidence of, 377
  in pregnancy, 238–239, 239(t)
  serologic tests for, 378, 378(t)
  treatment of, 378, 379(t)
  Treponema pallidum and, 377
Systemic lupus erythematosus (SLE), in
      pregnancy, 255

Tachycardia, fetal, baseline, defined, 134
Tanner's classification of sexual maturity, *15*
Task Force on Primary and Preventive Health
      Care, of American College of
      Obstetricians and Gynecologists, 5
Taxol (paclitaxel), for ovarian
      carcinoma, 599
TCU-380A (ParaGard), 340, *340*
Teletherapy, 522
Temperature, body, basal, in infertility
      evaluation, 495–497, *496, 497*
Teratogenesis, screening tests for, 57–58, 58(t)
Teratoma(s)
  cystic, benign, 590(t), 591, **602**
  immature, 596
Terminal hair, **481**
  defined, 473
Testosterone
  extraglandular, in hirsutism and virilization
      analysis, 474, 474(t)
  in hirsutism and virilization analysis,
      474, 474(t)
  in virilization, 474
Testosterone receptors, 475
Tetanus-diphtheria booster, 8(t)
Thalassemia(s)
  in pregnancy, 219, 220(t)
  sickle-cell, 220(t)
  α-thalassemia, 220(t)
  β-thalassemia, 220(t)
Thalassemia trait, 219
The Obstetrician-Gynecologist and Primary-
      Preventive Health Care, 5
Theca cells, in female reproductive cycle,
      446, *447*
Theca lutein cysts, 589
Thelarche, 456, 456(t), *457*
Thiazide, for hypertensive disorders, in
      pregnancy, 266(t)
Third-trimester bleeding, 285–292, **292–295**
  abruptio placentae, 289–291, *289,* 290(t)
  APGO objectives, 285
  causes of, 286, 286(t)

placenta previa, 286–289, 286(t), *287, 288*
  prevalence of, 286
  uterine rupture, 291–292
  vaginal bleeding, approach to, 292
  vasa previa, 291
Thrombocytopenia, in pregnancy,
      254–256, 255(t)
Thromboembolic disorders
  estrogen replacement therapy and, 492
  in pregnancy, 244–245, 245(t)
Thromboembolism, venous, during pregnancy,
      67–68, 67(t)
Thrombophlebitis
  septic pelvic, 187–188
    in pregnancy, 245
  superficial, in pregnancy, 244
Thyroid function, during pregnancy, 71, 71(t),
      236, 237(t)
Thyroid function studies, in pregnancy,
      236–237, 237(t)
Thyroid gland, fetal, 74
Tietze's syndrome, 427–428
Tobacco use, during pregnancy, 93
Tocodynamometer(s), in abnormal labor,
      117, *117*
Total abdominal hysterectomy, with bilateral
      salpingo-oophorectomy, for endometrial
      carcinoma, 582–583
Toxoplasmosis, in pregnancy, 242–243
Transformation zone (TZ), of cervix,
      549–551, *550*
Transfusion(s), in isoimmunization, 169
Transitory urinary retention, postpartum, 156
Transvaginal ultrasound, 434, *434*
  in endometrial hyperplasia evaluation, 578
Trauma
  abdominal, in pregnancy, 251–252
  to gravid abdomen, **257–258**
Travel, during pregnancy, 93–94
Treponema pallidum, syphilis due to, 377
Trichomonad(s), in bacterial vagninosis, 361, *361*
Trichomonas vaginalis, 360
Trichomonas vaginitis, 361–362, *361, 365*
Trichomoniasis, 360
  clinical aspects of physiologic vaginal
      secretions in, 357(t)
Triplet(s), incidence of, 271
Trisomy 13 (Patau syndrome), 51(t)
Trisomy 16, **59**
Trisomy 18 (Edwards syndrome), 51(t)
Trisomy 21 (Down syndrome), 51(t)
True labor, *vs.* false labor, 123(t)
Tubal ligation
  at laparotomy, techniques of, 352(t)
  pregnancy after, 353
  reversal, 353

Tubal pregnancy. *See* Ectopic pregnancy
Tubercle(s), genital, 42, *42*
Tuberculosis
  pelvic, 374
  in pregnancy, 226, 226(t)
Tumor(s)
  Brenner cell, 590(t), *591*, 596
  endometrioid, 590(t), *591*, 595
  functioning, ovarian, 597
  germ cell, ovarian, 590(t), *591*
    malignant, 596
  granulosa cell, 597
  granulosa theca cell, 590(t), 592
  hilus cell, Reinke crystalloid of, 478, *478*
  Krukenberg, 597–598
  lipid cell, 478
  malignant epithelial serous, 595
  malignant mucinous epithelial, 595
  mucinous, ovarian, 590(t), *591*
  ovarian
    borderline, 594–595
    removal of, **523**
  placental site, 531
  Sertoli-Leydig cell, 477–478, 590(t), 592
    management of, **600–601**
  sinus, endodermal, 596
  stromal cell, gonadal, 597
Tumor debulking, for ovarian carcinoma, 599
Turner syndrome
  features of, 458, 458(t)
  genetic defects in, 458, *459*
Twin(s), **275**
  amnion and chorion development in,
    271–272, *272*
  antenatal management of, 273–274, 273(t)
  incidence of, 271
  intrapartum management of, 274–275, *274*
Twin-twin transfusion syndrome, 272

Ulcerative colitis, in pregnancy, 249
Ultrasonography
  in breast cancer screening, 426
  described, 434
  in gynecology, 434–435, *434*
    Doppler ultrasound, 435
  during pregnancy, safety of, 435–436
  in pregnancy diagnosis, 81
  transabdominal, 434, *434*
  transvaginal, 434, *434*
    in endometrial hyperplasia evaluation, 578
Ultrasonohysterography, in endometrial
    hyperplasia evaluation, 578
Umbilical cord, postpartum care of, 148
Umbilical cord compression, 137–138
Urethral detachment, pelvic relaxation due to,
    385, *386*

Urethral gland, palpation of, 19, *20*
Urethritis, senile, 486
Urethritis/trigonitis, traumatic, **394–395**
Urethrocele(s), pelvic relaxation due to,
    385, *386*
Urinary calculi, in pregnancy, 222
Urinary incontinence
  APGO objectives, 384–385
  causes of, 386
  characteristics of, 387(t)
  clinical presentation of, 386–387, 387(t)
  differential diagnosis of, 389, *390*
  evaluation of, 387–388, *388*
  pelvic relaxation and, 385
  treatment of, nonsurgical, 389–391, *390*
Urinary retention, transitory, postpartum, 156
Urinary tract infections (UTIs), 393–394,
    394–395
  APGO objectives, 384–385
  causes of, 393
  clinical aspects of, 393
  evaluation of, 393
  postpartum, 186–187
  in pregnancy, 221–222
  prevalence of, 393
  recurrent, 393
  treatment of, **310**, 394
  vs. ovarian carcinoma, 587
Urinary urgency, treatment of, **29–30**
Urination, postpartum, 156
Urine, of newborns, 148–149
Urine pregnancy tests, in diagnosis of
    pregnancy, 80
Urogenital ridges, 40, *40*
Urogenital sinus, 41
Urogenital system, early development of, 40, *40*
Uterine atony
  defined, 174
  factors predisposing to, 174, 174(t)
  management of, 174–176, 174(t)
  postpartum hemorrhage due to,
    174–176, 174(t)
Uterine atopy, postpartum hemorrhage due to,
    180–181
Uterine body, wall of, layers in, 47–48, *48*
Uterine contractions, **128–129, 310–311**
  in abnormal labor, 119–120
  management of, **113–114**
  menstrual-associated prostaglandin release
    and, *449*
Uterine cramps, in menstural cycle, 448
Uterine factors, in spontaneous abortion, 193
Uterine fibroids, 564–571, **571–572**. *See also*
    Leiomyoma(s) (uterine fibroids)
Uterine inversion, postpartum hemorrhage due
    to, 179, *179*

Uterine prolapse, 385

Uteroplacental insufficiency, 132, 139

Uteroplacental unit, 132

Uterovaginal primordium, 41

Uterus
anatomy of, 46–47, 47, 48
bimanual examination of, 24, 24
formation of, 41, 41
inversion of, 111
involution of, 152
postpartum complications involving, 155
rupture of, obstetric hemorrhage due to, 291–292

UTIs. See Urinary tract infections (UTIs)

Vaccine(s). See also Immunization(s)
hepatitis B, 8(t)
influenza, 8(t)
pneumococcal, 8(t)

Vacuum extraction, 112, 322, 322

Vagina
anatomy of, 45–46, 47
cancer of
carcinoma in situ, 543
invasive, 544, 544, 544(t)
development of, 41–42
diseases of, 543. See also specific disease
lesions of, biopsy of, 437
neoplasia of, 543–544, 544, 544(t)
postpartum physiology of, 153
reproductive cycle changes in, 453

Vaginal birth after cesarean section (VBAC), 322

Vaginal bleeding
management of, 181
in second half of gestation, 292

Vaginal discharge
patient evaluation for, 28
during pregnancy, 70, 95
in vaginitis, causes of, 360

Vaginal dryness, in menopause, 486

Vaginal infections, 240(t)

Vaginal secretions
physiologic, 357(t)
in vaginitis, sources of, 360

Vaginitis, 356–357, 360–364, 364–365, 380(t).
See also Vulvitis
APGO objectives, 356
bacterial vaginosis, 360–361, 361, 361(t)
Candida, 362–363, 363(t)
chronic, 363–364
clinical presentation of, 357, 357(t)
cytolytic, 364
desquamative inflammatory, 364
monilial, 362–363, 363(t)
patient history in, 357

physical examination in, 357, 358, 365
symptoms of, 360
Trichomonas, 361–362, 361, 365
vaginal secretions in, 360

Vaginosis, bacterial. See Bacterial vaginosis

Vaporization, laser, in gynecology, 438

Varicose veins, during pregnancy, 95

Vasa previa, 291

Vascular spiders, during pregnancy, 69

Vasectomy, 348–349, 348
pregnancy after, 349

Vasomotor instability, in menopause, 485–486

Venereal Disease Research Laboratory (VDRL)
test, in syphilis detection, 378, 378(t)

Venereal warts, 376, 376

Venous thromboembolism, during pregnancy,
67–68, 67(t)

Vestibular glands, 536

Vestibule(s), 45

Vestibulitis, 534(t), 536, 536

VIN. See Vulvar intraepithelial neoplasia (VIN)

Vinca alkaloids, in cancer therapy, 519,
520, 521(t)

Violence, domestic. See Domestic violence

Virilization, 472–480, 480–481. See also
Androgen excess; Hirsutism, and
virilization
APGO objectives, 472
defined, 473, 473
testosterone and, 474

Vision
as factor in secondary sexual
maturation, 457
physiologic changes in, during
pregnancy, 70

Vitamin(s)
E, for PMS, 514
for PMS, 511, 514

Von Willebrand's disease, in pregnancy, 256

Voyeurism, defined, 605(t)

Vulva
anatomy of, 45, 45, 46
biopsies of, in gynecology, 437, 437
cancer of, 540–543
age as factor in, 540
carcinoma of Bartholin's gland, 543
epidermoid carcinoma, 545–546
evaluation of, 541, 542(t)
melanoma, 540
natural history of, 541
prevalence of, 540
prognosis of, 541–542
staging for, 542(t)
treatment of, 541
chancre of, 377, 377
condyloma lata of, 377, 377

Vulva (continued)
  diseases of, 533–543, **545–546**
    APGO objectives, 533
    benign vulvar lesions, 537
    common dermatoses, 534–536, 534(t), *536*
      lichen planus, 534(t), *535*
      lichen simplex chronicus, 534–535, 534(t)
      psoriasis, 534(t), *535*
      seborrheic dermatitis, 534(t), *535–536*
      vestibulitis, 534(t), 536, *536*
    lichen sclerosis, 537(t), *538*
    malignant carcinoma, 540–543. *See also*
      Vulva, cancer of
    neoplasia, 537–540, 537(t)
    Paget disease, 540, *540*
    squamous cell hyperplasia (hyperplastic
      dystrophy), 537–538, 537(t)
    symptoms of, 534
    vulvar intraepithelial neoplasia, 539–540
  physiologic changes in, during pregnancy, 70
Vulvar intraepithelial neoplasia (VIN), 539–540
  VIN-I, 539
  VIN-II, 539
  VIN-III, 539–540
Vulvar itching, causes of, 359, *359*, **364–365**
Vulvar pruritis, *Candida* infection and, 358
Vulvar varicosities, during pregnancy, 70
Vulvitis, 356–360, **364–365**. *See also*
      Vaginitis
  allergic causes of, 358
    secondary, 358
  APGO objectives, 356
  atrophic changes and, 359
  clinical presentation of, 357, 357(t),
      358, **365**
  dermatologic diseases and, 359–360
  differential diagnosis of, 358
  herpes, **382**
  KOH test in, 357, *358*, **365**
  patient history in, 357

  physical examination in, 357, *358*, **365**
  screening in, 358
Vulvovaginitis, cyclic, 364

Wart(s)
  genital, 381(t)
  venereal, 376, *376*
Weight
  as factor in secondary sexual maturation,
      456, 460
  low, premature ovarian failure due to, 489
Weight gain, during pregnancy, 92–93,
      92(t), 93(t)
Well-being, fetal, **283**
  assessment of, 87–89, *88*, 89(t)
  biophysical profile in, **97**
White blood cell (WBC) counts, during
      pregnancy, 67, 68(t)
WHO Prognostic Scoring System, for
      gestational trophoblastic disease,
      529, 530(t)
Women
  health care for, 2–27, **27–31**
    APGO objectives, 2–4
  older, in U.S. population, 8, *8*
  sterilization in, 349–353. *See also*
      Sterilization, in women
Women's Choice condom, 338
Wound infections, postpartum, 187

Xanax (alprazolam), for PMS, 514

Yuzpe, in postcoital/emergency contraception,
      343–344

Zidovudine, in HIV infection, 243, 244(t)
ZIFT (zygote intrafallopian tube transfer), 504
Zona basalis, 177
Zona spongiosa, 177
Zygote intrafallopian tube transfer (ZIFT), 504